65.00

✓

D1433775

Paediatric Anaesthesia

Edited by

EDWARD SUMNER MA, BM, BCh, FRCA

Consultant Paediatric Anaesthetist, Department of Anaesthesia,
Great Ormond Street Hospital for Children NHS Trust, London, UK

and

DAVID J HATCH MBBS, MRCS, LRCP, FRCA

Portex Professor of Paediatric Anaesthesia,
Institute of Child Health, London, UK

A member of the Hodder Headline Group
LONDON
Co-published in the USA by Oxford University Press Inc., New York

First published in Great Britain in 1989 by Baillière Tindall
Second edition published in Great Britain in 2000 by
Arnold, a member of the Hodder Headline Group,
338 Euston Road, London NW1 3BH

http://www.arnoldpublishers.com

Co-published in the USA by Oxford University Press Inc.,
198 Madison Avenue, New York, NY 10016
Oxford is a registered trademark of Oxford University Press

British Library Cataloguing in Publication Data
A catalogue record for this book is available from the British Library

Library of Congress Cataloging-in-Publication Data
A catalog record for this book is available from the Library of Congress

ISBN 0 340 71942 7

1 2 3 4 5 6 7 8 9 10

Publisher: Joanna Koster
Project Editor: Melissa Morton
Project Manager: Annette Bruno, Gray Publishing
Production Editor: Rada Radojicic
Production Controller: Priya Gohil

Produced and typeset by Gray Publishing, Tunbridge Wells, Kent
Printed and bound in Great Britain by The Bath Press

What do you think about this book? Or any other Arnold title?
Please send your comments to feedback.arnold@hodder.co.uk

Contents

Contributors

Frederic A Berry
Professor of Anesthesiology and Pediatrics, Department of Anesthesiology, University of Virginia Health System, Charlottesville, Virginia, USA

Ann E Black
Consultant Paediatric Anaesthetist, Department of Anaesthesia, Great Ormond Street Hospital for Children NHS Trust, London, UK

Peter D Booker
Senior Lecturer in Paediatric Anaesthesia, University of Liverpool; Honorary Consultant Paediatric Anaesthetist, Alder Hey Royal Liverpool Children's NHS Trust, Liverpool, UK

Liam J Brennan
Consultant Paediatric Anaesthetist and Director of Paediatric Day Surgery, Addenbrooke's NHS Trust, Cambridge, UK

Karen Brown
Associate Professor, Department of Anaesthesia, McGill University Health Centre, The Montreal Children's Hospital, Montreal, Canada

Jonathan de Lima
Honorary Consultant Paediatric Anaesthetist, Department of Anaesthesia, Great Ormond Street Hospital for Children NHS Trust, London, UK

Robert Lindsay Eyres
Deputy Director, Clinical Anaesthesia, Department of Paediatric Anaesthesia and Pain Management, Royal Children's Hospital, Melbourne, Victoria, Australia

Elspeth Facer
Consultant Paediatric Anaesthetist, Department of Anaesthesia, Great Ormond Street Hospital for Children NHS Trust, London, UK

Nishan G Goudsouzian
Director, Department of Pediatric Anesthesia and Critical Care, Massachusetts General Hospital; Professor of Anaesthesia, Harvard Medical School, Boston, Massachusetts, USA

David J Hatch
Portex Professor of Paediatric Anaesthesia, Institute of Child Health, London, UK

Josef Holzki
Chief of Paediatric Anaesthesia and Paediatric Intensive Care, Children's Hospital, Cologne, Germany

Richard Howard
Consultant in Paediatric Anaesthesia and Pain Management, Department of Anaesthesia, Great Ormond Street Hospital for Children NHS Trust, London, UK

Lucinda Huskisson
Consultant Paediatric Surgeon, Department of Paediatric Surgery, Bristol Royal Children's Hospital, Bristol, UK

Elizabeth Jackson
Consultant Paediatric Anaesthetist, Great Ormond Street Hospital for Children NHS Trust, London, UK

Ian James
Consultant Paediatric Anaesthetist, Director of Paediatric Intensive Care, Great Ormond Street Hospital for Children NHS Trust, London, UK

John P Keneally
Head, Department of Anaesthesia, New Children's Hospital, Westmead; Clinical Senior Lecturer, Department of Anaesthetics, University of Sydney, New South Wales, Australia

Peter C Laussen
Senior Associate in Anesthesia, Department of Anesthesia, Children's Hospital; Assistant Professor in Anesthesia, Harvard Medical School, Boston, Massachusetts, USA

Adrian Lloyd-Thomas
Consultant Paediatric Anaesthetist, Department of Anaesthesia, Great Ormond Street Hospital for Children NHS Trust, London, UK

Jane Lockie
Consultant Anaesthetist, The Middlesex Hospital, London, UK

Anne M Lynn
Associate Director, Department of Anesthesia and Critical Care, Children's Hospital and Medical Center; Professor, Anesthesiology and Pediatrics (adjunct), University of Washington School of Medicine, Seattle, Washington, USA

Angela Mackersie
Consultant Paediatric Anaesthetist, Great Ormond Street Hospital for Children NHS Trust, London, UK

Angus McEwan
Consultant Paediatric Anaesthetist, Great Ormond Street Hospital for Children NHS Trust, London, UK

George H Meakin
Senior Lecturer in Paediatric Anaesthesia, University of Manchester; Honorary Consultant Anaesthetist, Department of Anaesthesia, Royal Manchester Children's Hospital, Pendlebury, Manchester, UK

Andrea Messeri
Consultant, Department of Anaesthesia and Intensive Care Unit, 'A Meyer' Children's Hospital, Florence, Italy

Isabelle Murat
Professor of Anaesthesiology, Service d'Anesthésie-Réanimation, Hôpital d'enfants Armand Trousseau, Paris, France

Gunnar L Olsson
Paediatric Anaesthesia and Intensive Care, Karolinska Hospital, Astrid Lindgrens Children's Hospital, Stockholm, Sweden

Anna-Maria Rollin
Consultant Anaesthetist, Department of Anaesthesia, Epsom General Hospital, Epsom, Surrey, UK

Steven S Sasaki
Assistant Professor, Anesthesiology and Pediatrics, University of Washington School of Medicine, Department of Anesthesiology and Critical Care, Children's Hospital and Medical Center, Seattle, Washington, USA

Edward Sumner
Consultant Paediatric Anaesthetist, Great Ormond Street Hospital for Children NHS Trust, London, UK

Michael RJ Sury
Consultant Paediatric Anaesthetist, Great Ormond Street Hospital for Children NHS Trust, London, UK

Isabeau Walker
Consultant Paediatric Anaesthetist, Great Ormond Street Hospital for Children NHS Trust, London, UK

Mehernoor F Watcha
Director, Pediatric Anesthesia Research; Associate Professor, Department of Anesthesiology and Critical Care Medicine, Children's Hospital of Philadelphia, Pennsylvania, USA

David A Zideman
Consultant Anaesthetist, Department of Anaesthesia, Hammersmith Hospitals Trust; Honorary Senior Lecturer, Imperial College, University of London, London, UK

Preface

In producing the second edition of this book, we have tried to maintain the philosophy of the first edition while radically revising the content of every chapter. We are extremely grateful to the many well-known paediatric anaesthetists from around the world who have contributed to this work, many of whom were involved in the first edition in 1989. We have been aware of the major developments that have occurred in the past decade, not only in the practice of paediatric anaesthesia, but also in the organization of anaesthetic services in many countries, including the UK. We have been fortunate in obtaining the services of a number of new contributors, many of whom are equally well known, to help us to address these topics. It is hard to believe that neither pain management nor day-stay surgery deserved chapters of their own in the first edition; this reflects the major advances that have taken place in these fields. We have also included a chapter on sedation outside the operating room, another expanding area of practice, and have devoted separate chapters to the problems of postoperative recovery and immediate intensive care. More specialized areas such as transplantation, previously included, have been omitted from this edition, and only the most common neonatal problems are discussed, since these subjects are covered extensively elsewhere.

The aim of the book is to provide a readily accessible and readable source of information on modern paediatric anaesthesia to help anaesthetists, including trainees, to understand the problems that the specialty presents, together with suggested methods of manage-ment. It is hoped that general anaesthetists with an interest in children will find much of value within the book, and will be helped to identify those areas of practice that may be best managed in specialized centres. The specialist paediatric anaesthetist will find it a useful reference book.

The advice given is largely of a practical nature, with approximately one-third of the contributors having been chosen from the staff of the Great Ormond Street Children's Hospital in London, where over 10 000 anaesthetics are administered each year. The remainder, from Europe, Australia, USA and Canada, have been carefully selected not only because they are acknowledged experts in their field but also because of their ability to express themselves clearly and give sound, safe advice. Although unnecessary repetition has been avoided we have deliberately encouraged some overlap of content between chapters in order to allow the reader to learn of different approaches to the same topic.

ACKNOWLEDGEMENTS

The editors would like to thank all the chapter authors, both those who have radically updated their original contributions and those who have joined us for the first time, for their excellent contributions to this book. We are particularly grateful to Mrs Diana Newlands for once again ensuring that the grammar and style is uniform and readable.

CHAPTER 1

Development and disease in childhood

KAREN BROWN, JONATHAN DE LIMA, ANGUS MCEWAN AND
EDWARD SUMNER

DEVELOPMENTAL PHYSIOLOGY

METABOLISM AND THERMAL REGULATION

Neonates are true homeotherms; they attempt to maintain a pattern of temperature regulation in which core temperature is kept within narrow limits and overall thermal balance is maintained via a gradient for heat transfer from the body core to the environment. Obligatory heat gain from basal metabolism, feeding and muscle activity are exactly balanced by energy transfer to the environment via convective, radiative, conductive and evaporative heat loss.[1] Homeotherms also possess the ability to generate heat purely to maintain core temperature (facultative heat production) and this may be via either shivering or non-shivering thermogenesis.

Control over heat loss is exerted through behaviour, sweating and vasomotor control. The first two control heat transfer from the skin to the environment, while vascular changes effectively determine the movement of heat from the body core to more peripheral tissues. In this way, core temperatures are kept constant by changes in the temperature of an apparent 'outer body shell'.[2]

Several features distinguish thermal regulation in the neonate from that in adults. Basal metabolic rate calculated on a per kilogram basis is higher than that of adults, as evidenced by the higher oxygen consumption rates of neonates (6–8 ml kg^{-1} min^{-1} as opposed to 4–6 ml kg^{-1} min^{-1} in adults). This represents a biological necessity as human neonates have a surface area to mass ratio 2–2.5 times that of adults.[3]

Behavioural responses and tissue insulation against thermal stress in neonates and infants are limited. Hence, even light clothing (vest, napkin and nightdress) can more than double resistance to heat loss.[4] Although most babies maintain reasonably normal core temperatures in the face of cold stress, this is only accomplished at the expense of increased oxygen and caloric requirements. The response to cold stress is characterized by well-developed control over vasomotor tone allowing peripheral vasoconstriction to reduce heat transfer to the outer shell. Secondly, facultative heat generation is triggered. Of the two possible modes, shivering does not become an important mechanism of heat production until early childhood. Non-shivering thermogenesis, that is the production of heat through metabolism of brown fat, assumes greater importance in the neonate (including preterm babies) and young infants up to 2 years of age. In this way, metabolic heat production can be increased up to 2.5-fold during cold stress.[5]

In response to heat stress, active capillary vasodilation helps to move heat from core body tissues to the skin. This mechanism is well developed even in premature babies. The second response is sympathetically (cholinergic) activated sweating. Although the neonatal density of sweat glands is almost six times that of adult skin, peak response is only 30% of the maximum adult response.[6] The maturation of the sweat response is linked to gestational age and is little influenced by birth weight or postnatal age.

A further concept that is useful in understanding childhood thermal regulation is that of a 'thermoneutral environment'. This represents the range of ambient temperatures wherein thermoregulation is achieved by posture and blood flow alone (i.e. without metabolic expenditure) and hence with minimal oxygen consumption.[7] This neutral range is known to be narrow for all babies, particularly if naked, premature or small for gestational age. The aim

ought to be to nurse babies at the lower limit of the neutral range.[8]

RENAL PHYSIOLOGY

Metanephric development commences during the fifth week of intrauterine life and continues via progressive branching and division of the collecting system into metanephric excretory vesicles. These eventually form glomeruli and renal tubules.

The process continues until the 34th week of gestation, the most recently formed glomeruli being added to the outer cortex of the kidney. At birth, renal histology displays marked heterogeneity. It is some months after birth before a mature and homogenous renal morphology is apparent.[9]

Ultrafiltration through the primitive excretory system commences by the 9th week of fetal life and tubular resorption occurs by the 14th week. This results in 'urine' that is hypotonic and relatively free of sugar and protein. This fluid contributes to total amniotic fluid turnover (150 ml kg^{-1} day) but is not responsible for fetal waste removal.

Renal blood flow is low during fetal life, as is glomerular filtration. Major increases occur from 34 weeks' gestation and are dramatic within 48 h of umbilical cord clamping. The basis of the increase is probably both physiological (altered haemodynamics with birth and cord clamping) and morphological (completion of glomerulogenesis at 34 weeks).[9] Glomerular filtration rate (GFR) in the first week of life approximates to 34 ml min^{-1} 1.73 m^{-2} and rises to mature values at 12–18 months of age.

Infant tubular function is only sufficiently mature to regulate function under physiological conditions as evidenced by glycosuria, proteinuria and low tubular resorptive maxima for phosphate and bicarbonate.

Renal concentrating ability and maximum free water clearance mature in a variable period after birth. Although free water clearance increases significantly in the first 5 days of life, neonates are not able to compensate for acute, non-physiological water loads in the first week of life. Conversely, in the face of water restriction, neonates are only able to concentrate urine to half of the adult capacity. Maturation of this function follows the gradual accumulation of urea and sodium in the renal medullary interstitium in the first few months of life.[10]

Although renal acid excretion is operative *in utero* (via phosphate and ammonium urine acidification mechanisms), ammonium excretion capacity and therefore the ability to excrete an acid load take almost 12 months to mature.

Assessing renal function in neonates and infants remains problematic. Creatinine clearance gives a reasonable estimate of GFR and requires a timed urine collection and plasma determination. At birth, plasma creatinine concentrations reflect maternal serum values $(0.6–1.2 \text{ mg dl}^{-1})$ and these decrease within the first month to $0.1–0.2 \text{ mg dl}^{-1}$ as GFR rises. Creatinine values then increase steadily through childhood until the end of puberty.

Preterm neonates do not display the abrupt increase in both glomerular and tubular function of immediate postnatal life that characterizes their term counterparts. Instead, they show a much slower rate of maturation. Markedly reduced function persists at least until 18 months postconceptional age and only reaches normal values by 8 years of age.[11,12]

HEPATIC FUNCTION

Prior to the onset of the demands of extra-uterine life, the fetal liver functions primarily to produce plasma proteins in order to support continued cell proliferation. Further clusters of enzymic and metabolic processes develop with direct correlation to functional requirements.

Cord clamping brings about an abrupt interruption of transplacental glucose supply. The liver immediately compensates for this through glycogenolysis: 90% of stored glycogen is released during the first few hours of birth. The rest is consumed within the next 48 h. Enterally absorbed galactose then becomes the major energy substrate allowing the re-accumulation of glycogen from the second postnatal week. Hepatic glycogen stores are replenished by the third week in well-fed neonates.[13]

The fetal liver is capable of producing all major plasma proteins after the first trimester but concentrations are usually low. Albumin concentrations only rise to adult levels several months after birth as production gradually replaces synthesis of the primary fetal protein (α-feto-protein).

Hepatic metabolic biotransformation reactions (both phase I and phase II conversions) are minimally active *in utero*. Rapid maturation of multiple enzyme systems such as mono-oxygenase systems and conjugation reactions commence at birth and continue through infancy.[14] Neonatal bilirubin excretory capacity is tenuous at best. Poorly developed uridine diphospho-glucuronyl transferase (UDPGT) activity and reduced amounts of the glucuronical acid donor (UDP-glucuronic acid) readily allow 'spillover' of unconjugated bilirubin into hydrophobic tissue environments such as plasma membranes, meninges and brain. Further factors, including a depressed bilirubin binding capacity in serum and a lack of appropriate colonic flora, increase the risks of neonatal jaundice. Prematurity, acidosis, hypothermia and sepsis, quite apart from haemolysis owing to immune reactions and haemoglobinopathies, can easily result in clinically significant hyperbilirubinaemia and kernicterus.[15]

BRAIN DEVELOPMENT

An understanding of neural development is essential for understanding paediatric neurological dysfunction as well as forming the basis of rational anaesthetic and analgesic interventions in preterm and term neonates and infants.

By the fifth week of gestation, the neural tube has closed and three primitive vesicles (prosencephalon, mesencephalon and rhombencephalon) have formed. Rostral flexures, the primitive cerebral hemispheres and cerebellar placode are also now visible. Excess caudal segments undergo regression, giving rise to the cauda equina and filum terminale in a process termed retrogressive differentiation.[16]

Development is not a simple linear progression in cell numbers and connections but also involves remodelling, the pruning of connections and programmed cell death (apoptosis).

Most cells undergo some form of migration, often along glial fibres. Programmed migration of cortical neurons along radially placed glial fibres may be the embryological basis of functional modules even though the vertical stratification of the fetal cortex is gradually replaced by a more mature horizontal stratification. The adult pattern of six layers of cortical neurons starts to develop from 16 weeks' gestation.[16]

There is a tendency for motor nuclei to commence and complete histiogenesis before sensory nuclei, and motor histiogenesis is usually of shorter duration. Synaptogenesis commences by 23 weeks and pyramidal cells are differentiating by 25 weeks' gestation. Dendritic growth undergoes explosive expansion around 32 weeks and is associated with increased cellular metabolic demands.[16]

Myelination, a function of oligodendroglia, is a prominent feature of late gestation (34 weeks onwards) and postnatal life. It is particularly rapid from 38 weeks to 6 months of age and only reaches mature values in 4-year-old infants.[17]

Postnatal brain growth is prodigious. Weighing 335 g at birth, the brain doubles in size by 6 months and weighs 900 g by 12 months. Cortical maturation during this time proceeds in three phases. First to develop are the primary cortical areas such as the primary motor areas of Brodman (area 4) and the somatosensory cortex (area 41). The limbic system also matures early.

The association areas, such as the visual association area and Wernicke's area, are next to mature. These areas are connected by the corpus callosum to their contralateral homologous region

The last cortical regions to mature are the terminal zones. These include the anterior poles of the frontal lobe and angular gyrus and will eventually be concerned with motivational and cognitive function. They have no thalamic connections and their short association fibres may not become fully functional until late adolescence.

The development of pain processing parallels spinal cord development and involves transiently functional pathways. It almost certainly includes developmentally regulated changes in the roles played by chemotropic and neurotransmitter substances. Spinal cord development proceeds in a ventrodorsal fashion, commencing with the motor neurons and deep dorsal horn and finishing with the neurons of laminae I and II and the substantia gelatinosa.

Early in development, large myelinated cutaneous afferents (A-fibres) of dorsal root ganglion (DRG) cells enter the cord and occupy both the deep dorsal horn and superficial laminae. The peripheral extensions of these DRGs reach the skin between 11 and 20 weeks. Smaller C-fibre afferents (largely nociceptive) grow into the cord shortly after the larger fibres and mature later. Although not immediately functional in transmitting nociception, these C-fibres may alter the sensitivity of other (A-fibre) nociceptive afferents. The A-fibre afferents then withdraw during development to occupy only the deeper layers.[18] Spinal cord synapses are present as early as 6 weeks' gestation, although neurotransmitter vesicles only begin to form at 13 weeks. Thalamocortical tracts make synaptic connections at about 24 weeks' gestation and nociceptive nerve tracts are fully myelinated to the level of the thalamus by 30 weeks. As descending inhibitory controls mature, the early period of spinal reflex excitability gradually regresses.[17]

Inhibitory pathways mature at a later stage of development and classic inhibitory transmitters such as GABA play a complex role in early development that may include significant excitatory actions as well as trophic signalling. Opioid receptors appear early in fetal life, with μ- and κ-receptors appearing before δ- receptors. Binding sites for κ-receptors predominate in the immature cord and are initially widely distributed. During development they become selectively localized.[18]

The overall pattern of neural development results in neonates and preterm infants being predisposed to exaggerated and prolonged reflex responses before inhibitory controls eventually mature. These infants have increased and graded but diffuse central responses to noxious stimuli as sensitivity is achieved at the expense of precision.

Nociceptive responses continue to mature postnatally as higher integrating centres develop and cognitive and emotional skills evolve. By 6 months of age anticipatory responses to pain and other complex learned behaviours become evident.[17]

RESPIRATORY DISORDERS

RESPIRATORY ASSESSMENT

Children are at greater risk of perioperative complications than are adults. For example, laryngospasm is, reportedly, almost twice as likely to occur in healthy prepubertal children as in healthy adults[18]. The same is true of the incidence of bronchospasm: it is twice as likely in children.[19]

The Australian Incident Monitoring Study has published statistics on adverse respiratory events showing that sick children are more at risk of an incident during the process of sedation than are healthy children.[20] Overall, two-thirds of the perioperative respiratory incidents occurred in healthy children, a significantly higher proportion than that found in infants and adults.[21] Similarly, the American Society of Anesthesiologists Closed Claims Study of comparative complication risk reported a disproportionate representation of healthy children who experienced respiratory complications.[22] Therefore, although identification of the child at increased risk for perioperative respiratory morbidity is desirable, the preoperative assessment may be of limited use in identifying the healthy child who will experience complications during and following general anaesthesia. Nevertheless, studies have identified some factors associated with increased perioperative risk in children, of which age and a history of a respiratory tract infection are the most important.

Exposure to environmental tobacco smoke may also influence the incidence of postoperative hypoxaemia in children. Lyons has demonstrated a significantly higher incidence of desaturation in the recovery room in children habitually exposed to cigarette smoke than in those not exposed. He suggests that anaesthetists should consider advising parents to abstain from smoking for a period prior to their child's operation.[23]

Age

Being less than 1 year of age is a risk factor for respiratory morbidity and perioperative laryngospasm.[18,22,24] Unlike older children and adults, infants maintain their lung volume above the elastic equilibrium volume of their respiratory system. This dynamic hyperinflation is achieved by active mechanisms including laryngeal braking and persistent inspiratory activity in both the intercostal and phrenic musculature during expiration. These active mechanisms, coupled with a long expiratory time constant relative to the expiratory time, allow the maintenance of an end-expiratory lung volume above its passively determined functional residual capacity.[25–27] During anaesthesia these active mechanisms are attenuated,[28,29] predisposing the infant to lung collapse. In addition, vagal tone in the infant is high, as evidenced by an active Hering–Breuer reflex in infancy.[30] Stimulation of the rapidly adapting, vagal, irritant airway receptors by secretions or tracheal intubation tends to produce apnoea and laryngospasm in infants.[31]

Age less than 3 years is also an independent risk factor for postoperative respiratory complications.[32–34] Bivati et al.[32] reported that children undergoing tonsillectomy who were aged 3 years or younger had a relative risk of airway complications which was 2.3 times that of older children. McGill et al.[35] reported 11 cases of unexplained intra-anaesthetic pulmonary dysfunction characterized by poor expansion of the chest, an absence of breath sounds and tenacious mucous plugs. All 11 cases involved children aged 17 months to 5 years.

Why does the toddler represent a patient population at greater risk?

Numerous reports in the literature suggest that the toddler may be at increased risk for pulmonary collapse during anaesthesia.[22,32–36] Several maturational aspects of the respiratory system may predispose the toddler to lung collapse. It has been shown that the toddler has a more compliant chest wall compared with the older child. Indeed, the ratio of chest wall to lung compliance does not achieve unity (a value approaching that found in the adult) until after 3 years of age.[37] This is consistent with the fact that the magnitude of the decrease in functional residual capacity, associated with anaesthesia, is proportionally greater in the very young child.[36,38] Recent work also provides evidence of the adverse effects of prenatal exposure to tobacco on respiratory function in preterm infants. Since diminished airway function at birth has been shown to be predictive of subsequent wheezing during the first year of life, these changes may also increase the vulnerability of the toddlers' lungs to the adverse effects of anaesthesia.[39]

UPPER RESPIRATORY INFECTIONS

The child with a preoperative upper respiratory infection (URI) constitutes a common clinical dilemma. Should surgery be postponed, or not ? Various strategies based on a hierarchy of symptoms have been proposed (Table 1.1).[40,41]

However, a key factor may be simply the physician's skill in assessing the overall picture in each case: the tendency is for higher cancellation rates to correspond inversely with the number of years in anaesthetic practice. Administration of general anaesthesia in the presence of a URI carries with it an increased risk of perioperative respiratory complications.[21,22,35] All eleven patients suffering major lung collapse in the study reported by McGill *et al.*[35] had a history of a recent URI. A prospective study of healthy toddlers, aged 1–4 years, reported a higher incidence of postoperative desaturation ($<95\%$) in those who had signs and symptoms of a URI.[42] Similarly, a study of infants with a history of URI showed that they experienced a more rapid rate of desaturation during apnoea. Otherwise healthy

children who have a concomitant respiratory infection experienced a 2-fold increase in the incidence of perioperative laryngospasm[19,24] and a 10-fold increase in the incidence of bronchospasm.[19]

The mechanisms whereby viral respiratory infections increase the likelihood of respiratory morbidity are numerous. Viral airway infections are associated with bronchial hyperreactivity even in patients without pre-existing lung disease. The mechanisms underlying this bronchial hyperresponsiveness have been reviewed by Jacoby and Hirshman[43] and van der Walt *et al.*[21] There is no demonstrable intrinsic abnormality of smooth muscle. Much of the bronchial hyperresponsiveness is neurally mediated, and vagal mechanisms are important, as evidenced by the fact that the histamine-induced bronchoconstriction is abolished by pretreatment with nebulized isoproterenol and atropine.[44] It is noteworthy that pretreatment of adults with inhaled bronchodilators resulted in lower lung resistance after intubation compared with controls.[45] Since bronchoconstriction associated with tracheal intubation is also mediated by the rapidly adapting irritant receptors,[31] this undoubtedly underscores the higher incidence of bronchospasm associated with tracheal intubation in patients with a recent URI.

An increased release of acetylcholine to vagal stimulation has been postulated as a mechanism for the increased bronchoreactivity associated with a recent URI. Transient inhibition of the inhibitory muscarinic (M_2-subtype) receptors on the vagal nerve endings may result from the increase in viral neuraminidase. In addition, viral infections potentiate the bronchoconstriction to stimulation by tachykinins. The potentiation of the response to tachykinins is associated with the loss of the enzyme neutral endopeptidase, which breaks down tachykinins.[43]

The bronchial hyperresponsiveness results in a demonstrable increase in histamine and citric acid-induced bronchoconstriction and a 200% increase in airway resistance compared with controls.[44,45] Collier *et al.*,[46] in a longitudinal study of children, showed that indices of expiratory flow were decreased during a URI consistent with acute peripheral airway obstruction. Therefore, a recent upper respiratory infection may be associated with a predisposi-

Table 1.1 Signs and symptoms that may aid in the assessment of a child with respiratory tract infection

	Likely to cancel surgery	Less likely to cancel surgery
Cough	Productive	Non-productive
Fever	Y	N
History of asthma	Y	N
Administration of cough syrup	Y	N
Looks unwell	Y	N
Decreased appetite	Y	N
Decreased activity	Y	N
Wheezing on auscultation	Y	N

tion to earlier airway closure. In addition, both the quantity and quality of bronchial secretions may be altered during a respiratory tract infection.[43]

Toddlers spend much of their time suffering from the acute and subacute symptoms of a respiratory tract infection. There is evidence that bronchial hyperreactivity and the associated predisposition for closure of the small airways persists for up to 6 weeks following a URI.[44] Therefore, the maturational aspects of the respiratory system which predispose the toddler to a loss of lung volume during anaesthesia (see above) coupled with the URI-associated tendency to bronchorreactivity and airway collapse present a plausible explanation for the increased incidence of perioperative respiratory morbidity in the toddler.

OTHER RISK FACTORS FOR RESPIRATORY MORBIDITY

The presence of craniofacial anomalies, particularly midfacial hypoplasia or micro/retrognathia, and a history suggestive of chronic upper airway obstruction (see below) have been identified as additional risk factors for complications post-tonsillectomy and may also apply to other surgical procedures.[32–34,47]

Habitual benign snoring is present in 7–9% of otherwise healthy children, whereas obstructive sleep apnoea is reported in 1–2% of preschool children.[48,49] Chronic upper airway obstruction is suggested by the historical and physical findings outlined in Table 1.2.

Daytime mouth breathing, an observed apnoea, an impression that the child struggled to breathe during sleep and a history of shaking the child to make him or her resume breathing again were more frequently reported in children with obstructive sleep apnoea. However, history alone could not discriminate between obstructive sleep apnoea and benign snoring.[48]

Asthma

Wheezing associated with viral lower respiratory tract illness is common in children and asthma exacerbation frequently occurs with concomitant viral infections. The differential diagnosis of wheezing includes asthma, aspiration of a foreign body, especially in the toddler,

Table 1.2 Symptoms and signs suggestive of chronic upper airway obstruction

Symptoms	Signs
Mouth breathing	Orthodontic
Snoring every night	malformations
– very loud	Laboured breathing
– punctuated with	Paradoxical respiration
pauses and gasps	Diaphoresis during sleep
Unusual sleeping	Cyanosis
positions	Failure to thrive
– neck hyperextended	Crowded oropharynx
– seated	– adenotonsillar
Nocturnal enuresis	hypertrophy
Hyponasal speech-	
Increased intensity	
of the second	
heart sound	
Daytime somnolence	
Morning cephalgia	
Difficulty swallowing	

cystic fibrosis, ciliary dyskinesia, alpha-1 antitrypsin deficiency and bronchiolitis. Asthma affects 5–10% of children.[49–51] There is a widely held perception that the prevalence of asthma in children has increased. Asthma is a heterogeneous condition characterized by acute attacks of wheezing and shortness of breath associated with reversibility of airway obstruction. Recurrent cough and exercise-induced cough may represent asthma symptoms. Guidelines for classification of asthma severity are tabulated in Table 1.3. The pattern and severity of attacks vary with the individual. Pulmonary function tests typically show an obstructive pattern, characterized by low flows [a decrease in volume exhaled in the first second of expiration (FEV_1), FEV_1/forced vital capacity (FVC) and forced expiratory flow (FEF)$_{25-75}$ (see below)] and relatively normal lung volumes. An improvement in the indices of expiratory airflow following bronchodilator therapy supports the diagnosis of asthma and may indicate a need to alter medical therapy preoperatively in order to optimize lung function. The β-adrenergic agonists, cholinergic antagonists and methylxanthines remain the mainstay of

Table 1.3 Classification of asthma severity[a] in children prior to pharmacological intervention[b]

Mild asthma
    Intermittent, brief (<1 h) cough and wheeze up to 2 times week^{-1}
    Asymptomatic between exacerbations
    Good exercise tolerance. May not tolerate vigorous exercise
    Infrequent (<2 times month^{-1}) nocturnal symptoms
Moderate asthma
    Symptoms >1–2 times week^{-1}
    Exacerbations may last for several days
    Occasional emergency room care
    Exercise tolerance diminished
    Asthma symptoms present overnight 2–3 times week^{-1}
Severe asthma
    Continuous symptoms
    Limited activity level. Poor exercise tolerance
    Frequent exacerbations
    Overnight asthma symptoms almost every night. Chest tightness in early morning
    Occasional hospitalization and emergency room care

---

[a]The nature of asthma is variable. Symptoms may change with or without intervention and individuals may change categories at any time.
[b]Most of the symptoms resolve or are diminished with appropriate drug therapy.
(Reproduced with permission from Lenfant, 1991.[51])

asthma medication. It has been suggested that the degree of airway hyperresponsiveness correlates with the number of medications required to control them.[52]

Cystic fibrosis

Cystic fibrosis is a differential diagnosis of the wheezing child. Cystic fibrosis is a lethal autosomal recessive disease with an estimated incidence in the Caucasian population of 1 in 2500. Occasionally, cystic fibrosis may masquerade as a healthy child with a history of frequent respiratory tract infections. Bilateral nasal polyps are also consistent with a diagnosis of cystic fibrosis and may be the presenting symptom.[53] Although usually presenting in infancy, adult-onset cystic fibrosis has been reported.[54]

Cystic fibrosis arises from a mutation on the long arm of chromosome 7 in the gene for the chloride conductance channel and is associated with an abnormality of chloride conductance in epithelial cells on the mucosa. This abnormal chloride conductance underscores the use of the sweat chloride test in the diagnosis of cystic fibrosis. A sweat chloride in excess of 60 mEq l^{-1} is diagnostic.[54] The respiratory consequence of an altered chloride conductance in the lung epithelial cells results in dehydration of secretions predisposing the lung to airway obstruction and chronic infection. Treatment modalities include a daily programme of chest percussion and postural drainage, antibiotic, bronchodilator and oxygen therapy. The importance of the chest percussion and postural drainage regimen may influence the scheduling of elective surgery. A prospective study of 49 children with cystic fibrosis reported a significant correlation between the incidence of viral infections and every measure of disease progression.[55] Therefore, a concomitant URI in the child with cystic fibrosis may preclude elective surgery.

Recurrent lower respiratory infections may lead to necrotizing bronchitis and broncheictasis, although many children with cystic fibrosis retain relatively normal pulmonary function.[56] Pulmonary function testing (see below) is useful to document a deterioration in lung function. Initially, pulmonary function testing shows evidence of gas trapping with an increase in residual volume and the ratio of residual volume to total lung capacity. Progression of the disease in older children typically reveals a pattern of reduced FEV_1, reduced peak flows and reduced FEF_{25-75} (see below), suggestive of airways obstruction. An associated bronchoreactive component may be present and bronchodilators may be helpful in one-third of patients. Later in the disease progression, an abnormal carbon monoxide diffusing capacity is a reliable index of significant pulmonary dysfunction. Progressive hypoxaemia leading to pulmonary hypertension and cor pulmonale are present in the late stages of cystic fibrosis.[54]

RESPIRATORY CONSIDERATIONS IN THE CHILD WITH CARDIAC PROBLEMS

Cardiac malformations associated with a decrease in pulmonary blood flow (tetralogy of Fallot, Ebstein's anomaly) rarely have associated respiratory symptoms, whereas those characterized by an increase in pulmonary blood flow (ventricular septal defect, atrial septal defect) are frequently associated with tachypnoea and intercostal retractions. These conditions are described in detail in Chapter 13.

Respiratory resistance is reported to be higher and pulmonary compliance lower in cardiac lesions associated with an increased pulmonary blood flow.[57] A study of infants under the age of 2 years reported a negative relationship between lung compliance and the ratio of the right pulmonary artery to the aorta. Since a ratio in excess of 1 suggests an increase in pulmonary blood flow, it is likely that pulmonary vascular engorgement was largely responsible for the reduction in pulmonary compliance.[58]

Respiratory infection, in particular respiratory syncytial viral infection, in the infant with congenital heart disease is associated with significantly more severe illness and an increased mortality rate.[59]

RESPIRATORY CONSIDERATIONS IN THE EX-PREMATURE INFANT: APNOEA RISK

Barrington and Finer[60] examined 20 otherwise healthy premature infants and reported an apnoea frequency of 0.9 apnoeas per hour in the first 24 h of life, which decreased to 0.2 apnoeas in the first week of life. Central, obstructive and mixed apnoea were reported in otherwise healthy premature infants.[58] Demonstration of a correlation between the incidence of apnoea and the brainstem conduction times suggests that an immaturity of the central medullary respiratory control centre may underlie the apnoea of prematurity.[27]

In the early 1980s Steward[61] reported an increased incidence of postoperative apnoea in the expremature infant. Other investigators have reported postoperative apnoea in healthy term infants.[40,62] Although a recent prospective multicentre study reported that the incidence of postoperative apnoea in infants was inversely correlated with age, precise identification of the postconceptional age at increased risk remains to be defined.[63–65] Most studies support the notion that infants of less than 60 weeks' postconceptional age are at increased risk and both obstructive and central apnoeas have been reported in the postoperative period in infants.[66] Note that postoperative apnoea may occur immediately in the recovery room or be delayed by several hours.[62] A positive history for prematurity, anaemia, necrotizing enterocolitis, apnoea, respiratory distress syndrome, bronchopulmonary dysplasia and a diagnosis of small for gestational age are all reported to increase the incidence of postoperative apnoea. A history of respiratory syncytial virus infection in infants also increases the incidence of apnoea.[67] In addition, infants undergoing ventricular peritoneal shunt insertion/revision for hydrocephalus are at increased risk for postoperative apnoea. Since abnormalities of respiratory control have been demonstrated in patients with neural tube defects[68] postoperative apnoea in the neurosurgical patient, like the apnoea of prematurity, may be associated with an abnormality or immaturity of the medullary neural network.

The expremature infant with a history of intermittent positive pressure ventilation (IPPV), for the treatment of hyaline membrane disease[69] and apnoea,[70] has been shown to have increased airways resistance on subsequent testing. This delayed onset of increased airways resistance is consistent with the notion that the treatment of hyaline membrane disease with IPPV results in damage to the terminal airways which interferes with subsequent growth. It has been noted that infants aged greater than 33 weeks' postconceptional age and infants requiring IPPV for less than 5 days were less likely to develop airway injury and bronchopulmonary dysplasia.[70] Damage to the airways is a plausible aetiology for the increased frequency of respiratory morbidity and wheezing in these infants.

PREOPERATIVE RESPIRATORY FUNCTION TESTING

Chest X-ray

Biavati et al.[32] reported that the probability of postoperative (tonsillectomy) complications with a normal electrocardiogram (ECG) or chest X-ray (CXR) differed little from the probability of complications without knowing the result. Therefore, the value of the preoperative CXR and ECG in asymptomatic children has been questioned.[71] Indeed, there are few indications for a preoperative CXR in the routine preoperative workup of the healthy child. However, the preoperative CXR may be invaluable in the asymptomatic child requiring cervical node biopsy for the diagnosis of lymphoma for whom an anterior mediastinal mass has important anaesthetic implications.

Polysomnography

Polysomnography (or sleep studies) uses three- to six-channel recordings in order to quantify sleep state, breathing patterns and ventilation (including both oxygenation and carbon dioxide tensions) by non-invasive methods to aid in the diagnosis of respiratory control disorders. Interested readers are referred to Refs 49 and 72 for an in-depth discussion of its potential application in infants and children. Polysomnography is often used to assess obstructive sleep apnoea in the otherwise healthy child requiring tonsillectomy. Figure 1.1 shows a recording of a 3-year-old boy with obstructive sleep apnoea secondary to tonsillar hypertrophy. In children with obstructive sleep apnoea, partial airway obstruction (obstructive hypoventilation) may be present for hours. An important difference between adult and childhood sleep apnoea syndrome is the preservation of sleep architecture in children evidenced by normal proportions of active [rapid eye movement (REM)] and slow-wave (non-REM) sleep.[49]

Although polysomnography was not found to be cost-effective as a screening test for identification of the child at increased risk for postoperative (tonsillectomy) complications, it was useful preoperatively to confirm the diagnosis of obstructive sleep apnoea in high-risk patients.[32] Kurth *et al.*[66] reported that none of the premature infants who experienced postoperative apnoea had apnoea on the preoperative pneumogram, suggesting that the polysomnography was also of limited use as a screen for the infant at increased risk for postoperative apnoea.

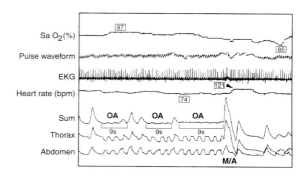

Figure 1.1 Polysomnograph recording of a 3-year-old boy during sleep. Note the series of obstructive apnoeas associated with paradoxical thoracic and abdominal movement associated with desaturation (SaO$_2$) to 85% and terminated by a movement/arousal (MIA). (Source: Jacob *et al.*, 1995.[73] Reproduced by permission of Wiley-Liss, Inc., a subsidiary of John Wiley & Sons, Inc.)

Pulmonary function testing

Pulmonary function testing is not routinely available for the clinical assessment of infants and young children because of technical difficulties inherent in the assessment of pulmonary function in infants. Both a lack of standardization and the inability of young children to co-operate with a maximal voluntary effort limit the use of pulmonary function testing in this age group,[74] although they represent the patient population at greatest risk for perioperative respiratory morbidity (see above). However, infant lung function measurements are being used in epidemiological studies to assess the effect of respiratory disease on lung maturation.[75] Interested readers are referred to Ref. 76 for a comprehensive discussion of pulmonary function testing in infants and young children.

Pulmonary function testing is available in children aged more than 6 years, who are able to co-operate with a vital capacity manoeuvre.[77] Pulmonary function testing in children is similar to that used in adults and includes an assessment of lung volumes, spirometry and flow–volume loops.

Lung volumes may be measured by body plethysmography or by gas dilution techniques. Total lung capacity (TLC), functional residual capacity (FRC), residual volume (RV) and the ratio of residual volume to total lung capacity (RV/TLC) are useful indices (Figure 1.2).

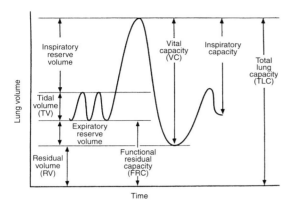

Figure 1.2 A spirogram of the lung volumes during tidal breathing and a vital capacity manoeuvre. See text for definitions.

Preoperative assessment of lung volumes in healthy adolescents with idiopathic scoliosis is important in order to evaluate the presence of an associated restrictive lung disease evidenced by a decrease in lung volumes (FRC, TLC and RV).

Spirometry measures the indices of airflow during exhalation usually involving a maximal expiratory effort. The rationale for the use of spirometry to assess the flow/pressure relationship of the respiratory system is based on the demonstration that at maximal flow, airflow becomes independent of effort and reflects the resistance of the airways and the driving pressure. The normal time required to exhale from a forced vital capacity to RV is less than 3 s, but may be prolonged in obstructive lung disease such as asthma. During a forced expiratory manoeuvre the volume exhaled in the first second of expiration (FEV_1) in the normal child is usually 75% of the forced vital capacity ($FEV_1/FVC = 0.75$). The peak expiratory flow rate (PEFR) occurs early in expiration and is an index of both the resistance of the large airways and patient effort. The forced expiratory flow defined as the slope of the expiratory flow between 25 and 75% of the FVC (FEF_{25-75}) is effort independent and an index of small airways resistance (Figure 1.3).

Interpretation of results of spirometry

Parameter	Restrictive	Obstructive
FVC	↓	Normal or ↓
FEV_1	Normal or ↓	↓
FEV_1/FVC	Normal or ↑	↓
FEF_{25-75}	Normal, ↓, ↑	↓

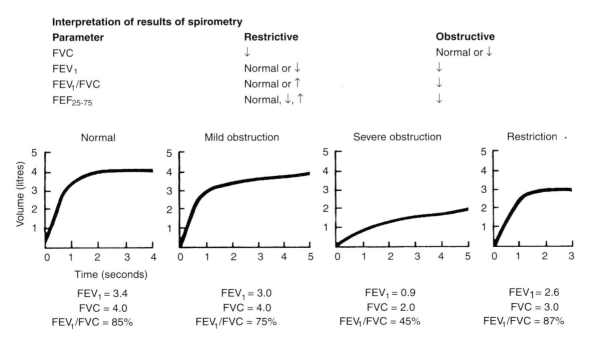

Figure 1.3 Stylized flow volume spirograms for normal, obstructive and restrictive conditions. See text for definitions.

Inspiratory and expiratory flow–volume loops are useful for assessing anatomic obstruction in children. Flow limitation in both inspiration and expiration suggests a fixed extrathoracic obstruction such as subglottic stenosis. Decreased inspiratory flows with near normal expiratory flows suggest a variable extrathoracic obstruction. Reduced expiratory flows with near normal inspiratory flows suggest a variable intrathoracic obstruction such as a mediastinal mass (Figure 1.4).[78]

Arterial blood gases

There is little indication for the use of arterial blood gas tensions in the preoperative assessment of the normal child. Oximetry is a useful screen for premorbid respiratory conditions and a saturation less than 95% while breathing room air is often indicative of an underlying cardiorespiratory process. When an estimate of carbon dioxide tension is indicated, capillary gases drawn from a warmed extremity (heel) provide a reasonable estimate of the carbon dioxide tension.

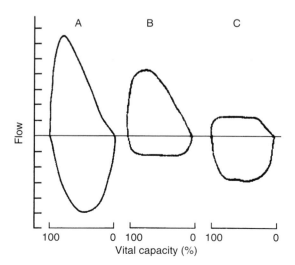

Figure 1.4 Stylized inspiratory/expiratory flow volume loops illustrating a normal loop configuration (A), inspiratory flow limitation associated with extra thoracic obstruction (B) and expiratory flow limitation associated with intrathoracic obstruction (C).

NEUROLOGICAL DISORDERS

EPILEPSY

A seizure is a paroxysmal disturbance of brain function resulting in motor, sensory, autonomic and psychic phenomena that may be associated with loss of consciousness. Repeated seizures are referred to as epilepsy. Both isolated seizures and epilepsy occur more commonly in childhood than in adult life. Epileptic seizures occur in 3–5% of children and 60% of epilepsy starts in childhood. Current antiepileptic drug treatment is ineffective in 20–25% of epilepsy cases.[80]

Epilepsy may be classified as generalized or partial (focal). In generalized seizures there is usually loss of consciousness associated with a generalized fit. In partial seizures epileptic activity may be restricted to one hemisphere and consciousness preserved (simple partial seizures), or if epileptic activity spreads to the opposite hemisphere consciousness may be impaired (complex partial seizure).

Any intracranial pathology may give rise to seizures. Most commonly this involves tumours or head injuries. In a large number of children no structural cause can be found for the epilepsy. In these cases, hypoglycaemia, hyperglycaemia, uraemia and syncope must be excluded as causes.

Grand mal or tonic–clonic epilepsy follows a number of stages. The prodromal phase lasting from hours to days usually takes the form of a mood change and aura. The tonic stage involves loss of consciousness and a generalized contracture of muscles, including the respiratory muscles, occasionally causing cyanosis. In the following clonic phase, jerking movements often result in biting of the tongue and incontinence. The postictal phase is characterized by the patient remaining unconscious and then drifting into sleep.

Petit mal or absence seizures occur in three distinct types. The first variety involves a very brief (10–15 s) episode in which the patient suffers an 'absence'. The second type is similar to the brief absence but is accompanied by jerking of some part of the body. The third type involves a true loss of consciousness but is short lived and not associated with any abnormal movement.

In children with partial seizures or focal epilepsy the discharge begins in a focus in the brain, but may then spread to other parts of the brain. The temporal lobe is a common site from which abnormal discharges may begin. Feelings of deja-vu are common and hallucinations of sight, smell or taste may occur. Jacksonian epilepsy represents another form of partial seizures. In this form the fit spreads from a well-defined area of a limb slowly to involve other parts of the limb or other areas. Prolonged paralysis following a Jacksonian seizure suggests a structural lesion.

Diagnosis depends on observation of the seizure or, if this is not possible, a good description. Electroencephalography (EEG) is useful in localizing a lesion or in confirming the diagnosis. Complex magnetic resonance imaging (MRI) sequences are now used in the evaluation of patients with epilepsy.

Drugs available for the treatment of epilepsy include phenobarbitone, phenytoin, carbamazepine, sodium valproate, ethosuxamide and primidone. Newer drugs introduced since 1994 include felbamate, gabapentin, lamotrigine, vigabatrin and vopiramate.[81] In general ,these drugs are well tolerated, although all may cause drowsiness. With the older drugs rickets or folate deficiency may occur and gingival hyperplasia is a specific problem of phenytoin. Other rare side-effects of phenytoin include lymphadenopathy and SLE type syndrome. Felbamate was found to have several side-effects and has fallen out of use. Gabapentin is well tolerated but lamotrigine has some side-effects, with rashes being quite common, and some severe reactions have been reported.

Surgery for epilepsy is gaining in popularity and various surgical procedures are available. These include lesionectomy, focal resections, either temporal or extratemporal, hemispherectomy and functional procedures such as callasotomy and subpial transections (see Chapter 16).

Anaesthetic implications of epilepsy

Anaesthetic management is aimed at minimizing the potential for perioperative seizures and the maintenance of drug therapy. Children presenting for epilepsy surgery almost always have some degree of neurological impairment. This ranges from learning difficulties to severe behavioural problems and/or severe developmental delay. These abnormalities may make these patients difficult to handle, particularly in the anaesthetic room. Careful use of sedative premedication may be indicated. These patients may be encountered during incidental surgery, for investigation of seizures (MRI) and for epilepsy surgery itself.

Children who are on antiepileptic medication frequently have induced liver enzymes and muscle relaxants that are metabolized in the liver have a very short duration of action. Vecuronium seems to be particularly short acting in these circumstances and a drug like atracuriun may be a better choice.

CEREBRAL PALSY

Cerebral palsy is defined as a non-progressive impairment of movement and abnormal posture that has been present since birth. There are a number of different forms but generally all types fall into one of three broad groups: spastic, dyskinetic or hypotonic. The pathophysiology remains unclear but suggested aetiological factors include intrauterine hypoxia, birth trauma, infectious agents or toxins including kernicterus. These children frequently suffer from epilepsy, developmental delay and poor speech, although intelligence may well be normal. Progressive spinal deformity is common and frequently compromises respiratory function. There may also be poor swallowing and gastro-oesophageal reflux. In severe forms the prognosis is poor and death usually results from intercurrent infection. In milder forms life expectancy may be almost normal.

These children commonly present for orthopaedic procedures aimed at correcting limb and spinal deformities and also for Nissen's fundoplication for severe reflux. Care should be taken to talk to these children in an appropriate manner as they may be of nearly normal intelligence although they do not appear capable of understanding. Chest infections may be more common and careful preoperative evaluation with physiotherapy may be required. Anaesthetic drugs may cause hypotension and are used with caution. Careful positioning on the operating table is required to prevent pressure sores.

TUMOURS OF THE CENTRAL NERVOUS SYSTEM

Tumours of the central nervous system (CNS) account for 20% of all malignant childhood cancer and come second only to leukaemia as a cause of cancer in children. The peak incidence of brain tumours is between 5 and 10 years of age, with an incidence of about 20–25 per million. Primary brain tumours are classified depending on the cell type involved (Table 1.4). The majority of tumours in children aged over 2 years are infratentorial (65%) and tend to occur in the midline. Childhood brain tumours are generally more differentiated than their adult counterparts[82] (see Chapter 16).

HYDROCEPHALUS

Hydrocephalus describes an excessive amount of cerebrospinal fluid (CSF) in the cranium and may be either congenital or acquired. Most congenital cases are associated with encephalocele and meningomyelocele.[83] Eighty per cent of neonates with encephalocele and 96% with meningomyelocele have hydrocephalus. Other congenital causes include X-linked aqueductal stenosis, aqueductal and arachnoid stenosis acquired from intrauterine viral infection and mass lesions.

Acquired causes are more common and include intraventicular haemorrhage, meningitis, tumours, cysts and arteriovenous malformations. It is particularly common in ex-premature babies.[84] Clinical features of hydrocephalus are mainly due to raised intracranial pressure (ICP). As the cranial sutures are not fused in infants papilloedema may be absent and the head may grow very large (see Chapter16)

Table 1.4 Common types of central nervous system tumours

Tumour type	Incidence	Example
Glial cell tumours	50–60%	Astrocytoma Optic nerve glioma Brain stem glioma Ependymoma
Neuroectodermal tumour		Gangliocytoma Medullo-blastoma
Cranio-pharyngioma	5–10%	
Germ cell tumour	<10%	Teratoma Dermoid Germinoma
Meningeal tumour	<5%	Meningioma Meningeal sarcoma
Lymphoma	<1%	

ARNOLD–CHIARI MALFORMATION

The Arnold–Chiari malformation represents an anomaly of the hindbrain characterized by the caudal displacement of the cerebellum and brainstem. It may take one of three forms. Type I involves elongation and displacement of the brainstem into the spinal canal with protrusion of the cerebellar vermis through the foramen magnum. Type II has, in addition, a lumbar meningomyelocele and hydrocephalus. Type III is associated with an occipital encephalocele.

Clinically, patients may present with difficulty swallowing, recurrent aspiration, stridor or apnoea. The gag reflex may be impaired and syringomyelia is a frequent association leading to sensory and motor deficits.

Management frequently involves surgical enlargement of the foramen magnum to allow decompression of the posterior fossa. Cervical laminectomy and dural opening may also be performed to allow decompresion of the cerebellar tongue. Associated syringomyelia may require drainage. Anaesthetic considerations include poor respiratory control with a risk of perioperative apnoea. Recurrent aspiration and bulbar nerve palsy presenting as stridor should be anticipated.

NEUROCUTANEOUS DYSPLASIAS

Neurofibromatosis

This term describes several distinct diseases that each display variable combinations of café au lait spots and tumours of the peripheral and central nervous system (neurofibromas and schwannomas). These children also have learning difficulties or developmental delay. The two more common forms, Nf1 (von Recklinghausen's disease) and Nf2 (bilateral acoustic or central neurofibromatosis) are inherited in an autosomal dominant fashion but severity within families cannot be predicted. Genetic counselling and monitoring for complications of the disease are the basis of ongoing care for affected families.[85]

Tuberous sclerosis

This autosomal dominant condition has a wide spectrum of presentation from skin manifestations only, through to severe debilitating epilepsy and severe developmental delay. Fibromas may occur almost anywhere, from the face and gums to brain, kidney and retina. Cardiac involvement with rhabdomyomas can cause outflow obstruction.

Sturge–Weber syndrome

Port wine staining of the face, meningeal angioma and choroidal angioma are features of this condition. These children may have epilepsy, developmental delay or hemiparesis depending on the sites of the lesions and glaucoma. Treatment is aimed at controlling the epilepsy and this may arrest the developmental delay. Surgical removal of the brain lesions is sometimes undertaken.

NEUROMUSCULAR DISEASE

The following section describes conditions that may confront the paediatric anaesthetist dealing with children who present with weakness, wasting or apparent hypertrophy of muscle groups. If these symptoms are combined with hypotonia and hyporeflexia or stiffness and myotonia, primary muscle disease should be suspected.

Myasthenia gravis describes disorders of the neuromuscular junction in which the pattern of weakness is typically one of fatigue and exhaustion with use. Paediatric cases involve several distinct pathophysiologies.

The myopathies are primary disorders of muscle characterized by lower motor neuron weakness and classified on the basis of ultrastructural changes on muscle biopsy. Most paediatric cases are genetically determined, but a few are acquired. Several glycogen storage diseases have primary manifestations in muscle and are considered here.

The muscular dystrophies are genetically determined disorders of muscle with similar lower motor neuron weakness but not associated with specific ultrastructural abnormalities. Muscle biopsy simply shows dystrophic changes. Classification has traditionally been based on clinical criteria but the recent elucidation of the molecular basis of these conditions has provoked a reclassification.[86]

The myotonic syndromes are inherited degenerative conditions characterized by muscle tension transiently outlasting voluntary muscle contraction. Weakness, dystrophic changes and extramuscular abnormalities are associated with particular named disorders.

Anaesthesia may be required for diagnostic procedures (in particular muscle biopsy), orthopaedic procedures or unrelated surgery. Specific diagnosis may not be available at the time of preoperative assessment (prediagnosis symptomatic phase). More worrying is that patients with mild or early disease may be entirely unsuspected of having major neuromuscular dysfunction at the time of anaesthesia.

An overall understanding of the pathophysiology, clinical features and associations of each condition is necessary for the safe conduct of anaesthesia in these children. The major concerns for the anaesthetist are: (1) unusual responses to drugs; (2) the risks of perioperative respiratory failure; (3) the risks of sudden cardiovascular decompensation; and (4) the association of some of these conditions with malignant hyperthermia (MH). Table 1.5 gives a general classification for these conditions together with the primary anaesthetic considerations for the major groups.

Table 1.5   Neuromuscular disorders

Muscle disease	Anaesthesia issues
Disorders of the neuromuscular junction	
Myasthenia gravis	
Neonatal transient	
Congenital	
Juvenile	Peri-operative anticholinesterase regime; post-operative ventilatory support
Myasthenic syndrome	
Muscle dystrophy	
The X-linked dystrophinopathies	Respiratory compromise; risk of sudden cardiac decompensation; avoid suxamethonium: monitor temperature
Duchenne MD	
Becker's MD	
The sarcoglycanopathies (limb girdle dystrophies) (previously Erb's and Leyden–Mobius dystrophies)	
Facio–Scapulo–Humeral dystrophy	
Emery–Dreifuss dystrophy	
Congenital MD	
The myotonias	
Myotonic dystrophy (Steinert's disease)	Sedative sensitivity; respiratory and cardiac compromise; myotonia with suxamethonium, A'cholinesterases,cold and surgical manipulation
Myotonia congenita	
Paramyotonia congenita	
Hyperkalaemic periodic paralysis	Flaccid paralysis with cold, hunger and emotional stress; avoid carbohydrate depletion
Schwartz–Jampel syndrome	MH risk
Recessive generalized myotonia	
Congenital myopathies	
Central core disease	MH risk
Nemaline myopathy	Respiratory compromise
Mitochondrial myopathies	
Glycogen storage diseases	
Muscle glycogenoses	
Type II (Pompe's disease)	Macrglossia; cardiomyopathy
Type V (McArdle's disease)	Rhabdomyolysis with severe activity
GSD associated with anaemia	Non-spherocytic haemolytic anaemia
Liver glycogenoses	
Type I, III, IV (Von Gierke, Forbes' and Andersen's diseases)	Hypoglycaemia; hepatomegaly

THE X-LINKED DYSTROPHINOPATHIES

These conditions result from absence or abnormality of dystrophin, a protein localized to muscle membrane and also expressed in cardiac and brain tissue. Dystrophin links the muscle cytoskeleton (via F-actin molecules) to the extracellular matrix via several dystrophin-related proteins (sarcoglycans, dystroglycans and syntrophins). Presumably this arrangement protects the muscle membrane from shearing forces during contraction. Dystrophin is a product of a large gene located on the X chromosome (Xp21).[87]

DUCHENNE MUSCULAR DYSTROPHY

This is the most common and most severe of the muscle dystrophies, with an incidence of 1 : 3300 male births. Its prevalence in the total population is 3 : 100 000. Being the result of a gene deletion, it tends to be a relatively homogeneous disorder with a predictable phenotype. The molecular defect is also present in skeletal, cardiac and smooth muscle.

Infants present between the ages of 2 and 6 years with clumsiness and a waddling gait. Pelvic girdle weakness results in the characteristic 'climbing-up-your-legs' manoeuvre termed Gower's sign. Pseudohypertrophy of muscles, particularly the calves, is the result of fatty infiltration and fibrosis. Weakness, limb contractures and kyphoscoliosis are progressive and eventually become disabling. Children often become wheelchair bound within 3–10 years and succumb to cardiorespiratory failure in their third decade.[88]

Some degree of mental impairment is also usual, with mean IQ being one standard deviation below normal.

Cardiac involvement in Duchenne muscular dystrophy (MD) is common (50–70%) and may present as rhythm disturbance such as atrial tachycardias, mitral valve prolapse, ventricular wall hypokinesia and sudden death. This cardiomyopathy does not usually become clinically apparent before 10 years of age. ECG abnormalities then become increasingly common and range from right axis deviation to atrioventricular and intraventricular conduction defects.

Progressive muscle weakness associated with scoliosis reduces ventilatory capacity and leads to inevitable respiratory complications with age. Smooth muscle involvement in the gastrointestinal tract increases the risk of gastric dilatation.

Diagnosis is based on clinical presentation and DNA analysis.[88]

BECKER'S DYSTROPHY

This is an allelic disorder of Duchenne MD, i.e. the gene defect lies in the same region of the X chromosome. Clinically, Becker's dystrophy has a later onset than Duchenne MD, with variable and less severe progression, although the clinical concerns remain identical. Survival rates are 50% at age 40 years.

The detection of the specific gene defect now allows early prenatal diagnosis of both X-linked dystrophinopathies from chorionic villous biopsy or amniocentesis.

ANAESTHESIA ISSUES IN THE DYSTROPHINOPATHIES

The dystrophinopathies impose significant anaesthesia risks on sufferers, making a comprehensive preoperative assessment essential. Respiratory muscle weakness, poor cough, kyphoscoliosis and postoperative immobility contribute to sputum retention, atelectasis and ventilation/perfusion mismatch. Aggressive perioperative respiratory care is essential to prevent hypoxaemia and pneumonia. Preoperative respiratory and cardiac function testing may help to plan the need for postoperative ventilation and decide the advisability of proceeding with elective surgery. Suggested minimal criteria for elective anaesthesia and surgery include FVC > 25% of predicted, PEFR > 30% predicted and LVEF > 0.5.[89]

Cardiac status should be thoroughly assessed prior to anaesthesia as general immobility and inanition may conceal significant dysfunction. Unexplained tachycardia or a non-specific murmur may be the first hints of a cardiomyopathy. ECG evidence of right ventricular strain or dilatation, arrhythmias and echocardiographic evidence of ventricular wall motion abnormalities should prompt intensive postoperative cardiac monitoring.

The potential for gastrointestinal involvement makes it wise to allow gastric drainage during all but the shortest anaesthetics as gastric dilatation will impede adequate ventilation and increase the risk of aspiration. Deformity and contracture require that extra care be taken with venous access, patient movement and positioning.

The use of muscle relaxants requires care and demands that neuromuscular function be strictly monitored.[90,91] The response to nondepolarizing agents is thought to be normal, although apparent sensitivity and prolonged action may occasionally result from altered drug kinetics in patients with severe muscle wasting.[92] The use of depolarizing agents is not advised as the response is unpredictable and may include rigidity, rhabdomyolysis and hyperkalaemic arrhythmias or arrest[93,94] (see Chapter 5).

The association of these dystrophinopathies with MH, although contentious, remains unproven. A small number of case reports with variable documentation must be balanced against several larger series that fail to demonstrate any increased susceptibility to MH.[95] It is perhaps wise to avoid known triggering agents in anaesthesia for muscle biopsy. Temperature must be monitored throughout and access to end-tidal carbon dioxide monitors or blood gas analysis is recommended. Preoperative anticholinergic agents should not be routinely used. It is likely that the risk of MH in Duchenne MD patients is no greater than that in the general population[96–98] (see also Chapter 5).

THE MYOTONIAS

This group of inherited conditions is characterized by delayed muscle relaxation and an electromyographic profile commonly referred to as the 'dive-bomber' effect (alluding to the audio amplification of the EMG signal). Although the exact pathophysiology differs between various myotonic syndromes they are all the result of defective sodium and chloride membrane channel function.

Myotonic dystrophy (Steinert's disease) is a multisystem disease, the genetic defect of which has been localized to chromosome 19. Defects of both sodium and chloride channels exist. Myotonia congenita, paramyotonia congenita and hyperkalaemic periodic paralysis result from defects on chromosome 17. Some of these latter conditions may be allelic disorders of a gene locus encoding a sodium channel. Extramuscular manifestations are less common.[95]

MYOTONIC DYSTROPHY

This is an autosomal dominant disorder with complete penetrance but variable expression within families. It is the most common dystro-phy of adult life, with an estimated prevalence of 3–5 : 100 000. The adult form of disease presents with myopathic weakness, myotonia and/or extramuscular symptoms including cataracts, infertility and colloid goitre. The onset is insidious and may go unrecognized for a long period before diagnosis. Diagnosis is based on clinical presentation and EMG recording. Muscle biopsy may reveal characteristic type I fibre atrophy with type II fibre hypertrophy.

The juvenile form of myotonic dystrophy may be initially diagnosed by an astute physician, on recognizing features in the mother of the affected offspring. Neonates present as 'floppy babies' and are generally hypotonic. Respiratory distress is common and unless immediate resuscitation and intubation are required, a weak cry with impaired swallowing and sucking may be noted.[88] Facial diplegia and a 'tent-shaped mouth' are typical. The prenatal impact of disease is evidenced by the occasional presentation with arthrogryposis. The natural history of this form of disease is one of progression to the adult form. By the end of the first decade most children display clinical myotonia with contraction to percussion and to voluntary movement. Sternomastoid wasting, dysarthria and distal muscle weakness follow. Adult features include frontal balding, cataracts (with specific morphology) and gonadal failure. Some degree of mental impairment is usual and endocrine abnormalities such as hypothyroidism and altered glucose tolerance are common.

Cardiac, respiratory and gastrointestinal involvement has significant implications for anaesthesia.[99]

Anaesthesia issues in myotonic dystrophy

Children with myotonic dystrophy most commonly require anaesthesia for surgical correction of talipes deformity, myringotomy and inguinal hernia repair. Careful preoperative evaluation of muscle tone, wasting and the degree of myotonia are necessary. Preoperative ECG and ventilatory function tests help to plan perioperative care.

Patients are known to be sensitive to a variety of sedatives, including the barbiturates, benzodiazepines, opioids and propofol. Inadvertently induced apnoea may prompt manoeuvres that trigger myotonia with subsequent inability to secure an airway effectively or ventilate the patient. Myotonia may also be triggered by cold, suxamethonium, anticholinesterases and surgical manipulation of muscle. It is unresponsive to neuromuscular blockade and regional anaesthesia but may respond to direct infiltration of muscles with local anaesthetic agents (see Chapter 9).

The use of non-depolarizing neuromuscular blocking drugs mandates monitoring neuromuscular junction function.[100] Hypotonic infants require greatly reduced doses while older children tend to respond normally.[101] In advanced cases, sensitivity to these drugs is related to the degree of muscle wasting.[90,102] Anticholinesterase drugs may have unpredictable actions; if necessary, they should be administered by titration.[103]

Impaired respiratory reserve in these patients results from progressive muscle weakness and recurrent aspiration. Reduced central sensitivity to carbon dioxide and kyphoscoliosis contribute to perioperative hypoxaemia and respiratory morbidity. Aggressive postoperative respiratory care should be planned in advance.[101]

Cardiac involvement is usual and present even in neonates. It does not necessarily correlate with the degree of skeletal muscle involvement. Conduction defects are common (up to 90% of cases if His bundle ECGs are analysed) and result in arrhythmias including flutter, bradycardias and ectopic activity. Sudden death may result from the development of third-degree heart block. Myocardial contractile function is also affected in the dystrophic process and cardiomyopathy with failure is a regular feature of late-stage disease.[104]

Gastrointestinal involvement results in oesophageal, gastric and intestinal adynamia. Gastric drainage should be a part of all but the shortest anaesthetics.[105]

NON-DYSTROPHIC MYOTONIA

Myotonia congenita

This condition, also known as Thomsen's disease, is inherited in an autosomal dominant pattern and has an incidence of about 2 : 50 000. It is characterized by muscle hyper-trophy and myotonia that is non-progressive and usually not disabling. Although it presents in childhood with stiffness especially after rest, symptoms may be concealed until later life. Cardiac, smooth muscle and extramuscular manifestations are not seen and life expectancy is normal. Treatment may be indicated for severe stiffness and blepharospasm and includes membrane-stabilizing drugs such as quinidine, procainamide and mexilitene. MH has been reported as the cause of death in at least one patient with myotonia congenita and several case reports of patients with this myotonia include documented positive caffeine–halothane contracture tests.[98,105] Despite these reports, it is unlikely that the risk of MH in patients with myotonia congenita is any greater than that in the general population.[95]

HYPERKALAEMIC PERIODIC PARALYSIS

This autosomal dominant condition is characterized by episodes of flaccid paralysis associated with hyperkalaemia. Precipitants include cold, hunger, infection, emotional stress and anaesthesia. Attacks can be aborted with insulin and glucose and prevented by a high sodium/low potassium/high carbohydrate diet.

Anaesthesia issues in myotonia

The preoperative assessment of children with non-dystrophic myotonia should aim to evaluate all the usual triggers of stiffness and facilitate avoidance of these in the perioperative period. Cold exposure, stress and prolonged fasting can all be alleviated with thoughtful planning. Intraoperative myotonia can be triggered by surgical manipulation of muscle and electrocautery. Direct infiltration of muscles with local anaesthetic agents may improve the surgical field.

Depolarizing neuromuscular agents are contraindicated and responses to non-depolarizing agents are normal if muscle wasting is not prominent.[100]

The Schwartz–Jampel syndrome may be associated with MH and warrants the avoidance of triggering agents.[107] Determining the exact association is complicated by the difficulties in interpreting the caffeine–halothane contracture test in the presence of myotonia.

Children with hyperkalaemic periodic paralysis should have plasma electrolytes monitored prior to anaesthesia. Preoperative potassium depletion with thiazide diuretics may prevent weakness, although it may worsen myotonia. It is important to avoid prolonged fasting in these children and to maintain the sodium and carbohydrate supply throughout the perioperative period. ECG monitoring may help in the early detection of intraoperative hyperkalaemia. Hyperkalaemia-induced weakness can be treated with intravenous calcium gluconate or glucose and insulin.[99] Postoperative monitoring needs to be vigilant.

MYASTHENIA GRAVIS

In adult practice myasthenia gravis is the prototypical antibody-mediated autoimmune disease. It is manifested by weakness and the rapid onset of fatigue in voluntary muscles and strongly associated with thymic abnormalities. The overall incidence is 1 : 20 000, with a quarter of these cases occurring under the age of 20 years. Ten per cent of cases occur in children under aged 16 years. Paediatric disease covers a broader spectrum of illness than does adult disease and is classified into the following three forms.[108]

Juvenile myasthenia gravis

This form of myasthenia most closely resembles the adult form. It too is directly attributable to an autoimmune process in which autoantibodies are directed toward the main immunogenic region of the α-subunit of the acetylcholine receptor. The reduction in the density of postjunctional receptors on the motor endplate results in typical weakness that worsens with activity.

Disease usually presents in early adolescence with a marked female preponderance (4 : 1). It may be either generalized or localized to extraocular muscles (usually asymmetric) and its course tends to be slowly progressive with intermittent fluctuations in severity. Unlike the adult form, juvenile myasthenia is not associated with the development of thymomas, although thymic hyperplasia is seen. As in adult disease, juvenile myasthenia may be associated with other conditions such as systemic lupus, thyroiditis and rheumatoid arthritis.

Congenital myasthenia gravis

Quite distinct from the adult disease, this diverse group of conditions does not have an autoimmune basis and may be inherited in an autosomal recessive or dominant pattern.

Signs of disease usually become apparent after the neonatal period and before 2 years of age. There is a male predominance and signs include weakness, particularly of ocular muscles, hypotonia and a weak cry. The course tends to be non-progressive, resulting in lifelong mild disease without marked fluctuation. Anticholinesterase therapy requirements tend to be low.

Neonatal transient myasthenia gravis

Some 10–15% of infants born to affected mothers suffer the consequences of transplacental transfer of maternal acetylcholine receptor antibodies. These neonates display signs of myasthenia from birth, including floppy limbs, ptosis, expressionless face and difficulty feeding. Choking and apnoea may occur in severe cases. The incidence of this form of disease is not well correlated with either the severity or the duration of maternal disease. The natural history of the condition is one of spontaneous resolution, although anticholinesterase therapy may be required for a variable period.

Anaesthesia issues in myasthenia gravis

Preoperative evaluation of children with myasthenia gravis must include assessment of the current pattern of weakness (with particular emphasis on respiratory and bulbar muscle dysfunction), the adequacy of anticholinesterase therapy and the existence of associated chronic debility (particularly respiratory disease and steroid dependence). Simplicity and strict monitoring should guide all pharmacological interventions.

Chronic anticholinesterase therapy predisposes to several drug interactions, including prolonged action of suxamethonium and ester local anaesthetics. Suxamethonium is best avoided as its dose–response curve is changed and phase II block appears earlier. Anticholinesterase therapy potentiates vagal actions, making preoperative atropinization advisable. Increased bronchial secretions make airway vigilance essential throughout the perioperative period.

Immediate preoperative anticholinesterase therapy need only be adjusted (reduced or ceased) for children with less severe symptoms and who require deep muscle relaxation for surgery. These adjustments may help to reduce bronchorrhoea and the incidence of phase II blockade. They will also reduce the likelihood of antagonism of non-depolarizing neuromuscular block intraoperatively and reduce possible confusion in the differential diagnosis of postoperative weakness.[109]

Non-depolarizing neuromuscular blockade can be safely used if doses are carefully titrated and neuromuscular function is monitored. Dose–response curves are variably shifted leftwards and deep relaxation may be achieved with only one-tenth of the usual dose.

Drugs of short and medium duration of action, such as atracurium and mivacurium, are well suited for titration and should be fully reversed before extubation. Monitoring with peripheral nerve stimulation allows assessment of the reversibility of blockade as well as the detection of residual neuromuscular weakness. Despite this, extubation requires clinical confirmation of the return of airway and respiratory muscle function. Head lift, measured inspiratory force and vital capacity can all be used to aid this assessment.[90]

Perioperative management must also include avoidance of factors that contribute to muscle weakness. These include hypothermia, hypokalaemia and other potentiators of neuromuscular blockade such as thiotepa, aminoglycoside drugs and membrane-stabilizing drugs. Supplementary steroid cover for dependent children ($1-2$ mg kg^{-1} hydrocortisone 6 hourly) should be considered and close postoperative observation instituted to allow the recognition and treatment of both a myasthenic and cholinergic crisis.[109]

THE MYOPATHIES

The following disorders of muscle function have traditionally been characterized by their histological morphology, although they are now increasingly defined by specific molecular and enzyme defects. Three broad groups of myopathy carry particular significance for anaesthesia.

The morphologically defined congenital myopathies, such as central core disease and nemaline myopathy are usually, although not always, non-progressive diseases which, in most other respects, are relatively benign.

The mitochondrial myopathies are a group of rare disorders that are characterized by electron-microscopic abnormalities. Both the clinical heterogeneity and a lack of specificity of morphological features make redefinition according to specific molecular defects more rational. A group of these is associated with both brain and muscle involvement and are termed mitochondrial encephalomyopathies.

The glycogen storage diseases (GSD) are inherited disorders of glycogen metabolism grouped on the basis of clinical features into muscle and liver glycogenoses. Muscle glycogenoses and their implications for anaesthesia are described here.

MORPHOLOGICALLY DEFINED CONGENITAL MYOPATHIES

Central core disease

This autosomal dominant inherited condition presents with proximal muscle weakness at or soon after birth. Bulbar muscles tend not to be involved and secondary skeletal changes such as hip dislocation, kyphoscoliosis, short neck and mandibular hypoplasia appear with continued development. It is named for its characteristic pathology, which shows type-I fibre dominance with cores of closely packed myofibrils extending along the entire length of the muscle fibre. Intelligence is normal and serum enzymes are not usually elevated. The genetic defect has been localized to chromosome 19 (close to the site of the MH gene) and, in some families, gene mutations at this site include those encoding the ryanodine receptor.[95] Central core disease is associated with MH on exposure to typical triggering agents and all precautions should be taken when planning anaesthesia.[88]

THE MITOCHONDRIAL DISORDERS

The mitochondrial disorders are a group of multisystem diseases that result from defects of the mitochondrial respiratory chain enzymes and the five complexes of oxidative phosphorylation. The genetic, clinical and biochemical heterogeneity that characterizes these disorders is most probably a function of mitochondrial genetic patterns. These patterns, unlike mendelian genetics, are exclusively maternally inherited, multiallelic (two to 10 copies of the DNA molecule per mitochondrion) and heteroplasmic (varying proportions of normal and mutant DNA coexist within a cell).

Historically, these disorders were considered to be primarily neuromuscular. Increasingly, expression of disease in other systems is being recognized and can be used as a clue to diagnosis. Ophthalmic symptoms (retinopathy, external ophthalmoplegia), neuropsychiatric symptoms, cardiomyopathy with conduction defects, renal tubular dysfunction and hepatic abnormalities are all recognized features.[110,111]

The neuromuscular presentation is often non-specific and includes both static and progressive myopathy, developmental delay, seizures and peripheral neuropathy. Congenital and late-onset forms exist and symptoms range from weakness to exercise intolerance and episodic paralysis.

Several progressive myopathies are closely associated with brain disease and are termed encephalomyopathies. A mitochondrial defect is implied by the appearance of 'ragged red fibres' (RRF) on light microscopy with modified Gomori trichrome staining.

Three distinctive syndromes have been identified: Kearnes–Sayre syndrome (KSS), myoclonus–epilepsy RRF syndrome (MERRF) and myopathy–encephalopathy–lactic acidosis–stroke syndrome (MELAS).[112] They share some features, including short stature, lactic acidosis and spongy brain degeneration.

Complex I is the largest enzyme complex of the respiratory chain and has the greatest number of mitochondrially encoded subunits. Deficiency of this complex may give rise to several phenotypes, including Leigh's syndrome, MERRF and MELAS syndromes. Leigh's syndrome is a subacute necrotizing encephalopathy characterized by psychomotor regression, hypotonia, lactic acidosis and brainstem dysfunction.[110]

Anaesthesia issues in mitochondrial myopathies

Without definitive anaesthetic experience in these rare conditions, general principles must serve to guide assessment of preoperative muscle weakness, metabolic (lactic) acidosis and cardiomyopathy.[112] It is appropriate to pay particular attention to adequate oxygen and glucose delivery throughout and to maintain a strict thermoneutral environment at all times. Bicarbonate may be required for acute exacerbations in acidosis.[110]

THE MUSCLE GLYCOGENOSES

The glycogenoses have been classified according to the chronological order of identified enzymic defects. More than 12 individual defects have been characterized, of which at least four have primary manifestations in muscle. The incidence of GSDs in Europe is estimated at 1 : 20 000 live births and all but two are transmitted in an autosomal recessive fashion. Signs and symptoms arise from abnormal accumulation of glycogen in tissues and a secondary reduction in free glucose. The four most common disorders (Von Gierke's, Pompe's, Forbes' and Hers' diseases) account for 94% of all GSDs.[108]

Type II (Pompe's disease)

Infantile, juvenile and adult forms exist. The infantile form manifests soon after birth with hypotonia and poor feeding. Macroglossia and hepatomegaly are notable and glycogen deposition in cardiac muscle leads to hypertrophic cardiomyopathy and cardiac failure. There is no effective therapy and cardiorespiratory failure ensues within 2 years. The juvenile form presents in early childhood as a progressive myopathy and also leads to respiratory failure by puberty.[114]

Type V (McArdle's disease)

This is the prototypical muscle glycogenosis and results from a deficiency of muscle phosphorylase that precludes rapid glycogenolysis. Although inherited in an autosomal recessive fashion, reports are more often of male patients. This may result from major symptoms being related to strenuous activity. The condition usually presents in adolescence with muscle pain, stiffness and cramps after exercise. Exaggerated tendency to fatigue may be accompanied by a 'second wind' phenomenon wherein pain and cramp may be alleviated by continued exercise. Muscle atrophy is not prominent on muscle biopsy and cardiac involvement is rare. Severe exercise can induce rhabdomyolysis with consequent myoglobinuria and acute renal failure. Diagnosis is suggested by elevated muscle enzymes and purine degradation products (ammonia, inosine, hypoxanthine) in response to exercise. Muscle biopsy and enzyme assay are required for definitive diagnosis. There is no consistently effective therapy, although a high protein diet may reduce symptoms.[115]

Anaesthesia issues in muscle glycogenoses

Preoperative evaluation is helped if there is a definitive diagnosis but this is unlikely if liver and/or muscle biopsy are planned. General principles must therefore guide assessment of blood glucose control, the pattern of muscle weakness (especially regarding respiratory compromise), cardiac involvement and mechanical effects of organomegaly (especially macroglossia and hepatomegaly).[116]

Hypoglycaemia on fasting is a feature of types I, III and IV, making intravenous glucose supplementation necessary. Progressive myopathy can severely reduce respiratory reserve (type II) and a history of recurrent pneumonia makes postoperative respiratory support very likely. Preoperative ECG may give clues (high-voltage QRS complexes, shortened PR interval) to possible cardiac involvement and prompt echocardiographic studies. ECG monitoring during induction of anaesthesia is mandatory. The possibility of impaired diaphragmatic excursion should be borne in mind if significant hepatomegaly is detected.

Without definitive data on the safety of neuromuscular blocking agents in these patients, it is wise to avoid depolarizing agents on the theoretical grounds of reducing the possibility of hyperkalaemia and rhabdomyolysis. Non-depolarizing agents can be safely used if doses are titrated and neuromuscular function is monitored.

The use of surgical tourniquets should be restricted to limb-saving procedures as muscle ischaemia is not tolerated well in some GSDs (type V) and may contribute to myoglobinuria and muscle atrophy.[116]

RENAL DISEASE

CHRONIC RENAL FAILURE

The sustained and progressive failure of a child's renal system jeopardizes normal somatic growth and psychomotor development through a variety of mechanisms. Understanding the pathophysiology of chronic renal failure is the basis of safe anaesthesia in these children when they present for diagnostic, therapeutic or incidental surgery.

Chronic renal failure is defined as a permanent reduction in GFR below a chosen level. Specifying this level in children is beset by problems of repeated measurements and estimations of GFR and the rapid changes in GFR associated with normal renal maturation. Suggested values for defining chronic renal failure include a GFR below 16 ml min^{-1} 1.73 m^{-2} for infants up to 4 months of age, and below 25 ml min^{-1} 1.73 m^{-2} for those up to 12 months; thereafter, the adult definition of a GFR below 30 ml min^{-1} 1.73 m^{-2} can be used.[117]

The aetiology of chronic renal failure comprises three main groups: (1) acquired glomerular disease; (2) developmental anomalies resulting from injury to the developing metanephros; and (3) hereditary renal disease. Developmental anomalies predominate as causes in early infancy but by later childhood the acquired glomerular diseases are slightly more prevalent. Table 1.6 lists causes of chronic renal failure in paediatric practice.[118–122]

Chronic renal failure has consequences for all body systems. Those of primary importance to the paediatric anaesthetist include changes to salt and water excretory mechanisms, electrolyte balance and acid–base homeostasis. Also important are the effects on the haematological, gastrointestinal and neurological systems.

Four patterns of salt and water excretion disturbances can be discerned, often characteristic of the underlying renal pathology. Primary damage to the medullary concentrating mechanism (such as in congenital renal dysplasia and obstructive lesions) leads to polyuria with a low urinary sodium content. These children are at risk of rapid dehydration if water is not continuously available.

In chronic glomerulonephritis, glomerular destruction with relative sparing of the tubular reabsorptive capacity (glomerulotubular imbalance) leads to salt and water retention. The clinical results are oliguria, hypertension and oedema.

In diseases that primarily disturb sodium resorption from the distal nephron, such as chronic pyelonephritis and sickle cell nephropathy, a 'salt-wasting' pattern is seen. Polyuria with high urinary sodium concentrations are noted and these children crave salt. Inadvertent sodium restriction will rapidly lead to hyponatraemic dehydration.

In end-stage renal failure glomerular filtration does not allow the excretion of the normal salt and water load, resulting in oedema, vascular congestion, hypertension and cardiac failure. Perioperative management must take account of the type of salt and water disturbance when planning preoperative fasting and perioperative fluid therapy.[123]

The possibility of acute electrolyte imbalances must always be borne in mind during preoperative assessment. Acute potassium loads such as in acute catabolic states, infection, haemolysis and acidosis may result in life-threatening hyperkalaemia. Calcium and dihydrogen phosphate homeostasis undergoes major alteration as reduced GFR reduces excretion of the phosphate ion. Reciprocal falls in serum calcium concentrations are compounded by the acidosis and disturbed vitamin D kinetics.

Acidosis in chronic renal failure arises principally from a reduced capacity to excrete hydrogen ions in the form of ammonium.

Table 1.6 Chronic renal failure aetiology in paediatric practice

Chronic renal failure aetiology	Estimated prevalence (%)	Typical age at presentation

Acquired glomerular disease
  Glomerulonephritis
  Membrano-proliferative GN
  Focal and segmental glomerulosclerosis
	40	5–15 years

Developmental anomalies
  Posterior urethral valves
  Bilateral severe reflux with pyelonephritis
	20
	Male : female
	ratio 3 : 1
		Antenatal, from
		birth to 5 years

Hereditary renal disease
  Nephronophthiasis
  Alport's disease
  Polycystic kidney disease (PKD)
  Lawrence–Moon–Biedl syndrome
  Cystinosis, oxalosis
	15	Below 5 years

Miscellaneous
  Haemolytic uraemic syndrome
  Papillary and cortical necrosis (birth asphyxia related)
  Vascular misadventure
  e.g. umbilical vein catheter-related thrombosis		

Body pH is maintained through buffering systems, primarily by bone salts. Despite a net reduction in acid excretion, urine pH is often appropriately acidic. Chronic acidosis leads to reduced appetite, vomiting, reduced bone mineralization and reduced growth hormone secretion.

A reduced secretion of erythropoietin together with reduced red cell survival and defective iron utilization commonly result in normochromic anaemia in chronic renal failure. Reduced platelet adhesiveness and reduced activation of platelet factor III commonly result in coagulopathy. Detection of this coagulopathy is facilitated by a skin bleeding time.

There is a reduction in the clearance of various gut hormones including gastrin, cholecystokinin and secretin, with the resultant increased risk of gastric ulcer together with gastro-oesophageal reflux in 70% of cases. All of these factors have major implications for feeding and caloric intake in paediatric patients, so many are provided with a percutaneous gastrostomy.[117] In early infancy cardiovascular manifestations of chronic renal failure directly reflect changes in circulating fluid volume, as determined by the disturbance of salt and water balance. In later childhood chronic disturbance of the several interacting mechanisms for blood pressure autoregulation may lead to overt hypertension.

There are four therapeutic strategies available in paediatric chronic renal failure. Firstly, the decision whether or not to treat an infant is an issue that must be faced by parents, neonatal physicians and paediatric nephrologists whenever a newborn is diagnosed as having unrecoverable renal function. It may also be an issue when renal disease progresses in concert with severe neurological damage. Conservative management, renal replacement therapies and transplantation are the other strategies. Conservative management of renal failure attempts to control the derangements in fluid and electrolyte homeostasis through nutritional management and pharmacological manipulation. It is aimed at optimizing somatic growth and development until complete or until dialysis and/or transplantation become necessary.[124] Three fundamental principles govern nutritional management. These are aggressive nutritional support, adequate caloric and electrolyte provision and sufficient supply of water.

Oral supplements that may be required include sodium chloride, bicarbonate and calcium. Supplements of renal endocrine function include calcitriol or vitamin D analogues to maintain normal serum calcium and parathyroid hormone levels. Recombinant human erythropoietin (rhuEPO) and iron supplements have significantly reduced the needs for blood transfusion and allow more frequent monitoring of blood chemistry in infants. The use of human growth hormone (rhuGH) in children with chronic renal failure may prove beneficial in helping these children to achieve adult height.[124]

Chronic renal dialysis is the standard treatment of end-stage renal failure in patients awaiting renal transplantation. Normally, dialysis is commenced when conservative management fails but the criteria for failure are not standard and are dependent on practice setting. Somatic growth and psychosocial developmental issues supersede laboratory values as indications to commence chronic dialysis. Peritoneal dialysis (PD) and haemodialysis (HD) are complimentary procedures in renal replacement therapy, although PD is used by a larger proportion of paediatric patients. The advantages of PD include its simplicity, efficacy, safety and the lesser disruption to a child's school life. Peritonitis remains a constant risk, estimated at 1 episode per 8–12 patient months.

The disadvantages of HD include cost, complexity and the risks of infection and disconnection. Regular hospital attendance is often more disruptive to psychosocial development than home-based PD regimes. In both PD and HD it is customary to increase dialysis to the point where protein intake and hence somatic growth can be maximized.[125]

Despite major advances in dialytic therapies, renal transplantation remains the optimal treatment for children with end-stage chronic renal disease.[126] Although limited by the availability of donor organs, the success of transplant programmes has increased because of new immunosuppressive agents, immunological conditioning and improved histocompatability testing. Compared with dialytic therapies, transplantation affords better somatic growth and neurological development. Problems following transplantation include rejection, immunosuppression, Cushing's syndrome, obesity, hirsuitism and risks of subsequent malignancy.[127]

Anaesthesia issues in chronic renal failure

Preoperative evaluation of children with chronic renal failure must include a general survey of somatic growth, evidence of uraemia and current fluid status. Both the quantity and quality of urine produced as well as the child's cardiovascular status ought to be assessed carefully. Laboratory investigations should include plasma urea and creatinine, electrolytes and full blood count. A skin bleeding time may help for major or prolonged surgery and when there is a history of bruisability. A recent ECG and chest X-ray should be obtained, especially when there is a significant history of hypertension or electrolyte imbalance.[128]

A careful assessment should allow appropriate planning of perioperative fasting, fluid and drug management. It should also facilitate identification and correction of factors that may further compromise renal function in the perioperative period. These factors include inadequately controlled cardiac failure, hypertension and hypovolaemia.[129]

Chronic renal failure results in altered drug kinetics via several mechanisms, including reduced excretory capacity, acidosis and altered protein binding. Anaesthetic agents should be chosen with care and carefully titrated, and have appropriate dose adjustments made. Drug interactions, particularly with antihypertensive medication, should be anticipated. Special efforts should be made to preserve limb veins for future fistulae and shunts.

Children receiving regular dialysis who require surgery must have their anaesthesia timed so as to optimize the efficiency of dialysis. Careful consideration should also be given to appropriate timing of dialysis after surgery. Children undergoing PD should be given adequate time to allow complete drainage of dialysate before induction of anaesthesia to prevent abdominal distension and compromised respiratory function. Care must be taken with venous access lines, A–V shunts and fistulae throughout. Haemodialysis venous lines should not be routinely used for perioperative intravenous access.

Anaesthesia in children following renal transplantation must take into account the immunosuppression and attendant risks of infection. Attention to asepsis must be observed in all procedures and the maintenance of full hydration is important. Avoiding blood transfusions where possible reduces the risk of alloimmunization. Steroid supplementation must be administered where appropriate and special care taken to avoid potential nephrotoxins. Hypoglycaemia with fasting has been noted in renal transplant children and is more common if β-blockers are being administered. Intravenous glucose supplements should be instituted during periods of fasting.[130]

GLOMERULONEPHRITIS

There is a large and diverse range of renal parenchymal inflammatory lesions. Their classification is complicated by the fact that renal histopathology is often neither specific nor constant for particular diseases.

Presentation may take one of three forms. The acute nephritic syndrome is characterized by haematuria, oliguria and hypertension, frequently accompanied by proteinuria and oedema. Acute post-streptococcal glomerulonephritis is a typical example and the most common glomerulonephritis of childhood. The nephrotic syndrome is defined as proteinuria in excess of 0.05 g kg^{-1} day, severe hypoalbuminaemia (less than 2.5 g dl^{-1}), hyperlipidaemia and oedema. Minimal lesion nephrotic syndrome represents three-quarters of all childhood nephrotics, while focal segmental glomerulosclerosis accounts for a further 10% of cases. Membranoproliferative glomerulonephritis may present with either the nephrotic or nephritic syndrome, the former conferring a worse prognosis. Interstitial nephritis is a third form of response to injury and is characterized by oliguria and hypertension and some degree of renal impairment, both glomerular and tubular. Acute and chronic recurrent pyelonephritis are major causes of interstitial nephritis. Other causes include Sickle cell uropathy, Alport's syndrome and analgesic uropathy.[123]

RENAL TUBULAR DISORDERS

Disorders of renal tubular function result in abnormalities of body water and electrolytes, acid excretion and/or abnormalities of mineral homeostasis. Unlike the common pathophysiological sequelae of disordered glomerular function recognized as renal failure, the clinical and biochemical manifestations of renal tubular disease vary according to the type and severity of the specific disordered mechanisms.

Renal tubular disorders may be inherited or acquired. They are classified as either generalized dysfunction (typified by the renal fanconi syndrome) or isolated transport disorders such as cystinuria.

The most common presentation is that of an infant who fails to thrive. Non-specific symptoms such as irritability, recurrent vomiting and mild weakness should prompt investigation of plasma and urine biochemistry. Earlier presentation in the neonatal period may result from excessive salt and water loss. These infants may have polyuria (full or 'leaking' nappies), polydipsia (not settling after feeds) or severe dehydration presenting as cardiovascular collapse or 'dehydration fever'. Milder disease may present in the toddler age group as chronic constipation (secondary to chronic dehydration), nocturia, salt craving and delayed milestones. If unrecognized at earlier stages, older children may present with bone pain, rickets, poor growth, weakness or fractures.

CYSTINURIA

This relatively prevalent disorder (1–8 : 15 000) results from defective transport of cystine and di-basic amino acids in the renal tubular and small intestinal epithelium. Urinary cystine forms calculi and patients present with the sequelae – obstruction, infection and chronic renal failure. Treatment consists of high fluid intake, urinary alkalinization and salt restriction. Captopril and penicillamine may also be of value in more severe cases.

SYSTEMIC HYPERTENSION

Hypertension is defined as a systolic blood pressure consistently above the 95th centile for age. The incidence of hypertension in paediatric practice is approximately 2.5% in the neonatal intensive care unit (NICU), 1–2% in children up to 10 years of age and up to 10% in adolescents. The North American pattern of disease is different, in that a large proportion of African–American young adults (25–30%) are hypertensive. After excluding those with hypertension secondary to the oral contraceptive pill, a vast majority of these adolescents has essential hypertension.[12]

Children with asymptomatic hypertension detected as an incidental finding usually have mild elevations of blood pressure. Diastolic readings are typically below 100 mmHg. Of these cases, 95% will have essential hypertension. The diagnosis of essential hypertension is suggested by the patient's age, race, blood-pressure level, dietary history and obesity. The paucity of symptoms and a strong family history of hypertension or coronary artery disease also strengthen the diagnosis.

In secondary hypertension the clinical manifestations of the underlying disease usually take precedence at presentation. Table 1.7 lists and classifies the aetiology of secondary hypertension. Renal abnormalities are the most common cause of secondary hypertension (75–80% of cases). One-third of these have chronic pyelonephritis, although the pathophysiological relationship between hypertension and pyelonephritis is far from clear. Renovascular disease as a cause of secondary hypertension is 10 times more common in children than in adults. The most common vascular pathologies are fibromuscular dysplasia and intimal dysplasia. Some of these cases are associated with neurofibromatosis. In 70% of cases bilateral abnormalities exist and in 50% intrarenal vessels are also abnormal. Extrarenal (mesenteric, aortic and intracranial) arterial abnormalities are also more common in these patients. Aortic coarctation is the cause of hypertension in 2% of all children with secondary hypertension. Accelerated hypertension is a progressive and sudden increase in chronic stable hypertension and represents a medical emergency. It may present with encephalopathy – vomiting, hyperpyrexia, ataxia and seizures and impending coma – or with arrhythmias and cardiac failure. Malignant hypertension is characterized by changes in the fundus of the eye, including

Table 1.7 Systemic hypertension aetiology

Systemic hypertension	Aetiology
Essential hypertension	
Secondary hypertension	
Renal	Chronic glomerulonephritis
	Congenital dysplastic kidneys
	Chronic pyelonephritis
	Hydronephrosis
	Polycystic kidney disease
	Medullary cystic kidney disease
	Chronic obstructive uropathy
Renovascular	Aortic coarctation
	Renal artery disease
	(fibromuscular dysplasia, intimal
	dysplasia,neurofibromatosis,
	William's syndrome, vasculitis,
	thrombosis,trauma,external
	compression)
	Renal vein thrombosis
Adrenal	Neuroblastoma, ganglioneuroma
	Phaeochromocytoma
	Cortical hyperplasia
	(adrenogenital syndrome)
	Cushing's disease
	Primary hyperaldosteronism
	(hyperplasia or adenoma)
	Adrenal carcinoma
Drug induced	Oral contraceptive pill
	Glucocorticoids
	Licorice
	Sympathomimetics,
	phencyclidine, amphetamines
	and anti-hypertensive withdrawal
Miscellaneous	Lead nephropathy, mercury
	poisoning
	Parenchymal or vascular
	damage from radiotherapy
	Guillain–Barre, familial
	dysautonomia, burns, leukaemia

papilloedema, peripheral arterial spasm, haemorrhage and exudates.

Pharmacological intervention in systemic hypertension must often accompany initial and surgical investigation and takes precedence in severe hypertension. Principles of management include titrating a single agent to achieve control or until maximum dosage is reached before adding a second agent. Reduction in blood pressure ought to be gradual, especially in severe cases so as to avoid unmasking failed autoregulatory mechanisms and risking cerebral, cardiac and renal hypoperfusion. Adequate control in severe cases may depend on concurrent rehydration.

The choice of drug must involve consideration of the patient's haemodynamic parameters such as effective circulating volume, GFR (thiazides become ineffective when GFR falls below 20–25 ml kg^{-1} min^{-1}) and possible intrarenal vascular stenosis (angiotensin-converting enzyme inhibitors may compromise renal function in this situation).[31]

Anaesthesia issues in hypertension

Assessment of children with hypertension must gauge the adequacy of blood-pressure control. Elective surgery should be delayed until moderate and severe hypertension is controlled. Accelerated hypertension is a medical emergency that takes precedence over all surgical intervention.

Cardiac and renal status should be evaluated to assess end-organ dysfunction and allow appropriate adjustment of anaesthetic technique and drug dosages. Careful review of the child's prescribed medication may alert the anaesthetist to possible drug interactions. Occasionally, side-effects of antihypertensive medication manifest during anaesthesia, such as bronchospasm and bradycardia due to β-blockers, or myocardial depression due to β-blockers and calcium antagonists. In general, it is wise to continue all antihypertensive medication throughout the perioperative period.

Chronic intravascular volume depletion, 'rebound phenomenon' after sudden drug withdrawal and some older antihypertensive agents (reserpine, guanethidine) may predispose to poor blood-pressure control, although care with intravenous fluid therapy and attentive postoperative analgesia should improve this.

ACUTE RENAL FAILURE

Acute renal failure is defined as a rapid reduction in renal function to the point where daily solute and nitrogenous load cannot be effectively excreted. It may be anuric (less than 1.5 ml of urine $kg^{-1} day^{-1}$), oliguric (urine flow less than 1 ml $kg^{-1} h^{-1}$) or non-oliguric.

The most common causes in paediatric practice are the haemolytic–uraemic syndrome, infection and trauma. Other important causes include burns, Henoch–Schonlein vasculitis and direct nephrotoxins including aminogycloside antibiotics, radiocontrast dyes and cancer chemotherapy agents. A pathophysiological classification is given in Table 1.8.

The clinical presentation and course are usually dominated by the causative disease but in many cases progression through recognizable stages can be seen. An initial period lasting for up to 12 days of progressive azotemia may be either oliguric or non-oliguric. A shorter diuretic phase but with continued increases in plasma creatinine often follows. A second diuretic phase is heralded by a progressive fall in creatinine and urea and, in uncomplicated cases, this is followed by a recovery phase.[132]

ENDOCRINE DISEASE

DIABETES MELLITUS

This is the most common endocrine disorder of childhood and insulin-dependent diabetes mellitus (type 1) is the most common form of diabetes in young people. It is associated with a reduced insulin production and a tendency to develop ketosis. The aetiology of diabetes is uncertain but genetic, environmental and immune-mediated processes are probably involved. Common symptoms include polydipsia, polyuria and weight loss. Hyperglycaemia and glycosuria with or without ketosis are present. Random blood glucose estimation above 16.6 mmol l^{-1} or fasting blood glucose above 11 mmol l^{-1} confirms the diagnosis.

The mainstay of treatment is insulin, which allows glucose to pass into cells while at the same time turning off gluconeogenesis and preventing ketosis. The majority of insulin used now is human insulin and a typical management regimen would be the concurrent use of long- and short-acting insulin to optimize blood sugar control during the day. Other

Table 1.8 Acute renal failure aetiology

Acute renal failure aetiology
Ischaemia
Hypovolaemia
Dehydration/shock
Burns
Sepsis
Renovascular
Renal artery stenosis
Renal vein thrombosis
Disseminated intravascular coagulation
Malignant hypertension
Inflammatory/immunological
Pyelonephritis
Bacterial endocarditis
Glomerulonephritis
Acute post-infectious GN
Membrane-proliferative GN
Henoch–Schonlein purpura
Systemic lupus erythematosus
Hypersensitivity reactions
Penicillins, sulphonamides
Anti-convulsants
Direct nephrotoxins
Chemotherapeutic agents (Ifosfamide, cisplatin)
Radiocontrast agents
Analgesics (salicylates, NSAIDs)
Antibiotics (aminoglycosides, amphotericin B)
Heavy metals, organic solvents
Myoglobin, haemoglobin
Obstruction
Retroperitoneal tumour/fibrosis
Calculi
Pelvi-ureteric/posterior urethral obstruction
Hepato-renal syndrome

aspects of management include diet, exercise and monitoring of blood glucose and urinary ketones.[133,134] Acute complications include hyperglycaemia with ketoacidosis and hypoglycaemia.

KETOACIDOSIS

The treatment of ketoacidosis involves restoration of circulating fluid volumes, normalization of blood glucose, correction of electrolyte abnormalities and correcting acidosis.

Fluid therapy is initially with normal saline with up to 20 ml kg^{-1} in the first hour with a similar amount in the second hour if required. Thereafter, half-normal saline (0.45%) may be used at a rate of 1.5 times normal maintenance. Insulin can be given at a rate of 0.1 U kg^{-1} h^{-1} by infusion. Blood glucose levels will begin to fall and as a result blood pH will increase. The insulin should be continued until the pH is greater than 7.3. When blood glucose falls below 13.9 mmol l^{-1} 5% glucose should be added to the intravenous fluids. Blood glucose levels of 6.6 mmol l^{-1} or lower warrants addition of 10% glucose to the infusion and, in addition, the insulin infusion rate may be halved to 0.05 U kg^{-1} h^{-1}. Serum potassium is initially high but tends to fall as insulin is given and potassium is driven back into the cells. Potassium should only be given when the serum levels are low or normal. Acidosis is corrected by a combination of fluid and insulin therapy. Some degree of cerebral oedema is reasonably common in ketoacidosis and a high degree of suspicion should be maintained.[135]

Perioperative management

The aim of management of children with diabetes who need elective or emergency surgery is the maintenance of blood glucose levels close to normal. Hypoglycaemia is dangerous because of the potential for coma, convulsions and brain damage. Hyperglycaemia with ketoacidosis must also be avoided but in some cases may need to be treated during surgery if the surgery is very urgent. It may mimic an acute abdomen. Close co-operation should be sought with the medical team.[136]

The following guidelines are based on recommendations by Alberti *et al.*[137] and Smail.[138] Table 1.9 outlines the preoperative regimen for diabetic children requiring elective surgery.[138]

Some authorities have advised using a separate infusion pump for the infusion of insulin. However, Alberti advises that the insulin be added to the bag of fluid. This author strongly supports this view as it avoids the possibility of infusing insulin without dextrose, thus exposing the patient to severe hypoglycaemia. If, however, a separate insulin infusion is to be used

Table 1.9 Preoperative regimen for elective surgery in children with diabetes.

1.	Admit morning before operation after usual insulin before breakfast
2.	Schedule operation for following morning (first on list if possible)
3.	Assess control, checking for intercurrent infection and ketosis
4.	Check blood urea and electrolytes
5.	Rapid-acting insulin only before supper
6.	Start infusion at bedtime (or 4–5 h after supper): – 500 ml 10% dextose – +N/5 saline – +10 mmol potassium chloride – +Insulin 12 U 500 ml^{-1} This should run at 50 ml kg^{-1} per 24 h If surgery is scheduled for the afternoon the child may have an early breakfast with rapid-acting insulin, with the infusion starting 4–5 h later
7.	Blood sugar should be checked every 2–3 h
8.	If blood sugar >10 mmol l^{-1} increase insulin in bag to 16 units If blood sugar <5 mmol l^{-1} reduce insulin in bag to 8 units

insulin should be infused at 0.05 U kg^{-1} h^{-1}. The fluid previously described (without insulin) must be given at the same time.

If blood glucose >10 mmol l^{-1} increase the infusion to 0.07 U kg^{-1} h^{-1} and if the blood glucose falls to <5 mmol l^{-1}, insulin should be reduced to 0.03 U kg^{-1} h^{-1}.

The infusion should be continued during and after surgery with regular checks of blood glucose and potassium. The infusion continues until the child is eating, when the usual insulin regimen used by the child should be restarted.

If the surgery is very minor and it is anticipated that the child will be eating and drinking very soon after surgery, a simpler approach can be used. Breakfast and the morning dose of insulin should be omitted, the surgery scheduled as early as possible, blood glucose checked every 2–3 h and the normal insulin regimen restarted postoperatively, provided the patient is eating and drinking well.

PITUITARY GLAND

The anterior pituitary produces at least six hormones: growth hormone (GH), follicle-stimulating hormone (FSH), luteinizing hormone (LH), thyroid-stimulating hormone (TSH), adrenocorticotrophic hormone (ACTH) and prolactin (PRL). The posterior pituitary under the control of the hypothalamus secretes two hormones: antidiuretic hormone (ADH) and oxytocin.

Pituitary tumours releasing excess hormone usually cause acromegaly (GH), Cushing's syndrome (ACTH) or lactation (PRL). Tumours frequently cause pressure on the optic chiasma or produce evidence of mass effect. Destruction of the anterior pituitary from any cause will result in panhypopituitarism and this will result in the atrophy of gonads, thyroid gland and adrenal cortex. The most common cause of pituitary failure in children is surgical excision of craniopharyngioma.

DIABETES INSIPIDUS

Neurogenic diabetes insipidus results from poor water conservation by the kidney because of low levels of ADH (vasopressin). It may be idiopathic or follow trauma but most frequently follows pituitary or hypothalmic surgery. The patient produces large amounts (> 5 ml kg^{-1} h^{-1}) of dilute urine (specific gravity < 1010). Thirst responses are usually intact and water intake matches water loss. If water intake is low for any reason such as preoperative starvation or postoperatively, then the serum osmolarity rises along with the serum sodium.[139]

Residual ADH production may occasionally be stimulated by chlorpropamide, clofibrate or carbamazapine, but the most common form of management is with desmopressin (DDAVP). This is usually given in a dose of 5–10 μg kg^{-1} nasally every 12 h, but it may also be given intravenously or intramuscularly in a dose of 0.4 μg. Parenteral use may result in hypertension.[139]

Diabetes insipidus may develop during surgery for craniopharyngioma or other intracranial surgery and so a urinary catheter should be inserted at the start of the procedure. Urine output and specific gravity, along with serum sodium and osmolality, are carefully monitored. Urine losses are generally replaced with hypotonic solutions because the urine is primarily water. If serum sodium or serum osmolality increase more fluid is required and DDAVP may be required. Management of these patients may be complex and should be closely supervised by an experienced endocrinologist.

PHAEOCHROMOCYTOMA

Phaeochromocytoma is a rare catecholamine-secreting neural crest tumour arising from the adrenal medulla which accounts for only 0.05% of hypertension in the paediatric age group.[140] Most cases are diagnosed preoperatively but some may present during surgery. Phaeochromocytomas may also arise from other chromaffin tissues but less than 2% are outside the abdomen, although extrarenal sites are more common in children. Ten per cent are bilateral and are rarely malignant. They may occur as part of multiple endocrine adenoma syndrome or associated with neurofibromatosis or thyroid carcinoma. The tumour secretes adrenaline or noradrenaline or both.

Patients usually present with hypertension, which is usually sustained but may be intermittent. Blood pressure may be very high and stroke and left ventricular failure are possible complications. A reversible catecholamine-induced cardiomyopathy has been reported.[141,142] Diagnosis is confirmed by demonstrating elevated levels of catecholamine in the blood or urine or of the metabolite vanillyl mandelic acid (VMA) in the urine. When the main catecholamine is noradrenaline, severe, prolonged vasoconstriction leads to a marked reduction in circulating blood volume. General anaesthesia in an unprepared patient leads to sudden and dramatic vasodilatation, effectively producing massive hypovolaemia which can be catastrophic.

Preparation for surgery depends primarily on α-adrenergic blockade for several days prior to surgery, usually with phenoxybenzamine. This long-acting drug is used with caution (1–2 mg kg^{-1} orally b.d.) at first as it blocks not only postsynaptic α_1 receptors but also presynaptic α_2 receptors, leading to an increase in noradrenaline release by loss of negative feedback. Phentolamine may be used in an emergency. β-Blockers may be added later if necessary to control tachycardia or dysrhythmias but are rarely needed in children. β-Blockers used in the absence of adequate α-blockade may precipitate heart failure or an increase in blood pressure. Treatment may also include a calcium channel blocker such as nifedipine (0.5 mg kg^{-1} day^{-1} orally) Adequate blockade is indicated by normal blood pressure and postural hypotension should be present. The haematocrit may fall, suggesting that volume expansion has taken place. In addition to other preoperative investigations, careful assessment of cardiovascular status should be performed, including an ECG and echocardiogram.

Volume loading in the immediate preoperative period is not thought to be necessary if effective α-blockade has been established over a long enough period, since spontaneous correction of blood volume occurs. For emergency surgery volume loading may be necessary.

Anaesthetic management is aimed at avoiding drugs which stimulate catecholamine release and minimize adrenergic responses. Sedative premedication, e.g. with midazolam, is helpful and vecuronium and fentanyl are logical drugs to use since neither stimulates histamine release.

Surgery for excision of pheochromocytoma necessitates invasive arterial and central venous pressure monitoring. Cardiovascular stability may be improved if draining veins from the tumour are ligated before extensive dissection. The period of hypertension during surgery can be controlled with an infusion of sodium nitroprusside. Phentolamine is less satisfactory because dysrhythmia and tachyphylaxis occur. Changes in ventricular rhythm can be treated with lignocaine and supraventricular tachycardia with amiodarone. Hypotension after tumour removal should be treated in the first instance with fluid rather than vasopressors but great care with fluid management should be taken to prevent cardiac failure. Blood loss may be high and should be anticipated.[140]

CONGENITAL ADRENAL HYPERPLASIA (ADRENOGENITAL SYNDROME)

The synthesis of cortisol and aldosterone is the result of a series of enzymic steps involving hydroxylases. Congenital adrenal hyperplasia (CAH) most commonly results from a deficiency of 21-hydroxylase. The low level of cortisol will stimulate the anterior pituitary to produce excess ACTH, leading to the production of large quantities of androgenic steroids.[143]

Presentation will depend on the severity and type of deficiency. Female infants may become virilized and show clitoral hypertrophy and possibly labial fusion. Up to 50% of CAH neonates develop a salt-losing crisis and present with vomiting, lethargy and hyponatraemia. If the defect is less severe, precocious puberty (males), primary amenorrhoea and ambiguous genitalia may point to the diagnosis.

Treatment of these children is aimed at reducing adrenal secretion by suppressing ACTH production with the use of glucocorticoids such as hydrocortisone and prednisone. Mineralocorticoids such as fludrocortisone and desoxycorticosterone may also be used. Female patients may need to undergo a feminizing genitoplasty to allow normal psychosexual development and sexual function.[144]

The anaesthetist will encounter these patients when they present for surgery for ambiguous genitalia or for other surgery. Steroid cover will be required and fluid and electrolyte balance will need to be checked carefully preoperatively.

ADRENOCORTICAL INSUFFICIENCY

Addison's disease represents primary failure of the adrenal cortex due to an acquired autoimmune process. Cortisol and mineralocorticoid secretion may also become inadequate following adrenal involvement in tuberculosis, meningococcal septicaemia, fungal infection, cancer or haemorrhage.

An adrenal crisis may present with nausea and vomiting, diarrhoea, abdominal pain, dehydration, hypotension, shock and coma, and this constitutes a medical emergency. The signs and symptoms of Addison's disease include weakness and fatigue, weight loss, vomiting and diarrhoea, dehydration and hypotension. Abnormal pigmentation over pressure points or a diffuse tanning is frequently present. There may be coexistent diabetes insipidus, hypothyroidism or hypoparathyroidism. Hyponatraemia and hyperkalaemia are present and hypoglycaemia is common. Blood gases may reveal a metabolic acidosis.

Occasionally, patients may present for emergency surgery while suffering an acute adrenal crisis. Management of such a crisis includes: (1) hydrocortisone 2 mg kg^{-1} i.v. given slowly over several minutes followed by 1–2 mg kg^{-1} every 4–6 h; (2) fluid therapy with normal saline 10–20 ml kg^{-1} initially. Further fluid management will depend on clinical findings; (3) 50% dextrose 1 ml kg^{-1} if hypoglycaemia is present, followed by a 10% dextrose infusion, the rate of which will depend on the degree of hypoglycaemia; and (4) management of hyperkalaemia with dextrose (50% 2 ml kg^{-1}) and insulin (0.1 U kg^{-1}).

The chronic condition presents few problems apart from providing steroid cover. Children receiving steroids on a long-term basis are at risk of developing a degree of adrenal suppression. These patients may be unable to increase their cortisol secretion in response to surgical stress. In order to prevent adverse reactions, hydrocortisone should be given perioperatively.[145] Dose regimens vary depending on the severity of surgery. Major surgery requires hydrocortisone 1–2 mg kg^{-1} i.v. at induction followed by 1–2 mg kg^{-1} i.v. every 6 h for 24–36 h and then tailed off during the following day. Minor surgery probably only requires a single intravenous dose at induction.

HYPOTHYROIDISM

Hypothyroidism may be congenital or acquired and a large number of different causes has been identified. The most common cause in childhood is chronic thyroiditis. Clinical findings may be apparent soon after birth but may take some time to manifest. Infants may be slow both physically and mentally. They may appear grey, pale or mottled with a slow pulse rate and low blood pressure. Myxoedema is common, as are a large tongue, nasal obstruction and poor muscle tone. The dry, coarse skin and hair are characteristic and a goitre may be present. Growth retardation and slow mental development are commonly seen. The presentation may be very mild and the diagnosis may be missed but it is important to make the diagnosis early as treatment can prevent permanent neurological deficits. Treatment with thyroxine needs to be started by the second or third month.

Anaesthetic for hypothyroid patients

The risks associated with anaesthesia and surgery for patients with untreated hypothyroidism are higher than for euthyroid patients and elective surgery should not be undertaken in the hypothyroid patient. If emergency surgery is required then urgent replacement therapy should be instituted. T3 can be given by slow intravenous infusion but must be given with great care as dysrythmias or hypertension may be precipitated. Patients are more sensitive to anaesthetic, opioid and sedative drugs and all of these must be used in reduced doses as they may precipitate a hypothyroid crisis. Hypothermia is more common and temperature should be carefully monitored and steps taken to prevent cooling. Hypotension is common and may require fluid or vasopressors to correct. Hydrocortisone should be given if adrenocortical suppression is suspected. The airway is the other area of concern, as the tongue is large and there may be nasal congestion. There may also be tracheal compression or deviation as a result of goitre.

INBORN ERRORS OF METABOLISM

A clear understanding of metabolic diseases is essential in paediatric medical practice, as early recognition and treatment of some conditions improve outcome. Even in lethal and untreatable disease, accurate diagnosis is important for genetic counselling. A more general understanding of the approach to diagnosis and management is helpful for the anaesthetist who may encounter children with diverse metabolic problems requiring anaesthesia for incidental surgery.

Diagnosis of inborn errors of metabolism may follow newborn screening, the investigation of clinical illness or recognition of a dysmorphic syndrome. In the UK metabolic screens include only that for phenylketonuria, although in Scotland galactosaemia also is part of routine screens.

Disorders of intermediary metabolism with rapid flux such as organic acidaemias and urea cycle disorders typically manifest as clinical illness in the newborn period. Poor feeding, vomiting and lethargy may progress to encephalopathy, apnoea, seizures and coma. It is worth noting that symptoms may precede established feeding and that metabolic acidosis may not be a prominent finding in some metabolic disorders.

Metabolic disorders may present in later infancy or early childhood only when unmasked by intercurrent illness. For example, fatty acid metabolic defects typically manifest at a time of acute infection and metabolic stress.

Still other metabolic diseases, such as storage diseases, present with insidious failure to thrive, developmental delay, neurological dysfunction and organomegaly. Several metabolic diseases, including Zellweger syndrome, pyruvate dehydrogenase deficiency and Smith–Lemli–Opitz syndrome are recognized on the basis of dysmorphic features.

Initial investigation of suspected metabolic disease must include plasma electrolytes, glucose and liver function tests. Acid–base analysis and infection screens will also be part of the initial investigation of any sick child. The second tier of investigation is aimed at the diagnosis of metabolic diseases that require urgent intervention. These tests may include blood ammonia and lactate levels (for suspected organic acidaemias, urea cycle disorders and congenital lactic acidosis), plasma insulin and cortisol (nesidioblastosis, hyperinsulinaemia, Addison's disease), urine and plasma amino acids, urine orotic acid and succinyl acetone (tyrosinaemia) and plasma carnitine.

Specialized investigations which are essential to long-term rather than acute management include DNA analysis and specific enzyme assays.[146]

Specific management of inborn errors of metabolism depends on the diagnosis and may range from careful dietary advice in phenylketonuria and galactosaemia to thoughtful genetic counselling for parents of non-surviving infants. The general principles of managing the acute metabolic problems must be understood by the practising anaesthetist. Initial care is supportive and involves careful rehydration and blood sugar control. Correction of severe acid–base derangements mandate close monitoring of pH and bicarbonate levels. In severely ill infants with signs of encephalopathy measures to limit cerebral oedema may be warranted. After basic supportive care, attempts should be made to reduce the load on affected metabolic pathways. This may include temporarily ceasing all exogenous protein sources and providing adequate caloric intake with intravenous glucose and insulin. A few disorders with severe acute presentations lend themselves to the removal of toxic metabolites. Ammonia (in organic acidaemias and urea cycle disorders), leucine (in maple syrup disease) and propionate (in propionic acidaemia) may be dialysed from plasma. Forced diuresis and veno-venous haemofiltration may also be useful. Intravenous carnitine infusions may be indicated in specific fatty acid transport defects but must be used with care as they are contraindicated in some fat oxidation defects.

Finally, if specific enzyme abnormalities are diagnosed an attempt to stimulate residual enzyme activity may be made by administering the appropriate cofactor.[115]

THE LIVER GLYCOGENOSES

This group of GSDs predominantly affects hepatic function, although a degree of muscle involvement is evident in some forms. Glycogenoses with primarily muscle manifestations are covered in the section dealing with myopathies.

Individual enzyme defects responsible for the glycogenoses (of which there are at least 12) have been determined and are the basis of classification. Each of the four most common liver GSDs have an incidence of between 1 : 100 000 and 1 : 500 000. Types I (Von Gierke's disease) and III (Forbe's or Cori's disease) are more prevalent than the others and are characterized by hepatomegaly and the inability to maintain normoglycaemia. [115] Diagnosis is made on liver biopsy; later cardiac involvement causes hypertrophic cardiomyopathy.

Treatment is aimed at maintaining blood sugar levels and may include parenteral nutrition, nocturnal gastric feeding with glucose polymer and the addition of uncooked cornstarch to the diet.[114] Vitamins, calcium supplements and uricosurics may be added. Liver and renal transplantation may be considered at the time of organ failure.

DISORDERS OF AMINO ACID METABOLISM

PHENYLKETONURIA

This is an inherited defect in phenylalanine hydroxylase (PAH) activity that leads to an accumulation of phenylalanine, impairing brain growth and development. The PAH gene has been mapped to chromosome 12q and over 200 mutations have been documented. There is a wide geographical variation in incidence, ranging from 1 : 5000 in Ireland to being very rare in Africans. Diagnosis should be made through neonatal screening and prenatal diagnosis may be made available to parents with an affected child.

There is wide clinical and biochemical heterogeneity in the disease and pathophysiological damage is related directly to phenylalanine accumulation without any apparent threshold. Abnormal dopamine and serotonin turnover together with altered protein synthesis and myelin stability lead to hypokinesia, dystonia and progressive mental retardation. Myoclonic epilepsy is common (25%) and hypopigmentation of skin, hair and irises may accompany the characteristic musty odour of phenylacetic acid.[147]

Management is based on lifelong dietary regulation in an attempt to prevent significant mental deterioration.[148]

Anaesthesia issues are those of handling potentially uncooperative and aggressive retarded children. Anticonvulsant medication should be continued throughout the perioperative period.

THE LYSOSOMAL ENZYME DEFICIENCIES

This group of disorders results from inherited deficiencies of various lysosomal enzymes and leads to accumulation of mucopolysaccharides, glycoproteins and sphingolipids in the skeleton, CNS and viscera. The mucopolysaccharidoses (MPS) represent the failure fully to degrade and eliminate dermatan, heparan and keratan sulfates and form the largest subgroup, although Gaucher's disease (a lipidosis) is the most prevalent single disorder.[115] The overall incidence of each group is in the region of 1 : 10 000 births.

THE MUCOPOLYSACCHARIDOSES

These disorders are inherited as recessive traits and all, except for Hunter's disease (which is X-linked), are autosomally transmitted. Individual gene mutations have been mapped to chromosomes 3, 5, 7 and 22 and although a clinical distinction can be made between specific enzyme defects, there is a wide spectrum of severity within each disease. The deposition of mucopolysaccharides begins before birth but clinical manifestations are usually delayed for several years. Diagnosis is based on clinical presentation, the presence of mucopolysaccharides in the urine and the demonstration of 'inclusive bodies' in leucocytes. *In vitro* enzyme assays of fibroblast or leucocyte cultures and occasionally serum enzyme assays establish a more exact diagnosis.[149]

Prenatal diagnosis is possible using direct enzyme assays on chorionic villous samples. The classification of this group of disorders and a summary of the clinical features and anaesthetic implications are given in Table 1.10.[150] At present, no treatment is fully effective for these conditions. Bone marrow transplantation offers mixed success but may at least halt disease progression. Gene therapy may prove to be the most hopeful long-term approach.

Type I disease (MPS-I) is caused by a deficiency of L-iduronidase. Three clinical forms are recognized based on onset and clinical course, with Hurler's syndrome being the prototypical mucopolysaccharide storage disease. It manifests at the end of the first year of life with dwarfing and increased head size. Coarse facies are characterized by macroglossia, patulous lips, hyperplastic gums and corneal clouding. Infants often have a short neck, thickened skin and hepatosplenomegaly. Thoracolumbar scoliosis producing a restrictive lung defect and some degree of mental retardation with sensorineural deafness are common. Coronary and valvular cardiac involvement often

Table 1.10 The mucopolysaccharidoses

MPS	Syndrome	Genetics/Biochemistry	Prevalence	Clinical features	Age at diagnosis	Life expectancy	Anaesthetic implications
I	Hurlers	Deficient ʟ-iduronidase Autosomal recessive Chromosomal mutation on chromosome 3,5,7 or 22	1 : 100 000	Skin and soft tissue thickening, increased head size and dwarfism. Coarse facies, skeletal abnormalities and kyphoscoliosis. Hepato-splenomegaly, cardiac-valvular and large vessel intimal thickening, mental retardation, sensorineural deafness and hydrocephalus. Corneal clouding and retinal degeneration	6–24 months	<10 years	Airway obstruction, difficult intubation, aspiration and secretions. Restrictive lung disease, sleep apnoea and RV strain. Ventricular dilatation/thickening and valvular incompetence. Common procedures: investigative radiology, ENT, venous access procedures
	Hurlers/Scheie	Autosomal recessive	1 : 100 000	Intermediate phenotype. Moderate intelligence	3–8 years	<20 years	As above
	Scheie	Autosomal recessive	1 : 600 000	Mild form. Intelligence and stature unaffected. Aortic valve involvement. Retinal degeneration and glaucoma	5–20 years	Normal	As above. Common procedures: carpal tunnel decompression, aortic valve replacement, ophthalmological
II	Hunters severe	X-linked recessive	1 : 70 000 (Israel)	Coarse facies, moderate dwarfism. Hydrocephalus may be severe, progressive vision and hearing loss. Retinitis pigmentosa, characteristic nodular ivory-coloured skin lesions. Cardiac valvular and coronary involvement.	2–4 years	10–15 years	As above
III	Mild Santilippo's	Types A–D (different enzyme defects)	1 : 24 000 in The Netherlands	Normal intelligence. Relatively benign Severe progressive mental retardation. Normal growth, milder somatic manifestations. Seizures and behavioural problems.	2–4 years 2–6 years	Normal 10–20 years	Aggressive behaviour. Seizure control
IV	Morquio's	Autosomal recessive	1 : 300 000	Severe skeletal abnormalities, dwarfism, pectus deformity and odontoid hypoplasia. Normal intelligence. Mild-mod facial coarsening and deafness	2–6 years	Normal	Atlanto-axial subluxation. Restrictive lung disease
VI	Maroteaux-Lamy	Autosomal recessive	Rare	Variable phenotype. Similar to Hurlers. Dwarfism with normal intelligence. Aortic valve involvement. Dural thickening-progressive myelopathy	4–8 years	Variable	
VII	Sly	Autosomal recessive	Rare	Variable phenotype may be present in the neonate. Similar to Hurlers	Neonate onwards	Variable	

progresses to cardiac failure and death in the first decade.

Scheie's syndrome is a less severe form of MPS-I with similar features to those described above, although these children may have normal stature, intelligence and lifespan. Common surgical presentations include carpal tunnel compression, aortic valve disease and glaucoma.

Hurler/Scheie syndrome represents an intermediate phenotype with moderate skeletal involvement and mental impairment. Aortic valve disease is more severe than in Scheie's syndrome and death usually ensues in the second decade.

Hunter's syndrome (MPS-II) has two clinical forms. The more severe results in moderate dwarfism and coarse facies by 2 years of age. Retinitis pigmentosa without corneal clouding together with nodular ivory-coloured skin lesions are characteristic. Hydrocephalus may be severe and valvular heart disease is common.

Sanfilippo's syndrome (MPS-III) involves any of four separate enzymic defects indistinguishable on clinical grounds. It is the most common MPS disorder in the UK. Although characterized by severe mental retardation, skeletal and visceral involvement in MPS-III is usually mild. Aggressive behaviour and seizures may become problematic.

Morquio's syndrome (MPS-IV) is characterized by severe skeletal involvement. Marked dwarfism, pectus deformity and flattened vertebrae result in kyphoscoliosis and upper cervical spine instability. Mild to moderate facial coarsening and hearing loss are also common, although intelligence is often normal.

Maroteaux–Lamy syndrome (MPS-VI) has a variable phenotype and children are often of normal intelligence. Moderate dwarfism and joint stiffness are prominent.[151]

The anaesthetic management of the mucopolysaccharidoses is described in Chapter 20.

THE MUCOLIPIDOSES

The mucolipidoses (ML) are closely related to the mucopolysaccharidoses. Similar facial features to those of Hurler's syndrome are noted and inheritance is also autosomal recessive. Three forms are recognized and distinguished from MPS disease by the absence of mucopolysacchariduria. Visceral, skeletal and cardiac involvement are also similar to MPS-I. Type III disease (ML-III) is a milder form sometimes referred to as pseudo-Hurler dystrophy. Table 1.11 summarizes some of the features of the disease.

Anaesthesia and MPS/ML disease

Owing to improved and newer therapies including bone marrow transplantation, children with these disorders are increasingly likely to present for surgery. Anaesthetic issues have been reviewed in three major series[151–153] and are summarized here and also in Chapter 20.

Airway management remains of primary concern. Upper airway obstruction needs to be anticipated and commonly results from hypoplastic upper airways and mucosal infiltration. Macroglossia, tonsillar and adenoidal enlargement and copious secretions also contribute to difficulties during gaseous induction and mask ventilation.[154] These tend to be more marked in MPS-I and II.[153]

Anaesthesia may be induced either by inhalation or intravenously, with or without preoperative light benzodiazepine sedation. Antisialogogue administration may aid gaseous induction of anaesthesia. Cases must be evaluated individually with respect to expected degrees of patient distress and co-operation. Ketamine anaesthesia may also be a useful technique in these patients. Upper airway manoeuvres including oral and nasopharyngeal airways and tongue traction may be necessary during induction. Theoretically, severe hepatosplenomegaly may make regurgitation and aspiration a greater risk.

Adequate preparation for difficult intubation is also essential, as the large head and short immobile neck together with micrognathia will make direct laryngoscopy awkward.[152] These considerations apply more to MPS-I and II than to III (Sanfilippo's syndrome) and IV (Morquio's syndrome). Intubation difficulties are compounded by the potential for atlanto–axial instability. Especially notable in MPS-IV is that a hypoplastic odontoid may result in significant cord compression during neck extension. Preoperative cervical spine radiology may help to delineate instability in these patients. Occasional patients will present with symptoms

Table 1.11 The mucolipidoses and lipidoses

Syndrome	Genetics/ biochemistry	Prevalence	Clinical features	Age at diagnosis	Life expectancy	Anaesthetic implications
The mucolipidoses: ML I, ML II	Deficiency of acetyl-glucosaminyl phospho-transferase		Typical coarse features seen in Hurler's disease but without excesive mucopolysacchariduria. Skeletal abnormalities, cardiac valvular involvement			Airway obstuction and difficult intubation, increasingly difficult with age. Restrictive lung disease and sleep apnoea
ML III Pseudo-Hurler's polydystrophy			Milder form, presents later – longer life span			
The lipidoses: Gaucher's disease type I chronic non-neuronopathic	Deficiency of gluco-cerebrosidase	1 : 2500 (Ashkenazi Jews)	Painless splenomegaly, anaemia, thrombocytopaenia and leucopaenia. Degenerative bone changes with 'bone crises'. Pulmonary disease		Enzyme therapy now available	Pulmonary hypertension. Anaemia and thrombocytopaenia.
Type II	Severe deficiency		Hepato-splenomegaly, early neurological involvement. Classic triad: trismus,strabismus and head retroflexion	5–15 years 3–6 months	12 months	Bulbar dysfunction – dysphagia and recurrent aspiration pneumonia
Type III			Variable phenotype with a variable course			As above
Krabbe's disease	Galactosyl-ceramide accumulation	1 : 50 000 (Swedes)	Irritability, vomiting and failure to thrive. Rapidly progressive mental and motor deterioration, spastic quadriparesis, deafness and blindness		2 years	
Farber's disease	Deficiency of ceramidase	Rare	Subcutaneous nodules around arthritic joints. Hoarseness and aphonia. Macroglossia, cardiomyopathy and mental retardation	2 weeks– 4 months		Laryngeal and epiglottic granulomas – avoid intubation. Postextubation stridor

of progressive myelopathy ('parameningitis cervicalis') requiring external or internal fixation of the cervical spine. Typically, a tracheal tube smaller than that predicted for age is appropriate and early recourse to other techniques of intubation, such as the two-operator technique and fibreoptic bronchoscopic intubation is recommended.[155] Nasal intubation is best avoided.[156] The laryngeal mask airway for short procedures is proving valuable.[157]

Difficulty with intubation may either increase or decrease with age, although a majority of cases will not change significantly. Interestingly, early reports of patients treated with bone marrow transplantation do not suggest any regression of the airway problems.[151]

Respiratory impairment is common, with both restrictive and obstructive lung defects leading to pulmonary hypertension.

Cardiac impairment must be suspected in all of these patients and ECG, chest X-ray and echocardiography may be helpful in preoperative assessment. The cardiac pathology includes ventricular dilatation or hypertrophy and valve-thickening leading to valvular incompetence. Intimal thickening may affect the coronary arteries and aorta. Although coronary disease is usually asymptomatic, subendocardial scarring has been reported in post-mortem studies.[158] Anaesthesia is tolerated by the majority of patients without cardiac morbidity, but the risk of intraoperative cardiac arrest remains significant.[159] Antibiotic prophylaxis must be given when significant valve disease is present.[156]

Preoperative neurological evaluation must take into account the possibility of raised intracranial pressure (especially in patients with MPS-I) and perioperative seizure control and aggressive behaviour (especially in patients with MPS-IV).

Finally, these patients benefit from careful postoperative observation, with particular attention directed towards respiratory function and aggressive treatment of sputum retention.

THE LIPIDOSES AND SPHINGOLIPIDOSES

These lysosomal abnormalities result in the visceral accumulation of various complex lipids. All of these lipids share the common moiety, ceramide, which comprises the amino-alcohol sphingosine and a fatty acid. The lipids and their precursors are primarily cell membrane components and enzyme defects of catabolic pathways lead to accumulation in tissues where turnover is highest. Hence, hepatosplenomegaly, neurological damage and a macular cherry-red spot are hallmarks of disease.

The most prevalent disorder is Gaucher's disease, the incidence of which is highest in Ashkenazi Jews (1 : 2500).[149] Clinical and anaesthetic features of the lipidoses are summarized in Table 1.12.

Gaucher's disease results from a deficiency of glucocerebrodase and has three clinical subtypes. Type I (chronic non-neuronopathic Gaucher's disease) presents with painless splenomegaly and a pancytopaenia. Degenerative bone changes may lead to vertebral fractures, femoral head necrosis and febrile 'bone crises'. Pulmonary involvement is common. The disorder can now be ameliorated with enzyme replacement therapy (ceredase). Type-II disease results from a more severe enzyme deficiency and CNS involvement is an early feature. Death often ensues within 12 months. Type-III disease runs a variable course after childhood or adolescent presentation with hepatosplenomegaly and skeletal and nervous system involvement. Surgical intervention in Gaucher's disease is commonly for liver or bone marrow biopsy. Preoperative evaluation must include haematological screening and awareness of the possibility of pulmonary hypertension.

Table 1.12 Modified child's severity scoring of liver disease

Clinical or biochemical parameter	1 point	2 points	3 points
Grade of encephalopathy	Absent	1 and 2	3, 4 and 5
Bilirubin (μmol l^{-1})	<25	25–40	>40
Albumin (g l^{-1})	>35	28–35	<28
Prothrombin time (s prolonged)	1–4	4–6	>6
Ascites	Absent	Slight	Moderate

LIVER DISEASE

The practical evaluation of a jaundiced infant is well served by consideration of its history, symptoms and signs. A full history disclosing parental blood types (ABO and Rh), ethnicity and any family history of jaundice may suggest haemolytic disease of the newborn (HDN) or G6PD deficiency. Fetal cord blood samples can be used to confirm feto–maternal isoimmunization. The early appearance of jaundice (i.e. within 24 h of birth), a rapid rise in serum bilirubin associated with hepatosplenomegaly and pallor are typical of haemolytic jaundice.

Jaundice in the presence of symptoms such as vomiting, lethargy or weight loss should prompt a search for sources of sepsis and investigation for infective hepatitis, galactosaemia and Crigler–Najer syndrome. Other consistent symptoms include weight loss, apnoeas and temperature instability.

Jaundice associated with prominent signs such as dark urine, pale stools or hepatomegaly may represent neonatal hepatitis or surgical conditions such as biliary atresia or a choledochal cyst.

The careful exclusion of major pathology allows the diagnosis of physiological jaundice or 'breast milk jaundice'. In the older child, sickle cell disease, viral hepatitis and Gilbert's, Dubin–Johnson and Rotor syndromes should all be considered.

HAEMOLYTIC DISEASE OF THE NEWBORN

Haemolysis due to maternal–fetal blood group incompatability may quickly give rise to neonatal jaundice as the mechanisms for the conjugation of bilirubin are immature in the newborn. Severe haemolytic disease may occasionally result in accretion of bile plugs within the biliary tree, leading to more prolonged conjugated hyperbilirubinaemia, termed the 'inspissated bile syndrome'.

NEONATAL HEPATITIS

Perinatally acquired infection may result in hepatitis. Common agents include herpes, cytomegalovirus (CMV), varicella, coxsackie, rubella, hepatitis B and human immunodeficiency virus (HIV).

The important laboratory findings are raised bilirubin, elevated transaminases and abnormal coagulation. Specific viruses may be cultured and viral serology may be diagnostic.

There is currently no specific treatment for viral hepatitis, although acylcovir may be given if herpes infection is the cause. Vitamin K, D and E are given along with calcium supplementation.

GIANT CELL HEPATITIS

This condition accounts for 70% of neonatal intrahepatic cholestasis, although the cause is still unknown. It is associated with prematurity and perinatal hepatic hypoxia. It results in poor feeding, vomiting and intermittently pale stools. Most patients recover without chronic liver damage but a small proportion will go on to develop hepatic fibrosis.[160]

BILIARY ATRESIA

The incidence of biliary atresia is approximately 1 : 10 000 births and is equally divided between males and females. Its pathology involves pansclerosis of all hepatic ductal elements during development. Dark urine and pale stools are characteristic and the liver is frequently enlarged and hard. Diagnosis may require exploratory laparotomy with on-table cholangiography. Without surgical correction deterioration continues with progression of ascites, portal hypertension, bleeding abnormalities and liver failure. Treatment is surgical and needs to be performed early. The most commonly performed surgical procedure is a hepatoportoenterostomy (Kasai procedure) carried out in a specialist centre.[161]

CHOLEDOCHAL CYST

Although less common than biliary atresia, the clinical presentation of this condition is very similar to biliary atresia. The diagnosis can be made with ultrasound scanning. Surgery should be carried out as soon as possible. Choledochal cysts may be associated with biliary atresia and the prognosis depends on this fact.

BREAST MILK JAUNDICE

This is common and occurs in up to 40% of breast-fed babies. This is a benign condition and kernicterus is thought not to occur with breast milk jaundice alone. It is a self-limiting condition and resolves by 3 months. It almost never needs any form of treatment but in some cases breast-feeding babies can be fed with formula milk for a short period.

ALPHA-1-ANTITRYPSIN DEFICIENCY

This is due to a deficiency in the protease inhibitor system. This predisposes the patients to chronic liver and lung disease. It should be suspected in low-birth-weight infants with neonatal cholestasis. Children with cirrhosis and no history of liver disease should also be suspected, as should those with recurrent pulmonary disease. Laboratory tests will reveal low levels of α_1-antitrypsin in the serum and liver function tests are likely to be abnormal. About 20% of children with homozygous α_1-antitrypsin deficiency will develop hepatic disease in childhood, which usually leads to portal hypertension and cirrhosis, and these children are more likely to develop liver cancer later in life. There remains no specific therapy and treatment is of the complications of liver disease. About half of all children who develop liver disease will go on to progressive liver failure and death without liver transplantation.

PORTAL HYPERTENSION

Prehepatic portal hypertension accounts for 5–10% of gastrointestinal bleeding in children. The cause is not always obvious but frequently will be due to sepsis, omphalitis, umbilical vein catheterization, pancreatitis and peritonitis. It may also be due to portal or splenic vein malformations or thrombosis. A number of cases is idiopathic. Clinical features of portal hypertension include splenomegaly and oeso-phageal varices which are associated with massive haematemesis and melena. The children are often completely well prior to the onset of the symptoms. Anaesthesia is often required for injection of varices via an endoscope. Large-bore venous access is required in case of unexpected haemorrhage.

Treatment may be either medical or surgical. The basis of surgical treatment is the formation of a portocaval anastamosis to bypass the obstruction. Various shunts have been attempted, including mesocaval shunt (superior mesenteric vein to inferior vena cava) and splenorenal shunt. Partial splenectomy may reduce the risk of rupture and surgical ligation of varices has also beeen tried as a last resort.

Prognosis depends to some extent on the availability of appropriate vessels for shunting and on the experience of the surgical team in dealing with these patients. Shunts are more successful in older patients and the problems of portacaval encephalopthy seen in adults are rare in children.[162]

REYE'S SYNDROME

Reye's syndrome describes an encephalopathy associated with fatty degeneration of the liver. The mechanisms are complex and poorly understood but involve mitochondrial damage by a salicylate or other toxin in the presence of viral infection.

Clinically, Reye's syndrome follows a viral illness and progresses to vomiting, lethargy and drowsiness. Convulsions, irregular respiration and dilated pupils are manifestations of progressive cerebral oedema, which is thought to be caused by the high serum ammonia levels. Hypoglycaemia, cardiac dysrhythmias and inappropriate ADH secretion may all complicate the course of the illness.

Treatment is largely supportive, with invasive monitoring, ventilation and measures to control raised intracranial pressure.[163]

Anaesthetic implications for children with liver disease

Jaundice should be regarded seriously and a clear diagnosis should ideally be made preoperatively. The complications and associated conditions of jaundice should be sought. Anaemia may be secondary to blood loss from the gastrointestinal tract, particularly from oesophageal varices. Bleeding disorders are common, may be unresponsive to vitamin K and may require clotting factors to be given preoperatively.

Hypoproteinaemia with resultant oedema, ascites and secondary hyperaldosteronism commonly presents with the features of cardiac failure.

Chest infections or areas of pulmonary collapse may also be more common and should be sought and treated. Respiratory excursion may be limited by hepatosplenomegaly and ascites.

Renal failure is a real risk during anaesthesia and surgery in patients with liver disease. A rising urea level in the presence of surgically correctable obstructive jaundice makes the surgical intervention urgent. Renal protection involves the aggressive treatment of hypovolaemia and cardiac failure. The aim of fluid therapy is to achieve a urine flow of $1 \ ml \ kg^{-1} \ h^{-1}$. The judicious slow infusion of $0.5–1 \ g \ kg^{-1}$ mannitol and the use of frusemide may be warranted. Dopamine may also be used to improve renal blood flow and as a natuiretic. Antibiotics should be given if the biliary tree is to be manipulated during surgery.

The development of encephalopathy is poorly understood but is thought to be related to toxic substances absorbed from the intestine. The absorption of these toxins from the gut can be reduced by the use of magnesium sulphate enemas, oral lactulose or oral neomycin.

Surgical risk is determined by the severity of the liver disease, which can be graded using the modified Childs' scoring method (see Table 1.11). Patients with 5–6 points have a low operative risk, those with 7–9 points have moderate risk and those with 10–15 points are at high risk from surgery. Only those in the low-risk group should be considered for elective surgery.[164]

ONCOLOGY

Important general medical considerations for children with cancer include direct effects and complications of the primary disease as well as the side-effects of various therapies. The anaesthetist may become involved in the care of the children at any stage of their management and should be able to recognize these effects and complications as they will have a bearing on any anaesthetic required.

During initial chemotherapy of any malignancy, massive tumour necrosis may occur. The resultant production of high levels of uric acid and phosphate may lead to nephropathy and renal failure. To reduce the risk of renal failure, uric acid production is reduced with allopurinol and a high urine output is promoted with liberal intravenous fluids. Patients given very large fluid loads may become fluid overloaded and risk pulmonary oedema. A child with acute renal failure who requires surgery has an increased risk of morbidity, particularly if fluid overload is present. Prior to surgery these patients require a careful assessment of their fluid balance, electrolytes and need for dialysis.

Infection is a constant threat during chemotherapy and a fever should be investigated with swabs and cultures. *Escherichia coli* and *Klebsiella* are common pathogens and both *Pneumosistis carinii* and fungal infections are more common than in the general population. Viral infection with *varicella* may be life-threatening and a high level of awareness is needed by all those looking after the child. Particular vigilance is required as the normal signs of infection may be masked because of immunosuppressive therapy. Careful sterile techniques must be used when inserting intravenous lines and particularly central lines. Exposure of chemotherapy patients to potential carriers of viral exanthems should be limited. Rectal administration of drugs to patients with severe neutropenia or mucositis may impose unacceptable risks of bacteraemia.

Thrombocytopaenia may result in bleeding from the nose, gastrointestinal tract or brain and may necessitate platelet transfusion. Haemoglobin levels are often low and should be kept at $8–10 \ g \ dl^{-1}$. This usually requires transfusion with irradiated or leucodepleted blood so as to prevent graft-versus-host disease. Platelet levels and coagulation studies should be checked preoperatively, particularly before major surgery. Intramuscular injections should be avoided if clotting is abnormal, as should epidural, caudal or spinal anaesthesia. The insertion of nasogastric tubes or nasopharangeal temperature probes may cause profuse bleeding. Care should be exercised during intubation to minimize trauma and bleeding. Meticulous care of the airway to avoid aspiration and good postoperative pain control will reduce the chances of postoperative chest infection.

Hepatic damage is usually the result of vincristine therapy and doses may need to be reduced if liver damage is apparent. Other drugs that have been implicated in liver damage are mercaptopurine and methotrexate.

The psychological aspects of dealing with children with cancer and their parents can be challenging. The children have often undergone multiple procedures and may be very frightened. The parents often know a great deal about their child's condition and require detailed explanations of planned procedures. Expectations for care are high and lapses in the care of the child are poorly tolerated. Procedures should be carefully explained.

LEUKAEMIA

Acute lymphoblastic leukaemia

Acute lymphoblastic leukaemia (ALL) is the most common of the childhood leukaemias, accounting for more than 80% of cases. ALL can occur at any age but the most common age is 4 years. Without treatment it is fatal in 3–4 months but management with chemotherapy is increasingly effective. Approximately 70% of children with ALL can now be expected to survive disease-free for 5 years. Prognosis within this group of children is not uniform and is worse if children present before 1 year or after 10 years of age. Higher initial white counts suggest a worse prognosis.

Clinically, anaemia is common and leads to pallor and tiredness. Repeated infection is more common and bleeding may be a presenting feature. Infiltration of bone marrow or other solid organs may cause discomfort and pain or dysfunction. The kidneys appear to be the most important organ involved.

Treatment involves an initial period which aims to induce remission and is generally followed by a maintenance period. Remission can almost always be induced with a combination of vincristine, prednisolone and asparaginase. This usually takes a period of about 4 weeks and is followed by maintenance using various regimens and drug combinations, but mercaptopurine and cyclophosphamide are common. Careful titration of drugs is required to minimize side-effects and to ensure that white cell counts do not drop too low.

Involvement of the CNS with leukaemic cells is common and symptoms include stiff neck, vomiting and lethargy. Diagnosis is made by demonstrating lymphoblastic cells in the spinal fluid. Specific therapy is needed to deal with this infiltration and involves the use of intrathecal drugs such as methotrexate. Cranial irradiation has been used in children but causes neurological damage and so tends to be avoided. Bone marrow transplantation is a modality which, although difficult and time-consuming, is used in some patients after relapse.

Acute non-lymphocytic leukaemia

This includes acute myeloblastic leukaemia, acute monoblastic leukaemias and others. Treatment is more difficult and prognosis is poor, being in the region of 25–35% long-term survivors.

Chronic myelocytic leukaemia

This occurs as an adult and juvenile form. The juvenile form tends to occur in young children and is difficult to treat. Bone marrow transplantation has been used successfully and is increasingly being tried.

LYMPHOMA

Hodgkin's lymphoma

There are several different histological types of Hodgkin's lymphoma and, although rare in children under 10 years of age, it does occur in children as young as 3 years. The classical presentation of Hodgkin's is of painless enlargement of lymph nodes and the most common sites for these are the cervical chain or mediastinum. Other features may include fever, night sweats, weight loss and pruritus. Laboratory findings may be normal but anaemia is common. Diagnosis is made by lymph-node biopsy. Patients with mediastinal masses are at great risk for respiratory obstruction after induction of anaesthesia (see Chapter 18).

Staging of the disease is important and influences prognosis. Table 1.13 outlines the Ann Arbor classification of Hodgkin's disease.[165]

Treatment is with combination chemotherapy or radiotherapy. Chemotherapy is now more popular because it has fewer long-term side-effects in the child and it has the added advantage of tackling concealed disease. The two most commonly used regimens are MOPP (mechlorethamine, vincristine, procarbazine and prednisolone) and ABVD (adriamycin, bleomycin, vinblastine and dacarbazine). The prognosis for these patients is encouraging, with a 5-year survival rate of 90% for those patients with limited disease. Those with more extensive disease (stage 3) have a 70% 5-year survival and even in stage 4 disease 5-year survival is reasonable.[165]

Non-Hodgkin's lymphoma

This may be broadly classified into lympho-blastic and non-lymphoblastic (Burkitt's lymphoma). The latter is common in central Africa, where the Epstein–Barr virus (EBV) is thought to play an aetiological role, but is much less common in developed countries.

Non-Hodgkin's lymphoma often presents with an abdominal tumour originating from the lymphoid tissue of the gut. However, it may also present with painless swelling of other lymph tissue causing compression of other structures. Non-Hodgkin's lymphomas are sensitive to both chemotherapy and radiotherapy and a number of different treatment protocols is used.

Prognosis is generally quite good, with an overall 2-year survival of about 70%. Where the lymphoma is confined to the gut cure is possible in 90% of patients.[166]

NEUROBLASTOMA

Neuroblastoma is the most common solid tumour of infancy. In childhood it is second only to the brain tumour in frequency. The tumour arises from the sympathetic chain or from the adrenal medulla and four stages of neuroblastoma exist. Presentation is frequently with an abdominal mass and although this can occur at any age the most common age for presentation is 2 years. Fever, weight loss and bone pain are also common and diarrhoea may occur. Laboratory studies demonstrate anaemia and thrombocytosis. However, in the presence of marrow infiltration thrombocytopenia will occur. Vanillylmandelic acid (VMA) and homovanillic acid (HMV) are elevated in the urine, as are other catecholamines. Hypertension may develop either from renal artery stenosis or from catecholamine secretion, although dysrhythmia is rare. Approximately 80% of cases have raised VMA; only 10–15% have symptoms and these should be treated preoperatively as for phaeochromocytoma.

Treatment of these patients is with a combination of surgery, chemotherapy and radiotherapy. A common approach is to perform an initial biopsy of the tumour followed by chemotherapy, which frequently reduces the size of the tumour, allowing surgical removal of the remaining tumour.[167,168]

In addition to those anaesthetic considerations applicable to all children with cancer undergoing therapy (see above), some specific features should be borne in mind. The large intrabdominal tumour may compress the inferior vena cava and compromise the circulation, while also predisposing the child to regurgitation during induction of anaesthesia. If the mass is in the thorax, compression of the

Table 1.13 Ann Arbor staging of Hodgkin's disease

Hodgkin's disease stage	
Stage 1	Single lymph node or node region or organ
Stage 2	Two lymph node regions involved on the same side of the diaphragm or localized involvement of an extra-lymphatic organ or site
Stage 3	Lymph node involvement on both sides of the diaphragm or localized involvement of extra-lymphatic organ or site or spleen
Stage 4	Disseminated involvement of one or more extralymphatic organs with or without associated lymph node involvement

trachea or lungs may occur, making airway management or intubation difficult. Massive blood loss during surgery is possible and preparations should be made for this possibility, including good intravenous access and invasive monitoring.[169,170]

WILM'S TUMOUR (NEPHROBLASTOMA)

Wilm's tumour is the next most common tumour of childhood after neuroblastoma. It originates in the kidney from whence it can invade the surrounding structures particularly the renal vessels, vena cava and aorta. Metastases occur to the lungs most commonly but also to the bone marrow, liver and brain (see also p. 393).

Clinical presentation is usually with an abdominal mass which can be enormous, occasionally splinting the diaphragm and restricting respiration. Laboratory findings are unremarkable but occasionally a coagulopathy is present as a result of acquired von Willebrand's disease, which is an uncommon association with Wilm's tumour. Prognosis depends on the extent of spread of the tumour and on the histological type but overall survival is 90%. Treatment usually consists of a combination of surgery, radiation therapy and chemotherapy.[171] Factor VIII may be required to correct the abnormal clotting.[172]

HAEMATOLOGY (NON-MALIGNANT)

SICKLE CELL DISEASE

The molecular basis of this inherited haemoglobinopathy was elucidated in 1957. The substitution of valine for a glutamic acid residue towards the N-terminal of the β-globin molecule results from a gene mutation on chromosome 11. The resultant haemoglobin molecule (HbS) shares codominant expression with normal HbA and two basic phenotypes are therefore apparent. The trait or carrier state (AS) is almost completely benign and confers relative resistance to malaria in malarial regions. The homozygous expression of an abnormal gene (SS) gives rise to sickle cell disease (SCD), a chronic haemolytic anaemia with variable severity. HbS may be combined with other haemoglobinopathies such as thalassaemia and haemoglobin C, D and E, thus increasing the spectrum of sickling disorders.

Disease prevalence follows an ethnic pattern in the UK. The highest incidence of disease is among those of Afro-Caribbean descent. It is suggested that in communities where more than 15% of the population is Afro-Caribbean, all antenatal women and neonates should be screened for sickle cell and related disorders.[173]

The essential pathophysiology of SCD is extravascular haemolysis due to reduced red cell deformability. This is a result of polymerization (gelation) of deoxyHbS in response to reduced oxygen tensions, lowered pH or hypertonic conditions. Haemoglobin polymerization is a reversible process but repeated cycles lead to the formation of irreversibly sickled cells. These cells have altered surface adhesion characteristics that lead to microvascular thrombosis and vaso-occlusion. The latter is the basis of most of the acute complications of SCD. Other associated abnormalities include altered serum coagulability and disordered splenic function which result in defective immune opsonization and ineffective phagocytosis. The latter effects are responsible for increasing patient susceptibility to infection with encapsulated micro-organisms. Fetal haemoglobin inhibits sickling and increased levels are associated with milder clinical disease.[174]

The natural history of SCD is one of chronic haemolysis punctuated by several well-recognized complications, many of which have a vaso-occlusive basis. The haemolytic anaemia is associated with reticulocytosis and hyperbilirubinaemia and is generally well tolerated. Acute haemolysis (sickling crises) may be precipitated by cold, dehydration, infection, acidosis, hypoxia and fatigue, and is characterized by pain of variable severity and duration. Apart from haemolytic crises, patients with SCD are prone to several other acute life-threatening complications, including an acute chest syndrome, splenic sequestration crises, overwhelming sepsis, aplastic crises and stroke. Significant morbidity in SCD also accrues from abdominal pain episodes, vaso-occlusive skin and bone involvement, cholelithiasis, retinopathy and uropathy.[175] Complications of SCD are summarized in Table 1.14.

Diagnosis of SCD is based on screening programmes within either preconceptional, antenatal or neonatal high-risk populations. Cellulose acetate haemoglobin electrophoresis is required and confirmatory tests use citrate agar. Liquid chromatography may be utilized in larger diagnostic centres. The emergency situation where definitive diagnostic tests and consultant hamatological review are not im-

mediately available may confront an anaesthetist. In these cases, history, physical examination, complete blood count and film, together with reticulocyte count, form the basis of rational risk management. The sodium metabisulfite test (Sickledex) may be helpful. A negative result effectively excludes SCD. A positive result indicates the presence of HbS but does not distinguish the trait from SCD. These tests are not screening tests and are not useful in neonates. False negatives may occur with SCD.

Table 1.14 Sickle cell disease complications

Sickle cell disease	Complications
Haemolytic (pain) crises	Major cause of hospitalization and morbidity
	Precipitated by cold, dehydration, hypoxia, infection, acidosis, stress, fatigue and menstruation
	Unpredictable frequency and variable duration
	Less frequent in patients with higher HbF concentrations
	Aggresive analgesia regimes and supportive measures required
	(Non-steroidal anti-inflamatory agents, opioids and patient controlled analgesia techniques are useful)
Overwhelming infection	High risk of invasive infection with *Strep. pneumoniae, H. influenza* due to altered splenic function
	Penicillin prophylaxis recommended from 4 months old to adolesence.
Aplastic crises	Often precipitated by Human Parvovirus B19 infection
	Confined to paediatric age group
	Usually self-limiting
	Requires urgent transfusion
Acute chest syndrome	Multifactorial pathophysiology including pneumococcal and atypical pneumonia, pulmonary sequestration, infarction and fat embolism
	Leading cause of death in patients with SCD
Stroke	MRI evidence of infarctive lesions in up to 17% of SCD patients
	Transcranial doppler ultrasound may identify children at risk
Acute splenic sequestration	Sudden splenic enlargement with circulatory collapse
	Often associated with infection
	Major cause of mortality under 2 years of age
Other complications	
Bone and skin involvement	Dactylitis (hand and foot syndrome)
	Femoral head necrosis
	Chronic leg ulceration
	Salmonella osteomyelitis
Hypersplenism and autosplenectomy	
Priapism	Incidence: up to 12% of children
Retinopathy	Vitreous haemorrhage, retinal detachment
Biliary disease	Gallbladder sludge, cholelithiasis and cholecystitis
Uropathy	Microangiopathic glomerulopathy and tubular dysfunction

Management of SCD patients has generally consisted of supportive care, treatment of complications and red cell transfusions, while attempting to avoid iron overload and allo-immunization. More recently, comprehensive health care has included counselling, monitoring for potential complications and antimicrobial prophylactic measures. Indications and techniques of transfusion therapy continue to undergo refinement and measures aimed at modulating fetal haemoglobin levels are proving effective. Bone marrow and cord blood transplantation offer the only possibility of cure but are limited by a lack of available donors.[173,176] Typical management strategies are summarized in Table 1.15.

Anaesthesia issues in sickle cell disease

Retrospective reviews of patient cohorts confirm that SCD patients are at greater risk of perioperative complications than their unaffected counterparts. The risks of anaesthesia and surgery have declined steadily since the 1970s and the reasons for this are probably mulitifactorial. Greater general awareness, the institution of exchange transfusion programmes and increased attention to perioperative oxygenation, hydration and monitoring have probably all contributed.

Safe anaesthesia in patients with SCD is based on careful preoperative evaluation of SCD complications (renal, cerebrovascular and pulmonary), assessing (and adjusting where necessary) the potential sickle cell mass and avoiding all possible sickle precipitants. This is best achieved in consultation with a haematologist and blood banking service.[177]

SCD complications with particular import for anaesthesia include glomerular and papillary renal insufficiency, which result in reduced urinary concentrating ability. Cerebrovascular

Table 1.15 Management strategies for sickle cell disease

Sickle cell disease	Management
Counselling	Genetic
	Pain management
Prophylactic measures	Folic acid supplements
	Pneumococcal, haemophilus and meningococcus vaccination
	Influenza and hepatitis vaccination
	Prophylactic penicillin from 4 months old
	Desferrioxamine iron chelation
Monitoring	Ophthalmological review for retinopathy
	Dental care for sepsis
	Renal function for uropathy
	Gall bladder ultrasonography for stones and sludge
	Transcranial doppler ultrasound for stroke risk
Pain management	Non-steroidal anti-inflammatory agents
	Opioids
	Patient-controlled analgesia
Chronic transfusion	Specific indications: anaemia with cardiac failure or cerebral symptoms
	Aplastic crisis
	Sequestration crisis
	Prevention of pain crisis
	Preoperative preparation
	Techniques: simple transfusion (leucodepletion filters/CMV seronegative)
	Partial exchange transfusion
	Erythrocytopheresis
Specific therapies	Splenectomy for hypersplenism/sequestration
	Foetal haemoglobin modulators, e.g. hydroxyurea
	Red cell hydration modulators, e.g. DDAVP, clotrimazole, urea

disease and stroke are devastating complications of SCD and a subgroup of susceptible patients may be identified on history and transcranial Doppler study.[178] These patients may receive particular protective benefit from a more aggressive transfusion regimen. Recurrent acute pulmonary complications may result in chronic pulmonary insufficiency with pulmonary hypertension. A history of respiratory events indicates an increased risk of perioperative acute chest syndrome. Painful crises may also complicate the perioperative course and are more common in older patients and those who have had more frequent and recent hospitalizations. Higher preoperative HbA levels appear to reduce the risk of perioperative pain crises. Other predictors of serious and life-threatening perioperative morbidity include a history of extensive transfusion, alloimmunization, more invasive surgery and the preoperative HbS value.[179] In order to reduce the potential sickle cell mass (HbS value), it has been traditional practice to exchange-transfuse patients with SCD prior to surgery. Although the optimal preoperative transfusion requirement, haematocrit and HbS level are yet to be determined, typical recommendations include: simple transfusion of SCD patients to a haematocrit of 30–36% if undergoing only minor surgery, and transfusion (by partial exchange if necessary) to a haematocrit of 30–36% and a HbS level = 30% if major surgery is planned. Patients with SC and SB type disease are recommended to undergo the more aggressive regime irrespective of the level of surgery. Planned cardiopulmonary bypass has usually been an indication for more complete removal of the sickle cell load (to < 5%). Sickle cell trait patients (HbAS) do not require preoperative transfusion, nor do neonates whose major haemoglobin is HbF.[177]

In 1995 the Cooperative Study of Sickle Cell Disease (CSSCD) completed its review of the natural history of SCD in 3765 patients over a 10-year period.[179] Following this analysis, a prospective study comparing conservative (preoperative Hb level of 10 g l^{-1} regardless of HbS level) and aggressive (Hb 10 g l^{-1} and HbS level 30%) transfusion regimes was completed. This study found the conservative guidelines to be as effective as aggressive regimens in preventing perioperative complications in SCD patients across all types of surgery. Furthermore, the

conservative approach reduced transfusion-related complications by 50%.[180]

Anaesthesia for children with SCD must be characterized by attention to detail. Dehydration and hyperosmolar states must be avoided in the perioperative period, as must hypothermia, hypoxia and acidosis. Attentive analgesia, early ambulation and monitoring for sickling, pain and chest crises must all be planned prior to surgery.[181] Aggressive postoperative respiratory care includes objective measures of oxygenation and obsessive recording of fluid balance.

GLUCOSE-6-PHOSPHATE DEHYDROGENASE DEFICIENCY

Glucose-6-phosphate dehydrogenase (G6PD) is a housekeeping enzyme that is expressed in all cells. It catalyses the conversion of glucose-6-phosphate to 6-phosphogluconate as the first and rate-limiting step of the hexose monophosphate shunt. This pathway generates NADPH and maintains glutathione in a reduced state, thereby protecting the cell from oxidative stress. Deficiencies in this cytoprotective mechanism are primarily manifest in erythrocytes as their membranes and the contained haemoglobin are continuously exposed to oxygen radicals and the peroxide molecule.

The enzyme is encoded on a gene locus located on the X-chromosome (Xq28) and over 60 different point (missense) mutations have been identified. Null (nonsense) mutations are probably lethal in early embryogenesis.

G6PD deficiency is the most common human genetic disorder, with more than 400 million people affected world-wide. Gene frequencies vary with ethnicity from 0.5% in northern European countries to 25% in central African and south-east Asian populations. This results in an incidence that varies from 1% in Mediterranean males to 5% in China and 10% among American black males. The geographical pattern closely resembles that of malaria endemicity, prompting the hypothesis of positive selection.[182]

The vast majority of individuals with G6PD deficiency are asymptomatic. Those with less than 60% of normal enzyme activity are prone to several well-recognized clinical syndromes. The most common presentation is that of acute haemolysis triggered by exposure to oxidants or infection. Drugs associated with haemolysis in G6PD deficiency are listed in Table 1.16. The pyrimidine glucosides vicine and convicine are probably the culprits in broad bean (*Vicia faba*)-induced haemolysis or favism. Symptoms usually develop 2–3 days after exposure and include fever, back pain, haemoglobinuria, pallor and tachycardia. The course and severity of the acute episode are variable but usually self-limiting. Management involves general supportive care and removing the trigger. As in all anaemic children, care should be exercised to avoid alloimmunization if red cell transfusions are necessary.

G6PD deficiency is an important cause of neonatal jaundice and is the leading cause of kernicterus in Africa and south-east Asia. Jaundice typically develops 1–4 days after birth and is more prominent in premature infants and those with infection. Anaemia may not be a prominent feature as some degree of hepatic dysfunction also contributes to the hyperbilirubinaemia. Management with photo-therapy and exchange transfusion follows conventional criteria but may be instituted earlier in the face of severe haemolysis.

Prevention of acute haemolysis is the main-stay of management of G6PD deficient individuals. Thorough counselling with a list of proscribed drugs and early intervention in the event of infection should reduce the morbidity of the disorder.[182]

Anaesthetic issues in G6PD deficiency

Uneventful anaesthesia can be anticipated if care is taken to avoid all possible oxidant drugs in the perioperative period. Of particular note, aspirin, the sulfonamides, ciprofloxacin and prilocaine are contraindicated. Special attention to asepsis during procedures is wise as some rare variants are associated with a leucocyte enzyme deficiency and hence an increased risk of bacterial infection.[181]

INHERITED COAGULATION DISORDERS

Children with either congenital or acquired disorders of haemostasis present a particular challenge to the anaesthetist. They may present for surgery with a known family history of a bleeding diathesis, an antenatal diagnosis, a personal history of bleeding or abnormal laboratory tests. In many cases, initial investigations, diagnosis and treatment are already in place and perioperative care is continued in consultation with a haematologist. The anaesthetist must understand the nature of the disorder and the currently available modes of therapy to facilitate a safe surgical course.

Eliciting the history, symptoms and signs of a coagulopathy and the ability to institute practical initial management are also vital in the

Table 1.16 Glucose 6 phosphate dehydrogenase deficiency: drugs implicated in haemolysis

Drug class	
Antimalarials	Primaquine, Chloroquine, Pamaquine
Analgesics/antipyretics	Acetylsalicylic acid
	Aminopyrine
	Phenacetin
Sulphonamides/sulphones	Sulphamethoxazole, Sulphanilamide
	Sulfasalazine, Sulphapyridine, Dapsone
Other antibacterials	Nitrofurans, Naladixic acid
	Chloramphenicol, Ciprofloxacin
Miscellaneous	Vitamin K (water sol analogues), Methylene blue
	Naphthalene, Tolbutamide

event of being confronted with a bleeding child previously unsuspected of having a bleeding disorder.

A positive family history, a history of petechiae and mucosal bleeding, spontaneous bruising or ecchymoses in response to minor trauma should prompt initial laboratory investigations. These include a full blood count and film, biochemical screen of renal and hepatic function and a coagulation screen: prothrombin time (PT), activated partial thromboplastin time (APTT) and thrombin time (TT). If either the PT or APTT is prolonged, dilution of the patient's plasma sample with an equal volume of normal plasma helps to differentiate between factor deficiency and the presence of an inhibitor. Based on these initial investigations, further studies may include specific factor assays, von Willebrand factor-related tests (vWF-related antigen, vWF ristocetin cofactor), a bleeding time and platelet function tests.[183] The presence of an inhibitor suggests an acquired coagulopathy, the diagnosis and management of which must take precedence over all but the most life-threatening surgery. These conditions, although rare, are often more difficult to manage.

HAEMOPHILIA

Haemophilia is an X-linked recessive disorder with a male prevalence of 1 : 10 000. The two most common forms, A and B, result from deficiencies of factor VIII and IX, respectively. Haemophilia A is four times more common than haemophilia B. The conditions arise from mutations of genes located at chromosome Xq2.8 and Xq2.6, respectively, and are clinically indistinguishable. Approximately one-third of cases arise as spontaneous mutations.

There is a wide spectrum of severity and some degree of consistency within families. Severity is correlated with circulating factor levels. In mild disease (factor levels 5–50 IU dl^{-1}), bleeding may only become apparent after trauma and surgery. Moderate disease (1–5 IU dl^{-1}) predisposes to spontaneous mucosal bleeds and soft tissue haematomas. Factor levels below 1 IU dl^{-1} constitute severe disease and place a child at risk of muscle haematomas and haemarthroses, especially when starting to walk (6–18 months). Up to 10% of these children will suffer major complications such as intracranial haemorrhage, gastrointestinal or retroperitoneal bleeding. Recurrent haemarthroses lead to chronic synovitis and arthropathy in what are termed 'target joints'. Neonatal presentation may include subgaleal haematoma, umbilical bleeding, haematuria and post-circumcision bleeding.[184]

Typical laboratory results in haemophilia show an elevated APTT with normal PT, TT and platelet count. Dilution with normal plasma (50 : 50 mix) corrects the APTT. Factor VIII and IX assays and vWF-related tests should confirm the exact diagnosis.

The overall aim in management is to prevent life-threatening haemorrhage and chronic joint disease in children with haemophilia, while at the same time minimizing the risks of complications related to blood product use. It is based on specific factor replacement titrated to the severity of disease. In cases of severe deficiency prophylaxis is indicated and is typically 20–25 U kg^{-1} three times a week for haemophilia A and twice a week for haemophilia B. Such regimens may require the insertion of a central line before the infant commences walking. Recombinant human factor VIII is a standard of care in paediatric practice.[185]

Factor replacement in the event of acute joint haemorrhage must aim to raise levels to at least 50% of normal. Soft tissue haematomas warrant raising levels to at least 40%. Life-threatening haemorrhage and major surgery require levels to be maintained at 80–100% of normal values.

Other therapies include DDAVP, which triggers the release of stored factor VIII and vWF from endothelial cells, and fibrinolytic inhibitors such as tranexamic acid. These can be used to reduce the total exposure to blood products or as sole therapy for minor surgery in mildly affected individuals.[185]

VON WILLEBRAND'S DISEASE

This heterogeneous group of disorders is the most common inherited coagulopathy, with an estimated prevalence of 1%. The genetic defects have been localized to chromosome 12 and are generally transmitted in an autosomal dominant pattern. They result in a quantitative or qualitative defect in the synthesis of a glycoprotein usually found in platelets, plasma and endothelial cells. This glycoprotein, termed von Willebrand's factor (vWF), is important in platelet adhesion and also acts as a carrier for factor VIII.

Three forms of von Willebrand's disease (vWD) are recognized. Type I, the most common, is also the mildest and presents with bruising only after trauma or surgery. Bleeding is typically mucosal, such as epistaxis or menorrhagia. Moderate disease (type II) may present with spontaneous skin and mucosal bleeding, e.g. gastrointestinal and dental. A subgroup of patients (type IIb) often has an associated thrombocytopenia. Type III disease causes more frequent and severe mucosal bleeding and may also lead to joint haemorrhage.[183]

vWD is characterized by a fluctuating severity and clinical picture over time. Variable laboratory results warrant serial testing in individuals suspected of the condition. As in the haemophilias, a prolonged APTT with normal PT and TT are suggestive. Factor VIII levels are often reduced and the bleeding time is prolonged. Diagnosis is confirmed by assaying vWF concentration (termed the vWF antigen test) or vWF activity based on platelet agglutination.

Management of children with vWD is based on judicious use of DDAVP, purified vWF concentrate or intermediate purity factor VIII concentrate. On occasions, platelet transfusion may be necessary. DDAVP given in a dose of 0.3 μg kg^{-1} either intravenously or intranasally results in a 3–6-fold rise in circulating levels of vWF. This is effective in a majority (62%) of children making it appropriate to identify these 'responders' with a trial early in the course of management. Tachyphylaxis limits the effectiveness of DDAVP to three doses in a 48-h period. Paradoxical intravascular platelet aggregation with an exacerbation of the thrombocytopenia precludes its use in type IIb disease.[183]

Anaesthesia in haemophilia and von Willebrand's disease

Careful assessment is made together with a haematologist and measurement of specific factor levels. For haemophilia A, the aim is to maintain levels above 80% of normal in the immediate surgical period and above 50% for the period of healing (7–14 days). Slightly lower levels are acceptable for haemophilia B. Consideration of the type and extent of surgery may alter the therapeutic goals. A half-life of 12 h requires factor VIII to be administered via twice-daily or continuous infusions in the immediate surgical period. Factor IX has a longer half-life (30 h) and may be infused daily.[186] Factor transfusion is indicated also for suture removal and plaster-cast removal.

Children with types I and II vWD undergoing minor surgery may be effectively managed with a combination of DDAVP and an antifibrinolytic agent. DDAVP is administered 60–75 min prior to surgery and tranexamic acid may be given orally (25–35 mg kg^{-1}) or intravenously (10 mg kg^{-1}). Tranexamic acid may also be effectively used as a mouthwash during dental surgery. Particular care must be exercised to avoid excessive water retention and hyponatraemia when administering DDAVP. Children with moderate to severe disease and all those undergoing major surgery should receive either vWF concentrate (0.2 U kg^{-1}) or an equivalent dose of intermediate-purity factor VIII concentrate. Failure of haemostasis intraoperatively should be treated with platelet transfusion.[187]

All children requiring regular blood product transfusion should be vaccinated against hepatitis B virus prior to exposure. It remains appropriate to check the serology of these children for hepatitis C and HIV and to maintain universal vigilant precautions for surgery. Anaesthesia management should aim to avoid intramuscular injections and preserve veins where possible.[181] Non-steroidal anti-inflammatory drugs (NSAIDs) are best avoided.

IMMUNE DISEASE

ANAESTHESIA AND THE CHILD WITH HIV

Since the diagnosis of the first paediatric cases of human T-lymphocyte virus infection in 1982, the pattern of this disease in childhood has become clearer and continues to raise new concerns. Paediatric acquired immunodeficiency syndrome (AIDS) refers to infection in those under 13 years, as older adolescents are more conveniently grouped with adult cases.

The responsible T-lymphotropic retrovirus preferentially infects and destroys T-cells (reducing CD4 T-cell counts), with direct adverse affects on cell-mediated immunity. The virus also directly infects cardiac myocytes and brain cells.

Eighty per cent of paediatric cases are acquired transplacentally (vertical transmission). The risk of transplacental transmission from HIV-positive pregnant women is estimated at 26–40% and correlated with maternal viral load without a threshold level. This risk is significantly reduced by perinatal antiviral therapy.[188]

The diagnosis of neonatal and paediatric infection is complicated by transplacental transfer of maternal antibodies (Ab). All neonates born to HIV Ab-positive mothers will be Ab positive (enzyme-linked immunosorbent assay or Western blot) for up to 15 months. Diagnosis of actual infection then depends on serial clinical assessments and more direct laboratory tests such as polymerase chain reaction (PCR) for proviral DNA, mononuclear cell cocultures. It is wise to consider all neonates born to HIV-positive mothers infected until proven otherwise.[189]

Vertically transmitted HIV infection is a disease of early childhood. Half of all infected infants show manifestations within 1 year of birth and 80% of cases are manifest by 3 years of age. Progress appears to be correlated to viral load (as determined by quantitative viral PCR assays) and, although early reports suggested that paediatric disease progressed more rapidly than does adult disease, there is now clearly a wide spectrum of survival.[190]

Non-specific manifestations include lymphadenopathy, parotid gland enlargement and craniofacial dysmorphology, sometimes termed AIDS embryopathy. Pulmonary disease remains the major cause of morbidity and mortality and includes a slowly progressive lymphoid interstitial pneumonitis (LIP) of uncertain pathophysiology. Dyspnoea, bronchospasm and hypoxaemia are typical presentations. Superinfection with opportunistic and commensal organisms may complicate the illness at any time. *Pneumocystis carinii*, CMV and *Mycobacterium avium* intracellulare are

common pathogens, as are *Streptococcus pneumoniae*, *Haemophilus influenza* and respiratory syncytial virus (RSV).

Cardiac involvement is being increasingly recognized as the retrovirus directly infects cardiac myocytes, resulting in myocarditis, ventricular dysfunction and rhythm disturbances. Pericardial effusion may also be present and autonomic neuropathy has been reported.

Neurological involvement results in progressive encephalopathy and developmental delay with motor dysfunction. Brain growth is poor, with resultant microcephaly and cerebral atrophy. These children are at risk of developing primary CNS lymphomas, stroke and meningitis.[191]

Similarly to adult disease, some children (5–10%) show renal involvement. Typically, focal glomerulosclerosis presents with a nephrotic syndrome. Failure to thrive is multifactorial but often results from chronic infectious diarrhoea and mucocutaneous candidiasis. Bone marrow suppression is common and results from direct viral infection, malnutrition, drug effects and chronic illness.

With increasing numbers of cases and longer survival rates a larger variety of secondary infections is being encountered.

Management of paediatric HIV disease relies heavily on the identification of maternal infection. Perinatal 'postexposure' prophylaxis with antiviral agents is proven to reduce vertical transmission rates (from 26% to 8%).

Childhood immunizations are usually well tolerated, although the response is generally suboptimal. Where possible, routine immunization should proceed when the child is on stable antiretroviral therapy.[188]

Anaesthesia issues in paediatric HIV

Children infected with HIV will increasingly present for surgery as management and their overall outlook improve. Central line placement, diagnostic procedures (lung/liver biopsy) and surgical drainage of infection are the most common procedures undertaken.

Evaluation must include assessment of overall disease stage as well as particular note of pulmonary and cardiac involvement. Chest radiology, ECG (up to 90% are abnormal) and echocardiography may all be valuable.

Laboratory evaluation of haematological, renal and liver function may reveal disturbances resulting from direct infection, chronic illness or drug side-effects. Careful note is made of all medications and steroid cover given where appropriate; possible nephrotoxins (acyclovir, gancyclovir, pentamidine, dapsone and amphotericin B) and causes of thrombocytopenia (zidovudine, diddeoxycitidine, bactrim and ketoconazole) should be identified.

The planning of perioperative care requires awareness of non-biological parents, legal guardianship issues and special arrangements for consent. At all times confidentiality must be respected and stigmatization avoided.

Universal precautions require that care be taken wherever risk of contamination with biological fluids exists, irrespective of HIV status. This reduces the occupational risks for health-care workers and the risk of cross-contamination between patients. Anaesthesia equipment should undergo routine cleaning and decontamination. Disposable breathing circuits add extra convenience and are preferred. Immunocompromised patients also require measures to prevent iatrogenic infection. Special attention to asepsis should be paid whenever performing invasive procedures.[192]

THE PRIMARY IMMUNODEFICIENCY SYNDROMES

These genetically determined disorders of immune function result from defects in one or a combination of the four major components of host defence; B-cells, T-cells, phagocytic cells and the complement proteins. Over 50 syndromes have been described, some of which have been mapped to specific chromosomal defects. Most are inherited in an autosomal recessive pattern, although a significant number is X-linked (chronic granulomatous disease, Wiskott–Aldrich syndrome, Bruton's agammaglobulinaemia), resulting in an overall male preponderance.[193]

Disease is characterized by an increased susceptibility to infection from the time of birth. The type of infection often suggests the nature of the immune defect. Defects in B-cells and hence antibody production result in infection with encapsulated micro-organisms such as *S. pneumoniae*, *Staphylococcus aureus*, *H. influ-*enza, *Neisseria meningitidis* and *Pseudomonas aeruginosa*. T-cell defects typically result in opportunistic infection with *Pneumocystis pneumonia* (PCP), fungal infections, CMV, *Varicella* and EBV.

Some specific diseases have well-recognized associations with non-immunological findings such as congenital heart disease, hypocalcaemia and dysmorphic facies in thymic hypoplasia (DiGeorge syndrome). Thrombocytopenic melaena and eczema are recognized as part of the Wiskott–Aldrich syndrome and oculocutaneous telangectasia with neurological deterioration is seen in ataxia–telangectasia syndrome.[194]

Table 1.17 gives a classification of primary immune disorders and examples of each.

Treatment of primary immune disorders is based on general supportive care and depends heavily on early detection of invading micro-organisms and the judicious use of specific antibiotics.

Intravenous preparations of immune serum globulin from pooled plasma represent a major advance in replacement therapy for patients with antibody deficiencies.

Bone marrow transplantation remains the most effective available treatment of severe T-cell defects and combined T- and B-cell defects. It requires major histocompatibility complex (MHC)-compatible marrow or MHC haploidentical parental marrow (with some form of post-thymic T-cell depletion) for success. Somatic-cell gene therapy may offer new therapeutic options for some conditions.

Therapy for phagocytic cell disorders relies on antibiotic treatment and prophylaxis. Vitamin C and γ-interferon may be of use in specific conditions. No specific therapies are available for most complement deficiencies, although danazol may reduce the frequency of acute attacks of angioedema in hereditary C1INH deficiency.

SEVERE COMBINED IMMUNODEFICIENCY

An absence of T- and B-cell function from birth can result from a variety of genetic defects and represents the most profound immunodeficiency recognized. Infants typically present in the first few days of life with a triad of diarrhoea, thrush and pneumonia (often interstitial). Failure to

Table 1.17 Primary immune disorders: classification

Primary immune defect	Examples	Particular anaesthesia issues
B-cell disorders	Selective IgA deficiency	Difficulties in blood cross-matching; atopy; autoimmune phenomenon
	X-linked agammaglobulinaemia (Bruton's disease)	
	Common variable immunodeficiency (CVID)	
T-cell disorders	Thymic hypoplasia (Di George syndrome)	Hypocalcaemia; congenital heart disease; micrognathia
	X-linked immnodeficiency with hyper IgM	
Combined disorders	Severe combined immunodeficiency (SCID)	
	Wiskott–Aldrich syndrome	Thrombocytopaenia
	Ataxia–Telangectasia syndrome	Neurological deterioration; muscle denervation.
Phagocytic cell disorders	Chediak–Higashi syndrome	Prolonged bleeding time
	Chronic granulomatous disease	Thoracic/upper abdominal granulomas
Complement disorders	C1q, C1r, C1s, C2 and C4 deficiencies	
	C1INH (C1 inhibitor) deficiency (hereditary angioedema)	Upper airway obstuction during acute attack

thrive and severe wasting soon follow and opportunistic infections (PCP, *Candida*, CMV, *Varicella*, EBV and *Parainfluenza* virus) often prove fatal. Investigation reveals lymphopenia, delayed cutaneous anergy and low serum immunoglobulins. These infants uniformly have a small, undescended thymus, a lack of peripheral lymph nodes and an underdeveloped Waldeyer's ring. The only available effective therapy is bone marrow stem-cell transplantation.[195]

Anaesthesia issues in primary immunodeficiency

With the success of bone marrow transplantation for primary immunodeficiency states, increasing numbers of these children are presented for anaesthesia and surgery. Common procedures include central venous access, surgical drainage of infected tissue, bone marrow aspiration and diagnostic bronchial lavage and biopsy.

Where possible, aggressive preoperative treatment of respiratory tract infection should be undertaken and includes physiotherapy, incentive spirometry and bronchodilator therapy. Careful assessment of cardiac function (in view of the possibility of right ventricular strain secondary to chronic respiratory disease) and of renal function (with respect to possible antibiotic-induced impairment) should be made. Careful planning of patient movement between the ward and operating theatre is required for children whose condition mandates reverse isolation. Avoiding transfers through an anaesthetic and recovery room may reduce exposure of immunocompromised patients to potential pathogens as well as reduce the spread of unusual pathogens from these patients to others.

All anaesthetic procedures must be undertaken with strict attention to asepsis and universal precautions regarding blood and body fluids. It is advisable to remove all indwelling percutaneous catheters and cannulae as soon as possible. Special care when transfusing blood products is essential and facilitated by preoperative consultation with the medical team caring for these children.[192] Particular anaesthetic considerations for specific syndromes are noted in Table 1.17.

BONE, JOINT AND CONNECTIVE TISSUE DISEASE

JUVENILE RHEUMATOID ARTHRITIS

Juvenile rheumatoid arthritis (JRA) is the most common paediatric connective tissue disorder and accounts for 5% of all cases of rheumatoid arthritis. As in adult disease, it represents a chronic, non-suppurative synovitis with an immunogenic basis that leads to bone and cartilage erosion with eventual joint deformity, ankylosis and subluxation. JRA is more often seronegative for rheumatoid factor (RhF) than is adult disease and probably has a significantly different pathophysiology. No specific autoantibodies have been detected, although HLA associations (DR5 and DR8) are documented and infectious agent involvement (HTLV I, *Rubella*, CMV, EBV) is postulated.

It rarely presents before 6 months and is bimodally distributed about two age group peaks at 1–3 years and 8–12 years. Three major groups can be identified based on the pattern of joint and systemic involvement at presentation.

POLYARTICULAR DISEASE

Forty per cent of juvenile cases have five or more joints involved at presentation, usually the small joints of the hands and feet (symmetrically) and various large joints. Systemic manifestations such as fever, anaemia, rash and lymphadenopathy are variable and usually less impressive than in systemic onset disease. Up to 70% of cases develop cervical spine involvement with the upper vertebrae undergoing ankylosis, occasionally fusing *en bloc*. A majority also develops temporomandibular joint synovitis, with up to 16% suffering reduced mouth opening.[196]

PAUCIARTICULAR DISEASE

Half of all children with JRA present with single joint involvement and no more than five joints involved within 6 months of presentation. The onset of this form is usually before the age of 4 years, with a female predominance. Symptoms are mild and systemic manifestations are rare. Typically, a swollen joint (most commonly a knee), possibly even with contracture, is found as an incidental finding in an otherwise well girl. Temporomandibular and cervical spine involvement is rare and the disease is prone to early remission.

SYSTEMIC ONSET DISEASE (STILL'S DISEASE)

This is the most dramatic form of JRA and comprises 10–15% of all cases. All age groups are affected, with an equal gender distribution.

These children tend to be quite ill. Systemic manifestations, sometimes severe, may precede the arthritis. High spiking temperatures associated with a migratory macular rash are the hallmark of the disease and are often combined with lymphadenopathy and splenomegaly. Anorexia, irritability, marked arthralgia and myalgia are common. A generalized serositis may be manifested by pericarditis, pleural effusion and peritonism. Occasionally, anaemia is profound and may be accompanied by leucocytosis and thrombocytosis. Myocarditis, vasculitis and transient pneumonitis may sometimes complicate the disease, although adult-like rheumatoid lung disease and nephritis are rare.[197] JRA tends to run a course of remissions and relapses: 45% of polyarticular and systemic onset cases have persistent active disease up to 10 years after presentation. One-quarter of these cases proceed to chronic joint disease with significant debility.

Management of these children is aimed at preserving joint function and controlling symptoms with both pharmacological and physical therapy. Aspirin and other NSAIDs remain the first-line therapeutic drugs. Systemic onset disease, polyarticular disease and progressive joint involvement may indicate the addition of second-line drugs such as hydroxychloroquine, gold salts, sulfusalazine and methotrexate.[198] Steroids have a very limited role in the management in JRA. Indications include acute severe febrile episodes, carditis and Coombs' positive haemolytic anaemia.[196]

Anaesthesia issues in juvenile rheumatoid arthritis

Evaluation of the extent and pattern of joint involvement preoperatively is essential for careful movement and positioning of JRA children. Evidence of temporomandibular disease, which may present as earache, limited mouth opening and, very occasionally, secondary mandibular hypoplasia, should be sought. Although cricoarytenoid involvement is estimated to occur in up to 26% of adults with RA, it has been less frequently mentioned in the paediatric literature. Hoarseness, stridor and a feeling of fullness on swallowing should alert the anaesthetist to the possibility of crico-arytenoid joint involvement.[199]

Radiological evidence of cervical spine involvement may be available but its significance when not combined with symptomatology is uncertain given the relatively high incidence of asymptomatic cervical ankylosis and atlantoaxial subluxation in these children. Cervical involvement with neurological symptoms or signs requires careful planning to avoid inappropriate neck movement.[200]

Cardiac and pulmonary disease should be suspected on clinical grounds (especially in systemic onset disease) and be further assessed with ECG, CXR and echocardiography. Chronic anaemia and coagulopathy related to aspirin or NSAID use need to be considered prior to undertaking major surgery. Hepatosplenomegaly may occasionally impinge on diaphragmatic excursion and predispose to basal atelectasis.

Awareness of the patient's drug therapy is useful as most anti-inflammatory agents used have a wide spectrum of side-effects, including platelet dysfunction secondary to cyclo-oxygenase inhibitors, bone marrow suppression due to hydroxychloroquin and leucopenia, nephritis and hepatitis from gold salts. The side-effects of systemic steroids in children preclude their general use in all but the most severe JRA cases; occasional children who are steroid dependent should receive supplemental corticosteroids.[201]

ARTHROGRYPOSIS MULTIPLEX CONGENITA

The term is descriptive and covers over 150 separate entities that are characterized by multiple joint contractures. Contractures together with muscle wasting, joint dislocation and waxy, featureless skin result in deformity often described as 'thin wooden doll-like'. It has an incidence estimated between 1 : 3000 and 1 : 10 000 live births and is the most frequent isolated skeletal malformation in children.

A variety of aetiological factors has been implicated in arthrogryposis multiplex congenita (AMC), some of which are given in Table 1.18. A majority of cases (94%) has a neurogenic basis. The wide spectrum of causative factors appears to implicate a common pathophysiological mechanism. Reduced early fetal movements and akinesia as early as the 7th fetal week jeopardize normal limb and joint development, leading to congenital contractures and muscle atrophy.[202]

The most common form of the condition is amyloplasia (classical AMC), which accounts for almost one-third of all newborn presentations. The typical positioning of these infants

Table 1.18 Arthrogryposis multiplex congenita

Arthrogryposis multiplex congenita	Aetiological factors
Neuropathic	
	Motor Cortex dysgenesis
	Pyramidal tract demyelination
	Anterior horn cell apoptosis
	Ventral root abnormalities
Myopathic	
	Central core disease
	Congenital muscular dystrophy
	Nemaline myopathy
	Myotonic dystrophy
	Congenital myasthenia
Connective tissue disease	
Mechanical	
	Bicornuate uterus
	Twins
	Fibroids
	Oligohydramnios

includes internal rotation of the shoulder, extension of the elbow and flexion of the wrist ('policeman's tip posture'). Equinovarus deformity of the feet and various knee and hip contractures or dislocations are also common.[203] The characteristic pathology appears to be a reduction in the number and size of anterior horn cells, together with a degree of pyramidal tract demyelination. Several anterior horn cell teratogens, including viral agents, toxic chemicals and hyperthermia, have been implicated. AMC of neurogenic origin is commonly associated with abnormalities of other organ systems. These include micrognathia (39%), congenital heart disease (23%), hypoplastic lungs (19%), cleft palate (11%) and scoliosis (12%). Apart from micrognathia and scoliosis, associated anomalies are less common in myopathic forms.[204]

Anaesthetic issues in arthrogryposis

Infants with AMC present most commonly for orthopaedic and related surgery. Soft tissue and contracture release operations and 'plaster-related' procedures form the bulk of anaesthesia requirements. These infants may also present for inguinal hernia repair, scoliosis, cardiac surgery and cleft palate repair.[205]

Preoperative assessment of potential airway difficulties must take into account temporomandibular contracture, micrognathia and other craniofacial anomalies. These may make slow gaseous induction a preferred technique and should prompt preparation of ancillary equipment (bougies, alternative laryngoscope blades, laryngeal mask, fibreoptic bronchoscope). Venous access is often complicated by abnormal or absent superficial veins and by difficulties in positioning limbs. Care must be taken to avoid applying undue forces through joints and prolonged skin pressure.[206]

Children with AMC are prone to hypermetabolic reactions under anaesthesia, although the risk of true MH probably relates more directly to any associated myopathy.[205,207]

Non-depolarizing neuromuscular blocking agents are used without event in these patients, while depolarizing agents are avoided as their action may be less predictable and is characterized by contracture and hyperkalaemia. In specific myopathic cases, suxmethonium may act as a trigger for MH.

Regional anaesthesia is difficult because of altered skin and bony landmarks. Children with significant truncal involvement and scoliosis may have a restrictive ventilatory defect, making postoperative monitoring and aggressive respiratory care essential.[208]

OSTEOGENESIS IMPERFECTA

This inherited connective tissue disease is characterized by fragile bones (hence 'brittle bone disease') and weakness of tissues rich in type-I collagen. It has an estimated incidence of 1 : 20 000 and is inherited in an autosomal dominant pattern. Penetrance is variable and mosaicism may occur.[209]

The molecular defects have been localized to two genes (COL1A1, COL1A2) that encode the pro-α-chains of type 1 collagen.

Osteogenesis imperfecta (OI) is now classified into four types, based on clinical and genetic considerations, replacing the older classification of 'congenita' and 'tarda' forms. Table 1.19 summarizes some of the information. Type-I disease (classical or tarda) is typified by mild to moderate skeletal fragility in children who appear relatively normal. Grey–blue sclera and premature deafness are common accompaniments. The lethal perinatal forms of disease (type II) rapidly lead to death from intracranial haemorrhage or respiratory failure. Type III and the more severe phenotypes of type IV correspond to the congenital forms of the older nomenclature. These children have moderate to severe bone fragility and deformity. Fractures often heal with bowing deformity and dentinogenesis imperfecta is relatively common. Midface hypoplasia, a small, pointed mandible and dwarfism are characteristic. Scoliosis is typically accompanied by chest-wall deformity and altered respiratory mechanics.[204]

Diagnosis is based on clinical presentation and skin biopsy. The typical X-ray finding is osteopenia and hyperplastic callous (which needs to be differentiated from osteosarcoma). There is no definitive biological test for the condition but collagen type-I : II ratios calculated from skin fibroblast cell cultures identify 90% of non-lethal variants of OI.

Table 1.19 Osteogenesis imperfecta: classification

Type	Genetics	Clinical features
Type I (Classical/'tarda')	Autosommal dominant null allele Quantitative defect in collagen I	Mild–moderate fragility without deformity. Blue sclera, bruisability, joint laxity, dwarfism and hearing loss are common
Type II	Aut. dom. (can be aut.rec. rarely) point mutations. Qualitative defects in collagen I	Extreme fragility, IUGR, *in utero* fractures, high perinatal mortality
Type III ('Congenita')	Aut. dom. Qualitative defects in collagen I. Parental gonadal mosaicism explains some cases	Progressive deforming disease. Severe osteoporosis. Macrocephaly, scoliosis and healing with deformity are common. White sclera
Type IV	Aut. dom. point mutations. Qualitative defects in collagen I	Moderate disease. White sclera

Clinical issues that confront the team looking after these children include the differential diagnosis of child abuse and orthopaedic intervention for fractures, particularly non-union and recurrent fractures. The treatment of deformity may require Sofield osteotomy and Ilizarov fixation. In addition, rapidly progressive kyphoscoliosis reduces respiratory reserve and a trefoil pelvis in type-III disease can cause rectosigmoid dysfunction with abdominal pain.

Skull deformity, in particular elevation of the posterior fossa and occipital condyles, can lead to basilar compression in up to 25% of cases. This is more common in type-IV disease and is often slowly progressive. Signs such as nystagmus, facial spasm and papilloedema may precede symptoms. Tetraplegia and respiratory arrest may follow brainstem compression.

Congenital cardiac defects may also be present and include mitral and aortic valve annulus dilation leading to regurgitation. Other anomalies reported to be associated with OI include hydrocephalus, inguinal and umbilical hernias, hyperhidrosis and premature arteriosclerosis. Diaphoresis and mild hyperthermia suggest that these children have a generally raised metabolic rate.

Management to date has focused on treatment of fractures and facilitating maximum growth and development in these children. Antisense oligonucleotides may prove of benefit in suppressing the expression of mutant collagen alleles.[210]

Anaesthesia issues in osteogenesis imperfecta

In all children with OI extreme care in handling and joint positioning is necessary to avoid fractures. Airway management in types III and IV disease may be complicated by micrognathia and midface hypoplasia, making preoperative evaluation and careful selection of face masks essential. The presence of dentinogenesis imperfecta and signs of basilar compression mandate caution during intubation and avoidance of excessive neck extension. The presence of kyphoscoliosis requires extra care with positioning and postoperative monitoring for respiratory dysfunction.

Patients with OI are known to be at risk of developing a hypermetabolic response to surgery. This may manifest as hypercarbia, pyrexia and acidosis and is probably unrelated to any risk of MH. It is unrelated to typical MH triggers and responds to simple supportive cooling measures. Temperature should always be measured and anticholinergic premedication used only when indicated.

An ill-defined platelet defect is known to occur in children with OI. Platelet counts are usually normal but aggregation is altered. Further investigation is indicated when a history of bruisability is obtained and prior to undertaking surgical procedures such as Sofield osteotomy that involve major blood loss.[211]

OTHER CONNECTIVE TISSUE DISORDERS

Marfan's syndrome

This inherited disease is transmitted in an autosomal dominant pattern with complete penetrance but variable expression. The molecular defect appears to be an abnormality in a glycoprotein called fibrillin, which results in degeneration of elastin fibres. The syndrome has an estimated incidence of 1 : 10 000–15 000.

The clinical hallmark of the condition is ectopia lentis (lens subluxation) and occurs at or soon after birth in 50–80% of cases. Patients tend to be tall with disproportionately long limbs. A high arched palate with dental crowding is common, as are pectus deformities. With continued growth, kyphoscoliosis may develop. Joint hypermobility is characteristic and hernias are common.[197]

Cardiovascular involvement is the main source of morbidity and takes the form of cystic medial necrosis of the aortic wall. Progressive aortic dilatation can be detected in up to 90% of all cases and begins in childhood. The process may include the aortic annulus leading to symptomatic regurgitation. Mitral valve prolapse is usually also detectable in most cases (80%). Bedside auscultation will reveal up to 60% of these abnormalities.[212]

Patients are at risk of spontaneous pneumothorax from rupture of pleural blebs and dural ectasia is also a notable feature of the condition. Diagnosis is based on clinical findings, echocardiography and ophthalmic examination. A consistent family history and exclusion of homocystinuria may make immunohistochemical analysis of fibrillin unnecessary.

Management is based on regular review (echocardiographic and ophthalmic) and restriction of any strenuous exercise that may trigger aortic dissection. β-Blockade in childhood may delay the progress of aortic dilatation. Induction of puberty has successfully reduced the final height without apparent adverse side-effects in some children. Careful management and timely surgical intervention for aortic disease should allow long-term survival of these children. To date, the median lifespan has been noted to be reduced by one-third.[213]

Anaesthesia issues in Marfan's syndrome

All children with Marfan's syndrome (irrespective of exact valve pathology) are at risk of bacterial endocarditis and should receive appropriate prophylaxis. Preoperative echocardiographic evidence of aortic involvement should prompt careful cardiovascular monitoring and particular avoidance of hypertension. Careful patient positioning and movement will avoid joint dislocation.

In most patients, forced vital capacity is less than predicted. Kyphoscoliosis and pectus deformities may lead to a marked reduction in total lung capacity and residual volume in some patients.[211] Active respiratory care is essential and minimizing peak airway pressure during positive pressure ventilation should help to reduce the risk of pneumothorax.[214]

DERMATOLOGICAL DISEASE

EPIDERMOLYSIS BULLOSA

Epidermolysis bullosa (EB) is a subgroup of the inherited mechanobullous diseases characterized by blister formation after minor trauma, especially shearing forces. It includes at least 20 variants, although four main varieties are sufficient to illustrate the spectrum of disease. Disease is classified into scarring (dystrophic) and non-scarring forms and also according to the pattern of inheritance. Recent advances in the genetic and molecular basis of disease have led to renewed understanding of the pathophysiology and the possibility of gene therapy in the future. The disease is known to be caused by gene mutations which lead to absent or abnormal cutaneous proteins: keratin 5 and 14, laminin 5 and collagen VII.[215] Table 1.20 summarizes some of this information.

EB simplex (Koebner's disease) is an autosomal dominant, non-scarring form that presents in the neonatal period with generalized intradermal blisters. These lesions heal rapidly and become limited to the hands and feet after 3 years of age. Infants are usually vigorous and

Table 1.20 Epidermolysis bullosa classification

Variant	Genetics		Molecular biology
Non scarring			
Intra-epidermal Lesion		Mutations in genes encoding keratin 5 and 14-chromosomes 17q and 12q	Keratin 5 and 14 are major structural proteins of basal keratinocytes. Severity of disease depends on site of mutation
EB Simplex			
Koebner disease	Aut. dom		
Weber–Cockayne	Aut. dom		
Dowling–Meara	Aut. dom		
Bart's disease			
Dermal-epidermal junction lesion		Mutations in genes encoding laminin 5 – laminin is an anchoring filament protein. Basement membrane hemidesmosomes are absent	
Junctional EB (letalis/herlitz)	Aut. rec		
Scarring (dystrophic/dermolytic)			
Dermal lesion			
Hyperplastic EB	Aut. dom	Mutations in genes encoding collagen VII chromosome 3p21	Aut. dom forms are 'missense' mutations
Cockayne–Torraine	Aut. dom		
Polydysplastic EB (mutilans)	Aut. rec		Aut. rec forms are 'nonsense' mutations

exacerbations become less frequent with age. Oral mucosal involvement is usually not prominent but in up to 20% of infants the nails become dystrophic. Localized forms of simplex disease also occur, such as in Weber–Cockayne disease. Here, lesions are limited to the hands and feet from the time of presentation.

Junctional EB (letalis) is the most severe form of disease and presents at birth with severe subepidermal blisters over the scalp and extremities, although the palms and soles are spared. The nails are lost soon after birth and oral mucosal lesions can be severe. Neonates that survive are afflicted by anaemia, scarring, chronic granulomas and recurrent infection often resulting in fatal septicaemia before 2 years of age.

Hyperplastic dystrophic EB is an autosomal dominant disorder that causes recurrent flat pink bullae, especially of the hands and feet. Scarring and milia formation are typical and up to 20% of cases have oral mucosal involvement.

The disease is relapsing and eventually mutilates the hands and feet.

Polydysplastic EB (mutilans) is the most incapacitating illness of infants who survive with EB. It is transmitted in an autosomal recessive pattern and has an incidence of 1 : 300 000. It presents in the newborn period with severe erosive subepidermal bullae and continuous mucous membrane involvement. Strictures, 'mitten hands' due to digital fusion and contractures are common, as are anaemia, growth retardation and malnutrition. Blepharitis and conjuncto-keratitis are also frequent accompaniments.

Bart's syndrome is a congenital localized absence of skin, usually on the legs. It may also be accompanied by nail changes and mouth lesions. Its prognosis is favourable.

Cockayne–Tourraine syndrome is a nondeforming disease of early infancy. Lesions on the hands, feet and sacral areas heal rapidly with soft wrinkled superficial scars. General health remains good and prognosis is favourable.

Diagnosis is based on clinical presentation and confirmed with histopathological and immunofluorescent staining of biopsied skin. In the past, prenatal diagnosis relied on fetal skin biopsy at 18–21 weeks. Molecular biology techniques now allow a much earlier diagnosis via chorionic villous sampling. This allows the planning of an elective caesarean section for infants thought to be at risk of blister formation through normal delivery.

Management of EB patients is essentially supportive. Antibacterials, topical and systemic antibiotics and attentive wound care are the mainstays. Nutritional support and avoidance of trauma are essential. Future therapies may include cultured epidermal allografts and gene therapy.[216] Anaesthetic issues in EB are discussed in Chapter 20.

Chronic illness in children with EB results in a wide variety of secondary health disturbances. Malnutrition, anaemia and impaired thermoregulation are common and should be borne in mind when planning anaesthesia. Renal impairment secondary to amyloidosis and electrolyte disturbances need to be investigated preoperatively.[217]

The previously reported association of EB with porphyria probably represented no more than the diagnostic confusion that existed between porphyria cutanea tarda and EB. Current histopathological, immunofluorescent and genetic diagnostic techniques allow clear distinctions to be drawn, making it unnecessary to withhold barbiturates from EB patients.[218] Malnutrition, recurrent sepsis and immobility in children with EB lead to muscle atrophy and general weakness.

STEVENS–JOHNSON SYNDROME

The Stevens–Johnson syndrome represents the more severe form of erythema multiforme (EM), a hypersensitivity reaction characterized by distinctive skin lesions. Patients with Stevens–Johnson syndrome display typical erythematous macules with superimposed vesicles that evolve into annular or target lesions. Blistering of at least two mucosal surfaces is characteristic. Most cases occur in those below 20 years of age, although it is rare below the age of 3 years.

Several aetiological agents have been implicated and include viral infection (a majority of EM minor cases are associated with the herpes simplex virus), *Mycoplasma* infection and drugs. Of particular note are the sulfonamides, penicillins and anticonvulsants. The condition is thought to be immune complex mediated as immunoglobulin M, complement and fibrin may be found in dermal vessels. Herpes-related disease may involve cell-mediated hypersensitivity.

Clinical illness is characterized by a prodrome of fever, malaise, sore throat and myalgias. A painful, erosive bullous eruption then involves skin and various mucous membranes. The oral mucosa, conjunctiva, larynx, tracheobronchial tree and gastrointestinal tract may each be involved in the blistering process.

Complications may ensue rapidly and include corneal ulceration, panophthalmitis, pneumothorax, gastrointestinal haemorrhage and anaemia. Management is supportive and may be best undertaken in a speciality burns unit or equivalent intensive care unit. Barrier isolation, strict asepsis and aggressive fluid and electrolyte therapy should follow the removal and treatment of any instigating agent.

Most cases resolve within 2–7 weeks. Up to one-quarter of cases may relapse and severe disease still carries a high (5–15%) mortality.[216]

Anaesthesia issues can be considered to be almost identical to those of the burned patient. Metabolic catabolism, malnutrition, anaemia and electrolyte abnormalities are common. Temperature homeostasis is often disturbed in proportion to the area of skin involvement. Superinfection and sepsis are always a threat and the 'toxic'-looking patient may be harbouring sites of sepsis other than the obviously injured skin. Skin care is paramount and should be dealt with as in epidermolysis bullosa patients. Airway management may be complicated by bullae that only become apparent on direct laryngoscopy.

THE EX-PREMATURE BABY

Premature births account for more than 6% of the total and are usually divided into (1) very low birth weight (VLB) (5–1500 g and 24–30 weeks' postconception); (2) moderate birth weight (1500–2500 g and 31–36 weeks); and (3) borderline prematurity (over 2500 g and 36 weeks' gestation). All preterm babies are at risk from respiratory failure and subsequent chronic lung disease, apnoea, necrotizing enterocolitis, retinopathy of prematurity, sepsis and anaemia.

There is no doubt that the prognosis for morbidity and mortality for the VLB group is improving, but neurological deficit remains a significant problem. Cognitive impairment and motor deficits correlate with cranial ultrasound findings of lesions within the brain and ventricular enlargement; 46% of infants with grade III and IV intracranial haemorrhage have neurological problems,[219] but overall only 5% of VLB infants have mental retardation. Babies born small for gestational age show more cognitive impairment than those of appropriate weight and, if bronchopulmonary dysplasia is a complication, the children are likely to have poorer motor skills.[220]

Intraventricular haemorrhage is the most common serious neurological disorder of the neonatal period as it affects approximately 40% of all infants below 35 weeks' gestation. It is associated with increasing prematurity, respiratory distress syndrome, hypoxia, acidosis, high ventilatory requirements and coagulation abnormalities. Surges of intracranial pressure have been measured during the practice of awake tracheal intubation. It is hoped that smooth induction of anaesthesia and intubation will contribute to lessening this complication in at-risk infants.

Surfactant therapy, high-frequency oscillation, inhaled nitric oxide therapy and extracorporeal membrane oxygenation are all claimed to improve oxygenation and minimize barotrauma, causing less chronic lung disease and possibly less intracranial haemorrhage.[221,222]

Many low-birth-weight babies require prolonged respiratory support in an intensive care setting and become oxygen dependent for prolonged periods.

The diaphragm is likely to fatigue easily and is a further factor causing reduced respiratory reserve. Animal studies show that halothane depresses the minute ventilation and FRC during spontaneous breathing in newborn lambs and doubles the arterial carbon dioxide tension ($PaCO_2$). Even nitrous oxide may have some of these effects in preterm babies. The units of gas exchange are smaller in the preterm lung (75 μm diameter) compared with the adult (250 μm) and thus have a greater tendency to collapse, but the FRC is partly maintained by the high respiratory rate, so that there is little time for the gas to escape and the FRC to fall. If the respiratory rate does fall, the FRC is reduced and during apnoea it may fall to very low levels. At least 30% of premature babies have apnoea during the first few weeks of life, a tendency worsened by changes in temperature and by general anaesthesia. It is not uncommon for apnoea to occur during induction of anaesthesia but what is more disturbing is the tendency to apnoea in the postoperative period for up to 12 h after surgery. The infants most at risk are preterm babies in the age group up to 46 weeks' postconceptional age; especially those with a history of previous apnoeic spells. Infants in this group are treated only for essential surgery and not on a day-stay basis; they are carefully monitored for apnoea for the first 24 h postoperatively. Theophylline 8 mg kg^{-1} i.v. may be given before the end of surgery in babies who have previously suffered from episodes of apnoea. This problem is also discussed in Chapters 10 and 11.

The ex-premature baby also has the risk for residual lung damage from intubation and mechanical ventilation earlier in life. This bronchopulmonary dysplasia (BPD) results from an unresolved acute lung injury associated with oxygen therapy and mechanical ventilation in infants with respiratory distress syndrome.[223] Complicating and exacerbating factors include L–R shunt from patent ductus arteriosus, loss of mucociliary function and low-grade, continuing pulmonary infection with secretion retention. Northway et al.[223] described grades I–IV of CXR changes with increasingly over-expanded lungs with focal areas of hyperlucency and dense strands of opacification. The effect is of ventilation–perfusion abnormality, stiff lungs, oxygen dependency beyond the first 28 days of life and occasionally continuing dependency on mechanical ventilation.

BPD is a major cause of mortality and morbidity in the VLB group, with possibly as high an incidence as 85% in infants below 800 g, but only 5% at 1300 g.[224] If factors known to cause BPD are not minimized [high inspiratory oxygen fraction (FiO_2) and barotrauma, chronic infection, PDA, etc.], then the condition progresses with abnormalities in all parts of the lung architecture.

Long-term treatment includes the use of appropriate, but minimal respiratory support (possibly allowing $PaCO_2$ to rise), levels of inspired oxygen and diuretic and bronchodilator therapy. Corticosteroids are used in BPD because of proven short-term improvement in pulmonary function,[225] although many dosage regimens exist as well as duration of treatment. Any baby still with oxygen dependency who presents for surgery poses an increased risk for respiratory support postoperatively using nasal continuous positive airway pressure or even intubation and mechanical ventilation. Intraoperatively higher FiO_2 than normal is usually required to achieve reasonable SpO_2.

Ex-preterm babies may also be anaemic because of a reduced ability to produce red cells and a greater fall in Hb levels than full-term babies, which is worsened by frequent blood sampling.[226] Iron and vitamin E deficiency make the anaemia worse. Top-up transfusions are usually given when the Hb level falls to 8 g dl^{-1} and erythropoietin therapy produces an earlier increase in reticulocyte formation. Anaemic babies are more likely to have worse respiratory and cardiac problems as well as an increased incidence of apnoea.[227]

Retinopathy of prematurity (ROP) (see also Chapter 15) is increasing in incidence despite advances in the delivery and monitoring of oxygenation. Although it may occur in term babies, those at greatest risk are babies below 35 weeks' gestation, weighing less than 2 kg, in whom the retina has not become fully vascularized. Pathology is divided into four stages of increasing vascular proliferation with scarring and retinal detachment, although early stages will regress.[228] Initially, oxygen causes constriction of the retinal arterioles and degeneration of the endothelium, i.e. retinal ischaemia, even in the presence of hyperoxia.

Oxygen is a major risk factor for ROP, but whether arterial oxygen tension (PaO_2) or oxygen content causes the problem is not known. Fetal oxygen saturations are low and

after birth are much higher, even with the infant breathing air. Other factors are also involved, such as $PaCO_2$ and concentration of HbA after blood transfusion, but it is wise to limit oxygen in the perioperative period to give a SpO_2 of 90–92% where possible. Intraoperative hyperoxia has been incriminated in the production of ROP.[229] It is not known whether hyperoxia worsens pre-existing ROP after 44 weeks' postconception, so it is wise to limit oxygenation even in this age group.

After a stay in a NICU with the need for continuous intravenous access in many cases, even with parenteral nutrition, subsequent vascular access may be very difficult.

REFERENCES

1 Hey, E.N. and Katz, G. Evaporative water loss in the new-born baby. *Journal of Physiology* 1969; **200**: 605–19.
2 Sessler, D.I. Temperature regulation. In: GA G (ed.). *Pediatric Anaesthesia*. 3rd edn. New York: Churchill Livingstone, 1994: 47–81.
3 Torrance, R.W. Heart size and body size. *Proceedings of the Physiological Society* 1997; 82P, Abstract C51.
4 Hey, E.N. and O'Connell, B. Oxygen consumption and heat balance in the cot-nursed baby. *Archives of Disease in Childhood* 1970; **45**: 335–41.
5 Hall, G.M. and Lucke, J.N. Brown fat – a thermogenic tissue of anaesthetic importance? *British Journal of Anaesthesia* 1982; **54**: 907–8.
6 Foster, K.G., Hey, E.N. and Katz, G. The response of the sweat glands of the newborn baby to thermal stimuli and to intradermal acetylcholine. *Journal of Physiology* 1969; **203**: 13–29.
7 Hey, E.N. The relation between environmental temperature and oxygen consumption in the new-born baby. *Journal of Physiology* 1969; **200**: 589–603.
8 Hey, E.N. and Katz, G. The optimum thermal environment for naked babies. *Archives of Disease in Childhood* 1970; **45**: 328–33.
9 Fetterman, G.H., Shuplock, N.A., Philipp, F.J. and Gregg, H.S. The growth and maturation of human glomeruli and proximal convolutions from term to adulthood. *Pediatrics* 1965; **35**: 601–19.
10 Arant, B.S. Developmental patterns of renal functional maturation compared in the human neonate. *Journal of Pediatrics* 1978; **92**: 705–12.
11 Vanpee, M., Blennow, M., Linne, T., Herin, P. and Aperia, A. Renal function in very birth weight infants: normal maturity reached during early childhood. *Journal of Pediatrics* 1992; **121**: 786–8.
12 Guillery, E.N. Fetal and neonatal nephrology. *Current Opinion in Pediatrics* 1997; **9**: 148–53.

13 Balistreri, W.F. and Bucuvalas, J.C. The liver and bile ducts. In: AM R, JI H and CD R (eds). *Rudolph's Pediatrics.* 20th edn. London: Prentice Hall, 1996: 1121–66.

14 Watkins, J.B. and Perman, J.A. Bile acid metabolism in infants and children. *Clinics in Gastroenterology* 1977; **6**: 201–16.

15 Robertson, W.O. Practice parameter: management of hyperbilirubinaemia in the healthy term newborn. *Pediatrics* 1994; **94**: 558–65.

16 Brown, J.K., Omar, T. and O'Regan, M. Brain development and the development of tone and muscle. In: KJ C, H F (eds). *Neurophysiology and the Neuropsychology of Motor Development.* Mackeith Press, 1997: 1–41.

17 Wolf, A.R. Development of Pain and Stress Responses. In: B D, I M and G B (eds). *Advances in Paediatric Anaesthesia. Paris: 4th European Congress of Paediatric Anaesthesia,* 1997: 33–56.

18 Olsson, G.L. and Hallen, B. Laryngospasm during anaesthesia. A computer-aided incidence study in 136 929 patients. *Acta Anaesthesiologica Scandinavica* 1984; **28**: 567–75.

19 Olsson, G.L. Bronchospasm during anaesthesia. A computer-aided incidence study of 136 929 patients. *Acta Anaesthesiologica Scandinavica* 1987; **31**: 244–52.

20 Malviya, S., Voepel-Lewis, T. and Tait, A.R. Adverse events and risk factors associated with the sedation of children by nonanesthesiologists. *Anesthesia and Analgesia* 1997; **85**: 1207–13.

21 Van Der Walt, J.H., Sweeney, D.B., Runciman, W.B. and Webb, R.K. Paediatric incidents in anaesthesia: an analysis of 2000 incidents reports. *Anaesthesia and Intensive Care* 1993; **21**: 655–8.

22 Holzman, R.S. Morbidity and mortality in pediatric anesthesia. *Pediatric Clinics of North America* 1994; **41**: 239–56.

23 Lyons, B., Frizelle, H., Kirby, F. and Casey, W. The effect of passive smoking on the incidence of airway complications in children undergoing general anaesthesia. *Anaesthesia* 1996; **51**: 324–6.

24 Schreiner, M.S., O'Hara, I., Markakis, D.A. and Politis, G.D. Do children who experience laryngospasm have an increased risk of upper respiratory tract infection? *Anesthesiology* 1996; **85**: 475–80.

25 Bryan, A.C. and England, S.J. Maintenance of an elevated FRC in the newborn. *American Review of Respiratory Disease* 1984; **129**: 209–10.

26 Stark, A.R., Cohlan, B.A., Waggener, T.B., Frantz, I.D., III and Kosch, P.C. Regulation of end-expiratory lung volume during sleep in premature infants. *Journal of Applied Physiology* 1987; **62**: 1117–23.

27 Henderson-Smart, D.J. and Read, J.C. Reduced lung volume during behavioral active sleep in the newborn. *Journal of Applied Physiology: Respiratory, Environmental and Exercise Physiology* 1979; **46**: 1081–5.

28 Ochiai, R., Guthrie, R.D. and Motoyama, E.K. Effects of varying concentrations of halothane on the activity of the genioglossus, intercostals, and diaphragm in cats: an electromyographic study. *Anesthesiology* 1989; **70**: 812–16.

29 Nishino, T., Shirahata, M., Yonezawa, T. and Honda, Y. Comparison of changes in the hypoglossal and the phrenic nerve activity in response to increasing depth of anesthesia in cats. *Anesthesiology* 1984; **60**: 19–24.

30 Rabbette, P.S., Costeloe, K.L. and Stocks, J. Persistence of the Hering–Breuer reflex beyond the neonatal period. *Journal of Applied Physiology* 1991; **71**: 474–80.

31 Nishino, T., Tagaito, Y. and Isono, S. Cough and other reflexes on irritation of airway mucosa in man. *Pulmonary Pharmacology* 1996; **9**: 285–92.

32 Biavati, M.J., Manning, S.C. and Phillips, D.L. Predictive factors for respiratory complications after tonsillectomy and adenoidectomy in children. *Archives of Otolaryngology and Head and Neck Surgery* 1997; **123**: 517–21.

33 McColley, S.A., April, M.M., Carroll, J.L., Naclerio, R.M. and Loughlin, G.M. Respiratory compromise after adenotonsillectomy in children with obstructive sleep apnea. *Archives of Otolaryngology and Head and Neck Surgery* 1992; **118**: 940–3.

34 Rosen, G.M., Muckle, R.P., Mahowald, M.W., Goding, G.S. and Ullevig, C. Postoperative respiratory compromise in children with obstructive sleep apnea syndrome: can it be anticipated? *Pediatrics* 1994; **93**: 784–8.

35 McGill, W.A., Coveler, L.A. and Epstein, B.S. Subacute upper respiratory infection in small children. *Anesthesia and Analgesia* 1979; **58**: 331–3.

36 Kinouchi, K., Tanigami, H., Tashiro, C., Nishimura, M., Fukumitsu, K. and Takauchi, Y. Duration of apnea in anesthetized infants and children required for desaturation of hemoglobin to 95%. *Anesthesiology* 1992; **77**: 1105–7.

37 Papastamelos, C., Panitch, H.B., England, S.E. and Allen, J.L. Developmental changes in chest wall compliance in infancy and early childhood. *Journal of Applied Physiology* 1995; **78**: 179–84.

38 Dobbinson, T.L., Nisbet, H.I.A., Pelton, D.A. and Levison, H. Functional residual capacity (FRC) and compliance in anaesthetized paralysed children Part II. Clinical results. *Canadian Journal of Anaesthesiology* 1973; **20**: 322–33.

39 Hoo, A.-F., Henschen, M., Dezateux, C. *et al.* Respiratory function among preterm infants whose mothers smoked during pregnancy. *American Journal of Respiration and Critical Care Medicine* 1998; **158**: 700–5.

40 Coté, C.J. and Kelly, D.H. Postoperative apnea in a full-term infant with a demonstrable respiratory pattern abnormality. *Anesthesiology* 1990; **72**: 559–61.

41 Tait, A.R., Reynolds, P.I. and Gutstein, H.B. Factors that influence an anesthesiologist's decision to cancel elective surgery for the child with an upper respiratory tract infection. *Journal of Clinical Anesthesia* 1995; **7**: 491–9.

42 DeSoto, H., Patel, R.I., Soliman, I.E. and Hannallah, R.S. Changes in oxygen saturation following general anesthesia in children with upper respiratory infection signs and symptoms undergoing otolaryngological procedures. *Anesthesiology* 1988; **68**: 276–9.

43 Jacoby, D.B. and Hirshman, C.A. General anesthesia in patients with viral respiratory infections: an unsound sleep? *Anesthesiology* 1991; **74**: 969–72.

44 Empey, D.W., Laitinen, L.A., Jacobs, L., Gold, W.M. and Nadel, J.A. Mechanisms of bronchial hyperreactivity in normal subjects after upper respiratory tract infection. *American Review of Respiratory Disease* 1976; **113**: 131–9.

45 Kil, H.-K., Rooke, G.A., Ryan-Dykes, M.A. and Bishop, M.J. Effect of prophylactic bronchodilator treatment on lung resistance after tracheal intubation. *Anesthesiology* 1994; **81**: 43–8.

46 Collier, A.M., Pimmel, R.L., Hasselblad, V., Clyde, W.A., Knelson, J.H. and Brooks, J.G. Spirometric changes in normal children with upper respiratory infections. *American Review of Respiratory Disease* 1978; **117**: 47–53.

47 Tom, L.W.C., DeDio, R.M., Cohen, D.E., Wetmore, R.F., Handler, S.D. and Potsic, W.P. Is outpatient tonsillectomy appropriate for young children? *Laryngoscope* 1992; **102**: 277–80.

48 Carroll, J.L., McColley, S.A., Marcus, C.L., Curtis, S. and Loughlin, G.M. Inability of clinical history to distinguish primary snoring from obstructive sleep apnea syndrome in children. *Chest* 1995; **108**: 610–18.

49 Davidson, S.L. and Marcus, C.L. Obstructive sleep apnea in infants and young children. *Journal of Clinical Neurophysiology* 1996; **13**: 198–207.

50 Bloomberg, G.R. and Strunk, R.C. Crisis in asthma care. *Pediatric Clinics of North America* 1992; **39**: 1225–41.

51 Lenfant, C. Asthma symposium. National Heart, Lung, and Blood Institute National Asthma Education Program Expert Panel Report: Guidelines for the diagnosis and management of asthma.. *Journal of Allergy and Clinical Immunology* 1991; **88**: 427–38.

52 Hill, M., Szefler, S.J. and Larsen, G.L. Asthma pathogenesis and the implications for therapy in children. *Pediatric Clinics of North America* 1992; **39**: 1205–21.

53 Lee, A.B.D and Pitcher-Wilmott, W. The clinical and laboratory correlates of nasal polyps in cystic fibrosis. *International Journal of Pediatric Otorhinolaryngology* 1982; **4**: 209–14.

54 Wilmott, R.W. and Fiedler, M.A. Recent advances in the treatment of cystic fibrosis. *Pediatric Clinics of North America* 1994; **41**: 431–45.

55 Wang, E.E.L., Prober, M.D.C.M., Manson, B., Corey, M. and Levison, H. Association of respiratory viral infections with pulmonary deterioration in patients with cystic fibrosis. *New England Journal of Medicine* 1984; **311**: 1653–8.

56 Corey, M., Levison, H. and Crozier, D. Five- to seven-year course of pulmonary function in cystic fibrosis. *American Review of Respiratory Disease* 1976; **114**: 1085–92.

57 Bancalari, E., Jesse, M.J., Gelband, H. and Garcia, O. Lung mechanics in congenital heart disease with increased and decreased pulmonary blood flow. *Journal of Pediatrics* 1977; **90**: 192–5.

58 Davies, C.J., Cooper, S.G., Fletcher, M.E., *et al.* Total respiratory compliance in infants and young children with congenital heart disease. *Pediatric Pulmonology* 1990; **8**: 155–61.

59 MacDonald, N.E., Hall, C.B., Suffin, S.C., Alexson, C., Harris, P.J. and Manning, J.A. Respiratory syncytial viral infection in infants with congenital heart disease. *New England Journal of Medicine* 1982; **307**: 397–400.

60 Barrington, K. and Finer, N. The natural history of the appearance of apnea of prematurity. *Pediatric Research* 1991; **29**: 372–5.

61 Steward, D.J. Preterm infants are more prone to complications following minor surgery than are term infants. *Anesthesiology* 1982; **56**: 304–6.

62 Andropoulos, D.B., Heard, M.B., Johnson, K.L., Clarke, J.T. and Rowe, R.W. Postanesthetic apnea in full-term infants after pyloromyotomy. *Anesthesiology* 1994; **80**: 216–19.

63 Fisher, D.M. When is the ex-premature infant no longer at risk for apnea? *Anesthesiology* 1995; **82**: 807–8.

64 Malviya, S., Swartz, J. and Lerman, J. Are all preterm infants younger than 60 weeks postconceptual age at risk for postanesthetic apnea. *Anesthesiology* 1993; **78**: 1076–81.

65 Coté, C.J., Zaslavsky, A., Downes, J.J., Kurth, C.D. and Welborn, L.G. Postoperative apnea in former preterm infants after inguinal herniorrhaphy. *Anesthesiology* 1995; **82**: 809–22.

66 Kurth, C.D., Spitzer, A.R., Broennie, A.M. and Downes, J.J. Postoperative apnea in preterm infants. *Anesthesiology* 1987; **66**: 483–8.

67 Pickens, D.L., Schefft, G.L., Storch, G.A. and Thach, B.T. Characterization of prolonged apneic episodes associated with respiratory syncytial virus infection. *Pediatric Pulmonology* 1989; **6**: 195–201.

68 Davidson Ward, S.L., Jacobs, R.A., Gates, E.P., Hart, L.D. and Keens, T.G. Abnormal ventilatory patterns during sleep in infants with myelomeningocele. *Journal of Pediatrics* 1986; **109**: 631–4.

69 Stocks, J., Godfrey, S. and Reynolds, E.O.R. Airway resistance in infants after various treatments for hyaline membrane disease: special emphasis on prolonged high levels of inspired oxygen. *Pediatrics* 1978; **61**: 178–83.

70 Lindroth, M., Svenningsen, N.W., Ahlstrom, H. and Jonson, B. Evaluation of mechanical ventilation in newborn infants. *Acta Paediatrica Scandinavica* 1980; **69**: 151–8.

71 Sane, S.M., Worsing, R.A., Wiens, C.W. and Sharma, R.K. Value of preoperative chest x-ray examinations in children. *Pediatrics* 1977; **60**: 669–72.

72 Beckerman, R.C., Brouillette, R.T. and Hunt, C.E. *Respiratory Control Disorders in Infants and Children.* Baltimore, MD: Williams & Wilkins, 1992.

73 Jacob, S.V., Morielli, A., Mograss, M.A., Ducharme, F.M., Schloss, M.D. and Brouillette, R.T. Home testing for pediatric obstructive sleep apnea syndrome secondary to adenotonsillar hypertrophy. *Pediatric Pulmonology* 1995; **20**: 241–52.

74 Hatch, D. and Fletcher, M. Anaesthesia and the ventilatory system in infants and young children. *British Journal of Anaesthesia* 1992; **68**: 398–410.

75 Hatch, D. Respiratory physiology in neonates and infants. *Current Opinion in Anaesthesiology* 1995; **8**: 224–9.

76 Stocks, J., Sly, P.D., Tepper, R.S. and Morgan, W.J. *Infant Respiratory Function Testing.* New York: John Wiley, 1996.

77 Pfaff, J.K. and Morgan, W.J. Pulmonary function in infants and children. *Pediatric Clinics of North America* 1994; 41: 401–23.

78 Miller, R.D. and Hyatt, R.E. Evaluation of obstructing lesions of the trachea and larynx by flow–volume loops. *American Review of Respiratory Disease* 1973; **108**: 475–81.

79 Fitzgerald, M. Neonatal Pharmacology of Pain. In: JM B and AH D (eds). *Handbook of Experimental Pharmacology.* Springer, 1997: 447–165.

80 Neville, B.G.R. Epilepsy in childhood. *British Medical Journal* 1997; **315**: 513–21.

81 Barron, T.F. and Hunt, S.L. A review of the newer antiepileptic drugs and the ketogenic diet. *Clinical Pediatrics* 1997; 513–20.

82 Capra, M. and Hewitt, M. Brain tumours in childhood. *Current Paediatrics* 1998; **8**: 88–91.

83 Guertin, S.R. Cerebrospinal fluid shunts. Evaluation, complications and crisis management. *Pediatric Clinics of North America* 1987; **34**: 203–16.

84 Jones, R.F.C., Stening, W.A. and Brydon, M. Endoscopic third ventriculostomy. *Neurosurgery* 1990; **26**: 86–92.

85 Ruggieri, M. and Huson, S.M. What's new in neurofibromatosis? *Current Paediatrics* 1997; **7**: 167–76.

86 Davies, K.E. Challenges in Duchenne muscular dystrophy. *Neuromuscular Disorders* 1997; **7**: 482–6.

87 Jones, K.G. and North, K.N. Recent advances in the diagnosis of childhood muscular dystrophies. *Journal of Paediatrics and Child Health* 1997; **33**: 195–201.

88 Ellis, F.R. Inherited muscle disease. *British Journal of Anaesthesia* 1980; **52**: 153–64.

89 Morris, P. Duchenne muscular dystrophy: a challenge for the anaesthetist. *Paediatric Anaesthesia* 1997; **7**: 1–4.

90 Azar, I. The response of patients with neuromuscular disorders to muscle relaxants: a review. *Anesthesiology* 1984; **61**: 173–87.

91 Buzello, W. and Huttarsch, H. Muscle relaxation in patients with duchenne muscular dystrophy. *British Journal of Anaesthesia* 1988; **60**: 228–31.

92 Tobias, J.D. and Atwood, R. Mivacurium in children with Duchenne muscular dystrophy. *Paediatric Anaesthesia* 1994; **4**: 57–60.

93 Smith, C.L. and Bush, G.H. Anaesthesia and progressive muscular dystrophy. *British Journal of Anaesthesia* 1985; **57**: 1113–18.

94 Miller, E.D., Sanders, D.B., Rowlingson, J.C. and Berry, F.A. Anaesthesia induced rhabdomyolysis in a patient with Duchenne's muscular dystrophy. *Anesthesiology* 1978; **48**: 146–8.

95 Rosenberg, H. and Shutack, J.G. Variants of malignant hyperthermia. Special problems for the paediatric anaesthesiologist. *Paediatric Anaesthesia* 1996; **6**: 87–93.

96 Brownell, A.K., Paasuke, R.T., Elash, A., *et al.* Malignant hyperthermia in duchenne muscular dystrophy. *Anesthesiology* 1983; **58**: 180–2.

97 Rosenberg, H. and Heiman-Patterson, T. Duchenne muscular dystrophy and malignant hyperthermia. *Anesthesiology* 1983; **59**: 362.

98 Oka, S., Igarashi, Y., Tagaki, A. and Nishida, M. Malignant hyperpyrexia and duchenne muscular dystrophy: case report. *Canadian Anaesthesists Society Journal* 1982; **29**: 627–9.

99 Russell, S.H. and Hirsch, N.P. Anaesthesia and myotonia. *British Journal of Anaesthesia* 1994; 210–16.

100 Mitchell, M.M., Ali, H.H. and Savarese, J.J. Myotonia and neuromuscular blocking agents. *Anesthesiology* 1978; **49**: 44–8.

101 Anderson, B.J. and Brown, T.C.K. Congenital myotonic dystrophy in children – a review of ten years experience. *Anaesthesia and Intensive Care* 1989; **17**: 320–4.

102 Nightingale, P., Healy, T.E. and McGuinness, K. Dystrophia myotonica and atracurium. *British Journal of Anaesthesia* 1985; **57**: 1131–5.

103 Buzello, W., Krieg, N. and Schlickewei, A. Hazards of neostigmine in patients with neuromuscular disorders. *British Journal of Anaesthesia* 1982; **54**: 529–34.

104 Bray, R.J. and Inkster, J.S. Anaesthesia in babies with congenital dystrophia myotonica. *Anaesthesia* 1984; **39**: 1007–11.

105 Aldridge, L.M. Anaesthetic Problems in myotonic dystrophy. *British Journal of Anaesthesia* 1985; **57**: 1119–30.

106 Haberer, J.P., Fabre, F. and Rose, E. Malignant hyperthermia and myotonia congenita (Thomsen's disease). *Anaesthesia* 1989; **44**: 166.

107 Seay, A.R. and Ziter, F.A. Malignant hyperpyrexia in a patient with Schwartz–Jampel syndrome. *Journal of Pediatrics* 1978; **93**: 83–4.

108 Duncan, P. Neuromuscular disease. In: J K, DJ S (eds). *Anaesthesia and Uncommon Pediatric Disease.* 2nd edn. Philadelphia, PA: WB Saunders, 1993: 672–94.

109 Baraka, A. Anaesthesia and myasthenia gravis. *Canadian Journal of Anaesthesia* 1992; **39**: 476–86.

110 Rahman, S. and Leonard, J.V. Mitochondrial disorders. *Current Paediatrics* 1997; **7**: 123–7.

111 Thomeer, E.C., Verhoven, W.M.A., Van de Vlasakker, C.J.W. and Klopenhhouwer, J.L. Psychiatric symptoms in MELAS; a case report. *Journal of Neurology, Neurosurgery and Psychiatry* 1998; **64**: 692–3.

112 Traeger, E and Rapid, I. Peroxisomal Disorders. In: AM R, JI H, CD R (eds). *Rudolph's Pediatrics.* 20th edn. London: Prentice Hall, 1996: 2033–9.

113 Wallace, J.J., Perndt, H. and Skinner, M. Anaesthesia and mitochondrial disease. *Paediatric Anaesthesia* 1998; **8**: 249–54.

114 Lee, P. Glycogen storage diseases. *Current Paediatrics* 1997; **7**: 108–13.

115 Stehling, L. Genetic Metabolic Diseases. In: J K, DJ S (eds). *Anesthesia and Uncommon Pediatric Diseases.* 2nd edn. Philadelphia, PA: WB Saunders, 1993: 461–80.

116 Cox, J.M. Anaesthesia and glycogen-storage disease. *Anesthesiology* 1968; **29**: 1221–5.

117 Proesmans, W.C. Chronic renal failure in infancy. *Baillière's Clinical Paediatrics* 1997; **5**: 617–35.

118 Friedman, A.L. Nephrology – Editorial overview. *Current Opinion in Pediatrics* 1997; **9**: 147.

119 Belman, A.B. Vesicoureteric reflux. *Pediatric Clinics of North America* 1997; **44**: 1171–90.

120 Alon, U.S. Nephrocalinosis. *Current Opinion in Pediatrics* 1997; **9**: 160–5.

121 Pan, C.G. Glomerulonephritis in childhood. *Current Opinion in Pediatrics* 1997; **9**: 154–9.

122 Springate, J.E. Toxic nephropathies. *Current Opinion in Pediatrics* 1997; **9**: 166–9.

123 Kalia, A. Chronic renal failure. In: AM R, JI H, CD R (eds). *Rudolph's Pediatrics.* 20th edn. London: Prentice Hall, 1996: 1344–7.

124 Friedman, A.L. Etiology, pathophysiology, diagnosis and management of chronic renal failure in children. *Current Opinion in Pediatrics* 1996; **8**: 147–51.

125 Warady, B.A. and Bunchman, T.E. An update on peritoneal dialysis and hemodialysis in the pediatric population. *Current Opinion in Pediatrics* 1996; **8**: 135–40.

126 Vester, U., Offner, G., Oldhafer, K. and Fangman, J. End stage renal failure in children younger than 6 years: renal transplantation is the therapy of choice. *European Journal of Pediatrics* 1998; **157**: 239–42.

127 Ettenger, R.B., Rosenthal, J.T., Marik, J.L., *et al.* Improved cadaveric renal transplant outcome in children. *Pediatric Nephrology* 1991; **5**: 137–42.

128 Aronson, S. Renal disease: dysfunction, failure, and transplantation. *Current Opinion in Anaesthesiology* 1993; **6**: 556–61.

129 Ecoffey, C. Anaesthesia for transplant surgery in paediatrics. In: D D, I M, G B (eds). *Advances in Paediatric Anaesthesia. Paris: 4th European Congress of Paediatric Anaesthesia,* 1997: 99–111.

130 Wells, T.G., Ulstrom, R.A. and Nevins, T.E. Hypoglycemia in pediatric renal allograft recipients. *Journal of Pediatrics* 1988; **113**: 1002–7.

131 Dillon, M. Therapeutic strategies in renovascular hypertension. *Ballière's Clinical Paediatrics* 1997; **5**: 675–85.

132 Cramolini, G.M. Diseases of the renal system. In: J K, DJ S (eds). *Anesthesia and Uncommon Diseases.* 2nd edn. Philadelphia, PA: WB Saunders, 1993: 238–46.

133 Chase, P.H. Diabetes Mellitus. In: Hathaway, W.E., Hay, W.W., Groothius, J.R. and Paisley, J.W. (eds). *Current Pediatric Diagnosis and Treatment.* 11th edn. Norwalk, CT: Appleton & Lange, 1993: 881–4.

134 Sperling, M.A. Diabetes mellitus. *Pediatric Clinics of North America* 1979; **26**: 149–54.

135 Krane, E.J. Subclinical brain swelling in children during treatment of diabetic ketoacidosis. *New England Journal of Medicine* 1985; **312**: 1147–9.

136 Gavin, L.A. Perioperative treatment of the diabetic patient. *Endocrinology and Metabolism Clinics of North America* 1992; **21**: 1147–52.

137 Alberti, K.G.M.M., Gill, G.V. and Elliot, M.J. Insulin delivery during surgery in the diabetic patient. *Diabetes Care* 1982; **5**: 65–77.

138 Smail, P.J. Children with diabetes who need surgery. *Archives of Disease in Childhood* 1986; **61**: 413–14.

139 Robinson, A.G. DDAVP in the treatment of central diabetes insipidus. *New England Journal of Medicine* 1976; **294**: 507–11.

140 Turner, M.C., Lieberman, E. and Dequattro, V. The perioperative management of children with phaechromocytoma. *Clinical Pediatrics* 1992; **31**: 583–9.

141 Radke, W.E., Kazmier, F.J. and Rutherford, H.D. Cardiovascular complications of phaechromocytoma crisis. *American Journal of Cardiology* 1975; **35**: 701–5.

142 Imperato-McGinley, J., Gautier, T. and Ehlers, K. Reversibility of cathecholamine induced dilated cardiomyopathy in a child with phaechromocytoma. *New England Journal of Medicine* 1987; **316**: 793–9.

143 Hutton, P. and Cooper, G. Endocrine and metabolic disease. In: Hutton, P. and Cooper, G. (eds). *Guidelines in Clinical Anaesthesia.* Oxford: Blackwell Scientific, 1985: 228–9.

144 Perrin, C., White, M.D. and Maria, I. Congenital adrenal hyperplasia. *New England Journal of Medicine* 1987; **316**: 1580–7.

145 Symreng, T., Karlberg, B.E. and Kagedal, B. Physiological cortisol substitution of longterm steroid treated patients undergoing major surgery. *British Journal of Anaesthesia* 1981; **53**: 949–54.

146 Walter, J.H. Investigation and initial management of suspected metabolic disease. *Current Paediatrics* 1997; **7**: 103–7.

147 Ramaswami, U. and Smith, I. Phenylketonuria. *Current Therapeutics* 1997; **7**: 251–5.

148 Spronsen, F., Verkerk, P.H. and van Houten, M. Does impaired growth of PKU patients correlate with the strictness of dietary treatment? *Acta Paediatrica* 1997; **86**: 816–18.

149 Brady, R.O. Disorders of lipid metabolism. In: AM R, JI H, CD R (eds). *Rudolph's Pediatrics.* 20th edn. London: Prentice Hall, 1996: 333–43.

150 Besley, G.T. and Wraith, J.E. Lysosomal disorders. *Current Paediatrics* 1997; **7**: 128–34.

151 Mahoney, A., Soni, N. and Vellodi, A. Anaesthesia and the mucopolysaccharidoses: a review of patients treated by bone marrow transplantation. *Paediatric Anaesthesia* 1992; **2**: 317–24.

152 Baines, D. and Keneally, J. Anaesthetic implications of the mucopolysaccharidoses: a 15 year experience in a children's hospital. *Anaesthesia and Intensive Care* 1983; **11**: 198–202.

153 Herrick, I.A. and Rhine, E.J. The mucopolysaccharidoses and anaesthesia: a report of clinical experience. *Canadian Journal of Anaesthesia* 1988; **35**: 67–73.

154 Baines, D.B., Street, N. and Overton, J.H. Anaesthetic implications of mucolipidosis. *Paediatric Anaesthesia* 1993; **3**: 303–6.

155 Kempthorne, P.M. and Brown, T.C.K. Anaesthesia and the mucopolysaccharidoses: a survey of techniques and problems. *Anaesthesia and Intensive Care* 1983; **11**: 203–7.

156 King, D.H., Jones, R.M. and Barnett, M.B. Anaesthetic considerations in the mucopolysaccharidoses. *Anaesthesia* 1984; **39**: 126–31.

157 Beushausen, T., Fouckhardt-Bradt, B. and Ohrdorf, W. Anaesthetic Implications of mucolipidosis. *Paediatric Anaesthesia* 1994; **4**: 202.

158 Brosius, F.C. and Roberts, W.C. Coronary artery disease in the Hurler syndrome. *American Journal of Cardiology* 1981; **47**: 649–53.

159 Sjogren, P., Pedersen, T. and Steinmetz, H. Mucopolysaccharidoses and anaesthesia risks. *Acta Anaesthesiologica Scandinavica* 1987; **31**: 214–18.

160 Jacquemin, E., Lykavieris, P. and Chaoui, N. Transient neonatal cholestasis: origin and outcome. *Journal of Pediatrics* 1998; **133**: 563–7.

161 Barkin, R. and Lilly, J.R. Biliary atresia and the Kasai operation: continuing care. *Journal of Pediatrics* 1980; **96**: 1015–19.

162 Bernard, O. Portal hypertension in children. *Clinical Gastroenterology* 1995; **14**: 33–7.

163 Heubi, J.E. Reye's syndrome: current concepts. *Hepatology* 1987; **7**: 155–64.

164 Child, C.G. and Turcotte, J.G. Surgery and portal hypertension. *Major Problems in Clinical Surgery* 1964; **1**: 1–85.

165 Donaldson, S.S. and Link, M.P. Hodgkins disease: treatment of the young child. *Pediatric Clinics of North America* 1991; **39**: 457–73.

166 Wilson, J.F. The pathology of non-Hodgkin's lymphoma in childhood. *Human Pathology* 1987; **18**: 1008–14.

167 Keily, E.M. The surgical challenge of neuroblastoma. *Journal of Paediatric Surgery* 1994; **29**: 128–33.

168 Grosfield, J.L. Neuroblastoma: a 1990 review. *Paediatric Surgery International* 1990; **6**: 9–13.

169 Creagh-Barry, P. and Sumner, E. Neuroblastoma and anaesthesia. *Paediatric Anaesthesia* 1992; **2**: 147–52.

170 Kain, Z.N., Shamberger, R.S. and Holzman, R.S. Anaesthetic management of children with neuroblastoma. Journal of Clinical Anaesthesia 1993; 5: 486–91.

171 Jenkins, R.D.T. The treatment of Wilm's tumour. Pediatric Clinics of North America 1976; 23: 147.

172 Nicolin, G.L. and Mitchell, C.D. Wilms tumour. Current Paediatrics 1998; 8: 83–7.

173 Adetunji, Y. and Barton, C.J. Sickle cell disorders. Current Paediatrics 1995; 5: 186–9.

174 Vijay, V., Cavenagh, J.D. and Yate, P. The anaesthetist's role in acute sickle cell crisis. British Journal of Anaesthesia 1998; 80: 820–8.

175 Hoppe, C., Styles, L. and Vichinsky, E. The natural history of sickle cell disease. Current Opinion in Pediatrics 1998; 10: 49–52.

176 Styles, L.A. and Vichinsky, E.P. New therapies and approaches to transfusion in sickle cell disease in children. Current Opinion in Pediatrics 1997; 9: 41–5.

177 Esseltine, D.W., Baxter, M.R. and Bevan, J.C. Sickle cell states and the anaesthetist. Canadian Journal of Anaesthesia 1988; 35: 385–403.

178 Newberger, P.E. Haematology and oncology. Current Opinion in Pediatrics 1998; 5: 47–8.

179 Koshy, M., Weiner, S.J., Miller, S.T., Sleeper, L.A. and Vichinsky, E. Surgery and anaesthesia in sickle cell disease. Blood 1995; 86: 3676–84.

180 Vichinsky, E., Haberkern, C.M., Neumayr, L., Earles, A.N., Black, D. and Koshy, M. A comparison of conservative and aggressive transfusion regimens in the perioperative management of sickle cell disease. New England Journal of Medicine 1995; 333: 206–13.

181 Hain, W.R. and Jones, S.E. Diseases of the blood. In: J K and DJ S (eds). Anesthesia and Uncommon Pediatric Diseases. 2nd edn. Philadelphia, PA: WB Saunders, 1993: 646–71.

182 Layton, M., Ramachandran, M., O'Saughnessy, D. and Luzzatto, L. Glucose-6-Phosphate dehydrogenase deficiency. Current Paediatrics 1995; 5: 190–4.

183 Leisner, R. Coagulation Disorders in Children. Current Paediatrics 1995; 5: 175–80.

184 Conway, J.H. and Hilgartner, M.W. Initial presentations of Pediatric Haemaphiliacs. Archives of Pediatrics and Adolescent Medicine 1994; 148: 589–94.

185 Manco-Johnson, M.J. Genetic bleeding disorders. In: AM R, JI H, CI R (eds). Rudolph's Pediatrics, 20th edn. London: Prentice Hall, 1996: 1245–8.

186 Pascuci, R.C. Hemophilia and Fracture. In: L S (ed.). Common Problems in Pediatric Anesthesia. 2nd edn. St Louis, MO: Mosby, 1992: 487–91.

187 Wood, C.E. and Goresky, G.V. Hypospadias and von Willebrands Disease. In: L S (ed.). Common Problems in Pediatric Anesthesia. 2nd edn. St. Louis, MO: Mosby, 1992: 127–40.

188 Lambert, J.S. Pediatric HIV infection. Current Opinion in Pediatrics 1996; 8: 606–14.

189 Husson, R.N., Comeau, A.M. and Hoff, R. Diagnosis of human immunodeficiency virus infection in infants and children. Pediatrics 1990; 86: 1–9.

190 Hoyt, L. HIV Infection in women and children. Postgraduate Medicine 1997; 102: 165–76.

191 Shapiro, H.M., Grant, I. and Weinger, M.B. AIDS and the central nervous system. Anesthesiology 1994; 80: 187–99.

192 Schwartz, D., Scharwt z, T., Cooper, E. and Pullerits, J. Anaesthesia and the child with HIV infection. Canadian Journal of Anaesthesia 1991; 38: 5: 626–33.

193 Smart, B.A. and Ochs, H.D. The molecular basis and treatment of primary immunodeficiency disorders. Current Opinion in Pediatrics 1997; 9: 570–6.

194 Buckley, R H. Approaches to the child with suspected immune dysfunction. In: AM R, JI H and CD R (eds). Rudolph's Pediatrics. 20th edn. London: Prentice Hall, 1996: 437–50.

195 Buckley, R. and Schiff, R.I. Human severe combined immunodeficiency: genetic, phenotypic and functional diversity in one hundred eight infants. Journal of Pediatrics 1997; 130: 378–87.

196 Welt Kredich, D. Juvenile rheumatoid arthritis. In: AM R, JI H, Rudolph (eds). Rudolph's Pediatrics. 20th edn. London: Prentice Hall, 1996: 479–82.

197 Smith, M. Skin and connective tissue disease. In: J K, DJ S (eds). Anesthesia and Uncommon Pediatric Diseases. 2nd edn. Philadelphia, PA: WB Saunders, 1993: 501–62.

198 Gottlieb, B., Keenan, G.F., Lu, T. and Ilowite, N.T. Discontinuation of methotrexate treatment in juvenile rheumatoid arthritis. Pediatrics 1997; 100: 994–9.

199 Jacobs, J.C. and Hui, R.M. Cricoarytenoid arthritis and airway obstruction in juvenile rheumatoid arthritis. Pediatrics 1977; 59: 292–3.

200 Espada, G., Babin, i.J.C., Maldonado-Cocco, J.A. and Garcia-Morteo, O. Radiologic review: the cervical spine in juvenile rheumatoid arthritis. Seminars in Arthitis and Rheumatism 1988; 17: 185–95.

201 Smith, M. Rheumatoid arthritis and cervical laminectomy. In: L S (ed.). Common Problems in Pediatric Anesthesia. 2nd edn. St Louis, MO: Mosby, 1992: 493–8.

202 Krishna, G. Arthrogryposis. In: L S (ed.). Common Problems in Pediatric Anesthesia. 2nd edn. St Louis, MO: Mosby, 1992: 127–34.

203 Audenaert, S.M. Arthrogryposis is not a diagnosis. Paediatric Anaesthesia 1994; 4: 201–2.

204 Salem, M.R. and Klowden, A.J. Anesthesia for orthopedic surgery. In: GA G (ed.). Pediatric Anaesthesia. 3rd edn. New York: Churchill Livingstone, 1994: 607–56.

205 Baines, D.B., Douglas, I.D. and Overton, J.H. Anaesthesia for Patients with arthrogryposis congenita: what is the risk of malignant hyperthermia? Anaesthesia and Intensive Care 1986; 14: 370–2.

206 Zamudio, I.A. and Brown, T.C.K. Arthrogryposis multiplex congenita (AMC): a review of 32 years experience. Paediatric Anaesthesia 1993; 3: 101–6.

207 Hopkins, P.M., Ellis, F.R. and Halsall, P.J. Hypermetabolism in arthrogryposis multiplex congenita. Anaesthesia 1991; 46: 374–5.

208 Oberoi G.S., Kaul H.L., Gill I. and Batra R.K. Anaesthesia in arthrogryposis multiplex congenita: case report. Canadian Journal of Anaesthesia 1987; 34: 288–90.

209 Lund A.M., Nicholls A.C., Scharwtz M. and Skovby F. Parental mosaicism and autosomal dominant mutations causing structural abnormalities of collagen I in families with osteogenisis imperfecta type III/IV. Acta Paediatrica 1997; 86: 711–18.

210 Tosi L.L. Osteogenesis imperfecta. Current Opinion in Pediatrics 1997; 9: 94–9.

211 Hall R.M., Henning R.D., Brown T.C.K. and Cole W.G. Anaesthesia for children with osteogenesis imperfecta – a review. *Paediatric Anaesthesia* 1992; **2**: 115–21.

212 Pyeritz R.E. and McKusick V.A. The Marfan syndrome: diagnosis and management. *New England Journal of Medicine* 1979; **300**: 772–7.

213 Godfrey M. Marfan's Syndrome. In: AM R, JI H, CI R (eds). *Rudolph's Pediatrics.* 20th edn. London: Prentice Hall, 1996: 392–4.

214 Wells D.G. and Podolakin W. Anaesthesia and Marfan's syndrome: case report. *Canadian Journal of Anaesthesia* 1987; **34**: 311–14.

215 Paller, A.S. The genetic basis of heriditary blistering disorders. *Current Opinion in Pediatrics* 1996; **8**: 367–71.

216 Eichenfield, L.F. and Honig, P.J. Blistering disorders in childhood. *Pediatric Clinics of North America* 1991; **38**: 966–76.

217 Spargo, P.M. and Smith, G.B. Epidermolysis bullosa. *Anaesthesia and Analgesia* 1988; **67**: 296–9.

218 Broughton, R., Crawford, M.R. and Vonwiller, J.B. Epidermolysis bullosa – a review of 15 years experience. *Anaesthesia and Intensive Care* 1988; **16**: 260–4.

219 Whitaker, A.H., Feldman, J.F., Van Rossem, R., *et al.* Neonatal cranial ultrasound abnormalities in low birth weight infants: relation to cognitive outcomes at six years of age. *Pediatrics* 1996; **98**: 719–27.

220 McCarton, C.M., Wallace, I.F., Divon, M. and Vaughn, H.G., Jr. Cognitive and neurologic development of the premature, small for gestational age infant through age 6: comparison by birth weight and gestational age. *Pediatrics* 1996; **98**: 1167–78.

221 Kresch, M.J., Lin, W.H. and Thrall, R.S. Surfactant replacement therapy. *Thorax* 1996; **51**: 1137–54.

222 Gerstmann, D.R., Minton, S.D., Stoddard, R.A., *et al.* The Provo multicenter early high-frequency oscillatory ventilation trial: improved pulmonary and clinical outcome in respiratory distress syndrome. *Pediatrics* 1996; **98**: 1044–57.

223 Northway, W.H., Rosan, R.C. and Porter, D.Y. Pulmonary disease following respiratory therapy of hyaline-membrane disease. *New England Journal of Medicine* 1967; **276**: 357–68.

224 Avery, M.E., Tooley, W.H., Keller, J.B., *et al.* Is chronic lung disease in low birthweight babies preventable? A survey of eight centers. *Pediatrics* 1987; **79**: 26–30.

225 Rush, M.G. and Hazinski, T.A. Current therapy of bronchopulmonary dysplasia. *Clinics in Perinatology* 1992; **19**: 563–90.

226 Chessells, J.M. Blood formation in infancy. *Archives of Disease in Childhood* 1979; **54**: 831–4.

227 Welborn, L.G., Hannallah, R.S., Luban, N.L., *et al.* Anemia and postoperative apnea in former preterm infants. *Anesthesiology* 1991; **74**: 1003–1005.

228 The Committee for the Classification of Retinopathy of Prematurity: an international classification of retinopathy of prematurity. *Archives of Ophthalmology* 1984; **102**: 1130.

229 Betts, E.K., Downes, J.J., Schaffer, D.B., *et al.* Retrolental fibroplasia and oxygen administration during general anaesthesia. *Anesthesiology* 1977; **47**: 518–20.

CHAPTER 2

Immediate preoperative preparation

GEORGE MEAKIN AND ISABELLE MURAT

INTRODUCTION

Anaesthesia and surgery in childhood are associated with considerable emotional stress for both patients and their families. In addition, stressful experiences in hospital are known to make a deeper and more lasting impression on children, who may show regressive behavioural changes after they return home. It should therefore be a priority for paediatric anaesthetists to ensure, as far as possible, the emotional well-being of their patients in the perioperative period. In this chapter the psychological effects of hospitalization and surgery on children and their parents are described, along with the psychological and medical preparation of children for anaesthesia and surgery. The chapter concludes with sections on preoperative fasting and premedication.

PSYCHOLOGICAL FACTORS

Childhood disease can be viewed in a psychological as well as a biological context. Indeed, for many elective paediatric surgical procedures, the attendant psychological disruption appears to match or surpass the pathophysiological insult. Familiarity with developmental theories and the psychological effects of hospitalization can help health professionals to prepare children for surgery more effectively.

They are many ways to alleviate the anxiety of children and their families before anaesthesia and surgery. Preadmission hospital visits, organized guided tours and videotapes are an important part of organized preoperative care in many centres. The preoperative visit of the anaesthetist is probably the most important single element of good psychological preparation. Premedication with an anxiolytic drug may improve patient compliance at induction of anaesthesia and may reduce the incidence of postoperative behavioural disturbances.

PSYCHOLOGICAL FACTORS RELATED TO AGE

Various personality theories can aid in the understanding of how children of different ages respond to stress.[1,2] Freud's psychoanalytic theory emphasizes the evolution and development of personality, and explains why the defence mechanisms of younger children are incompletely equipped to process anxiety arising from the unknown or imagined. In Piaget's cognitive theory, children are grouped into age categories according to their ability to understand the environment. The first 2 years of life are termed the sensory-motor period. During this period, children learn basic things about their relationship with the environment. The period between age 2 and about 7 years is called preoperational period, and is subdivided into the preconceptual (up to about 4 years) and the intuitive (4–7 years) periods. In the preconceptual period, children can use language symbols and represent things by drawing them. During the intuitive substage, children can give reasons for their action and belief, but thinking still depends on immediate perception rather than on mental representation of relevant concepts. This stage is followed at the age of about 7 years by the period of concrete operations. Children now have the capacity to put objects in order or classify them, and are able to make comparisons. Adolescence is called the period of formal operations. The main features are the ability to accept assumptions for the sake of argument, and to make hypotheses and set up propositions to test them. Besides the psychoanalytic and cognitive theories, paediatric anaesthetists should be familiar with the behavioural model and the family system model. The behavioural model is based on learning theory and emphasizes that most behaviour is learned. The family system model emphasizes that the behaviour and values of parents have a considerable impact on the child.

PARENTAL ANXIETIES

The child's parents may often be preoccupied with feelings of guilt, concerned over their loss of control and afraid because of uncertainty.[3,4] Parents may be anxious about adverse surgical or anaesthetic outcomes (e.g. death, brain damage, postoperative pain), or adverse interactions with medical staff, especially when they, or another family member, have had a previous bad experience. It should be remembered that parents often focus on minor aspects of the perioperative events, such as the amount of hair removed in preparation for a large brain tumour resection. Mothers have been shown to be more anxious than fathers, and anxiety is greatest for children aged less than 1 year undergoing their first surgical episode.[5] This subgroup of parents may need additional support and attention before anaesthesia and surgery. Parental anxiety has been shown to be a factor predicting the child's behaviour at induction of anaesthesia and 1 week after surgery.[6] Thus preoperative support for parents benefits not only the parents themselves but also the child.[7]

CHILDHOOD ANXIETIES

For the child, the first anxious moment in the perioperative experience occurs when they learn that they are to have an operation.[8] The exact details of the announcement depend on the cognitive level of the child (and the parents). Whatever the detail, it must be entirely truthful. Communication should be gentle, simple and age appropriate. Throughout most of childhood, separation anxiety remains a major problem. Children aged between 2 and 6 years are five times more likely to have preoperative anxiety reactions than older children.[9] Risk factors include lack of preoperative familiarity with the surgical facility and dependency behaviour. Older children are more concerned with loss of self-identity, autonomy, control and function. Concerns about mutilation and torture are part of the fear of the unknown. These concerns are strikingly evident in young boys undergoing hypospadias repair. For this reason, the American Academy of Pediatrics recommends that surgery should be planned between 6 and 12 months of age.[10] Frank and forthright disclosure of anticipated events during hospitalization reduces much of this type of fear. Needles remain a major focus of anxiety for children and this has probably resulted in decades of inadequate postoperative analgesia.[11]

PSYCHOLOGICAL EFFECTS OF HOSPITALIZATION

At the beginning of the twentieth century, concern in hospital care for children was mainly disease orientated and custodial. Changes started in the 1940s with the recognition of the importance of maintaining an adequate mother–child relationship throughout hospitalization. Hospital rules have changed dramatically over the past 50 years and, nowadays, parents are allowed to stay with their children in hospital. However, allowing parents to stay with their children is not the complete answer; the hospital environment should also be supportive, compassionate and understanding, and parents should be encouraged to participate in caring for their child whenever possible.[12] Children between 6 months and 4 years of age are most likely to be upset following hospitalization, as demonstrated by Vernon and colleagues.[13] In this study, separation from parents was an important factor in the behavioural disturbances in young children and long-term behavioural changes were correlated with the length of hospitalization.

PSYCHOLOGICAL EFFECTS OF ANAESTHESIA AND SURGERY

As more became known about children's psychological needs, increasing attention was turned towards possible psychological sequelae of anaesthesia and surgery. The first study to address specifically the question of the psychological effects of surgery on children was published by Levy in 1945.[14] He noticed that the highest incidence of postoperative emotional sequelae was seen between the ages of 1 and 3 years. These problems included prolonged night terrors, negativism and a variety of phobias and anxiety reactions. In 1952, Jackson examined emotional trauma in children after tonsillectomy.[15] The incidence of psychological disturbances was 9% (vs 20% in Levy's study) and children between 1 and 3 years of age were at increased risk. In 1953, Eckenhoff reported an overall incidence of 17% of behavioural changes, with the highest incidence (40%) in the 2–3-year-old age group.[16] This incidence has not decreased since the 1950s, in spite of the increasing tendency to perform surgery on a day-case basis.[17] The changes are mostly transient, but in some children they persist for several weeks, months or even years. The incidence is apparently not affected by anaesthetic technique, but has been shown to be reduced by premedication with midazolam (see below).

In a large recent prospective multicentre survey of 551 children,[18] the overall incidence of problematical behavioural changes was 47% and that of beneficial changes 17%. The former were most common in children aged 1–3 years and the incidence decreased significantly from 46% on the day of the operation to 9% 4 weeks later. The most common behavioural changes were seeking attention, crying, waking up at night, problems when going to bed and fear of being alone. Predictors of postoperative behavioural changes were age, mild pain at home following surgery, severe pain and a previous bad experience of health care, which has adversely affected the attitude of the child towards doctors or nurses. Pain on the day of operation predicted the occurrence of behavioural problems up to the fourth week. This emphasizes the importance of effective prevention of postoperative pain as well as the importance of avoiding unpleasant experiences in all contacts that children could have with health care.

THE PREOPERATIVE VISIT

The major purpose and process of the clinical interview is the exchange of information. McGraw has proposed the following rules when interviewing children.[1]

1 Don't talk to a child in a condescending way, but as a physician talks to a patient.
2 Do not convey to a child the notion that their feelings, concerns or ideas are 'childish'.
3 Do not laugh at what a child says unless you are quite sure they intend to be humorous.
4 Never tease children unless you know them very well, and they know they have permission to tease in return.
5 Initial encounters with young children are often made easier when introduced in a whisper, which young children may find reassuring. In addition, squatting or kneeling

to be at eye level with a child may present a less imposing image.

6 With children greater than 3–4 years of age, discuss their care in terms they can understand; never discuss their illness or treatment in their presence unless discussing it with them as well. During a medical interview, children are most often listening intently to what is being said, even when appearing not to do so.

A familiar and supportive environment is helpful and can be accomplished through the use of tours, special books, videos and toys. It is also important to reassure the parents, because the parent's anxiety is reflected in the child. It was demonstrated several years ago that a preadmission visit contributes to a lessening of maternal anxiety during and after the child's hospitalization.[7,19] The preadmission visit was also associated with a reduction in the incidence of negative posthospital behaviour, particularly in children aged 6–7 years. However, the effects of a behavioural-based preoperative preparation programme vary with the child's age, the timing of intervention and a history of previous hospitalization.[20] The preparation programme was more effective when performed 5–7 days prior to surgery compared with the day before surgery and also more effective in children 6 years or older than in the younger ones. It has also been reported that most American parents prefer to have comprehensive information concerning their child's perioperative period.[21,22] Detailed anaesthetic information of what might go wrong does not increase parental anxiety and has the advantage of allowing parents a fully informed choice. These studies emphasize the importance of planning the preoperative visit several days before surgery to give the parents enough time to understand what was said. In France, the preoperative visit is mandatory and has to be performed several days before surgery, but this is not the case in most European countries.

The preoperative visit should be performed by an anaesthetist and not by a paediatrician, as proposed by some,[23] in order that the anaesthetic procedure can be explained clearly to the child and the parents. It is important not to lie to the child (needles hurt, propofol stings, etc.). The sensations and emotions the child will or might experience should be described as clearly as possible. The anaesthetist should be honest about unpleasant events that may occur at induction or in the postoperative period (chest tube, gastric tube, i.v. line, etc.). All children aged 3 years or older should be told that they will go to sleep before the surgery, and that they will wake up after the surgery. In children aged 3–6 years, explanations per se appear to be more important than the accuracy of the content.[1] Indeed, children who were given explanations, whether accurate or not, experienced fewer postoperative behavioural changes than those who were not.[24] Children aged 7–12 years have an increased need for explanation and participation. Adolescents require clear explanations and assurances, and they should be allowed some decision making. The method of anaesthetic induction should be discussed with the child. Most children aged less than 8 years prefer inhalational induction rather than i.v. induction. Contact between the anaesthetist and the child before the day of surgery positively affects the quality of the anaesthetic induction and the overall experience of the child. Simple procedures, such as allowing the child choices, for example to 'help hold the mask in place', are often effective in avoiding difficult inductions. Patients who experience smooth anaesthetic inductions have a 50–70% reduction in the incidence of postoperative emotional consequences.[25]

During the preoperative visit, the anaesthetist should anticipate questions from both children and parents regarding postoperative pain and its relief.[21,22,26,27] Although there is a general tendency towards improving postoperative pain management, the occurrence of moderate to severe pain still appears to be a realistic fear for children and a common outcome after surgery.[28] It is been demonstrated that unrelieved pain is associated with both negative physical effects, including postoperative complications, slower wound healing, infection and suppressed insulin response, and psychological effects, such as development of maladaptive behaviours and distrustful attitudes toward health-care providers. Moreover, the expected benefits of effective pain management include earlier mobilization, shortened hospital stay and reduced costs. Patient-controlled analgesia (PCA) is a useful way of providing pain relief for children after major surgery providing the patients are selected appropriately. In order to benefit from PCA a child must: (1) have the ability to push the button; (2) understand the relationship between pushing the button and medication delivery; (3) trust that the amount of medication being delivered is in a safe range; and (4) understand that expected outcome is pain control, not elimination of pain. In some cases children as young as 4–5 years of age are able to use a PCA pump correctly, but in general patients should be aged 8 years or over to benefit fully from the technique. The method should be explained to both children and parents during the preoperative visit. Parents should be instructed not to press the button, which has to be activated only by the child.

In addition to personal contact with the anaesthetist, other methods may be helpful to prepare children for anaesthesia. Viewing a peer modelling film was associated with a decrease in the children's hospital physiological anxiety response preoperatively, and with a lower incidence of undesirable posthospital behaviour.[19] A videotape showing induction of anaesthesia procedure, information about paediatric anaesthesia and a discussion of the risks of injury and death during anaesthesia was demonstrated to be helpful for parents in reducing concern before outpatient surgery.[29]

IS PARENTAL PRESENCE AT INDUCTION OF ANAESTHESIA BENEFICIAL?

It has long been recognized that forced separation from the mother is a traumatic and disorganizing experience, especially for the younger child.[30] Thus, it has become routine in many hospitals to allow a parent to remain with the child during induction of anaesthesia.[31,32] However, wide discrepancies exist between countries and practices. In the UK, a parent is allowed to be present at induction of anaesthesia in most paediatric centres as a part of routine practice.[33,34] By contrast, only 50% of paediatric anaesthetists in the USA allow parents to be present at their child's induction.[35] In a recent survey, Kain[36] reported that the majority of US anaesthetists did not allow parental presence at induction because they did not feel that it was useful. In France, parental presence is limited to some small units and not usual practice in most busy centres.

While allowing parents to be present at induction of anaesthesia avoids distress on separation from parents, other potential benefits such as reducing the child's anxiety during induction or affecting long-term behaviour after surgery remain unproved.[37,38] Furthermore, recent reports indicate that parental presence may not always be beneficial.[6,39,40] Bevan et al.,[6] in a randomized trial, found that parental presence had no effect on the behaviour of the child during induction. Further, when parental behaviour was introduced as a covariable, the most upset children were those who were accompanied by extremely anxious parents. Children of calm parents did not differ in their mood as a result of having a parent accompany them during induction. Vessey et al.[39] determined the features of induction most upsetting to parents participating in induction of anaesthesia of their children. The most important factors were (1) separation from the child after induction; (2) watching/feeling the child go limp during induction; and (3) seeing the child upset before induction. More recently, Kain et al.[40] conducted a randomized, controlled trial to determine whether or not parental presence during induction is an effective behavioural intervention. When the intervention group (parent present) was compared with the control group (parent absent), there were no overall significant differences in any of the behavioural or physiological measures of anxiety tested during induction of anaesthesia. Only children who were older than 4 years, those whose parent was not anxious or who had a low baseline level of activity benefited from parental presence during induction.

From these studies, it is clear that the individual child, parent and anaesthetist must be considered when the question of parental presence at induction arises. In a recent survey on practices across the UK, all departments permitted parental presence at induction for elective surgery, but the decision about whether a parent should be present for induction of anaesthesia was left to the individual anaesthetist.[34] When parental presence is encouraged, parents should be selected carefully. The following exclusion criteria were proposed by Hannallah and Epstein:[41] infants of less than 1 year of age, serious pre-existing disease, emergency, adolescent not wishing parents to be present at induction, extremely anxious parents and any mandatory indication for premedication. In addition, the hospital should have adequate nursing resources to provide an escort for the parent and the theatre suite should be equipped with induction rooms. The latter factor limits parental presence at induction in many hospitals. For example, a recent survey indicates that only 25% of Australian hospitals have adequate facilities.[42]

Special concerns with repeated anaesthesia

Children with cancer, leukaemia and chronic disease such as cystic fibrosis or sickle cell anaemia often require repeated anaesthesia for minor or major procedures. In order to minimize distress, anxiety and fears associated with repeated anaesthesia, the preoperative visit should be personalized. Ideally, a long-term relationship has to be established with the same anaesthetist and founded on mutual trust. Unfortunately, this is not always feasible, but the anaesthetist should be aware of the child's history before their first meeting. The first contact and the first anaesthetic are of primary importance for the ongoing relationship. An initial bad experience will remain an obstacle to the development of a trustful relationship. Conversely, a good relationship may contribute to improving the child's compliance with treatment. The psychological adjustment of children and adolescents with cancer has not been well addressed in the literature.[43] The need for systemic assessment of pain throughout the course of an illness has been emphasized recently, and general anaesthesia is one of the choices for alleviating pain during medical procedures in children with cancer or chronic diseases.[44-46] Those children who have had multiple procedures usually know the process of anaesthesia induction, and they should have the choice of the technique whenever possible. They have a tendency to ritualize the induction down to the smallest detail in order to feel secure. They are usually very concerned with postoperative pain relief as well as the discomfort of bowel paralysis after laparotomy. Assurance should be given of adequate postoperative pain relief and the chosen technique (PCA, epidural catheter, etc.) should be described and explained. Children with chronic disease often show considerable interest in and knowledge of technical details, and they are usually good candidates for PCA techniques.

IMMEDIATE CLINICAL EVALUATION

MEDICAL HISTORY

On the morning of surgery, the anaesthetist should address the question of ongoing or recent illness that may have consequences for the proposed anaesthetic.[47] During the winter, upper respiratory tract infection (URTI) is a common condition in preschool children, and several studies have focused on the increased anaesthesia-related morbidity in children with a recent history of URTI.[48-53] In 1979, McGill *et al.*[48] reported 11 cases of acute pulmonary complications during induction of anaesthesia in children. All but one child had URTI within a few days of surgery. In 1988, DeSoto *et al.*[50] observed that the incidence of oxygen desaturation after anaesthesia for ENT procedures was significantly increased in children with URTI compared with those without URTI; Kinouchi *et al.*[54] demonstrated that the presence of URTI was an additional factor increasing the susceptibility of small children to hypoxaemia. Finally, Cohen *et al.*[49] surveyed more than 20 000 anaesthesia records and clearly demonstrated that the presence of URTI-increased anaesthesia morbidity in children. The risk of perioperative respiratory complications was 4–7 times higher in symptomatic children, and 11 times higher when a tracheal tube was used. The children's age, physical status score, site of operation and emergency status did not explain this elevated risk. These studies explain why it is common practice to postpone elective surgery in children with URTI. However, cancelling surgery at the last minute may be emotionally unsettling, inconvenient and costly, and may have an impact on the efficiency of the operating department. In a recent American survey,[55] 34.5% of the respondents reported that they seldom (1–25% of the time) cancelled cases because of URTI, and 20.9% stated that they usually (76–99% of the time) cancelled in the event of URTI. Factors that were considered most important in making the decision included the urgency of surgery and the presence of asthma. This survey contradicts the traditional dogma of routine cancellation, and reflects the wide range of opinions and approaches to this enduring clinical dilemma. In general, the presence of an elevated temperature, cough and chest signs indicative of infection involving the lower respiratory tract should prompt a postponement of elective surgery. Ideally, when elective surgery is cancelled because of the presence of URTI 3–4 weels should elapse before anaesthesia is carried out.

Medications

Information on current and past medications should be obtained. This should include the use of aspirin or other non-steroidal agents. Although there is no evidence that recent immunization affects the outcome of anaesthesia, some children exhibit systemic toxic reactions to the vaccines which commonly occur 2–3 days after diphtheria–tetanus–pertussis (DTP) and haemophilus influenza B (HiB) vaccines, but may be as late as 2 weeks after measles–mumps–rubella vaccine (MMR).[56] In general, it is advisable to avoid elective surgery during these periods. If surgery is unavoidable and a toxic reaction is present the guidelines for current URTI should be followed.

Known allergies

Allergies to drugs and other substances should be noted. Allergic or immediate reactions to natural latex have been reported with increasing frequency since their first description in 1979. As an example, the incidence of such reactions in surgical patients in France was as low as 0.5% in 1984–1989, increasing to 12% in 1991–1992 and 19% in 1993–1994.[57] In children, the overall incidence of anaphylaxis is similar to that observed in adults (1 : 7500 vs 1 : 6000 anaesthesia), but latex anaphylaxis is responsible for 75% of anaphylactic reactions, whereas anaphylaxis to myorelaxants still remains the major cause of anaphylaxis in adults.[58] A group

of high-risk patients has been described. This includes patients with spina bifida and bladder exstrophy, and should be extended to all patients undergoing multiple surgical procedures, especially those operated on in the neonatal period.[59,60] Atopy and frequent exposure to latex are independent risk factors for sensitization to latex, but act synergistically so that the cumulative risk is very high. In the two large paediatric series,[58,59] 62% and 77% of children with latex allergy had a history of drug allergy or atopy, respectively. Susceptible patients should benefit from a 'latex-free' environment when surgery is planned.[61] The role of the preoperative visit is crucial to identify at-risk patients.[62]

Previous anaesthetic experiences

Information about difficulties or complications encountered in previous anaesthetic experiences should be obtained, especially those related to intubation or respiratory or cardiovascular compromise. Also important are events that may have been influenced by anaesthesia, such as nausea and vomiting.

Family history

Anaesthetic-related complications such as malignant hyperthermia or prolonged paralysis after an anaesthetic (pseudocholinesterase deficiency) are sought. A family history of bleeding tendencies, muscular dystrophy or drug use is also significant.

PHYSICAL EXAMINATION

Emphasis of the examination should be on the airway (adequate mouth opening, loose teeth, etc.), cardiovascular, respiratory and neurological systems and the body system that is pertinent to the specific operation. Most of the abnormal conditions are described in Chapter 1; only some common clinical conditions will be discussed here.

Cardiovascular system

Previously unrecognized heart murmurs are not uncommonly discovered[63] but most of them are functional or 'innocent' murmurs. Innocent murmurs are most commonly recognized around 3–4 years of age, and their incidence declines with increasing age. They are generally no longer detectable when auscultation is performed after changing body position (i.e. standing to supine position). In general, the child with a murmur who has normal S1 and S2 and normal exercise tolerance is acyanotic and will tolerate general anaesthesia without complications. If there is any unanswered question regarding a cardiac abnormality, preoperative echocardiography and evaluation by a paediatric cardiologist should be suggested. Prophylaxis against bacterial endocarditis should be planned in children with known cardiac abnormalities (Appendix 4).[63]

Respiratory system

Significant abnormalities of the airway, such as reduced neck and jaw mobility, micrognathia, glossoptosis or reduced mouth opening should be recognized as they may be responsible for difficult tracheal intubation. Reactive airway diseases are common during infancy and childhood. They should be as well controlled as possible before planned anaesthesia. Children with obstructive sleep apnoea related to hypertrophied adenoids and tonsils should be meticulously evaluated before surgery. Adenotonsillectomy usually results in marked long-term improvement but children should be closely monitored in the perioperative period. Major spinal deformities are often associated with restrictive lung disease that requires careful evaluation for planning the perioperative period.

Neuromuscular system

Children on anticonvulsant therapy should receive their medication on the morning of surgery. If a prolonged fasting period is anticipated postoperatively, plans must be made for maintenance anticonvulsant therapy. Children with functioning ventricular shunts do not need special preparation. However, one should look for signs of elevated intracranial pressure (vomiting, irritability, sleepiness or personality changes) in children requiring shunt placement or revision of an obstructed shunt. Undiagnosed myopathies may lead to

severe adverse anaesthetic interactions (e.g. hyperkalaemic cardiac arrest after suxamethonium). Neuromuscular examination is usually suggested in children presenting with blepharoptosis (drooping eyelids), which may be an early sign of muscular weakness.

Following the preoperative assessment, the anaesthetist should make a formal assessment of the risk of anaesthesia using the ASA grading system. In addition, it may be advisable to note any special precautions that are considered necessary for the safe conduct of anaesthesia.

PREOPERATIVE INVESTIGATIONS

In recent years, the value of screening tests in otherwise healthy surgical patients has been re-examined.[64] Preoperative laboratory tests are now most often used for specific diagnostic purposes or to establish important baseline values. Although there are no uniform guidelines for the use of preoperative laboratory tests in paediatric patients, the following discussion of some specific tests may help to address common questions.[47,65]

Haemoglobin determination

Although severe anaemia can usually be suspected in children during a careful preoperative clinical evaluation, mild degrees of anaemia can be missed without laboratory testing.[66] When anaemia is defined as a haemoglobin (Hb) value < 10 g dl^{-1}, its incidence appears to be about 0.5%.[67] This prevalence might be higher in patients with low socioeconomic backgrounds.[68] Therefore, it has been proposed that 'routine' preoperative haemoglobin testing is indicated only for: (1) infants < 1 year of age; (2) children at risk of sickle cell disease who have never been tested; and (3) children with systemic disease.[65,69,70] In addition, Hb concentration should be measured to establish a reference point in anticipation of significant surgical blood loss.[71]

Urinalysis

Routine microscopic and chemical testing of urine is insufficiently sensitive and too non-specific to be of clinical value in detecting asymptomatic disease that would have an impact on perioperative management. Indeed, routine urinalysis adds little to the preoperative evaluation of the healthy child.[68] It may be indicated in patients with renal or urinary tract abnormalities.

Chest radiograph

Many studies have clearly demonstrated that preoperative chest radiography revealed few clinically important abnormalities that were not suggested by history and clinical evaluation.[72,73] Therefore, in 1983, the American Academy of Pediatrics recommended the abandonment of routine preoperative chest radiography.[74]

Coagulation screening

Coagulation screening remains the most debated of all laboratory tests. Although an undiagnosed coagulopathy could result in serious surgical morbidity, commonly used screening tests, such as bleeding time, prothrombin time, activated partial thromboplastin time and platelet count, do not reliably predict abnormal perioperative bleeding.[75–77]

Laboratory testing should be considered in patients in whom either the history or medical condition suggests a possible haemostatic defect (see below), in patients undergoing surgical procedures that might induce haemostatic disturbances (e.g. cardiopulmonary bypass), when a normal coagulation system is particularly needed for adequate haemostasis (e.g. adenoidectomy and tonsillectomy),[78] and in patients in whom even minimal postoperative bleeding could be critical (e.g. patients undergoing neurosurgery). In addition to bleeding tendency, parents should be asked about recent ingestion of aspirin or other non-steroidal anti-inflammatory drugs. Adequate history of bleeding tendency might be difficult to obtain from parents with poor language skills, or in young children below 2–3 years of age. With these patients, routine coagulation screening should be performed if possible defects are suspected. Even with careful history taking, mild forms of von Willebrand's disease, platelet dysfunction or factor deficiency (e.g. factor XI) may easily be missed. In the case of minor surgery and a negative history of clotting disorders, no tests are suggested in children over 3 years of age. It is accepted that there will be a few patients who will have more bleeding than anticipated because of a haemostatic defect, despite a negative family history. In cases in which the decision is made to obtain preoperative coagulation tests, a small number of patients with negative bleeding history will have prolonged partial thromboplastin times. Surgery in these patients should be postponed until the defect is defined, although in the majority of cases the defect is found not to be related to a clinical bleeding disorder.

PREOPERATIVE FASTING

Preoperative fasting has been a prerequisite for elective surgery since the demonstration by Mendelson of a link between feeding and pulmonary aspiration of gastric contents in parturients.[79] However, recent work has shown that prolonged fasting does not reduce the risk of aspiration pneumonitis during anaesthesia and has highlighted the need to avoid regurgitation of gastric contents. This has led to a reduction in fasting times and a greater appreciation of the several risk factors for regurgitation and aspiration.[80,81] Reduced fasting increases patient comfort and hydration and reduces the potential for hypoglycaemia during anaesthesia in neonates aged less than 48 h.[82]

PATHOPHYSIOLOGY OF REGURGITATION

Regurgitation may be defined as the passive flow of gastric contents from the stomach into the oesophagus. Normally, this is prevented by the lower oesophageal sphincter (LOS), an indistinct portion of the lower oesophagus with a high resting tone. The stomach is very distensible and in the adult human can accommodate 1600 ml of air or 1000 ml of food with little increase in pressure.[83] Thus, it would appear that the small residual gastric volumes found normally at induction of anaesthesia do not increase the risk of regurgitation.[84] Infants may be at greater risk of regurgitation as a result of a relative lack of intra-abdominal oesophagus resulting in an abnormal LOS.[85,86] Anaesthetic factors that may increase the risk in this age group include inadvertent inflation of the stomach during ventilation with a face mask and partial airway obstruction during mask anaesthesia. Thus, endotracheal anaesthesia should reduce the risk of regurgitation in infants. Specific conditions which predispose to perioperative regurgitation in both infants and children include pre-existing gastro-oeso-phageal reflux, bowel obstruction, physical injury, narcotics, obesity, prone, lateral or head down position, ascites and emergency surgery. In these cases manoeuvres to reduce the risk of regurgitation and aspiration, such as a nasogastric tube, antacids, rapid sequence induction or awake intubation should be considered.

PATHOGENESIS OF ASPIRATION PNEUMONITIS

Mendelson described two aspiration syndromes in his study of 44 016 parturient patients.[79] The first was inhalation of solid food leading to complete airway obstruction and death in three patients and massive atelectasis in two patients. The other syndrome was aspiration of liquid gastric contents resulting in chemical pneumo-nitis (Mendelson's syndrome). This occurred in 40 patients, all of whom recovered. Mendelson also demonstrated that the acidity of the aspirate was the important factor in the development of aspiration pneumonitis in rabbits, and Teabeaut showed that the syndrome did not appear unless the pH was less than 2.5.[87] In rhesus monkeys, the syndrome occurs only when the pH of the aspirate is less than 2.5 and its volume is greater than 0.4 mg kg^{-1}.[88,89] When these criteria are applied to the gastric aspirates of children fasted prior to anaesthesia, up to 76% are found to be at risk of pulmonary aspiration syndrome.[90,91] The fact that pulmonary aspiration is rare in children (1–9 per 10 000 anaesthetics) may be interpreted as evidence of the significant role of regurgitation in its pathogenesis.[92,93]

MINIMUM FASTING PERIOD

Preoperative fasting does not guarantee an empty stomach; its aim is to ensure the minimum residual gastric volume at induction of anaesthesia. The duration of fast required to achieve the minimum gastric volume depends on the nature of the last intake. In adults, solid food leaves the stomach in a linear fashion with time and 10–30% may be left after 6 h.[94] Liquid contents leave the stomach in an exponential fashion. The half-time for water is about 12 min, which implies that 95% of ingested water will leave the stomach in 1 h. In babies, breast milk leaves the stomach more rapidly than formula. The half-time for breast milk is about 25 min, while that for formula is 51 min.[95,96]

There is now a large body of evidence to show that free intake of clear fluids (defined as those through which it is possible to read newsprint) up to 2 h preoperatively does not affect the pH or volume of gastric contents at induction of anaesthesia in children[97–101] or adults.[102,103] Although many of these studies can be criticized for lacking adequate controls and/or sample sizes, a meta-analysis of 12 adult studies did not change the main conclusion that intake of clear fluids up to 2 h preoperatively was safe.[104] While there have been relatively few studies in infants, these suggest that infants may be allowed clear fluids up to 2 h and breast milk 4 h preoperatively.[105,106] There is also evidence that infants aged less than 3 months may safely be given infant formula (cow's milk) up to 4 h preoperatively.[105] By contrast, there is little evidence to support a reduction in the present 6-h fasting time for cow's milk or solid food in older infants and children. In the only paediatric study in which solid food was allowed within 6 h of anaesthesia, food residue was found in the aspirates 13 of 32 children fed within 4 h of operation and three of 18 children fed 4–6 h preoperatively.[107] No food residue was found in the aspirates of 20 children fasted for longer than 6 h. Children given solid food within 6 h of an operation may therefore be at increased risk of airway obstruction due to aspiration of food particles. Table 2.1 reflects current practices in many hospitals regarding fasting times for infants and children.

COMPLIANCE

Compliance with fasting guidelines is a potential problem whether preoperative fluids are allowed

Table 2.1 Preoperative fasting times for different types of liquids and solids

	Minimum fasting period (h)			
	Clear fluids	Breast milk	Formula or cow's milk	Solids
Children	2	–	6	6
Infants aged 3–12 months	2	4	6	6
Infants aged < 3 months	2	4	4	6

or not. Although one study suggested that liberalization of fluid could lead to non-compliance for solid food this has not been confirmed.[108] On the contrary, parents of children allowed clear fluid up to 2 h preoperatively reported less difficulty in adhering to preoperative feeding instructions, rated their children as less irritable and rated the overall peroperative experience as better than did the parents of controls.[99] Furthermore, when children inadvertently ingested clear fluid within 2 h of their operation this resulted in only moderate delays to surgery (30–60 min) and no cancellations. While most anaesthetists are now convinced that a clear drink 2 h before surgery is safe, concerns about reduced flexibility in the timing of operations have led some to recommend a 3-h fluid fast.[109,110] In the authors' experience this is a difficult policy to implement since it is has no physiological basis and may lead to non-compliance by medical and nursing staff. An alternative method, which is also suitable for day-case patients, is to instruct nursing staff (or parents) to give the last clear drink 2 h before the scheduled starting time of the operating list (e.g. before 07.00 h for 09.00 h list; 12.00 h for 14.00 h list). Children scheduled late on operating lists may then be allowed a further clear drink at the discretion of the anaesthetist.

EMERGENCY ANAESTHESIA

Pulmonary aspiration is about five times more common during emergency anaesthesia than with elective anaesthesia.[111] Fasting reduces the residual gastric volume of children presenting for emergency surgery, but does not affect pH.[112] In children presenting for emergency trauma surgery, the gastric volume at induction of anaesthesia has been shown to be more clearly related to the interval between food and injury than to the total fasting period.[113] However, neither of these relationships was reliable enough to define a safe fasting period. These studies suggest that, in general, fasting for 6 h should reduce the risk of aspiration in children presenting for emergency surgery. However, a short duration of fast does not contraindicate anaesthesia in the presence of a clear surgical indication for early operation. The use of drugs to increase gastric motility is discussed on p. 179. Anaesthetic management of all emergency cases should proceed on the assumption that the child has a full stomach.

PREMEDICATION

Historically, premedication was a necessity for the safe conduct of anaesthesia.[114] Writing in 1938, Waters recommended that children, like the adult patients of that time, should be premedicated with morphine and hyoscine.[115] As most muscle relaxation was provided by volatile anaesthetics, morphine was used to decrease the amount of volatile anaesthetic required and improve cardiovascular stability. The use of hyoscine as a drying agent was also extremely important at a period when ether was the principal volatile anaesthetic agent. With the introduction of muscle relaxants and newer anaesthetic agents with less propensity for airway irritation, the necessity for this type of premedication in children has largely disappeared. Although premedicants may still be indicated to improve the safety of paediatric anaesthesia (e.g. the use of H_2 receptor antagonists such as cimetidine in patients at increased risk of gastroesophageal reflux during induction of anaesthesia) they are much more likely to be used to reduce the stress of anaesthesia and surgery and the attendant risk of postoperative behavioural disturbances.

Patients of different ages vary in their response to the psychological stress of anaesthesia and surgery. Infants aged less than 6 months have not yet developed a fear of strangers and appear relatively undisturbed when separated from their mothers. Accordingly, sedative premedication is not indicated in young infants, who may also be particularly sensitive to its respiratory and cardiovascular depressant effects. Preschool children appear to be the most vulnerable to emotional upset. They can experience separation anxiety and anticipate pain on the basis of past experiences, but often they cannot understand the explanations offered by doctors and nurses. Sedative premedication is particularly useful in this group, reducing both the level of anxiety at induction of anaesthesia and the incidence of postoperative behavioural changes. Fear of needles is common to children of all ages;[116,117] accordingly, when prescribing a premedicant, the intramuscular route should be avoided whenever possible. Similarly, local anaesthetic creams or gels should be applied to the skin over intended venepuncture sites when intravenous induction of anaesthesia is planned.

A survey of the UK-based members of the Association of Anaesthetists in 1991 revealed that 84% of respondents used sedative premedicants in children, although only 15% used them frequently in day-case patients.[118] Major changes since the previous survey in 1978 were a reduction in the use of anticholinergic drugs and the greater use of oral premedicants. The most commonly used drug in children was trimeprazine, being used by 67% of respondents, followed by 12% using diazepam and 7% using papaveretum. Recently, midazolam has become popular in many centres in the UK, following the trend in the USA. In a postal survey of 5396 US anaesthetists undertaken in 1997, more than 80% of respondents stated that they used midazolam when premedicating children; the remaining correspondents used mainly ketamine (4%) and transmucosal fentanyl (3%).[119] Decreased anxiety and increased co-operation were rated as the most important indications for premedication. About 80% of respondents premedicated their paediatric patients using the oral route; others used the intranasal route (8%), the intramuscular route (6%) or the rectal route (3%).

LOCAL ANAESTHETICS

The availability of effective local anaesthetic preparations has greatly facilitated intravenous induction of anaesthesia in children. Not only are these preparations effective in reducing the pain of venepuncture at induction of anaesthesia, but their use provides considerable emotional reassurance to children in the immediate preoperative period. Careful consideration should be given to the use of these preparations in infants who derive no psychological benefit and who may be at increased risk of complications.

EMLA cream 5% is a eutectic mixture of local anaesthetics containing 25 mg g^{-1} of prilocaine and 25 mg g^{-1} of lignocaine in an oily base.[120] This mixture of crystalline bases of lignocaine and prilocaine has a lower melting point than the melting point of the individual drugs and is a liquid at room temperature. The high concentration of active bases in the mixture (up to 80%), a small relatively uniform droplet diameter (1 μm) and the fact that the drugs are present in a liquid phase all promote skin penetration. The efficacy of EMLA cream in reducing the pain of venepuncture and venous cannulation in children has been established in several randomized placebo controlled trials.[121-123] EMLA has also been shown to be as effective as intradermal infiltration of lignocaine in producing analgesia prior to venous cannulation in children.[124] Interestingly, in this last study, patient co-operation did not improve with pain-free conditions, emphasizing the significance of the emotional component of anticipated pain in children.[7]

EMLA cream is supplied in 5 g tubes containing sufficient local anaesthetic cream for two applications. A thick layer of the cream (about 2 g) is applied under an occlusive dressing at least 60 min before induction of anaesthesia. Analgesic efficacy may decline if the skin application time is longer than 5 h. EMLA is not licensed for infants under 1 year of age. Local skin reactions such as pallor, erythema and itching are common following EMLA but are generally mild and transient. More serious complications include aspiration of the occlusive dressing with resulting respiratory obstruction and ingestion of the cream, giving rise to the possibility of local anaesthetic toxicity.[125] The application of a secondary protective dressing of crêpe bandage may help to prevent such incidents. Absorbed prilocaine may cause methaemoglobinaemia. The highest reported concentration of methaemoglobin occurred in an infant of 3 months who became cyanosed after application of 5 g of the cream for 5 h. His methaemoglobin concentration was 28%, although this may have been partly due to concomitant sulfonamide therapy. Engberg and colleagues measured plasma methaemoglobin concentrations in 22 infants aged 3–12 months after application of 2 g of EMLA for 2–4 h.[126] Methaemoglobin concentrations remained in the normal range (< 2%). Small but significant increases in methaemoglobin concentrations have been found in children aged 1–6 years following routine administration of 5 g of EMLA.[127] Although the mean maximum methaemoglobin concentration was well within safe limits (0.85%) the finding of an increased concentration 24 h later suggests that cumulative effects may occur in children receiving the cream daily.

Amethocaine: There are pharmacological and experimental grounds for considering amethocaine to be a more appropriate local anaesthetic than lignocaine or prilocaine for the provision of percutaneous analgesia.[128,129] Specifically, the relatively high lipid solubility of amethocaine should aid penetration of the epidermis, resulting in rapid onset of action. High affinity for neural tissue and a high degree of protein binding should favour prolonged clinical activity, while rapid clearance of amethocaine by esterases in the skin and plasma should make systemic toxicity unlikely.

Doyle and colleagues evaluated a self-adhesive patch preparation of amethocaine for topical analgesia prior to venous cannulation in 189 children.[130] Satisfactory analgesia was found in 80% of children after application times of 45–60 min. Subsequently, Lawson and colleagues compared an amethocaine gel preparation with EMLA for alleviation of the pain of venous cannulation in 148 children.[131] They found that the amethocaine gel had a more rapid onset of action and greater efficacy than EMLA. This preparation, now available commercially as *Ametop gel*, contains 40 mg ml^{-1} of amethocaine base (4% w/w). It is supplied in 1.5 g tubes designed to deliver about 1 g of amethocaine gel to the proposed venepuncture site, which is then covered by an occlusive dressing. Onset of analgesia occurs in about 30 min. Side-effects appear to be few, but precautions against ingestion or misapplication of the gel, such as those suggested for EMLA, would seem advisable. Slight erythema at the application site as a result of local vasodilation in about 40% of patients is said to make venous cannulation easier. Ametop gel is licensed for infants and children over 1 month of age.

TRANQUILLIZERS

This group of drugs includes the phenothiazines, butyrophenones and benzodiazepines. These drugs characteristically relieve tension and anxiety without producing undue sedation. The phenothiazines and butyrophenones are classified as major tranquillizers (or neuroleptics), while the benzodiazepines are classed as minor tranquillizers.

Benzodiazepines

Benzodiazepine derivatives are widely used for premedicating children. They are given to allay anxiety and diminish recall of perianaesthetic events. At the doses used for premedication, sedation and cardiovascular or respiratory depression are minimal. The drugs are believed to facilitate the binding of the inhibitory neurotransmitter γ-aminobutyric acid (GABA) to its receptors in the central nervous system (CNS).[132]

Midazolam is a short-acting water-soluble benzodiazepine with an elimination half-life of about 2 h, which is suitable for premedicating paediatric patients undergoing either day-case or inpatient surgery. It may be administered by a variety of routes each having its own advantages and disadvantages. It is well absorbed intramuscularly in a dose of 0.1–0.2 mg kg^{-1}, but the pain and anxiety associated with intramuscular injection generally precludes the use of this route in children.[133–135] If parenteral administration is desired and the child has an intravenous line *in situ*, midazolam 0.1–0.2 mg kg^{-1} can be given intravenously. Rectal instillation of 0.4–0.5 mg kg^{-1} is reliable and painless but some children (and their parents) may find the procedure distressing.[136,137] Intranasal administration of midazolam 0.2 mg kg^{-1} elicits a rapid response, although the burning sensation produced causes the child to cry in the majority of cases.[138,139] Sublingual midazolam in a dose of 0.2 mg kg^{-1} appears to be well tolerated and is effective within 10 min.[140] Oral administration of mid-azolam is widely used and is acceptable and effective in children.[141–148] The usual dose for children weighing over 20 kg is 0.5 mg kg^{-1} (maximum 20 mg), which is given 30–45 min preoperatively; children weighing less than 20 kg may be given 0.75 mg kg^{-1}. Anxiolytic and sedative effects are apparent within 20 min[148] and peak at 30–45 min.[143]

In addition to promoting smooth and satisfactory induction of anaesthesia, midazolam premedication has been shown to reduce the incidence of postoperative behavioural disturbances in children undergoing day-case and inpatient surgery.[149–151] In one of these studies, the incidence of postoperative behavioural disturbances in paediatric surgical outpatients premedicated with midazolam was 17% compared with 52% in a comparable group treated with a placebo.[150] This effect of midazolam may be due to its powerful anterograde amnesic properties.[152]

The short duration of action of midazolam means that the effect of the drug may wear off if surgery is delayed beyond 1 h. Recovery from anaesthesia and discharge from hospital following day-case surgery may also take slightly longer in children given midazolam compared with a placebo, although these delays should not seriously disrupt ward routine.[150] A further disadvantage of the use of oral midazolam is its bitter taste, which can be difficult to disguise, and the absence of an approved oral formulation. An acceptable 0.1% midazolam syrup can be made up by the hospital pharmacy by adding the appropriate volume of midazolam injection to syrup BP which contains methyl hydroxybenzoate as an antimicrobial preservative; this formulation has been shown to be stable at room temperature for up to 6 weeks.[153] Alternatively, 0.5 mg kg^{-1} of midazolam can be mixed with a dose of 15–20 mg kg^{-1} of paracetamol syrup (Calpol) and used immediately.

Diazepam is a long-acting benzodiazepine with a half-life of 20–50 h in adults. Absorption from the gastrointestinal tract is reliable and peak plasma concentrations occur in 1–2 h. It is available for use in children as a flavoured syrup containing 2 mg in 5 ml. The usual dose for premedication is 0.2–0.3 mg kg^{-1}, which should be given 60–90 min preoperatively. In a randomized, controlled trial, diazepam 0.25 mg kg^{-1} with droperidol 0.25 mg kg^{-1} produced less satisfactory anxiolysis scores at induction of anaesthesia compared with mid-azolam 0.5 mg kg^{-1}.[154] Diazepam in tablet form provides a useful alternative to midazolam for premedicating older children.

Lorazepam is about five times more potent than diazepam and produces a greater degree of amnesia.[155] Despite having a shorter half-life than diazepam (10–20 h) its duration of action is longer, possibly reflecting a greater affinity of lorazepam for benzodiazepine receptors.[156] Following oral administration maximal blood concentrations occur in 2–4 h and persist at therapeutic levels for 24–48 h. The usual dose for premedication is 50 μg kg^{-1}, which should be given 2 h preoperatively.[157] The relatively slow onset and long duration of action of lorazepam may be an advantage if surgery is delayed, but make it unsuitable for use in day-case patients.

Temazepam is a short-acting, water-insoluble benzodiazepine which is supplied as 10 mg capsules and a mint-flavoured alcohol based elixir containing 10 mg per 5 ml. The usual dose for premedication is 1 mg kg^{-1} (maximum 20 mg) given 1 h before anaesthesia. In view of its short duration of action, temazepam would appear to be an alternative to midazolam as a premedicant for paediatric day-case anaesthesia. However, a randomized controlled trial failed to show a significant difference in preinduction sedation scores between 29 children given temazepam and 27 children given a placebo.[158] Also, a report that temazepam elixir (but not the capsules) significantly increases gastric volume at induction of anaesthesia is a possible cause for concern.[107]

Phenothiazines

Phenothiazine derivatives have also been widely used as premedicants in children. Their clinical effects include sedation, anxiolysis, antiemesis, H_2 receptor blockade and anticholinergic properties. As these drugs produce their CNS effects by competitive antagonism of dopaminergic receptors in the basal ganglia and limbic portions of the brain, their use can be associated with extrapyramidal side-effects.

Trimeprazine is a long-acting phenothiazine derivative with sedative, anticholinergic and antiemetic properties. Its anticholinergic and antihistaminic actions are probably responsible for an observed increase in pH and decrease in the volume of gastric contents at induction of anaesthesia in children premedicated with trimeprazine.[107] Trimeprazine is available as a palatable peach-flavoured syrup containing 30 mg per 5 ml (Vallergan Forte). The recommended dose for premedication is 2 mg kg^{-1}, which should be given 90 min prior to anaesthesia.

Although popular as a premedicant for children in the UK since its introduction by Cope and Glover in 1959,[159] trimeprazine began to lose favour in the 1980s following reports of respiratory and cardiovascular depression after its use in doses up to 4 mg kg^{-1}.[160,161] Largely in response to these reports, the manufacturers reduced the recommended dose for premedication from 4 to 2 mg kg^{-1}, which is often insufficient to produce sedation.[162,163] In a recent study, children premedicated with trimeprazine 3 mg kg^{-1} were found to have significantly worse anxiolysis scores both on arrival at the anaesthetic room and at induction of anaesthesia compared with children premedicated with midazolam 0.5 mg kg^{-1}.[154] In addition, significantly more children who received trimeprazine were distressed or crying at induction of anaesthesia than children who were given midazolam. In another study, more children premedicated with trimeprazine 2 mg kg^{-1} or a placebo were distressed or crying on arrival at the anaesthetic room compared with children premedicated with midazolam 0.5 mg kg^{-1}.[164] These studies suggest that trimeprazine is a less effective oral premedicant for children than midazolam.

Promethazine (Phenergan) has sedative, antihistaminic, antimotion sickness and anticholinergic effects. In the USA it was commonly administered with narcotic premedicants in a dose of 0.5–1.0 mg kg^{-1} 1 h preoperatively to control nausea and vomiting.[165] It has never achieved great popularity as a paediatric premedicant in the UK, although it is sometimes used as a sedative and drying agent.

Butyrophenones

Droperidol is a substituted butyrophenone closely resembling haloperidol and certain phenothiazine derivatives. It is the most commonly used drug of this class for premedication. Droperidol has good sedative and antiemetic properties, but is only weakly anxiolytic; hence, in paediatric trials the preoperative calming effects of droperidol alone were not significantly different from those of a placebo.[166,167] It has mainly been used in combination with other premedicant drugs for its antiemetic effect.[145,154,166–169] The usual dose is 0.05–0.1 mg kg^{-1} orally, given 1 h preoperatively. In view of its poor anxiolytic properties and the high incidence of extrapyramidal reactions occurring after its use in some studies (2–8%), there has been a suggestion that its use as a premedicant in children should in future be limited.[170]

BARBITURATES

Short and ultra-short-acting barbiturates have been widely used for paediatric premedication in the USA. Their main clinical effect is to induce sleep by depressing the reticular activating system, but those children who remain awake may be more difficult to manage at induction of anaesthesia as a result of restlessness or confusion.[171] As most anaesthetists now prefer their paediatric patients to be awake and calm preoperatively, the use of these agents as premedicants has declined.

Pentobarbitone is a short-acting barbiturate that produces effective sedation in 1–2 h after oral or rectal administration of 2–5 mg kg^{-1}. It has frequently been used in combination with an opioid prior to inpatient surgery. In a comparative study of patients with congenital cyanotic heart disease, premedication with oral midazolam 0.75 mg kg^{-1} produced greater anxiolysis at the time of separation from parents and at induction of anaesthesia compared with premedication with oral or rectal pentobarbitone 2 mg kg^{-1} followed by i.m. morphine 0.2 mg kg^{-1} and atropine 0.2 mg kg^{-1}.[148] The authors concluded that oral midazolam was as effective as the older two-step premedication regimen using pentobarbitone and morphine, and avoided the need for a distressing intramuscular injection.

Thiopentone was the first ultra-short-acting barbiturate to be used as a premedicant for children. A suppository of approximately 30 mg kg^{-1} produces sleep in two-thirds of children in 15 min.[172] At this dose termination of effect is partially dependent on elimination, which for thiopentone is relatively slow (mean elimination half-time in children 6.1 h).[173] Delayed recovery from anaesthesia is a particular disadvantage in patients undergoing short surgical procedures.

Methohexitone is another ultra-short-acting barbiturate which has been used rectally to premedicate children. Its mean elimination half-time in children is 3.2 h, and hence recovery is faster than that after thiopentone.[174] Following a dose of 25 mg kg^{-1} of methohexitone 10% rectally, sleep occurs in 8–9 min, while peak plasma concentrations occur in 14–15 min.[175] Aspiration of any drug remaining after the child is asleep will reduce postoperative drowsiness.[176] Children should be observed closely following the administration of rectal methohexitone as unpredictable absorption of the drug can lead to airway obstruction or apnoea; other disadvantages of this method include defecation and hiccups. In a large prospective study the incidence of these complications was 4%, 10% and 13%, respectively.[177] When used in day-case patients full recovery from anaesthesia may be prolonged by 15–30 min, but discharge times from hospital should not be affected.[178]

OPIOIDS

The clinical effects of opioids include analgesia, euphoria and sedation; they may also cause respiratory depression, nausea, dryness of the mouth and pruritus. They produce these effects by acting on specific opioid receptors in the brain and spinal cord. In the past, long-acting opioids such as morphine, papaveretum and pethidine were used frequently as premedicants in children with the aim of providing sedation and supplementing anaesthesia. With the recent emphasis on the production of anxiolysis and a desire to avoid painful injections there has been a decline in the use of these drugs. However, some anaesthetists are using short-acting opioids (e.g. fentanyl) by the transmucosal oral or nasal routes for their sedative effects.

Morphine The usual dose of morphine for premedication in children is 0.2 mg kg^{-1} intramuscularly which should be given 1 h preoperatively. Morphine may have special value for premedicating children with congenital heart disease, since it minimizes oxygen consumption and decreases the demands on the cardiovascular system during induction of anaesthesia.[179,180] However, intramuscular injection of morphine causes a transient decrease in oxygen saturation in these patients which does not occur after ingestion of oral midazolam.[148] Premedication with morphine increases the incidence of both preoperative and postoperative vomiting.[181,182] Although useful in special situations such as tetralogy of Fallot, where it may reduce the incidence of infundibular spasm, morphine should not be given as a routine premedicant to infants aged less than 6 months as these patients do not usually require preoperative sedation and are especially susceptible to its respiratory depressant effects. This effect is probably due to an increase in the permeability of the infant's blood–brain barrier to morphine.[183,184]

Papaveretum is a mixture of the water-soluble alkaloids of opium, which is standardized to contain 50% anhydrous morphine; the other opioids do not exert much sedative or analgesic effect.[155] The clinical effects of 20 mg of papaveretum are equivalent to 13.0 mg of morphine. The usual dose for premedication in children is 0.4 mg kg^{-1}, which is often given in combination with 8 μg kg^{-1} of hyoscine (*omnopon–scopolamine*) by intramuscular injection, 90 min preoperatively. Papaveretum should not be used to premedicate infants aged less than 6 months. It is also contraindicated in postmenarchal girls because of its possible teratogenicity.

Pethidine is another long-acting opioid drug that has been used to premedicate children. The usual dose is 1.5 mg kg^{-1} intramuscularly, 1 h preoperatively. Compared with morphine, pethidine produces less sedation and euphoria and less respiratory depression especially in infants; however, pethidine, like morphine, should not be used to premedicate young infants. Vomiting is a common complication.[185] Pethidine has also been used in a dose of 1.0–

2.0 mg kg^{-1} as an oral premedicant, either alone or in combination with other drugs. In a double blind, placebo-controlled trial, oral midazolam 0.5 mg kg^{-1} with or without atropine 0.02 mg kg^{-1} produced better anxiolysis scores at separation from parents and induction of anaesthesia compared with oral pethidine 1.5 mg kg^{-1} and atropine 0.02 mg kg^{-1}.[143] Moreover, in this study oral pethidine with atropine did not produce better sedation scores than placebo and the combination of pethidine, midazolam and atropine did not provide any significant clinical benefits compared with premedication with midazolam alone.

Fentanyl was the first in a series of synthetic opioids characterized by rapid onset and short duration of action related to high lipid solubility. Oral transmucosal fentanyl citrate (OTFC) administered as a lollipop has been shown to increase sedation, reduce anxiety and improve the quality of induction of anaesthesia in children undergoing a variety of surgical procedures.[186–190] Most studies have been undertaken in the USA where OTFC is available as a licensed propriety medication for use in children aged 2 years and over (Oralet®, Abbott Laboratories). In a dose-finding study, the optimum dose of OTFC lollipops was 15–20 μg kg^{-1}.[187] Signs of sedation appeared at around 20 min and peaked at 30–45 min. A high incidence of emesis and pruritis and occasional cases of oxygen desaturation are serious drawbacks to the use of OTFC in children. Some concern has also been expressed, particularly in the USA, about the association of the word 'lollipop' with the administration of addictive drugs. As with other opioids fentanyl should not be used to premedicate infants aged less than 6 months.

Sufentanil is a potent, short-acting opioid which has been used to premedicate children. The usual dose for premedication is 2 μg kg^{-1}, which is administered intranasally;[191] peak plasma concentrations occur in 15–30 min.[192] In a randomized, double-blind trial comparing the efficacy and safety of intranasal midazolam 0.2 mg kg^{-1} and sufentanil 2 μg kg^{-1} as premedicants in children, maximum anxiolysis occurred 10 min after drug administration in both groups.[139] Although intranasal sufentanil appeared less unpleasant to receive than fentanyl, most patients cried during instillation of the drops (> 75%). Both drugs produced good to excellent conditions for induction of anaesthesia, but the response to midazolam was less variable. Midazolam-treated patients remained well oxygenated [98% with arterial oxygen saturation (Sa,o_2) > 95%] and their lungs were easy to ventilate (96%). By contrast, 55% of sufentanil-treated patients had Sa,o_2 < 95% and the lungs of 37% were not easy to ventilate. The authors concluded that premedication with nasal midazolam is preferable to sufentanil for most patients.

OTHER SEDATIVE DRUGS

Chloral hydrate was synthesized in 1832 and apart from alcohol is the oldest hypnotic. It is rapidly hydrolysed in the body to trichlorethanol, which is the main active principle. In a comparative dose-finding study in children, premedication with chloral hydrate 75 mg kg^{-1} provided anxiolysis that was as good or better than that obtained with midazolam 0.5 mg kg^{-1}. However, many younger children found the taste of chloral hydrate unacceptable and the authors felt unable to recommend it.[146] *Triclofos*, the phosphoric ester of trichlorethanol, is also metabolized to trichloroethanol, so the two drugs have a similar action. The advantage of triclofos is that it can be made up as a pleasantly flavoured syrup. The dose for premedication is up to 70 mg kg^{-1}.[193]

Ketamine is a phencyclizine derivative with powerful analgesic, amnesic and anaesthetic activity. It is highly lipid soluble and rapidly absorbed after intravenous, intramuscular, intranasal or oral administration. As a premedicant, intramuscular injection of ketamine 2 mg kg^{-1} is occasionally useful for the very apprehensive or combative child who will not take an oral premedicant and refuses to co-operate at induction of anaesthesia. This dose provides adequate sedation for mask acceptance in such children after approximately 3 min and is not associated with excessive salivation or emergence delirium.[194] Ketamine has also been used successfully as an oral premedicant in doses of 5–6 mg kg^{-1}; onset of sedation occurs in 10–15 min and peaks at 20–25 min.[195,196] However, this dose of ketamine may be associated with increased salivation, hyperventilation, random limb movements, hallucinations and serious emergence reactions, the latter being more likely after short surgical procedures.[197–199] Children premedicated with ketamine require close observation in a quiet environment where resuscitation equipment is readily available.

Clonidine is an α_2-agonist which has been used as an oral premedicant in children. Its clinical effects include sedation, analgesia, reduction in the sleep dose of induction agents, reduction in oral secretions and antiemesis.[200,201] In a randomized, double-blind study, a dose of 4 μg kg^{-1} of clonidine given 90–120 min preoperatively produced better quality of separation from parents and mask acceptance than a dose of 2 μg kg^{-1} or a placebo.[202] However, despite the coadministration of oral atropine 0.3 mg kg^{-1}, premedication of children with clonidine 4 μg kg^{-1} was associated with a significant lowering of arterial pressure, heart rate and respiratory rate until 10 h postoperatively. Significant perioperative haemodynamic effects have also been reported in adults premedicated with clonidine.[203] Further studies are required to determine the safety and optimal dose of clonidine as a premedicant in children.

ANTICHOLINERGICS

Anticholinergic drugs may be given preoperatively to prevent reflex bradycardia and reduce airway secretions. As noted earlier, the indications for these drugs as premedicants has declined significantly in recent years as a result of the use of newer anaesthetic agents and techniques.

Atropine is the anticholinergic drug used most commonly to premedicate children.[118] The predominant choice of atropine could be based on the potent vagolytic action of this drug,[204] since prevention of bradycardia is the most important indication for its use in this age group. The dose for premedication is 0.02 mg kg^{-1} intramuscularly, which should be given 45 min preoperatively; alternatively, twice this dose (0.04 mg kg^{-1}) may be given orally 90 min preoperatively.[205,206] Because modern inhalational anaesthetics are less irritant to the airways, many anaesthetists omit premedication with atropine, preferring instead to give 0.02 mg kg^{-1} of the drug intravenously when indicated: e.g. at induction of anaesthesia if suxamethonium is to be given, or during

anaesthesia if bradycardia occurs. Occasionally, premedication with atropine will be indicated for children with excessive secretions, or an expected difficult airway. Even in these circumstances, the intramuscular route should rarely be necessary as atropine is well absorbed and effective when given by the oral route.[207,208] *Hyoscine* is a less effective vagolytic than atropine but a better sedative, antisialogue and amnesic. It is less well absorbed orally. Given that the older imperatives of premedication were to provide sedation and dry secretions, hyoscine was the logical choice for coadministration with papaveretum in the traditional *omnopon–scopolamine* mixture (see above). Hyoscine should be avoided in small children, in whom it may cause confusion. *Glycopyrrolate* (dose 0.1 mg kg^{-1}) is not very popular for routine premedication, probably as a result of a very long and uncomfortable drying effect.[209]

GASTRIC MOTILITY DRUGS AND H_2 BLOCKERS

Children at increased risk of vomiting or regurgitation (e.g. those with full stomach, obesity or pre-existing gastro-oesophageal reflux) may benefit from drugs which promote gastric emptying or elevate the pH of residual gastric contents. However, while such prophylaxis is considered prudent, the avoidance of regurgitation by proper anaesthetic management, including a rapid sequence induction with cricoid pressure, is at least as important for the prevention of aspiration pneumonitis.

Metoclopramide is a dopamine receptor antagonist with antiemetic and prokinetic properties. Its antiemetic effect is the result of direct action on the chemoreceptor trigger zone and the vomiting centre. It also increases lower oesophageal sphincter tone, relaxes the pyloric sphincter and promotes gastric emptying by increasing gastric and intestinal peristalsis. These peripheral effects are believed to result mainly from enhanced release of acetylcholine from cholinergic neurons.[210] A dose of 0.15 mg kg^{-1} is effective when given orally 1–4 h preoperatively[211,212] or intravenously shortly before induction.[213]

Cimetidine is an H_2 receptor antagonist that reduces gastric volume and acidity through inhibition of gastric secretion. A single oral dose of 6 mg kg^{-1} is effective when administered 1.5–2 h preoperatively; alternatively a dose of 3 mg kg^{-1} can be administered intravenously 1 h preoperatively. Since cimetidine has no effect on acid already present in the stomach, best results will be obtained by combining this drug with metoclopramide to promote gastric emptying. *Ranitidine* closely resembles cimetidine, but is much longer acting.[155] The recommended doses for premedication are 2 mg kg^{-1} orally, 2 h preoperatively, and preferably also 2 mg kg^{-1} on the previous evening. Ranitidine may also be given in a dose of 1 mg kg^{-1} intravenously, 45–60 min preoperatively.

IMMEDIATE PREPARATION AND TRANSPORT

There should be an agreed protocol for the preparation and transport of children to and from the operating theatres. Details will vary between institutions, but all should incorporate adequate patient checks. Most commonly, patients are dressed in a theatre gown and transported on a hospital trolley accompanied by a porter and a nurse. The use of a trolley is considered essential in older children who have received sedative premedication, although infants and small children may be carried by their parents. Less commonly, unpremedicated children are encouraged to walk to the operating room wearing their own clothes, or even ride to the operating theatres on electric cars, etc. Claims that these methods produce greater patient satisfaction are unsubstantiated, while considerable disruption to the operating room schedule may result. Some hospital theatre complexes (especially in the USA) are equipped with patient holding areas to reduce delays between cases and provide a suitable environment for administering premedication. As children's wards become increasingly informal this approach may become more popular.

JEHOVAH'S WITNESSES

The beliefs of Jehovah's Witnesses must be respected, but in our society we do not accept that a child's life be put at risk for want of blood or blood products. The Witnesses' Law forbids the use of these which include red and white cells, platelets and plasma. Cardiopulmonary bypass using the child's own blood and not involving a break in the flow of blood and organ transplants is accepted.

Jehovah's Witnesses do, however, seek the very best possible care for their children consistent with their beliefs and do know that there are many legitimate and effective ways of managing serious medical conditions without the use of blood products, such as with the use of synthetic colloids, erythropoietin, haemodilution and ultrafiltration after cardiopulmonary bypass.

When time allows, decisions about the treatment of these children are taken only after full discussion with the parents and also the child, who may be a competent minor and wish to have a say in what happens. The medical and nursing staff should guarantee that every possible alternative to the use of blood will be explored and that it will only be given in a life-threatening situation. Even if the staff accept that blood must be used to save the life, they may well feel uncomfortable having contravened a religious belief.

If ample time can be allowed for full discussion, experience has shown that agreement can be reached in the vast majority of cases, sometimes with the help of the chaplaincy, social services departments or a department of counselling.

The Witnesses have a liaison committee which acts between the patients and the hospital staff and although they will explore all alternatives to blood products, they do accept that the doctor has the duty to behave in the child's best interests. In most areas they provide a 24-h service which is useful for the parents and the hospital staff. It is extremely unusual that a legal route involving the courts has to be taken.

Further counselling is provided in the relatively unusual situation that blood products must be used.

REFERENCES

1 McGraw, T. Preparing children for the operating room: psychological issues. *Canadian Journal of Anaesthesia* 1994; **41**: 1094–103.

2 Forman, M.A., Kerschbaum, W.E., Hetznecker, W.H. and Dunn, J.M. Some conceptual models of child development. In: Behrman, R.E., Vaughn, V.C. III and Nelson, W.E. (eds). *Nelson Textbook of Pediatrics*. Philadelphia, PA: WB Saunders, 1987: 36.

3 Zuckerberg, A.L. Perioperative approach to children. *Pediatric Clinics of North America* 1994; **41**: 15–29.

4 Maligalic, R.M.L. Parents' perceptions of the stressors of pediatric ambulatory surgery. *Journal of Post Anesthesia Nursing* 1994; **9**: 278–82.

5 Litman, R.S., Berger, A.A. and Chhibber, A. An evaluation of preoperative anxiety in a population of parents of infants and children undergoing ambulatory surgery. *Paediatric Anaesthesia* 1996; **6**: 443–7.

6 Bevan, J.C., Johnston, C., Haig, M.J., *et al.* Preoperative parental anxiety predicts behavioural and emotional responses to induction of anaesthesia in children. *Canadian Journal of Anaesthesia* 1990; 3**7**: 177–82.

7 Visintainer, M.A. and Wolfer, J.A. Psychological preparation for surgical pediatric patients: the effect on children's and parents' stress responses and adjustment. *Pediatrics* 1975; **97**: 590–4.

8 Seeman, R.G. and Rockoff, M.A. Preoperative anxiety: the pediatric patient. *International Anesthesiology Clinics* 1986; **24**: 1–15.

9 Vetter, T.R. The epidemiology and selective identification of children at risk for preoperative anxiety reactions. *Anesthesia and Analgesia* 1993; **77**: 96–9.

10 American Academy of Pediatrics. Timing of elective surgery on the genitalia of male children with particular reference to the risks, benefits, and psychological effects of surgery and anesthesia. *Pediatrics* 1996; **97**: 590–4.

11 Rice, L.J. Needle phobia: an anesthesiologist's perspective. *Pediatrics* 1993; **122**: s9–13.

12 Mahaffy, P.R. The effects of hospitalization on children admitted for tonsillectomy and adenoidectomy. *Nursing Research* 1965; **14**: 12–19.

13 Vernon, D.T.A, Schulman, J.L. and Foley, J.M. Changes in children's behavior after hospitalization. *American Journal of Diseases of Children* 1966; **111**: 581–93.

14 Levy, D.M. Psychic trauma of operations in children and a note on combat neurosis. *American Journal of Diseases of Children* 1945; **69**: 7–25.

15 Jackson, K. Psychological preparation as a method of reducing emotional trauma of anesthesia in children. *Anesthesiology* 1951; **12**: 293–300.

16 Eckenhoff, J.E. Relationship of anesthesia to postoperative personality changes in children. *American Journal of Diseases of Children* 1953; **86**: 587–91.

17 Campbell, I.R., Scaife, J.M. and Johnstone, J.M. Psychological effects of day-case surgery compared with inpatient surgery. *Archives of Disease in Childhood* 1988; **63**: 415–17.

18 Kotiniemi, L.H., Ryhanen, PT. and Moilanen, I.K. Behavioural changes in children following day-case surgery: a 4-week follow-up of 551 children. *Anaesthesia* 1997; **52**: 970–6.

19 Ferguson, B.F. Preparing young children for hospitalization: a comparison of two methods. *Pediatrics* 1979; **64**: 656–64.

20 Kain, Z.N., Mayes, L.C. and Caramico, L.A. Preoperative preparation in children: a cross-sectional study. *Journal of Clinical Anesthesia* 1996; **8**: 508–14.

21 Kain, Z.N., Wang, S.M., Caramico, L.A., Hofstadter, M. and Mayes, L.C. Parental desire for perioperative information and informed consent: a two-phase study. *Anesthesia and Analgesia* 1997; **84**: 299–306.

22 Litman, R.S., Perkins, F.M. and Dawson, S.C. Parental knowledge and attitudes toward discussing the risk of death from anesthesia. *Anesthesia and Analgesia* 1993; **77**: 256–60.

23 Fisher, Q.A., Feldman, M.A. and Wilson, M.D. Pediatric responsibilities for preoperative evaluation. *Journal of Pediatrics* 1994; **125**: 675–85.

24 Bothe, A. and Galdston, R. The child's loss of consciousness: psychiatric view of pediatric anesthesia. *Pediatrics* 1972; **50**: 252–63.

25 Meyers, E.F. and Muravchick, S. Anesthesia induction techniques in pediatric patients: a controlled study of behavioral consequences. *Anesthesia and Analgesia* 1977; **56**: 538–42.

26 Romsing, J. and Walther, L.S. Postoperative pain in children: a survey of parents' expectations and perceptions of their children's experiences. *Paediatric Anaesthesia* 1996; **6**: 215–18.

27 Sikich, N., Carr, A.S. and Lerman, J. Parental perceptions, expectations, and preferences for the postanaesthetic recovery of children. *Paediatric Anaesthesia* 1997; **7**: 139–42.

28 Palermo, T.M. and Drotar, D. Prediction of children's postoperative pain: the role of presurgical expectations and anticipatory emotions. *Journal of Pediatric Psychology* 1996; **21**: 683–98.

29 Karl, H.W., Pauza, K.J., Heyneman, N. and Tinker, D.E. Preanesthetic preparation of pediatric outpatients: the role of a videotape for parents. *Journal of Clinical Anesthesia* 1990; **2**: 172–7.

30 Jones, S.T. Reducing children's psychological stress in the operating suite. *Ophthalmic Plastic and Reconstructive Surgery* 1985; **1**: 199–203.

31 Kain, Z.N. Parental presence during induction of anaesthesia. *Paediatric Anaesthesia* 1995; **5**: 209–12.

32 Gauderer, M.W., Lorig, J.L. and Eastwood, D.W. Is there a place for parents in the operating room? *Journal of Pediatric Surgery* 1989; **24**: 705–6.

33 Braude, N., Ridley, S.A. and Sumner, E. Parents and paediatric anaesthesia: a prospective survey of parental attitudes to their presence at induction. *Annals of the Royal College of Surgeons of England* 1990; **72**: 41–4.

34 McCormick, A.S. and Spargo, P.M. Parents in the anaesthetic room: a questionnaire survey of departments of anaesthesia. *Paediatric Anaesthesia* 1996; **6**: 183–6.

35 Hannallah, R.S. Who benefits when parents are present during anaesthesia induction in their children? *Canadian Journal of Anaesthesia* 1994; **41**: 271–5.

36 Kain, Z.N., Ferris, C.A., Mayes, L.C. and Rimar, S. Parental presence during induction of anaesthesia: practice differences between the United States and Great Britain. *Paediatric Anaesthesia* 1996; **6**: 187–93.

37 Hannallah, R.S. and Rosales, J.K. Experience with parents' presence during anaesthesia induction in children. *Canadian Anaesthetists Society Journal* 1983; **30**: 286–9.

38 Schulman, J.L., Foley, J.M., Vernon, D.T.A. and Allan, D. A study of the effect of the mother's presence during anesthesia induction. *Pediatrics* 1967; **39**: 111–14.

39 Vessey, J.A., Bogetz, M.S., Caserza, C.L., Liu, K.R. and Cassidy, M.D. Parental upset associated with participation in induction of anaesthesia in children. *Canadian Journal of Anaesthesia* 1994; **41**: 276–80.

40 Kain, Z.N., Mayes, L.C., Caramico, L.A., *et al.* Parental presence during induction of anesthesia. A randomized controlled trial. *Anesthesiology* 1996; **84**: 1060–7.

41 Hannallah, R.S. and Epstein, B.S. The pediatric patient. In: Wetchler, B.V. (ed.). *Anesthesia for Ambulatory Surgery*. 2nd edn. Philadelphia, PA: Lippincott, 1991: 131–95.

42 Baines, D. and Overton, J.H. Parental presence at induction of anaesthesia: a survey of N.S.W. hospitals and tertiary paediatric hospitals in Australia. *Anaesthesia and Intensive Care* 1995; **23**: 191–5.

43 Varni, J.W. and Katz, E.R. Psychological aspects of childhood cancer: a review of research. *Journal of Psychosocial Oncology* 1987; **5**: 93–119.

44 Zeltzer, L.K., Jay, S.M. and Fisher, D.M. The management of pain associated with pediatric procedures. *Pediatric Clinics of North America* 1989; **36**: 941–64.

45 Hall, S.C. and Stevenson, G.W. Anesthetic considerations in the pediatric cancer patient. *Seminars in Surgical Oncology* 1990; **6**: 148–55.

46 Jay, S., Elliott, C.H., Fitzgibbons, I., Woody, P. and Siegel, S. A comparative study of cognitive behavior therapy versus general anesthesia for painful medical procedures in children. *Pain* 1995; **62**: 3–9.

47 American Academy of Pediatrics, Section on Anesthesiology. Evaluation and preparation of pediatric patients undergoing anesthesia. *Pediatrics* 1996; **98**: 502–8.

48 McGill, W.A., Coveler, L.A. and Epstein, B.S. Subacute respiratory infection in small children. *Anesthesia and Analgesia* 1979; **58**: 331–3.

49 Cohen, M.M. and Cameron, C.B. Should you cancel the operation when a child has an upper respiratory tract infection? *Anesthesia and Analgesia* 1991; **72**: 282–8.

50 DeSoto, H., Patel, R.I., Soliman, I.E. and Hannallah, R.S. Changes in oxygen saturation following general anesthesia in children with upper respiratory signs and symtoms undergoing otolaryngological procedures. *Anesthesiology* 1988; **68**: 969–72.

51 Konarzewski, W.H., Ravindran, N., Findlow, D. and Timmis, P.K. Anaesthetic death of a child with a cold. *Anaesthesia* 1992; **47**: 624.

52 Williams, O.A., Hills, R. and Goddard, J.M. Pulmonary collapse during anaesthesia in children with respiratory tract symptoms. *Anaesthesia* 1992; **47**: 411–13.

53 Levy, L., Pandit, U.A., Randel, G.I., Lewis, I.H. and Tait, A.R. Upper respiratory tract infections and general anaesthesia in children. Peri-operative complications and oxygen saturation. *Anaesthesia* 1992; **47**: 678–82.

54 Kinouchi, K., Tanigami, H., Tashiro, C., Nishimura, M., Fukumitsu, K. and Takauchi, Y. Duration of apnea in anesthetized infants and children required for desaturation of hemoglobin to 95%. The influence of upper respiratory infection. *Anesthesiology* 1992; **77**: 1105–7.

55 Tait, A.R., Reynolds, P.I. and Gutstein, H.B. Factors that influence an anesthesiologist's decision to cancel elective surgery for the child with an upper respiratory tract infection. *Journal of Clinical Anesthesia* 1995; **7**: 491–9.

56 Van der Walt, J.H. and Roberton, D.M. Anaesthesia and recently vaccinated children. *Paediatric Anaesthesia* 1996; **6**: 135–41.

57 Laxenaire, M.C. Drugs and other agents involved in anaphylactic shock occurring during anaesthesia. A French multicenter epidemiological inquiry. *Annales Francaises d'Anesthesie et de Reanimation* 1993; **12**: 91–6.

58 Murat, I. Anaphylactic reactions during paediatric anaesthesia: results of the survey of the French Society of Paediatric Anaesthesia (ADARPEF) 1991–1992. *Paediatric Anaesthesia* 1993; **3**: 339–43.

59 Kwittken, P.L., Sweinberg, S.K., Campbell, D.E. and Pawlowski, N.A. Latex hypersensitivity in children: clinical presentation and detection of latex-specific immunoglobuline E. *Pediatrics* 1995; **95**: 693–9.

60 Porri, F., Pradal, M., Lemiere, C., *et al.* Association between latex sensitization and repeated latex exposure in children. *Anesthesiology* 1997; **86**: 599–602.

61 Task force on allergic reactions to latex. Committee report. *Journal of Allergy and Clinical Immunology* 1993; **92**: 16–18.

62 Delorme, M., Gall, O., Constant, I. and Murat, I. Latex hypersensitivity: a foreseeable accident? *Cahiers d'Anesthesiologie* 1995; **43**: 467–70.

63 Dajani, A.S., Tambert, K.A., Wilson, A.F. *et al.* Prevention of bacterial endocarditis: recommendation of the American Heart Association. *Journal of the American Medical Association* 1977; **227**: 1791–801.

64 MacPherson, D.S. Preoperative laboratory testing: should any tests be 'routine' before surgery. *Medical Clinics of North America* 1993; **77**: 289–308.

65 Hannallah, R.S. Preoperative investigations. *Paediatric Anaesthesia* 1995; **5**: 325–9.

66 Hackmann, T., Steward, D.J. and Sheps, S.B. Anemia in pediatric day-surgery patients: prevalence and detection. *Anesthesiology* 1991; **75**: 27–31.

67 Roy, W.L., Lerman, J. and McIntyre, B.G. Is preoperative haemoglobin testing justified in children undergoing minor elective surgery? *Canadian Journal of Anaesthesia* 1991; **38**: 700–3.

68 O'Connor, M.E. and Drasner, K. Preoperative laboratory testing of children undergoing elective surgery. *Anesthesia and Analgesia* 1990; **70**: 176–80.

69 Welborn, L.G., Hannallah, R.S., Luban, L.N.C., Fink, R. and Ruttinam, V.E. Anemia and postoperative apnea in former preterm infants. *Anesthesiology* 1991; **74**: 1003–6.

70 Patel, R.I. and Hannallah, R.S. Preoperative screening for pediatric ambulatory surgery: evaluation of a telephone questionnaire method. *Anesthesia and Analgesia* 1992; **75**: 258–61.

71 Steward, D.J. Screening tests before surgery in children. *Canadian Journal of Anaesthesia* 1991; **38**: 693–5.

72 Wood, R.A. and Hoekelman, R.A. Value of the chest X-ray as a screening test for elective surgery in children. *Pediatrics* 1981; **67**: 447–52.

73 Brill, P.W., Ewing, M.L. and Dunn, A.A. The value (?) of routine chest radiography in children and adolescents. *Pediatrics* 1973; **52**: 125–7.

74 American Academy of Pediatrics, Committee on Hospital Care. Preoperative chest radiographs. *Pediatrics* 1983; **71**: 858.

75 Paqueron, X., Favier, R., Richard, P., Maillet, J. and Murat, I. Severe postadenoidectomy bleeding revealing congenital alpha 2 antiplasmin deficiency in a child. *Anesthesia and Analgesia* 1997; **84**: 1147–9.

76 Janvier, G., Winnock, S. and Freyburger, G. Value of the activated partial thromboplastin time for preoperative detection of coagulation disorders not revealed by a specific questionnaire. *Anesthesiology* 1991; **75**: 920–1.

77 Burk, C.D., Miller, L., Handler, S.D. and Cohen, A.R. Preoperative history and coagulation screening in children undergoing tonsillectomy. *Pediatrics* 1992; **89**: 691–5.

78 Kang, J., Brodsky, L., Danziger, I., Volk, M. and Stanievich, J. Coagulation profile as a predictor for post-tonsillectomy and adenoidectomy hemorrhage. *International Journal of Pediatric Otorhinolaryngology* 1994; **28**: 157–65.

79 Mendelson, C.L. The aspiration of stomach contents into the lungs during obstetric anesthesia. *American Journal of Obstetrics and Gynaecology* 1946; **53**: 191–205.

80 Phillips, S., Daborn, A.K. and Hatch, D.J. Preoperative fasting for paediatric anaesthesia. *British Journal of Anaesthesia* 1994; **73**: 529–36.

81 Cote, C.J. NPO after midnight for children – a reappraisal. *Anesthesiology* 1990; **72**: 589–92.

82 Larsson, L.E., Nilsson, K., Niklasson, A., Andreasson, S. and Ekstom-Jodal, B. Influence of fluid regimens on perioperative blood glucose concentrations in neonates. *British Journal of Anaesthesia* 1990; **64**: 419–24.

83 Nimmo, W.S. Effect of anaesthesia on gastric motility and emptying. *British Journal of Anaesthesia* 1984; **56**: 29–36.

84 Hardy, J.F. Large volume gastro-oesophageal reflux: a rationale for risk reduction in the perioperative period. *Canadian Journal of Anaesthesia* 1988; **35**: 162–73.

85 Carre, I.J. Clinical significance of gastro-oesophageal reflux. *Archives of Disease in Childhood* 1984; **59**: 911–12.

86 Hamilton, J.R. Disorders of the gastrointestinal tract. In: Behrman, R E. and Vaughan, V.C. III (eds). *Nelson Textbook of Pediatrics*. Philadelphia, PA: WB Saunders, 1990: 887–9.

87 Teabeaut, J.R. Aspiration of gastric contents – an experimental study. *American Journal of Pathology* 1952; **28**: 51–62.

88 Roberts, R.B. and Shirley, M.A. Reducing the risk of acid aspiration during cesarian section. *Anesthesia and Analgesia* 1974; **53**: 859–68.

89 Raidoo, D.M., Rocke, D.A., Brock-Utne, J.G., Marszalek, A. and Engelbrecht, H.E. Critical volume for pulmonary acid aspiration: reappraisal in a primate model. *British Journal of Anaesthesia* 1990; **65**: 248–50.

90 Cote, C.J., Goudsouzian, N.G., Liu, L.M.P., Dedrick, D.F. and Szyfelbein, S.K. Assessment of risk factors related to the acid aspiration syndrome in pediatric patients – gastric pH and residual volume. *Anesthesiology* 1982; **56**: 70–2.

91 Manchikanti, L., Colliver, J.A., Marrero, T.C. and Roush, J.R. Assessment of age-related acid aspiration risk factors in pediatric, adult and geriatric patients. *Anesthesia and Analgesia* 1985; **64**: 11–17.

92 Tiret, L., Nivoche, Y., Hatton, F., Desmonts, M. and Vourc'h, G. Complications related to anaesthesia in infants and children. *British Journal of Anaesthesia* 1988; **61**: 263–9.

93 Olsson, G.L. and Hallen, B. Pharmacological evacuation of the stomach with metoclopramide. *Acta Anaesthesiologica Scandinavica* 1982; **26**: 417–20.

94 Heading, R.C. Gastric motility and emptying. In: Sircus, W. and Smith, A.N. (eds). *Scientific Foundations of Gastroenterology*. London: Heinemann, 1980: 287–96.

95 Cavell, B. Gastric emptying in preterm infants. *Acta Paediatrica Scandinavica* 1979; **68**: 527–31.

96 Cavell, B. Gastric emptying in infants fed human milk or infant formula. *Acta Paediatrica Scandinavica* 1981; **70**: 639–41.

97 Sandhar, B.K., Goresky, G.V., Maltby, J.R. and Shaffer, E.A. Effect of oral liquids and ranitidine on gastric fluid volume and pH in children undergoing outpatient surgery. *Anesthesiology* 1989; **71**: 327–30.

98 Splinter, W.M., Steward, D.A. and Muir, J.G. The effect of preoperative apple juice on gastric contents, thirst, and hunger in children. *Canadian Journal of Anaesthesia* 1989; **36**: 55–8.

99 Schreiner, M.S., Triebwasser, A. and Keon, T.P. Ingestion of liquids compared with preoperative fasting in pediatric outpatients. *Anesthesiology* 1990; **72**: 593–7.

100 Splinter, W.M. and Schaefer, J.D. Unlimited clear fluid ingestion two hours before surgery does not affect volume or pH of stomach contents. *Anaesthesia and Intensive Care* 1990; **18**: 522–6.

101 Nicolson, S.C., Dorsey, A.T. and Schreiner, M.S. Shortened preanesthetic fasting interval in pediatric cardiac surgical patients. *Anesthesia and Analgesia* 1992; **74**: 694–7.

102 Phillips, S., Hutchinson, S. and Davidson, T. Preoperative drinking does not affect gastric contents. *British Journal of Anaesthesia* 1993; **70**: 6–9.

103 Soreide, E., Holst-Larsen, H., Reite, K., Mikkesen, H., Soreide, J.A. and Steen, P.A. Effects of giving water 20–450 ml with oral diazepam premedication 1–2 h before operation. *British Journal of Anaesthesia* 1993; **71**: 503–6.

104 Soreide, E., Stomskag, K.E. and Steen, P.A. Statistical aspects in studies of preoperative fluid intake and gastric content. *Acta Anaesthesiologica Scandinavica* 1995; **39**: 738–43.

105 Van der Walt, J.H., Floate, J.A., Murrell, D., Jacob, R. and Bentley, M. A study of preoperative fasting in infants aged less than three months. *Anaesthesia and Intensive Care* 1990; **18**: 527–31.

106 Litman, R.S., Wu, C.L. and Quinlivan, J.K. Gastric volume and pH in infants fed clear fluids and breast milk prior to surgery. *Anesthesia and Analgesia* 1994; **79**: 482–5.

107 Meakin, G., Dingwall, A.E. and Addison, G.M. Effects of fasting and oral premedication on the pH and volume of gastric aspirate in children. *British Journal of Anaesthesia* 1987; **59**: 678–82.

108 Splinter, W.M., Stewart, J.A. and Muir, J.G. Large volumes of apple juice peroperatively do not affect gastric pH and volume in children. *Canadian Journal of Anaesthesia* 1990; **37**: 36–9.

109 Strunin, L. How long should patients fast before surgery? Time for new guidelines. *British Journal of Anaesthesia* 1993; **70**: 1–3.

110 Stack, C.G. and Stokes, M.A. Preoperative fasting for paediatric anaesthesia. *British Journal of Anaesthesia* 1995; **75**: 375.

111 Olsson, G.L., Hallen, B. and Hambreaeus-Jonzon, K. Aspiration during anaesthesia: a computer aided study of 185358 anaesthetics. *Acta Anaesthesiologica Scandinavica* 1986; **30**: 84–92.

112 Schurizek, B.A., Rybro, L., Boggild-Madsen, N.B. and Juhl, B. Gastric volume and pH in children for emergency surgery. *Acta Anaesthesiologica Scandinavica* 1986; **30**: 404–8.

113 Bricker, S.R.W., McLuckie, A. and Nightingale, D.A. Gastric aspirates after trauma in children. *Anaesthesia* 1989; **44**: 721–4.

114 Ullyot, S.C. Paediatric premedication. *Canadian Journal of Anaesthesia* 1992; **39**: 533–6.

115 Waters, R.M. Pain relief for children. *American Journal of Surgery* 1938; **39**: 470–5.

116 Smith, R.M. Children, hospitals and parents. *Anesthesiology* 1964; **25**: 461–65.

117 Blom, G.E. The reactions of hospitalized children to illness. *Pediatrics* 1958; **22**: 590–600.

118 Mirakhur, K. Preanaesthetic medication: a survey of current usage. *Journal of the Royal Society of Medicine* 1991; **84**: 481–3.

119 Kain, Z.N., Mayes, L.C., Bell, C., Weisman, S., Hofstadter, M.B. and Rimar, S. Premedication in the United States: a status report. *Anesthesia and Analgesia* 1997; **84**: 427–32.

120 Gajraj, N.M., Pennant, J.H. and Watcha, M.F. Eutectic mixture of local anaesthetics (EMLA®) cream. *Anesthesia and Analgesia* 1994; **78**: 574–83.

121 Hallen, B. and Uppfeldt, A. Does lidocaine–prilocaine cream permit painfree insertion of i.v. catheters in children? *Anesthesiology* 1982; **57**: 340–2.

122 Ehrenström Reiz, G.M.E. and Reiz, S.L.A. EMLA – an eutectic mixture of local anaesthetics for topical anaesthesia. *Acta Anaesthesiologica Scandinavica* 1982; **26**: 596–8.

123 Hallen, B., Olssen, G.L. and Uppfeldt, A. Pain-free venepuncture. *Anaesthesia* 1984; **39**: 969–72.

124 Soliman, I.E., Broadman, L.M., Hannallah, R.S. and McGill, W.A. Comparison of the analgesic effects of EMLA (eutectic mixture of local anesthetics) to intradermal lidocaine infiltration prior to venous cannulation in unpremedicated children. *Anesthesiology* 1988; **68**: 804–6.

125 Norman, L. and Jones, P.L. Complications of the use of EMLA. *British Journal of Anaesthesia* 1990; **64**: 403–6.

126 Engberg, G., Danielson, K., Henneberg, S. and Nilsson, A. Plasma concentrations of prilocaine and lidocaine and methaemoglobin formation in infants after epicutaneous application of 5% lidocaine–prilocaine (EMLA). *Acta Anaesthesiologica Scandinavica* 1987; **31**: 624–8.

127 Frayling, I.M., Addison, G.M., Chattergee, K. and Meakin, G. Methaemoglobinaemia in children treated with prilocaine–lignocaine cream. *British Medical Journal* 1990; **301**: 153–4.

128 McCafferty, D.F., Woolfson, A.D., McLelland, K.H. and Boston, V. *In vivo* and *in vitro* assessment of the percutaneous absorption of local anaesthetics. *British Journal of Anaesthesia* 1988; **60**: 64–9.

129 McCafferty, D.F., Woolfson, A.D. and Boston, V. *In vivo* assessment of percutaneous local anaesthetic preparations. *British Journal of Anaesthesia* 1989; **62**: 17–21.

130 Doyle, E., Freeman, J., Im, N.T. and Morton, N.S. An evaluation of a new self-adhesive patch preparation of amethocaine for topical anaesthesia prior to venous cannulation in children. *Anaesthesia* 1993; **48**: 1050–2.

131 Lawson, R.A., Smart, N.G. and Morton, N.S. Evaluation of an amethocaine gel preparation for percutaneous analgesia before venous cannulation in children. *British Journal of Anaesthesia* 1995; **75**: 282–5.

132 Moher, H. and Richards, J.G. The benzodiazepine receptor: a pharmacological control element of brain function. *European Journal of Anaesthesiology* 1988; **2**: 15–24.

133 Rita, L., Seleny, F.L., Mazurek, A. and Rabins, S. Intramuscular midazolam for pediatric preanesthetic sedation: a double blind controlled study with morphine. *Anesthesiology* 1985; **63**: 528–31.

134 Taylor, M.B., Vine, P.R. and Hatch, D.J. Intramuscular midazolam premedication in small children. *Anaesthesia* 1986: **41**: 21–6.

135 Payne, K.A., Heydenrych, J.J., Kruger, T.C. and Samuels, G. Midazolam premedication in paediatric anaesthesia. *South African Medical Journal* 1986; **70**: 657–9.

136 Saint-Maurice, C., Meistelman, C., Rey, E., Esteve, C., De Lauture, D. and Olive, G. The pharmacokinetics of rectal midazolam for premedication in children. *Anesthesiology* 1986; **65**: 536–8.

137 De Jong, P.C. and Verburg, M.P. Comparison of rectal to intramuscular administration of midazolam and atropine for premedication of children. *Acta Anaesthesiologica Scandanavica* 1988; **32**: 485–9.

138 Wilton, N.C.T., Leigh, J., Rosen, D.R. and Pandit, U.A. Preanesthetic sedation of preschool children using intranasal midazolam. *Anesthesiology* 1988; **69**: 972–75.

139 Karl, H.W., Keifer, A.T., Rosenberger, J.L., Larach, M.G. and Ruffle, J.M. Comparison of the safety and efficacy of intranasal midazolam or sufentanil for preinduction of anesthesia in pediatric patients. *Anesthesiology* 1992; **76**: 209–15.

140 Karl, H.W., Rosenberger, J.L., Larach, M.G. and Ruffle, J.M. Transmucosal administration of midazolam for premedication of pediatric patients. Comparison of the nasal and sublingual routes. *Anesthesiology* 1993; **78**: 885–91.

141 Vetter, T.R. A comparison of midazolam, diazepam and placebo as oral anesthetic premedicants in younger children. *Journal of Clinical Anesthesia* 1993; **5**: 58–61.

142 McMillan, C.O., Spahr-Schopfer, I.A., Sikich, N., Hartley, E. and Lerman, J. Premedication of children with oral midazolam. *Canadian Journal of Anaesthesia* 1992; **39**: 545–50.

143 Weldon, B.C., Watcha, M.F. and White, P.F. Oral midazolam in children; effect of time and adjunctive therapy. *Anesthesia and Analgesia* 1992; **75**: 51–5.

144 Parnis, S.J., Foate, J.A., Van der Walt, J.H., Short, T. and Crowe, C.E. Oral Midazolam is an effective premedication for children having day-stay anaesthesia. *Anaesthesia and Intensive Care* 1992; **20**: 9–14.

145 Payne, K.A., Coetzee, A.R., Mattheyse, F.J. and Dawes, T. Oral midazolam in paediatric premedication. *South African Medical Journal* 1991; **79**: 372–75.

146 Saarnivaara, L., Lindgren, L. and Klemola, U.-M. Comparison of chloral hydrate and midazolam by mouth as premedicants in children undergoing otolaryngological surgery. *British Journal of Anaesthesia* 1988; **61**: 390–6.

147 Feld, L.H., Negus, J.B. and White, P.F. Oral midazolam preanesthetic medication in pediatric outpatients. *Anesthesiology* 1990; **78**: 831–4.

148 Levine, M.F., Spahr-Schopfer, I.A., Hartley, E., Lerman, J. and Macpherson, B. Oral midazolam premedication in children: the minimum time interval for separation from parents. *Canadian Journal of Anaesthesia* 1993; **40**: 726–29.

149 Payne, K.A., Coetzee, A.R., Mattheyse, F.J. and Heydenrych, J.J. Behavioural changes in children following minor surgery – is premedication beneficial? *Acta Anaesthesiologica Belgica* 1992; **43**: 173–9.

150 McCluskey, A. and Meakin, G.H. Oral administration of midazolam as a premedicant for paediatric day-case anaesthesia. *Anaesthesia* 1994; **49**: 782–5.

151 Kain, Z.N., Mayes, L., Wang, S.M., Hofstadter, M.B. and Bagnall, A. Effect of premedication on postoperative behavioural outcomes in children. *Anesthesiology* 1997; **87**: A1032.

152 Twersky, R.S., Hartung, J., Berger, B.J., McClain, J. and Beaton, C. Midazolam enhances anterograde but not retrograde amnesia in pediatric patients. *Anesthesiology* 1993; **78**: 51–5.

153 Mehta, A.C., Hart-Davies, S. and Bedford, C. Chemical stability of midazolam syrup. *Hospital Pharmacy Practice* 1993; **3**: 224–6.

154 Patel, D. and Meakin, G. Oral midazolam compared with diazepam–droperidol and trimeprazine as premedicants in children. *Paediatric Anaesthesia* 1997; **7**: 287–93.

155 Vickers, M.D., Schnieden, H. and Wood-Smith, F.G. (eds). *Drugs in Anaesthetic Practice.* 7th edn. London: Butterworths, 1991.

156 Stoelting, R.K. and Miller, R.D. (eds). *Basics of Anesthesia.* 2nd edn. New York: Churchill Livingstone, 1991: 129–30.

157 Fragen, R.J. and Caldwell, N. Lorazepam premedication: lack of recall and relief of anxiety. *Anesthesia and Analgesia* 1976; **55**: 792–6.

158 Padfield, N.L., Twohig, M.McD. and Fraser, A.C.L. Temazepam and trimeprazine compared with placebo as premedication in children. An investigation extending into the first two weeks at home. *British Journal of Anaesthesia* 1986; **58**: 487–93.

159 Cope, R.W. and Glover, W.J. Trimeprazine tartrate for premedication of children. *Lancet* 1959; **i**: 858–60.

160 Mann, N.P. Trimeprazine and respiratory depression. *Archives of Disease in Childhood* 1981; **56**: 481–2.

161 Loan, W.B. and Cuthbert, D. Adverse cardiovascular response to oral trimeprazine in children. *British Medical Journal* 1985; **290**: 1548–9.

162 Zorab, J.S.M. Trimeprazine premedication in children. *Anaesthesia* 1991; **46**: 1088.

163 Glover, W.J., Hatch, D.J. and Sumner, E. Trimeprazine premedication in children. *Anaesthesia* 1992; **47**: 441–2.

164 Mitchell, V., Grange, C., Black, A. and Train, J. A comparison of midazolam with trimeprazine as an oral premedicant for children. *Anaesthesia* 1997; **52**: 416–21.

165 Liu, L.M. and Ryan, J.F. Premedication and induction of anesthesia. In: Cote, C.J., Ryan, J.F., Todres, I.D. and Goudsouzian, N.G. (eds). *A Practice of Anesthesia for Infants and Children.* 2nd edn. Philadelphia, PA: WB Saunders, 1993: 135–49.

166 Davies, D.R. and Doughty, A.G. Premedication in children. A trial of intramuscular droperidol, droperidol–phenoperidine, papaveretum–hyocine and normal saline. *British Journal of Anaesthesia* 1971; **43**: 65–75.

167 McGarry, P.M.F. A double-blind study of diazepam, droperidol and meperidine as premedication in children. *Canadian Anaesthetists' Society Journal* 1970; **17**: 157–65.

168 Van Der Walt, J.H., Nicholls, B., Bentley, M. and Tomkins, D.P. Oral premedication in children. *Anaesthesia and Intensive Care* 1987; **15**: 151–7.

169 Phillips, G.H., Mian, T., Becber, U., Stone, P.A. and Jones, H.M. Oral premedication in children. A comparison of trimeprazine with a trimeprazine, droperidol and methadone mixture. *Anaesthesia* 1990; **45**: 870–2.

170 Dupre, L.J. and Stieglitz, P. Extrapyramidal syndromes after premedication with droperidol in children. *British Journal of Anaesthesia* 1980; **52**: 831–3.

171 Binning, R., Watson, W.R., Samrah, M. and Martin, E. Premedication for adenotonsillectomy. *British Journal of Anaesthesia* 1962; **34**: 812–16.

172 Mark, L.C. and Papper, E.M. Preanesthetic preparation of children. *Journal of the Medical Society of New Jersey* 1949; **46**; 520–3.

173 Sorbo, S., Hudson, R.J. and Loomis, J.C. The pharmacokinetics of thiopental in pediatric surgical patients. *Anesthesiology* 1984; **61**: 666–70.

174 Björkman, S., Gabrielsson, J., Quaynor, H. and Corbey, M. Pharmacokinetics of i.v. and rectal methohexitone in children. *British Journal of Anaesthesia* 1987; **59**: 1541–7.

175 Liu, L.M.P., Gaudreault, P., Friedman, P.A., Goudsouzian, N.G. and Liu, P.L. Methohexital plasma concentrations in children following rectal administration. *Anesthesiology* 1985; **62**: 567–70.

176 Kestin, I.G., McIllvaine, W.B., Lockhart, C.H., Kestin, K.J. and Jones, M.A. Rectal methohexitone for induction of sleep in children with and without rectal aspiration after sleep. *Anesthesia and Analgesia* 1988; **67**: 1102–4.

177 Audenaert, S.M., Montgomery, C.L., Thompson, D.E. and Sutherland, J.M. A prospective study of rectal methohexital: efficacy and side effects in 648 cases. *Anesthesia and Analgesia* 1995; **81**: 957–61.

178 Goresky, G.V. and Steward, D.J. Rectal methohexitone for induction of anaesthesia in children. *Canadian Anaesthetists Society Journal* 1979; **26**: 213–15.

179 McQuiston, W.O. Anesthetic problems in cardiac surgery in children. *Anesthesiology* 1949; **10**: 590–600.

180 Moffit, E.A., Mcgoon, D.C. and Ritter, D.G. The diagnosis and correction of congenital cardiac defects. *Anesthesiology* 1970; **33**: 144–60.

181 Smith, B.L. and Manford, M.L.M. Postoperative vomiting after paediatric adenotonsillectomy: a survey of incidence following differing pre- and postoperative drugs. *British Journal of Anaesthesia* 1974; **46**: 373–8.

182 Booker, P.D. and Chapman, D.H. Premedication in children undergoing day-care surgery. *British Journal of Anaesthesia* 1979; **51**: 1083–7.

183 Way, W.L., Costley, E.C. and Leong Way, E. Respiratory sensitivity of the newborn infant to meperidine and morphine. *Clinical Pharmacology and Therapeutics* 1965; **6**: 454–61.

184 Kupferberg, H.J. and Leong Way, E. Pharmacologic basis for the increased sensitivity of the newborn rat to morphine. *Journal of Pharmacology and Experimental Therapeutics* 1963; **141**: 105–12.

185 Dundee, J.W., Moore, J. and Clarke, R.S.J. Studies of drugs given before anaesthesia. V: Pethidine 100 mg alone and with atropine or hyoscine. *British Journal of Anaesthesia* 1964; **36**: 703–10.

186 Ashburn, M.A., Streisand, J.B., Tarver, S.D., *et al.* Oral transmucosal fentanyl citrate for premedication in paediatric outpatients. *Canadian Journal of Anaesthesia* 1990; **37**: 857–66.

187 Streisand, J.B., Stanley, T.H., Hague, B., Van Vreeswijk, H., Ho, G.H. and Pace, N.L. Oral transmucosal fentanyl citrate premedication in children. *Anesthesia and Analgesia* 1989; **69**: 28–34.

188 Feld, L.H., Champeau, M.W., van Steenis, C.A. and Scott, J.C. Preanesthetic medication in children: a comparison of oral transmucosal fentanyl citrate versus placebo. *Anesthesiology* 1989; **71**: 374–7.

189 Stanley, T.H., Leiman, B.C., Rawal, N., *et al.* The effects of oral transmucosal fentanyl citrate premedication on preoperative behavioral responses and gastric volume and acidity in children. *Anesthesia and Analgesia* 1989; **69**: 328–35.

190 Goldstein-Dresner, M.C., Davis, P.J., Kretchman, E., *et al.* Double-blind comparison of oral transmucosal fentanyl citrate with oral meperidine, diazepam, and atropine as preanesthetic medication in children with congenital heart disease. *Anesthesiology* 1991; **74**: 28–33.

191 Henderson, J.M., Brodsky, D.A., Fisher, D.M., Brett, C.M. and Herzka, R.E. Preinduction of anesthesia in pediatric patients with nasally administered sufentanil. *Anesthesiology* 1988; **68**: 671–5.

192 Haynes, G., Brahen, N.H. and Hill, H.F. Plasma sufentanil concentration after intranasal administration to paediatric outpatients. *Canadian Journal of Anaesthesia* 1993; **40**: 286.

193 Boyd, J.D. and Manford, M.L.M. Premedication in children. A controlled clinical trial of oral triclofos and diazepam. *British Journal of Anaesthesia* 1973; **45**: 501–6.

194 Hannallah, R.S. and Patel, R.I. Low-dose intramuscular ketamine for anesthesia pre-induction in young children undergoing brief outpatient procedures. *Anesthesiology* 1989; **70**: 598–600.

195 Gutstein, H.B., Johnson, K.L., Heard, M.B. and Gregory, G.A. Oral ketamine preanesthetic medication in children. *Anesthesiology* 1992: **76**: 28–33.

196 Alderson, P.J. and Lerman, J. Oral premedication for paediatric ambulatory anaesthesia; a comparison of midazolam and ketamine. *Canadian Journal of Anaesthesia* 1994; **41**: 221–6.

197 Donahue, P.J. and Dineen, P.S. Emergence delirium following oral ketamine. *Anesthesiology* 1992; **77**: 604.

198 Gingrich, B.K. Difficulties encountered in a comparative study of orally administered midazolam and ketamine. *Anesthesiology* 1994; **80**: 1415.

199 Rowbottam, S.J., Stewart, K.G., Sudhaman, D.A. and Aitken, A.W. Oral ketamine. *Anaesthesia* 1991; **46**: 1084–5.

200 Nishina, K., Mikawa, K., Maekawa, N., Takao, Y. and Obara, H. Clonidine decreases the dose of thiamylal required to induce anesthesia in children. *Anesthesia and Analgesia* 1994; **79**: 766–8.

201 Mikawa, K., Nishina, K., Maekawa, N., Asano, M. and Obara, H. Oral clonidine premedication reduces vomiting in children after strabismus surgery. *Canadian Journal of Anaesthesia* 1995; **42**: 977–81.

202 Mikawa, K., Maekawa, N., Nishina, K., Takao, Y., Yaku, H. and Obara, H. Efficacy of oral clonidine premedication in children. *Anesthesiology* 1993; **79**: 926–31.

203 Wright, P.M.C., Carabine, U.A., McClune, S., Orr, D.A. and Moore, J. Preanaesthetic medication with clonidine. *British Journal of Anaesthesia* 1990; **65**: 628–32.

204 Orkin, L.R., Bergman, P.S. and Nathanson, M. Effect of atropine, scopolamine and meperidine on man. *Anesthesiology* 1956; **17**: 30–7.

205 Murrin, K.R. A study of oral atropine in healthy adult subjects. *British Journal of Anaesthesia* 1973; **45**: 475–80.

206 Mirakhur, R.K. Comparative study of the effects of oral and i.m. atropine and hyoscine in volunteers. *British Journal of Anaesthesia* 1978; **50**: 591–8.

207 Crean, P.M., Laird, C.R.D., Keilty, S.R. and Black, G.W. The influence of atropine premedication on the induction of anaesthesia with isoflurane in children. *Paediatric Anaesthesia* 1991; **1**: 37–9.

208 Saarnivaara, L., Kautto, U.M., Iisaldo, E. and Pihlajamaki, K. Comparison of pharmacokinetic parameters following oral or intramuscular atropine in children. Atropine overdose in two small children. *Acta Anaesthesiologica Scandinavica* 1985; **29**: 529–36.

209 Mirakhur, R.K., Dundee, J.W. and Jones, C.J. Evaluation of the anticholinergic actions of glycopyrronium bromide. *British Journal of Clinical Pharmacology* 1978; **5**: 77–84.

210 Reynolds, J.C. and Putnam, P.E. Prokinetic agents. *Gastroenterology Clinics of North America* 1992; **21**: 567–96.

211 Manchikanti, L., Grow, J.B., Colliver, J.A., *et al.* Bicitra (sodium citrate) and metoclopramide in outpatient anesthesia for prophylaxis against aspiration pneumonitis. *Anesthesiology* 1985; **63**: 378–84.

212 Manchikanti, L., Marrero, T.C. and Roush, J.R. Preanesthetic cimetidine and metoclopramide for acid aspiration prophylaxis in elective surgery. *Anesthesiology* 1984; **61**: 48–54.

213 Wyner, J. and Cohen S.E. Gastric volume in early pregnancy; effect of metoclopramide. *Anesthesiology* 1982; **57**: 209–12.

CHAPTER 3

Inhalation agents in paediatric anaesthesia

FREDERIC BERRY

INTRODUCTION

Over the past few decades the practice of anaesthesia has undergone profound change. Even the expectations of what an anaesthetic is all about have been transformed: the continuing development of volatile agents and regional anaesthesia alongside that of various adjuvant drugs, including, for example, muscle relaxants, narcotics, hypnotics and local anaesthetics, means that the paediatric anaesthetist has a much broader choice both of agent and of technique in achieving his or her goals, which include:

1 minimal upset before and during induction of anaesthesia;
2 maintenance of an anaesthetic state appropriate for the procedure in hand;
3 rapid and pain-free recovery from the anaesthetic;
4 safety;
5 reduction of the stress response.

Inhalation agents are amongst the mainstays of paediatric anaesthetic practice. In routine cases anaesthesia can often be induced before an intravenous cannula is inserted, causing minimal disturbance to the child. They can be used either alone or, depending on the situation, in combination with the various adjuvants. This chapter aims to define the areas where inhalation agents can play a major role in the continuing development of paediatric anaesthesia.

BALANCED ANAESTHESIA

Lundy introduced the concept of 'balanced anaesthesia' in 1926, whereby a mixture of several drugs, each in small doses, was advocated, to reduce the side-effects and disadvantages of a high dose of any one drug.[1] Nitrous oxide was the basic anaesthetic, but because of its limited ability to provide sufficient anaesthesia by itself, various adjuvants were introduced, such as barbiturates, scopolamine, opioids and, later, muscle relaxants. Volatile anaesthetics were developed and added to the mix. Moreover, safety has been continually enhanced by the development of ever more sophisticated monitoring systems: it is possible now to monitor not only the important functions of the patient but also the concentrations of the various gases. In addition to the patient and end-tidal gas monitors, there are also monitors of the anaesthetic machine and the delivery of the anaesthetic gases. All of these factors have greatly reduced the morbidity and mortality of paediatric anaesthesia. The use of the various anaesthetic monitors has given the anaesthetist the ability not only to provide the anaesthetized state sufficient for surgery or whatever the anaesthetic requirement is, but also to control the neuromuscular system, the cerebral circulation, the circulatory system to maintain perfusion and minimize blood loss, and the control of ventilation. So, today, the concept of 'balanced anaesthesia' remains unchanged, but inevitably it embraces a much broader spectrum of drugs and techniques. For example, some anaesthetists prefer the use of topical analgesic cream to site an intravenous cannula, followed by an intravenous infusion with propofol or thiopentone, succinyl choline or a short-acting nondepolarizing muscle relaxant for intubation followed by various concentrations of volatile anaesthetics for maintenance. Others prefer to use an inhalational induction with an agent such as sevoflurane to sufficient depth to allow topicalization of the larynx with lignocaine

and intubation without relaxants. The combinations are almost endless. In short, today's anaesthetists have at their disposal sufficient means to administer anaesthetics appropriate for any procedure from the simplest to the most complex. Nevertheless, the key to successful management of the paediatric patient is not in the monitors or in the various anaesthetic agents but in the knowledge and expertise of the anaesthetist, who must be prepared to benefit from current advances while retaining the best practice of past experience.

UNIQUE CHARACTERISTICS OF THE PAEDIATRIC PATIENT AND INHALATION ANAESTHETICS

Many factors determine the uptake of inhaled anaesthetics.[2] These include the various tissue volumes of the body, alveolar ventilation, inspired anaesthetic concentration, cardiac output and the solubility of the anaesthetic agent. Likewise, there are many factors that are responsible for the more rapid induction and awakening of the neonate and infant with the inhalation anaesthetics.[3] Table 3.1 gives the percentages of total body volume of the various tissue components. It is evident that the newborn and neonate have a higher percentage of the vessel-rich group and a lower fat and muscle group compared with the older child and adult. The vessel-rich group is composed of the heart, the brain and various viscera. This means the anaesthetic will be delivered more rapidly to the brain and therefore the infant will have a more rapid induction and recovery from anaesthesia. The other factor of major importance in the neonate and infant is the relatively high oxygen consumption. The oxygen consumption of the neonate and infant is approximately 7–9 ml kg^{-1} of oxygen per minute, compared with 2–3 ml kg^{-1} min^{-1} in the adult. Because of this the neonate and infant will have a cardiac output and a rate of alveolar ventilation approximately three times those of the adult. Oxygen consumption is reduced during anaesthesia. Eger has elegantly shown the effects of ventilation on the rate of rise of the alveolar concentration of anaesthetics relative to their inspired concentration (Figure 3.1).[5] It is obvious that when drugs such as nitrous oxide and sevoflurane which are relatively insoluble are used, the changes in ventilation are not as important as with more soluble agents such as halothane. However, even though the effects are less, during an inhalation induction on a small child, speed is vital as the infant or small child goes through the excitement phase. Anaesthetic agents are less soluble in the brain, heart and liver in the neonate compared with the mature state. This is thought to be due to a decrease in water content and an increase in lipid content with increasing age.[3] In addition, there is an increase in muscle mass as well as in the protein concentration of muscle during the first several decades of life, which results in an increase in the solubility of inhaled anaesthetics as maturation occurs. In short, the solubility of anaesthetics in the neonate and the small infant is lower than that in the older child and adult and this also adds to the more rapid induction and recovery from anaesthesia.

Table 3.1 Tissue volumes

| Age group | Volume (% of total body volume) | | |
	Vessel-rich group	Muscle group	Fat group
Newborn	22.0	38.7	13.2
1 year	17.3	38.7	25.4
4 years	16.6	40.7	23.4
8 years	13.2	44.8	21.4
Adult	10.2	50.0	22.3

Reproduced with permission from Eger *et al.* (1971).[4]

METABOLISM OF ANAESTHETICS IN INFANTS AND CHILDREN

The metabolism of the various volatile anaesthetics and their potential for organ damage has been the subject of much clinical research. The story of methoxyflurane anaesthesia is a classic.[6] Methoxyflurane is the anaesthetic that caused high output renal failure by the metabolism of methoxyflurane to fluoride, which caused the nephrotoxicity. Table 3.2 gives the various percentages of the metabolism of the inhaled anaesthetics. Current thinking is that the less metabolized the anaesthetic, the lower the incidence and severity of organ toxicity. Sevoflurane has proved to be an excellent induction agent for the paediatric patient. There are factors, however, which have caused concerns with the metabolism of sevoflurane. Although sevoflurane is metabolized to fluoride, at the present time the major issue is that of com-

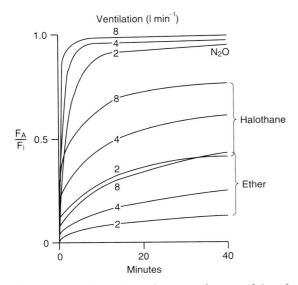

Figure 3.1 Effects of ventilation on the rate of rise of the alveolar concentration (F_A) relative to the inspired anaesthetic concentration (F_I). (Reproduced with permission from Eger, 1994.[5])

Table 3.2 Metabolism of inhaled anaesthetics

Drug	% Metabolized
Halothane	15–20
Sevoflurane	3
Isoflurane	0.2
Desflurane	0.02
N_2O	0.004

After Table 15.8 in Barash *et al.* (1997).[7]

pound A, or olefin. Compound A is formed in the anaesthetic circuit by the metabolism of sevoflurane by the carbon dioxide absorbant within the circuit. The experimental work and potential clinical implications of compound A will be discussed later in the chapter.

For several reasons, metabolism of anaesthetic agents in neonates and paediatric patients occurs to a lesser degree than it does in adults. The two issues in metabolism are tissue solubility, which results in a reservoir of anaesthetic agent in the body to be metabolized, and the amount of anaesthetic agent that is metabolized. Anaesthetic agents are less soluble in the neonate and young infant than in the adult.[3] The incidence of halothane-induced hepatitis was noted in paediatric patients below puberty to be much lower than in adults. This was observed in spite of the fact that for a long time, halothane was and may still be the most popular inhalation agent in children, many of whom underwent multiple exposures to halothane because of repeated anaesthetics for burns, papillomatosis, radiation therapy, etc. The exact reason for this finding is not clear. The result is that less drug is metabolized, with a reduction in the metabolic products that may be responsible for the problems of hepatic toxicity from halothane. As regards the issue of fluoride concentrations and toxicity, it is known that children exposed to methoxyflurane have lower peak serum fluoride concentrations than those of adults. In summary, then, it would appear that the paediatric patient is less susceptible to the metabolism of the various inhalation agents than the older patient.[3]

ANAESTHETIC REQUIREMENTS OF PAEDIATRIC PATIENTS: MAC

Attempts to quantify the anaesthetic requirement for the various volatile anaesthetics resulted in the development of the concept of MAC, which is defined as the minimum alveolar concentration of an anaesthetic at which 50% of patients fail to move in response to a well-defined surgical stimulus.[8–10] Some investigators have used the similar concept of the median effective dose (ED_{50}).[11] It is evident from the definition of MAC that the anaesthetic concentration required to stop all patient movement will be higher, and this has been estimated at about a 25% increase. The volatile anaesthetics, nitrous oxide and the opioids all contribute to MAC. While the various volatile anaesthetics can provide the complete anaesthetic requirement, nitrous oxide is a weak anaesthetic agent and 105% nitrous oxide is required in order to achieve 1 MAC. It is obvious that this can only be achieved in a hyperbaric environment. Remifentanil can also provide complete anaesthesia, but it is the only current opioid that can do so. Most clinicians administer anaesthetic concentrations in excess of 1 MAC, both to control blood pressure and to achieve anaesthesia.

The MAC values vary greatly with age, for reasons that are not entirely clear, but it has been suggested that they are related to the amount of water content in the brain. Other possible explanations have included the increased oxygen consumption and metabolic rate. However, the exact explanation has never been determined. The MAC values in the first 1 or 2 years of life vary greatly and have been determined by several investigators.[8–12] Figure 3.2 is a composite of several studies on the

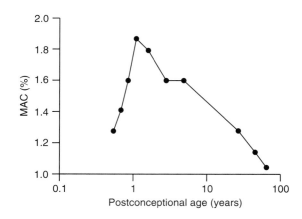

Figure 3.2 Minimum alveolar concentration (MAC) of isoflurane as a function of postconceptional age. The postconceptional age is calculated by adding 40 weeks to the mean postnatal age for each age group. (Reproduced with permission from Gregory, 1994.[3])

MAC value for isoflurane. This is quite similar to the changing anaesthetic requirements with halothane and other volatile anaesthetics and it provides a concept that is quite useful. The anaesthetic requirement in the first month of life is similar to the mature value for the various volatile anaesthetics. The anaesthetic requirement at 6 months to 1 year is approximately 50% greater than the mature value, while the anaesthetic requirement for the premature infants of 7–8 months' gestational age is somewhat lower, in the range of a decrease of 20–30%. Care must be taken in translating MAC values into anaesthetic practice, because of the time requirements for determining the MAC values. These values were determined after 15 min of equilibration at various end-tidal volatile anaesthetic concentrations. It is evident as one observes end-tidal gas concentrations during induction and immediately thereafter that these concentrations vary considerably according to uptake, distribution, fresh gas flow, etc. For the least soluble anaesthetics such as sevoflurane, desflurane and nitrous oxide, the uptake and equilibration are much faster and the difference between the inspired and the end-tidal concentration narrows more rapidly than with the more soluble anaesthetics such as halothane. However, there still is a considerable time lag for this to equilibrate. Regardless of these limitations, the concept of MAC as it applies to anaesthetic requirement is quite useful for the anaesthetist as it determines the anaesthetic concentrations that are required to produce the desired anaesthetic state.

Table 3.3   MAC-sparing effect of nitrous oxide

Halothane	60%
Isoflurane	40%
Sevoflurane	24%
Desflurane	20%

more soluble agents (Table 3.3).[10,13] Nitrous oxide does have cardiovascular effects in neonates and in children, but its effects are relatively mild compared with the other inhalation anaesthetics. Its major effect, particularly in the neonate, is that it will decrease the baroreflex and it has been reported to increase pulmonary vascular resistance. These changes in pulmonary vascular resistance may be more important in cardiac patients than in children who have normal cardiovascular and pulmonary systems. Nitrous oxide is an insoluble anaesthetic agent and will rapidly equilibrate in the bloodstream (Table 3.4). At the end of 5 min, the end-tidal concentration of nitrous oxide (F_A) will be approximately 90% of inspired (F_I) (Figure 3.3). This insolubility has clinical significance at the end of anaesthesia, since the nitrous oxide will offload in the same manner. This rapid clearing of nitrous oxide at the end of surgery is what is responsible for a condition known as 'diffusion hypoxia' caused by the more rapid efflux of nitrous oxide from the blood into the lungs than absorption of nitrogen from them, which dilutes the oxygen in the alveoli. When the patient is breathing air, alveolar gas may become hypoxic, producing a

SPECIFIC INHALATION AGENTS: NITROUS OXIDE

Nitrous oxide is a weak inhalation agent which by itself cannot predictably produce surgical anaesthesia since the minimum alveolar anaesthetic concentration (MAC) is 105%. Nitrous oxide, however, is an excellent adjunct as an induction agent and to reduce the MAC of volatile anaesthetics. Surprisingly, the MAC-sparing effect of nitrous oxide is significantly less for sevoflurane and desflurane than for the

Table 3.4   Characteristics of inhalation anaesthesia

	Partition coefficients		MAC mature	Vapour pressure
	Blood/ gas	Brain/ blood	(%)	(mmHg) at 20°C
Desflurane	0.45	1.3	6.0	669
Sevoflurane	0.65	1.7	2.0	170
N_2O	0.47	1.1	1.05	–
Isoflurane	1.4	1.6	1.15	240
Halothane	2.4	1.9	0.75	244

After Table 1 in Eger (1997).[14]

decrease in oxygen saturation. The use of 100% oxygen at the end of surgery for 2–3 min minimizes and in most cases eliminates the issue of diffusion hypoxia.

CONCERNS WITH NITROUS OXIDE

The blood partition coefficient for nitrous oxide is 34 times that for nitrogen. Therefore, the nitrous oxide will rapidly equilibrate in any pocket of trapped gas and will cause an expansion of this gas. This may be important if there is pneumocephalus following cranial surgery, since the nitrous oxide will equilibrate

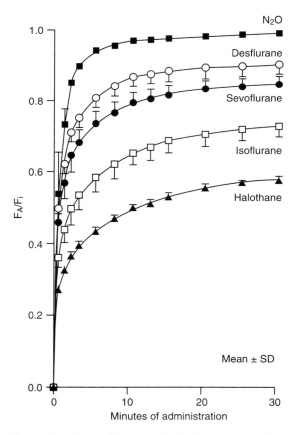

Figure 3.3 Rate of increase in alveolar concentration (F_A) towards the inspired concentration (F_I) of inhaled anaesthetics is depicted as the ratio F_{A+}/F_I. The rate of increase of the ratio is inversely related to the blood–gas partition coefficients of the agents. (Reproduced with permission from Yasuda *et al.*, 1991.[15])

with any air pockets within the cranium and has the potential for increasing intracranial pressure (ICP). This would be a rare occurrence, but one that the anaesthetist needs to be aware of. It may also be important if there are obstructed loops of bowel. In abdominal cases, if there is any gas within the intestinal system, this gas will expand and may interfere with both the surgery and the closure of the abdomen. Therefore, one strategy to minimize this possibility is to check the preoperative X-ray to see the content of gas within the bowel. If there is considerable gas, nitrous oxide may be used be for the induction of anaesthesia but consideration should be given to discontinuing it immediately thereafter. If there is no evidence of distention, then after induction a 50 : 50 concentration of nitrous oxide with oxygen is administered until the lumen of the bowel can be observed. If minimal gas is present, then the concentration of nitrous oxide has little significance. However, if there are moderate amounts of gas within the bowel, 50% nitrous oxide will double the quantity of gas in the bowel and the anaesthetist must decide whether this might interfere with the surgery. After the peritoneum is closed, nitrous oxide can be added in order to reduce the concentration of volatile anaesthetic.

Nitrous oxide has also been a concern because of its potential for fetal and haematopoietic effects. Methionine synthetase is important for cell division, and since nitrous oxide can interfere with this enzyme, concerns have been raised that its use during pregnancy may be associated with an increased incidence of fetal abnormalities.[16–18] There is no evidence at the present time to substantiate this possibility, but it raises concerns if during surgery an unsuspected pregnancy is discovered in a teenage female patient. Rare cases of neurological problems have been reported in the adult literature that are thought to be caused by the effects of the prolonged use of nitrous oxide on methionine synthetase. Methionine synthetase is involved in the metabolism of vitamin B_{12} and the concern in susceptible adult patients is that pernicious anaemia with neurological sequelae may develop in association with nitrous oxide. This is extremely rare.

VOLATILE INHALATION ANAESTHETICS: INDUCTION, MAINTENANCE AND RECOVERY

The volatile anaesthetics are the most frequently used primary anaesthetic agents in paediatric anaesthesia. The three volatile agents used most frequently are halothane, isoflurane and sevoflurane. The strategies for premedication and induction have changed over the last several years following the introduction of sevoflurane with its ease of administration. Halothane combined with nitrous oxide has been the gold standard for a long period, and in many parts of the world remains the most frequently used volatile anaesthetic. However, in many countries, sevoflurane is well on its way to being the primary induction agent. The final criteria for which agent will emerge as the primary volatile anaesthetic will depend upon cost, ease of use and toxicity. Some of these areas have yet to be defined completely. Isoflurane, when it was introduced, required a very gradual induction with a base of nitrous oxide and slowly increasing concentrations. Isoflurane is quite irritating to the airway and speed of induction is directly related to the skill of the practitioner. Desflurane is more irritable than isoflurane and therefore, when used for an inhalation induction, can certainly be an ordeal for the patient, the family and the anaesthetist.

After a sevoflurane or halothane induction, some clinicians switch to either isoflurane or desflurane because of their reported low metabolism and, in the case of desflurane, its low solubility resulting in rapid awakening.[14] Desflurane can be administered with low fresh gas flow rates, i.e. less than 1 l, because of its relative lack of metabolism. Desflurane is a very expensive anaesthetic and requires a special vaporizer. Table 3.3 lists the partition coefficients of the various anaesthetic agents and it is obvious that halothane is the most soluble and nitrous oxide and desflurane are the least soluble. Sevoflurane is slightly more soluble than desflurane and, after long cases, its recovery time is greater than that of desflurane.

Isoflurane lies between halothane and sevoflurane in its solubility and in its recovery characteristics.

HALOTHANE

Halothane remains one of the most popular volatile anaesthetics for children, despite its myocardial irritability and the rare but recognized risk of hepatotoxicity. As mentioned previously, even though it has a relatively high degree of biotransformation (20%), the incidence of halothane hepatitis is extremely low, with an estimated incidence of between 1 in 82 000 and 1 in 200 000.[19,20] This compares with an estimated incidence of between 1 in 6000 and 1 in 22 000 in adults.[21] Halothane is a good agent for induction either by itself or when used with nitrous oxide. It has a mildly pungent odour, but it is well tolerated, especially if given with high-flow nitrous oxide (7 l nitrous oxide, 3 l oxygen). The halothane is increased in increments of 0.5% as tolerated. Halothane is also a very popular agent because of its very low cost, even when higher flow rates are necessary, and this remains a crucial factor in many parts of the world. The other advantage of both halothane and isoflurane is that they have a lower incidence of delirium on recovery from anaesthesia. Because of the slower wake-up, the child recovering from anaesthesia has less chance of going through a period of delirium, as occurs with sevoflurane and desflurane. The greater solubility of halothane also makes it particularly useful for airway endoscopy procedures and the difficult airway patient. The more soluble the anaesthetic agent, the longer it takes for the anaesthetic to equilibrate. However, at the same time, when an adequate depth of anaesthesia is obtained because of the greater solubility, the patient can be maintained at that level with greater success than with the insoluble agents, in which there may be rapid arousal with interruption of ventilation. Isoflurane can also be used for endoscopy. Sevoflurane and desflurane are so insoluble that except for relatively short periods of endoscopy, i.e. 5–10 min, there is difficulty in maintaining an adequate level of anaesthesia without the use of intravenous agents.

ISOFLURANE

Isoflurane is an expensive, moderately soluble inhalation anaesthetic. It has a very pungent odour and requires considerable skill for an inhalation induction. However, isoflurane is a good maintenance anaesthetic and allows a more rapid recovery from anaesthesia than halothane. All of these recovery rates are greatly assisted by the ability to monitor end-tidal gases or to develop the clinical skills that are required for a more rapid awakening. Isoflurane has a relatively low level of metabolism, much less than halothane and sevoflurane and similar to desflurane. For that reason, even though hepatitis has been reported with isoflurane, at least theoretically, it should not occur as often.

SEVOFLURANE

First reports of the use of sevoflurane appeared in the early 1970s, but only in the early 1990s has it been widely introduced into clinical practice, where it has been found to be an excellent anaesthetic agent, particularly for the inhalation induction of anaesthesia in children.[22] It has much greater cardiovascular stability than halothane, and less risk of hepatotoxicity. Sevoflurane is an expensive agent and there has been a great deal of controversy about the appropriate fresh gas flow that should be administered because of the concerns about compound A. Sevoflurane is almost odourless and when used with nitrous oxide can result in a relatively rapid pleasant inhalation induction. Because of its lack of pungency a higher overpressure, i.e. 8%, with nitrous oxide can be administered at the beginning of the anaesthetic than with halothane. Nitrous oxide is an excellent induction agent to use with sevoflurane since it takes advantage of the second gas effect.[20,23] This effect occurs when the first gas, i.e. nitrous oxide, is rapidly taken up in the alveolus, thereby increasing the concentration of the second gas, i.e. sevoflurane, in the alveolus and this diffusion gradient then speeds the induction. This author uses a fresh gas flow rate of 4 l of nitrous oxide and 2 l of oxygen, holds the mask (Figure 3.4) approximately 1–2 inches away from the face as the child breathes the mixture for about 15–20 s, and

then gently brings the mask into contact with the face. The induction time is 1–2 min. Co-operative children can hold their own mask. If the surgery is short, i.e. under 30 min, then sevoflurane is continued as the primary anaesthetic with a total gas flow rate of less than 1 l, i.e. nitrous oxide 400 ml and oxygen 200 ml.

One disadvantage of sevoflurane that has become evident is that in a significant number of children there is a period of delirium upon awakening from the anaesthetic.[24,25] It was originally thought that perhaps the child was in pain and that the delirium was due to this factor. However, in studies comparing halothane with sevoflurane with similar analgesics there was an increase in the occurrence of delirium with sevoflurane. In another study, the children had received regional anaesthesia and, in spite of this, delirium still occurred. The major problem with the delirium of a child awaking from anaesthesia is the potential for injury. There is also a potential problem for the other families in the recovery room, since they may wonder whether this is the way that their own child recovered. For this reason, this author practises a technique of recovery from anaesthesia called the 'peaceful awakening from anaesthesia'. This technique reduces but does not eliminate delirium: when the anaesthetic is discontinued there is no more stimulation of either the airway or the child and all movements are made as gently and as peacefully as possible. In addition, intraoperative narcotics and local or regional analgesics are administered so that the child can awaken as pain-free as possible. If suctioning of the oropharynx or the stomach is required, this is done while the child is still anaesthetized and/or paralysed. Unless the abdomen is obviously distended, this author never suctions the stomach and in the case of secretions, rarely ever suctions secretions from the oropharynx. Once the anaesthetic is discontinued, then no more suctioning is used, even if there are secretions or blood in the oropharynx and nasopharynx. In order to remove these secretions, the child is laid on its side so that they will drain by gravity. The child is taken to the postanaesthesia care unit (PACU) and the PACU nurses are instructed not to suction or disturb the child except to take vital signs with the pulse oximeter and the blood pressure cuff. No attempt is made to arouse the children by shaking them, jiggling the tube, calling their name loudly, etc. They are allowed to recover from anaesthesia spontaneously and peacefully. This minimizes the problems of postextubation laryngospasm as well as the issues of delirium. This does not eliminate delirium but it reduces it. If the child does develop a degree of delirium, this is explained to the parents and they are brought in to attempt to comfort their child. It is very important for the anaesthetist to explain to the parent the problems of delirium and the fact that this will be a short-lived phenomenon and that the parent is there to help moderate this problem. It is not yet clear whether this problem occurs if sevoflurane is only used for induction or if it is seen exclusively after its use for maintenance of anaesthesia.

Toxic effects of sevoflurane

Between 3% and 5% of sevoflurane is metabolized, with the production of fluoride ions. Metabolism occurs by defluorination via cytochromes P450 31 and P450 2E1 to hexafluoroisopropanol + inorganic fluoride, which is then conjugated with glucuronic acid and excreted in urine. Trifluoroacetic acid is not produced during hepatic metabolism, so that the risk of hepatotoxicity is theoretically small.

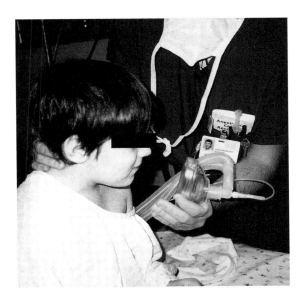

Figure 3.4 Technique of inhalation induction.

Methoxyflurane was discovered to produce a high output renal failure because the metabolism of methoxyflurane released fluoride in a sufficient concentration to cause renal damage. Peak fluoride levels transiently in excess of the level of 50 mM l^{-1}, regarded as toxic in adults, have been reported after sevoflurane anaesthesia, but fluoride levels remain high for much shorter periods after sevoflurane than after methoxyflurane, so that the area under the curve is significantly smaller. There have been no clinical reports of renal toxicity after sevoflurane, even in renally impaired patients or after long anaesthetics, despite the fact that several million patients world-wide have received the drug. Investigators have recently intensified their efforts in determining the biochemical markers of possible renal injury caused by the various anaesthetic agents. Measurements of blood urea nitrogen, creatinine and creatinine clearance are all very gross measurements of renal damage and renal function. Recent investigation into biochemical markers of potential renal injury have focused on measurements of urinary albumen and protein, which would demonstrate glomerular injury, and the various enzymes within the tubular cells, which would indicate or suggest injury to tubular cells.[26] Kharasch has suggested that *in situ* renal production of fluoride may be more important than hepatic metabolism.[27] Kharasch found that enzymatic sevoflurane defluorination by kidney microsomes was minimal, compared with methoxyflurane. Cytochrome P450 2E1 is not found in the human kidney.

Compound A

Sevoflurane is partially degraded by soda-lyme, particularly when fresh, and to an even greater extent by Baralyme® to produce small amounts of a sevo-olefin called compound A [fluoromethyl-2,2-difluoro-1-(trifluoromethyl) vinyl ether],[14] which causes mild renal changes in rats at concentrations above those found clinically. However, these changes depend on a beta lyase found in higher concentrations in rats than humans. Levels of compound A are higher with increases in temperature and reduction in flow rates below 2 l min^{-1}. Paediatric patients produce less carbon dioxide than adults, so that a given flow rate will produce a lower concentration of compound A in a child. However, this may be offset by the increase in MAC in children and the fact that many paediatric anaesthetist rely more heavily on inhaled anaesthetics alone rather than a balance with intravenous agents. Compound A in experimental animals and in human volunteers in long exposures at relatively high concentrations has been shown to produce biochemical markers of renal injury. In rats, compound A at high concentrations for prolonged exposures has proved to be lethal. The exposure in these rats was 3 h at a concentration of 331 ppm h^{-1}. Eger *et al.* suggest that the concentrations required for producing biochemical markers of renal injury in the volunteers are between 80 and 168 ppm h^{-1}.[26] There is a considerable debate over the problems of compound A in humans. The first issue to be answered is whether or not compound A produces a significant renal injury in humans. There is disagreement on this subject. The other issue to be discussed later is fresh gas flow rate, since the Food and Drug Administration (FDA) has recommended at least a 2 l fresh gas flow to minimize the concerns about compound A.

Alteration of function of the proximal tubule is thought to result in a release of γ-glutathione-S-transferase (γ-GST). Potential injury to distal tubules is thought to be reflected in an increase in π-glutathione-S-transferase (πST). Several studies which have attempted to demonstrate alterations in biochemical markers have resulted in different results. Eger's study of 1.25 MAC sevoflurane given for 4 h at 2 l^{-1} min^{-1} demonstrated a statistically significant increase in the biochemical markers and the authors concluded that compound A produced dose-related glomerular and tubular injuries with a threshold between 80 and 168 ppm h^{-1} of exposure to compound A.[26] Another study under similar conditions did not demonstrate any significant change in the biochemical markers.[28] The vast majority of studies which have measured compound A have shown that the levels vary between 20 and 60 ppm h^{-1} and rarely achieve threshold levels for potential injury. Sevoflurane produces fluoride, but there is no evidence that this has any adverse effect on renal function.

Early in the clinical release of sevoflurane in the USA, it was suggested that there was insufficient experience with sevoflurane in patients with impaired renal function to be sure about the potential harmful effects of sevoflurane on renal function.[29] At that time, it was recommended that sevoflurane not be used in patients with impaired kidney function until further studies might provide the proper information. Since that time (1995), there have been no case reports or studies in patients with impaired renal function to support this caution.

What fresh gas flow rate for sevoflurane?

Sevoflurane is a very expensive anaesthetic when used at moderate to high fresh flow rates (2–6 l min^{-1}). A recent study on the cost of anaesthetics comparing propofol, sevoflurane, desflurane and isoflurane revealed several interesting findings.[30] First of all, the cost of using propofol as the anaesthetic was considerably more than that of the inhalation anaesthetics: the cost was approximately US$0.30 min^{-1} of anaesthesia, whereas the costs for the inhalation agents (sevoflurane, desflurane and isoflurane) were quite similar, at approximately US$0.15 min^{-1} when the fresh gas flow was 1.5–2 l min^{-1}. One of the goals of anaesthesiologists in their attempts at cost containment is to reduce the cost of the anaesthetics as much as possible within the limits of safety. When sevoflurane was released in the USA several years ago, because of the concerns of renal toxicity and compound A, a flow rate of at least 2 l min^{-1} was recommended by the FDA. Since that time, there have been numerous studies to show that lower fresh gas flow rates are safe. For that reason, many clinicians have been using lower flow rates both to conserve the anaesthetic and to maintain the humidity within the circle system, and thereby to help to maintain the patient's temperature. The major concern about compound A and sevoflurane has been the prolonged exposure. Most paediatric cases are under the 2–4 h exposure that has resulted in alteration of the biochemical markers in some human volunteer studies but not in others.[26,28] In addition, infants and children seem to resist the metabolic effects of the degradation of various anaesthetics more than adults and it is only speculation that the same may be true for compound A. There are no studies to refute or support this idea. Therefore, it is this author's practice to use a high fresh gas flow initially to achieve induction, as described previously; then, after a period of 4–5 min, to reduce the fresh gas flow rates to 1 l min^{-1} or less and monitor the various concentrations of oxygen and the anaesthetic agents in the circuit.

High fresh gas flow rates: compound A and carbon monoxide

Several years ago, it was noted by several astute clinicians that their patients were being exposed to elevated levels of carbon monoxide.[31] The issue was clarified as it was discovered that oxygen had been left flowing through the anaesthetic machine at 5–10 l min^{-1} for 24–48 h, which resulted in dehydration of the CO_2 absorbant.[32] This, in turn, was responsible for the production of the carbon monoxide. The problem is greatest with desflurane, followed in descending order of severity by enflurane and isoflurane. It does not appear to be a clinically significant problem with halothane or sevoflurane. Dehydration of CO_2 absorbant has also been associated with increased amounts of compound A from the anaesthetic circuit. The manufacturers of the absorbant strongly suggest that if at any time a CO_2 absorber is found to be dehydrated by prolonged exposures to high flow rates (24–48 h) the absorbant should be replaced.[33] Some clinicians have suggested that the CO_2 absorbant be rehydrated by injecting water into the absorbant.[34]

DESFLURANE

Desflurane is the least soluble and the least metabolized of the volatile anaesthetics. It is also very expensive, in the same category as sevoflurane and isoflurane. It requires a special vaporizer, since it has a boiling point of 22.8°C and a vapour pressure of 88.53 kPa (664 mmHg). It is very pungent and not useful for the inhalational induction of anaesthesia, but may be useful for maintenance. A recent case report of a suspected malignant hyper-

thermia episode heightened awareness about volatile agents and malignant hyperthermia.[35]

EFFECTS OF INHALATIONAL ANAESTHETICS ON THE RESPIRATORY SYSTEM

All inhalational anaesthetics produce a dose-related depression of tidal and minute volume, with resultant increases in carbon dioxide. Ventilatory responses to carbon dioxide and vasoconstrictor response to hypoxia are also depressed. The effects of individual agents on respiratory frequency are, however, different, with halothane causing an increase, enflurane a decrease and isoflurane producing little change.

A recent study by Brown *et al.* compared the respiratory effects of sevoflurane and halothane in infants and young children between 6 months and 2 years old.[36] During anaesthesia at 1 MAC with nitrous oxide, minute ventilation and respiratory frequency were lower with sevoflurane than with halothane. Since the difference in end-tidal carbon dioxide level was only modest, this finding may not be clinically relevant at these concentrations. The study also demonstrated differences in parameters of breath timing and the shape of the flow wave-form, suggesting different effects of these agents on ventilatory control. Greater reduction in respiratory frequency with sevoflurane than halothane has also been reported in older children, but only at or above 1.5 MAC.[37] At the lighter levels of anaesthesia required when using the laryngeal mask airway, especially in combination with effective local or regional analgesia, respiratory depression is unlikely to be clinically significant.

Sevoflurane's remarkable lack of pungency and upper airway irritation has already been mentioned, and this has been mainly responsible for its replacing halothane as the induction agent of choice in children in those countries which can afford it. The pungency of desflurane makes it entirely unsuitable for inhalational induction.

EFFECTS OF INHALATIONAL ANAESTHETICS ON THE CENTRAL NERVOUS SYSTEM

For many years isoflurane has been accepted as the most suitable inhalational anaesthetic for neuroanaesthesia because of its minimal effects on cerebral blood flow, autoregulation and cerebral reactivity to carbon dioxide. Recent studies in adults have shown that cerebral autoregulation and carbon dioxide reactivity remain intact during sevoflurane anaesthesia,[38,39] that both sevoflurane and isoflurane decrease middle cerebral artery blood flow velocity, and that neither significantly alters ICP, or causes epileptiform EEG activity.[40] Sevoflurane may therefore be suitable for neurosurgery, although it may adversely increase cerebrospinal fluid volume and/or intracranial elastance. In one study in children sevoflurane produced cerebrovascular effects similar to those of halothane during induction.[41]

EFFECTS OF INHALATIONAL ANAESTHETICS ON THE CARDIOVASCULAR SYSTEM

Information about the circulatory effects of the inhalational agents has come from two sources: (1) experiments on healthy volunteers in whom no surgery was performed and (2) clinical studies. There have been clinical studies on the effects of inhalational anaesthetics on the circulation of infants and children. The major areas that will be discussed are the effects of inhalational anaesthetics on blood pressure, cardiac output and the baroreceptors. The studies on human volunteers have been very valuable since they demonstrated the effects of volatile anaesthetics when the full compensatory system of the circulation was assumed to be intact and functional. This compensatory system includes the sympathetic nervous system, the cardiovascular reserve, the baror-

eceptors and the peripheral circulation. Patients who have cardiovascular disease may have any or all of the various compensatory mechanisms of the body stressed almost to their limit, so that the circulation may be susceptible to depression from much lower concentrations of the volatile anaesthetics. The object of this chapter is not to give a complete compendium on the management of the circulation. However, children with cardiovascular disease who are on the various β-blockers, calcium-channel blockers, vasodilators, diuretics, etc., may have limited cardiovascular reserve. These children often test the knowledge and skills of the anaesthetist. However, in the vast majority of situations, the skilled clinician can choose a relatively safe technique.

BLOOD PRESSURE

All of the volatile anaesthetics in current use, i.e. halothane, isoflurane, desflurane and sevoflurane, will decrease arterial blood pressure in a dose-related manner (Figure 3.5). Halothane increases venous compliance but the major reason for the decrease in blood pressure is a decrease in cardiac output. The reduction in blood pressure associated with desflurane, isoflurane and sevoflurane is primarily due to a reduction in peripheral vascular resistance. Studies have been carried out in neonates

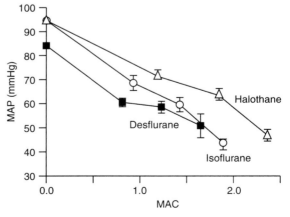

Figure 3.5 Mean arterial pressure (MAP) in humans decreases as the dose of the anaesthetic is increased, shown here as multiples of MAC. (Reproduced with permission from Weiskopf *et al.*, 1991.[42])

which demonstrate that their blood pressure is reduced more by volatile anaesthetics than in the adult, without any particular effects on the heart rate.[3] This would suggest that the inhalational anaesthetics have a greater effect on the baroresponse, which is more marked in preterm infants and neonates than in adults.

HEART RATE AND RHYTHM

There are also differences in the effect of the anaesthetics on heart rate. Halothane and isoflurane will decrease the heart rate, whereas sevoflurane has relatively little effect at MAC 1 and 2 levels during an induction. MAC 1 and 2 levels of desflurane are thought to stimulate the sympathetic nervous system via irritive receptors in the airway, which increase the sympathetic response resulting in a more rapid heart rate.[14] This also occurs with rapid concentration changes during maintenance anaesthesia with desflurane and less so with isoflurane when sudden increases in inspired concentration are necessary because of light anaesthesia. The increase in heart rate due to the stimulation of the sympathetic nervous system via the irritant receptors of the airway is usually short lived because the cells have a rapid adaptation to the irritation and, in addition, the higher concentrations of the anaesthetic will blunt the response. These increases in heart rate can also be blunted by the use of β-blockers and opioids.

Cardiac arrhythmias, both atrial and ventricular, are much more likely to occur with halothane than with isoflurane[43] or other inhalational anaesthetic agents. This is of particular concern in the field of dental surgery, where a recent study has shown the incidence of arrhythmias during halothane anaesthesia to be 44% compared with 24% with sevoflurane.[44]

CARDIAC OUTPUT

Halothane decreases the cardiac output more than any other of the inhalational agents because of its direct myocardial depression (Figure 3.6). Nitrous oxide has the least effect on cardiac output, with isoflurane, desflurane and sevoflurane only moderately decreasing cardiac output.[46]

There have been several paediatric studies comparing sevoflurane and halothane.[47–48] One

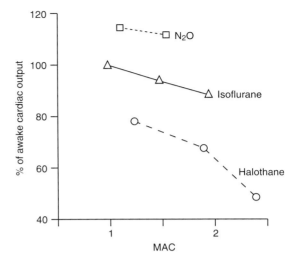

Figure 3.6 Percentage change from awake values of cardiac output in anaesthetized, normocapnic volunteers. (Reproduced with permission from Eger, 1981.[45])

of the major reasons for the interest in the haemodynamic effects of the volatile agents is that one of the chief causes of intraoperative complications in infants and children is the cardiovascular depression by the volatile anaesthetics. In one study, the children were between 2 and 12 years old.[47] The effects of the anaesthetics on myocardial contractility were determined with an echocardiogram. Nitrous oxide was used in the study for the initial induction of anaesthesia, but it was discontinued shortly after induction and after the patient was unconscious, so that all of the echo cardiographic data were recorded with an end-tidal nitrous oxide concentration of less than 0.5%. The patients were studied at end-tidal concentrations of 1 and 1.5 MAC of sevoflurane and halothane. Heart rates with sevoflurane decreased slightly at 1 MAC and returned to the baseline level with 1.5 MAC. The systolic and diastolic blood pressure were reduced with both anaesthetics at both MAC values but had returned towards control at 1.5 MAC. The authors found less direct myocardial depression during inhalation induction with sevoflurane compared with halothane, as measured by the stress velocity index and stress-shortening index. Contractility remained within normal limits with sevoflurane but was depressed by halothane. In a study of infants under 1 year of age, the circulatory effects of sevoflurane and halothane were compared echocardiographically. These infants were studied awake and at 1 MAC and 1.5 MAC concentrations for halothane and sevoflurane. They were premedicated with rectal midazolam. Nitrous oxide was used in a 50 : 50 concentration with oxygen. Halothane significantly decreased blood pressure and cardiac index as well as heart rate. The systolic blood pressure decreased with sevoflurane, indicating a decrease in peripheral vascular resistance. Sevoflurane did not alter the heart rate but there was a slight decrease in cardiac index (Figure 3.7). The authors suggest that the use of nitrous oxide in this study might explain why halothane and sevoflurane had more cardiovascular depressant effects than the study in older children in whom nitrous oxide had been discontinued after induction. Regardless of the effects of nitrous oxide, sevoflurane has much less effect on cardiac contractility than does halothane in infants and children. Similar studies had demonstrated that halothane caused a greater decrease in cardiac

output and cardiac index than isoflurane.[46] It has been suggested that one of the major effects of halothane in infants is that it causes an 18–30% decrease in heart rate and that the heart rate plays an important role in the decrease in cardiac output in these infants. Piat *et al.*, in a study of 34 children under 10 years old randomized to receive either sevoflurane or halothane in nitrous oxide, showed that heart rate increased and systolic blood pressure was maintained between induction and intubation in the sevoflurane group. By contrast, in the halothane group heart rate was unchanged and systolic blood pressure was significantly reduced.[49] In many of the studies with sevoflurane, heart rate has been shown to be stable. Lerman has shown that under 3 years of age, at 1 MAC sevoflurane, heart rate is unchanged, but that in children older than 3 years, the heart rate increases 10% above the awake values.[50] As far as the cardiovascular system is concerned, it would appear that sevoflurane is an excellent agent for the induction of anaesthesia in infants and children, having little effect on heart rate, and only a minor effect on cardiac contractility, which is compensated for by a decrease in systemic vascular resistance so that cardiac output remains relatively unchanged.

SOME INTERACTIONS OF DRUGS WITH VOLATILE ANAESTHETICS

Two major interactions of volatile anaesthetics with agents used in surgery will be discussed. These are (1) the use of adrenaline solutions and (2) the use of non-depolarizing muscle relaxants.

VOLATILE ANAESTHETICS AND ADRENALINE SOLUTIONS

The propensity for halothane to cause cardiac arrhythmias has already been mentioned. Shortly after its introduction it was noted that adrenaline injected into the tissue for haemostasis could cause ventricular dysrhythmias (Table 3.5). The initial studies in adults com-

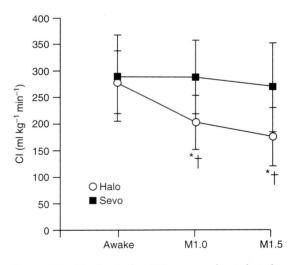

Figure 3.7 Cardiac index (CI) measured in infants by echocardiography–Doppler scanning who received sevoflurane (SEVO) or halothane (HALO) at all concentrations of anaesthetics. MAC 1.0 and MAC 1.5 were minimum alveolar concentrations of both anaesthetics adjusted for age. Data are mean ± SD. *$p < 0.05$ vs Awake; $p < 0.05$ HALO vs SEVO.

paring enflurane, isoflurane and halothane demonstrated that at 1.25 MAC, 50% of the patients would have ventricular dysrhythmias when adrenaline was given in a dose of 2.1 μg kg^{-1}.[51] When lignocaine was mixed with the adrenaline and during halothane at 1.25 MAC, the dose of adrenaline to produce ventricular dysrhythmias was 3.7 μg kg^{-1}. It was evident that adding lignocaine to the adrenaline reduced the incidence of ventricular dysrhythmias. In the presence of 1.25 MAC enflurane, the dose of adrenaline was 10.9 μg kg^{-1} and for isoflurane 6.7 μg kg^{-1} to produce dysrhythmias in 50% of the patients. These initial studies caused apprehension about what would be the dose response in children. Several studies were done which revealed that, for whatever reason, children had a higher threshold for dysrhythmias than adults. The report by Ueda *et al.* in spontaneously breathing children concluded that 7.8 μg kg^{-1} of adrenaline given with lignocaine was safe during halothane anaesthesia.[52] Karl *et al.* felt that at least 10 μg kg^{-1} of adrenaline could safely be used during halothane anaesthesia in normocarbic and hypocarbic paediatric patients who did not have congenital heart disease.[53] Some of the patients in their series had lignocaine administered with the adrenaline while others did not. It is evident from comparing the studies that there is a different interaction between adrenaline and halothane in children compared with adults. The reason for this difference is not clear. It is felt by most

authors that the addition of lignocaine to the adrenaline solution increases the margin of safety since the lignocaine will reduce the frequency of ventricular dysrhythmias. As a practical matter, it would appear that the dosage recommendation for children should be up to 10 μg kg^{-1} of adrenaline and that if arrhythmias develop they should be treated with intravenous lignocaine 1–1.5 mg kg^{-1}. If the dysrhythmias continue, then consideration should be given to the use of a β-blocker and if the patient is hypercarbic, to the control of ventilation. Another solution is to switch from halothane to isoflurane. There have been no studies in children of desflurane and sevoflurane with adrenaline and the incidence of dysrhythmias. In summary, it would appear that the use of adrenaline in the paediatric patient is only important when halothane is being administered and only then if large amounts are being administered.

ANAESTHESIA FOR ENDOSCOPY

ANAESTHESIA FOR ENDOSCOPY: SEVOFLURANE OR HALOTHANE?

The question of what is the best agent for endoscopy has been asked in recent years as has the question of whether or not halothane should be eliminated as an anaesthetic agent for children because of its very rare but documented problem with halothane hepatitis. The question of which anaesthetic is best for endoscopy, either for diagnosis or for the removal of a foreign body of the airway, depends on several factors. The anaesthetic choice depends on the needs of the surgeon, the length of the surgery and sometimes on the experience of the anaesthetist. Whichever technique is used, effective topical analgesia of the airway with lignocaine is essential. One technique is to paralyse the patient and use a jet ventilator. In these situations, it does not matter which agent is used for endoscopy. However, many surgeons prefer the patient to be breathing spontaneously during the endoscopic pro-

Table 3.5 Cardiac dysrhythmic dose of adrenaline during anaesthesia

Anaesthetic		Adrenaline (μg kg^{-1} min^{-1})[a]
Halothane	0.7 MAC	1.3 ± 0.2
	1.1	1.1 ± 0.3
Isoflurane	0.7	5.7 ± 1.1
	1.1	6.0 ± 1.0
Desflurane	0.8	6.9 ± 0.7
	1.2	6.6 ± 0.9
Sevoflurane	1.3	8.8 ± 1.18

[a]Mean ± SEM.
After Table 15.7 in Barash *et al.* (1997).[7]

cedure. This is because in the case of a diagnostic laryngoscopy they would like to see the movement of the vocal cords, or in the case of a foreign body it may be blown further down the airway with the use of a ventilator. The endoscopic procedure for the removal of a foreign body is often accompanied by various periods of interruption of ventilation as the bronchoscope is introduced down one bronchus or the other. The result is that there may be a reduction or even a complete interruption in anaesthetic delivery to the patient. With a very insoluble agent such as sevoflurane, the patient may lighten, whereas with a more soluble agent such as halothane the level of the anaesthetic is more stable. For that reason, the majority opinion today seems to be that halothane should remain in the armamentarium; for many, it is the anaesthetic of choice for endoscopy if the anaesthetic technique is going to involve spontaneous ventilation and if the duration of the anaesthetic is uncertain. One alternative strategy being adopted is to induce anaesthesia with sevoflurane and then to change to isoflurane for the endoscopy.

THE ROLE OF HALOTHANE

Since the introduction of sevoflurane, with its generally accepted superiority over halothane as an induction agent, the question of whether there remains a role for halothane in paediatric anaesthesia is increasingly debated. Many, if not most paediatric anaesthetists feel that halothane's slower recovery profile makes it a safer agent to use for manouevres involving the upper airway, such as diagnostic laryngoscopy or bronchoscopy. However, this advantage may be more than offset by the fact that since halothane is disappearing from adult practice, the next generation of anaesthetists will have had little or no experience with the agent. At the time of writing the expense of sevoflurane, together with uncertainties about emergence delirium and possible toxicity, suggest that it would be irresponsible to advocate the discontinuation of halothane production.

SUMMARY

Inhalation anaesthetics provide the basis for most paediatric anaesthesia. The best anaesthetists – those for whom anaesthesia is both an art and a science – will combine their knowledge and experience of the various inhalation anaesthetics and adjuvants with knowledge and experience of how to manage and meet, sensitively, the needs of the child within the context of the family.

ACKNOWLEDGEMENT

The author acknowledges the excellent editorial assistance of Robert Bland.

REFERENCES

1 Lundy, J.S. Balanced anesthesia. *Minnesota Medicine* 1926; **9**: 399–404.
2 Stevens, W.C. and Kingston, H.G.G. Inhalation anesthesia. In: Barash, P.G., Cullen, B.F. and Stoelting, R.K. (eds). *Clinical Anesthesia*. 3rd edn. Philadelphia, PA: Lippincott-Raven, 1997: 359–83.
3 Gregory, G.A. Pharmacology. In: Gregory, G.A. (ed.). *Pediatric Anesthesia*. 3rd edn. New York: Churchill Livingstone, 1994: 13–45.
4 Eger, E.I. II, Bahlman, S.H. and Munson, E.S. The effect of age on the rate of increase of alveolar anesthetic concentration. *Anesthesiology* 1971; **35**: 365–72.
5 Eger, E.I. II. Uptake and distribution. In: Miller, R.D. (ed.) *Anesthesia*. 4th edn. New York: Churchill Livingstone, 1994: 101–24.
6 Mazze, R., Trudell, J. and Cousins, M. Methoxyflurane metabolism and renal dysfunction: clinical correlations in man. *Anesthesiology* 1971; **35**: 247–52.
7 Barash, P.G., Cullen, B.F. and Stoelting, R.K. (eds). *Clinical Anesthesia*. 3rd edn. Philadelphia, PA: Lippincott-Raven, 1997.
8 LeDez, K.M. and Lerman, J. The minimum alveolar concentration (MAC) of isoflurane in preterm neonates. *Anesthesiology* 1987; **67**: 301–7.
9 Katoh, T. and Ikeda, K. Minimum alveolar concentration of sevoflurane in children. *British Journal of Anaesthesia* 1992; **68**: 139–41.
10 Fisher, D.M. and Zwass, M. MAC of desflurane in 60% nitrous oxide in infants and children. *Anesthesiology* 1992; **76**: 354–6.
11 Nicodemus, N.F., Nassiri-Rhimi, C. and Bachman, L. Median effective doses (ED$_{50}$) of halothane in adults and children. *Anesthesiology* 1969; **31**: 344–8.

12 Deming, M.V. Agents and techniques for induction of anesthesia in infants and young children. *Anesthesia and Analgesia* 1952; **31**: 113.

13 Taylor, R.H. and Lerman, J. Minimum alveolar concentration of desflurane and haemodynamic responses in neonates, infants and children. *Anesthesiology* 1991; **75**: 975–9.

14 Eger, E.I. II. New inhaled anesthetics. *Anesthesiology* 1994; **80**: 906–922.

15 Yasuda, N., Lockhart, S.H., Eger, E.I. II, *et al.* Comparison of kinetics of sevoflurane and isoflurane in humans. *Anesthesia and Analgesia* 1991; **72**: 316–24

16 Berry, A.J. and Katz, J.D. Hazards of working in the operating room. In: Barash, P.G., Cullen, B.F. and Stoelting, R.K. (eds). *Clinical Anesthesia.* 3rd edn. Philadelphia, PA: Lippincott-Raven, 1997: 69–91.

17 Aldridge, L.M. and Tunstall, M.E. Nitrous oxide and the fetus. *British Journal of Anaesthesia* 1986; **58**: 1348–56.

18 Duncan, P.G., Pope, W.D., Cohen, M.M. and Greer, N. Fetal risk of anesthesia and surgery during pregnancy. *Anesthesiology* 1986; **64**: 790–4.

19 Wark, H.J. Postoperative jaundice in children. The influence of halothane. *Anaesthesia* 1983; **38**: 237–42

20 Warner, L.O., Beach, T.P., Garvin, J.P. and Warner, E.J. Halothane and children: the first quarter century. *Anesthesia and Analgesia* 1984; **63**: 838–40.

21 Ray, D.C. and Drummond, G.B. Halothane hepatitis. *British Journal of Anaesthesia* 1991; **67**: 84–99.

22 Sarner, J.B., Levine, M., Davis, P.J., Lerman, J., Cook, D.R. and Motoyama, E.K. Clinical characteristics of sevoflurane in children: a comparison with halothane. *Anesthesiology* 1995; **82**: 38–46.

23 Epstein, R.M., Rackow, H., Salanitre, E. and Wolf, G.L. Influence of the concentration effect on the uptake of anesthetic mixtures: the second gas effect. *Anesthesiology* 1964; **25**: 364–71.

24 Weldon, B.C., Abele, A., Simeon, R., *et al.* Postoperative agitation in children: sevoflurane vs halothane. *Anesthesiology* 1997; **87**: A1057.

25 Westrin, P. and Beskow, A. Sevoflurane causes more postoperative agitation in children than does halothane. *Anesthesiology* 1997; **87**: A1061.

26 Eger, E.I. II, Gong, D., Koblin, D.D., *et al.* Dose-related biochemical markers of renal injury after sevoflurane versus desflurane anesthesia in volunteers. *Anesthesia and Analgesia* 1997; **85**: 1154–63.

27 Kharasch, E.D., Hankins, D.C. and Thummel, K.E. Human kidney methoxyflurane and seroflurane metabolism. Intrarenal fluoride production as a possible mechanism of methoxyflurane nephrotoxicity. *Anesthesiology* 1995; **82**: 689–99.

28 Ebert,T.J., Messana, L.D., Uhrich, T.D. and Staacke, T.S. Absence of renal and hepatic toxicity after four hours of 1.25 minimum alveolar anesthetic concentration sevoflurane anesthesia in volunteers. *Anesthesia and Analgesia* 1998; **86**: 662–7.

29 Mazze, R.I. and Jamison, R. Renal effects of sevoflurane. *Anesthesiology* 1995; **83**: 443–5.

30 Boldt, J., Jaun, N., Kumle, B., Heck, M. and Mund, K. Economic considerations of the use of new anesthetics: A comparison of propofol, sevoflurane, desflurane, and isoflurane. *Anesthesia and Analgesia* 1998; **86**: 504–9.

31 Moon, R.E. Cause of CO poisoning, relation to halogenated agents still not clear. *Journal of Clinical Monitoring* 1995; **11**: 66–7.

32 Fang, Z.X., Ege, E.I., Laster, M.J., Chortkoff, B.S., Kandel, L. and Ionescu, P. Carbon monoxide production from degradation of desflurane, enflurane, isoflurane, halothane, and sevoflurane by soda lime and Baralyme. *Anesthesia and Analgesia* 1995; **80**: 1187–93.

33 McGovern, J.F. Desflurane degradation to carbon monoxide. Letter to editor. *Anesthesiology* 1998; **88**: 547.

34 Baxter, P.J. and Kharasch, E.D. Rehydration of desiccated Baralyme prevents carbon monoxide formation from desflurane in an anesthesia machine. *Anesthesiology* 1997; **86**: 1061–5.

35 Lowes, R. and Mayhew, J.F. A suspected malignant hyperthermia episode during desflurane anesthesia. *Anesthesia and Analgesia* 1998; **86**: 449–50.

36 Brown, K., Aun, C., Stocks, J., Jackson, E., Mackersie, A. and Hatch, D. A comparison of the respiratory effects of sevoflurane and halothane in infants and young children. *Anesthesiology* 1998; **89**: 86–92.

37 Yamakage, M., Tamiya, K., Horikawa, D., Sato, K. and Namiki, A. Effects of halothane and sevoflurane on the paediatric respiratory pattern. *Paediatric Anaesthesia* 1994; **4**: 53–6.

38 Gupta, S., Heath, K. and Matta, B.F. Effect of incremental doses of sevoflurane on cerebral pressure autoregulation in humans. *British Journal of Anaesthesia* 1997; **79**: 469–72.

39 Inada, T., Shingu, K., Uchida, M., Kawachi, S., Tsushima, K. and Niitsu, T. Changes in the cerebral arteriovenous oxygen content difference by surgical incision are similar during sevoflurane and isoflurane anaesthesia. *Canadian Journal of Anaesthesia* 1996; **43**: 1019–244.

40 Artru, A.A., Lam, A.M., Johnson, J.O. and Sperry, R.J. Intracranial pressure, middle cerebral artery flow velocity, and plasma inorganic fluoride concentrations in neurosurgical patients receiving sevoflurane or isoflurane. *Anesthesia and Analgesia* 1997; **85**: 587–92.

41 Berkowitz, R.A., Hoffman, W.E., Cunningham, F. and McDonald, T. Changes in cerebral blood flow velocity in children during sevoflurane and halothane anesthesia. *Journal of Neurosurgical Anesthesiology* 1996; **8**: 194–8.

42 Weiskopf, R., Cahalan, M. and Eger, E.I. II. Cardiovascular actions of desflurane in normocarbic volunteers. *Anesthesia and Analgesia* 1991; **73**: 143–56.

43 Rodrigo, M.R.C., Moles, T.M. and Lee, P.K. Comparison of the incidence and nature of cardiac arrhythmias occurring during isoflurane and halothane anaesthesia. *British Journal of Anaesthesia* 1986; **58**: 394–400.

44 Paris, S.T., Cafferkey, M., Tarling, M., Hancock, P., Yate, P.M. and Flynn, P.J. Comparison of sevoflurane and halothane for outpatient dental anaesthesia in children. *British Journal of Anaesthesia* 1997; **79**: 280–4.

45 Eger, E.I. II. Isoflurane: a review. *Anesthesiology* 1981; **55**: 559–76.

46 Murray, D.J., Forbes, R.B. and Mahoney, L.T. Comparative hemodynamic depression of halothane versus isoflurane in neonates and infants: an echocardiographic study. *Anesthesia and Analgesia* 1992; **74**: 329–37.

47 Holzman, R.S., van der Velde, M.E., Kaus, S.J., *et al.* Sevoflurane depresses myocardial contractility less than halothane during induction of anesthesia in children. *Anesthesiology* 1996; **85**: 1260–7.

48 Wodey, E., Pladys, P., Copin, C., *et al.* Comparative hemodynamic depression of sevoflurane versus halothane in infants: an echocardiographic study. *Anesthesiology* 1997; **87**: 795–800.

49 Piat, V., Dubois, M.-C., Johanet, S. and Murat, I. Induction and recovery characteristics and hemodynamic responses to sevoflurane and halothane in children. *Anesthesia and Analgesia* 1994; **79**: 840–4.

50 Lerman, J., Sikich, N., Kleinman, S. and Yentis, S. The pharmacology of sevoflurane in infants and children. *Anesthesiology* 1994; **80**: 814–24.

51 Johnston, R.R., Eger, E.I. II and Wilson, C. A comparative interaction of adrenaline with enflurane, isoflurane, and halothane in man. *Anesthesia and Analgesia* 1976; **55**: 709–12.

52 Ueda, W., Hirakawa, M. and Mae, O. Appraisal of adrenaline administration to patients under halothane anesthesia for closure of cleft palate. *Anesthesiology* 1983; **58**: 574–6.

53 Karl, H.W., Swedlow, M.D., Lee, K.W. and Downes, J.J. Adrenaline–halothane interactions in children. *Anesthesiology* 1983; **58**: 142–5.

CHAPTER 4

Intravenous agents

PETER BOOKER

INTRODUCTION

The pharmacology of individual drugs used in paediatric anaesthesia can only be discussed sensibly once the most important differences among infants, children and adults affecting their response to intravenous drug administration have been fully understood.

Information about the pharmacology of intravenous anaesthetic drugs obtained from studies in healthy children cannot usually be extrapolated to critically ill infants.

Pharmacological studies tend to examine the effects of giving a single drug to an individual, whereas in clinical practice this is unusual, as drug interactions are often usefully employed. Co-administration of interacting drugs may make it possible to use lower doses of each drug and so reduce the incidence of undesirable side-effects. Studies of drug interactions in anaesthesia have revealed that the mechanism can be pharmacokinetic as well as pharmacodynamic. The nature of the interaction may differ according to the end-point studied, as the various effects produced by one or more drugs are propagated through many different receptor complexes at different sites within the central nervous system (CNS).

Although the recognized age groupings, neonate, infant and child, represent convenient labels for comparative purposes, physiological maturation and development of vital organ function is a continuous and uninterrupted process. Nevertheless, in general it may be assumed that pharmacological maturation takes place within the first year of life, although this does not imply that children more than 1 year old should be given a weight-related adult dose of drug. The dosage of many anaesthetic drugs, when related to body weight, may need to be higher in young children than in adults.

PHARMACOKINETICS

Pharmacokinetics is the study of drug absorption, distribution and elimination, made possible by measurement of the concentration of drug and metabolite(s) in plasma and urine. Changes in drug concentration with time can be used to derive certain pharmacokinetic values that not only describe drug handling in the body, but also can be used to predict optimum dosage scheduling and rate of drug elimination. Pharmacokinetics uses mathematical models; in the simplest, the body is considered to be a single compartment within which the drug is uniformly and rapidly distributed. The apparent volume of distribution (V_d) of a drug at equilibrium is the total amount of drug in the body divided by its concentration in plasma. Hence, if a drug is concentrated mainly in extravascular tissues, the V_d will be much larger than actual bodily compartments. V_d can also be calculated by multiplying the tissue volume by the relative solubility (partition coefficient) of the drug in tissue and plasma. Hence, the V_d for a given drug is dependent on the partition coefficient of the drug, the regional blood flow to tissues and the proportion bound to plasma proteins and other tissues. Thus, it is not altogether surprising that the V_d of various drugs may be different, in terms of litres per kilogram, in the infant compared with the adult, because regional blood flow and relative proportions of water, fat and protein all change with age (Table 4.1).

Another important measured pharmacokinetic parameter, clearance, reflects the ability of the body to eliminate the drug. Clearance represents the volume of blood from which the drug is completely eliminated in unit time. For most intravenous anaesthetic drugs, clearance will depend mostly on hepatic function, although renal excretion of drug and/or metabolites may also be important. Hence, maturation of hepatic and renal function will have significant effects on clearance values for many drugs throughout infancy. Drug concentrations in a body compartment usually decrease exponentially, so that the same fraction of drug is eliminated in any given time period. The rate of this exponential process may be expressed as its elimination half-life ($t_{1/2}$), which is the time necessary for a 50% reduction in drug concentration. Both apparent volume of distribution and clearance (Cl) will determine how long it takes for the plasma concentration of a drug to decrease. These three pharmacokinetic values, $t_{1/2}$, V_d and Cl, can be related by the equation:

$$t_{1/2} = 0.693 \times V_d/Cl.$$

Consequently, a prolongation of the elimination half-life may reflect an increase in the volume of distribution, a reduction in clearance or both.

A more accurate pharmacokinetic representation of events after intravenous injection of anaesthetic drugs uses a two-compartment model, in which distribution of drug from plasma into tissue is taken into account. The rate and extent of this initial decrease in plasma concentration are mainly dependent on the tissue perfusion and lipid solubility of the drug. In the two-compartment model, the change in plasma drug concentration with time can be represented by two exponential decay curves, as shown in Figure 4.1. The first and faster decay represents redistribution from a central to a peripheral compartment, and the second slower phase represents elimination. Although each phase has its own half-life (distribution half-life, $t_{1/2a}$, and elimination half-life, $t_{1/2b}$), it should be appreciated that the process of distribution of drugs between compartments continues throughout the elimination phase. Similarly, the elimination processes begin as soon as the drug reaches the relevant tissues.

Although the pharmacokinetics of some drugs is consistent with a two-compartment model, for many anaesthetic drugs models of greater complexity offer a better description of events and the decline in plasma concentration can be resolved into three exponential

Table 4.1 Comparison of relative organ mass[14] and regional blood flow between the neonate and adult

Organ	Organ mass (% of body weight)		Regional blood flow (% of cardiac output)	
	Neonate	Adult	Neonate	Adult
Muscle	25.0	40.0	5	11[181,182]
Heart	0.5	0.4	3	4[182]
Liver	5.0	2.0	25[a]	25[183,184]
Kidneys	1.0	0.5	3	17[185]
Brain	12.0	2.0	14	14[186,187]

[a]Signifies animal data.

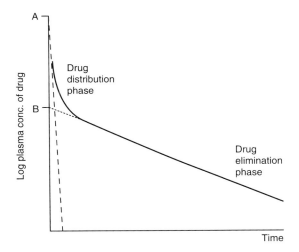

Figure 4.1 Diagrammatic representation of a bi-exponential decline in the plasma concentration of a drug after intravenous injection. The initial rapid fall in concentration due to drug distribution is defined by a regression line which intercepts the y-axis at A. Point B represents the concentration of drug when the slower elimination phase of the decline in plasma concentration is extrapolated to zero time. Both phases have characteristic slopes a and b and half-lives ($t_{1/2a}$ and $t_{1/2b}$).

components. Alternatively, non-compartmental methods of pharmacokinetic analysis can be used to estimate drug clearance and volume of distribution at steady state. Nevertheless, however sophisticated the mathematical modelling, the pharmacokinetic data that are produced remain relatively specific for the individuals studied under the particular conditions of the study. This is because there is often great interpatient variability in both pharmacokinetic and pharmacodynamic processes and, for many drugs, the relationship between drug concentration in plasma and drug effect is very tenuous. Pharmacokinetic data can be used, nonetheless, to predict the optimal frequency of drug administration, loading dose, infusion rate, dosage modifications required in patients with vital organ dysfunction and determination of the effects of other drugs on drug disposition. Hence, drug dosage regimens can be guided by pharmacokinetic information but must always be reviewed in the light of clinical experience.

DEVELOPMENTAL FACTORS AFFECTING DRUG DISTRIBUTION

Anaesthetic drugs exert their effects by binding reversibly to various receptor proteins such as ion channels and/or intracellular proteins. However, before a drug can exert an effect it must pass from its site of administration and reach its site(s) of action. Plasma concentrations of a drug do not always relate to clinical effect, as drug plasma concentration does not necessarily correlate with concentration of the drug near the receptor. This is because a drug molecule given intravenously must cross several phospholipid membranes to reach its receptor. Small molecules tend to cross membranes more rapidly than large ones, but a highly ionized molecule, whatever its size, will be unable to pass passively through a lipid membrane and will have to use active or facilitated transport mechanisms. In contrast, lipid-soluble drugs, which are mostly unionized at physiological pH, can cross lipid membranes in significant quantities by passive diffusion down concentration gradients. The degree of drug ionization depends on the dissociation constant (pK_a) of the drug and on the local pH. Most intravenous anaesthetic drugs are weak bases (B) which combine with hydrogen ions (H^+) in solution to form a charged molecule:

$$B + H^+ \rightleftharpoons BH^+.$$

The equilibrium will shift to the right in an acid pH. When the local pH = pK_a of the drug, 50% of the drug will be ionized. Hence, small changes in pH can affect the distribution of a drug with a pK_a close to 7.4 (Table 4.2). The degree of ionization is only one of many physicochemical factors affecting the ability of a drug to diffuse passively through lipid membranes. The relative solubility of drug in blood and tissue, the blood–tissue partition coefficient, is another individual drug constant that can be assessed *in vitro* by measuring drug solubility in organic and aqueous solvents. Other important factors influencing anaesthetic drug distribution, some of which have already been alluded to, include regional tissue perfusion, permeability of the blood–brain barrier, the relative size of body compartments into which the drug is distributed and the degree of protein binding. All these factors are subject to developmental change.

REGIONAL BLOOD FLOW

The initial phase of distribution reflects regional blood flow. Hence, a major determinant of drug distribution is cardiac output and how it is distributed to the various tissues of the body. Cardiac output in the healthy term neonate during the first week of life, when measured by Doppler ultrasound, is 230–240 ml kg^{-1} min^{-1}, although such measurements have inherent inaccuracies of at least ± 18%. Indexing cardiac output to body surface area rather than weight provides a better means of comparing grouped data. Hence, the 1-month-old infant has a cardiac output of about 2.6 l min^{-1} m^{-2}, which increases to 3.2 l min^{-1} m^{-2} by 1 year of age and 4.0 l min^{-1} m^{-2} by 2–15 years of age.[1–4]

Organs that are well perfused, such as the brain, heart and liver, are the tissues first exposed to the drug. The second phase of distribution involves other relatively well-perfused tissues, such as skeletal muscle, with much slower tertiary distribution to relatively underperfused tissues of the body usually only assuming importance with long-term drug infusions. Acute changes in the neonatal circulation that affect organ blood flow take place in the first few days and weeks after birth, secondary to functional closure of the ductus venosus and

ductus arteriosus. In addition, differences in relative organ mass and regional blood flow change with growth and development during the first few months of life. Renal and hepatic blood flow achieve adult levels by about 12 months of age. The most important differences in regional perfusion between the neonate and adult are summarized in Table 4.1. Although cerebral mass as a proportion of body weight is much higher in the infant than in the adult, the proportion of cardiac output perfusing the brain is similar in both the neonate and adult. After the neonatal period, mean cerebral blood flow per unit volume of brain does not vary significantly with age, but values throughout infancy and childhood exceed those in adults.[5] As highly lipophilic drugs in cerebral arterial blood diffuse rapidly across the blood–brain barrier to achieve concentration equilibrium with brain tissue, the rate of entry of drug is determined largely by cerebral blood flow. Hence, onset times for intravenous anaesthetic agents tend to be shorter in infancy and childhood than in adults.

BLOOD–BRAIN BARRIER

Although the blood–cerebrospinal fluid (CSF) and blood–brain barriers are not identical, developmental changes in the blood–CSF barrier probably reflect analogous changes in the blood–brain barrier. There appears to be continuous development of the blood–CSF barrier from early fetal life. The permeability of the fetal barrier is high, but infants 2–12 months of age demonstrate similar CSF/

Table 4.2 Physical characteristics of some commonly used anaesthetic drugs[71,117,169,188,189]

Drug	pK_a	% drug ionized at pH 7.4	Plasma protein binding (%)	Octanol/buffer partition coefficient at pH 7.4
Morphine	7.9	76	35	1.4
Midazolam	6.2	<5	96	34
Remifentanil	7.1	32	70	17.9
Thiopentone	7.6	39	78	600
Propofol	11.0	99	98	5000
Ketamine	7.5	55	47	60
Fentanyl	8.4	91	85	960
Alfentanil	6.5	11	92	130

plasma ratios of fentanyl to older children.[6] Significant increases in the permeability of the blood–CSF barrier can be induced by a variety of pathological conditions, including infection and hypoxia.[7]

Passive diffusion is the dominant process at the blood–CSF barrier and the analogy with the blood–brain barrier is probably valid for lipophilic anaesthetic drugs, which passively diffuse across the blood–brain barrier to achieve equilibrium very quickly. However, the kinetics of their penetration into brain tissue becomes more complicated if they are bound to plasma proteins. The blood–brain barrier is composed of non-fenestrated endothelial cells, which are interconnected by a continuous network of complex tight junctions that functionally fuse the plasma membranes of adjacent endothelial cells.[8] These tight intercellular junctions represent a barrier to passive diffusion of drugs with low lipophilicity, protein macromolecules and smaller hydrophilic molecules such as glucose.[9] In preterm neonates, immaturity of transcellular protein-specific transfer mechanisms in the choroid plexus means that drugs bound to plasma proteins may be able to penetrate into the immature brain.[10]

BODY WATER CONTENT

Water constitutes at least 80% by weight of a preterm and 75% of a term newborn infant.[11] After birth, total body water (TBW) gradually decreases to achieve adult proportions (57 ± 2%) by 1 year of age (Figure 4.2). From this point there is a linear relationship between TBW and lean body mass until old age. At equilibrium, ionized water-soluble drugs will be uniformly distributed throughout the TBW and any changes in TBW will have a significant effect on the distribution volume of water-soluble drugs that have a small V_d, such as pancuronium. Conventionally, TBW is divided into two discrete compartments: intracellular and extracellular fluid. The former makes up about 35% of body weight at birth, but quickly rises to 40% by 3 months of age. The proportion of body weight contributed by intracellular water then falls in line with the decrease in TBW until about 1 year of age, when it increases again to the adult value of 40% by 4 years of age. In contrast, the contribution of

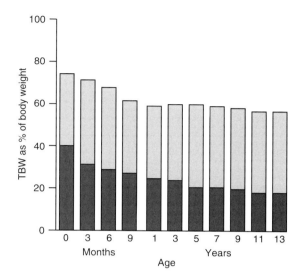

Figure 4.2 Changes in distribution of body water during childhood. TBW: Total body water; ▨: intracellular water; ▧: extracellular water. (Adapted with permission from Friis-Hansen, 1983.[11])

extracellular water to body weight decreases more gradually from about 40% at birth to about 20% by 6 years of age. Furthermore, the proportion of TBW and the relative amount of intracellular and extracellular water in each organ also change with age.

BODY FAT CONTENT

Fat constitutes about 12% of body weight in the term neonate, rapidly increasing to about 25% by 6 months, and 30% by 1 year of age, before declining for the next 7 years.[12,13] Girls substantially increase their fat content from 8 years onwards, compared with boys who only slightly increase their fat content from the start of puberty (Figure 4.3). Superimposed on these overall changes in fat content is the disproportionate growth of different organs. The CNS in the neonate constitutes a higher proportion of body weight and has a higher proportion of both extracellular water and fat than in the adult.[14] These changes in body and organ lipid content have obvious implications for the apparent volume of distribution for highly lipid-soluble drugs such as fentanyl. Moreover, any increase in adipose tissue, which is often

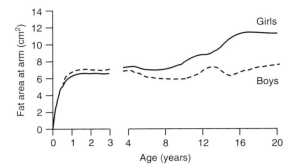

Figure 4.3 Development of fat area at arm, approximated from repeated measurements of biceps and triceps skinfold thickness and arm circumferences. (Data with permission from Gasser, 1996.[13])

relatively poorly perfused, increases the potential for producing a 'reservoir' of drug, which diffuses back into the circulation along concentration gradients after administration has ceased.

PROTEIN BINDING

The low inherent solubility of highly lipophilic drugs in plasma water makes reversible protein binding essential for their transport in plasma, but only the unbound fraction can readily diffuse across biological membranes to reach receptor sites or be eliminated from the body. Alterations in the degree of protein binding may, therefore, affect the apparent volume of distribution of certain drugs. Although albumin has a greater binding capacity than α_1-acid glycoprotein (AAG), AAG has a much greater drug affinity, particularly for weakly basic drugs. Neonates and young infants may have very low concentrations of albumin and AAG.[15] However, plasma protein binding is rarely of clinical significance even when drugs are extensively bound, as any concentration gradient that encourages passive diffusion of unbound drug from plasma to tissue also results in dissociation of protein-bound drug. Hence, as the total drug concentration in plasma decreases, the concentration of unbound drug tends to stay constant. Similarly, drug dissociation from binding to plasma proteins is so fast that hepatic clearance and glomerular filtration of drugs are relatively insensitive to changes in the concentrations of plasma proteins. However, low concentrations of binding proteins may become clinically relevant if a fast injection of an extensively bound drug is given at high dose, when pharmacodynamic effects may be transiently greater than would otherwise be expected. For instance, the induction dose of thiopentone is significantly lower in neonates than in older age groups and one of the reasons for this may be the decreased binding of thiopentone to plasma albumin. *In vitro* studies of thiopentone binding have shown that neonatal serum binds thiopentone significantly less than adult serum, possibly because of competitive binding of available receptor binding sites by bilirubin and/or structural differences between adult and fetal albumin.[16]

DEVELOPMENTAL FACTORS AFFECTING DRUG ELIMINATION

Metabolism and excretion together constitute the body's mechanisms for elimination of drugs and both processes demonstrate marked age-related variation.

HEPATIC METABOLISM

Most anaesthetic drugs are lipophilic compounds dependent on biotransformation to more water-soluble metabolites for elimination from the body. The principal site for drug metabolism is in the liver, where complex groups of enzymes are concentrated in the membranes of the hepatocyte endoplasmic reticulum. The numerous biotransformation reactions are conventionally classified into two main types, phase I and phase II, which often occur sequentially. Phase-I reactions convert the parent drug by oxidation, reduction or hydrolysis, to a more polar metabolite by introducing or revealing a functional group such as a hydroxyl or ammonium radical. Some phase-I metabolites are renally excreted, while others may then undergo a phase-II conjugation reaction. Phase-II conjugation reactions include glucuronidation, methylation and sulphation, which serve to increase further the polarity of a metabolite and promote its renal excretion. Many microsomal enzymes are polymorphically expressed and subject to considerable variability in activity during development.

The cytochrome P450 enzymes are quantitatively the most important hepatic microsomal oxidative enzymes. The oxidative biotransformation of drugs involves multiple hepatic P450 enzymes that have distinct substrate specificities and maturational sequences, which result in varying rates of maturation of drug metabolism. For instance, the cytochrome P450 enzymes involved in the oxidation of midazolam and alfentanil (CYP3A4) have low levels of activity during the first month of life but increase to adult levels by 6–12 months of postnatal age. Adult activity may then be exceeded between 1–4 years of age before declining progressively to reach adult levels again at the conclusion of puberty.[17] Other P450 enzyme systems will achieve adult activity levels at different rates. Furthermore, some of the cytochrome P450 enzymes, including CYP3A4, demonstrate significant interpatient variability in hepatic enzyme content even in the adult. Competition for the same P450 enzyme by more than one drug may result in slower rates of elimination. This effect will be exacerbated if concentrations of enzyme are low as, for example, CYP3A4 during the first month of life.

Conjugation reactions are responsible for the majority of anaesthetic drug biotransformations and several enzymes involved in these reactions are also polymorphically expressed, such that developmental and interindividual variation can be quite substantial. For instance, sulphotransferase activity (involved in paracetamol sulfation) usually achieves adult levels rapidly and may even exceed them during infancy and early childhood. In contrast, glucuronosyltransferase enzyme activity (involved in morphine glucuronidation) is deficient in the neonate and may take from 6 to 18 months to achieve adult levels. Moreover, differential development of glucuronidation pathways is common. For example, in the neonate, morphine glucuronidation to morphine-6-glucuronide is more impaired than glucuronidation to morphine-3-glucuronide.[18]

Hepatic drug clearance is a function not only of microsomal metabolic activity but also of hepatic blood flow. Hepatic blood flow will influence the hepatic clearance of a drug differently if metabolic activity is low or high. For drugs with a high intrinsic hepatic clearance, overall changes in hepatic clearance will be proportional to changes in liver blood flow. In contrast, changes in enzyme activity such as occur during maturation will influence hepatic clearance only if the drug has a low intrinsic clearance, whereas highly extracted drugs, such as propofol, will be essentially unaffected.

EXTRAHEPATIC METABOLISM

Important drug biotransformations also take place outside the liver. For instance, CYP34A enzymes are found in the small intestine, accounting for the relatively low bioavailability of orally administered midazolam. Other important extrahepatic drug biotransformations include esterase reactions in plasma and many other tissues. Non-specific esterase activity in plasma and other tissues may be reduced in neonates,[19] although this does not appear significantly to compromise metabolism of drugs such as remifentanil.[20] Furthermore, remifentanil that crosses the placenta continues to be rapidly metabolized by the term fetus.[21]

RENAL EXCRETION

Renal excretion of drugs and their metabolites may be necessary to avoid the potential toxicity associated with accumulation of these compounds. However, highly lipophilic drugs are usually only partially ionized at physiological pH and may also be bound to plasma proteins. These drugs are not readily filtered at the glomerulus. The lipophilic nature of renal tubular membranes also facilitates the reabsorption of hydrophobic compounds following glomerular filtration. Thus, the termination of action of anaesthetic drugs never depends solely on renal excretion. Nevertheless, the kidney is a major route of elimination not only for water-soluble drugs, but also for water-soluble metabolites of lipophilic drugs. The two basic processes involved in the renal elimination of drugs are glomerular filtration and tubular excretion.

The glomerular filtration rate (GFR) of term neonates at birth, when related to their surface area, is about 10% of that of the adult, but it increases rapidly in the early postnatal period, rising to 100% of the figure expected for size by 1 year of age. The maturational changes in GFR are due to a combination of increasing systemic arterial blood pressure and decreasing renal vascular resistance. Furthermore, the porosity of the glomerular membrane and the area available for filtration increase as glomeruli differentiate morphologically. Changes in the intrarenal distribution of blood may also lead to an increase in GFR, as blood flow to the outer cortex is enhanced compared with flow to the inner cortex and medulla. This developmental change in GFR increases the clearance of drugs and metabolites eliminated by filtration, such as glycopyrrolate. Hence, as would be expected, there are no significant age-dependent differences in glycopyrrolate clearance after the age of 6 months.[22] Similarly, tubular function in the neonate is relatively poor, but improves dramatically as renal mass and renal blood flow increase. Proximal tubular secretion assumes adult values by about 6 months of age. The glucuronide metabolites of drugs such as morphine and propofol are dependent on proximal tubular secretion for their elimination.

GENERAL FACTORS AFFECTING DRUG PHARMACOKINETICS

Certain pathophysiological factors may have a significant influence on drug distribution and/or elimination, and although they are not subject to developmental influence, may occur more frequently in paediatric than in adult anaesthetic practice.

HYPOVOLAEMIA AND HYPOTENSION

Hypovolaemia and/or hypotension will result in reduced tissue perfusion that can have profound effects on drug pharmacokinetics. The distribution of drugs between the blood and poorly perfused tissues will be restricted, which may result in greater relative distribution to those tissues such as the brain whose perfusion is maintained. Conversely, sick neonates may have impaired cerebral autoregulation,[23] such that systemic hypotension may result in subnormal cerebral blood flow and hence reduced uptake of lipophilic drugs. In hypotensive children, the drug may become sequestered in poorly perfused fat, only to return to the vascular compartment when perfusion is restored to normal. If hepatic blood flow is significantly reduced, elimination of drugs that have a high intrinsic hepatic clearance, such as propofol, may be compromised. However, lipophilic drugs are not the only type of drug to be affected by hypoperfusion. If renal perfusion is reduced, elimination of drug and/or metabolites may be significantly compromised. Moreover, children with congenital cardiac disease, who have poor peripheral perfusion secondary to myocardial dysfunction, may have a decreased apparent volume of distribution and reduced clearance of water-soluble drugs.[24]

HYPOXIA

Hypoxia can cause renal arteriolar vasoconstriction, which adversely affects both glomerular and tubular function. Similarly, decreased microsomal concentrations of cytochrome P450 enzyme systems may follow birth asphyxia. Experimental studies examining the effects of hypoxia on the hepatic metabolism of certain drugs have produced conflicting results. The limited clinical data that are available suggest that water-soluble drug elimination in infants with cyanotic congenital heart disease is not significantly different from that in a matched acyanotic group.[24]

HYPOTHERMIA

Hypothermia is commonly induced during cardiac surgery for infants and young children and thus the effects of temperature on drug pharmacokinetics can have important clinical significance. Experimental *in vitro*[25] and animal[26] work suggests that hypothermia may significantly reduce hepatic microsomal metabolism of certain drugs. The apparent volume of distribution and clearance of fentanyl in children may be reduced by profound hypothermia (18–25°C).[26] In contrast, alfentanil pharmacokinetics in adults undergoing cardiopulmonary bypass (CPB) is not significantly affected by moderate hypothermia to 28°C.[27] Reduced blood and tissue esterase activity secondary to hypothermia causes a 20% decrease in remifentanil clearance.[28] *In vitro* animal work has suggested that the affinity of opioid receptors for morphine, but not for naloxone, may decline with decreasing temperature.[29]

CARDIOPULMONARY BYPASS

Onset of CPB will cause an immediate and substantial decrease in the plasma concentration of both water-soluble and lipophilic drugs as a result of haemodilution. The decrease in total drug concentration is particularly large with fentanyl and thiopentone, where a significant proportion of drug undergoes hydrophobic binding to the extracorporeal circuit.[30] Haemodilution of plasma proteins may affect the protein binding of drugs such as alfentanil, midazolam and propofol, causing a decrease in bound drug concentration and an increase in apparent volume of distribution, although free drug concentration will remain relatively unchanged. Drug distribution and elimination during CPB is also affected by changes in acid–base balance, reduction in systemic flow and altered regional blood flow. Many highly lipophilic opioids with a high apparent volume of distribution maintain relatively stable total drug concentrations during initiation of CPB, as their rapid re-equilibration minimizes any dilutional effect. In the post-CPB period, fentanyl and alfentanil have decreased clearance, prolonged elimination half-life and an increased volume of distribution compared with pre-CPB values.[30,31] Propofol pharmacokinetics are not changed significantly during CPB and slight prolongation of its elimination after CPB does not prevent rapid recovery.

ACID–BASE BALANCE AND PACO2

Alterations in blood pH lead to significant changes in the degree of ionization of drugs with a pK_a close to physiological pH. For instance, 61% of thiopentone is unionized at a pH of 7.4, whereas at a pH of 7.1, 76% of the drug is unionized. This decrease in ionization of thiopentone alters its tissue distribution and increases its apparent volume of distribution. More importantly, acidosis increases the potency of thiopentone and accentuates the drug-induced depression in myocardial contractility.[32]

Drugs with very high lipid solubility tend to have cerebral venous concentrations less than 50% of arterial concentrations after a single passage through the brain, secondary to their rapid diffusion across the blood–brain barrier. Hence, the rate of lipophilic drug entry is largely determined by cerebral blood flow. Alterations in $PaCO_2$ that cause significant alterations in global and regional cerebral blood flow will therefore affect the uptake and distribution of many anaesthetic drugs in the brain.

DRUG–RECEPTOR INTERACTIONS

The identification of specific drug receptors implies the existence of endogenous ligands that exert their normal physiological action by binding to these receptors, as occurs with opioids and benzodiazepines. The affinity of the drug molecule for the receptor and the proportion of receptors occupied determine the relative potency of a drug at its site of action. However, it is not necessary for all receptors to be occupied to obtain maximum effect, as a large proportion of receptors can be 'spare'. The formation of a drug–receptor complex leads to the production of a pharmacological signal that may initiate a further cascade of physicochemical reactions before a measurable response is produced. The total number of receptors in a given volume of tissue varies in response to the presence of an agonist or antagonist and such downregulation may explain opioid tolerance.

Human and animal experimental studies have confirmed that significant change in receptor binding, density and initiation of secondary messenger systems can occur during development. Post-mortem human experimental studies, using quantitative tissue autoradiography techniques with radioligands for opioid receptors, have shown that although opioid receptor affinity does not change during development, opioid receptor distribution[33] and binding capacities[34] show significant variation with postnatal age. In addition, animal experiments have suggested that benzodiazepine binding sites may not only show quantitative and qualitative age-related changes, but also are distributed within the brain differently in the term neonate compared with the adult.[35]

PHARMACOLOGY OF INDIVIDUAL DRUGS

This section does not attempt to be all-inclusive and is restricted to discussing only those intravenous drugs that are commonly used in current paediatric anaesthetic practice to induce or maintain anaesthesia.

THIOPENTONE

Thiopentone may still be the most commonly used intravenous induction agent for children requiring inpatient anaesthesia, but its popularity is on the wane. Propofol is now preferred to thiopentone for day-case anaesthesia in children. The reason for this fundamental change in paediatric anaesthetic practice resides in the different pharmacokinetic properties of the two drugs.

Pharmacokinetics

Thiopentone has a rapid onset of action as passive diffusion into brain tissue from cerebral capillaries is facilitated by the drug's high lipid solubility. Hence, peak concentrations are reached in the brain and other well-perfused organs within one circulation time. After injection, the concentration of thiopentone in arterial blood declines rapidly, through distribution to well-perfused tissue, followed by a slower decline in concentration lasting for 40–50 min. Hence, pharmacokinetic data are usually consistent with a three-compartment model, and do not appear to vary significantly with

age after the neonatal period.[36] The recovery of consciousness following a single sleep dose of thiopentone is therefore entirely due to redistribution of drug into muscle, as although thiopentone is extensively metabolized by the liver to inactive metabolites, elimination of drug normally plays an insignificant role in the termination of effect. Hence, although thiopentone clearance is greater in young children than in adults, recovery time following a single injection is not age related.

Thiopentone has a low hepatic extraction ratio consistent with capacity-limited elimination. Hence, thiopentone given by infusion leads to delayed recovery, as the relevant hepatic oxidative enzyme systems will quickly become saturated. One clinical study has demonstrated that immature hepatic function in the neonate causes significantly reduced clearance of drug and a greatly prolonged elimination time.[37] This same study calculated a relatively large apparent volume of distribution for thiopentone, probably attributable to reduced plasma protein binding and a relatively low blood pH in the group of babies studied (see subsection *Acid–base balance and* $PaCO_2$).

Pharmacodynamics

In common with other induction agents, the dose of thiopentone required to induce anaesthesia (ED_{50}) in healthy children is reduced by premedication with sedative drugs.[38] The ED_{50} of thiopentone also varies with age (Figure 4.4), primarily owing to developmental changes in many of the factors affecting drug distribution (see section *Developmental factors affecting drug distribution*). Furthermore, the brain concentration of thiopentone needed to induce anaesthesia in neonates may be lower than in older infants, because the neonate has relatively immature cerebral cortical function, rudimentary dendritic arborizations and relatively few synapses.[39]

Infants and children recover more quickly after receiving propofol for induction of anaesthesia than after receiving an equipotent dose of thiopentone.[40] The difference between the two drugs is usually demonstrated in the completeness of recovery rather than in the time to extubation.[41] Recovery of psychomotor skills is usually significantly faster in children receiving

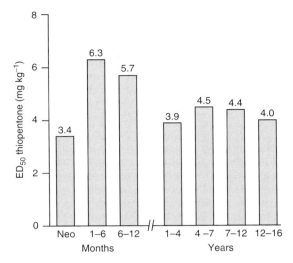

Figure 4.4 Dose of thiopentone required to induce anaesthesia reliably in 50% of healthy, unpremedicated patients at various ages.[198,199]

propofol than in those receiving thiopentone,[42] although by 4 h after awakening there may be no significant differences between the groups.[43] Moreover, one study has shown that children may wake up feeling more apprehensive after induction of anaesthesia with propofol than after thiopentone.[44] Recovery from anaesthesia is more dependent on the maintenance agent than on the induction agent for anaesthesia lasting for longer than 30 min.[40] For children requiring minor day-case surgery, therefore, thiopentone is not the induction agent of choice, although for children requiring more major surgery it still retains some advantages over its current competitors.

The reduction in mean arterial blood pressure produced in healthy children by inducing anaesthesia using propofol is significantly greater than that produced by an equipotent dose of thiopentone.[45] Thiopentone has little direct effect on vascular smooth muscle tone and causes cardiovascular depression by centrally mediated inhibition of sympathetic nervous activity and direct myocardial depression, the latter probably related to its effects on trans-sarcolemmal and sarcoplasmic reticulum calcium flux.[46]

One advantage of thiopentone over propofol is that it does not cause pain on injection, even when injected into small veins. Thiopentone is much less expensive than propofol, particularly if bulk solutions are used until depleted. A recent study has confirmed that the prepared solution of thiopentone can be used safely for up to 6 days even when stored at room temperature and much longer if refrigerated.[47] In contrast to propofol, the alkaline, bacteriostatic environment of the prepared thiopentone solution (pH 10.5) means that significant bacterial colonization is extremely unlikely.[48]

PROPOFOL

Compared with thiopentone, propofol offers improved recovery from anaesthesia of short duration, which can lead to a reduction in discharge time after day-case surgery, if appropriate discharge criteria are used.[41] This significant advance in the management of children having day-care surgery relates to the favourable pharmacokinetic properties of propofol.

Pharmacokinetics

Propofol is almost insoluble in water and is currently available as a 1% isotonic emulsion containing soybean oil and purified egg phosphatide. Propofol's high lipid solubility facilitates the passive diffusion of drug from cerebral capillaries into brain tissue and results in peak concentrations being achieved in the brain within one circulation time. After injection, the concentration of propofol in arterial blood declines rapidly within 1–3 min, as it is distributed to all well-perfused tissues. This initial distribution of propofol is comparable to that of thiopentone and plasma concentrations of both drugs decline at similar rates. Similarly, pharmacokinetic data for propofol, as for thiopentone, are usually consistent with a three-compartment model.[49] However, the subsequent decrease in arterial propofol concentration is more rapid than that of thiopentone because, while distribution to relatively poorly perfused tissue is occurring, metabolism of propofol is progressing at a high rate. Although awakening after a single rapid injection of propofol is mostly due to drug redistribution, rapid metabolism ensures more complete clinical recovery, compared with thiopentone, over the following few hours.

Propofol has a large steady-state volume of distribution, indicating extensive redistribution into muscle and fat. The capacity of these sites is large, although their rate of equilibration with the central compartment is slow. When an infusion of propofol is terminated, the concentration in the central compartment is much higher than in these peripheral compartments, and so redistribution continues to occur. Thus, propofol concentration in the central compartment declines both from metabolism and from continuing redistribution. The capacity of the peripheral compartments is so large, however, that redistribution from the central compartment can still occur even after prolonged drug administration, allowing a rapid decline in propofol concentrations. Eventually, the concentration in the central compartment becomes lower than that in the peripheral compartment and drug will then begin to move back into the central compartment. However, the rate of this transfer is so slow that the concentration of propofol in the central compartment remains subtherapeutic. The complete elimination of propofol from the body may take many hours or even days but has little effect on clinical recovery.

Propofol is extensively metabolized by the liver to inactive glucuronide conjugates, although extrahepatic metabolism may also be significant in some individuals.[50] In contrast to thiopentone, propofol has a hepatic extraction ratio close to 1.0 and elimination is mainly dependent on hepatic blood flow. Children aged below 3 years have a higher clearance of propofol than older children, on account of increased hepatic blood flow,[49] but as elimination of drug following a single injection normally plays a relatively minor role in termination of effect, time to awakening is similar in all ages.

Propofol is extensively bound to plasma proteins (Table 4.2) and the reduced albumin concentration in young infants may increase the drug's apparent volume of distribution. Moreover, the central compartment volume into which propofol is initially distributed, consisting of plasma and highly perfused organs such as brain and liver, is 30–80% higher in young children than in older children and adults, when related to body weight.[49] This is probably due to age-related differences in regional blood flow and fat distribution. Hence, giving a single injection of propofol to a young child will result in a lower plasma concentration than that obtained in an adult if the dose of drug has been related to body weight. Likewise, the ED_{50} of propofol is significantly higher in young children than in older children and adults (Figure 4.5). Short-term infusions of propofol given to infants result in similar pharmacokinetic values to those found in young children,[51] although its potential pharmacokinetic advantages over other anaesthetic agents may be less clinically significant in this age group. Furthermore, the ability of the neonatal liver to form glucuronide conjugates is severely reduced, so that a decrease in propofol clearance should be expected. These pharmacokinetic differences should not influence the duration of clinical effect if the drug is given by a single injection, but it would seem advisable to avoid the use of long-term propofol infusion in neonates and young infants.

Pharmacodynamics

Premedicated children require a significantly lower dose of propofol to induce anaesthesia than do unsedated children.[52] Studies of unpremedicated children suggest that although there are significant age-related differences in the ED_{50} of propofol, these are not as pronounced as are seen for thiopentone (Figure 4.5). Children between 6 and 12 years of age have similar ED_{50} requirements of propofol to adults (approx. 1.5 mg kg^{-1}),[53] although infants 1–6 months of age require 3.0 mg kg^{-1}.[54]

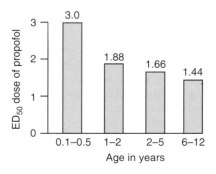

Figure 4.5 Dose of propofol required to induce anaesthesia reliably in 50% of healthy, unpremedicated patients at various ages (mg kg^{-1}).[53,54]

Following induction of anaesthesia in healthy children using propofol, a transient 10–20% decrease in mean arterial blood pressure is often observed. This degree of induced hypotension is significantly greater than that produced by an equipotent dose of thiopentone.[45] This is because although propofol depresses myocardial contractility less than thiopentone,[55] it causes direct relaxation of systemic vascular smooth muscle.[56] Experimental animal studies have suggested that propofol has little effect on normal pulmonary vascular tone, but significantly decreases increased pulmonary vascular tone.[57] In addition, propofol causes prolongation of the QT interval and a relatively high incidence of bradycardia and junctional rhythm, even in children premedicated with atropine.[58] Reduction of heart rate following propofol injection may be due to depression of baroreceptor reflexes and appears to be more common in children under 2 years of age.[45] During strabismus surgery, the incidence of bradycardia resulting from the oculocardiac reflex is higher in children receiving a propofol infusion than in those having isoflurane.[59] Propofol appears to suppress the haemodynamic response to tracheal intubation better than thiopentone.[60,61]

Induction of anaesthesia using propofol causes apnoea for more than 20 s in 20–50% of unpremedicated healthy children.[62,63] The ventilatory response to carbon dioxide is depressed for longer after a single induction dose of propofol than after an equipotent dose of thiopentone.[64] Propofol given by infusion to spontaneously breathing children causes a significant decrease in minute ventilation and carbon dioxide retention.[65] Pharyngeal and laryngeal reactivity are also depressed by propofol more than by thiopentone,[66] which can be advantageous when inserting a laryngeal mask airway. Ease of laryngeal mask airway insertion is aided if the dose of propofol administered is increased to 33% more than the ED_{50}.[63] This higher dose of propofol does not appear to accentuate the decrease in mean arterial pressure or incidence of apnoea following induction of anaesthesia in healthy children. Propofol can be used to facilitate tracheal intubation in children without the use of muscle relaxants, although the addition of alfentanil significantly improves intubating conditions and attenuates the stress response to intubation.[67,68]

Spontaneous excitatory movements may occur during induction of anaesthesia and recovery when using propofol in younger children and infants, although they are not usually associated with cortical epileptic activity and may be caused by preferential depression of subcortical areas of the brain. Propofol produces dose-dependent CNS depression: low doses may increase the activity of an epileptiform focus, whereas higher doses lead to suppression of electroencephalographic activity.[69] The significant decrease in mean arterial blood pressure that occurs after induction of anaesthesia using propofol means that it should be used with caution in patients with reduced intracranial compliance. Propofol anaesthesia may be advantageous for many patients undergoing elective neurosurgery, however, as it causes significant reductions in cerebral blood flow, cerebral oxygen consumption and intracranial pressure.

If propofol is injected into a small vein, about 40% of children will experience pain. This appears to be related to the aqueous concentration of propofol in the emulsion directly stimulating venous nociceptive receptors and/or stimulating the release of kininogens.[70] The addition of 1% lignocaine to propofol emulsion in a 1 : 10 dilution reduces the pH of the solution from 8.0 to 6.3 and increases the proportion of propofol in lipid phase, so reducing injection pain significantly.[71] The use of large veins, warming the solution to 37°C[72] and addition of alfentanil[73] are among other strategies that reduce the incidence of injection pain.

Propofol has useful antiemetic properties: it significantly reduces the frequency of postoperative vomiting in ambulatory patients, compared with patients receiving either thiopentone or an inhalational anaesthetic.[74] Propofol has no effect on adrenal steroidogenesis, has a similar cerebral protective action to that of the barbiturates,[75] but unlike thiopentone does not depress T-lymphocyte function.[76] An aseptic technique should be used when aspirating propofol and the ampoule contents should be discarded within 6 h of opening, as propofol supports the growth of many pathogenic bacteria.[48]

The incidence and severity of anaphylaxis or anaphylactoid reactions following either single or multiple exposure of patients to propofol is comparable to that following thiopentone administration. Propofol should not be given to patients with a history of allergy to muscle relaxants or eggs, or those with multiple drug allergies.[77] Propofol can cause histamine release, although even when used in conjunction with atracurium it does not appear to cause significant changes in respiratory mechanics in susceptible individuals.[78] Repeated administration of propofol does not appear to cause the development of clinically significant tolerance.[79]

KETAMINE

Ketamine hydrochloride is a 'dissociative' anaesthetic agent that has been in widespread clinical use for over 30 years. It produces a cataleptic state characterized clinically by a functional and electrophysiological dissociation between thalamic, cortical and limbic systems in the brain. Ketamine is unique among anaesthetic agents not only for its mechanism of action, but also because it produces intense analgesia, has relatively little effect on cardiorespiratory function and can be given by intravenous, intramuscular or enteral routes. Ketamine is currently available as a mixture of two enantiomers in equal proportion: the $S(+)$-enantiomer of ketamine has approximately four times the potency of the $R(-)$-enantiomer and a different pharmacological profile.[80] In the neonatal rat, all of the actions of ketamine can be accounted for by its action as a non-competitive antagonist at N-methyl-D-aspartate (NMDA) receptors.[81] Positron emission tomographic studies in humans have shown that ketamine distribution in the brain correlates with regional distribution of NMDA receptor complexes.[82] Hence, although ketamine also reduces opening times at other ion channels, and interacts with opioid receptors, these are probably not crucial for its anaesthetic action. In contrast to thiopentone and propofol, ketamine does not significantly affect $GABA_A$ receptor function.[83]

Pharmacokinetics

Although ketamine hydrochloride is water soluble, it is approximately 45% non-ionized at a pH of 7.4 (Table 4.2) and readily crosses the blood–brain barrier. In adults, peak plasma concentrations occur within 1 min of an intravenous injection and within 5 min of an intramuscular injection. In common with thiopentone and propofol, ketamine is initially distributed to highly perfused organs such as the brain and, subsequently, to less well-perfused tissues such as muscle. Pharmacokinetic data are usually analysed using a two-compartment model. Ketamine has a relatively high hepatic extraction ratio, so that both redistribution and elimination play a part in the termination of clinical effect. The duration of anaesthesia induced by a single injection of ketamine 2 mg kg^{-1} intravenously or 10 mg kg^{-1} intramuscularly varies between 10 and 20 min, although analgesic effects will persist for somewhat longer. Tolerance may develop acutely with repeated administration.[84]

There is relatively little information on the pharmacokinetics of ketamine in children. Plasma ketamine concentrations are similar in children 4–9 years of age and adults during the first 3 h following a single intravenous injection, although concentrations decrease at a faster rate in children thereafter.[85] This is because although the volume of distribution at steady state for ketamine is similar in children and adults, clearance in children is slightly increased,[86] probably because of the relatively high hepatic blood flow seen in this age group. The pharmacokinetic profile of ketamine in infants receiving the drug by infusion appears to be very similar to that found in adults.[87] Neonates, however, have reduced clearance and a higher apparent volume of distribution than older children and adults.[88] The decreased clearance rate in neonates relates to the reduced hepatic microsomal activity in this age group. Ketamine is extensively metabolized in the liver, initially undergoing N-demethylation via a cytochrome P450 system to form norketamine, which has a potency of about one-third that of the parent drug.[89] Norketamine is further metabolized either by oxidative metabolism to form the less potent dehydronorketamine, or by hydroxylation followed by conjugation with glucuronide to form water-soluble products that are then excreted by the kidney.[88] All of these metabolic pathways are subject to developmental influences to a greater or lesser extent (see subsection *Hepatic metabolism*) and it is therefore not surprising that the elimination half-life for ketamine is prolonged in early infancy.

Pharmacodynamics

Ketamine is a relatively poor hypnotic, but produces dose-related anterograde amnesia and profound analgesia. The drug takes more than one arm–brain circulation time before CNS depression is noticeable, although the precise time of onset of action may be difficult to determine as the child may gaze into the distance with open eyes for several minutes. Spontaneous involuntary muscle movements may occur and muscle relaxation is often poor. Induction of anaesthesia with ketamine is associated with a decrease in electroencephalographic amplitude and frequency, followed by intermittent high-amplitude polymorphic delta activity,[90] although overt epileptiform seizures are not produced.[91] Children with increased intracranial pressure may be more prone to ketamine-induced apnoea,[92] thought to be secondary to the drug's sympathomimetic and direct vasodilator effects on cerebral blood flow. However, recent clinical studies have demonstrated that ketamine does not increase cerebral blood flow or intracranial pressure in anaesthetized patients with reduced intracranial compliance.[93,94]

Although sensory and perceptual illusions and vivid dreams commonly occur after ketamine anaesthesia, the incidence of these psychic phenomena is relatively low in young children and can be minimized by the concurrent administration of midazolam. There is no evidence that emergence in a quiet, dark environment reduces the incidence of emergence reactions, which usually disappear upon awakening, although recurrent illusions have been reported several weeks after administration.[95] The incidence of postoperative nausea and vomiting following ketamine is relatively high and administration of a prophylactic antiemetic such as ondansetron is recommended.

Ketamine is one of the few anaesthetic agents that does not cause transient hypotension in healthy patients, although it does cause a significant decrease in contractility in the isolated heart.[96] Ketamine has sympathomimetic actions, caused primarily by direct stimulation of neuronal pathways in the CNS.[80,97] In addition, ketamine inhibits extraneuronal uptake of catecholamines,[98] although plasma concentrations of adrenaline and noradrenaline do not change significantly from baseline and do not correlate with the significant increases in heart rate and arterial blood pressure that usually occur after bolus administration.[80] Experimental[99] and clinical studies in sick, preterm neonates[100] have shown that ketamine is better than fentanyl- or isoflurane-based techniques at maintaining mean arterial blood pressure. A study involving critically ill adults, however, found that a single dose of ketamine causes a significant decrease in blood pressure, contractility and cardiac output in some patients.[101] A study in children recovering from cardiac surgery has shown that ketamine usually produces insignificant changes in cardiac index and systemic vascular resistance, but a significant increase in pulmonary vascular resistance, particularly in susceptible individuals.[102] Similar findings have been demonstrated in acyanotic children undergoing cardiac catheterization.[103]

Ketamine is a potent bronchodilator and may be used to treat asthmatic children refractory to more conventional forms of therapy.[104] Ketamine inhibits bronchial constriction by inhibition of extraneuronal uptake of catecholamines,[98] by inhibiting calcium influx through calcium channels in bronchial smooth muscle cells,[105] and by inhibitory effects on nicotinic receptors in intramural ganglia of the vagus in the tracheobronchial tree.[106] *In vitro* animal work has suggested that ketamine inhibits both neurogenically mediated bronchial smooth muscle contraction and bronchoconstriction caused by direct stimulation, the latter effect being particularly prominent in the neonate.[107] Salivary and tracheobronchial secretions are increased by ketamine, and prophylactic administration of an antisialogogue is strongly recommended.

Ketamine does not affect functional residual capacity in spontaneously breathing healthy young children.[108] It does increase intrinsic positive end expiratory pressure.[109] Although these effects help to maintain normal oxygenation and prevent atelectasis in spontaneously breathing patients, energy expenditure by the inspiratory muscles tends to increase. Ketamine is a mild respiratory depressant and the ventilatory response to carbon dioxide is significantly reduced 5 min after a single injection of intravenous ketamine 2 mg kg^{-1} given over 1 min.[110] However, when ketamine is given by infusion, although the carbon dioxide response curve is shifted to the right, the slope does not change and resting ventilatory variables including minute ventilation are usually maintained at control levels. This suggests a correlation between the plasma concentration of ketamine and its respiratory depressant effects, a hypothesis substantiated by clinical studies demonstrating that episodes of desaturation or apnoea, if they occur at all during ketamine anaesthesia, tend to occur within a few minutes of induction.[111,112] Hence, it is recommended that ketamine should be given intravenously at a slow rate, rather than by rapid injection, unless the patient is to be artificially ventilated. Ketamine anaesthesia is associated with greater retention of protective pharyngeal and laryngeal reflexes than occurs with other anaesthetic agents, although tracheal soiling and aspiration have been reported following induction of anaesthesia with ketamine.[97] The report of a child having a respiratory arrest following intramuscular ketamine[113] has served to emphasize that ketamine anaesthesia should only be administered in situations where appropriate equipment and trained staff are readily available. In spite of this, and because of its favourable characteristics, ketamine has become a mainstay for anaesthesia in developing countries. There is also a renewed interest in the drug for paediatric anaesthesia, for induction in cardiac patients, for short procedures and, because it is well absorbed from mucous membranes, for rectal use as premedication or for induction of anaesthesia.

MIDAZOLAM

Midazolam has powerful hypnotic and amnesic properties and can be used to induce anaesthesia but, unlike most other induction agents, it has a variable and relatively slow onset of action, although this can be decreased to less than 1 min if dose and injection time are increased. Nevertheless, some children may remain conscious even after a dose of 0.6 mg kg^{-1} has been given.[114] The introduction of propofol has meant that the role of midazolam in current paediatric anaesthetic practice has been substantially curtailed and it is usually given only for premedication or sedation, or with ketamine.

Pharmacokinetics

The benzodiazepine midazolam is water soluble at a pH below 4, but at physiological pH its imidazole ring closes and the molecule then becomes extremely lipophilic. This high lipid solubility of midazolam, which ensures rapid diffusion through the blood–brain barrier, and a rapid receptor association–dissociation rate, means that CNS effects tend to follow plasma drug concentration. Following intravenous injection, midazolam is initially distributed to highly perfused tissues such as the brain, before plasma concentrations decrease as a result of redistribution to less well-perfused tissues. Pharmacokinetic data are usually compatible with a two- or three-compartment model.[115,116] There is some evidence that the pharmacokinetics of midazolam is dose dependent.[117,118] This may be due to saturation of plasma protein binding sites or to microsomal enzyme activity, but it probably only assumes clinical relevance if the drug is being given by continuous infusion.

Oxidative microsomal enzymes in the liver, and to a lesser extent in the small intestine, hydroxylate midazolam to a variety of metabolites including 1- and 4-hydroxyl metabolites, which are then conjugated to glucuronides and excreted in urine. The hydroxyl metabolites are pharmacologically active, although they have a shorter half-life and less potency than the parent drug. As midazolam has a hepatic extraction ratio of about 50%, its metabolic clearance is dependent on both hepatic blood flow and enzymic activity. Clearance in neonates is substantially less than that in infants, children and adults (Table 4.3) and is due to reduced concentrations of hepatic microsomal enzymes, in particular the cytochrome P450 CYP3A4 oxidative enzymes (see subsection *Hepatic metabolism*). This dependence on CYP34A activity for midazolam elimination also explains

Table 4.3 Age-related differences in pharmacokinetic parameters for induction/hypnotic drugs

Drug	Age group	Apparent volume of distribution (ml kg^{-1})	Elimination half-life (min)	Clearance (ml min^{-1} kg^{-1})	Main references
Thiopentone	Neonate	3600	2160	1	37
	Child	2100	366	7	36
	Adult	2200	720	3	36
Propofol	Child (1–3)	9500	188	53	49
	Child (3–11)	9700	398	34	190
	Adult	4700	312	28	75
Ketamine	Neonate	3720	184	14	88
	Infant	3360	204	17	87
	Child	2800	125	22	86
	Adult	3010	155	17	80
Midazolam	Neonate	1000	391	2	191
	Infant	2020	198	9	192
	Child	1290	70	9	117
	Adult	1750	135	9	193

Mean values only are given, with the understanding that all parameters have large interpatient variation.

some of the wide interpatient variation in the drug's pharmacokinetics observed in most studies. A more than 20-fold variation in constitutive CYP34A may occur between individuals.

Pharmacodynamics

Rapid intravenous administration of midazolam causes a 17% decrease in mean arterial blood pressure in adults with coronary artery disease, secondary to a 12% decrease in systemic vascular resistance and a 9% decrease in cardiac index.[119] Induction of anaesthesia using midazolam does not cause a clinically significant decrease in mean arterial pressure in normovolaemic children.[120] In common with most anaesthetic induction agents, intravenous midazolam may cause apnoea in some children, although this is usually of short duration (< 10 s). A study of children undergoing circumcision given midazolam 0.5 mg kg^{-1} intravenously showed time to eye opening in excess of 30 min after a 35-min procedure.[121] This recovery time could be reduced to 10 min by the administration of the benzodiazepine receptor antagonist flumazenil 0.025 mg kg^{-1}. No resedation, adverse haemodynamic effects

or reversal of anxiolysis were seen, although the elimination half-life of flumazenil is significantly shorter than that of midazolam in all age groups.[116] Delayed recovery after midazolam has generally restricted its usefulness in anaesthesia, but it remains the agent of choice to prevent or reduce adverse psychic phenomena resulting from ketamine administration.

MORPHINE

Although morphine remains the gold-standard opioid for postoperative pain relief in all age groups, its use in the operating theatre as a major component of the anaesthetic technique is becoming less popular. Adult[122] and infant[123] studies have shown that low doses of fentanyl are more effective than morphine in preventing significant increases in the concentrations of stress hormones that occur in response to surgical stimulation. Morphine is an agonist at all opioid receptors, but its actions on the μ-receptor account for the majority of its analgesic, respiratory depressant and sedative effects.

Pharmacokinetics

After rapid intravenous injection, plasma concentrations of morphine usually decline in a tri-exponential manner, as the rate of distribution of drug alters with time. Morphine is poorly lipid soluble so diffusion across the blood–brain barrier is comparatively slow. Similarly, morphine concentrations in the brain decline relatively slowly during its elimination phase and, therefore, there is usually little correlation between plasma concentration and clinical effects. Hence, morphine has a slower onset of action and longer duration of action than the newer synthetic opioids. There are no significant age-related changes in the apparent volume of distribution.[124] In contrast, clearance of morphine is largely dependent on biotransformation in the liver and varies significantly with age.

Morphine is unusual in that the active metabolites rather than the parent drug produce the majority of clinical effects. Morphine is metabolized predominantly in the liver, although some contribution from enzymes in kidney and gut also may occur. Morphine-6-glucuronide (M6G) and morphine-3-glucuronide (M3G) are the most abundant and clinically significant metabolites.[18] They are formed when the phase-II enzymes, uridine diphosphate glucuronosyltransferases, facilitate transfer of a glucuronic acid group to hydroxyl groups on the substrate. M6G has potent antinociceptive activity[125] but causes less respiratory depression than morphine,[126] while M3G antagonizes the antinociceptive and respiratory depressant effects of morphine and M6G.[127] M6G excretion is highly dependent on renal function and M6G accumulation may cause prolonged respiratory depression in patients with severe renal dysfunction, in the absence of the parent drug.[128] The developmental changes in the clearance of morphine relate to changes in both the level of glucuronidation and the renal excretion of parent drug. In adults, renal clearance of morphine accounts for less than 10% of total body clearance, while in term neonates it may account for the majority.[129] Differential development of the relevant transferase isoenzymes causes the M3G : M6G ratio to be about half that found in adults.[18] In general, infants from the age of 2 months have a clearance rate of morphine similar to that in adults.[124]

Pharmacodynamics

Experimental studies have suggested that the maturational changes in the ventilatory depressant effects of morphine relate to changes in drug sensitivity rather than to age-related changes in pharmacokinetics.[130] Maturational changes in the ventilatory sensitivity to fentanyl are much smaller in magnitude. Developmental changes in blood–brain barrier permeability may account for this age-related change in morphine pharmacodynamics.[131] One clinical study in infants demonstrated great interpatient variation in the respiratory depressant effects of known plasma concentrations of morphine, although metabolite concentrations were not measured.[132] However, as plasma morphine: M6G concentration ratios change with age, and correlation between plasma and CSF morphine concentrations is relatively poor even after prolonged infusions,[133] age-related differences in the relationship between plasma morphine concentrations and carbon dioxide responsiveness should not be expected.

Fast intravenous injection of morphine in critically ill adults causes a 15–20% decrease in heart rate, cardiac index and mean arterial pressure,[134] due mainly to a decrease in systemic vascular resistance and an increase in venous capacitance.[135] Morphine is one of the few opioids that may cause significant histamine release from cutaneous mast cells in a high proportion of patients.[136,137] This large increase in plasma histamine concentration is probably a major contributory factor in the haemodynamic changes associated with morphine administration,[138] although it can be substantially ameliorated by the use of histamine receptor antagonists.[139]

Morphine has useful sedative and anxiolytic properties and, like other potent opioids, significantly reduces the minimum alveolar concentration (MAC) of inhalational agents in a dose-dependent manner.[140,141] However, analgesic doses of morphine do not affect the end-tidal concentration of isoflurane or sevoflurane associated with awakening.[142,143] Morphine is less likely to cause muscle rigidity than fentanyl derivatives,[144] but has similar emetogenic properties,[145] secondary to its effects on dopamine and 5-hydroxytryptamine-3 receptors associated with the chemoreceptor trigger zone.

FENTANYL

Fentanyl is a highly lipophilic synthetic μ-opioid receptor agonist at least 50 times more potent than morphine. In low doses fentanyl has little sedative effect, although in very high doses (50–100 μg kg^{-1}) its hypnotic properties are pronounced. Cardiovascular effects are not dose dependent and high-dose fentanyl is effective in attenuating the stress response to surgical stimulation. For this reason, it is often used in cardiac anaesthesia as the principal anaesthetic agent.

Pharmacokinetics

Following rapid intravenous injection, plasma concentrations of fentanyl decline in a tri-exponential manner.[146] Its high lipid solubility means that it is rapidly and extensively distributed throughout most tissues of the body, so that its apparent volume of distribution at steady state is relatively large (Table 4.4). Its duration of action is somewhat dose dependent. In small doses fentanyl has a short duration of action and rapid recovery, because the plasma and brain concentrations decrease to below therapeutic levels during the rapid distribution phase. However, if a very high dose of the drug is given, the duration of action is significantly prolonged. In these circumstances, the distribution phase is complete while the plasma concentration of fentanyl is still relatively high. Fentanyl that is removed from plasma by elimination is immediately replaced by fentanyl returning from the peripheral compartment. Recovery from the effects of the drug then depends on its relatively slow clearance. Similarly, fentanyl is an unsuitable drug to give by prolonged infusion if rapid clinical recovery is required after stopping the infusion (Figure 4.6).

Fentanyl is metabolized in the liver by dealkylation, hydroxylation and amide hydrolysis to inactive metabolites. Although it has a high intrinsic hepatic clearance in adults, an experimental study in neonatal lambs has suggested that the hepatic extraction ratio in neonates may be relatively low.[148] Significant pharmacokinetic differences between infants and adults have been consistently demonstrated (Table 4.4), such that prolongation of pharmacodynamic effect may be expected for infants less than 6 months of age receiving a single injection or short-term infusion. However, prolonged infusions of fentanyl may quickly lead to

Table 4.4 Age-related differences in pharmacokinetic parameters for opioids

Drug	Age group	Apparent volume of distribution (ml kg^{-1})	Elimination half-life (min)	Clearance (ml min^{-1} kg^{-1})	Main references
Morphine	Neonate	2800	390	8	124
	Infant	2000	100	14	188
	Child	2800	120	24	124
	Adult	3200	177	15	194
Fentanyl	Neonate	5100	320	18	195
	Infant	3400	150	24	188
	Child	2250	195	12	188
	Adult	4000	219	13	194
Alfentanil	Neonate	750	330	2	188
	Infant	550	55	10	188
	Child	500	50	8	188
	Adult	750	94	8	194
Remifentanil	Neonate	325	4	90	20
	Child	213	5	59	196
	Adult	390	15	40	169

Mean values only are given, with the understanding that all parameters have large interpatient variation.

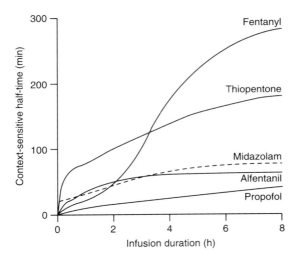

Figure 4.6 Context-sensitive half-times related to infusion duration for commonly used intravenous anaesthetic drugs, calculated from pharmacokinetic models. (Adapted with permission from Hughes *et al.*, 1992.[176])

tolerance, somewhat attenuating this potential pharmacological problem in the very young.[149]

Pharmacodynamics

In common with most other opioids, fentanyl may be used as an adjunct to inhalational or intravenous hypnotic agents to induce and/or to maintain anaesthesia. In adults, fentanyl has been shown to reduce the dose of propofol required to induce anaesthesia, and does so in an additive rather than a synergistic fashion.[150] Similarly, fentanyl has been shown to reduce the MAC of sevoflurane[151] and isoflurane[152] by at least 50%. However, in all age groups, administration of fentanyl can be associated with concentration-dependent adverse effects, including bradycardia, chest-wall rigidity and respiratory depression. In neonates, fentanyl has been shown to produce significant depression of baroreflex control of heart rate, probably secondary to decreased vasomotor centre activity.[153] These adverse cardiovascular effects can be ameliorated by giving the initial loading dose as a short infusion, by prior administration of atropine[154] or by concurrent administration of pancuronium.[155,156] A fall in blood pressure after bolus administration of

fentanyl is not unusual in the absence of surgical stimulus, especially in small children with cardiovascular compromise.

Although fentanyl 3 μg kg^{-1} h^{-1} has been used successfully in neonates with congenital diaphragmatic hernia to blunt pulmonary hypertensive responses to bronchocarinal and surgical stimulation,[157] this dose may not always be adequate to prevent pulmonary hypertensive crises in susceptible infants.[158] Fentanyl 25 μg kg^{-1}, given over 2 min prior to tracheal suction, has been shown to abolish pulmonary vasoconstrictive responses in susceptible infants almost completely.[159] Neonates and infants undergoing major general surgery require less than 10 μg kg^{-1} h^{-1} to prevent significant changes in cardiovascular indices[153] or stress hormone concentrations[160] in response to surgical stimulation, but older children probably require a higher dose.[161] Moreover, infants and children undergoing cardiac surgery may require fentanyl in a dose equivalent to 15–20 μg kg^{-1} h^{-1} to blunt hormonal[162] and cardiovascular[156,163] responses to surgical stimulation effectively. This higher dose requirement may be partially explained by the 70% decrease in plasma concentration that occurs on initiation of bypass,[164] secondary to haemodilution and binding of circulating drug to the bypass circuit (see subsection *Cardiopulmonary bypass*, p. 355).

ALFENTANIL

Alfentanil is about one-seventh as potent as fentanyl, but has similar pharmacodynamic effects. There are important pharmacokinetic differences between alfentanil and fentanyl; alfentanil is a more logical opioid to use if an infusion is being considered.

Pharmacokinetics

Although alfentanil has lower lipid solubility than fentanyl (Table 4.2), more alfentanil in plasma is present in the unionized form so that diffusion across the blood–brain barrier is extremely rapid and the onset of action is faster. When given as a rapid intravenous injection, plasma concentrations decline rapidly in a bi-exponential fashion.[165] The comparatively low lipid solubility of alfentanil results in a relatively small apparent volume of distribution that does not change significantly with age (Table 4.4). However, neonates and young infants have significantly reduced clearance and prolonged elimination compared with older infants and children. This is because, in the first few months of life, concentrations of the hepatic microsomal cytochrome P450 enzymes involved in the oxidation of alfentanil (CYP3A4), are greatly reduced (see subsection *Hepatic metabolism*).

Pharmacodynamics

Alfentanil may be used as an adjunct to a hypnotic drug such as midazolam or propofol to induce anaesthesia. Clinical studies in adults have demonstrated synergistic pharmacodynamic interactions between midazolam and alfentanil[166] and between propofol and alfentanil.[167] Moreover, alfentanil, in common with other opioids, can reduce the MAC of inhalational agents such as isoflurane by 50%.[168] Conditions for laryngoscopy and intubation are usually excellent without the need for a muscle relaxant, in children receiving alfentanil 10 μg kg^{-1} followed 30 s later by a sleep dose of propofol.[67] Unless the operative procedure is expected to take only a few minutes, the initial loading dose of alfentanil should be followed by an infusion, starting at a rate of 1 μg kg^{-1} min^{-1}. Extra bolus injections and/or changes in infusion rate are governed by cardiovascular response to surgical stimulus and by the progress of the surgery. If the infusion is terminated at the end of surgery, recovery time will depend largely on the duration of the infusion and the termination of effect of concurrently administered anaesthetic drugs (see section *Total intravenous anaesthesia*).

The clinical effects of giving alfentanil as a rapid injection to infants and children are similar to those seen following fentanyl administration. Significant bradycardia and hypotension are frequently observed in infants, despite the use of pre-emptive atropine,[169] but are less common or severe in older children.[67] Giving the loading dose as a short-term infusion over 5–10 min can attenuate drug-induced bradycardia and hypotension. The incidence of other adverse effects, such as postoperative nausea and vomiting, is similar in both drugs.[161]

REMIFENTANIL

Remifentanil is a very short-acting, selective μ-opioid receptor agonist with an analgesic potency about 25 times greater than that of alfentanil.[170] Its unusual metabolism means that it is uniquely suited to administration by infusion.

Pharmacokinetics

Remifentanil is metabolized, by cleavage of its ester linkage, by non-specific blood and tissue esterases, and the rate of its metabolism is approximately the same in all patients, irrespective of age, plasma cholinesterase deficiency, hepatic or renal dysfunction. The primary (carboxylic acid) metabolite of remifentanil is 4600 times less potent than the parent compound and is renally excreted. In common with fentanyl and alfentanil, the pharmacokinetics of remifentanil can be represented using a three-compartment model. Remifentanil has an initial distribution phase half-life of less than 1 min, a second distribution phase half-life of about 3 min and a terminal elimination half-life of 11–15 min.[170] Preliminary pharmacokinetic and theoretical data suggest that the dosage regimen for remifentanil should be unaffected by age (Table 4.4).

Recovery following an opioid infusion is often longer than that predicted from pharmacokinetic data based on an intravenous bolus injection, and the concept of 'context-sensitive half-time' described later helps to explain the observed discrepancy between the terminal half-life of a drug and the time for plasma concentration to decrease after stopping the infusion. The duration of the context-sensitive half-time for alfentanil and fentanyl increases as the duration of infusion increases (Figure 4.6). In contrast, remifentanil shows no significant increase in either pharmacokinetic or pharmacodynamic context-sensitive half-times even after infusions lasting for many hours (Table 4.5).

Pharmacodynamics

Clinical studies in adults have shown that remifentanil may be used to attenuate the pressor response to intubation, but causes bradycardia and hypotension in 50% of patients

Table 4.5 Elimination half-lives and context-sensitive half-times as measured for alfentanil and remifentanil after a 3-h infusion in adult volunteers[197]

	Elimination half-life (min)	Measured pharmacokinetic context-sensitive half-time (min)	Measured pharmacodynamic context-sensitive half-time (min)
Remifentanil	11.8 (5.1)	3.2 (0.9)	5.4 (1.8)
Alfentanil	76.5 (12.6)	47.3 (12.0)	54.0 (48.1)

Data are shown as mean (SD).

unless a vagolytic agent is given concurrently.[171] Remifentanil, when used in combination with isoflurane, may provide significantly better attenuation of surgical stress responses than alfentanil when given in equipotent dosage.[172] An infusion of remifentanil at 0.05 μg kg^{-1} min^{-1} reduces isoflurane MAC by 50%.[173] Remifentanil has greater synergistic sedative and analgesic effects with propofol than fentanyl or alfentanil.[174]

Dose-dependent effects on central nervous, cardiovascular and respiratory systems are similar to those seen with alfentanil. Paediatric clinical studies have confirmed that remifentanil causes a decrease in heart rate, blood pressure and respiratory rate similar to that induced by alfentanil.[175] The incidence of postoperative emesis and pruritus was similar in both alfentanil and remifentanil groups, although the postoperative hypoxaemia seen in 21% patients receiving alfentanil was not observed in any patient receiving remifentanil.

Although the short and predictable duration of action of remifentanil has an inherent attraction for anaesthetists, these very qualities also produce unique disadvantages. For continued clinical effect the drug needs to be given by continuous infusion and, therefore, there is a risk of a rapid loss of analgesic and anaesthetic effects if the infusion is interrupted accidentally. The provision of postoperative analgesia also requires careful management, as alternative methods of analgesia need to be commenced before stopping the remifentanil infusion. Although remifentanil can be used for postoperative analgesia in patients requiring artificial ventilation, other longer acting and cheaper opioids and/or regional techniques are usually more appropriate in patients breathing spontaneously.

TOTAL INTRAVENOUS ANAESTHESIA

Although the concept of inducing and maintaining anaesthesia using only drugs given intravenously has been available for many years, the technique remains relatively unpopular, despite its environmental advantages. This is because intravenous anaesthesia has not yet acquired the same controllability as inhalational anaesthesia, mainly because a reliable pharmacodynamic end-point remains undefined. Computer-controlled infusions delivering intravenous anaesthetic drugs according to pharmacokinetic model-driven algorithms have not yet advanced sufficiently to allow both satisfactory anaesthesia and rapid recovery.[176] Nevertheless, an improved understanding of the biochemical functioning of the brain and the introduction of short-acting drugs into clinical practice may lead to practical closed-loop feedback systems in the near future.

Drugs administered intravenously to induce anaesthesia characteristically produce a rapid onset of unconsciousness and allow a rapid recovery. The short duration of action results from a rapid decrease in plasma concentration caused by drug redistribution from brain to other tissues. However, when the same drug is administered by infusion, the total body clearance of the drug determines the steady-state plasma concentration and has an important influence on recovery time after the infusion is stopped. Nevertheless, distribution between central and peripheral compartments remains important in governing drug disposition even after prolonged infusions. Clinical recovery from the drug often relates to the duration of the infusion and cannot necessarily be predicted from knowledge of its elimination half-life. This has led to the introduction of the concept of 'context-sensitive half-time'.

CONTEXT-SENSITIVE HALF-TIME

Hughes and colleagues introduced the concept of context-sensitive half-time to describe recovery from anaesthetic infusions of varying duration.[147] The 'half-time' is the time required for the drug concentration in the central compartment to decrease by 50% after stopping its administration. The 'context' refers to the duration of drug infusion before its discontinuation. For instance, propofol has context-sensitive half-times of less than 25 min after 3 h of infusion, increasing to 50 min after a 12-h infusion. Drug infusion rates do not need to be kept constant, however, and if they can be titrated against effect, so that the concentration of drug in plasma has only to decline by 10–20% to permit awakening, clinical recovery times can be reduced.

Once an infusion of anaesthetic drug is stopped, the well-perfused peripheral compartment will usually have had time to equilibrate with the central compartment and, therefore, will be unable to accept additional drug from the central compartment to hasten the decline in plasma drug concentration. In contrast, a more poorly perfused peripheral compartment (fat) will not have had time to equilibrate with plasma and the concentration gradient between central and fat compartments will cause drug to continue to move into the fat compartment. Eventually, the declining plasma drug concentration and the rising fat compartment drug concentration equilibrate; thereafter, continuing decline of the central compartment drug concentration occurs by elimination mechanisms. This type of drug behaviour is exemplified by propofol.

Nevertheless, although context-sensitive half-time may be a better predictor of recovery time than terminal half-life, any pharmacokinetic or pharmacodynamic interaction between two or more anaesthetic drugs makes accurate predictions of recovery time for an individual patient much less likely.

DRUG INTERACTIONS

A single drug is seldom used to maintain anaesthesia because no one drug is able to provide all components of anaesthesia without either seriously compromising vital organ function or postponing postoperative recovery. Interactions between drugs usually allow a reduction in the dose of each drug that would otherwise be required to produce optimal operating conditions. Drug interactions can be between inhalational and intravenous drugs and between different intravenous drugs, although only the latter will be discussed here. These interactions can be pharmacokinetic and/or pharmacodynamic in nature.

Pharmacokinetic interactions

Performance of computer-controlled infusions suggests that propofol may affect its own distribution and elimination, possibly because of changing regional blood flow.[174] Similarly, the α_2-agonist dexmedetomidine has been shown to decrease thiopentone requirements by reducing its distribution volume, probably secondary to effects on cardiac output and regional blood flow.[177] Fentanyl and alfentanil increase the volume of the central compartment and clearance of propofol by unknown mechanisms. Propofol, midazolam and dexmedetomidine inhibit the oxidative metabolism of alfentanil *in vitro*, possibly owing to competition for the same P450 cytochrome enzyme CYP3A4.[178,179]

Pharmacodynamic interactions

Most opioids decrease propofol requirements for induction and maintenance of anaesthesia in a synergistic manner, although they may also potentiate its hypotensive effects.[174] Similarly, the plasma propofol concentration at which patients awake postoperatively will be reduced after opioid administration. Remifentanil offers the combination of fastest recovery time with greatest reduction in propofol requirements for maintenance of anaesthesia.[174] Adult studies have also shown that α_2-agonists such as dexmedetomidine can significantly reduce the operative requirements for volatile anaesthetic agents and/or opioids,[180] although whether they will make a significant impact on paediatric anaesthetic practice is still unclear.

In clinical practice, however, the 'purity' of a total intravenous anaesthesia (TIVA) technique is less inherently attractive than other less environmentally friendly alternatives. The synergistic combination of volatile anaesthetic agents in low-dose and intravenous agents remains more practical and, hence, more popular. This situation will probably remain unchanged until such time as intraoperative monitoring of brain performance, as opposed to brain activity, becomes a realistic proposition.

REFERENCES

1 Walther, F.J., Siassi, B., Ramadan, N.A., Ananda, A.K. and Wu, P.Y.K. Pulsed Doppler determinations of cardiac output in neonates: normal standards for clinical use. *Pediatrics* 1985; **76**: 829–33.

2 Hudson, I., Houston, A., Aitchison, T., Holland, B. and Turner, T. Reproducibility of measurements of cardiac output in newborn infants by Doppler ultrasound. *Archives of Disease in Childhood* 1990; **65**: 15–19.

3 Sholler, G.F., Celermajer, J.M., Whight, C.M. and Bauman, A.E. Echo Doppler assessment of cardiac output and its relation to growth in normal infants. *American Journal of Cardiology* 1987; **60**: 1112–16.

4 Sholler, G.F., Celermajer, J.M. and Whight, C.M. Doppler echocardiographic assessment of cardiac output in normal children with and without innocent precordial murmurs. *American Journal of Cardiology* 1987; **59**: 487–8.

5 Settergren, G., Lindblad, B.S. and Persson, B. Cerebral blood flow and exchange of oxygen, glucose, ketone bodies, lactate, pyruvate and amino acids in anaesthetized children. *Acta Paediatrica Scandinavica* 1980; **69**: 457–65.

6 Hastings, L.A., Monitto, C.L., Lenox, C. and Yaster, M. CSF and plasma fentanyl levels in children undergoing ventriculoperitoneal shunt surgery. *Anesthesiology* 1997; **87**: A1063.

7 Anagnostakis, D., Messaritakis, J., Damianos, D. and Mandyla, H. Blood–brain barrier permeability in 'healthy' infected and stressed neonates. *Journal of Pediatrics* 1992; **121**: 291–4.

8 Laterra, J., Stewart, P.A. and Goldstein, G.W. Development of the blood–brain barrier. In: Polin, R.A. and Fox, W.W. (eds). *Fetal and Neonatal Physiology*. London: W.B. Saunders, 1998: 2103–10.

9 Van Bree, J.B., De Boer, A.G., Danhof, M. and Breimer, D.D. Drug transport across the blood–brain barrier. I Anatomical and physiological aspects. *Pharmaceutical Science* 1992; **14**: 305–10.

10 Davis, S.L. and Lagercrantz, H. Basic Neurophysiology. In: Gluckman, P.D. and Heymann, M.A. (eds). *Pediatrics*

and *Perinatalogy. The Scientific Basis*. London: Arnold, 1996: 329–55.

11 Friis-Hansen, B. Water distribution in the foetus and newborn infant. *Acta Paediatrica Scandinavica* 1983; **305**: 7–11.

12 Friis-Hansen, B. Body composition during growth. *In vivo* measurements and biochemical data correlated to differential anatomical growth. *Pediatrics* 1971; **47**: 264–74.

13 Gasser, T. Development of fat tissue and body mass index from infancy to adulthood. *Pediatric Nephrology* 1996; **10**: 340–2.

14 Widdowson, E.M. Changes in body composition during growth. In: Davis, J.A. and Dobbing, J. (eds). *Scientific Foundations of Paediatrics*. London: William Heinemann Medical Books, 1981: 330–42.

15 Booker, P.D., Taylor, C. and Saba, G. Perioperative changes in a_1-acid glycoprotein concentrations in infants undergoing major surgery. *British Journal of Anaesthesia* 1996; **76**: 365–8.

16 Kingston, H.G.G., Kendrick, A., Sommer, K.M., Olsen, G.D. and Downes, H. Binding of thiopental in neonatal serum. *Anesthesiology* 1990; **72**: 428–31.

17 Leeder, J.S. and Kearns, G.L. Pharmacogenetics in pediatrics. Implications for practice. *Pediatric Clinics of North America* 1997; **44**: 55–77.

18 Hartley, R., Green, M., Quinn, M.W., Rushforth, J.A. and Levene, M.I. Development of morphine glucuronidation in premature neonates. *Biology of the Neonate* 1994; **66**: 1–9.

19 Ecobichon, D.J. and Stephens, D.S. Perinatal development of human blood esterases. *Clinical Pharmacology and Therapeutics* 1973; **14**: 41–7.

20 Davis, P.J., Ross, A.K., Henson, L.G. and Muir, K.T. Remifentanil pharmacokinetics in neonates. *Anaesthesiology* 1997; **87**: A1065.

21 Hughes, S.C., Kan, R.E., Rosen, M.A., *et al*. Remifentanil: ultra-short acting opioid for obstetric anaesthesia. *Anesthesiology* 1996; **85**: A894.

22 Rautakorpi, P., Ali-Melkkilä, T., Kaila, T., Olkkola, K.T., Iisalo, E. and Kanto, J. Pharmacokinetics of glycopyrrolate in children. *Journal of Clinical Anesthesia* 1994; **6**: 217–20.

23 Lou, H.C., Lassen, N.A. and Friis-Hansen. B. Impaired autoregulation of cerebral blood flow in the distressed newborn infant. *Journal of Pediatrics* 1979; **94**: 118–21.

24 Weekes, L.M., Keneally, J.P., Goonetilleke, P.H. and Ramzan, I.M. Pharmacokinetics of alcuronium in children with acyanotic and cyanotic cardiac disease undergoing cardiopulmonary bypass surgery. *Paediatric Anaesthesia* 1995; **5**: 369–74.

25 McAllister, R.G., Jr and Tan, T.G. Effect of hypothermia on drug metabolism. *In vitro* studies with propranolol and verapamil. *Pharmacology* 1980; **20**: 95–100.

26 Koren, G., Barker, C., Goresky, G., *et al*. The influence of hypothermia on the disposition of fentanyl – human and animal studies. *European Journal of Clinical Pharmacology* 1987; **32**: 373–6.

27 Petros, A., Dunne, N., Mehta, R., *et al*. The pharmacokinetics of alfentanil after normothermic and hypothermic cardiopulmonary bypass. *Anesthesia and Analgesia* 1995; **81**: 458–64.

28 Russell, D., Royston, D., Rees, P.H., Gupta, S.K. and Kenny, G.N.C. Effect of temperature and cardiopulmon-

ary bypass on the pharmacokinetics of remifentanil. *British Journal of Anaesthesia* 1997; **79**: 456–9.

29 Puig, M.M., Warner, W., Tang, C.K, Laorden, M.L. and Turndorf, H. Effects of temperature on the interaction of morphine with opioid receptors. *British Journal of Anaesthesia* 1987; **59**: 1459–64.

30 Gedney, J.A. and Ghosh, S. Pharmacokinetics of analgesics, sedatives and anaesthetic agents during cardiopulmonary bypass. *British Journal of Anaesthesia* 1995; **75**: 344–51.

31 den-Hollander, J.M., Hennis, P.J., Burm, A.G.L., Vletter, A.A. and Bovill, J.G. Pharmacokinetics of alfentanil before and after cardiopulmonary bypass in pediatric patients undergoing cardiac surgery. *Journal of Cardiothoracic and Vascular Anesthesia* 1992; **6**: 308–12.

32 Thurston, T.A., Maldonado, G. and Mathew, B.P. Acidosis accentuates thiopental-induced myocardial depression *in vitro*. *Anesthesia and Analgesia* 1996; **83**: 636–8.

33 Kinney, H.C. and White, W.F. Opioid receptors localize to the external granular cell layer of the developing human cerebellum. *Neuroscience* 1991; **45**: 13–21.

34 Reddy, S.C., Panigraphy, A., White, W.F. and Kinney, H.C. Developmental changes in neurotransmitter receptor binding in the human periaqueductal gray matter. *Journal of Neuropathology and Experimental Neurology* 1996; **55**: 409–18.

35 Clark, A.S., Robinson, S. and Henderson, L.P. Dynamics of GABA(A) receptor binding in the ventromedial hypothalamus during postnatal development in the rat. *Brain Research and Developments in Brain Research* 1997; **103**: 195–8.

36 Sorbo, S., Hudson, R.J. and Loomis, J.C. The pharmacokinetics of thiopental in pediatric surgical patients. *Anesthesiology* 1984; **61**: 666–70.

37 Garg, D.C., Goldberg, R.N., Woo-Ming, R.B. and Weilder, D.J. Pharmacokinetics of thiopental in the asphyxiated neonate. *Developments in Pharmacology and Therapeutics* 1988; **11**: 213–18.

38 Duncan, B.B.A., Zaimi, F., Newman, G.B., Jenkins, J.G. and Aveling, W. Effect of premedication on the induction dose of thiopentone in children. *Anaesthesia* 1984; **39**: 426–8.

39 Pomeroy, S.L. and Segal, R.A. Development of the nervous system. In: Polin, R.A. and Fox, W.W. (eds). *Fetal and Neonatal Physiology*. London: W.B. Saunders, 1998: 2083–103.

40 Runcie, C.J., Mackenzie, S.J., Arthur, D.S. and Morton, N.S. Comparison of recovery from anaesthesia induced in children with either propofol or thiopentone. *British Journal of Anaesthesia* 1993; **70**: 192–5.

41 Hannallah, R.S., Britton, J.T., Schafer, P.G., Patel, R.I. and Norden, J.M. Propofol anaesthesia in paediatric ambulatory patients: a comparison with thiopentone and halothane. *Canadian Journal of Anaesthesia* 1994; **41**: 12–16.

42 Schroter, J., Motsch, J., Hufnagel, A.R., Bach, A. and Martin, E. Recovery of psychomotor function following anaesthesia in children: a comparison of propofol and thiopentone/halothane. *Paediatric Anaesthesia* 1996; **6**: 317–24.

43 Jones, R.D., Visram, A.R., Chan, M.M., Bacon-Shone, J., Mya, G.H. and Irwin, M.G. A comparison of three induction agents in paediatric anaesthesia – cardiovas-

cular effects and recovery. *Anaesthesia and Intensive Care* 1994; **22**: 545–55.

44 Larsson, S., Asgeirsson, B. and Magnusson, J.M. Propofol–fentanyl anaesthesia compared to thiopental–halothane with special reference to recovery and vomiting after paediatric strabismus surgery. *Acta Anaesthesiologica Scandinavica* 1992; **36**: 182–6.

45 Aun, C.S.T., Sung, R.Y.T., O'Meara, M.E., Short ,T.G. and Oh, T.E. Cardiovascular effects of intravenous induction in children: comparison between propofol and thiopentone. *British Journal of Anaesthesia* 1993; **70**: 647–53.

46 Komai, H. and Rusy, B.F. Effect of thiopental on Ca^{2+} release from sarcoplasmic reticulum in intact myocardium. *Anesthesiology* 1994; **81**: 946–52.

47 Haws, J.L., Herman, N., Clark, Y., Bjoraker, R. and Jones, D. The chemical stability and sterility of sodium thiopental after preparation. *Anesthesia and Analgesia* 1998; **86**: 208–13.

48 Crowther, J., Hrazdil, J., Jolly, D.T., Galbraith, J.C., Greacen, M. and Grace, M. Growth of micro-organisms in propofol, thiopental and a 1 : 1 mixture of propofol and thiopental. *Anesthesia and Analgesia* 1996; **82**: 475–8.

49 Murat, I., Billard, V., Vernois, J., *et al*. Pharmacokinetics of propofol after a single dose in children aged 1–3 years with minor burns. *Anesthesiology* 1996; **84**: 526–32.

50 Jones, R.D., Chan, K., Andrew, L.J., Lawson, A.D. and Wong, P. Comparative pharmacokinetics of propofol in chinese adults and children. *Methods and Findings in Experimental Clinical Pharmacology* 1992; **14**: 41–7.

51 Reed, M.D., Yamashita, T., Marx, C.M., Myers, C. and Blumer, J.L. A pharmacokinetically based propofol dosing strategy for sedation of the critically ill, mechanically ventilated pediatric patient. *Critical Care Medicine* 1996; **24**: 1473–81.

52 Patel, D.K., Keeling, P.A., Newman, G.B. and Radford, P. Induction dose of propofol in children. *Anaesthesia* 1988; **43**: 949–52.

53 Aun, C.S.T., Short, S.M., Leung, D.H.Y. and Oh, T.E. Induction dose–response of propofol in unpremedicated children. *British Journal of Anaesthesia* 1992; **68**: 64–7.

54 Westrin, P. The induction dose of propofol in infants 1–6 months of age and in children 10–16 years of age. *Anesthesiology* 1991; **74**: 455–8.

55 Azari, D.M. and Cork, R.C. Comparative myocardial depressive effects of propofol and thiopental. *Anesthesia and Analgesia* 1993; **77**: 324–9.

56 Park, W.K., Lynch, C.I. and Johns, R.A. Effects of propofol and thiopental in isolated rat aorta and pulmonary artery. *Anesthesiology* 1992; **77**: 956–63.

57 Uezono, S. and Clarke, W.R. The effect of propofol on normal and increased pulmonary vascular resistance in isolated perfused rabbit lung. *Anesthesia and Analgesia* 1995; **80**: 577–82.

58 Saarnivaara, L., Hiller, A. and Oikkonem, M. QT interval, heart rate and arterial pressures using propofol, thiopentone or methohexitone for induction of anaesthesia in children. *Acta Anaesthesiologica Scandinavica* 1993; **37**: 419–23.

59 Snellen, F.T., Vanacker, B. and Van Aken, H. Propofol–nitrous oxide versus thiopental sodium–isoflurane–nitrous oxide for strabismus surgery in children. *Journal of Clinical Anesthesia* 1993; **5**: 37–41.

60 Schrum, S., Hannallah, R.S., Verghese, P.M., Welborn, L.G., Norden, J.M. and Ruttiman, U. Comparison of propofol and thiopental for rapid anesthesia induction in infants. *Anesthesia and Analgesia* 1994; **78**: 482–5.

61 Valtonen, M., Iisalo, E., Kanto, J. and Tikkanen, J. Comparison between propofol and thiopentone for induction of anaesthesia in children. *Anaesthesia* 1988; **43**: 696–9.

62 Hannallah, R.S., Baker, S.B., Casey, W., McGill, W.A., Broadman, L.M. and Norden, J.M. Propofol: effective dose and induction characteristics in unpremedicated children. *Anesthesiology* 1991; **74**: 217–19.

63 Allsop, E., Innes, P., Jackson, M. and Cunliffe, M. Dose of propofol required to insert the laryngeal mask airway in children. *Paediatric Anaesthesia* 1995; **5**: 47–51.

64 Blouin, R.T., Conard, P.F. and Gross, J.B. Time course of ventilatory depression following induction doses of propofol and thiopental. *Anesthesiology* 1991; **75**: 940–4.

65 Kulkarni, P. and Brown, K.A. Ventilatory parameters in children during propofol anaesthesia: a comparison with halothane. *Canadian Journal of Anaesthesia* 1996; **43**: 653–7.

66 McKeating, K., Bali, I.M. and Dundee, J.W. The effects of thiopentone and propofol on upper airway integrity. *Anaesthesia* 1988; **43**: 638–40.

67 McConaghy, P. and Bunting, H.E. Assessment of intubating conditions in children after induction with propofol and varying doses of alfentanil. *British Journal of Anaesthesia* 1994; **73**: 596–9.

68 Steyn, M.P., Quinn, A.M., Gillespie, J.A., Miller, D.C., Best, C.J. and Morton, N.S. Tracheal intubation without neuromuscular block in children. *British Journal of Anaesthesia* 1994; **72**: 403–6.

69 Bevan, J.C. Propofol-related convulsions. *Canadian Journal of Anaesthesia* 1993; **40**: 805–8.

70 Doenicke, A.W., Roizen, M.F., Rau, J., Kellerman, W. and Babl, J. Reducing pain during propofol injection: the role of the solvent. *Anesthesia and Analgesia* 1996; **82**: 472–4.

71 Eriksson, M., Englesson, S., Niklasson, F. and Hartvig, P. Effect of lignocaine and pH on propofol-induced pain. *British Journal of Anaesthesia* 1997; **78**: 502–6.

72 Fletcher, G.C., Gillespie, J.A. and Davidson, J.A. The effect of temperature upon pain during injection of propofol. *Anaesthesia* 1996; **51**: 498–9.

73 Nathanson, M.H., Gajraj, N.M. and Russell, J.A. Prevention of pain on injection of propofol: a comparison of lidocaine with alfentanil. *Anesthesia and Analgesia* 1996; **82**: 469–71.

74 Weir, P.M., Munro, H.M., Reynolds, P.I., Lewis, I.H. and Wilton, N.C. Propofol infusion and the incidence of emesis in pediatric outpatient strabismus surgery. *Anesthesia and Analgesia* 1993; **76**: 760–4.

75 Biebuyck, J.F., Gouldson, R., Nathanson, M., White, P.F. and Smith, I. Propofol: an update on its clinical use. *Anesthesiology* 1994; **81**: 1005–43.

76 Devlin, E.G., Clarke, R.S., Mirakhur, R.K. and McNeill, T.A. Effect of four intravenous induction agents on T-lymphocyte proliferation to PHA *in vitro*. *British Journal of Anaesthesia* 1994; **73**: 315–17.

77 Laxenaire, M.C., Mata-Bermejo, E., Moneret-Vautrin, D.A. and Gueant, J.-L. Life-threatening anaphylactoid reactions to propofol (Diprivan®). *Anesthesiology* 1992; **77**: 275–80.

78 Habre, W., Matsumoto, I. and Sly, P.D. Propofol or halothane anaesthesia for children with asthma; effects on respiratory mechanics. *British Journal of Anaesthesia* 1996; **77**: 739–43.

79 Setlock, M.A., Palmisano, B.W., Berens, R.J., Rosner, D.R., Troshynski, T.J. and Murray, K.J. Tolerance to propofol generally does not develop in pediatric patients undergoing radiation therapy. *Anesthesiology* 1996; **85**: 207–11.

80 Geisslinger, G., Hering, W., Thomann, P., Knoll, R., Kamp, H.D. and Brune, K. Pharmacokinetics and pharmacodynamics of ketamine enantiomers in surgical patients using a stereoselective analytical method. *British Journal of Anaesthesia* 1993; **70**: 666–71.

81 Brockmeyer, D.M. and Kendig, J.J. Selective effects of ketamine on amino acid-mediated pathways in neonatal rat spinal cord. *British Journal of Anaesthesia* 1995; **74**: 79–84.

82 Hartvig, P., Valtysson, J., Lindner, K.J., *et al.* Central nervous system effects of subdissociative doses of (S)-ketamine are related to plasma and brain concentrations measured with positron emission tomography in healthy volunteers. *Clinical Pharmacology and Therapeutics* 1995; **58**: 165–73.

83 Hirota, K. and Lambert, D.G. Ketamine: its mechanism(s) of action and unusual clinical uses. *British Journal of Anaesthesia* 1996; **77**: 442–4.

84 Byer, D.E. and Gould, A.B.J. Development of tolerance to ketamine in an infant undergoing repeated anesthesia. *Anesthesiology* 1981; **54**: 255–6.

85 Grant, I.S., Nimmo, W.S., McNicol, L.R. and Clements, J.A. Ketamine disposition in children and adults. *British Journal of Anaesthesia* 1983; **55**: 1107–10.

86 Malinovsky, J.-M., Servin, F., Cozian, A., Lepage, J.-Y. and Pinaud, M. Ketamine and norketamine plasma concentrations after intravenous, nasal and rectal administration in children. *British Journal of Anaesthesia* 1996; **77**: 203–7.

87 Hartvig, P., Larsson, E. and Joachimsson, P.-O. Postoperative analgesia and sedation following pediatric cardiac surgery using a constant infusion of ketamine. *Journal of Cardiothoracic and Vascular Anesthesia* 1993; **7**: 148–53.

88 Greeley, W.J., Boyd, J.L.I. and Kern, F.H. Pharmacokinetics of analgesic drugs. In: Anand, K.J.S. and McGrath, P.J. (eds). *Pain in Neonates*. New York: Elsevier Science Publishers, 1993: 107–55.

89 Leung, L. and Baille, T. Comparative pharmacology of ketamine in the rat and its two principal metabolites norketamine and (2)-6-hydroxynorketamine. *Journal of Medicinal Chemistry* 1986; **29**: 2396–9.

90 White, P.F., Schüttler, J., Shafer, A., Stanski, D.R., Horai, Y. and Trevor, A.J. Comparative pharmacology of the ketamine isomers. *British Journal of Anaesthesia* 1985; **57**: 197–203.

91 Reich, D.L. and Silvay, G. Ketamine: an update on the first twenty-five years of clinical experience. *Canadian Journal of Anaesthesia* 1989; **36**: 186–97.

92 Lockhart, C.H. and Jenkins, J.J. Ketamine-induced apnea in patients with increased intracranial pressure. *Anesthesiology* 1972; **37**: 92–3.

93 Albanèse, J., Arnaud, S., Rey, M., Thomachot, L., Alliez, B. and Martin, C. Ketamine decreases intracranial pressure and electroencephalographic activity in traumatic brain injury patients during propofol sedation. *Anesthesiology* 1997; **87**: 1328–34.

94 Mayberg, T.S., Lam, A.M., Matta, B.F., Domino, K.B. and Winn, H.R. Ketamine does not increase cerebral blood flow velocity or intracranial pressure during isoflurane/nitrous oxide anesthesia in patients undergoing craniotomy. *Anesthesia and Analgesia* 1995; **81**: 84–9.

95 Meyers, E.F. and Charles, P. Prolonged adverse reactions to ketamine in children. *Anesthesiology* 1978; **49**: 39–40.

96 Davies, A.E. and McCans, J.L. Effects of barbiturate anesthetics and ketamine on the force–frequency relation of cardiac muscle. *European Journal of Pharmacology* 1979; **59**: 65–73.

97 White, P.F., Way, W.L. and Trevor, A.J. Ketamine – its pharmacology and therapeutic uses. *Anesthesiology* 1982; **56**: 119–36.

98 Lundy, P.M., Lockwood, P.A., Thompson, G. and Frew, R. Differential effects of ketamine isomers on neuronal and extraneuronal catecholamine uptake mechanisms. *Anesthesiology* 1986; **64**: 359–63.

99 Van der Linden, P., Gilbart, E., Engelman, E., Schmartz, D., De Rood, M. and Vincent, J.L. Comparison of halothane, isoflurane, alfentanil and ketamine in experimental septic shock. *Anesthesia and Analgesia* 1990; **70**: 608–17.

100 Friesen, R.H. and Henry, D.B. Cardiovascular changes in preterm neonates receiving isoflurane, halothane, fentanyl and ketamine. *Anesthesiology* 1986; **64**: 238–42.

101 Waxman, K., Shoemaker, W.C. and Lippermann, M. Cardiovascular effects of anesthetic induction with ketamine. *Anesthesia and Analgesia* 1980; **59**: 355–8.

102 Wolfe, R.R., Loehr, J.P., Schaffer, M.S. and Wiggins, J.W. Hemodynamic effects of ketamine, hypoxia and hyperoxia in children with surgically treated congenital heart disease residing > 1200 meters above sea level. *American Journal of Cardiology* 1991; **67**: 84–7.

103 Berman, W., Fripp, R.R., Rubler, M. and Alderete, L. Hemodynamic effects of ketamine in children undergoing cardiac catheterization. *Pediatric Cardiology* 1990; **11**: 72–6.

104 Rock, M., De La Rocha, S., L'Hommidieu, C. and Truemper, E. Use of ketamine in asthmatic children to treat respiratory failure refractory to conventional therapy. *Critical Care Medicine* 1986; **14**: 514–16.

105 Hirota, K., Sato, T., Rabito, S.F., Zsigmond, E.K. and Matsuki, A.. Relaxant effect of ketamine and its isomers on histamine-induced contraction of tracheal smooth muscle. *British Journal of Anaesthesia* 1996; **76**: 266–70.

106 Wilson, L.E., Hatch, D.J. and Rehder, K. Mechanisms of the relaxant action of ketamine on isolated porcine trachealis muscle. *British Journal of Anaesthesia* 1993; **71**: 544–50.

107 Hodgson, P.E., Rehder, K. and Hatch, D.J. Comparison of the pharmacodynamics of ketamine in the isolated neonatal and adult porcine airway. *British Journal of Anaesthesia* 1995; **75**: 71–9.

108 Shulman, D., Beardsmore, C.S., Aronson, H.B. and Godfrey, S. The effect of ketamine on the functional residual capacity in young children. *Anesthesiology* 1985; **62**: 551–6.

109 Shulman, D.L., Bat-Yishay, E. and Godfrey, S. Respiratory mechanics and intrinsic PEEP during ketamine and halothane anesthesia in young children. *Anesthesia and Analgesia* 1988; **67**: 656–62.

110 Hamza, J., Ecoffey, C. and Gross, J.B. Ventilatory response to CO_2 following intravenous ketamine in children. *Anesthesiology* 1989; **70**: 422–5.

111 Joly, L.-M. and Benhamou, D. Ventilation during total intravenous anaesthesia with ketamine. *Canadian Journal of Anaesthesia* 1994; **41**: 227–31.

112 Hickey, P.R., Hansen, D.D., Cramolini, G.M., Vincent, R.N. and Lang, P. Pulmonary and systemic hemodynamic responses to ketamine in infants with normal and elevated pulmonary vascular resistance. *Anesthesiology* 1985; **63**: 287–93.

113 Smith, J.A. and Santer, L.J. Respiratory arrest following intramuscular ketamine injection in a 4-year-old child. *Annals of Emergency Medicine* 1993; **22**: 613–15.

114 Salonem, M., Kanto, J., Iisalo, E. and Himberg, J.-J. Midazolam as an induction agent in children. *Anesthesia and Analgesia* 1987; **66**: 625–8.

115 Persson, P., Nilsson, A., Hartvig, P. and Tamsen, A. Pharmacokinetics of midazolam in total intravenous anaesthesia. *British Journal of Anaesthesia* 1987; **59**: 548–56.

116 Jones, R.D.M., Chan, K., Roulson, C.J., Brown, A.G., Smith, I.D. and Mya, G.H. Pharmacokinetics of flumazenil and midazolam. *British Journal of Anaesthesia* 1993; **70**: 286–92.

117 Payne, K., Mattheyse, F.J., Liebenberg, D. and Dawes, T. The pharmacokinetics of midazolam in paediatric patients. *European Journal of Clinical Pharmacology* 1989; **37**: 267–72.

118 Bornemann, L.D., Min, B.H., Crews, T., et al. Dose dependent pharmacokinetics of midazolam. *European Journal of Clinical Pharmacology* 1985; **29**: 91–5.

119 Massaut, J., d'Hollander, A., Barvais, L. and Dubois-Primo, J. Haemodynamic effects of midazolam in the anaesthetized patient with coronary artery disease. *Acta Anaesthesiologica Scandinavica* 1983; **27**: 299–302.

120 Cole, W.H. Midazolam in paediatric anaesthesia. *Anaesthesia and Intensive Care* 1982; **10**: 36–9.

121 Jones, R.D.M., Lawson, A.D., Andrew, L.J., Gunawardene, W.M.S. and Bacon-Shone, J. Antagonism of the hypnotic effect of midazolam in children: a randomised, double-blind study of placebo and flumazenil administered after midazolam-induced anaesthesia. *British Journal of Anaesthesia* 1991; **66**: 660–6.

122 Pathak, K.S., Anton, A.H. and Sutheimer, C.A. Effects of low-dose morphine and fentanyl infusions on urinary and plasma catecholamine concentrations during scoliosis surgery. *Anesthesia and Analgesia* 1985; **64**: 509–14.

123 Anand, K.J.S., Hansen, D.D. and Hickey, P.R. Hormonal–metabolic stress responses in neonates undergoing cardiac surgery. *Anesthesiology* 1991; **73**: 661–70.

124 Kart, T., Christrup, L.L. and Rasmussen, M. Recommended use of morphine in neonates, infants and children based on a literature review: part 1 – pharmacokinetics. *Paediatric Anaesthesia* 1997; **7**: 5–11.

125 Osborne, R., Joel, S., Trew. D. and Slevin. M. Analgesic activity of morphine-6-glucuronide. *Lancet* 1988; **i**: 828.

126 Peat, S.J., Hanna, M.H., Woodham, M., Knibb, A.A. and Ponte, J. Morphine-6-glucuronide: effects on ventilation in normal volunteers. *Pain* 1991; **45**: 101–4.

127 Gong, Q.L., Hedner, J., Bjorkman, R. and Hedner, T. Morphine-3-glucuronide may functionally antagonise morphine-6-glucuronide induced antinociception and ventilatory depression in the rat. *Pain* 1992; **48**: 249–55.

128 Osborne, R., Joel, S., Grebenik, K., Trew, D. and Slevin, M. The pharmacokinetics of morphine and morphine glucuronides in kidney failure. *Clinical Pharmacology and Therapeutics* 1993; **54**: 158–67.

129 Farrington, E.A., McGuiness, G.A., Johnson, G.F., Erenberg, A. and Leff, R.D. Continuous intravenous morphine infusion in postoperative newborn infants. *American Journal of Perinatology* 1993; **10**: 84–7.

130 Bragg, P., Zwass, M.S., Lau, M. and Fisher, D.M. Opioid pharmacodynamics in neonatal dogs: differences between morphine and fentanyl. *Journal of Applied Physiology* 1995; **79**: 1519–24.

131 Lynn, A.M., McRorie, T.I., Slattery, J.T., Calkins, D.F. and Opheim, K.E. Age-dependent morphine partitioning between plasma and cerebrospinal fluid in monkeys. *Developments in Pharmacology and Therapeutics* 1991; **17**: 200–4.

132 Lynn, A.M., Nespeca, M.K., Opheim, K.E. and Slattery, J.T. Respiratory effects of intravenous morphine infusions in neonates, infants and children after cardiac surgery. *Anesthesia and Analgesia* 1993; **77**: 695–701.

133 Greene, R.F., Miser, A.W., Lester, C.M., Balis, F.M. and Poplack, D.G. Cerebrospinal fluid and plasma pharmacokinetics of morphine infusions in pediatric cancer patients and rhesus monkeys. *Pain* 1987; **30**: 348.

134 Rouby, J.J., Eurin, B., Glaser, P., et al. Hemodynamic and metabolic effects of morphine in the critically ill. *Circulation* 1981; **64**: 53–9.

135 Samuel, I.O., Morrison, J.D. and Dundee, J.W. Central haemodynamic and forearm vascular effects of morphine in patients after open heart surgery. *British Journal of Anaesthesia* 1980; **52**: 1237–46.

136 Doenicke, A., Moss, J., Lorenz, W. and Hoernecke, R. Intravenous morphine and nalbuphine increase histamine and catecholamine release without accompanying hemodynamic changes. *Clinical Pharmacology and Therapeutics* 1995; **58**: 81–9.

137 Withington, D.E., Patrick, J.A. and Reynolds, F. Histamine release by morphine and diamorphine in man. *Anaesthesia* 1993; **48**: 26–9.

138 Flacke, J.W., Flacke, W.E., Bloor, B.C., Van Etten, A.P. and Kripke, B.J. Histamine release by four narcotics: a double-blind study in humans. *Anesthesia and Analgesia* 1987; **66**: 723–30.

139 Grossmann, M., Abiose, A., Tangphao, O., Blaschke, T.F. and Hoffman, B.B. Morphine-induced venodilation in humans. *Clinical Pharmacology and Therapeutics* 1996; **60**: 554–60.

140 Steffey, E.P., Eisele, J.H., Baggot, J.D., Woliner, M.J., Jarvis, K.A. and Elliott, A.R. Influence of inhaled anesthetics on the pharmacokinetics and pharmacodynamics of morphine. *Anesthesia and Analgesia* 1993; **77**: 346–51.

141 Concannon, K.T., Dodam, J.R. and Hellyer, P.W. Influence of a mu- and kappa-opioid agonist on isoflurane minimal anesthetic concentration in chickens. *American Journal of Veterinary Research* 1995; **56**: 806–11.

142 Katoh, T., Suguro, Y., Kimura, T. and Ikeda, K. Morphine does not affect the awakening concentration of sevoflurane. *Canadian Journal of Anaesthesia* 1993; **40**: 825–8.

143 Gross, J.B. and Alexander, C.M. Awakening concentrations of isoflurane are not affected by analgesic doses of morphine. *Anesthesia and Analgesia* 1988; **67**: 27–30.

144 Hartley, R. and Levene, M.I. Opioid pharmacology in the newborn. *Bailliere's Clinical Paediatrics* 1995; **3**: 467–93.

145 Weinstein, M.S., Nicolson, S.C. and Schreiner, M.S. A single dose of morphine sulphate increases the incidence of vomiting after outpatient inguinal surgery in children. *Anesthesiology* 1994; **81**: 572–7.

146 Davis, P.J. and Cook, D.R. Clinical pharmacokinetics of the newer intravenous anesthetic agents. *Clinical Pharmacokinetics* 1986; **11**: 18–35.

147 Hughes, M.A., Glass, P.S.A. and Jacobs, J.R. Context-sensitive half-time in multicompartment pharmacokinetic models for intravenous anesthetic drugs. *Anesthesiology* 1992; **76**: 334–41.

148 Kuhls, E., Gauntlett, I.S., Lau, M., et al. Effect of increased intra-abdominal pressure on hepatic extraction and clearance of fentanyl in neonatal lambs. *Journal of Pharmacology and Experimental Therapeutics* 1995; **274**: 115–19.

149 Arnold, J.H., Truog, R.D., Scavone, J.M. and Fenton, T. Changes in the pharmacodynamic response to fentanyl in neonates during continuous infusion. *Journal of Pediatrics* 1991; **119**: 639–43.

150 Ben-Shlomo, I., Finger, J., Bar-Av, E., Perl, A.Z., Etchin, A. and Tverskoy, M. Propofol and fentanyl act additively for induction of anaesthesia. *Anaesthesia* 1993; **48**: 111–13.

151 Katoh, T. and Ikeda, K. The effects of fentanyl on sevoflurane requirements for loss of consciousness and skin incision. *Anesthesiology* 1998; **88**: 18–24.

152 McEwan, A.I., Smith, C., Dyar, O., Goodman, D., Smith, L.R. and Glass, P.S.A. Isoflurane minimum alveolar concentration reduction by fentanyl. *Anesthesiology* 1993; **78**: 864–9.

153 Murat, I., Levron, J.C., Berg, A. and Saint-Maurice, C. Effects of fentanyl on baroreceptor reflex control of heart rate in newborn infants. *Anesthesiology* 1988; **68**: 717–22.

154 Yaster, M. The dose response of fentanyl in neonatal anesthesia. *Anesthesiology* 1987; **66**: 433–5.

155 Hickey, P.R., Hansen, D., Wessel, D.L., Lang, P. and Jonas, R.A. Pulmonary and systemic hemodynamic responses to fentanyl in infants. *Anesthesia and Analgesia* 1985; **64**: 483–6.

156 Hickey, P.R. and Hansen, D.D. Fentanyl– and sufentanil–oxygen–pancuronium anesthesia for cardiac surgery in infants. *Anesthesia and Analgesia* 1984; **63**: 117–24.

157 Vacanti, J.P., Crone, R.K., Murphy, J.D., et al. The pulmonary hemodynamic response to perioperative anesthesia in the treatment of high-risk infants with congenital diaphragmatic hernia. *Journal of Pediatric Surgery* 1984; **16**: 672–9.

158 Hickey, P.R. and Retzack, S.M. Acute right ventricular failure after pulmonary hypertensive responses to airway

instrumentation: effect of fentanyl dose. *Anesthesiology* 1993; **78**: 372–6.

159 Hickey, P.R., Hansen, D., Wessel, D.L., Lang, P., Jonas, R.A. and Elixson, E.M. Blunting of stress responses in the pulmonary circulation of infants by fentanyl. *Anesthesia and Analgesia* 1985; **64**: 1137–42.

160 Anand, K.J.S., Sippell, W.G. and Aynsley-Green, A. Randomised trial of fentanyl anaesthesia in preterm babies undergoing surgery: effects on the stress response. *Lancet* 1987; **i**: 62–6.

161 Sfez, M., Le Mapihan, Y., Gaillard, J.L. and Rosemblatt, J.M. Analgesia for appendectomy: comparison of fentanyl and alfentanil in children. *Acta Anaesthesiologica Scandinavica* 1990; **34**: 30–4.

162 Ellis, D.J. and Steward, D.J. Fentanyl dosage is associated with reduced blood glucose in pediatric patients after hypothermic cardiopulmonary bypass. *Anesthesiology* 1990; **72**: 812–15.

163 Newland, M.C., Leuschen, P., Sarafian, L.B., *et al.* Fentanyl intermittent bolus technique for anesthesia in infants and children undergoing cardiac surgery. *Journal of Cardiothoracic Anesthesia* 1989; **3**: 407–10.

164 Koren, G., Goresky, G., Crean, P., Klein, J. and MacCleod, S.M. Pediatric fentanyl dosing based on pharmacokinetics during cardiac surgery. *Anesthesia and Analgesia* 1984; **63**: 577–82.

165 Meistelman, C., Saint-Maurice, C., Lepaul, M., Levron, J.C., Loose, J.P. and MacGee, K. A comparison of alfentanil pharmacokinetics in children and adults. *Anesthesiology* 1987; **66**: 13–16.

166 Vinik, H.R., Bradley, E.L., Jr and Kissin, I. Midazolam–alfentanil synergism for anesthetic induction in patients. *Anesthesia and Analgesia* 1989; **69**: 213–17.

167 Vuyk, J., Engbers, F.H.M., Burm, A.G.L., *et al.* Pharmacodynamic interaction between propofol and alfentanil when given for induction of anesthesia. *Anesthesiology* 1996; **84**: 288–99.

168 Westmoreland, C.L., Sebel, P.S. and Gropper, A. Fentanyl or alfentanil decreases the minimum alveolar anesthetic concentration of isoflurane in surgical patients. *Anesthesia and Analgesia* 1994; **78**: 23–8.

169 den Hollander, J.M., Hennis, P.J., Burm, A.G.L. and Bovill, J.G. Alfentanil in infants and children with congenital heart defects. *Journal of Cardiothoracic Anesthesia* 1988; **2**: 12–17.

170 Bürkle, H., Dunbar, S. and Van Aken, H. Remifentanil: a novel, short-acting, m-opioid. *Anesthesia and Analgesia* 1996; **83**: 646–51.

171 Thompson, J.P., Hall, A.P., Russell, J., Cagney, B. and Rowbotham, D.J. Effect of remifentanil on the haemodynamic response to orotracheal intubation. *British Journal of Anaesthesia* 1998; **80**: 467–9.

172 Cartwright, D.P., Kvalsvik, O., Cassuto, J., *et al.* A randomised, blind comparison of remifentanil and alfentanil during anesthesia for outpatient surgery. *Anesthesia and Analgesia* 1997; **85**: 1014–19.

173 Lang, E., Kapila, A., Shlugman, D., Hoke, J.F., Sebel, P.S. and Glass, P.S. Reduction of isoflurane minimal alveolar concentration by remifentanil. *Anesthesiology* 1996; **85**: 721–8.

174 Vuyk, J. Pharmacokinetic and pharmacodynamic interactions between opioids and propofol. *Journal of Clinical Anesthesia* 1997; **9**: 23–6S.

175 Davis, P.J., Lerman, J., Suresh, S., *et al.* A randomized multicenter study of remifentanil compared with alfentanil, isoflurane, or propofol in anesthetized pediatric patients undergoing elective strabismus surgery. *Anesthesia and Analgesia* 1997; **84**: 982–9.

176 Short, T.G., Aun, C.S.T., Tan, P., Wong, J., Tam, Y.H. and Oh, T.E. A prospective evaluation of pharmacokinetic model controlled infusion of propofol in paediatric patients. *British Journal of Anaesthesia* 1994; **72**: 302–6.

177 Bührer, M., Mappes, A., Lauber, R., Stanski, D.R. and Maitre, P.O. Dexmedetomidine decreases thiopental dose requirement and alters distribution pharmacokinetics. *Anesthesiology* 1994; **80**: 1216–27.

178 Chen, T.L., Ueng, T.H., Chen, S.H., Lee, P.H., Fan, S.Z. and Liu, C.C. Human cytochrome P450 mono-oxygenase system is suppressed by propofol. *British Journal of Anaesthesia* 1995; **74**: 558–62.

179 Kharasch, E.D., Hill, H.F. and Eddy, A.C. Influence of dexmedetomidine and clonidine on human liver microsomal alfentanil metabolism. *Anesthesiology* 1991; **75**: 520–4.

180 Aantaa, R. and Scheinin, M. Alpha$_2$-adrenergic agents in anaesthesia. *Acta Anaesthesiologica Scandinavica* 1993; **37**: 1–16.

181 Wu, P.Y.K., Wong, W.H., Guerra, G., *et al.* Peripheral blood flow in the neonate. 1. Changes in total, skin and muscle blood flow with gestational and postnatal age. *Pediatric Research* 1980; **14**: 1374–8.

182 Cook, D.R. and Davis, P.J. Pediatric anesthesia pharmacology. In: Lake, C.L. (ed.). *Pediatric Cardiac Anesthesia.* Stamford: Appleton and Lange, 1998: 123–64.

183 Edelstone, D.I. and Holzman, I.R. Oxygen consumption by the gastrointestinal tract and liver in conscious newborn lambs. *American Journal of Physiology* 1981; **240**: G297–304.

184 Lautt, W.W. and Greenway, C.V. Conceptual review of the hepatic vascular bed. *Hepatology* 1987; **7**: 952–63.

185 Seikaly, M.G. and Arant, B.S., Jr. Development of renal hemodynamics: glomerular filtration and renal blood flow. *Clinics in Perinatology* 1992; **19**: 1–13.

186 Greisen, G. Cerebral blood flow and energy metabolism in the newborn. *Clinics in Perinatology* 1997; **24**: 531–46.

187 Madsen, P.L., Holm, S., Herning, M. and Lassen, N.A. Average blood flow and oxygen uptake in the human brain during resting wakefulness: a critical appraisal of the Kety–Schmidt technique. *Journal of Cerebral Blood Flow Metabolism* 1993; **13**: 646–55.

188 Olkkola, K.T., Hamunen, K. and Maunuksela, E.L. Clinical pharmacokinetics and pharmacodynamics of opioid analgesics in infants and children. *Clinical Pharmacokinetics* 1995; **28**: 385–404.

189 Wachtel, R.E. and Wegrzynowicz, E.S. Kinetics of nicotinic acetylcholine ion channels in the presence of intravenous anaesthetics and induction agents. *British Journal of Pharmacology* 1992; **106**: 623–7.

190 Katarina, B.K., Ved, S.A., Nicodemus, H.F., *et al.* The pharmacokinetics of propofol in children using three different data analysis approaches. *Anesthesiology* 1994; **80**: 104–22.

191 Burtin, P., Jacqz-Aigrain, E., Girard, P., *et al.* Population pharmacokinetics of midazolam in neonates. *Clinical Pharmacology and Therapeutics* 1994; **56**: 615–25.

192 Mathews, H.M.L., Carson, I.W., Lyons, S.M., *et al.* A pharmacokinetic study of midazolam in paediatric patients undergoing cardiac surgery. *British Journal of Anaesthesia* 1988; **61**: 302–7.

193 Jacqz-Aigrain, E. and Burtin, P. Clinical pharmacokinetics of sedatives in neonates. *Clinical Pharmacokinetics* 1996; **31**: 423–43.

194 Scholz, J., Steinfath, M. and Schulz, M. Clinical pharmacokinetics of alfentanil, fentanyl and sufentanil. *Clinical Pharmacokinetics* 1996; **31**: 275–92.

195 Koehntop, D.E., Rodman, J.H., Brundage, D.M., Hegland, M.G. and Buckley, J.J. Pharmacokinetics of fentanyl in neonates. *Anesthesia and Analgesia* 1986; **65**: 227–32.

196 Davis, P.J., Ross, A., Stiller, R.L., *et al.* Pharmacokinetics of remifentanil in anesthetized children 2–12 years of age. *Anesthesia and Analgesia* 1995; **80**: S93.

197 Kapila, A., Glass, P.S.A., Jacobs, J.R., *et al.* Measured context-sensitive half-times of remifentanil and alfentanil. *Anesthesiology* 1995; **83**: 968–75.

198 Westrin, P., Jonmarker, C. and Werner, O. Thiopental requirements for induction of anesthesia in neonates and in infants one to six months of age. *Anesthesiology* 1989; **71**: 344–6.

199 Jonmarker, C., Westrin, P, Larsson, S. and Werner, O. Thiopental requirements for induction of anesthesia in children. *Anaesthesiology* 1987; **67**: 104–7.

CHAPTER 5

Relaxants in paediatric anaesthesia

NISHAN GOUDSOUZIAN

INTRODUCTION

Until the 1970s, the practice of paediatric anaesthesia depended in part on two neuromuscular blocking drugs, succinylcholine and tubocurarine. Nowadays, by contrast, at least 10 such relaxants are clinically available, with the promise of another short-acting relaxant currently under evaluation. The different properties of each drug allow for a more carefully tailored anaesthesia course. To meet the demands for prolonged surgical relaxation, an intermediate- or short-acting agent might be given in sequential doses or via infusion; alternatively, a long-acting agent might be substituted. Because some of the newer agents have no appreciable cumulative properties, the anaesthetist can time recovery to the conclusion of surgery or can quickly and easily reverse residual effects. There are even added extraclinical decisions: since the cost of the newer drugs is two to three times higher than that of the older ones, anaesthetists can at times choose freely only within the limits of their own hospital's fiscal restraints.

This chapter reviews and classifies the neuromuscular blocking agents available to the modern paediatric anaesthetist and makes suggestions for their practical use.

SHORT-ACTING RELAXANTS

SUCCINYLCHOLINE

Succinylcholine (SCh) is still the relaxant with the fastest onset and the shortest duration of action. The short duration of SCh is due to its rapid hydrolysis by plasma cholinesterase (pseudocholinesterase, butirylcholinesterase). Plasma cholinesterase is synthesized by the liver and is present in serum as a tetrameric glycoprotein consisting of four identical subunits, each made of nine sugar chains.[1] The enzyme hydrolyses SCh (succinyldicholine) by first-order pharmacokinetic elimination to succinylmonocholine and choline.

Early in 1955 it was observed that infants require more SCh than adults relative to body weight.[2] Later, it was confirmed with twitch recording that 1 mg kg^{-1} SCh in small infants produced neuromuscular block equal to that produced by 0.5 mg kg^{-1} in older children.[3] Since the extracellular volume occupies a larger percentage of body weight in the infant (40% vs 18% in adults), it may be assumed that the drug is distributed in a larger volume and that the net result is a lower concentration reaching the myoneural junction. Consequently, in infants the initial dose should be 1.5 to 2 times larger than that given to older children.

When SCh is administered to infants and children via continuous intravenous infusion, tachyphylaxis and phase-II block develop as in adults. Clinical evaluations have shown that tachyphylaxis may occur in children after the administration of 3 mg kg^{-1} over an interval of 23 min and phase II block after a total of 4 mg kg^{-1} has been given.[4] A longer infusion period (100 min) may lead to the development of bradyphylaxis because of decreased requirements subsequent to the establishment of phase-II block.[5] Interestingly, in some very young infants (5 days to 4 months of age) marked resistance to the neuromuscular effects of SCh has been detected with a three-fold difference in dosage requirement. These infants go on to recover within the short span of 5 min after discontinuation of infusion.[6] It was originally suggested that such infants might have a high level of plasma cholinesterase but investigators have found that cholinesterase activity and dibucaine numbers are similar and very rarely lower in infants than in adults.[7] Differences in distribution volume may be partially responsible, but the three-fold difference in requirement remains something of a mystery. There probably exists an inherent resistance of the myoneural junction to SCh in very young infants but this has yet to be demonstrated with certainty.

The duration of action of SCh is related to plasma cholinesterase activity: whenever there is a decreased activity of the enzyme the duration of action of SCh is prolonged. The most common cause of decreased plasma cholinesterase activity in children is the presence of the atypical enzyme. The latter can be present in the usual concentrations, but has markedly diminished hydrolytic activity. In heterozygous patients, who comprise 4% of Caucasians, the prolongation is only for a few minutes and is usually undetected. In homozygotes (incidence 1 : 2000) who have two atypical genes (fluoride or silent), prolonged paralysis that may extend for a few hours can occur.[1,8]

Side-effects

Most of the side-effects associated with SCh are benign in nature and resolve spontaneously, but they are not the same in children as in adults. The most frequently observed side-effects of SCh are bradyarrhythmias which usually manifest as premature atrial or nodal contractions lasting for a few beats and then disappearing spontaneously.[9] In adults most arrhythmias are seen after a second intravenous dose but in children they can frequently occur after a single dose; they are not seen following intramuscular administration of the drug. These arrhythmias are most reliably prevented by intravenous atropine 0.01 mg kg^{-1} just prior to SCh administration.[9–11] These types of arrhythmias were more frequently noted when halothane was the mainstay of paediatric anaesthesia;[11] they seem to be less frequent with thiopentone or with the newer anaesthetic agents such as isoflurane or sevoflurane.[12,13]

In healthy children SCh does not cause any significant hyperkalaemia; only a slight potassium increase of 0.23 nmol l^{-1} has been reported.[14] In the presence of burns, tetanus and paraplegia, marked hyperkalaemia can occur; in children with cerebral palsy it does not.[15,16]

Although fasciculations occur frequently in adults following intravenous SCh, they rarely develop in children less than 4 years of age. Some gross muscle movements are occasionally present in children.[17] Children, in general, do not demonstrate the rise in intragastric pressures seen in their older counterparts.[18]

Masseter spasm has been frequently associated with the use of SCh, especially in the presence of halothane.[19] This increase in masseter muscle tone is usually a transient phenomenon lasting only for a few minutes and can be present in the absence of twitch response.[20] This increase in muscle tone is usually mild and can be overcome by manually opening the mouth. Very occasionally it will be so severe that extreme force will be required, interfering with tracheal intubation. Very rarely also, some of these patients will be found to have a rise in serum phosphokinase levels, and some will prove positive on biopsy for malignant hyperthermia.[21,22] Most of the patients with trismus, however, will have a normal intraoperative or postoperative course.[23] These observations have left paediatric anaesthetists in a quandary about how to proceed when a child develops trismus. Some have advocated treating the patient as susceptible to malignant hyperthermia and cancelling the procedure.[24] Others have advocated continuation of the course, changing the technique to avoid further triggering agents and carefully observing for early signs of malignant hyperthermia (such as increased CO_2 production or tachycardia) and being prepared for early confirmation of diagnosis by measuring arterial and venous blood gases and early treatment with dantrolene.[25]

Whereas adults are usually free of the risk of myoglobinuria following SCh administration, children may show a slight but significant increase in serum myoglobin concentrations.[26,27] This increase is even greater when halothane is being used but can be easily prevented by the prior administration of small doses of non-depolarizing relaxants, alfentanil, or relatively large doses of thiopentone.[28,29]

Malignant hyperthermia, when it occurs, is frequently associated with the use of SCh, together with halothane anaesthesia.

Intraocular pressure may rise after SCh whether the patient fasciculates or not. The rise in pressure begins about 1 min after administration of the drug, reaches its peak in about 3 min and subsides in 7 min.[30] In the clinical situation it is advisable to wait at least this long before tonometry in children. Although the use of SCh without untoward side-effects has been reported in several cases of open eye injury,[31] many anaesthetists feel it prudent to refrain from its use in situations of penetrating ocular wounds unless the eye is not salvageable. The mechanism of the rise in intraocular pressure is unclear. Initially, it was assumed to be due to tonic contracture of the extraocular muscles. It has been observed,

however, that it even occurs when the extraocular muscles are detached from the globe. It is assumed to be due to the cyclopegic action of SCh with deepening of the anterior chamber and increased outflow resistance of the acqueous humour.[32]

Clinical uses of succinylcholine

Because SCh has the fastest onset of the currently available neuromuscular blocking agents, it remains the most suitable, despite its side-effects, for rapid tracheal intubation. Although satisfactory intubating conditions can be achieved in most cases with 1 mg kg^{-1} in children, the inclination is to use at least twice the dose that causes 95% depression of twitch response (ED_{95}), i.e. at least 1.5 mg kg^{-1} to achieve a faster and more reliable onset. In infants, a higher dose of 3 mg kg^{-1} is advisable.[33,34] If the main inhalation anaesthetic is halothane, pretreatment with atropine 0.01 mg kg^{-1} i.v. is advisable to decrease the incidence of arrhythmias. The intramuscular dose in children is 4 mg kg^{-1}, whereas in infants it is 5 mg kg^{-1}.[35]

Because of the multiple side-effects of SCh, several paediatric hospitals have discontinued the routine use of SCh in children.[36] In the USA the Federal Drug Administration has issued a specific warning restricting the use of SCh in children.[37] They recommend that the use of SCh be limited to emergency intubation or instances where it is necessary to secure the airway, e.g. laryngospasm, difficult airway, full stomach, or for an intramuscular route when a suitable vein is inaccessible. The recommendation was prompted by several case reports of hyperkalemic cardiac arrests, with the high mortality rates (55%) that have occurred in children. Most of these children had undiagnosed Duchenne's muscular dystrophy or an occult myopathy.[38]

It is widely thought that rapid intubation can avoid aspiration, but there are as yet no data to confirm this statement, albeit logical. In cases where the child had a recent meal but there is no obvious distention or active regurgitation, a controlled induction with a non-depolarizing relaxant with a fast onset such as rocuronium would be as safe as SCh. Relatively large doses of non-depolarizing relaxants in the presence of an adequate level of anaesthesia and cricoid pressure will accomplish the same result. Since, in frightened children, adequate preoxygenation might be difficult to provide, it is very reasonable once the relaxant has been given and the patient is showing evidence of relaxation, such as slackening of abdominal muscles, to ventilate the patient with low inspiratory pressures in the presence of cricoid pressure until the relaxant takes full effect.

There will still be some emergency situations where a short relaxant might arguably be safer, such as when treating a combative patient with blood or excessive secretions in the pharynx, or a patient with marked abdominal distention, where it might be argued that SCh is safer because of its rapid onset.

MIVACURIUM

Mivacurium chloride is currently the only available non-depolarizing, short-acting relaxant. It is a bisquaternary benzylisoquinolinium diester structurally related to atracurium. Its two active isomers (*cis–trans* and *trans–trans*) are practically equipotent with half-lives of about 2 min. These active isomers are hydrolysed by plasma cholinesterase to inactive monoquaternary esters or alcohols.[39]

In the past, 0.2 mg kg^{-1} of doses of mivacurium were used for tracheal intubation. This dose provided complete suppression of the twitch response in about 2 min with the recovery to 25 and 95% occurring in 11 and 19 min, respectively.[40,41] When mivacurium became available for clinical use, clinicians noted that the standard recommended intubating 0.2 mg kg^{-1} dose did not provide adequate intubating conditions in all patients, especially after an intravenous induction. Therefore, the tendency has been to increase the dose of the drug to 0.3–0.4 mg kg^{-1}. Following propofol and fentanyl induction, the intubating conditions following 0.3 mg kg^{-1} were classified as good to excellent in all children.[42] By increasing the dose to 0.4 mg kg^{-1} the onset time (time to maximum depression) can be decreased to 1.5 min.[42] The onset times of mivacurium are thus usually twice as long as SCh, with the duration of blockade being twice as long. Equipotent doses of mivacurium last 30% shorter in children than

in adults, despite comparable plasma cholinesterase activity.[43,44]

Mivacurium, like other benzylisoquinolinium relaxants, has a tendency to release histamine upon rapid administration. In children this effect is less marked than in adults. It is usually limited to reddening along the tract of the vein or generalized flushing. Increasing the initial dose from 0.2 to 0.3 and 0.4 mg kg^{-1} will increase the incidence of flushing and the diminution in arterial blood pressure. These hypotensive episodes, however, are usually mild, self-limiting and counteracted by the stimulation of tracheal intubation.[40]

Mivacurium's main advantage is when given by continuous infusion, where the recovery of the twitch response is practically the same as after a single dose. Once the twitch response is detected, complete recovery occurs in 15 min.[45] In children the mivacurium infusion requirements are practically double those seen in adults. During halothane anaesthesia to maintain 95% neuromuscular blockade children require 10–12 μg kg^{-1} min^{-1} and in the absence of potent inhalational agents it is 13–16 μg kg^{-1} min^{-1}.[45,46] In infants this value is even higher.[47]

A word of caution should be noted in using mivacurium infusion (or any infusion) by the 'piggy-back' technique: there is always the possibility that the intravenous flow will stop and the mivacurium will back up into the main intravenous infusion; upon clearing the infusion the patient may receive a bolus dose of the drug and become reparalysed. This effect will be more dangerous if this event occurs outside the operating theatre where respiratory support might not always be available immediately.[48]

INTERMEDIATE-ACTING RELAXANTS

The availability of the non-depolarizing relaxants with intermediate duration has made a significant impact on the practice of paediatric anaesthesia. The major advantage of these agents lies in the fact that at clinical doses they cause only minimal changes in the pulse rate and blood pressure. Since they are also free from the side-effects of SCh and have a comparatively short duration of action (20–40 min), they can be used satisfactorily in many short procedures.

ATRACURIUM AND CISATRACURIUM

Atracurium and cisatracurium are imidazoline bisquaternary compounds that have the characteristic chemical feature of spontaneous hydrolysis at the alkaline pH of the blood and tissue fluids (Hofmann elimination). In blood and tissues the quaternary compound breaks down and the degradation products include laudanosine and methylacrylate.[49] Cisatracurium is one of the 10 isomers of atracurium, which has the least histamine-releasing effect. In the original formula atracurium constituted 15% of the mixture.[50]

For intubating purposes, two to three times the ED_{95} (0.3–0.6 mg kg^{-1}) of atracurium or two to four times the ED_{95} of the cisatracurium dose (0.1–0.2 mg kg^{-1}) are given to produce rapid and effective blockade in most children and adolescents. Such doses provide adequate conditions for intubation within 2 min. The period of absence of twitch response after such doses usually lasts for 15–30 min. Hence, in the clinical situation, the intubating dose provides complete neuromuscular relaxation from such an interval, followed by another 20 min of intermediate blockade (twitch response 5–25%) and complete recovery in 1 h.[49]

Children generally require more of these two relaxants than do adults to obtain the same degree of neuromuscular blockade. The difference, however, is relatively small and is masked in most analyses by the wide range of individual responses. The effect of potentiation by volatile anaesthetics is also apparent, but it is less marked than that observed with the long-acting neuromuscular blocking agents.[51]

Some investigators have observed that the atracurium requirement of infants seems to be less than that of older children.[52] This difference, however, is a small one, and has not appeared in other studies.[49] In infants the distribution volume of atracurium is larger than in children (176 vs 139 ml kg^{-1}) and the clearance is more rapid; this explains the shorter

duration of action detected in some studies of infants.[53]

When comparing the pharmacokinetics of atracurium in normal children and in those with impaired hepatic function, no significant differences in the volume of distribution, clearance or half-lives were detected. Laudanosine, one of the degradation products of atracurium, can cause convulsions in animals at high concentrations (17 mg ml^{-1}). In patients with impaired liver function the plasma laudanosine concentration tends to be higher than in normal patients; however, concentrations high enough to cause convulsions are never achieved in clinical situations.[54,55]

The side-effects of atracurium are minimal. At clinical doses up to 0.6 mg kg^{-1}, the compound does not cause significant haemodynamic changes. Mild cutaneous flushing can be detected, especially in older children or adolescents. Occasionally, it is associated with a rise in plasma histamine concentrations.[56] Very few cases of anaphylactoid reactions or bronchospasm have been reported with the use of atracurium,[57–59] and their incidence does not seem to be different from that found with other relaxants.

Cisatracurium is one of the potent isomers of atracurium; it is three times more potent than atracurium. Since it undergoes non-enzymic hydrolysis, doubling its dose prolongs its effect for about 25 min, indicating the non-cumulative nature of the drug.[50,60] In paediatric patients, the clearance of cisatracurium is faster than in adults. These faster effects are associated with a shorter duration than in adults.[61,62,62a] The higher potency of cisatracurium offers a major advantage of the drug. Since a lower amount of relaxant is administered and since histamine release is usually related to the molar concentration of the drug, no cutaneous flushing or change in plasma histamine concentration is seen at doses up to five times the ED95 in adults (0.25 mg kg^{-1}) and cardiovascular changes almost never occur.

The cardiovascular stability observed from cisatracurium has led to the virtual cessation of the use of atracurium when the former is available. Cisatracurium has the same desirable characteristics of atracurium, i.e. non-cumulative Hofmann elimination independent of hepatic or renal function. Both are suitable for use by infusion; a useful approximate guide to dosage is to administer the intubating dose over 1 h.[61]

VECURONIUM

Vecuronium, like pancuronium, is a steroidal muscle relaxant, being a monoquaternary homologue in which the methyl group of the 2-beta nitrogen is absent. It has virtually no cardiovascular effect. It is excreted mostly in bile and a small amount (10–25%) is excreted in urine.[63]

In comparing recovery times with atracurium, vecuronium is similar to other intermediate-acting relaxants following an intubating dose (0.08–0.1 mg kg^{-1}). Recovery of twitch height to 25% of control occurs in about 25 min in children and complete recovery in 40–60 min.[64]

The dose requirements of vecuronium vary according to age. There is a biphasic distribution pattern. The infant dose is about half that given to a child. Thereafter, the dose increases, reaching its peak at 3–4 years. Then, it decreases gradually until at adolescence the requirement is similar to an adult dose.[65] This biphasic distribution also applies to the duration of action of vecuronium.[66] These observations have led some investigators to conclude that vecuronium is a long-acting relaxant in infants.[67] The pharmacokinetic explanation is that the plasma level required for a given degree of paralysis is lower in infants than in children, but this effect is partially compensated for by the larger distribution volume in infants.[68] The decreased required plasma concentration with the increased distribution volume leads to a relatively slow diminution in plasma concentration, which is reflected in a prolonged mean residence time.[68]

In studies with vecuronium, clearance has been found to be faster in children than in adults, a factor which partly explains the drug's shorter duration of action in the younger patients.[69] Their requirement, however, tends to be the same as that of older children. Further, vecuronium's shorter duration of action relative to pancuronium can be explained by its higher rate of plasma clearance.

Vecuronium has been popular for some time in intensive care units to maintain patients in phase with respirators, its main advantage being the absence of cardiovascular effects and the virtual absence of metabolites with central nervous effects. In adults, however, several cases have been described of residual weakness following the discontinuation of the relaxant.[70] These patients characteristically had renal failure and a high plasma concentration of 3-desacetyl vecuronium.[71] Children seem to be an exception in this respect: in one study where the rate of vecuronium infusion was adjusted by accelerometry for about 2.5 days, all of them recovered in 1 h.[72]

ROCURONIUM

Rocuronium is a 3-hydroxy derivative of vecuronium but because of its low potency and higher dose requirements it has a faster onset. In general, the onset of action of rocuronium is twice as fast as that of vecuronium, whereas its duration of action is similar. In animals it is primarily eliminated by the liver and about 10% is excreted by the kidneys.[73]

In children a standard intubating dose of 0.6 mg kg^{-1} causes 90% and 100% suppression of the twitch response in 0.8 and 1.3 min, respectively. At this dose a slight increase in heart rate of about 15 beats min^{-1} can be detected. As with the other intermediate relaxants, the recovery to 25% of control occurs in about 30 min and to 90% in 45 min.[74] Potency is greater in infants than in children.[75] In infants aged 2–11 months the onset is faster: 90 and 100% depression of the twitch response after the same 0.6 mg kg^{-1} dose occurs in 37 and 64 s, whereas the recovery to 25% occurs after an interval 15 min longer than in children.[76]

Although rocuronium has a fast onset in adults and children, it is not as fast as SCh. In infants, however, the 60-s neuromuscular depression is similar to SCh.[76] In addition, the onset of action of rocuronium can be accelerated by increasing the dose up to 3–4 times the ED$_{95}$. For example, by increasing the dose to 1.2 mg kg^{-1} the 90% block occurs in 33 s, which is not very different from 2 mg kg^{-1} SCh (30 s).[77,78]

When the intubating conditions of elective cases were compared among 0.6 mg kg^{-1} rocuronium, 0.1 mg kg^{-1} vecuronium and 0.5 mg kg^{-1} atracurium, it was found that all of the children receiving rocuronium could be intubated within 60 s, whereas with vecuronium

Table 5.1 Doses that cause 95% depression of the twitch response (ED$_{95}$) in neonates, infants, children and adults

	Neonates (μg kg^{-1})	Infants (μg kg^{-1})	Children (μg kg^{-1})	Adults (μg kg^{-1})
Short-acting relaxants				
Succinylcholine	620	729	423	290
Mivacurium		65–94	82–110	58–120
Intermediate-acting relaxants				
Atracurium	120	156–175	170–350	110–280
Cisatracurium			41	50
Rocuronium		255	402	350
Vecuronium	47	42–47	56–80	27–56
Long-acting relaxants				
Doxacurium		25	27–32	14–19
Metocurine		180	108–340	280
Pancuronium		55–92	55–93	50–70
Pipecuronium	46	33–48	49–79	42–59
Tubocurarine	340	320	320–600	290–510

The data are derived from the various references in the text. The lower values are in the presence of potent inhalational anaesthetics. The higher values are those determined during the N$_2$O–O$_2$ narcotic technique.

this value was 120 s and with atracurium 180 s.[79] The 1-min intubating conditions can be improved further by increasing the dose to 0.9 mg kg^{-1}.[80] Increasing the dose will increase the tendency to tachycardia. In almost all cases, however, this tachycardia is mild (11–18%) and is not accompanied by changes in blood pressure.

As with vecuronium the clearance of rocuronium in infants (4 ml kg^{-1} min^{-1}) is slower than in children (7 ml kg^{-1} min^{-1}), with the volume of distribution being larger in infants. Consequently, the mean residence time is longer in infants than in children (56 vs 26 min). Again, children have faster clearance and lower distribution volumes than adults, giving a shorter mean residence time and shorter neuromuscular block.[81,82]

With liver disease the increased volume of distribution of rocuronium leads to increased elimination half-life.[83] In renal failure the clearance is also prolonged, which results in an increase of about 10 min in the duration of action of rocuronium.[84] Although the duration of action of rocuronium is prolonged in these conditions, the onset time remains rapid.[84]

Intramuscular rocuronium

It is desirable to have a non-depolarizing muscle relaxant which is clinically effective when given intramuscularly. Rocuronium was investigated in this respect and it was found that 1 mg kg^{-1} rocuronium in infants or 1.8 mg kg^{-1} in children by deltoid injection would give satisfactory relaxation.[85] Further studies, however, found that such doses were ineffective to provide adequate intubating conditions in 3.5–4 min because of the slow absorption, despite the biovailability of an intramuscular dose being about 80%. Following these intramuscular doses the maximum neuromuscular depression occurs in 6–8 min.[86,87]

THE USE OF INTERMEDIATE RELAXANTS IN CHILDREN

Relaxants with intermediate duration are very useful in children because of the large number of short surgical procedures (e.g. hernia repairs, orchidopexies and tonsillectomies) that are performed. Because of their short duration of action, these drugs can be given in one intubating dose (atracurium 0.4–0.6 mg kg^{-1}, cisatracurium 0.1–0.15 mg kg^{-1}, vecuronium

0.08–0.12 mg kg^{-1}, rocuronium 0.6 mg kg^{-1}), and a relatively light anaesthetic level maintained throughout the procedure. Reversal does not seem to be mandatory in all patients. In fact, if more than 45 min has elapsed since the final dose of any of these drugs, one may reasonably assume that neuromuscular function has nearly recovered. This can, of course, be adequately confirmed by observing four equal twitches during train-of-four stimulation. It is, none the less, essential that an evaluation of clinical recovery be made in all cases. Respiratory patterns should be observed and strong movement of all four limbs should be in evidence. Most important, especially in infants, is the return of facial movement and crying.

Because of their desirable properties, these relaxants have varied uses. They are particularly useful in children with irritable airways. Paediatricians are frequently confronted with children who have repeated airway infection. Ideally, one would like to operate when such children are completely free of residual infection, but this becomes a practical impossibility. With these relaxants one can maintain the patient at a relatively light level of anaesthesia, provide adequate surgical relaxation, reverse the effect of the relaxant, and have the child's reflexes fully recovered at the end of the surgical procedure. A similar situation pertains to children presenting for bronchoscopy or oesophagoscopy.

For all their advantages these agents do have some drawbacks, the main one being a delayed onset of action after an intubating dose. Complete paralysis does not occur until at least 2 min after administration (1 min with rocuronium), which is considerably longer than the 45-s span found with SCh. It should be realized, however, that complete peripheral neuromuscular relaxation is not an absolute prerequisite for ventilation or tracheal intubation. In an adequately anaesthetized patient who receives a non-depolarizing relaxant, ventilation can be assisted before the occurrence of complete peripheral paralysis, presumably because of early paralysis of the laryngeal and pharyngeal muscles. Furthermore, after relaxants have been given, these patients do not develop laryngospasm if difficulty is experienced during the intubation attempt. Although priming might seem logical in some situations it has

very limited use in paediatric practice. One example might serve to illustrate: in the child presenting with a 'full stomach', where rapid intubation is desirable, it is wishful thinking to suppose a co-operative subject. It is clearly unrealistic to administer a small dose of relaxant and then wait for 5 min while the child is experiencing some muscle weakness. Such a child is liable to be upset, to flail about and retch or vomit, creating a situation much worse than the one that the anaesthetist is trying to avoid.

Moreover, these relaxants are acidic compounds (pH values between 3 and 4) and as such can be easily deactivated in alkaline media. This fact is especially important for atracurium, since its mode of elimination is alkaline hydrolysis (Hofmann elimination). In a slowly running intravenous system in which thiopentone (pH 10–11) is injected with atracurium, precipitation and loss of the relaxant's potency might conceivably occur. Consequently, if these drugs are to be used in tandem the clinician should ensure that the thiopentone is washed through the intravenous tubing before the introduction of atracurium. A further point to be noted is the unsuitability of these agents for intramuscular administration, where SCh holds the advantage.

LONG-ACTING MUSCLE RELAXANTS

At least seven long-acting neuromuscular blocking agents have been used in children. Tubocurarine has been the mainstay for a long time but is no longer universally available. In the late 1970s pancuronium became more popular because of its vagolytic properties. Cardiac output in children, and especially in infants, is rate dependent, the young heart being less compliant than the adult; hence, the Frank Starling mechanism is less efficient. Consequently, mild tachycardia is a desirable condition in children, and even more so in infants. Because cardiac output can generally be well maintained with pancuronium, this has for many years been the drug of choice in children,

Table 5.2 Suggested intubating doses of relaxant in infants, children and adults

	Infants (mg kg^{-1})	Children (mg kg^{-1})	Adults (mg kg^{-1})
Short-acting relaxants			
Succinylcholine	3	1.5–2	1
Mivacurium	0.3	0.2–0.3	0.2
Intermediate-acting relaxants			
Atracurium	0.5	0.5–0.6	0.4–0.5
Cisatracurium	0.1	0.1–0.2	0.1–0.15
Rocuronium	0.5	0.6–1	0.6
Vecuronium	0.07–0.1	0.1	0.1
Long-acting relaxants			
Doxacurium		0.05	0.05
Metocurine		0.3	0.4
Pancuronium	0.08	0.1	0.1
Pipecuronium	0.07–0.1	0.1	0.08–0.1
Tubocurarine	0.2–0.5	0.3–0.6	0.6

especially for cardiac surgery. Metocurine, fazadinium and gallamine do not enjoy wide popularity nowadays. Doxacurium and pipecuronium have the advantage in not having any side-effects, but their cost has limited their use.

TUBOCURARINE

Tubocurarine can generally be used in children without the worry of marked cardiovascular side-effects. A large intubating dose, however, may cause histamine release, especially in adolescents. Such an occurrence manifests as a transient rash and mild hypotension, but clears spontaneously.[88]

Since neonates and small infants have twice the adult ratio of extracellular fluid to body weight, there exists in them a greater distribution volume for tubocurarine.[89,90] Furthermore, the elimination half-life is longer in neonates than in older children and adults, suggesting that in neonates the duration of action of multiple doses or of a large initial dose might be prolonged. One study, however, observed that the plasma concentration causing 50% depression of twitch response was markedly lower in neonates than in adults,[89] whereas another study found no significant differences in the effect of plasma concentration response lines among adults, children, infants and neonates.[90] No specific reason can be found for these divergent findings. The anaesthetic agent or

the condition of the patients might be a factor. Selection of the study population was also different: one used general surgical patients and the other neurosurgical patients who might have been fluid restricted. In reviewing these studies one should also realize that tubocurarine and metocurine bind less to plasma proteins in neonates. Hence, the free fraction of the muscle relaxant is higher in neonatal than in adult blood, as a result of the lower α_1 acid glycoprotein levels present there.[91] Consequently, these drugs will be more effective in neonates at a lower plasma concentration.

A feature common to most studies on infants is the wide individual variation; some infants are sensitive to relaxants and some are markedly resistant.[92] One can assume the lower requirement in some infants to be a sign of underdevelopment of the myoneural junction, but it is more difficult to explain the resistant individual. A correlation can perhaps be drawn from animal studies in which developing muscle cells are shown to have immature fetal and/or extrajunctional receptors which are resistant to tubocurarine.[93]

PANCURONIUM

Pancuronium is a bisquaternary ammonium steroidal compound. For most practical purposes it has been used at a dose of 0.1 mg kg^{-1} and it has been advocated for a variety of cardiac surgical procedures in infants. For example, infants presenting for ligation of patent ductus arteriosus tolerate the anaesthetic technique of fentanyl–air–oxygen pancuronium satisfactorily.[94] The vagolytic effects of pancuronium counteract the bradycardiac effects of fentanyl, and its relaxant properties counteract the muscle stiffness caused by fentanyl. Pancuronium has also been found to be useful for correction of cyanotic and acyanotic congenital cardiac anomalies. In the presence of pancuronium infants tolerate large doses of fentanyl (75 μg kg^{-1}) or sufentanil 10 μg kg^{-1}.[95]

In contrast to those for tubocurarine, the pharmacokinetic data for pancuronium do not differ between children and adults. Pancuronium is mostly excreted by the kidney and since renal function does not change after infancy, changes in pharmacokinetic data are not seen after the early stages of life.[96]

In neonatal intensive care units pancuronium can be employed to achieve an easier ventilation pattern, especially for premature infants who actively expire against the positive pressure of the ventilator, increasing the risk of pneumothorax.[97] Since pancuronium increases the heart rate, blood pressure, plasma adrenaline and noradrenaline levels,[98] there has been some concern that it might be a contributing factor in cerebral haemorrhage.[99] In patients at risk, it should be noted that nasotracheal intubation or intratracheal suctioning in the presence of pancuronium causes a smaller change in intracranial pressure than such activity in patients not receiving any relaxant.[100] Adequate sedation is required prior to the introduction of the relaxant. Thus, the best approach to neonatal intubation seems to be the administration of a relaxant with sedation in the intensive care unit or a general anaesthetic in the operating theatre. Vecuronium might offer an advantage over pancuronium in that it does not significantly increase the blood pressure, which is related to cerebral blood flow.

There are several methods for maintaining the respirator in phase with the paediatric patient, such as sedation and adjustment of the respirator. If these methods fail, neuromuscular relaxation for a short time might be appropriate. In considering the demands of neonatal intensive care, it is also interesting to note that prolonged blockade with pancuronium can be adequately reversed with the usual doses of atropine and neostigmine.[101]

PIPECURONIUM AND DOXACURIUM

These drugs are practically devoid of side-effects at doses up to three times the ED$_{95}$. They do not have any cardiovascular or histaminergic properties. The ED$_{95}$ of doxacurium is approximately 30 μg kg^{-1}, making it the most potent neuromuscular blocking agent available.[102,103] Although it is approximately twice as potent as vecuronium, its duration of action is similar to that of tubocurarine or metocurine. Doxacurium is a benzylisoquinolinium compound, structurally related to atracurium, whereas pipecuronium has a steroidal molecule related to pancuronium.[104] They are both metabolized. These drugs are the drugs of choice in situations where no changes in cardiovascular parameters are desirable. Metocurine, although having the potential for histamine release, does not cause appreciable changes in pulse rate or blood pressure at large intubating doses.[105]

For practical purposes all of the long-acting relaxants have a similar duration of action. An intubating dose gives complete paralysis (no twitch response) for 1 h and satisfactory surgical relaxation (twitch 5–25%) for another 30 min in children. Pancuronium appears in some studies to have a slightly shorter duration of action, although it may be masked at times by wide individual variations.

It is a common finding that the duration of action following equipotent doses of relaxants is slightly shorter in children than in adults. Although there are several variations in the results, children generally have a larger volume of distribution and faster clearance, which results in shorter mean residence times and faster recovery. Relaxants last longer in neonates and infants. Here again, the increased distribution volume is noted but clearance is diminished. Consequently, a longer duration than in children is the rule. It is extremely difficult to discern at what age this transition from an infantile pattern to a childhood pattern occurs, or indeed why. The mode of excretion or metabolism of the drug may be a factor, as may the degree of sickness of the patient or even differences in sample size between the various studies.

The choice of long-acting relaxant depends on the clinical circumstances and on the preference of the anaesthetist. One can, however, make good use of these agents by matching particular side-effects to the given situation. If a mild tachycardia is desirable, pancuronium is preferred; a good indication for its use is in the presence of halothane or fentanyl when the tachycardia will counteract the slowing of the heart rate and help to maintain the blood pressure. If a slow heart rate or mild hypotension is desirable, tubocurarine, where available, is a better choice; it can be especially useful if a narcotic N_2O–O_2 relaxant technique is to be used. If no particular change in heart rate or blood pressure is desired then doxacurium or pipecuronium is a good choice. These differences, however, are minor, and the side-effects of these drugs are minimal and they can be used interchangeably. Most of these side-effects can be averted by administering the drugs slowly or in incremental doses. Only very rarely do these side-effects have to be treated by pharmacological means.

REVERSAL OF LONG-ACTING RELAXANTS

With the intermediate-acting relaxants few children need to be reversed if monitored adequately. However, for long-acting relaxants almost all do, the main reason being the long recovery time – over 1 h in most children – from 5 to 95% of control twitch height.

Contrary to previous reports the neostigmine requirement (mg kg^{-1}) of infants and children is less than that of adults.[106] In clinical trials infants have been shown to require only about half as much neostigmine as do adults for reversal of tubocurarine-induced neuromuscular blockade. In contrast to tubocurarine, the distribution half-lives and distribution volumes of neostigmine were also similar for infants, children and adults. Based on these data, the recommended dose of neostigmine to reverse tubocurarine blockade in infants and children was set at 20 μg kg^{-1}. In the experimental settings from which these observations were drawn the twitch height before the attempted reversal was at least 10% of control and the return of the twitch was therefore prompt. This desirable situation is not always possible at the end of surgical procedures; therefore, higher doses of neostigmine (60 μg kg^{-1}) will sometimes be required. It always remains of great importance for the anaesthetist to assess the adequacy of reversal, both by clinical signs and by the neuromuscular monitor. The presence of four equal twitches during train-of-four stimulation is a very satisfactory and easily discernible end-point, although the post-tetanic twitch count is more sensitive.[107] Clinical signs of recovery include adequate airway, satisfactory respiratory excursions, facial expressions, leg-lifting and, most important in an infant, crying.[108,109]

In contrast to neostigmine, the dose of edrophonium required to antagonize tubocurarine-induced neuromuscular blockade in infants and children is similar to or possibly greater than in adults. Under controlled circumstances optimal antagonism has been obtained by administering 1 mg kg^{-1} edrophonium.[110,111] The onset and duration of antagonism were observed to be similar in the three age groups, while clearance was highest in infants and lowest in adults. Theoretically, this rapid clearance may allow the possibility of recurarization. As with neostigmine, to prevent the vagomimetic effects of edrophonium it is preferable to give atropine 10–20 μg kg^{-1} before its administration. If atropine is given 30 s before, heart rate and systolic blood pressure remain constant.

Whether edrophonium offers a specific advantage over neostigmine is a matter of opinion. Edrophonium has a more rapid onset of action, but whether the difference of a few minutes justifies the higher cost of edrophonium and risk of recurarization is questionable. The two agents produce dissimilar patterns of recovery of the train-of-four. The train-of-four ratios (T4/T1) at the same twitch height tensions (T1) are greater with edrophonium than with neostigmine, indicating a greater prejunctional effect of edrophonium.[111]

In dealing with reversal of the muscle relaxant effects in infants there are some important physiological considerations that should be taken into account. An important consideration is that the oxygen consumption (per kg body weight) is higher in infants and children than in adults. Consequently, a slight decrease in respiratory mechanics may lead to earlier hypoxaemia and CO_2 retention, which in turn lead to acidosis, with potentiation of the action of relaxant. In this respect, the neonate is the most vulnerable, for the following reasons.

1 Immaturity of the neuromuscular system, which is evidenced by lower train-of-four values, tetanus twitch ratios and prominent fade during tetanic stimulation.[93]
2 Longer elimination half-lives or mean residence times of relaxants.[68,69]
3 The presence of a greater number of fast muscles in the respiratory muscles. These fast muscles are liable to be fatigued earlier than the slow muscles.[112]
4 The closing volume of the neonate which is within the tidal volume; therefore airway closure occurs at the end of every normal expiration.[113] If the respiration is mildly impaired as a result of residual neuromuscular weakness, more alveoli will collapse, resulting in hypoxia and acidosis, which might potentiate and prolong the action of muscle relaxant, creating a vicious circle.

A factor in favour of the anaesthetist in this respect is the observation that higher doses of relaxants are required to block the central muscles of the body, such as the diaphragm, than the peripheral muscles of the hand.[114] Consequently, if the strength of the hand muscles is adequately recovered with a train-of-four near normal, it can reasonably be assumed that the central muscles, including the diaphragm, are fully recovered.

One of the issues frequently debated is whether the neuromuscular effects of all non-depolarizing relaxants should be reversed in all situations even if the patient looks fully recovered both clinically and by monitoring. Reversal was mandatory about 20 years ago when all available relaxants were long acting and the techniques of evaluation were in their infancy. With the advent of reliable monitors and their use in conjunction with clinical observations and measurements of respiratory adequacy, one can confidently judge the degree of reversal and the condition of the child. It can be claimed that even in the presence of adequate signs of reversal 75% of the receptors are still occupied by the relaxant, but the system still functions satisfactorily with the receptors partially occupied. This partial occupation is time

dependent, so it can be theorized that it is of much shorter duration with short- and intermediate-acting relaxants. Children have the additional advantage of recovering more quickly than adults from residual neuromuscular block.[115]

Recent studies in adult volunteers have shown differences in respiratory mechanics or fine motor co-ordination between train-of-four of 75% and 95%, but whether these differences are important in the recovery period of the average patient is a matter of debate.[116,117] Since the mid-1980s, clinicians have used a train-of-four of 75% as a satisfactory end-point for recovery from relaxation and no major clinical issues have arisen in following this principle. In the absence of aggravating factors such as hypothermia, acidosis or hypoxia, if a minor residual relaxation is present the patient will recover spontaneously without any side-effects. Although not all patients are monitored in the recovery period with neuromuscular monitors, as long as oxygenation is adequate, as demonstrated clinically and by pulse oximetry, one can be confident that the patient will recover from any minor residual neuromuscular effect.

RELAXANTS IN CERTAIN CLINICAL SITUATIONS

In the presence of certain diseases, many of which are described in Chapter 1, the response of the patient to a given relaxant may be different from that expected, whereas in some other states an otherwise minor or insignificant side-effect could be catastrophic. The following are some pathological situations in which deviations from the norm are likely to occur.

PROGRESSIVE MUSCULAR DYSTROPHY

The Duchenne form is the most common and severe type of the childhood muscular dystrophies, caused by an X-linked recessive gene.[118] The gene has been isolated and is located in the short arm of the X chromosome.[119] In these patients, the intracellular protein dystrophin is

Table 5.3 Approximate recovery characteristics from the various groups of muscle relaxants

	Clinical duration intubating dose → 25% recovery	Recovery 5–95%	Recovery index 25–75%
Succinylcholine			
Children	6	8	3
Adults	8	8	4
Mivacurium			
Children	10	12	6
Adults	15	14	8
Intermediate-acting relaxants			
Children	25	30	10
Adults	30	30	12
Long-acting relaxants			
Children	40	50	25
Adults	60	60	35

practically absent.[120] The absence of this protein weakens the attachment of intracellular calcium to the extracellular basal lamina and hence the stability of the myofibrillar membrane during contraction.[119] In the milder forms, such as facioscapulohumeral, limb-girdle and Becker dystrophy, lower than normal levels of dystrophyns or abnormal dystrophyns are present.

Duchenne's dystrophy usually becomes apparent at 2–6 years of age, with the onset of clumsy, waddling gait and frequent falling. It affects first the proximal muscles of the pelvis and the shoulder; these muscles enlarge from fatty infiltration and become extremely weak (pseudohypertrophy). Eventually, the weakness progresses to all the muscles of the body; the young victim loses the ability to walk and develops contractures. These patients also have myocardial involvement that can manifest during anaesthesia as tachycardia, ventricular fibrillation or cardiac arrest.[121]

In these patients SCh causes rhabdomyolysis, as evidenced by myoglobinurea, increased creatine phosphokinase, hyperkalaemia and, occasionally, metabolic acidosis. During anaesthesia a moderate rise in body temperature has been seen and biopsied muscles have shown increased sensitivity to halothane and caffeine, suggesting some association between muscular dystrophy and malignant hyperthermia.[122] These two diseases, however, have completely different courses and outcomes.

Because of their prominent cardiac and muscular effects, depolarizing muscle relaxants such as SCh should be avoided in these patients, especially in combination with halothane. Non-depolarizing agents can, however, be safely used. In general, these patients are slightly more sensitive to non-depolarizers than normal patients and the duration of action is usually moderately prolonged.[123–126] They have weakness of the respiratory muscles that may lead to respiratory failure and, consequently, adequacy of reversal should be thoroughly evaluated before any attempt at extubation; if there is any doubt the patient should be ventilated postoperatively.

MYOTONIA

Myotonic dystrophy (dystrophia myotonica) is an autosomal dominant disease that results from abnormal regulation of sodium channels, causing facial weakness (expressionless face), wasting of the sternomastoids, ptosis, dysarthria and a progressive distal muscle weakness with wasting.[127,128] A characteristic feature of its victims is an inability to relax the hand muscles after stimulation, hence the name myotonia.

SCh may exacerbate myotonia, causing respiratory and jaw muscle rigidity, leading to hypoxia and the inability to relax jaw muscles. Occasionally, increased myotonia has been seen following neostigmine, presumably from the stimulating effect of acetylcholine. These patients are also known to be extremely sensitive to thiopentone and opioids. Consequently, the dose of these drugs should be carefully titrated.

Safe practice demands the avoidance of SCh and the use of one of the non-depolarizing agents instead. Of those currently available, atracurium and, recently, cisatracurium, seem to be the most favoured because of their predictably rapid recovery rate obviating the need for reversal agents in most clinical situations.[129,130]

Myotonia is generally a disease of adulthood, although some variants occur in infants and children. Myotonia congenita (Thomsen's disease) is characterized by general myotonia and hypertrophy of voluntary muscles. Congenital dystrophica myotonica is manifested in the neonatal period and appears as generalized hypotonia and facial diplegia. Affected infants may have difficulty in swallowing and breathing and are mentally underdeveloped. They improve in the first decade of life, but later develop the adult form. Another subvariant of this disease is paramyotonia, where the symptoms appear after exposure to cold.

MYASTHENIA GRAVIS

Myasthenia usually affects women in their 20s. In about 15% of newborns born to myasthenic mothers the passage of antibodies across the placenta leads to neonatal myasthenia.[131,132] The symptoms of myasthenia appears in the newborn within 3 days of birth, usually persist for a few days and may last for up to 8 weeks. Other rare forms are the congenital and juvenile types, and 10% of all cases are in children under 16 years of age. The disease has an autoimmune background with a reduction in the number of acetylcholine receptor sites at the neuromuscular junction. Thymectomy is a common form of treatment for the young as an adjunct to oral anticholinesterase therapy (pyridostigmine).

There is no agreement about the best anaesthetic regimen to follow. It varies according to the status of the patient, the drug regimen and the patient's response. More important is the extent of surgery. Respiratory failure with secretion retention may follow surgery and provision should be made for respiratory

support postoperatively if necessary. Small doses of opioid analgesics should be used if assisted ventilation is not planned. Intubation can be achieved by volatile anaesthetics, although competitive neuromuscular blocking drugs can be used if treated with great caution. A dose of 5% of normal is used. Initially, the block should be closely monitored with a peripheral nerve stimulator and the subsequent dose adjusted accordingly. At the end of the operation the action of the drug is reversed with the usual dose of atropine and neostigmine. These patients may require respiratory support postoperatively, even after simple surgery where no muscle relaxants have been used, because of the changing requirements of anticholinesterases.

Again, there is no specific treatment for congenital myasthenia; the treatment is tailored to the patient. The critical period to watch in these infants is during feeding. If necessary, these infants can be tested by relatively large but frequently used reversal agents, such as glycopyrrolate 10 μg kg^{-1} and neostigmine 50 μg kg^{-1}. If the child's condition improves, pyridostigmine 5 mg kg^{-1} can be given orally before each feeding. If the patient becomes resistant to pyridostigmine, tracheal intubation and ventilation can be carried out and the dose of pyridostigmine titrated.

MALIGNANT HYPERTHERMIA

The combination of SCh and halothane seems to be the one most likely to trigger malignant hyperthermia.[133,134] Depolarizing relaxants and halogenated agents should, therefore, be avoided in patients thought to be at risk of this syndrome.[135] The safest general anaesthetic technique is the use of a narcotic–nitrous oxide oxygen combination with a non-depolarizing relaxant. Non-depolarizing agents devoid of side-effects may offer an advantage in not masking tachycardia, which is one of the first signs of malignant hyperthermia (see Chapter 20).[136]

BURNS

Since the early reports of cardiac arrest in burned patients receiving SCh, extensive investigations have sought to define and understand the effects of relaxants in these unfortunate patients.[15,137,138] In such patients, SCh is known to cause hyperkalaemia, which predisposes to cardiac arrest. It seems to be the case that the more extensive the burn the more likely the hyperkalaemic response. Although most cases of cardiac arrest have occurred 20–50 days after the burn injury, abnormal elevations of plasma potassium levels can occur within a few days of the burn. The hyperkalaemia probably results from the development of new acetylcholine receptors along the surface of the muscle membrane in the postburn phase.[138] Such receptors are thought to be supersensitive to the usual doses of agonists such as acetylcholine or SCh, so instead of the discrete potassium movement at the end-plate, there is a more general leakage along the entire muscle membrane.

In burned patients the pharmacodynamic effects of non-depolarizing muscle relaxants are markedly altered. These patients may require two to three times the usual intravenous dose (except with mivacurium), with the resultant increased plasma concentration to produce the desired clinical effect. This resistance peaks about 2 weeks after the burn, persists for many months in patients with major burns and decreases gradually with healing. It seems to correlate with both the magnitude of the burn and the period of healing. The resistance can be partially explained by the increased drug binding as a result of increased plasma α_1 acid glycoprotein levels normally found in the presence of a burn.

Although no cases of cardiac arrest have been reported in the first few days following a burn, the use of SCh at that time should be avoided because of the ever-present possibility of hyperkalaemia. Patients can usually tolerate a non-depolarizing relaxant, although in most cases they will require up to three times the usual dose. The relaxant effect can, however, be reversed by the usual dose of anticholinesterase.

REFERENCES

1 Davis, L., Britten, J.J. and Morgan, M. Cholinesterase. Its significance in anaesthetic practice. *Anaesthesia* 1997; **52**: 244–60.

2 Stead, A.L. The response of the newborn infant to muscle relaxants. *British Journal of Anaesthesia* 1955; **27**: 124–30.

3 Cook, D.R. and Fischer, C.G. Neuromuscular blocking effects of succinylcholine in infants and children. *Anesthesiology* 1975; **42**: 662–5.

4 DeCook, T.H. and Goudsouzian, N.G. Tachyphylaxis and phase II block development during infusion of succinylcholine in children. *Anesthesia and Analgesia* 1980; **59**: 639–43.

5 Bevan, J.C., Donati, F. and Bevan, D.R. Prolonged infusion of suxamethonium in infants and children. *British Journal of Anaesthesia* 1986; **58**: 839–43.

6 Goudsouzian, N.G. and Liu, L.M.P. The neuromuscular response of infants to a continuous infusion of succinylcholine. *Anesthesiology* 1984; **60**: 97–101.

7 Vassallo, S.A., Denman, W. and Goudsouzian, N.G. Plasma cholinesterase activity and dibucaine number in infants and children. *Paediatric Anaesthesia* 1994; **4**: 313–17.

8 Whittaker, M. Plasma cholinesterase variants and the anaesthetist. *Anaesthesia* 1980; **35**: 174–9.

9 Goudsouzian, N.G. Turbe del ritmo cardiaco durante intubazione tracheal nei bambini. *Acta Anaesthesiologica Italica* 1981; **32**: 293–9.

10 Hannallah, R.S., Oh, T.H., McGill, W.A. and Epstein, B.S. Changes in heart rate and rhythm after intramuscular succinylcholine with or without atropine in anesthetized children. *Anesthesia and Analgesia* 1986; **65**: 1329–32.

11 Shorten, G.D., Bissonnette, B., Hartley, E., Nelson, W. and Carr, A.S. It is not necessary to administer more than 10 μg.kg^{-1} of atropine to older children before succinylcholine. *Canadian Journal of Anaesthesia* 1995; **42**: 8–11.

12 McAufliffe, G., Bissonnette, B. and Boutin, C. Should the routine use of atropine before succinylcholine in children be reconsidered? *Canadian Journal of Anaesthesia* 1995; **42**: 724–9.

13 Rieger, A., Hass, I., Striebel, H.W., Brummer, G. and Eyrich, K. Marked increases in heart rate associated with sevoflurane but not with halothane following suxamethonium administration in children. *European Journal of Anaesthesia* 1996; **13**: 616–21.

14 Kenally, J.P. and Bush, G.H. Changes in serum potassium after suxamethonium in children. *Anaesthesia and Intensive Care* 1974; **2**: 147–50.

15 Martyn, J.A.J., White, D.A., Gronert, G.A., *et al.* Up- and down-regulation of skeletal muscle acetylcholine receptors. Effects of neuromuscular blockers. *Anesthesiology* 1992; **76**: 822–43.

16 Dierdorf, F., McNiece, W.L., Rao, C.C., *et al.* Effect of succinylcholine on plasma potassium in children with cerebral palsy. *Anesthesiology* 1985; **62**: 88–90.

17 Cozanitis, D.A., Erkola, O., Klemola, U.M. and Mukela, V. Precurarisation in infants and children less than three years of age. *Canadian Journal of Anaesthesia* 1987; **34**: 17–20.

18 Salem, M.R., Wong, A.Y. and Lin, Y.H. The effect of suxamethonium on the intragastric pressure in infants and children. *British Journal of Anaesthesia* 1972; **44**: 166–9.

19 Schwartz, L., Rockoff, M.A. and Koka, B.V. Masseter spasm with anesthesia: incidence and implications. *Anesthesiology* 1984; **61**: 772–5.

20 Van Der Spek, A.F.L., Fang, W.B., AshtonMiller, J.A., *et al.* Increased masticatory muscle stiffness during limb muscle flaccidity associated with succinylcholine administration. *Anesthesiology* 1988; **69**: 11–16.

21 Ellis, F.R. and Halsall, P.J. Suxamethonium spasm: a differential diagnostic conundrum. *British Journal of Anaesthesia* 1984; **56**: 381–3.

22 O'Flynn, R.P., Shutack, J.G., Rosenberg, H. and Fletcher, J.E. Masseter muscle rigidity and malignant hyperthermia susceptibility in pediatric patients. *Anesthesiology* 1994; **80**: 1228–33.

23 Saddler, J.M., Bevan, J.C. and Plumley, M.H. *et al.* Jaw muscle tension after succinylcholine in children undergoing strabismus surgery. *Canadian Journal of Anaesthesia* 1990; **37**: 21–5.

24 Rosenberg, H. Editorial: Trismus is not trivial. *Anesthesiology* 1987; **67**: 453–5.

25 Berry, F.A. and Lynch, C. Succinylcholine and trismus. *Anesthesiology* 1989; **70**: 161–2.

26 Ryan, J.F., Kagen, L.J. and Hyman, A.I. Myoglobinemia after a single dose of succinylcholine. *New England Journal of Medicine* 1971; **285**: 824–7.

27 Lawrence, A.S. Serum myoglobin release following suxamethonium administration to children. *European Journal of Anaesthesia* 1988; **5**: 31–8.

28 Asari, H., Inoue, K., Maruta, H. and Hirose, Y. The inhibitory effect of intravenous *d*-tubocurarine and oral dantrolene on halothane-succinylcholine-induced myoglobinemia in children. *Anesthesiology* 1984; **61**: 332–3.

29 Noguchi, I., Suzuki, G. and Amemiya, Y. Effects of different doses of thiopentone on the increase in serum myoglobin induced by suxamethonium in children. *British Journal of Anaesthesia* 1993; **71**: 291–3.

30 Craythorne, N.W.B., Rottenstein, H.S. and Dripps, R.D. The effect of succinylcholine on intraocular pressure in adults, infants and children during general anesthesia. *Anesthesiology* 1960; **21**: 59–63.

31 Libonati, M.M., Leahy, J.J. and Ellison, N. The use of succinylcholine in open eye surgery. *Anesthesiology* 1985; **62**: 637–40.

32 Kelly, R.E., Dinner, M., Turner, L.S., Haik, B., Abramson, D.H. and Daines, P. Succinylcholine increases intraocular pressure in the human eye with extraocular muscles detached. *Anesthesiology* 1993; **79**: 948–52.

33 Meakin, G., McKiernan, E.P., Morris, P., *et al.* Dose–response curves for suxamethonium in neonates, infants and children. *British Journal of Anaesthesia* 1989; **62**: 655–8.

34 Meakin, G., Walker, R.W.M. and Dearlove, O.R. Myotonic and neuromuscular blocking effects of increased doses of suxamethonium in infants and chidlren. *British Journal of Anaesthesia* 1990; **65**: 816–18.

35 Liu, L.M.P., DeCook, T.H., Goudsouzian, N.G., *et al.* Dose response to intramuscular succinylcholine in children. *Anesthesiology* 1981; **55**: 599–602.

36 O'Flynn, R.P., Shutack, J.G. and Rosenberg, H. Limitation of succinylcholine use: a fact of life. *Anesthesiology* 1995; **83**: A1087.

37 Goudsouzian, N.G. Recent changes in the package insert for succinylcholine chloride: should this drug be contraindicated for routine use in children and adolescents? (Summary of the discussions of the Anesthetic and Life Support Drug Advisory Meeting of the Food and Drug Administration, FDA Building, Rockville, MD, June 9, 1994). *Anesthesia and Analgesia* 1995; **80**: 207–8.

38 Larach, M.G., Rosenberg, H., Gronert, G.A. and Allen, G.C. Hyperkalemic cardiac arrest during anesthesia in infants and children with occult myopathies. *Clinical Pediatrics* 1997; **36**: 9–16.

39 Goudsouzian, N.G. Mivacurium in infants and children. *Paediatric Anaesthesia* 1997; **7**: 183–90.

40 Goudsouzian, N.G, Alifimoff, J.K., Eberly, C., *et al.* Neuromuscular and cardiovascular effects of mivacurium in children. *Anesthesiology* 1989; **70**: 237–42.

41 Woelfel, S.K., Brandom, B.W., McCowan, F.X. and Cook, D.R. Clinical pharmacology of mivacurium in pediatric patients less than two years old during nitrous oxide–halothane. *Anesthesia and Analgesia* 1993; **77**: 713–20.

42 Shorten, G., Crawford, M., St. Louis, P., *et al.* The neuromuscular effects of mivacurium chloride during propofol anesthesia in children. *Anesthesia and Analgesia* 1996; **82**: 1170–5.

43 Cook, D.R., Gronert, B.J. and Woelfel, S.K. Comparison of the neuromuscular effects of mivacurium and suxamethonium in infants and children. *Acta Anaesthesiologica Scandinavica* 1995; **106**: 35–40.

44 Mangat, P.S., Evans, D.E.N., Harmer, M. and Lunn, J.N. A comparison between mivacurium and suxamethonium in children. *Anaesthesia* 1993; **48**: 866–9.

45 Alifimoff, J.K. and Goudsouzian, N.G. Continuous infusion of mivacurium in children. *British Journal of Anaesthesia* 1989; **63**: 520–4.

46 Meretoja, O.A. and Olkhola, K.T. Pharmacodynamics of mivacurium in children using a computer-controlled infusion. *British Journal of Anaesthesia* 1993; **71**: 232–7.

47 Goudsouzian, N.G., Denman, W., Schwartz, A., Shorten, G., Foster, V. and Samara, B. Pharmacodynamic and hemodynamic effects of mivacurium in infants anesthetized with halothane and nitrous oxide. *Anesthesiology* 1993; **79**: 919–25.

48 Litman, R.S., Younan, M.M., Patt, R.B. and Ward, D.S. Postoperative recurrent paralysis in an infant after mivacurium infusion. *Canadian Journal of Anaesthesia* 1994; **4**: 758–9.

49 Goudsouzian, N.G. Atracurium in infants and children. *British Journal of Anaesthesia* 1986; **58**: 23–8S.

50 Lien, C.A., Belmont, M.R., Abalos, A., *et al.* The cardiovascular effects and histamine-releasing properties of 51W89 in patients receiving nitrous oxide opioid/barbiturate anesthesia. *Anesthesiology* 1995; **82**: 1131–8.

51 Brandom, B.W., Cook, D.R., Woelfel, S.K., *et al.* Atracurium infusion requirements in children during halothane, isoflurane, and narcotic anesthesia. *Anesthesia and Analgesia* 1985; **64**: 471–6.

52 Meakin, G., Shaw, E.A., Baker, R.D. and Morris, P. Comparison of atracurium-induced neuromuscular blockade in neonates, infants and children. *British Journal of Anaesthesia* 1988; **60**: 171–5.

53 Brandom, B.W., Stiller, R.L., Cook, D.R., *et al.* Pharmacokinetics of atracurium in anaesthetized infants and children. *British Journal of Anaesthesia* 1986; **58**: 1210–13.

54 Parker, C.J.R. and Hunter, J.M. Pharmacokinetics of atracurium and laudanosine in patients with hepatic cirrhosis. *British Journal of Anaesthesia* 1989; **62**: 177–83.

55 Lawhead, R.G., Matsumi, M., Peters, K.R., Landers, D.F., Becker, G.L. and Earl, R.A. Plasma laudanosine levels in patients given atracurium during liver transplantation. *Anesthesia and Analgesia* 1993; **76**: 569–73.

56 Goudsouzian, N.G., Young, E.T., Moss, J., *et al.* Histamine release during the administration of atracurium or vecuronium in children. *British Journal of Anaesthesia* 1986; **58**: 1229–33.

57 Pollock, E.M.M., MacLeod, A.D. and McNicol, L.R. Anaphylactoid reaction complicating neonatal anaesthesia. *Anaesthesia* 1986; **41**: 178–80.

58 Woods, I., Morris, P. and Meakin, G. Severe bronchospasm following the use of atracurium in children. *Anaesthesia* 1985; **40**: 207–8.

59 Cohen, A.Y. and Frank, G. Periorbital edema after atracurium administration. *Anesthesiology* 1987; **66**: 431–2.

60 Eastwood, N.B., Boyd, A.H., Parker, C.J.R. and Hunter, J.M. Pharmacokinetics of 1*R*-cis 1′*R*-cis atracurium besylate (51W89) and plasma laudanosine concentrations in health and chronic renal failure. *British Journal of Anaesthesia* 1995; **75**: 431–5.

61 Meretoja, O.A., Taivainen, T. and Wirtavuori, K. Pharmacodynamic effects of 51W89, an isomer of atracurium, in children during halothane anaesthesia. *British Journal of Anaesthesia* 1995; **74**: 6–11.

62 Brandom, B.W., Woelfel, S.K., Gronert, B.J., Cook, D.R., Ference, A. and Dayal, B. Effects of 51W89 (cisatracurium) in children during halothane nitrous oxide anesthesia. *Anesthesiology* 1995; **83**: A921.

62a Brandom, B.W. and Westman, H.R. Effects of 0.86 mg kg^{-1} cisatracurium in an infant. *Anesthesiology* 1996; **85**: 688–9.

63 Bencini, A.F., Scaf, A.H.J., John, Y.J., *et al.* Hepatobiliary disposition of vecuronium bromide in man. *British Journal of Anaesthesia* 1986; **58**: 988–95.

64 Goudsouzian, N.G., Martyn, J.J.A., Liu, L.M.P. and Gionfriddo, M. Safety and efficacy of vecuronium in adolescents and children. *Anesthesia and Analgesia* 1983; **62**: 1083–8.

65 Meretoja, O.A., Wirtavuori, K. and Neuvonen, P.J. Age dependence of the dose–response curve of vecuronium in pediatric patients during balanced anesthesia. *Anesthesia and Analgesia* 1988; **67**: 21–6.

66 Meretoja, O.A. Vecuronium infusion requirements in pediatric patients during fentanyl N_2O–O_2 anesthesia. *Anesthesia and Analgesia* 1989; **68**: 20–4.

67 Meretoja, O.A. Is vecuronium a long-acting neuromuscular blocking agent in neonates and infants? *British Journal of Anaesthesia* 1989; **62**: 184–7.

68 Fisher, D.M., Castagnoli, K. and Miller, R.D. Vecuronium kinetics and dynamics in anesthetized infants and children. *Clinical Pharmacology and Therapeutics* 1985; **37**: 402–6.

69 Steinbereithner, K., Fitzal, S., Schwarz, S., Gilly, H., Semsroth, M. and Weindimayr-Goettel. Pharmacocinetique et pharmacodynamique du vecuronium chez l'enfant. *Cahiers d'Anesthesiologie* 1984; **32**: 5.

70 Segredo, V., Caldwell, J.E., Matthay, M.A., Sharma, M.L., Gruenke, L.D. and Miller, R.D. Persistent paralysis in critically ill patients after long-term administration of vecuronium. *New England Journal of Medicine* 1992; **327**: 524–8.

71 Kupfer, Y., Namba, T., Kaldawi, E. and Tessler, S. Prolonged weakness after long-term infusion of vecuronium bromide. *Annals of Internal Medicine* 1992; **117**: 484–6.

72 Hodges, U.M. Vecuronium infusion requirements in paediatric patients in intensive care units: the use of acceleromyography. *British Journal of Anaesthesia* 1996; **76**: 23–8.

73 Khuenl-Brady, K., Castagnoli, K.P., Canfell, P.C., *et al.* The neuromuscular blocking effects of pharmacokinetics of ORG 9426 and ORG 9616 in the cat. *Anesthesiology* 1990; **72**: 669–74.

74 Woelfel, S.K., Brandom, B.W., Cook, D.R. and Sarner, J.B. Effects of bolus administration of ORG-9426 in children during nitrous oxide–halothane anesthesia. *Anesthesiology* 1992; **76**: 939–42.

75 Taivainen, T., Meretoja, O.A., Erkola, O., Rautoma, P. and Juvakoski, M. Rocuronium in infants, children and adults during balanced anaesthesia. *Paediatric Anaesthesia* 1996; **6**: 271–5.

76 Woelfel, S.K., Brandom, B.W., McGowan, F.X., Gronert, B.J. and Cook, D.R. Neuromuscular effects of 600 mg.kg^{-1} of rocuronium in infants during nitrous oxide–halothane anaesthesia. *Paediatric Anaesthesia* 1994; **4**: 173–7.

77 Woolf, R.L., Crawford, M.W. and Choo, S.M. Dose–response of rocuronium bromide in children anesthetized with propofol. *Anesthesiology* 1997; **87**: 1368–72.

78 Vuksanaj, D., Skjonsby, B. and Dunbar, B.S. Neuromuscular effects of rocuronium in children during halothane anaesthesia. *Paediatric Anaesthesia* 1996; **6**: 277–81.

79 Scheiber, G., Ribeiro, F.C., Marichal, A., Bredendiek, M. and Renzing, K. Intubating conditions and onset of action after rocuronium, vecuronium, and atracurium in young children. *Anesthesia and Analgesia* 1996; **83**: 320–4.

80 Fuchs-Buder, T. and Tassonyi, E. Intubating conditions and time course of rocuronium-induced neuromuscular block in children. *British Journal of Anaesthesia* 1996; **77**: 335–8.

81 Wierda, J.M.K.H., Meretoja, O.A., Taivainen, T. and Proost, J.H. Pharmacokinetics and pharmacokineticdynamic modelling of rocuronium in infants and children. *British Journal of Anaesthesia* 1997; **78**: 690–5.

82 Vuksanaj, D. and Fisher, D.M. Pharmacokinetics of rocuronium in children aged 4–11 years. *Anesthesiology* 1995; **82**: 1104–10.

83 Magorian, T., Wood, P., Caldwell, J., *et al.* The pharmacokinetics and neuromuscular effects of rocuronium bromide in patients with liver disease. *Anesthesia and Analgesia* 1995; **80**: 754–9.

84 Szenohradszky, J., Fisher, D.M., Segredo, V., *et al.* Pharmacokinetics of rocuronium bromide (ORG 9426) in patients with normal renal function or patients undergoing cadaver renal transplantation. *Anesthesiology* 1992; **77**: 899–904.

85 Reynolds, L.M., Lau, M., Brown, R., Luks, A. and Fisher, D.M. Intramuscular rocuronium in infants and children. *Anesthesiology* 1996; **85**: 231–9.

86 Kaplan, R.F., Lobel, G., Goudsouzian, N., *et al.* A multicenter study to confirm the efficacy and safety of IM

rocuronium in pediatric patients. *Anesthesiology* 1997; **87**: A1046.

87 Reynolds, L.M., Lau, M., Brown, R., Luks, A., Sharma, M. and Fisher, D.M. Bioavailability of intramuscular rocuronium in infants and children. *Anesthesiology* 1997; **87**: 1096–105.

88 Nightingale, D.A. and Bush, C.H. A clinical comparison between tubocurarine and pancuronium in children. *British Journal of Anaesthesia* 1973; **45**: 63–7.

89 Fisher, D.M., O'Keeffe, C. and Stanski, D.R., *et al.* Pharmacokinetics and pharmacodynamics of *d*-tubocurarine in infants, children and adults. *Anesthesiology* 1982; **57**: 203–8.

90 Matteo, R.S., Lieberman, I.G., Salanitre, E. *et al.* Distribution, elimination, and action of *d*-tubocurarine in neonates, infants, children, and adults. *Anesthesia and Analgesia* 1984; **63**: 799–804.

91 Wood, M.. and Wood, A.J.J. Changes in plasma drug binding and a-acid glycoprotein in mother and newborn infant. *Clinical Pharmacology and Therapeutics* 1981; **4**: 522–8.

92 Goudsouzian, N.G., Donlon, J.V., Savarese, J.J., *et al.* Reevaluation of d-tubocurarine dosage and duration in the pediatric age group. *Anesthesiology* 1975; **43**: 416–23.

93 Goudsouzian, N.G. and Standaert, F.G. The infant and the myoneural junction. *Anesthesia and Analgesia* 1986; **65**: 1208–17.

94 Robinson, S. and Gregory, G.A. Fentanyl-air-oxygen anesthesia for ligation of patent ductus arteriosus in preterm infants. *Anesthesia and Analgesia* 1981; **60**: 331–4.

95 Hickey, P.R. and Hansen, D.D. Fentanyl and sufentanil-oxygen-pancuronium anesthesia for cardiac surgery in infants. *Anesthesia and Analgesia* 1984; **63**: 117–24.

96 Meistelman, C., Agoston, S., Kersten, U.W., *et al.* Pharmacokinetics and pharmacodynamics of vecuronium and pancuronium in anesthetized patients. *Anesthesia and Analgesia* 1986; **65**: 1319–24.

97 Greenough, A., Wood, S., Morley, C.J., *et al.* Pancuronium prevents pneumothoraces in ventilated premature babies who actively expire against positive pressure inflation. *Lancet* 1984; **i**: 1–3.

98 Cabal, L.A., Siassi, B., Artal, R., *et al.* Cardiovascular and catecholamine changes after administration of pancuronium in distressed neonates. *Pediatrics* 1985; **75**: 284–7.

99 Reynolds, E.O.R., Hope, P.L. and Whitehead, M.D. Muscle relaxation and periventricular hemorrhage. *New England Journal of Medicine* 1985; **313**: 955–8.

100 Finer, N.N. and Tomney, P.M. Controlled evaluation of muscle relaxation in the ventilated neonate. *Pediatrics* 1981; **67**: 641–6.

101 Goudsouzian, N.G., Crone, R.R. and Todres, I.D. Recovery from pancuronium blockade in the neonatal intensive care unit. 1981; *British Journal of Anaesthesia* **53**: 1303.

102 Goudsouzian, N.G., Alifimoff, J.K., Liu, L.M.P. *et al.* Neuromuscular and cardiovascular effects of doxacurium in children anaesthetized with halothane. *British Journal of Anaesthesia* 1989; **62**: 263–8.

103 Sarner, J.B., Brandom, B.W., Cook, D.R. *et al.* Clinical pharmacology of doxacurium chloride (BW A938U) in children. *Anesthesia and Analgesia* 1988; **67**: 303–6.

104 Pittet, J.F., Tassonyi, E., Morel, D.R. *et al.* Neuromuscular effects of pipecuronium bromide in infants and children during nitrous oxide–alfentanil anesthesia. *Anesthesiology* 1984; **72**: 432–5.

105 Goudsouzian, N.G., Liu, L.M.P. and Savarese, J.J. Metocurine in infants and children: neuromuscular and clinical effects. *Anesthesiology* 1978; **49**: 266–9.

106 Fisher, D.M., Cronnelly, R., Miller, R.D., *et al.* The neuromuscular pharmacology of neostigmine in infants and children. *Anesthesiology* 1983; **59**: 220–5.

107 Viby-Mogensen, J., Howardy-Hansen, P. and Chraemmer-Jorgensen, B. Post Tetanic Count (PTC); a new method of evaluating an intense non-depolarising neuromuscular blockade. *Anesthesiology* 1981; **55**: 458–61.

108 Mason, L.J. and Betts, E.K. Leg lift and maximum inspiratory force: clinical signs of neuromuscular blockade reversal in neonates and infants. *Anesthesiology* 1980; **52**: 441–2.

109 Shimada, Y., Yoshiya, I., Tanaka, K., *et al.* Crying vital capacity and maximal inspiratory pressure as clinical indicators of readiness for weaning of infants less than a year of age. *Anesthesiology* 1979; **51**: 456–9.

110 Fisher, D.M., Cronnelly, R. and Sharma, M. *et al.* Clinical pharmacology of edrophonium in infants and children. *Anesthesiology* 1984; **61**: 428–33.

111 Meakin, G., Sweet, P.T., Bevan, J.C., *et al.* Neostigmine and edrophonium as antagonists of pancuronium in infants and children. *Anesthesiology* 1983; **59**: 316–21.

112 Keens, T.G., Bryan, A.C., Levison, H., *et al.* Developmental pattern of muscle fiber types in human ventilatory muscles. *Journal of Applied Physiology* 1978; **44**: 909–13.

113 Mansell, A., Bryan, C. and Levison, H. Airway closure in children. *Journal of Applied Physiology* 1972; **33**: 711–14.

114 Laycock, J.R.D., Baxter, M.K., Bevan, J.C., Sangwan, S., Donati, F. and Bevan, D.R. The potency of pancuronium at the adductor pollicis and diaphragm in infants and children. *Anesthesiology* 1988; **68**: 908–11.

115 Bevan, D.R., Kahwaji, R., Ansermino, J.M., *et al.* Residual block after mivacurium with or without edrophonium reversal in adults and children. *Anesthesiology* 1996; **84**: 362–7.

116 Kopman, A.F. Surrogate endpoints and neuromuscular recovery. *Anesthesiology* 1997; **87**: 1029–31.

117 D'Honneur, G., Lofaso, F., Drummond, G.B., *et al.* Susceptibility to upper airway obstruction during partial neuromuscular block. *Anesthesiology* 1988; **88**: 371–8.

118 Smith, C.L. and Bush, G.H. Anaesthesia and progressive muscular dystrophy. *British Journal of Anaesthesia* 1985; **57**: 1113–18.

119 Morris, P. Duchenne muscular dystrophy. A challenge for the anaesthetist. *Paediatric Anaesthesia* 1997; **7**: 1–4.

120 Hoffman, E.P., Fischbeck, K.H., Brown, R.H., *et al.* Characterization of dystrophin muscle-biopsy specimens from patients with Duchenne's or Becker's muscular dystrophy. *New England Journal of Medicine* 1988; **318**: 1363–8.

121 Sethna, N.F. and Rockoff, M.A. Anesthesia-related complications in children with Duchenne muscular dystrophy. *Anesthesiology* 1988; **68**: 462–5.

122 Brownell, A.K.W., Paasuke, R.T., Elash, A., *et al.* Malignant hyperthermia in Duchenne Muscular Dystrophy. *Anesthesiology* 1983; **58**: 180–2.

123 Iaizzo, P.A. and Lehmann-Horn, F. Anesthetic complications in muscle disorders. *Anesthesiology* 1995; **82**: 1093–6.

124 Ririe, D.G., Shapiro, F. and Sethna, N.F. The response of patients with Duchenne's muscular dystrophy to neuromuscular blockade with vecuronium. *Anesthesiology* 1998; **88**: 351–4.

125 Buzello, W. and Huttarsch, H. Muscle relaxation in patients with Duchenne's muscular dystrophy: use of vecuronium in two patients. *British Journal of Anaesthesia* 1988; **60**: 228–31.

126 Tobias, J.D. and Atwood, R. Mivacurium in children with Duchenne muscular dystrophy. *Paediatric Anaesthesia* 1994; **4**: 57–60.

127 Aldridge, L.M. Anaesthetic problems in myotonic dystrophy. *British Journal of Anaesthesia* 1985; **57**: 1119–26.

128 Ptacek, L.J., Johnson, K.J. and Griggs, R.C. Genetics and physiology of the myotonic muscle disorders. *New England Journal of Medicine* **328**: 482–9.

129 Nightingale, P., Healy, T.E.J. and McGuinness, K. Dystrophia myotonica and atracurium. *British Journal of Anaesthesia* 1985; **57**: 1131–5.

130 Stirt, J.A., Stone, D.J., Weinberg, G., *et al.* Atracurium in a child with myotonic dystrophy. *Anesthesia and Analgesia* 1985; **64**: 369–70.

131 Oosterhuis, H.J.G.H. Myasthenia gravis: a survey. *Clinical Neurology and Neurosurgery* 1981; **83**: 105–35.

132 Wise, G.A. and McQuillen, M.P. Transient neonatal myasthenia. *Archives of Neurology* 1970; **22**: 556–65.

133 Gronert, G.A. Malignant hyperthermia. *Anesthesiology* 1980; **53**: 395–423.

134 Strazis, K.P. and Fox, A.W. Malignant hyperthermia: a review of published cases. *Anesthesia and Analgesia* 1993; **77**: 297–304.

135 Rosenberg, H. and Shutack, J.G. Variants of malignant hyperthermia. Special problems for the paediatric anaesthesiologist. *Paediatric Anaesthesia* 1996; **6**: 87–93.

136 Michel, P.A. and Fronefield, H.P. Use of atracurium in a patient susceptible to malignant hyperthermia. *Anesthesiology* 1985; **62**: 213.

137 Martyn, J., Goldhill, D.R. and Goudsouzian, N. Clinical pharmacology of muscle relaxants in patients with burns. *Journal of Clinical Pharmacology* 1986; **26**: 680–6.

138 Kim, C., Fuke, N. and Martyn, J.A.J. Burn injury to rat increases nicotinic acetylcholine receptors in the diaphragm. *Anesthesiology* 1988; **68**: 401–6.

CHAPTER 6

Basic techniques for anaesthesia

ISABEAU WALKER AND JANE LOCKIE

In 1937 Philip Ayre commented that it was the duty of anaesthetists to adapt the anaesthetic to the patient, not the patient to the anaesthetic.[1] This philosophy is as true today as it was then.

ENVIRONMENT AND PERSONNEL

One of the first requirements for paediatric anaesthesia is an appropriately trained anaesthesia team. Theory is no substitute for experience when faced with a small infant for surgery. As pointed out in Chapter 23, 'occasional paediatric practice' is to be discouraged by both surgeons and anaesthetists.[2] In the UK, there is currently much debate about where children should be treated (district general hospital or specialist centre).[3,4] Wherever children are cared for they should receive a high standard of service. Fundamental to this is a suitably trained anaesthetist with appropriate continuing experience. Patients encountered in routine paediatric practice range from the premature infant weighing less then 1 kg to the adolescent of 70 kg. The anaesthetist should be prepared and competent to deal with these children with obviously quite different requirements. Theatre nurses and anaesthetic assistants should also be trained and experienced in working with children (and their parents). As much as personnel, the environment should be child friendly, with attention paid to items such as toys, decorations on the walls and a safe environment for inquisitive youngsters. In general hospitals, where both adults and children are admitted, there should be a designated paediatric theatre that is kept stocked with specialized paediatric equipment. Alternatively, there could be a mobile paediatric trolley, which is stocked and checked on a daily basis. In a general hospital, where there is a centralized recovery room, one or more spaces should be allocated to children and be fully provided with equipment of appropriate size for children of all ages. There should be decorations and pictures to maintain a child's interest in the areas of the theatre suite in which they are conscious. The anaesthetic and recovery rooms should have sufficient space to allow a parent to participate whilst the child is conscious. Parents should have clear instructions as to their role whilst the child is in the theatre suite.[5]

The report of a joint working group of the British Paediatric Association[6] suggested that every hospital that admits children should have a named consultant anaesthetist responsible for the anaesthetic services for children. Their responsibilities should include all aspects of the paediatric anaesthetic service in that hospital.[7] They should also be involved in policies regarding transfer of children and provision of intensive care, and are ideally placed to coordinate training and provision of paediatric resuscitation services within the hospital.

EQUIPMENT

The speciality of paediatric anaesthesia has advanced to such an extent that it would now be unthinkable to embark upon an anaesthetic in a small child without the appropriate equipment available or to allow the 'ingenuity of the anaesthetist to bridge the gap'.[8] The lead paediatric anaesthetist in each department has a particular responsibility in this area, and it would be sensible to establish inventories against which all items can be regularly checked. Obviously, all equipment should be well maintained and adequately sterilized or cleaned as appropriate. The current position of high-quality reliable equipment is partly due to the presence and efforts of the International Standards committees working with manufacturers

to produce reliably manufactured equipment with agreed dimensions at key interfaces.

ANAESTHESIA MACHINES

Most children can be anaesthetized with the standard continuous flow anaesthesia machine, the details of which are described elsewhere.[9] The primary function of the machine is to deliver a known concentration of oxygen and anaesthetic gas easily, safely and accurately. In addition, it is useful to be able to deliver air in situations where nitrous oxide is to be avoided and hyperoxia is undesirable (e.g. during bowel surgery or for infants born at less than 30 weeks' gestation and at risk for retinopathy of prematurity or during laser surgery). Most modern anaesthesia machines are equipped with antihypoxia devices whereby oxygen delivery is linked to nitrous oxide delivery so that a minimum 25% oxygen is always ensured. However, these devices do not take other gases into account (such as air), thus emphasizing the importance of an in-line oxygen analyser at all times. The anaesthetic machine should be equipped with full monitoring (as discussed in Chapter 7) and appropriate variable suction equipment. The machine should be checked according to standard local guidelines prior to the start of any anaesthetic.

BREATHING SYSTEMS

There have been several important factors influencing the development of anaesthetic breathing systems. These include the safety and ease of use, appropriate and efficient use of fresh gas and, more recently, the economical use of expensive volatile agents with minimal pollution of the operating theatre. In addition, it has long been recognized that breathing systems used in adults are not always suitable for use in children. Ayre first discussed this in 1937,[1] when he was concerned at the poor condition of infants and small babies when using a closed system, noting their 'ashy-grey pallor and rapid breathing'. As a result, he introduced the T-piece system with a continuous supply of oxygen close to the patient's airway and an absence of valves. This provided a system with minimal dead space and minimal resistance to breathing. Jackson Rees later modified the Ayre's T-piece in 1950 by increasing the length of the expiratory limb to avoid air entrainment and adding an open-ended reservoir bag to monitor respiration. Although it has some drawbacks, the Jackson Rees modification of the Ayre's T-piece has remained in popular use in paediatric anaesthesia around the world.

THE IDEAL PAEDIATRIC BREATHING SYSTEM

There are important physiological considerations in children that have a bearing on the choice of breathing system used, particularly during spontaneous ventilation. The tidal volume of infants is small in absolute terms (7 ml kg^{-1}) and may be further reduced under anaesthesia (to as little as 4 ml kg^{-1}).[10] Thus, apparatus dead space can assume great importance and should be kept as small as possible to reduce rebreathing of carbon dioxide-containing gases and minimize the work of breathing.[11,11a]

Similarly, resistance in a breathing circuit should be low to avoid respiratory muscle fatigue. Several factors are important in determining resistance in a breathing circuit. Firstly, the diameter of the breathing tubes has an important effect.[12] During laminar flow through tubes, the Hagen–Poiseuille equation applies:

$$Q = \frac{\pi p r^4}{8ln}$$

where Q is flow, p the pressure change across the tube, r the radius, l the length and n the viscosity of the gas. Thus, for a given flow rate, the pressure across the tube and hence the resistance is related to the fourth power of the radius. The use of relatively large-bore tubing will reduce resistance during spontaneous ventilation. In practice, tubing with an internal diameter of 15 mm is used in paediatric breathing systems. In fact, any increase in size may be detrimental, as the compressible volume and the

inertia of the gases within the system would be increased, thus increasing the work of breathing. Larger tubing is also bulky to handle when dealing with small children. Lightweight, plastic 15-mm corrugated tubing is popular, but cannot be sterilized, so if reused, should be protected by a disposable breathing filter. Corrugated hosing may promote turbulent flow within the breathing system. Smooth-bore silicone hoses are now available which offer a lower resistance to gas flow. They have a reinforcing spiral on the external surface to resist kinking.

Unidirectional valves within a breathing system add extra resistance. Ideally, they should be light and of large diameter to reduce resistance to a minimum.[10] If the valves become wet the resistance will increase, so unidirectional valves within a breathing system should be kept dry. The presence of an expiratory pressure relief valve within a breathing system will add to the resistance and may be detrimental in small infants.

In summary, the ideal paediatric breathing system should have minimal dead space, minimal resistance with either no valves or very low resistance valves, have small internal gas volumes and be constructed in such a way as to minimize gas turbulence.[9] In practice, the vast majority of older children and adolescents can be anaesthetized using standard adult breathing systems. However, for smaller children, especially in infants weighing 10 kg or less, breathing systems designed for children should be used.[13]

CLASSIFICATION OF BREATHING SYSTEMS

The traditional classification of anaesthesia breathing systems into open, closed, semi-open and semi-closed is rather confusing terminology and does not add much to an understanding of the functional differences between systems. Conway[14] suggested that a more rational approach to the classification of breathing systems would be to define them in two broad classes: systems that do not contain the means to absorb carbon dioxide and those equipped with carbon dioxide absorption equipment. Miller has extended this classification further to subdivide each group into unidirectional flow systems (those with one-way valves) and bidirectional flow systems in which rebreathing of expired gases may occur.[15] The advantage of this classification is that it allows prediction of the fresh gas flow required when using the different breathing systems and inclusion of newer breathing systems, as will be discussed below[16].

NON-ABSORBER BREATHING SYSTEMS

Of the non-absorber breathing systems, the bidirectional flow systems will be described, as they are the systems in most common use in anaesthesia. They are known as rebreathing systems as they allow some rebreathing of anaesthetic gases to occur. They rely on the flushing action of the fresh gas to clear exhaled carbon dioxide from the system to avoid an increase in inhaled carbon dioxide or compensatory increase in ventilation. They differ in the arrangement of their component parts: the fresh gas inlet, the reservoir bag, the pressure relief valve (if present) and the patient breathing connector. They include the classical Mapleson systems A–F (Figure 6.1).[17,18] These may be subdivided into afferent, efferent and junctional reservoir systems, depending on the position of the reservoir bag in relation to the fresh gas flow from the anaesthetic machine. Thus, the Magill system becomes an afferent reservoir system, the Mapleson D–F and coaxial Bain system efferent reservoir systems and the Mapleson B and C junctional reservoir systems. The Humphrey ADE system is a hybrid system where there is a possibility to switch between afferent and efferent reservoir systems.

An understanding of the functional characteristics of the different breathing systems is important in order to make economical use of the anaesthetic gases whilst avoiding excessive rebreathing. In addition, the mechanics of the different breathing systems should be considered when anaesthetizing small infants. The breathing systems in common use will be described below.

Afferent reservoir breathing systems: Magill and Lack systems

The Mapleson A system, the original Magill system, consists of a reservoir bag at the machine end of the breathing system, a length of corrugated breathing hose and a pressure relief valve at the patient end of the breathing system. When used for spontaneous ventilation in adults, it makes efficient use of the fresh gas and a fresh gas flow of the order of the minute ventilation (70 ml kg^{-1} min^{-1}) is appropriate. The fresh gas is drawn in from the reservoir on the afferent limb of the breathing system. During expiration, initial dead-space gas passes into the breathing hose and is conserved; alveolar gas is preferentially vented from the expiratory valve. It is inefficient when used for positive pressure ventilation, however, since the fresh gas is vented via the expiratory valve during inspiration and high fresh gas flows are required to prevent rebreathing (more than twice minute ventilation). It is not suitable for use for children under 20 kg owing to the large apparatus dead space and the resistance of the pressure relief valve. The presence of the pressure relief valve at the patient end of the breathing system is also cumbersome and difficult to scavenge, and may drag on the tracheal tube and displace it.

Lack[19] modified the Magill breathing system by extending the connection to the pressure relief valve. The valve is positioned at the machine end of the breathing system where it can easily be scavenged. The coaxial version is bulky but the parallel version of the Lack system is convenient to use, especially when supplied with lightweight plastic breathing hose. It is more economical during spontaneous ventilation than the Magill system, requiring a minimum fresh gas flow of only 50 ml kg^{-1} min^{-1}. Separation of inspiratory and expiratory limbs reduces mixing of fresh gas and exhaled gas and reduces the functional dead space. It is suitable for spontaneous ventilation in children from about 15 kg. A minimum fresh gas flow of 3 l min^{-1} should be used (Table 6.1).

Enclosed afferent reservoir breathing system

The enclosed afferent reservoir (EAR) breathing systems are new breathing systems that are capable of being used efficiently with low fresh gas flows during spontaneous ventilation and controlled ventilation. They have a set of bellows on the afferent limb of the breathing system, enclosed within a plastic container. A

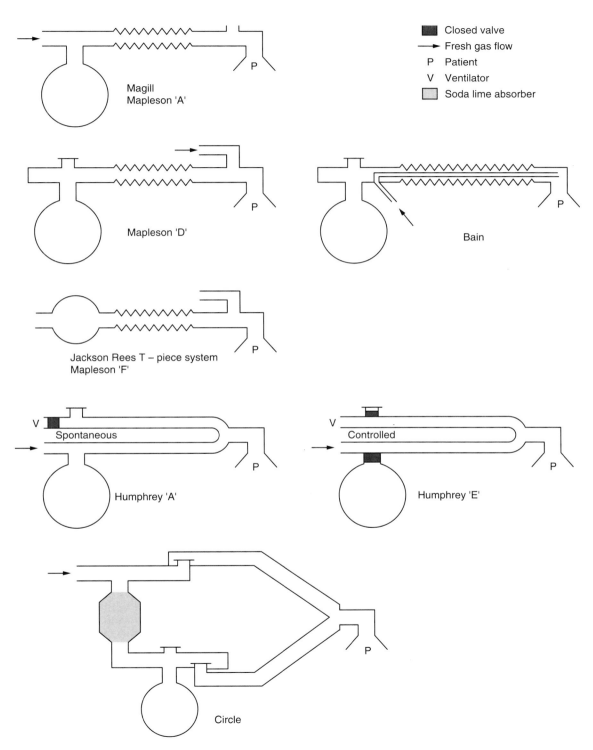

Figure 6.1 Anaesthesia breathing systems.

Table 6.1 Breathing systems: recommended gas flow rates as a fraction of normal minute ventilation

	Recommended fresh gas flow rates as a fraction of normal minute ventilation	
	Spontaneous ventilation	Controlled ventilation
1. Non-absorber breathing systems		
A. Unidirectional breathing systems		
Non-rebreathing valves	1	1
B. *Bidirectional breathing systems*		
Efferent reservoir (Mapleson D, E, F)	> 2	1
Junctional reservoir (Mapleson B, C)	> 1.5	1.5
Simple afferent reservoir (Mapleson A)	< 1	> 2
Enclosed afferent reservoir	< 1	0.7
2. Absorber breathing systems		
A. *Unidirectional breathing systems*		
Circle absorber	High to low	High to low
B. *Bidirectional breathing systems*		
To-and-fro canister	High to low	High to low

From Miller (1995).[15]

one-way valve on the expiratory limb is linked to the container. During spontaneous ventilation the patient breathes from the bellows and the system behaves like a Magill system. Ventilation is controlled by increasing the pressure within the container and compressing the bellows. At the same time, the expiratory valve is closed, avoiding venting fresh gas as occurs in the standard Magill system. The Ohmeda version of the EAR system has been investigated in children from 10 kg in weight.[20] It has been found to be highly efficient in both controlled and spontaneous ventilation. It requires a fresh gas flow close to alveolar ventilation, predicted by the formula [0.6 × weight$^{0.5}$ (kg)], regardless of the mode of ventilation.

Efferent reservoir breathing systems: Mapleson D, E and F systems

The Mapleson D, E (Ayre's T-piece) and F (Jackson Rees T-piece) systems are functionally similar. The Bain system is a coaxial version of the Mapleson D. In all cases, the fresh gas enters at the patient end of the breathing system and flushes out expired gases to provide a low functional dead space. During expiration a mixture of fresh gas and exhaled gases passes down a length of corrugated tube to the efferent limb of the breathing system. Here there is a reservoir bag and pressure relief valve in the case of the Mapleson D system, an open-ended reservoir bag in the case of the Jackson Rees T-piece, and an open tube in the case of the Ayre's T-piece. These systems are all relatively inefficient during spontaneous ventilation and require high fresh gas flows of at least two to three times the minute ventilation to avoid significant rebreathing. They are much more efficient during controlled ventilation where normocarbia may be maintained with a fresh gas flow close to minute ventilation (particularly if slow ventilation rates with long expiratory pauses and large tidal volumes are used).[15]

The Jackson Rees T-piece system

The Jackson Rees T-piece [21] is still the most popular breathing system for paediatric anaesthesia, particularly infant and neonatal anaesthesia. It has largely superseded the open-ended Ayre's T-piece in clinical use. It is available in lightweight disposable plastic and closely approximates to the ideal paediatric breathing system (Figure 6.2). The low-volume, low-resistance expiratory limb without valves offers minimal resistance to breathing. The open-ended reservoir bag allows easy assessment of spontaneous breathing and may be used to provide controlled ventilation, although this is a technique that may require some practice. It is possible to gain an idea of lung compliance by the feel of the bag, although the 'educated hand' may not always be reliable in detecting changes in lung compliance.[22] The bag may be partially occluded to apply continuous positive airway pressure (CPAP) to reduce the tendency to airway closure during spontaneous ventilation. The reservoir bag may be removed and the T-

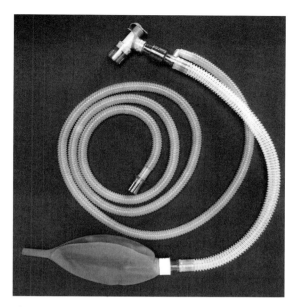

Figure 6.2 A disposable version of the Ayres T-piece with Jackson Rees modification.

piece used in conjunction with an automatic ventilator, as described later. One of the main drawbacks of the Jackson Rees T-piece system is the difficulty in scavenging gases from the open reservoir bag during spontaneous ventilation. As a minimum, the T-piece should be used in an operating suite with effective air conditioning (preferably the equivalent of 25 air changes per hour). The open end of the T-piece may be placed into a shroud to which the scavenging system is attached (such as the Stellenbosch collector).[9] Alternatively, a paediatric adjustable pressure relief valve and standard 30-mm scavenging outlet may be placed at the end of the expiratory limb, with a closed bag to replace the open-ended reservoir bag (such as the Intersurgical paediatric APL valve). The valve should have a lower pressure release than the standard adult pressure relief valves (no more than 35 cmH_2O). This is particularly important since there is no pressure relief valve in the T-piece itself. The valve will increase expiratory resistance but the addition of a low level of CPAP may be beneficial, as described above.

There have been many studies to determine the minimum fresh gas flows required using the T-piece. The fresh gas flow depends on the size of the child (which relates to the volume of carbon dioxide produced), the respiratory pattern, and the volume of the expiratory limb of the breathing system and the mode of breathing. Small infants breathing spontaneously have rapid respiratory rates with a sinusoidal pattern and no expiratory pause. The lack of expiratory pause means that there is less time for the fresh gas to flush out the expiratory reservoir before the next breath and thus a requirement for high fresh gas flows. Similarly, during controlled ventilation, if there is an end-expiratory pause, fresh gas flow required will be reduced. The volume of the expiratory limb must exceed the tidal volume of the patient, otherwise high fresh gas flows will be required to avoid entrainment of room air during spontaneous ventilation.

Since it is difficult to predict the minute volume of small infants, formulae based on weight have been suggested to predict minimum fresh gas flow during both spontaneous and controlled ventilation. Froese and Rose[23] suggested that during spontaneous ventilation a flow rate of $(1000 + 100$ ml $kg^{-1})$ ml min^{-1} would avoid rebreathing. They suggested a flow rate of $(1000 + 100$ ml $kg^{-1})$, with a minimum fresh gas flow of 3 l min^{-1}, and moderate hyperventilation $(1.5 \times FGF)$ to avoid rebreathing in ventilated children of 10–30 kg. Lindahl *et al.*[24] suggested an alternative formula for fresh gas flow during spontaneous ventilation, taking into account the respiratory rate: $15 \times$ respiratory rate $(min^{-1}) \times$ weight (kg) (ml min^{-1}). Hatch suggested that during controlled ventilation lower minute ventilation should be used than that suggested by Froese and Rose (tidal volume 10 ml kg^{-1}): respiratory rate of 20 breaths min^{-1} (i.e. minute ventilation 200 ml kg^{-1} min^{-1}), but with a more generous fresh gas flow $(1000 + 200$ ml $kg^{-1})$.[25] This formula can be applied to children from 3 to 20 kg. Most authors recommend a minimum fresh gas flow of 3 l min^{-1}. In practical terms, an approximate fresh gas flow can be selected and adjusted to obtain an appropriate end-tidal carbon dioxide tension without excessive rebreathing (inspired carbon dioxide less than 0.5 kPa). The presence of rebreathed air in the non-respiratory air passages has the additional advantage of providing some humidity and heat to the upper airway. Note that end-tidal carbon dioxide measurements may be underestimated in small infants (less than 8 kg) ventilated with a T-piece due to dilution of expired gases by fresh gas.[26] The sampling site for the capnograph should be as close to the tracheal tube as possible to allow for early detection of rebreathing using a T-piece.[27] The Jackson Rees T-piece is commonly used in children up to about 25–30 kg in weight but its main advantages are for infants less than 10 kg in weight. It is particularly wasteful of fresh gases during spontaneous ventilation in larger children and an alternative system should be used.

Bain system

The Bain system[28] is a coaxial version of the Mapleson D breathing system. It has an inner tube carrying fresh gas to the patient end of the breathing system and an outer corrugated tube carrying gases to the reservoir bag and the expiratory valve. These are located at the machine end of the breathing system with easy attachment for the scavenging valve. Care must be taken that the inner tube is not disconnected at the proximal end of the breathing system or excessive rebreathing will result. It is made of lightweight plastic and is streamlined and easy to use. It is disposable but may be reused if protected by a breathing filter. There is a 2-l reservoir bag that may be removed for connection to a ventilator such as the Penlon Nuffield Anaesthetic Ventilator. It makes economical use of fresh gas during positive pressure ventilation ($70 \text{ ml kg}^{-1} \text{ min}^{-1}$ for normocarbia), but high fresh gas flows are required during spontaneous ventilation. This system is not suitable for spontaneous ventilation in children weighing less than 20 kg owing to the resistance of the expiratory valve. It is not used for controlled ventilation of infants because of the high compliance of the expiratory limb relative to small tidal volumes.

Hybrid systems: the Humphrey ADE

The Humphrey ADE system is a hybrid system incorporating the Mapleson A, D and E principles[29] (Figure 6.1). Parallel breathing hoses are connected to the anaesthetic machine via a cylindrical manifold with a lever, reservoir bag and pressure relief valve. With the lever in the upright position, the reservoir bag and the

expiratory valve are included in the inspiratory limb of the breathing system (Mapleson A configuration). With the lever down, the bag and valve are excluded, fresh gas passes directly to the patient via the inspiratory limb of the breathing system and exhaled gases are directed into the expiratory limb which is now opened to atmosphere via a port at the ADE block (Mapleson E mode). A ventilator such as the Penlon Nuffield Anaesthetic Ventilator may be connected to this port. There is an overpressure relief valve that is connected in both modes. In the A configuration, during spontaneous ventilation, the breathing system is very economical and performs as a Lack breathing system; with controlled ventilation in the E configuration it is as economical as the Bain system. It has been evaluated in children using 15-mm tubing and a 500-ml reservoir bag.[30] During controlled ventilation in the E mode it behaves like a standard T-piece, with similar fresh gas requirements. In the A mode, it is suitable for spontaneous ventilation in children from 10 kg with a minimum fresh gas flow of 3 l min^{-1} recommended. It has the advantage of being more economical and easy to scavenge than the standard paediatric T-piece during spontaneous ventilation. The expiratory valve is of low resistance and does not add appreciably to the work of breathing. Nevertheless, the possibility of the expiratory valve sticking and the potential consequences should be borne in mind. Hand ventilation (only possible when the system is in the A mode) is probably more convenient than learning to use the open-ended bag of the T-piece system.

ABSORBER BREATHING SYSTEMS

Breathing systems with carbon dioxide absorption

The breathing systems described above require high fresh gas flows in order to flush exhaled carbon dioxide from the system, up to 90% of the administered volatile agent being eliminated unchanged into the atmosphere.[31] If carbon dioxide is removed from exhaled gases, fresh gas flows can be reduced to very low levels. The benefits of carbon dioxide absorption techniques were recognized from the early days of anaesthesia, namely, reduced loss of heat and moisture, economical use of anaesthetic gases and reduction of operating theatre pollution.[32]

Circle absorption systems

There has been a resurgence of interest in low-flow anaesthetic techniques using carbon dioxide absorption over the past few years, mainly because of economic concerns, environmental factors, advances in monitoring technology and the introduction of new, expensive volatile anaesthetics.[33] Although anaesthetic drugs are relatively inexpensive compared with the total cost of hospital drugs, the use of low-flow anaesthesia has been found to reduce the use of volatile agents by more than 50% in both adults and children over 5 years.[31,34] Halogenated anaesthetic agents are ozone depleting and anaesthesia accounts for 3–12% of global nitrous oxide release, a greenhouse gas which contributes to global warming. Concerns about the safety of low-flow anaesthesia, namely accidental hypoxia, overdosage or underdosage of volatile agents and increased risks of hypercapnia are no longer an issue with the availability of modern anaesthesia monitors of inhaled and exhaled gas concentration and oxygen saturation.[32] The reaction of carbon dioxide with soda lime is exothermic and produces water, and the advantages of maintaining body temperature and increasing humidification of inspired gases have been well recognized. Probably one of the most significant factors in stimulating interest in low-flow anaesthesia has been the introduction of the new expensive volatile agents such as isoflurane and sevoflurane. This is particularly so in paediatric anaesthesia, as halothane, which is relatively inexpensive, has in many centres been largely replaced by sevoflurane for inhalational induction and either sevoflurane or isoflurane for the maintenance of anaesthesia.

Space does not permit a full description of the equipment required and technique of low-flow anaesthesia, but this is comprehensively reviewed elsewhere.[9,32,33] There is a requirement for full monitoring, as described above: oximetry, capnography, inspired oxygen concentration, tidal volume (ventilator bellows and spirometer), and volatile agent and nitrous oxide analyser. A leak-free circle circuit with a carbon dioxide absorber is required. Accurate

flow meters calibrated to 1 l min^{-1} are required. Ventilation is usually controlled with a ventilator of the ascending bellows type.[33]

There are several concerns regarding the use of circle systems in small children. The volume of the breathing system is large and has unidirectional valves that may increase the resistance to breathing. Lightweight 15-mm diameter hose should be used. Modern unidirectional valves are of low resistance, but must be kept dry to avoid an increase in flow resistance. In fact, the resistive load of a paediatric circle has been found to be similar to that of a Jackson Rees T-piece,[35] with a greater impedance to spontaneous breathing seen with the T-piece.[36] The paediatric circle was found to be a reliable alternative to the Jackson Rees T-piece for children greater than 10 kg breathing spontaneously. Children below the age of about 8 years are traditionally anaesthetized with uncuffed tracheal tubes to minimize airway trauma, the size chosen to allow a small leak around the tube. However, the presence of a significant leak in the breathing system may be such as to make low-flow anaesthesia impossible. Fröhlich et al.[37] investigated the loss of gas from the breathing system in children aged 2–6 years anaesthetized with uncuffed tubes or laryngeal masks and concluded that airway sealing with both groups was tight enough to perform low-flow anaesthesia. The airway leak was less than 100 ml min^{-1} in most children, although there were a few with much higher airway leaks, especially in the tracheal tube group. A standard formula for selection of the tracheal tube was used [internal diameter = age (years)/4 + 4], emphasizing the need to have a tube size above and below that predicted by the formula, the final selection of tube size being made on clinical grounds. Many surgical procedures in children are of short duration, so it may not be possible to obtain the benefits of low-flow anaesthesia. Most workers suggest a period of 10 min high flow at the start of low-flow anaesthesia to prime the breathing system, denitrogenate the patient and allow for rapid uptake of volatile agents. Appreciable savings are still seen with low-flow anaesthesia in shorter procedures.[38] Circle absorbers have a beneficial effect in maintaining body temperature, but body temperature may increase significantly in children less than 5 years of age and should be monitored carefully.[34] Sevoflurane is degraded in the presence of carbon dioxide absorbents to produce compound A, which is nephrotoxic in rats in concentrations greater than 50–100 ppm. This has not been shown to be a problem in clinical practice, including in limited studies in children.[39] The production of compound A is related in part to fresh gas flow and the Food and Drug Administration (FDA) in America currently recommends that a minimum fresh gas flow of $2 \, l \, min^{-1}$ should be used when using sevoflurane. They also recommend that it should be avoided in patients with renal impairment.[40,40a] In the UK the Committee on Safety of Medicines has made no such recommendations. This topic is addressed more fully in Chapter 3.

AUTOMATIC VENTILATORS

Intermittent positive pressure ventilation is commonly used in paediatric practice and there are reliable ventilators available for children of all ages. The majority of children can be ventilated using standard adult anaesthesia ventilators providing the ventilator is of low internal compliance and equipped with paediatric breathing hoses. The ventilator should be capable of delivering small tidal volumes and rapid respiratory rates, and have an adjustable inspiratory flow rate and inspiratory:expiratory ratio so that peak airway pressures can be kept as low as possible.[41] When using an adult ventilator to ventilate an infant with a small tidal volume, adjustments must be made for the volume loss in distending the ventilator tubing and the leak around an uncuffed tracheal tube (see below). Ventilators may be used in conjunction with specialized breathing systems such as a circle system, Jackson Rees T-piece or Bain system. Examples of ventilators commonly used in paediatric practice will be discussed.

CLASSIFICATION OF VENTILATORS

There are numerous different ways of classifying ventilators, for instance, that described by Mushin and simplified to consider the inspiratory phase and the cycling mechanism at the end of the inspiratory phase.[41] Ventilators may act as either pressure generators (low-powered ventilators) or flow generators (high-powered ventilators). Cycling from inspiration to expiration may be determined by time, volume, pressure or flow. Most modern anaesthesia ventilators are time cycled. In addition, they may be volume controlled, in which case the ventilator delivers a preset tidal volume irrespective of inspiratory pressure, or pressure controlled, in which case the ventilator delivers gases to a preset inspiratory pressure. The tidal volume delivered in pressure-controlled mode will be markedly affected by lung compliance; the tidal volume delivered in volume-controlled mode will be less affected by lung compliance, but high pressures may develop if lung compliance falls. Pressure-controlled ventilation is commonly used in paediatric practice as a measure to prevent barotrauma. For ease of description, ventilators can also be classified according to the principles upon which they work: 'mechanical thumbs', 'intermittent blowers', 'minute volume dividers' and 'bag squeezers'.[9]

MANUAL VENTILATION

The end of an Ayre's T-piece may be occluded intermittently to provide positive pressure ventilation in infants and neonates. This incidentally also forms the basis of T-piece occluder ventilators such as the Sechrist infant ventilator (the 'mechanical thumb'). Since this mode of ventilation depends on the fresh gas supply to determine the inspiratory flow rate, it is very wasteful of fresh gas in larger children. Very high fresh gas flow rates are required during inspiration in order to generate adequate tidal volumes. T-piece occluders allow little variation in waveform or pattern of ventilation. The addition of a 500-ml reservoir bag to the T-piece allows it to be used much more efficiently. The ability to hand ventilate using the Jackson Rees T-piece is regarded as an essential technique in paediatric anaesthesia. An experienced anaesthetist may gain important information about changes in lung compliance resistance, for instance during cleft palate surgery when the Boyle Davies gag may occlude the tracheal tube. Hand ventilation may be used during surgical procedures such as tracheoesophageal fistula ligation where the anaesthetist co-operates closely with the surgeon to allow maximum access to the fistula with intermittent lung inflation. The ability to hand ventilate is an essential part of respiratory monitoring, but should not be used as the only form of respiratory monitoring as it may not always reliably detect changes in pulmonary compliance.[13]

The Nuffield anaesthetic ventilator and the Newton valve

The Nuffield anaesthetic ventilator is an 'intermittent blower' type of ventilator (Figure 6.3). It is driven by a source of compressed oxygen or air and does not require an electrical supply. In its usual form it acts as a time-cycled constant flow generator. It has a compact control unit with independent inspiratory and expiratory timers, a flow control knob, a pressure manometer and an on–off switch. The control unit directs the flow of driving gas into the patient valve. The patient valve contains a spring-loaded piston with a ventilator connection, a patient connection with inspiratory and expiratory ports and an exhaust port. During the inspiratory phase, gas flows into the patient valve from the control unit, the inspiratory port is opened, and the driving gas passes to the efferent limb of the patient breathing circuit via a suitable length of connecting hose. During the expiratory phase, the flow of driving gas stops, and the piston moves to close the inspiratory port and open the expiratory port to allow exhalation. The inspiratory flow may be varied between 0.25 and 1.0 l s^{-1} by adjusting the flow control knob on the front of the control unit. The flow rate and the inspiratory time determine the tidal volume; the pressure that is developed in the patient valve is displayed on the manometer on the front of the control

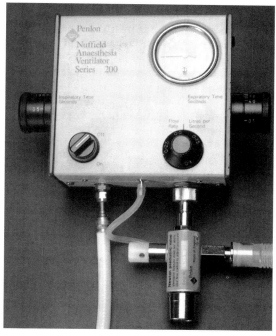

Figure 6.3 Penlon Nuffield anaesthesia ventilator with paediatric Newton valve.

module. The inspiratory and expiratory times may be varied independently to give a wide range of respiratory frequency from 10 to 85 breaths min^{-1}. However, it is not possible to reduce the inspiratory flow to low enough levels to generate the small tidal volumes required to ventilate small children safely. In this unmodified form, the Nuffield ventilator may only be used to ventilate adults and children above about 25 kg in weight.

The Newton valve is an ingenious device that replaces the patient valve of the Nuffield ventilator to convert it from a time-cycled flow generator to a time-cycled pressure generator suitable for neonates and infants.[42] The moving piston is removed from the valve that is simplified to consist of a ventilator connection, a patient connection and a fixed orifice gas outlet. The Newton valve thus simply acts as a constant 'fixed leak' to reduce inspiratory flows to the patient. The ventilator may now be used to deliver very small tidal volumes at low inspiratory pressures. It is ideal for ventilation of children in conjunction with a T-piece breathing circuit; the ventilator is connected to the expiratory limb of the T-piece and the flow control knob rotated from the minimal setting until adequate chest movement (and thus tidal volume) is obtained. The inspiratory pressure is indicated on the pressure manometer, but the tidal volume can no longer be calculated from the flow and inspiratory time settings. The modified ventilator is capable of delivering volumes between 10 and 300 ml at frequencies from 10 to 85 min^{-1}. It is suitable for use in neonates and children up to 20 kg and allows for easy conversion from controlled to manual ventilation and visa versa. (Figure 6.3)

The Nuffield ventilator with the Newton valve has proved to be very satisfactory in neonatal and paediatric practice but it does have some disadvantages. The size of the orifice in the valve is designed to reduce inspiratory flows significantly, and is also large enough to allow unimpeded flow of gases from the patient during expiration. However, low levels of positive end expiratory pressures (PEEP) are generated, which may become more significant when high inspiratory flows are used in larger children.[43] The ability to generate PEEP may be exploited by the addition of a PEEP valve to the gas outlet; the level of PEEP is indicated on the pressure manometer. The leak of driving gas from the valve makes the ventilator rather noisy in operation, but this is reduced when the scavenging valve is connected to the gas outlet. The driving gas may dilute out the anaesthetic gases and, for this reason, the 22-mm hose connecting ventilator to the breathing circuit should be at least 90 cm in length.[42] Of more concern is the situation when lung compliance is reduced or resistance rises. Since the ventilator functions as a pressure generator, tidal volume may be markedly reduced but the peak inspiratory pressure may not change, and potential airway obstruction will not be detected by a pressure alarm. It is difficult to monitor expired volume, as there is a continuous flow of gas in the T-piece in addition to the expired volume. Since the driving gas is separate from the fresh gas, it is also possible to have satisfactory chest movement but with no fresh gas flowing and significant rebreathing of expired gases. The use of a capnometer, which has become routine in most countries, is thus even more important with this ventilator than most others.

The Servo 900 series ventilator

The Servo 900C is a sophisticated ventilator designed for use in intensive care. It can be adapted for use in theatre to ventilate children of all sizes. It is a pneumatically driven, electronically controlled, time-cycled minute volume divider. For use in theatre, fresh gas from the anaesthetic machine is fed into the low-pressure gas supply and stored in spring-loaded bellows inside the ventilator. The pressurized gas in the bellows provides the inspiratory gas flow for the patient. The pressure within the bellows is adjusted using a key on the front of the ventilator; the working pressure is usually set to 60 cmH$_2$O. The fresh gas supply keeps the bellows full; fresh gas flow should be set just in excess of the delivered minute volume in order to keep the working pressure at 60 cmH$_2$O. The ventilator has controls for minute volume, respiratory rate and PEEP. A significant advantage over the Nuffield ventilator is the presence of sophisticated electronic alarms (expired minute volume, high and low airway pressure, and inspired oxygen). In addition, there are controls to vary the inspiratory waveforms (inspiratory time and flow pattern). For use with older children, the ventilator is used as a straightforward minute volume divider: the appropriate minute volume and respiratory rates are selected from which the tidal volume can be deduced (tidal volume = minute volume/rate). When used in infants with small tidal volumes, the amount of ventilation lost in compression of the ventilator tubing becomes significant compared with the tidal volume of the child. In fact, in some adult ventilators, the compression volume may be as large as 0.45 ml kPa^{-1}. With a peak inflation pressure of 20 cmH$_2$O (2 kPa), 90 ml is lost in compression per breath, which is significantly larger than the tidal volume of the average neonate.[10] Some of the delivered ventilation may also be lost with the leak around an uncuffed tracheal tube. The ventilator may be used successfully to ventilate neonates but a higher than expected minute ventilation may be required to compensate for these losses. An appropriate respiratory rate is selected and the minute volume is increased or decreased to achieve the desired inspiratory pressure, chest movement and end-tidal carbon dioxide. Paediatric hoses should be used to reduce the compressive losses to a minimum.

The MIE Carden ventilator

The MIE Carden 'Ventmasta' is a compact, versatile anaesthetic breathing system/ventilator that is integrated with the MIE anaesthetic machine. It consists of an electronic control unit and valve block, a Perspex canister containing a rising bellows arrangement and a mode block which allows the bellows to be attached to different breathing systems. The integrated ventilator is pressure preset and allows the ventilator to be used safely in small children. The system can be used as an enclosed Mapleson A system for spontaneous or for controlled ventilation, or used as a 'bag squeezer' in conjunction with a Bain system or a circle absorber system. The system has been found to be very efficient for fresh gas use during both spontaneous and controlled ventilation in children from 10 kg when employed as an enclosed Mapleson A system (i.e. without soda lime).[44] A fresh gas flow of $0.6 \times$ weight$^{0.5}$ has been recommended.

Ohmeda 7800 and 7900 ventilators

These are microprocessor-based, electronically controlled, pneumatically driven ventilators of the 'bag squeezer' type. They have a bellows-type ventilator used in conjunction with a circle breathing system. The 7800 ventilator is available as a stand-alone ventilator or in conjunction with an Ohmeda anaesthetic machine; the 7900 is only available integrated with an Ohmeda anaesthesia machine.

The 7800 is a time-cycled, volume-controlled ventilator, primarily designed for adult use, but it has been successfully used to ventilate children of all ages, including premature infants, providing they have a reasonably normal lung compliance.[45] In the study by Bagwell *et al.*, tidal volume was set to provide an appropriate chest expansion and inspiratory pressure (about 20 cmH$_2$O), I : E ratio of 1 : 2, fresh gas flow of 3 l min^{-1} and respiratory rate of 20 breaths min^{-1}. They used standard adult breathing systems, bellows and carbon dioxide absorption canisters. Not surprisingly, tidal volumes required for neonates in terms of body weight

(150–200 ml kg^{-1}) were very high, reflecting the volume wasted to compression in the ventilator, absorber and breathing system relative to the size of the child. Tidal volumes required for older children were proportionately less (25 ml kg^{-1} for infants greater than 10 kg). It is thus difficult to use a strict volume (ml kg^{-1}) formula to determine tidal volume in this situation. A study using an infant lung model suggested that the peak inspiratory pressure was the main determinant of delivered minute volume rather than the precise compliance of the individual breathing system. Adult or paediatric breathing systems may therefore be used.[46] For infants with low lung compliance, high inspiratory pressures will be required. It is important to set the inspiratory pressure limit to a suitable level to avoid accidental barotrauma when using this ventilator for small children.

A possible drawback of a bellows type ventilator used in conjunction with a circle system is the effect of a change in fresh gas flow on minute ventilation. This effect may be particularly significant in a small infant.[13] Fresh gas added to the breathing system during the inspiratory phase of respiration may make a contribution to the total minute ventilation. For an infant with a set minute ventilation of 2 l min^{-1} on the ventilator, an I : E ratio of 1 : 2, and fresh gas flow of 6 l min^{-1}, the actual delivered minute ventilation is 2 l min^{-1} + 1/3 × 6 l min^{-1}, that is 4 l min^{-1}. If the fresh gas flow is reduced to 3 l min^{-1}, by the same reasoning, the delivered minute ventilation is reduced to 2 l min^{-1} + 1/3 × 3 l min^{-1}, that is, 3 l min^{-1}. Delivered minute ventilation is significantly changed without a change in the ventilator settings. These effects are proportionally less in older children with large set minute ventilation relative to the fresh gas flow[13].

The Ohmeda 7900[47] ventilator has significant advantages for use in paediatric anaesthesia. The ventilator may be used in two modes: volume controlled (as for the 7800), and pressure controlled, a mode usually only seen in intensive care ventilators and the preferred mode to avoid pulmonary barotrauma in children. In the pressure-controlled mode, the target inspiratory pressure is selected and the ventilator delivers a high initial flow to achieve that pressure. Once the inspiratory pressure is reached, the ventilator keeps the inspiratory pressure at that level for the selected inspiratory time; the maximum tidal volume possible at that pressure is delivered. In this way, high inspiratory pressures may be avoided for infants with poorly compliant lungs. The ventilator has flow sensors on the inspiratory and expiratory limbs of the breathing system and is capable of measuring very small tidal volumes. It has the additional advantage of a 'volume compensation' mechanism so that the tidal volume set on the ventilator is that which is delivered to the breathing system. The ventilator compensates for compression loss in the absorber and bellows and the tidal volume required may be predicted accurately. It does not compensate for compression losses in the actual breathing system or around the tracheal tube; tidal volume may have to be adjusted slightly to take this into account. The volume compensation mechanism does, however, take changes in fresh gas flow into account. If fresh gas flow is reduced as described above, the ventilator will compensate in five or six breaths, so the minute volume remains the same.

AIRWAY EQUIPMENT

FACEMASKS

Facemasks are used during spontaneous respiration or they may be used to deliver positive pressure ventilation. They are also used for preoxygenation or for inhalational induction of anaesthesia. Therefore, the ideal paediatric facemask should be non-threatening to the conscious patient, easy to apply to the face and easy to achieve a good seal on the face to allow positive pressure ventilation The facemask connects directly to the breathing system via a 22-mm connector.

Clear plastic facemasks with inflatable cushioned rims are now in widespread use. A selection of these masks is shown in Figure 6.4. The amount of air in the cushion can be adjusted. The presence of the cushion reduces the downward pressure on the patient's face. Clear masks also offer the advantages of seeing the child directly, helping to detect cyanosis,

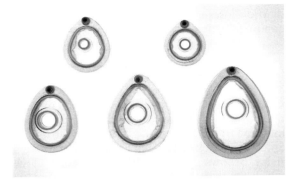

Figure 6.4 Paediatric facemasks.

regurgitation or occasionally the lip caught on the airway. They are less threatening to the patient than black rubber masks. They are available in round or teardrop shapes to provide a good fit. They are easier to position than the traditional Rendell–Baker Soucek facemasks described below. Cushion masks are available impregnated with scents such as bubble gum, cherry or mint, to aid acceptance of inhalational induction or preoxygenation. They are also suitable for use in latex-allergic patients.

LOW DEAD-SPACE MASKS

The tidal volume/dead-space ratio of children (V_t/V_d) is similar to that of adults, at 0.3. As the tidal volume of the child will be much smaller than the adult (and decreases under anaesthesia) the dead space of equipment becomes more relevant. The Rendell–Baker Soucek masks were designed to have a low dead space and are applied directly to the face without a cushioned rim. Anaesthesia is a dynamic, not a static situation. The dead-space volume of equipment as measured by displacement of water does not actually reflect the dynamic situation where gases are flowing through the system. The dead space as measured by volume displacement of water markedly overestimates the increase in physiological dead space. This may be due to the effects of gas streaming, and not all of the gas within the facemask needs to be displaced with each breath.[48] As these low dead-space masks are difficult to position and in practice the larger dead space of the cushioned masks is not clinically significant, their use is declining.

NASAL MASKS

Nasal masks, for example the Goldman nasal mask, are used in children undergoing dental anaesthesia. The mask fits only over the nose of the patient. The mouth is thus free for dental work. A pharyngeal pack is required to prevent soiling of the airway and to prevent excessive mouth breathing, which would dilute out the anaesthetic gases. It takes experience to use a nasal mask and other methods of airway maintenance are becoming more widely used for dental anaesthesia. Both the laryngeal mask and nasopharyngeal airway have been described as giving superior airway management in dental anaesthesia.[49,50]

FACEMASKS FOR FIBREOPTIC INTUBATION

Specialized facemasks are available to aid fibreoptic intubation. They have an off-centre connector to the breathing system to allow the scope to pass through the facemask centrally (Figure 6.5) (see also Chapter 15).

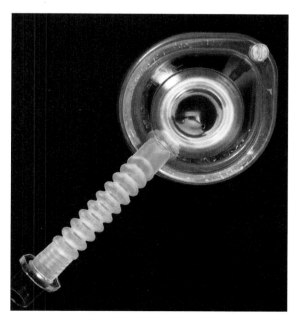

Figure 6.5 Facemask for fibreoptic intubation.

AIRWAYS

OROPHARYNGEAL AIRWAYS

Guedel oropharyngeal airways should be available but should not be regarded as a substitute for correct positioning of the anaesthetist's fingers whilst maintaining the airway. Correct positioning of the anaesthetist's fingers on the mandible, not the floor of the mouth, avoids forcing the soft tissues of the tongue on to the palate above, which will cause airway obstruction. It may also improve the airway to open the patient's mouth gently. If these measures are insufficient to provide a clear airway then the Guedel airway is a useful adjunct. The airway should not be inserted until an adequate depth of anaesthesia is reached, as coughing or laryngospasm may be provoked. Guedel airways are for single use and are available in sizes 000 to 2 and up to size 4 for adults (Figure 6.6).

The appropriate size of airway can be assessed by placing the airway against the side of the child's face, as shown in Figure 6.7. The correct size should lie from the angle of the mandible to the centre of the incisors. Selecting the correct size is important. An incorrectly sized airway will exacerbate airway obstruction if too short by impinging on the back of the tongue or in the case of an airway that is too long may cause laryngospasm. The Guedel airway is usually inserted without rotation in a young child as this may lead to damage to the pharyngeal structures and tonsils.

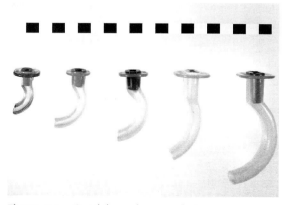

Figure 6.6 Guedel oropharyngeal airways.

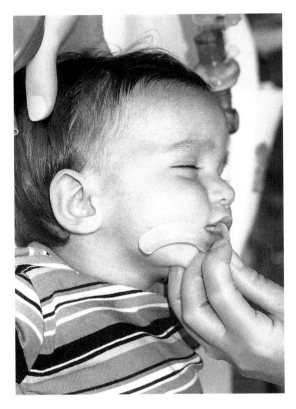

Figure 6.7 Sizing a Guedel airway.

NASOPHARYNGEAL AIRWAYS

Nasopharyngeal airways can be used for alleviating airway obstruction by opening the nasopharynx. They are useful for children with loose teeth where an oropharyngeal airway may be hazardous. They can be tolerated in place during recovery for longer than an oral airway and may therefore be useful in children with sleep apnoea who may obstruct their airways even at very light levels of anaesthesia. Nasopharyngeal airways may also be used for the provision of nasal CPAP in small infants. A nasopharyngeal airway can be constructed by shortening a tracheal tube of the appropriate size. The size chosen should be 1 mm less than a tracheal tube size for that patient, i.e. for nasopharyngeal airways the formula: age (in years)/4 + 3.5 is used above 2 years of age.

The length is assessed by measuring the distance from the tip of the nose to the external auditory meatus. They are also available as flanged soft rubber airways. During insertion care should be taken to avoid nasal mucosal or adenoidal damage, and they should be well lubricated prior to insertion.

Nasopharyngeal airways may be particularly useful for dental anaesthesia, where they have been shown to provide better airway maintenance than the Goldman nasal mask.[50]

THE LARYNGEAL MASK AIRWAY

One of the great advances in anaesthesia has been the introduction of the laryngeal mask airway (LMA) (Figure 6.8). Although invented and developed originally by Dr Brain[51] for adults, the range now includes sizes suitable for paediatric use. The paediatric sizes are scaled-down adult sizes. Infants and small children have anatomical differences in their airway from adults but cadaveric studies have shown that the pharyngeal shape (most relevant for laryngeal mask use) is similar.[51] The available sizes, suggested weight ranges and cuff volumes are shown in Table 6.2[52] (Figure 6.8).

The laryngeal mask consists of an oropharyngeal tube with a bowl-shaped mask part designed to sit around the laryngeal inlet. Laryngeal masks are reusable. There should be a registration card to record each sterilization and use up to 40 times the manufacturer's recommended maximum number of uses.

The LMA should be prepared for use by deflating all the air from the cuff and applying a small quantity of water-soluble lubricant to the back of the cuff.

Table 6.2 Appropriate sizes of laryngeal mask airway for different paediatric age groups

Size of LMA	Suggested weight of patient (kg)	Cuff volume (ml)
1	< 5	2–5
1.5	5–10	5–7
2	10–20	7–10
2.5	20–30	12–14
3	Not chosen by weight	15–20
4	Not chosen by weight	25–30
5	Not chosen by weight	35–40

From Brimacombe *et al.* (1996).[52]

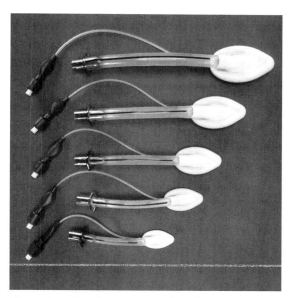

Figure 6.8 Paediatric laryngeal mask airways.

Reinforced laryngeal masks are available for procedures involving the head and neck[52] (Figure 6.9). These consist of a normal mask with a long flexometallic tube (slightly narrower than the usual LMA tube of the corresponding size). This tube is resistant to kinking but can still be occluded by the patient biting on the tube. Their passage may be assisted by the use of a semirigid bougie. There is a small metal spring in the pilot cuff of the LMA sufficient to distort images if used for MRI scanning.[52] LMAs are also available with a special colour-coded pilot cuff for MRI compatibility.

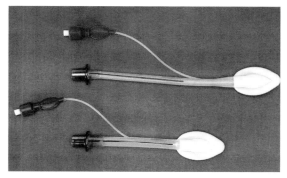

Figure 6.9 Size 2 laryngeal mask airways, reinforced and standard designs.

When correctly positioned the LMA does not pass through the glottis; therefore, a larger tube part can be used. The large diameter of the tube part of the LMA poses less resistance to respiration than a tracheal tube.

Laryngeal masks are becoming very widely used. Their use is described in the section on airway management below. The laryngeal mask is safe for use in latex-sensitive patients.

THE INTUBATING LARYNGEAL MASK AIRWAY (ILMA)

This relatively new device has begun to be used in adult practice. A size 3 is currently available which could be useful for larger children. Instead of the usual soft grille in the bowl of the mask there is a stiffer bar to lift the epiglottis. The tube part of the mask is made of a curved metal tube that has a handle to facilitate introduction into the mouth, but remains outside the patient when in position. A straight silicone tracheal tube is then introduced 'blind' through the ILMA. The anatomical differences between smaller children and adults, particularly the long epiglottis in children, may make this device more difficult to use even if developed for smaller children.

TRACHEAL TUBES AND CONNECTORS

Despite the vastly increased use of the LMA, the gold standard for airway management remains the tracheal tube. The narrowest part of the child's upper airway is the cricoid ring. The cricoid cartilage is round and the lumen of the airway is therefore round in cross-section at this point. A cylindrical tracheal tube, also round in cross-section, should therefore easily give a snug fit. The tube will be in light contact with the airway over a reasonable length without the need for a cuff. The cricoid ring is the only part of the airway entirely surrounded in cartilage. It is thus less yielding than the vocal cords to a tube that is too big. Also, because of the surrounding cartilage, any oedema of the airway will cause narrowing into the lumen of the airway at this point. A consequent increase in resistance and reduction in flow will occur as a result of oedema. For example, a 6-month-old infant with an internal diameter at the cricoid ring of 4 mm and with 1 mm of oedema around the circumference of the ring will have a 75% decrease in the area of the cricoid ring. Thus, airway oedema from damage by too large a tracheal tube must be avoided. The size of the tracheal tube is therefore very important, especially in children below about 8 years of age. An excellent description of this will be found in Eckenhoff's paper.[53]

Size of tracheal tube

From the discussion above it is obvious that the external diameter of the tracheal tube to avoid oedema is important. The largest internal diameter possible, however, will provide least resistance to gas flow. An ideal tube, therefore, should be relatively thin walled. Tube sizes are chosen from a formula for the internal diameter. Thick-walled tubes, e.g. armoured tubes, may not follow the general rules. Although the formulae are a useful guide, tube sizes 0.5 mm above and below the predicted sizes should also be prepared. Above the age of 2 years a useful formula is:

$$\text{Internal diameter (in mm)} = \frac{\text{Age (in years)}}{4} + 4.5$$

[The original formula plus 4 was for thicker walled, red-rubber tubes; the above formula is for polyvinyl chloride (PVC) tubes.]

Although there has been some recent interest in the use of cuffed tubes in children, as discussed below, most paediatric centres still use uncuffed tubes in the first 8 years of life. A correctly sized uncuffed tube should have a small audible leak around the tube when 20 cm of water pressure is applied from the breathing system. This is clinically the best guide to a correctly sized tube, although interobserver variation has been demonstrated.[54] A tube with no leak or a tube with an excessive leak should be changed accordingly up or down half a size following this test.

There is no easily remembered guide to tube sizes below 2 years of age. The age and weight of the baby will be relevant: normal-sized, full-term neonates of 3–3.5 kg will usually take a size 3.5 tube; smaller babies of 2–3 kg will take a size 3 tube; babies smaller than 2 kg may require a 2.5 tube; from 3 months to about

1 year a size 4 will be required and by 2 years a size 4.5.

Some have suggested that an approximate guide to tracheal tube size is to use the size of the index finger as a guide to the external diameter of the tube. This has been shown to be unreliable and the same authors have confirmed that the formula for above 2 years of age gives good sizing.[55] Length of the child was shown by Keep and Manford to be the best guide to the appropriate size but this is not widely used as length is slightly less convenient to measure than the child's weight.[56]

Length of tracheal tubes

The length of the tracheal tube is critical in paediatric practice as bronchial intubation occurs all too easily. The following formulae are useful:

Length = age/2 + 12 cm for oral tubes.

Length = age/2 + 15 cm for nasal tubes.

Uncuffed tubes also have a black marker, which if lined up with the vocal cords should give the correct length through the cords. Another guide is that the number of centimetres of tube through the cords should be the same as the internal diameter of the tube. The correct position of the tube should be confirmed by capnography, auscultation and, if for longer term ICU use, by chest X-ray as well.

Cutting tracheal tubes to length requires reinsertion of the connector. The connector can be damaged by rotational forces causing narrowing of the lumen and even total obstruction. Even with uncut tubes the connector should be slightly advanced into the tube as they are transported from the manufacturer with a loose connection. Some institutions therefore use uncut tubes and this allows the tube to be positioned in the patient rather than being committed to a precut length. This will leave a length of tube protruding from the child's mouth. Care must be taken, as the tube will be easily kinked in the length outside the mouth. This is more likely to happen where a warming device is used, as the warmth softens the tube.

Use of cuffed tubes in small children

Recently, there has been renewed interest in using cuffed tubes in small children. It has been shown that using small cuffed tubes in children may be satisfactory and indeed reduces the number of postoperative airway problems by eliminating the need for repeat laryngoscopy for incorrect tube sizes. High-volume, low-pressure cuffs are used to minimize the possibility of ischaemic damage to the mucosa of the cricoid region. Cuffed tubes may be particularly useful for those with non-compliant lungs.[57,58] For cuffed tubes the formula: Age (in years)/4 + 3 is used.

Suction catheters

The narrower lumens of paediatric tubes can easily become obstructed. This is especially likely to occur where excessive lubricant has been used on the tube. Suction catheters need to be available and the size is French gauge of suction catheter = twice the internal diameter in mm of the tracheal tube.[59]

Type and size of tube for children above 8 years

In the older child (above about 8 years old) and adult the narrowest part of the airway is the rima glottidis, that is the ligamentous vocal cords anteriorly and the vocal processes of the arytenoid cartilages posteriorly. These structures are not round in cross-section. Thus, a tube which is round in cross-section and small enough to fit through the narrowest part of the rima glottidis easily will have a large leak around it. An inflatable cuff will be required to create a good fit below the vocal cords. Cuffed tubes have a cuff to be inflated with air and the cuff will lie below the vocal cords. The size of tube will not relate to formulae above this age, but the size of the patient (both height and weight) will be considered.

Types of tube

The availability of PVC tubes has superseded the use of other reusable tubes in most parts of the world. These tracheal tubes are implant tested for allergens and the implant test number is stated on the tube.[60] The sizes range from 2 to 10. The size relates to the internal diameter in mm. There is a radiopaque line to demonstrate the length and position of the tube on X-rays. Where PVC tubes are unavailable red-rubber tubes can be used. Tubes are connected to the breathing system by a standard 15-mm ET tube connector. The end of the connector introduced to the tube is variable in size to fit the tracheal tube size. Plain PVC tubes are used in most anaesthesia, but in some situations modification of the tube is necessary.

RAE tubes were first described by Drs Ring, Adair and Elwyn.[61] These preformed shaped tubes are widely used for surgery to the head and neck. The wall of the trachea can obstruct the bevel in a standard tube if the head is flexed. RAE tubes have two Murphy eyes (side holes) to allow ventilation if the tube is advanced too far into the trachea or if the head is flexed. Occasionally, RAE tubes of the appropriate size are too long. The tube can be withdrawn slightly, a swab taped under the tube at the chin and then the tube secured. The bent shape is designed to improve fixation to the chin with the connector well away from the face.

Cole shouldered ET tubes are still used in some neonatal units.[62] The tube has a wide diameter in the mouth and only narrows to the correct diameter of the child's airway at the part of the tube that will be through the cords. Cole tubes are generally discouraged in anaesthesia as damage to the larynx can occur if the tube slips downwards. However, Cole tubes are occasionally extremely useful as their extra stiffness may help to intubate a baby with a difficult airway.

Special tubes for laser work

As PVC tubes are readily ignited by lasers special tubes are required (see Chapter 17).

Armoured tracheal tubes

For neurosurgery procedures, prone patients and other situations where there may be a lot of head and neck movement, armoured tubes are used. These have a coil of stainless steel embedded in the wall of the tube. It should be remembered that tube sizes are chosen by internal diameter and armoured tubes are thicker walled. The join of the tube with the connector may kink, as the wire stops just short of the connector insertion. As these tubes are so flexible they frequently require a malleable introducer or stylet to aid intubation.

Cricothyroid puncture

Equipment for cricothyroid puncture should be available in the dreadful event of total airway obstruction where a tracheal tube is not able to be passed and a clear airway cannot be obtained with other airway manoeuvres or by inserting a laryngeal mask. Rigid bronchoscopes will occasionally be needed, e.g for children with possible intrathoracic tracheal compression (see Chapter 17).

Tracheal tube connectors

Fortunately, the huge range of connectors previously encountered is largely obsolete. Plastic standard 15-mm connectors are now used to connect the tube to the breathing system in all theatre situations, despite the increased resistance from turbulent flow at the site of the connector joint with the tube. This seems to have little clinical significance. The connectors are specifically sized at the tracheal tube end to fit individual tube sizes. Torsional forces when inserting the connector can cause the plastic of the connector to bend and impinge or even totally occlude the lumen of the tube.[63] Several systems with connectors of 8.5-mm diameter exist for intensive care use. A huge variety of fixation methods also exists.It is safest to use a standard method in each unit rather than having a variety according to the individual clinician's preference. Nasal tubes are usually used in intensive care and fixation of nasal tubes tends to be more secure.

Catheter mounts

Catheter mounts to join the tube connector to the breathing system are not often used in paediatric anaesthesia because of the large increase in dead space.

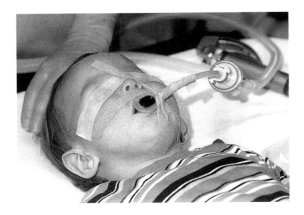

Figure 6.10 Fixation of the tracheal tube.

Tube fixation in anaesthesia

Secure tube fixation cannot be overemphasized. Positioning a Guedel airway alongside a plain oral tracheal tube may help to stabilize the tube. The authors' current practice is to use two pieces of strong sticky tape, cut in 'trouser shape', both connected to the tube and one side connected to the mandible the other to the maxilla. Several points of fixation, to the chin, to the forehead and fixing the breathing system to a board, will help to prevent transmitted movement to the larynx (Figure 6.10).

LARYNGOSCOPES

There is a bewildering choice of laryngoscopes for all types of anaesthesia. The anatomical considerations of the paediatric airway should be taken into account.

POSITION OF THE LARYNX

The larynx is more cephalad in the infant than in the adult. In adults the rima glottis is at the level of the interspace between the fourth and fifth cervical vertebrae. In infants it is opposite the third to fourth interspace.

SHAPE OF THE EPIGLOTTIS

The epiglottis is relatively long, stiff and U- or V-shaped. It approximates a 45° angle from the anterior pharyngeal wall. In the adult the epiglottis lies at a lesser angle to the base of the tongue. The reason for this difference in angle is that the infant hyoid bone is attached to the thyroid cartilage. An excellent review of the infant larynx will be found by Eckenhoff.[53]

The relatively high larynx with long epiglottis means that infants younger than 6 months are easier to intubate with the straight-bladed laryngoscope. The long epiglottis will be lifted by the blade of the laryngoscope. The laryngoscope is usually advanced into the mouth as far back as possible and then gradually withdrawn until the cords come into view. The straight-bladed laryngoscope therefore does not sit in the vallecula as a curved blade does and so the straight blade is in contact with the posterior surface of the epiglottis. The posterior surface of the epiglottis is innervated by the vagus nerve and therefore this technique may be associated with bradycardia during laryngoscopy.

The head should be level with the bed and in very small babies with large heads the shoulders may have to be raised. A head ring may be used to stabilize a wobbly head.

Older children above 6 months to 1 year become intubatable with the standard curved blade advancing along the tongue and into the vallecula, pulling the epiglottis and tongue forwards along the line of the laryngoscope handle.

The blades essentially differ in cross-section and longitudinal shape (Figures 6.11–6.14). Therefore, a sensible choice of blade can be made with the above considerations in mind. Intraoral manipulation, e.g. of a nasal tube, is restricted by the use of a blade with a C shape in cross-section. Similarly, a Cole tube may be difficult to position through a laryngoscope with this cross-sectional shape. In the infant with a cleft palate this type of blade may be most appropriate to prevent the laryngoscope continually slipping into the cleft.

The adjustable hook on the Magill Anderson scope may allow easier manipulation of the handle and can allow the anaesthetist to manipulate the larynx with the fifth digit of

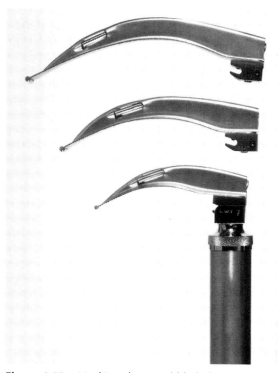

Figure 6.11 Laryngoscope blades in cross section.

Figure 6.12 Mackintosh curved-blade laryngoscope, adult and child.

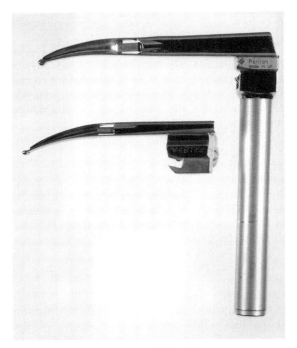

Figure 6.13 Seward straight-blade laryngoscopes.

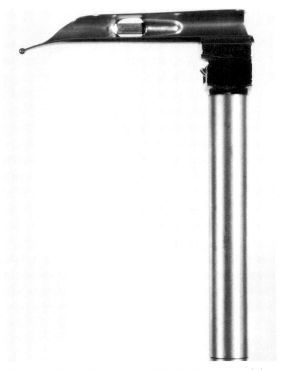

Figure 6.14 Wisconsin straight-blade neonatal laryngoscope.

their left hand. In special circumstances other types of blade will be required. Very short blades may not improve the intubating conditions for babies. Polio blades (with a large angle between the blade and the handle) and McCoy blades (with a hinged blade to lift up the epiglottis) are now available in paediatric sizes and may be helpful in some circumstances.

Laryngoscopes are reusable and care must be taken to clean them thoroughly between cases. Some authors have found contamination with blood. Disposable blades have recently become available.

For other reviews of paediatric airway equipment see Refs 10 and 60.

VASCULAR ACCESS

TOPICAL ANAESTHESIA

The use of topical local anaesthetic creams prior to cannulation is now the standard of care in paediatric anaesthetic practice.[64] It has meant that intravenous induction of anaesthesia is becoming the method of choice in many centres.[65] There are two local anaesthetic creams commercially available at present. EMLA cream (eutectic mixture of local anaesthetic) is a 5% mixture of lignocaine and prilocaine in a 1 : 1 ratio, formulated into an oil-in-water emulsion. It should be applied to intact skin under an occlusive dressing for at least 1 h to be effective. A thick deposit is said to be more effective than a thin layer and efficacy increases with application time. After 30–60 min skin blanching may be seen as a result of vasoconstriction, which can make intravenous cannulation more difficult. Skin erythema due to vasodilatation is seen if EMLA cream is left on for a long period but, in general, local skin reactions are mild and transient. Topical nitroglycerine ointment (0.2 ml of a 0.4% preparation) promotes venodilatation and has been shown to increase the ease of cannulation of EMLA-treated skin in children.[66] Metabolites of prilocaine may convert haemoglobin to methaemoglobin and cause cyanosis.[67] EMLA cream should not be used in children with congenital methaemoglobinaemia and should be avoided in infants under 1 year who are taking methaemoglobin-inducing drugs (paracetamol, phenytoin and nitroprusside).[65] Methaemoglobin is converted back to haemoglobin by the enzyme methaemoglobin reductase, which does not reach full activity until after the age of 3 months. It has been suggested that EMLA cream should be avoided in children younger than 3 months of age.[68]

Amethocaine is an effective local anaesthetic for topical use. It is highly lipid soluble and highly protein bound, thus forming a depot at the site of action. A 4% gel formulation of amethocaine is now commercially available (Ametop gel). It penetrates the skin more effectively, and has a shorter onset time and a more prolonged duration of action than EMLA.[69] It should be applied as a thin layer to the skin under an occlusive dressing for at least 45 min prior to cannulation. There is a high incidence of erythema (37% in the study by Lawson), so the gel should be removed after 90 min and the skin site marked. It has a prolonged duration of action (4–6 h), far in excess of EMLA cream (30–60 min). It is less toxic than EMLA as it is metabolized by non-specific esterases in the skin and systemically and may be used in infants from 6 weeks of age. It has a vasodilatory action that may result in the high incidence of erythema reported. It is an ester local anaesthetic. These drugs have a fairly high incidence of allergic reactions, which may prove to be the main disadvantage of Ametop gel.[64]

In general, when using local anaesthetic cream, it is sensible for the anaesthetist to identify and mark suitable veins during the preoperative visit. Neither cream will be effective if it not applied over a vein. It should not be forgotten that foot veins are useful in children if the veins on the hands do not look very promising. There have been case reports of children licking off the local anaesthetic cream, swallowing the occlusive dressing or inadvertently rubbing the cream in their eyes.[65] A bandage should be placed over the occlusive dressing to prevent this.

PERIPHERAL VENOUS CANNULATION

An 'open vein' is mandatory for all children undergoing anaesthesia. It is used for drug and fluid administration and possibly for sampling of venous blood. Intravenous access should be obtained prior to induction of anaesthesia in emergency cases, in children requiring fluid resuscitation, neonates and obviously in those for whom intravenous induction is planned. In healthy children for whom an elective gaseous induction technique is planned, it is acceptable to obtain intravenous access after induction, assuming there is second competent individual to manage the airway.

There is a wide variety of cannulae available, usually made of inert material with low frictional resistance such as Teflon, polyurethane or silicone. A 22G cannula is sufficient for fluid and drug administration in most infants. Smaller 24G cannulae may be useful if venous access is difficult, but may necessitate the use of infusion pumps for viscous fluids such as blood. Larger cannulae will be required if rapid transfusion of fluid is anticipated in older children. It is a sensible precaution to obtain two sites of intravenous access for all but minor surgery, especially if there has been some difficulty with the first line. Access will be considerably more difficult to obtain if this line tissues and the child is draped and covered on the operating table. It is useful to have a dedicated peripheral line for drug administration when PCA or NCA is being used. It is also sensible to obtain venous access above the level of the surgery. For example, there is no point in replacing massive blood loss during the excision of a Wilm's tumour via a long saphenous line at the ankle.

The site chosen for cannulation depends on the age of the child.[70] Neonates have little subcutaneous fat and their veins, although fragile, are usually easily visible. Transillumination of the tissues with a 'cold light' may aid cannulation in the very small premature infant. The veins in chubby toddlers are often more easily felt than seen. Veins in older children, as in adults, are more superficial. The hand and foot veins (including the ventral aspect of the wrist) are commonly used in children of all ages, with an assistant either squeezing the wrist or using one hand for this and the other to insert the cannula. Hand veins are the most convenient to cannulate in the awake patient. Scalp veins may be used in children under 1 year in age. They are not ideal for several reasons. It is difficult to secure a scalp vein cannula and it may be dislodged during airway manipulations such as intubation. The veins are fragile and tissue easily; forehead veins should be avoided as unsightly facial scars may result. Vessels over the fontanelle should be avoided, as should inadvertent cannulation of the superficial temporal artery. The long saphenous vein is extremely useful in paediatric anaesthesia. It is a large vein and lies immediately anterior to the medial malleolus, and is often more easily felt then seen. Forearm veins are useful in older children, as in adult practice.

The presence of an experienced assistant to help with obtaining intravenous access is invaluable. If the child is awake, a parent to comfort and distract the child will be helpful. Small children may be cuddled on the parent's lap, which may make it possible to obscure the cannulation process from the child's view; however, some may prefer to watch. The assistant should gently immobilize the site of cannulation to prevent the child withdrawing, and gently squeeze the limb to cause venous distension (but not arterial occlusion) (Figure 6.15). It is sensible to hold the limb below the level of the heart to avoid emptying the veins.[71] A child's skin is extremely mobile in relation to the underlying vein and a crucial function of the assistant is to stretch the skin lightly to fix the vein. A transfixion technique is often useful, especially for larger veins, as the elastic tissues

of the child are much more 'forgiving' than those of the adult. Loosening the cap of the cannula will make it easier to detect when a vein has been entered. If a vessel is transfixed, the needle should be withdrawn from the cannula, and the cannula slowly pulled back until there is a free flow of blood. The cannula is then advanced up the vessel, possibility with some gentle rotation or the use of saline flush.[70]

After venous access has been achieved, the cannula should be secured firmly. It is sensible to use a short extension tube with a three-way tap to minimize interference with the cannulation site. Of the numerous techniques used to secure cannulae, it has been suggested that taping the hub of the cannula and the intravenous tubing to which it is attached will reduce the risk of inadvertent dislodgement.[72] The use of non-sterile tape is not associated with any increase in infective complications compared with sterile dressings.[73] Burettes are usually used for fluid administration in paediatric practice so that fluid volumes can be accurately monitored. As the burettes cannot be pressurized to increase the rate of fluid administration (unlike a bag of fluid as used in adult practice), it is important to consider access to lines after the child is draped in theatre. A long extension with a three-way tap should be attached to long saphenous vein lines, so that fluid may be pushed in by syringe if required. The dead space of lines should be taken into consideration and all lines flushed after drug administration. This is particularly important if undiluted drugs are used; the injection port of a venflon will contain sufficient suxamethonium, for instance, to reparalyse an infant on the ward if not flushed after initial administration. Attention to air in intravenous lines is important; air bubbles may have important clinical effects on small infants with right to left shunting.

It has been suggested that peripheral cannulae can remain *in situ* for up to 6 days with careful handling.[74] However, they are often associated with complications, particularly in the neonatal population. Common problems include phlebitis, extravasation and bacterial colonization. Far more worrying have been case reports of damage to the tibial growth plate as a consequence of extravasation injuries involving the long saphenous vein, such that leg lengthening procedures were required years after the

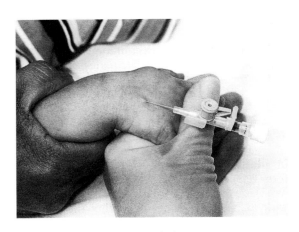

Figure 6.15 Venous cannulation.

original injury.[75] Peripheral lines should be monitored carefully and consideration given to obtaining central access for certain drugs and hyperosmolar fluids. Extravasation injuries should be assessed urgently, preferably by a plastic surgeon. Locally administered hyaluronidase will facilitate the clearance of the extravasated fluid.

CENTRAL VENOUS CANNULATION

Insertion of short-term percutaneous central venous cannulae is indicated for the infusion of inotropic or resuscitative drugs or hyperosmolar fluids, or for central venous pressure monitoring. Tunnelled central lines are commonly used for the administration of long-term therapy in children, for instance, chemotherapy and long-term total parenteral nutrition. The veins commonly used for central access are the internal jugular vein, the femoral vein, the subclavian vein and the external jugular veins. Antecubital fossa veins are used for the insertion of peripherally inserted central (PICC) lines, which are useful when medium-term intravenous access is required, for instance for limited parenteral nutrition or antibiotic administration.[76]

For percutaneous central access the Seldinger technique using a guidewire is commonly used. There are many commercially available central venous percutaneous access kits for use in children, with single-, double- and triple-lumen catheters of varying lengths (including 5, 8, 12 and 16 cm). Catheters are available from 4 Fr for use in neonates. Venous access is initially obtained, often with the use of a short 20G cannula. The guidewire is inserted through the cannula, the cannula removed and the vein dilated leaving the guidewire in place. The catheter is then passed over the guidewire into the vein. It is important to secure the catheter in place with sutures, particularly in the toddler population. This procedure should be undertaken under general anaesthesia except in exceptional circumstances.

The incidence of complications is higher in children than in adults. Possible complications include local and systemic infection, venous or arterial bleeding, arterial puncture, thrombosis, phlebitis, pulmonary thromboembolism, hydrothorax, haemothorax, pneumothorax, cardiac tamponade, arrhythmias, air embolism and catheter embolism.[77] The incidence of complication depends on the site (lowest with femoral vein cannulation and highest with subclavian vein cannulation) and the experience of the operator. An audit of paediatric anaesthetic practice in a paediatric centre in 1990 indicated that 86% of percutaneous lines were inserted into the internal jugular vein, 10% into the femoral and 3.5% into the subclavian veins. The early complication rate was 14.7%, mainly due to failure to cannulate a vessel at the chosen site, particularly in children under 5 kg. Failure to obtain venous access at any site was seen in 1% of cases. The major complication rate was 0.9% (mainly pneumothorax). Late complications were mainly associated with sepsis.[78]

The approach to the internal jugular vein is usually from the right side of the neck, a direct route to the right atrium that avoids damage to the thoracic duct. A sterile technique is mandatory. The child is placed in a head-down position with a roll under the shoulders and the neck turned to the left. Gentle pressure on the liver will further distend the neck vessels. The triangle formed by the two heads of sternocleidomastoid is identified. A short 20G cannula with a 2-ml syringe attached is inserted at the apex of the triangle and directed towards the ipsilateral nipple, gently aspirating as the cannula is advanced. The vein should be entered after 1–3 cm, depending on the size of the child. A transfixion technique may be used. Anterior and posterior approaches to the internal jugular vein may also be used.[77] Ultrasound has been used to evaluate the internal jugular vein anatomy of children up to 6 years undergoing cardiac surgery. Anomalous venous anatomy was found in 18% of children. In the majority, the internal jugular vein was anterolateral to the internal carotid artery. In 10% the vein ran medially to overlie the artery, in 4% the vein was unusually small and in 2% the vein ran widely lateral to the artery. In 2% of cases the vein could not be identified at all. A portable battery operated ultrasound scanner was used to visualize the internal jugular vein and mark its projection on the overlying skin. The time and number of needle insertions required to obtain venous access were reduced compared with the conventional blind insertion technique.[79] The use of ultrasound should certainly be considered if veins have been used previously and there is any doubt about their patency. The subclavian vein may be used as an alternative to the internal jugular vein. A cannula will enter the subclavian vein if passed underneath the clavicle from the junction of the lateral and middle thirds towards the suprasternal notch. There is a higher incidence of complications using the subclavian than the internal jugular route in children.

The tips of central venous catheters should be placed in or above the right atrium. Case reports of fatal right atrial perforation have been described, leading to the suggestion that catheter tips should be placed in the superior vena cava and that their position should be checked by radiological means.[80] Electrocardiographic (ECG) monitoring has been used to guide central line placement. An ECG electrode is attached to the catheter system, the typical intra-atrial tracing is identified when the catheter tip is in the right atrium and the catheter is withdrawn until the trace changes. The technique can be used in theatre, thus making radiological control unnecessary.[81] Long-term silastic central venous catheters (see below) are often placed with the tip of the catheter in the right atrium.[82] This may facilitate sampling from the line, reduces the risk of thrombus formation and is associated with a lower incidence of catheter migration.[83]

Femoral venous cannulation has a high success rate, a low complication rate and an infection rate comparable to catheters inserted at other non-femoral sites[84]. A sandbag is placed under the buttock to stretch the groin crease and make the vein more superficial. The vein lies immediately medial to the femoral artery. An aseptic technique should be used. Common complications of the technique include inadvertent arterial puncture (14%) and catheter-related sepsis (1–4%).[84] Swelling of the leg may occur, mainly in younger patients (3–4 Fr catheters should be used in babies). More serious complications of femoral vein catheterization have been described, including septic arthritis of the hip joint.[70] Cannulation of the epidural venous plexus via the ascending lumbar vein (a branch of the common iliac vein) has also been described, with fatal consequences.[85] It should always be possible to aspirate blood from a correctly placed central

venous catheter. Loss of the ability to aspirate blood and a central course of a femoral line over the spinal canal on X-ray, rather than the expected path to the right of the midline, should alert one to the possibility of this unusual complication.

The axillary vein has been suggested as a route for access to the central circulation using 24G silastic microcatheters.[86] If the axillary vein is inadvertently punctured with a short rigid cannula during attempts at axillary artery cannulation, the cannula should probably be withdrawn as these catheters may erode through the vein into the pleural space.[87]

Intraosseus infusion was used as the method of choice for fluid administration in the 1940s but fell out of use with the advent of disposable intravenous catheters in the 1950s.[88] The bone marrow is essentially a non-collapsible vein and the intraosseous route provides rapid, safe and effective access to the circulation for drugs and fluids.[89] Intraosseous access is a simple technique to perform and is used during paediatric resuscitation in children under the age of about 6 years if venous access is not achieved within 90 s. Its use in anaesthetic practice is more controversial. The intraosseous route can be safely used to administer any fluid or drug required during resuscitation (except for bretylium). The use of neuromuscular blocking drugs, atropine, crystalloids, colloids and blood has been described. Chemically irritant drugs such as thiopentone should not be given through an intraosseous needle. It is possible to draw bone marrow from an intraosseous needle for estimation of haemoglobin, electrolytes and blood gases. There are many complications associated with intraosseous needles, although all are rare. They include subperiosteal or subcutaneous infusion, growth plate injury, cellulitis, osteomyelitis, fractures and compartment syndrome requiring amputation.[88] It may be an invaluable technique in the 'veinless' child for whom other access has proved impossible.[90] It is particularly useful for fluid administration before a definitive line can be obtained. Intraosseous lines are easily dislodged and should not be relied upon as the sole venous access for a surgical procedure.[91]

The preferred site for intraosseous access is the flat anteromedial aspect of the proximal tibia, 1–3 cm below the tibial tuberosity. A purpose-designed disposable intraosseous needle should be used. The needle is inserted through the skin and passed through the bony cortex of the tibia. The needle is directed away from the epiphyseal plate in a caudal direction. It is advanced with a firm twisting motion until there is a sudden 'give'. Confirmation of position in the bone marrow is made if the needle can stand upright without support, marrow can be aspirated (although this is not always possible) and fluid flows freely through the needle (by gravity) without evidence of subcutaneous infiltration[77] (Figure 6.16).

Intensive treatment of children with oncological, haematological and complex medical conditions requires reliable intravenous access for extended periods, often for several years. Access is required for the administration of chemotherapy agents, blood products, total parenteral nutrition, therapeutic drugs and blood sampling. Tunnelled silastic catheters are used, which may have external catheters (Broviac or Hickman lines) or be fully implanted systems (Portacath). They are commonly single- or double-lumen catheters. They may be inserted percutaneously by interventional radiologists or anaesthetists, or by open procedure by surgeons. A full description of technique is beyond the scope of this chapter. There are important points to note, however. A survey of practice in an Australian centre indicated that one-third of all lines were removed because of infection,[83] whereas only one-third of lines were removed because they were no longer required. A recent survey of line use in UK Children's Cancer Study Group (UKCCSG) oncology centres indicated that 26% of central lines inserted over a 6-month

period were reinsertions, although the reasons for line failure were not noted.[82] The most common source of bloodstream infection associated with lines appears to be micro-organisms colonizing the hub of the catheters. Medical staff handling lines should be aware of this fact, and pay careful attention to sterile technique, which should include cleaning catheter hubs with 2% chlorhexidine prior to use. Lines should be carefully flushed after drug administration and are commonly flushed with heparin-containing solutions. Wide-bore implanted catheters used for dialysis (Permacaths) are instilled with concentrated heparin after use. The heparin must be aspirated before the line is next flushed as it is otherwise possible inadvertently to anticoagulate fully a small infant, for instance. Care should also be taken when administering anaesthetic drugs through these lines as they may have a dead space of up to 2 ml, depending on the size of the child and the length of the catheter.[92] All anaesthetic drugs should be carefully flushed with at least 10 ml of saline after administration and it is probably sensible practice to avoid the use of muscle relaxants via this route.

ARTERIAL CANNULATION

Arterial cannulation is indicated when direct arterial monitoring is required, such as when the planned surgical procedure has the potential for extensive blood loss or circulatory insufficiency, for critically ill patients and where repeated blood gas estimation is required.

Percutaneous arterial lines may be placed in the radial, femoral, axillary, brachial, dorsalis pedis and posterior tibial arteries. The radial artery is the preferred site as it is easily accessible. Small cannulae should be used (24G in the neonate, 22G in older children) and a strict aseptic technique employed. The vessel may be transfixed or punctured directly, or a Seldinger technique employed; fine wires are available for use with a 22G cannula. Adverse side-effects include transient or permanent ischaemic damage to the hand. The incidence is increased by the use of large cannulae relative to the size of the vessel and with prolonged duration of cannulation. A Doppler flow study in newborn infants demonstrated complete occlusion of the radial artery

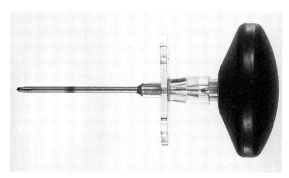

Figure 6.16 Intraosseous needle.

in 63% of infants after removal of a radial artery catheter. Blood flow resumed in the artery 1–29 days after catheter removal in all cases.[93] In older children the postocclusion rate varies from 8 to 38%. Severe thrombotic sequelae including ischaemic necrosis of the hand and fingers have been reported [75]. It may be helpful to evaluate the collateral blood supply to the hand before radial artery cannulation is attempted, using a modified Allen test or Doppler flow studies, although the Allen test is more useful in children. Distal circulation should be carefully monitored after insertion of an arterial line and the line removed if there are concerns. Thrombolysis, anticoagulation or vascular repair should be considered in the event of thrombotic complications.[75] A continuous infusion of heparinized saline (1–2 ml h^{-1}, 1 IU heparin ml^{-1}) improves the patency of radial artery catheters. It is particularly important to label arterial lines clearly in the operating room. The administration of drugs such as antibiotics via the arterial route will have disastrous effects. For this reason, cannulae with injection ports should not be used for arterial lines.

Catheterization of more central arteries such as the femoral artery or axillary artery is an alternative in small infants or critically ill infants with poor peripheral perfusion. There is good collateral blood supply around both of these vessels, so problems secondary to distal ischaemia are uncommon. Arterial spasm may occur, particularly in smaller infants, and is related to the size of the cannula used. The cannula should be removed in this situation. Serious complications such as limb shortening have been described, but mainly after cardiac catheterization, when larger cannulae are used as a routine. In this situation, arterial occlusion has been reported in up to one-third of patients.[94]

The technique for femoral arterial catheterization is similar to that for venous cannulation, with the artery easily palpated lateral to the vein. Catheterization is performed under sterile conditions using a 20G or 22G gauge cannula depending on the age of the child. An audit of femoral arterial lines in critically ill infants and children indicated a high success rate for insertion and a low complication rate. Complications included haematoma formation or minor bleeding at the puncture site, often associated with inadvertent venous puncture. Distal pulses were reduced in 7% of cases, all in children younger than 1 year. There was no evidence of distal ischaemia and all pulses returned to normal within 10 days. It is important to monitor the distal circulation in all children with an arterial line *in situ*.[84]

Percutaneous cannulation of the axillary artery is well described. It has been recommended particularly in critically ill children with vascular collapse where more peripheral arteries may not be palpated or may not give an accurate reflection of central pressures.[95] The tip of the cannula lies in close proximity to the heart and great vessels, so particular care should be taken when flushing lines. Complications of axillary artery cannulation include direct injury to the brachial plexus or axillary sheath haematoma. The incidence appears to be low.

CONSERVATION OF HEAT

Temperature control is an important consideration in paediatric anaesthesia. There are situations in which hypothermia may be beneficial, for instance in patients at risk of ischaemic neurological injury[96] and during hypothermic cardiopulmonary bypass. However, in the main, mild intraoperative hypothermia is undesirable and has been shown to be associated with many adverse effects. It increases sympathetic stimulation, promotes shivering and increases patient discomfort. It has been associated with impaired immune function and delayed wound healing, impaired coagulation and platelet activity, increased blood loss and transfusion requirements, decreased drug metabolism and delayed discharge from recovery, even when temperature is not a discharge criterion.[97]

HEAT LOSS

Hypothermia during anaesthesia occurs in two distinct phases. There is an initial large decrease in body temperature, with a slower reduction in temperature thereafter. The initial fall in temperature may be up to 1°C and is the result of anaesthesia-induced vasodilatation with mixing of cool peripheral blood and warmer core blood. The temperature then falls at a rate of 0.5°C h^{-1} in the absence of active warming.[98,99] Most of the continuing losses occur as a result of loss of heat to the environment, although anaesthesia also results in a decrease in metabolic heat production and adaptive responses to heat loss (see below).

Heat loss to the environment takes place by the mechanisms of radiation, convection, evaporation and conduction. Approximately 90% of all heat is lost through the skin, with the remaining loss from the respiratory tract and from surgical incisions. Evaporative losses from wounds may become significant with large incisions,[97] particularly in small children.

Radiant heat loss from the skin is proportional to the temperature difference between the patient and the environment and accounts for 40–50% of the body's total heat loss in the operating room. Convective heat losses represent 25–35% of heat loss from a patient lying uncovered in a modern air-conditioned operating theatre.[100] Evaporative losses may occur from the skin, respiratory tract or open body cavities as described above. Evaporative losses will obviously be greater if the child is allowed to become wet (e.g. during cystoscopy with bladder irrigation). Evaporative heat and water losses may be significant in premature neonates, especially if nursed under radiant heaters. Conductive losses are probably the least significant source of heat loss in a modern operating theatre, although care should be taken to prewarm under-patient gel mattresses.

MEASUREMENT OF BODY TEMPERATURE

Continuous monitoring of body temperature should be part of standard monitoring in paediatric anaesthetic practice. Different tissues have different temperatures but temperature measurements are usually described in terms of 'central' (core) or 'peripheral' (skin) temperature. Thermocouple thermometers or thermistors are commonly used to monitor core temperature. Nasopharyngeal temperature probes are widely available but may underestimate core temperature in the presence of a

significant leak around the tracheal tube. Oesophageal stethoscopes and urinary catheters may have temperature probes incorporated into them. Bladder temperature measurement is invasive and is inaccurate at low urinary flows. Rectal thermometers may be used, but may be inaccurate in the presence of faeces. Traditionally, tympanic membrane temperature is taken as a measure of hypothalamic temperature, the area of the brain responsible for thermoregulation. Care should be taken to avoid tympanic membrane perforation with the use of a thermistor temperature probe. The recently introduced infrared tympanic thermometer is atraumatic and is useful for intermittent temperature measurement, particularly during recovery. Liquid crystal thermometers are for intermittent use and too inaccurate for use in theatre. Measurement of forehead temperature with these thermometers in children has not been shown to reflect accurately changes in core temperature.[101]

PHYSIOLOGICAL RESPONSE TO COLD

Under normal conditions, thermoregulatory responses maintain the core body temperature to within 0.2°C of a set value of approximately 37°C. The thermoregulatory system consists of afferent thermal sensors, central regulation and efferent responses. Afferent thermal sensory inputs come from the skin, deep tissues, spinal cord, non-hypothalamic parts of the brain and the hypothalamus in roughly equal proportions. The hypothalamus integrates the various inputs and triggers specific thermoregulatory responses at fixed threshold temperatures.[97] These responses are aimed at modulating metabolic heat production or altering environmental heat loss. A fall in temperature results in vasoconstriction, shivering and appropriate behavioural responses. Shivering thermogenesis involves an increase in heat production by vigorous contraction of many muscle groups and a 2–3-fold increase in metabolic rate. Infants have a limited ability to shiver but respond by generalized increase in motor activity. Non-shivering thermogenesis is particularly important in infants. It involves the activation of metabolism of specialized adipose tissue rich in mitochondria known as brown fat. It is possible by this means to double the metabolic rate. Brown fat is under sympathetic control and is present at birth, develops for a few weeks after birth and recedes following infancy. Thermoregulatory responses are poorly developed in the preterm neonate, which is said to behave more like a poikilothermic animal.[102] The response to an increase in temperature results in vasodilatation and sweating.

General anaesthesia produces a marked inhibition of thermoregulation. Clearly, behavioural responses are inhibited, but there is also an increase in the threshold for sweating and vasodilatation and a reduction in the threshold for shivering and vasoconstriction, although these responses are still seen at extremes of temperature.[97] Non-shivering thermogenesis is abolished even at low temperatures. Surprisingly, responses to maintain core temperature under anaesthesia appear to be more effective in children than adults, even though children are often considered to be more susceptible to cold environments. This may be due to intense thermoregulatory vasoconstriction or differences in body morphology.[103]

HEAT CONSERVATION: PREVENTION OF HYPOTHERMIA

It is clear that active measures must be taken to conserve heat when anaesthetizing children. Radiation loss from the skin is the predominant source of heat loss during surgery and may be reduced by raising the ambient temperature of the operating theatre. An ambient temperature of 21°C is adequate in larger children, but smaller children and neonates may require an ambient temperature of about 26°C to maintain normothermia. This may result in an extremely uncomfortable working environment for the surgeons. A sensible compromise is to maintain the room temperature at 21°C and concentrate on warming the microclimate around the anaesthetized child.

Simply avoiding exposure of the child is an important means of reducing heat loss and should be remembered even during difficult line insertions in the anaesthetic room. The material used appears to be less important than the total area of skin covered.[104] The relatively large head of small infants represents a large surface area for heat loss and should remain covered if possible. Increasing the number of blankets or

prewarming blankets appears to be of limited benefit.[97]

A number of active patient-warming devices is commercially available. These include electric undermattresses, warm-air undermattresses and forced warm-air convective heating blankets. Forced warm-air heating blankets are the most effective of these.[105] They are so effective at warming the microclimate around the patient that careful monitoring of temperature is mandatory to avoid hyperthermia. These devices should always be used with the sheet provided. This prevents thermal injury and filters the air blown across the patient. Even in the presence of active warming it is difficult to prevent the initial drop in temperature due to vasodilatation after induction of anaesthesia. It has been suggested that preinduction skin warming will reduce the distributive heat loss.[106]

Humidification and warming of dry anaesthetic gas make a minor contribution to heat loss associated with anaesthesia. Nevertheless, humidification of gases should be considered as part of the overall strategy to prevent hypothermia during anaesthesia. Humidification is also important to maintain the integrity of the respiratory epithelium, to maintain ciliary function and mucous clearance and prevent pulmonary complications from thick secretions.[107] Humidification may play a more significant role in the maintenance of body temperature in small infants than in adults as they have greater minute ventilation relative to body weight. Several humidifiers are available. Active humidifiers, such as heated water vapour humidifiers, are commonly used in the intensive care unit. They are the most efficient humidifiers, but the equipment is expensive and complex to avoid the possibility of thermal burns to the airway and overhumidification. In addition, water may condense in the breathing tubing to contaminate the airway and the water bath may act as a source of infection.

The disposable heat and moisture exchangers (HME) are much more convenient to use than water bath humidifiers, are less expensive and are capable of providing physiological levels of humidity.[107,108] They are passive humidifiers and may be classified into condenser, hygroscopic or hydrophobic filters. The condenser humidifiers were the first to be introduced, with the disposable versions containing rolled corrugated microporous paper. They work on the simple principle that water in expired gases condenses on the humidifier material and evaporates during the inspiratory phase. The hygroscopic filters include a chemical means to trap water vapour. The filter material is coated with a hygroscopic substance such as calcium or lithium chloride. The hydrophobic HMEs rely on the principle of condensation only but contain a water-repellent ceramic membrane that is pleated to give a very large surface area for condensation and evaporation. They have been shown to be very efficient as humidifiers and are also efficient bacterial and viral filters. Modern filters have been designed which are composites of hygroscopic and hydrophobic principle.[107] As they act as efficient filters for micro-organisms, it has been recommended that HME filters are used as a routine during every anaesthetic to prevent contamination of the breathing system, particularly where disposable breathing systems are reused.[109] The design of modern HME filters is such they have a small dead space and low resistance. Small-sized filters are available for use in infants and babies but care must be taken to avoid secretions in the filter or an increase in respiratory resistance will ensue.

The reaction of carbon dioxide with soda lime is exothermic and results in the production of water. Circle breathing systems provide an effective means of warming and humidifying anaesthetic gases. However, soda lime has been shown not to have a bactericidal effect so a filter should be used to prevent contamination of the breathing tubing. The rebreathing systems (Mapleson A, D and E) also contribute to airway humidification by allowing rebreathing of fully saturated expired gases.

Rapid fluid administration results in cooling, which may be prevented by the use of prewarmed fluids. There is a number of commercially available devices for use as fluid warmers. The 'Hotline' fluid warmer actively warms fluid in the delivery tubes by a countercurrent mechanism and has been found to be very efficient even at the low flows used for small children.[110]

INDUCTION OF ANAESTHESIA

In addition to the preoperative preparation of the patient described elsewhere, immediately prior to induction the following should be confirmed: patient identification, preparation, starvation, presence of allergies and consent for all procedures, both anaesthetic and surgical. The equipment should have been checked. The drugs and equipment that the anaesthetist is planning to use should have been prepared according to the child's weight. A useful check that the recorded weight is correct is the formula:

$$2 \times age\ (in\ years) + 8$$

to estimate the weight (in kg).[59]

The use of an induction or anaesthetic room has advantages. The advantages include a more child-friendly environment, less noise during induction and hopefully a slightly more peaceful environment for the anaesthetist and the patient. The anaesthesia team is not required to hide behind surgical facemasks, as is the case if a prepared theatre area is used for anaesthetic induction.

Disadvantages are the need for duplicate monitoring equipment and the possibility of the period of disconnection of monitoring whilst going into theatre coinciding with a patient event. In practice this is very rare. The increased number of connections and reconnections of equipment may also compromise the patient.

MONITORING DURING INDUCTION

Where possible, monitoring equipment should be applied before induction commences (Figure 6.17). Children are much more accepting of this than might be expected and indeed they may be less fearful than the elderly of 'high-tech' equipment. The minimum is a pulse oximeter, which should not upset the child unduly and for sicker children additional monitoring should always be applied. It is common practice in the UK to allow one parent to the anaesthetic room until their child is asleep. The parent should have a clear explanation of their role and should

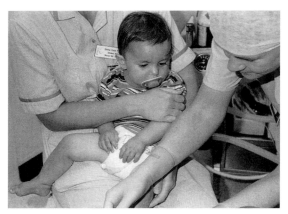

Figure 6.17 Application of monitoring prior to induction of anaesthesia.

be accompanied by a ward nurse or other staff to escort them out of the room, once their child is asleep. The parental presence is generally felt to be helpful but the high maternal anxiety of witnessing the induction should not be underestimated.[111] The anaesthetist should communicate with both the child and parent as much as possible throughout the induction period. It is best to avoid using the terms like 'put to sleep' as children may associate this with family pets not recovering.

It is important that parents realize that accompanying their child is an option for them, and is not compulsory. It is ultimately the decision of the individual anaesthetist but increasingly parents expect to be present for any procedure.

Types of induction

The most common choices for induction in children are either intravenous or inhalational. Both intramuscular and rectal inductions have also been described. These are not widely practised and will only be mentioned briefly.

TECHNIQUE OF INTRAVENOUS INDUCTION

The use of topical anaesthetic creams (see above) has improved the acceptance of intravenous induction. Generally, an indwelling intravenous cannula is used for induction. Very

small 27-gauge needles are available and may be useful if inadequate time for topical anaesthesia has elapsed or if the child has difficult veins and a small vein on the wrist is to be used. The drugs and needles should be prepared before the child arrives in the induction room and should be kept out of sight. The child is distracted by the parent or ward nurse whilst the limb to be used for venepuncture is held. The limb is compressed sufficiently to obstruct venous return but not arterial supply. The skin is also held slightly stretched to help with visualization and ease cannulation of the veins. Good assistants are invaluable; alternatively, the anaesthetist may hold a small child's hand in their own hand and cannulate with the other. Although the upright position may be unsafe for some sick or heavily premedicated infants, the child may be in the parent's lap, in which case it may be possible to wrap their arm or leg around the parent to access the child's limb from behind the parent, keeping the cannulation out of sight. Asking the child to cough just at the point of insertion of the cannula can also distract some children. A quick venepuncture seems to be the least painful, even with topical anaesthetic cream. Following cannulation some children wish to look at the cannula. The anaesthetist can now follow with the intravenous induction agent. The cannula should be both taped securely and held gently by the anaesthetist during injection of the induction agent to stop the cannula becoming dislodged half way through induction. Following induction the child is laid flat (if they are not already lying flat on the trolley) and either anaesthesia is continued with inhalational agents or intravenous anaesthesia is continued by infusion. Any monitoring not applied preinduction should be immediately connected.

CHOICE OF AGENT FOR INTRAVENOUS INDUCTION

Propofol is becoming the most common choice of drug for intravenous induction. The main disadvantage is pain on injection. The addition of lignocaine at a dose of 0.2 mg per 4 mg of propofol improves this. Other measures include warming the drug or mixing it with thiopentone.[112] It is a particularly suitable choice of intravenous agent where a laryngeal mask is to be used. Unfortunately, it is not licensed for those less than 3 years of age. The advantages of propofol, good-quality recovery with low incidence of nausea and vomiting, frequently override the licensing consideration. The dose for induction is in the region of 4 mg kg^{-1}.

Thiopentone gives a very smooth induction without pain on injection. The dose is 5–6 mg kg^{-1}. It remains cheaper than propofol, and is a shorter acting agent in children than in adults.

Ketamine may be chosen for shocked patients, or those with cardiovascular instability or severe asthma. Further discussion of these drugs is in Chapter 4

TECHNIQUE OF INHALATIONAL INDUCTION

To achieve anaesthesia by inhalational induction sufficient vapour must be inhaled by the child to increase the brain concentration. The speed of induction will depend on the minute ventilation of the child and on the properties of the inhalational agent. Agents with low blood gas solubility give a more rapid induction. A higher minute ventilation, for example, in a crying child produces faster induction. The anaesthetic gases are delivered via the breathing system to the patient's face. Some anaesthetists use the breathing system connected directly to the facemask, while others prefer initially to hold the breathing circuit in their hand until the child is unconscious. Nitrous oxide is generally used in a concentration of 70% nitrous oxide with 30% oxygen. Inhalational induction is currently performed with sevoflurane or halothane, depending on availability. The properties of the inhalational agents are discussed fully in Chapter 3. Sevoflurane is the agent of choice as it causes less cardiovascular depression than halothane, and gives a smooth induction.[113] The technique of starting with an immediate high concentration, overpressure as opposed to incremental increases, is successful with both these agents. The author currently uses 8% sevoflurane until the eyelash reflex has disappeared and then switches to isoflurane for the maintenance of anaesthesia.[114] Isoflurane is a cheaper alternative for maintenance. If the child is asleep on arrival in the induction room it is probably better to waken them than to

attempt to induce without disturbing them. This avoids the child either waking up during the induction or becoming very distressed afterwards.

Isoflurane and enflurane are less suitable for inhalational induction. Both have a pungent odour and need to be used with slow incremental increases in concentration to avoid airway irritability.

A number of modifications has been suggested to improve the acceptance of inhalational induction. These include altering the smell of the agents. Initially, people used a variety of pleasant-smelling oils. However, there was concern about the potential toxicity of these oils. Facemasks impregnated with non-toxic smells are now available but the introduction of inhalational anaesthetics to the inspired gases will generally become the dominant smell. Sevoflurane is said to be the most pleasant smelling; certainly, induction with sevoflurane does seem to be associated with less struggling than with other agents.[114]

INTRAVENOUS INDUCTION VERSUS INHALATIONAL INDUCTION

A smooth inhalational induction carried out by an anaesthetist quietly talking to a calm child is very satisfactory. Similarly, a slick intravenous cannulation using topical anaesthesia, followed by the administration of an intravenous induction agent whilst talking to the child is satisfactory induction. Sadly, these two ideal situations cannot always be achieved. What are the advantages and disadvantages of these two types of induction?

SAFETY

Hypoxia

Audits[115,116] of hypoxia during induction have shown an increased incidence of hypoxia during intravenous induction. However, in these audits preoxygenation of the patients was not used.

Therefore, only the children having inhalational induction received supplemental oxygen during induction. Subsequent work has shown that preoxygenation during intravenous induction with propofol can reduce the hypoxia.[117]

The length of time to desaturate is dependent on age.[118] Even with preoxygenation small children will begin to desaturate extremely quickly. Any episode of coughing or laryngospasm may result in hypoxia. Coughing or laryngospasm is more likely during inhalational induction. The choice of inhalational drug significantly alters this. Sevoflurane or halothane is currently the best choice to avoid this.[114]

The practice of inducing anaesthesia by inhalation and then obtaining venous access with the child asleep works well where there are two experienced anaesthetists. It is not a good choice of technique where an inexperienced person has to look after the airway, whilst the more experienced looks for venous access. This is particularly so where difficulty with venous access is anticipated. Difficulty obtaining access can lead to hypoxia at worst and the anaesthetist being distracted from finding a vein at best. There are two alternatives. The first is to give an intramuscular muscle relaxant following induction and intubate the paralysed child. Alternatively, the child is intubated under deep inhalational anaesthesia, prior to establishing intravenous access. This practice is not appropriate, however, for some sick patients, such as those with unstable cardiac disease. For either type of induction the child should be examined carefully preoperatively to find the best site for venous access.

In the child with the difficult airway or partial airway obstruction an inhalational induction is regarded by most anaesthetists as the safest option so that spontaneous respiration is maintained; intravenous induction is more likely to lead to apnoea. The depth of anaesthesia can be controlled by adjusting the concentration of the inhalational agent. Definitive airway management takes place without muscle relaxants. In this circumstance intravenous access should precede induction to allow the administration of drugs and fluids. Although halothane in oxygen is the best described method in this situation, there are now several case reports of the successful use of sevoflurane.[119,120]

Overdosage of drugs

Intravenous induction can cause inadvertent overdose when the required dose is miscalculated. It is good practice to draw up in the syringe only that dose of anaesthetic agent that you calculate that patient will require plus a small extra amount to cover interpatient variability. Similarly, high concentrations of volatile agent can be equally depressant on the cardiovascular or respiratory systems. This can occur unexpectedly during induction or if a much higher concentration of volatile agent than the patient requires is continued after induction. Thus, overdosage of drugs is possible with either technique

Psychological effects

The childhood memory of an inhalational induction is often vivid, even into adulthood. It can be the cause of recurrent nightmares.[121] Children having an inhalational induction, even if they appear calm at the time, have more negative memories of induction of anaesthesia and hospitalization, compared with children who have had an intravenous induction.[122]

Intravenous induction is well accepted with the use of topical anaesthetic and has the advantage that the experience the child most fears (i.e. 'the needle') is complete before they go off to sleep. Intravenous access is usually obtained on the first attempt with practice and may lead to less needle phobia in the long term. Recent work suggests that even a calm, premedicated child having a smooth perioperative course may have nightmares and behavioural problems following their hospital episode. A recent study has shown that premedication with midazolam may even make this worse.[123]

Children's choice

Where children are offered either type of induction many will choose intravenous. Others will be afraid of needles and request an inhalational induction. The anaesthetist can have quite an influence over their choice. Needle-phobic children may have their fears further reinforced by the avoidance of needles, so that as they get older it may be beneficial to spend time with them and aim for intravenous induction.

Environmental pollution

During induction the technique of holding, the breathing system in the anaesthetist's hand will lead to high concentrations of anaesthetic in the induction room. The parent or nurse holding the child should be encouraged to keep their face away from the breathing circuit. Pollution during paediatric anaesthesia and therefore occupational exposure has been shown to be higher during paediatric anaesthesia. It has also been shown that induction is the time of maximum pollution. Gas flow should be turned off when the breathing system is not applied to the patient.[124]

Failure

It is less common to fail to induce anaesthesia by the inhalational route; however, the time taken may be prolonged if the child is not co-operative and the anaesthetist has difficulty maintaining contact with the child's face. Failure can be due to an incorrect gas delivery system or an inability to keep the end of the breathing system close enough to the patient's face. For successful intravenous induction there has to be secure venous access. If the attempt at cannulation fails, the choice is to attempt to repeat the cannulation or to convert the induction to an inhalational one. Where the topical cream has worked well, the choice will usually be to make a second attempt at intravenous line insertion.

Pain on injection

Although pain-free intravenous cannulation is possible with topical anaesthesia, the child may experience pain from the injection, particularly with propofol. Inhalational induction is not painful but a significant number of children find it unpleasant.

Positioning the child for induction

It can sometimes be easier to reach one limb of the child to obtain intravenous access than to have unobstructed access to the face for inhalational induction. The period of time required for immobilization is short for intravenous cannulation, but will be 2 min for inhalational induction. A small child of up to about 15 kg can be seated on the parent's or nurse's lap for either type of induction but the speed of induction should be explained to the parent. They should be advised to support the child's head. It also saves time and embarrassment to state which way round on the trolley you wish the parent to place their child when induction is complete. Unconscious children over about 15 kg can prove difficult to lift on to the trolley, as well as potentially damaging the backs of anaesthesia personnel. Children with cardiovascular instability should not be induced sitting up and in any child there should be a reasonably swift transition to the supine position as soon as anaesthesia is induced.

Movements during induction

Movements during induction are distressing for the parents. Such movements are most common during inhalational induction, but also occur with propofol. The movements induced by propofol can look unnatural, but can be avoided by giving a large bolus of propofol quickly. Padded sides on the induction and recovery trolley can help to prevent injury from these abnormal movements.

The choice of induction is a balance of the risks and benefits. The previous experience of the child, the 'normal' practice in the hospital and the individual anaesthetist's preference are all factors which will influence the choice. As a variety of patients with different conditions and requirements will be met, a paediatric anaesthetist should be able to carry out both intravenous and inhalational induction smoothly and efficiently. The anaesthetist should be able to judge the situations where a particular type of induction is indicated.

Intramuscular induction

Intramuscularly administered drugs can be used for induction of anaesthesia. Ketamine in a dose of up to 10 mg kg^{-1} has been used. Intramuscular injections are very infrequently used in paediatrics as the pain of injection cannot be alleviated by topical anaesthesia. This method of induction is very rarely used.

Rectal induction

Rectally administered barbiturates can be used to induce anaesthesia, e.g. methohexitone 10% in a dose of 15 mg kg^{-1}. The drug can be introduced into the rectum via a soft catheter. Anaesthetic induction will be slower than with other techniques. Rectal thiopentone can also be used but may lead to prolonged recovery.

RAPID SEQUENCE INDUCTION IN CHILDREN

In the UK the accepted technique for dealing with the patient with a full or potentially full stomach is to perform a rapid sequence induction. This technique is believed to prevent aspiration of gastric contents:

1 the patient is preoxygenated;
2 anaesthesia is induced and muscle relaxation achieved rapidly with a predetermined dose of thiopentone, immediately followed by suxamethonium;
3 cricoid pressure is applied throughout the induction;
4 inflation of the lungs is avoided, as this may also inflate the stomach;
5 the patient remains oxygenated from the store of oxygen in the functional residual capacity, and by apnoeic oxygenation from the facemask;
6 the patient is intubated and the cuff of the tracheal tube inflated until there is an airtight seal;
7 the patient's lungs are inflated to check for a seal;
8 finally, the cricoid pressure is released.

Whilst rapid sequence induction is widely practised in the UK, it is not practised in the remainder of Europe, nor in many other parts of the world. Assuming that rapid sequence induction is a useful technique (which it may not be), there are aspects in the child that merit further consideration.

1. WHO SHOULD BE CONSIDERED AT RISK?

Children with a full or potentially full stomach

Children who require emergency surgery where insufficient time has elapsed from the last oral intake are considered at highest risk. But the question as to what constitutes a safe time interval is vexed. It has been shown in animals that a gastric pH < 2.5 and a stomach volume > 0.4 ml kg^{-1}, if aspirated, can give rise to aspiration pneumonia. However, the majority of children presenting for emergency surgery have a gastric pH < 2.5 and will have a volume > 0.4 ml kg^{-1}, even after a period of starvation.[125] Even amongst starved children, presenting for elective surgery, 21% have gastric pH < 2.5 and volume > 0.4 ml kg^{-1} g. This study found that a low pH and high gastric volume did not correlate with anxiety.

Thus, there is no time which constitutes a safe interval between last ingestion, ingestion to injury interval and anaesthesia. Bricker *et al.* observed that the most likely time for vomiting is on emerging from anaesthesia.[125]

It has been shown in children that metoclopramide is effective in increasing gastric emptying and that sodium citrate is effective at increasing the pH of the gastric contents. Neither of these measures is widely used in children.

Children with gastro-oesophageal reflux

Children with known gastro-oesophageal reflux are another interesting group where practices vary. Wetzel[126] observed that in the USA these children are treated as being at high risk for aspiration, and anaesthetized with a rapid sequence induction. In contrast, in the UK inhalational induction with or without cricoid pressure is practised.

2. PREOXYGENATION

Distressed children become hypoxic following induction of anaesthesia more quickly than those who are calm. The small child will desaturate much more quickly than the older child or adult following preoxygenation.[118] This is because although their functional residual capacity may be similar in ml kg^{-1}, their oxygen consumption is greater. Therefore, the safe duration of apnoea is shorter and preoxygenation may not prevent hypoxia following induction. Hypoxia may ensue before the relaxants have worked sufficiently to allow intubation. If attempts at preoxygenation distress the child, further attempts may even be counterproductive by increasing oxygen consumption. Thus, in paediatric practice most anaesthetists only attempt preoxygenation in co-operative children. Paediatric anaesthetists also gently inflate the lungs after induction with oxygen via a facemask, with cricoid pressure applied until they are ready to intubate. Hypoxia is a very potent stimulator of vomiting during induction and some paediatric anaesthetists would argue that a smooth inhalational induction with cricoid pressure applied as the child loses consciousness is a better way of preventing aspiration than a rapid sequence induction. It should be noted that if oral atropine is used as premedication for inhalational induction, one of its side-effects is to decrease the lower oesophageal sphincter pressure. This decrease in pressure does not occur with intramuscular atropine.

3. CRICOID PRESSURE

The cricoid cartilage is well formed in children, including neonates, and cricoid pressure, as described by Sellick, has been shown to be effective in cadaveric studies.[127] These authors also showed that nasogastric tubes should be left *in situ* as they allow the stomach to decompress, and do not make cricoid pressure ineffective. Nasogastric tubes should be aspirated in several positions to increase emptying of the stomach but they cannot be relied on to empty the stomach.

The cricoid cartilage should be palpated before anaesthesia is induced so that the assistant knows where to apply pressure. Poorly applied cricoid pressure can make intubation much more difficult.

It should be remembered that children with trauma might have a neck injury, and therefore great care should be taken in positioning the head. In children, as opposed to adults, the top three cervical vertebrae are most likely to be injured. It should also be kept in mind that a normal X-ray does not rule out spinal instability.

4. USE OF UNCUFFED TUBES

One of the tests of a correctly fitting tube in children under 8 years is that a small leak is audible at 20 cmH$_2$O. It is thus theoretically possible for any regurgitated stomach contents to make their way past this 'seal'. In practice, the area of the tube in contact with the larynx and the application of positive pressure ventilation prevent this occurrence. Although most paediatric anaesthetists use uncuffed tubes in young children, there has been some recent interest in revisiting the use of cuffs, leaving them deflated unless the leak is excessive or where the risk of aspiration is particularly high. There has been little evidence to suggest that the use of cuffed tubes during anaesthesia causes significant airway damage.

Thus, in summary there is no standard technique for dealing with the child with the potential to aspirate, and the attempt to practice a rapid sequence induction may be counterproductive.

AIRWAY MANAGEMENT

One of the most important skills for an anaesthetist is airway management. This is especially important for paediatric practice. Infants and young children are more vulnerable to upper airway obstruction during anaesthesia than adults.[128] Much of the excess morbidity associated with paediatric anaesthesia, compared with adult, is due to airway problems[8]. Thus, most anaesthetized children require intervention to ensure a clear airway. This may be necessary at any time, including recovery from anaesthesia.

The choice of airway management depends on the age of the patient, the type of procedure to be undertaken and particular patient characteristics. The proposed mode of ventilation is also important. The choices for airway management are: a facemask, with or without the addition of an airway, a laryngeal mask airway (LMA), a tracheal tube, or other more complex options such as tracheostomy.

The modes of ventilation which can be used are spontaneous, intermittent positive pressure ventilation (IPPV) or assisted spontaneous respiration. Positive end-expiratory pressure (PEEP) or continuous positive airway pressure (CPAP) can be added to all of these modes.

AIRWAY OPENING MANOEUVRES AND THE APPLICATION OF A FACEMASK

The least invasive, but not necessarily the simplest, technique for airway management is with a facemask and airway opening manoeuvres. The child should be supine. Below the age of about 6 years the airway is easier to maintain without a pillow supporting the head. The facemask is applied to the face with the thumb and forefinger whilst the other fingers gently lift the chin. The anaesthetist must avoid pressing on the floor of the mouth, as the tongue will be compressed against the roof of the mouth, causing airway obstruction. The fingers should only be placed on the mandible (Figure 6.18). This technique of airway management is used initially in all types of anaesthesia. Additional airway adjuncts, such as oropharyngeal or nasopharyngeal airways, may be necessary. A sufficient depth of anaesthesia must be obtained before attempted insertion of these airways.

Occasionally, partial airway obstruction will occur during induction. Stridor may be heard or observation of the patient shows that the respiratory effort exceeds the movement of the reservoir bag. This can be improved by applying a small amount of positive pressure via the breathing circuit and extending the head on the neck to stretch the trachea. These manoeuvres prevent the trachea collapsing inwards.

Positive pressure ventilation can also be achieved with a facemask with a good seal. The duration of positive pressure ventilation through a facemask is limited, as gastric distension occurs. Any degree of airway obstruction will exacerbate this and good technique is therefore important. Gastric distension will cause splinting of the diaphragm and therefore decreased compliance of the lungs. Positive pressure ventilation via a face-

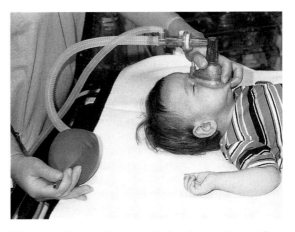

Figure 6.18 Application of the facemask avoiding compression of the soft tissues of the floor of the mouth.

mask is in practice limited to the time waiting for muscle relaxation prior to intubation, or in resuscitation situations prior to definitive airway management. A gastric tube may be required following facemask ventilation to empty the air from the stomach.

Anaesthesia may be maintained during a short procedure using a facemask, with the patient breathing spontaneously. This is unsuitable for children younger than about 6 months, as anaesthesia reduces their tidal volume and airway closure occurs during spontaneous respiration. The exception in the very young is during an extremely short procedure. Above the age of 6 months procedures of up to about 20 min can be maintained in this way. The anaesthetist's hands are not free for any other tasks and surgical access to the face is limited.

USE OF THE LARYNGEAL MASK

Since its introduction into clinical practice the laryngeal mask has gained widespread popularity. The design is shown in Figure 6.8 and the sizes appropriate for paediatric age groups are given in Table 6.2. The laryngeal mask, when in position, sits around the glottis. It does not go through the vocal cords. The aim of positioning the mask is to obtain a seal around the glottis. No special equipment is required for positioning.[52] Initially, the LMA was used for cases where a facemask would be suitable. With increasing confidence the number and types of use have increased enormously. For example, the LMA is now used for longer procedures where breathing is spontaneous and for cases where positive pressure ventilation is needed. Some authors have shown a learning curve in the use of the LMA, while others found similar results for experienced and inexperienced users.[129–132]

A clinically patent airway is obtained in up to 98% of cases, although fibreoptic study of LMA[130] positioning in paediatric patients has shown that the epiglottis lies within part of the mask or is downfolded in 49% of patients. In 19% of patients there was partial airway obstruction, and in 2% complete obstruction. This is a higher incidence than in adults. Other radiological studies have shown that even when the position seems less than ideal, clinical airway patency is acceptable. Mason and Bingham's study[131] has shown a 97.5% success in its use. One of the causes of failure in their study was inadequate depth of anaesthesia.

It should be remembered that the catheter mount which is commonly used in adults to attach the LMA to the breathing circuit will greatly increase the dead space in children.

Insertion technique

Many insertion techniques are described, with and without introducers. The likelihood of a clinically satisfactory placement is unaffected by the insertion technique.

Two main techniques have gained widespread acceptance in paediatric practice; the first technique is that described by Dr Brain.[52] The mask should be completely deflated. The anaesthetist opens the patient's mouth and introduces the mask with a downward force. The mask should then follow the contours of the oropharynx. When resistance is felt the cuff of the mask is inflated via the pilot cuff and the mask is seen to slightly move upwards. An alternative insertion technique is described by McNichol.[133] The mask is introduced partially inflated and upside down, and then rotated through 180° into position. With either technique the black line along the posterior part of the tube will confirm the correct final orientation of the mask.

Anaesthetic depth required for mask insertion

1 *Intravenous induction.* Propofol provides very good conditions for the insertion of the laryngeal mask. The dose of propofol (4 mg kg^{-1}) to allow induction of anaesthesia and insertion of the laryngeal mask is greater in children than in adults.[134] Where thiopentone is used for induction, anaesthesia needs to be deepened with a volatile agent, as the pharyngeal structures are still responsive. The incidence of desaturation following intravenous induction can be avoided by preoxygenating the child during induction.

2 *Inhalational induction.* A suitable depth of anaesthesia for insertion of the laryngeal mask can be obtained in children following inhalational induction. Jaw relaxation and small centrally placed pupils give a good guide that anaesthesia is sufficiently deep for LMA insertion.

3 *Awake LMA insertion.* This has been described using topical local anaesthesia in the management of Treacher–Collins syndrome. Awake LMA insertion is not widely practised. The new intubating LMA (ILMA) has been inserted awake and offers an alternative to awake fibreoptic intubation.

Other uses of the laryngeal mask airway

The LMA can be invaluable in dealing with the difficult paediatric airway. Many children who have airways that are otherwise difficult or impossible to maintain can be managed with the LMA (see Chapter 17).

There is a vast experience using the LMA in prone patients, for example in the short procedures of radiotherapy treatment with the patient prone. If the device is dislodged it is easier to slip the LMA back into position than a tracheal tube. Even in patients requiring marked head and neck movement during the procedure the laryngeal mask can maintain a stable position. Some authors suggest the use of an antisialogue premed with the LMA, but this is not widely practised.

The laryngeal mask can also be used for positive pressure ventilation. Gastric distension does not occur at airway pressures up to 20 cm H_2O positive pressure.[135] Other research has shown a slight increase in abdominal girth using positive pressure and an LMA; however, muscle relaxants were not used in this study.[136] This technique is becoming more widely used.

The LMA has been described for resuscitation situations, including neonatal resuscitation.[137] A more rapid establishment of ventilation can occur than with bag and mask ventilation.

Contraindications to the laryngeal mask airway

The LMA cannot be expected to protect the airway from gastric contents, and is therefore contraindicated in those at risk of aspiration. However, airway protection from secretions and blood from the mouth may be better with an LMA than with an uncuffed tracheal tube, for example during tonsillectomy or adenoidectomy.

Removal of the laryngeal mask airway

The LMA is removed when swallowing returns and the child will open their mouth. The old adage that 'it doesn't matter whether you extubate deep or awake, so long as you do one or the other' also holds true for laryngeal masks. The depth of anaesthesia required to tolerate the LMA *in situ* is less than for a tracheal tube, therefore the child may never be sufficiently 'deep'. It has been shown that fewer complications occur on awakening if the LMA is left *in situ* until the child responds to voice. Others have shown lower complication rates if the mask is removed deep, but in some studies halothane was used prior to extubation, whereas isoflurane is currently more likely to be used for maintenance.[138–140] Again, the usual practice of the hospital has an influence on the success of the technique. It may be that where there is possible airway soiling it is better to leave the mask *in situ* until the patient is wide awake. Bite blocks should be used with the laryngeal mask, to prevent airway obstruction if the patient bites on the tube part of the LMA. A rolled-up swab with tape around it provides a very satisfactory block. Dental damage can occur in children with loose teeth during

removal of an LMA if the mouth is not adequately open.

Studies comparing airway maintenance between the facemask and LMA during maintenance of anaesthesia have shown that the LMA requires fewer airway manoeuvres and provides a more reliable airway. In comparison with tracheal intubation the LMA produces fewer airway problems in children with non-compliant lungs and compares favourably with an ET tube in ENT procedures including adenotonsillectomy.

Laryngospasm remains a possibility during airway maintenance with the LMA if there is an inadequate depth of anaesthesia.

INTUBATION

The most reliable method for maintaining a clear airway in anaesthesia is the tracheal tube. Anaesthesia may proceed with spontaneous respiration or IPPV.

The types of tube available are described above. The tracheal tube will be introduced through the vocal cords into the trachea. To allow the tube through the cords anaesthesia must be sufficiently deep or muscle relaxants are given. Awake intubation in infants is no longer a recommended technique. A suitable laryngoscope will be required, a straight blade for young infants and a curved blade for those above six months. The position of the patient is the single most important factor in facilitating intubation. The head should be slightly extended on the neck and the neck should be flexed. Small children will have relatively larger heads and therefore this position is easier to obtain without a pillow. Older children and adults require a pillow for the ideal intubating position.

Usually a muscle relaxant will be given intravenously to facilitate intubation following induction of anaesthesia

The use of intramuscular relaxants for intubation

Occasionally, the situation arises where intubation is required in a child who does not have any intravenous access. Intramuscular relaxants can be used. Suxamethonium is traditionally used for the speed of onset. Interestingly, Liu *et al* found that the dose required was 4 mg kg^{-1}, although many use only 2 mg in clinical practice.[141,142] The same authors also showed that clinical help was obtained before maximum twitch depression on nerve stimulation. Rocuronium has also been used intramuscularly and gives intubating conditions in 2.5 min for infants at a dose of 1 mg kg^{-1} and in 3 min for older children with a dose of 1.8 mg kg^{-1}.[142] The same authors found the deltoid muscle the most reliable for speed of onset of intramuscularly administered drugs. The use of muscle relaxants is discussed in detail in Chapter 5.

Intubation can also be facilitated by a combination of propofol with alfentanil. This is a good combination where spontaneous respiration is planned for the procedure as suxamethonium, which would otherwise be used but has many side-effects, can be avoided.

Where deep inhalational anaesthesia is used for intubation a sufficient depth of anaesthesia must be reached prior to laryngoscopy. Ideally, intravenous access should also be established. Intubation can be obtained with sevoflurane in 100–335 s.[143] The most reliable guide to time of intubation was found to be small, centrally placed pupils.[144] Others have found smooth intubating conditions with sevoflurane 5% in oxygen at 200 s. Sevoflurane has also been used for inhalational induction in croup.[119,120]

COMPLICATIONS

Although a tracheal tube provides a reliable airway, problems can occur. The length of the tube is critical to avoid bronchial intubation. The tube may become blocked by blood or secretions. Constant vigilance by the anaesthetist is still required even with a tracheal tube in place. The position should be confirmed by capnography, auscultation and patency by monitoring the airway pressures.

EXTUBATION

The timing and method of extubation are as important as intubation to avoid airway problems such as laryngospasm. Prior to extubation the pharynx should be suctioned to ensure that there are no secretions or debris in the mouth. Extubation can be performed awake or deep but never between the two. Deep extuba-

tion means that the volatile is continued in 100% oxygen when the surgical procedure is complete and after pharyngeal suctioning the tube is removed with the child in the lateral position. The airway will be unprotected until the airway reflexes return. The child must be breathing spontaneously at this time. Any airway problems that do occur are likely to do so in the recovery room, probably when the anaesthetist is starting the next case. Alternatively, the child can be woken up with the tracheal tube in place and the trachea extubated when they open their eyes. It may be helpful for both types of extubation to apply a positive pressure to the airway during extubation to blow any secretions from around the tube upwards into the pharynx. Awake extubation is problematic in patients where coughing is undesirable, e.g. neurosurgical patients, but in most other situations is more satisfactory. An oral airway, facemask and assistant are all required for safe extubation.

LARYNGOSPASM

This is defined as glottic closure due to a reflex constriction of the laryngeal muscles. It is much more common in paediatric anaesthesia than in adults. Olsson and Hallen[145] showed the incidence to be twice that of adults in older children, and three times in younger children. Airway complications are further increased in children with upper respiratory tract infections, and in those passively exposed to cigarette smoke.[146,147] In the paediatric patient the oxygen consumption is greater and so the consequences of laryngospasm in children are more serious. The oxygen consumption is highest in the youngest patients.

Laryngospasm seems to occur during anaesthesia for two reasons: firstly, a lack of inhibition of glottic reflexes because of central nervous system depression and, secondly, increased numbers of stimuli – such as manipulation of the airway, secretions or blood irritating the cords, and stimulation of visceral nerve endings at an inadequate depth of anaesthesia.

Laryngospasm may be partial or complete. Partial spasm will be diagnosed by a characteristic stidulous noise and a mismatch between the patient's respiratory effort and the disappointingly small movements of the reservoir bag. Methods for overcoming laryngospasm include the application of positive pressure to the airway, deepening anaesthesia, administering muscle relaxants or a bolus dose of propofol. Recently, it was found that a bolus dose of propofol works extremely quickly, without the risks of bradycardia or other side-effects from suxamethonium. The exact mechanism of action of propofol is not clear, but it could be due to increasing the depth of anaesthesia or a direct effect on glottis. Where there is complete laryngospasm there will be silence. The application of positive pressure may not be helpful in these circumstances and indeed may make the situation worse by forcing the false cords against the tightly closed true cords. It is much better to relax the cords before hypoxia is severe. Suxamethonium can be given either intravenously or intramuscularly. Severe bradycardia can occur. A bolus dose of propofol 1–2 mg kg^{-1} is an alternative.

THE ANAESTHESIA PLAN

It is important to have a clear anaesthesia plan prior to embarking on an anaesthetic in a child. The appropriate equipment and competent assistant should be available. The parent should be appraised of his or her role in the proceedings and should be appropriately supported by a member of the nursing staff. Preoperative checks must be completed. The method of induction should be chosen, although some flexibility is always advisable. An analgesia plan should be formulated and preferably instituted before the start of surgery. Multimodal analgesia is sensible, with a combination of simple analgesics (non-steroidal analgesics) and local anaesthetic techniques (local blocks or central blocks), with opioids used if appropriate. The type of surgery and local facilities must be taken into account. It is important to consider the side-effects of the analgesia technique. For instance, it is only appropriate to use an opioid in a caudal block for hypospadias repair if the child is to remain catheterized at the end of the procedure, since there is a significant incidence of retention of urine. The incidence of

nausea and vomiting is age related and antiemetics should be used in older children if an opioid-based technique is employed. Methods of pain relief will be discussed fully in a later chapter. The choice of spontaneous ventilation versus controlled ventilation for maintenance of anaesthesia depends on the nature of the surgery, the duration of the procedure and the age of the child. It is perfectly acceptable to have a child breathing spontaneously for a procedure of moderate duration, provided the surgery is peripheral and does not interfere with respiratory mechanics. The child should be breathing through a low-resistance breathing system with a secure airway (e.g. a laryngeal mask and a T-piece system), ideally with moderate CPAP applied. Controlled ventilation should probably be employed when using a circle system for younger children and infants.

The importance of the continuous presence of an ever-vigilant anaesthetist cannot be overemphasized. Complications associated with anaesthesia in children occur as commonly during maintenance of anaesthesia as during induction or the immediate postoperative period.[148] The importance of secure fixation of tubes and lines is obvious when a small child is covered by surgical drapes and relatively inaccessible, as is access to a three-way tap for rapid administration of fluids if a non-compressible paediatric burette for fluid administration is used. Monitoring of the child, equipment, the progress of surgery, blood loss and fluid replacement must be continuous, and effected by both clinical means and the appropriate monitoring technology where applicable. Monitoring should be continued after extubation and into the recovery phase, until the child's clinical condition is stable. Monitoring will be discussed fully in a later chapter. Finally, it is important to keep a clear, complete and contemporaneous record. This should include a record of the preoperative assessment, results of investigations and consent for invasive procedures. Details of induction and maintenance technique should be noted, with a record of cardiorespiratory variables, fluid balance and temperature. Electronic recording methods will be a great advance in this area.

REFERENCES

1 Ayre, P. Anaesthesia for an intracranial operation. *Lancet* 1937; **i**: 561–3.

2 Campling, E.A., Devlin, H.B. and Lunn, J.N. *Report of the National Enquiry into Perioperative Deaths.* London: NCEPOD, 1989.

3 McNicol, R Paediatric anaesthesia – who should do it? The view from the specialist hospital. *Anaesthesia* 1997; **52**: 513–15.

4 Rollin, A.-M. Paediatric anaesthesia – who should do it? The view from the district general hospital. *Anaesthesia* 1997; **52**: 515–16.

5 Thornes, R. Just for the Day: Children admitted to hospital for day treatment. Caring for Children in the Health Services (NAWCH). London: NAWCH Ltd, 1991.

6 British Paediatric Association. The transfer of infants and children for surgery: Report of the Joint Working Group, 1993.

7 Sumner, E. Editorial: Paediatric anaesthesia *Paediatric Anaesthesia* 1994; **4**: 1–2.

8 Cohen, D. and Godinez, R. Pediatric anaesthetic apparatus. *International Anesthesiology Clinics* 1992; **30**: 25–35.

9 Ward, C. (ed.). *Ward's Anaesthetic Equipment.* London: WB Saunders, 1998.

10 Hatch DJ. Paediatric anaesthetic equipment. *British Journal of Anaesthesia* 1985; **57**: 672–84.

11 Charlton, A.J., Lindahl, S.G.E. and Hatch, D.J. Ventilatory responses of children to changes in deadspace volume. *British Journal of Anaesthesia* 1985; **57**: 562–8.

11a Conway CM. Anaesthetic breathing systems. British Journal of Anaesthesia 1985; **57**: 649–57.

12 Hatch, D.J. Anaesthesia and the ventilatory system in infants and young children. *British Journal of Anaesthesia* 1992; **68**: 398–410.

13 Coté, C.J. Pediatric breathing circuits and anesthesia machines. *International Anesthesiology Clinics* 1992; **30**: 51–61.

14 Conway, C.M. Anaesthetic breathing systems. *British Journal of Anaesthesia* 1985; **57**: 649–57.

15 Miller, D.M. Breathing systems reclassified. *Anaesthesia and Intensive Care* 1995; **23**: 281–3.

16 Meakin, G. and Perkins, R.J. Anaesthetic breathing systems for children. *Paediatric Anaesthesia* 1996; **6**: 346.

17 Mapleson, W.W. The elimination of rebreathing in various semiclosed anaesthetic systems. *British Journal of Anaesthesia* 1954; **26**: 323–32.

18 Willis, B.A., Pender, J.W. and Mapleson, W.W. Rebreathing in a T-piece: volunteer and theoretical studies of the Jackson–Rees modification of Ayre's T-piece during spontaneous respiration. *British Journal of Anaesthesia* 1975; **47**: 1239–46.

19 Lack, J.A. Theatre pollution control. *Anaesthesia* 1976; **31**: 259–62.

20 Meakin, G., Jennings, A.D., Beatty, P.C.W. and Healy, T.E.J. Fresh gas requirements of an enclosed afferent reservoir breathing system in anaesthetised, spontaneously ventilating children. *British Journal of Anaesthesia* 1992; **68**: 333–7.

21 Jackson Rees, G. Anaesthesia in the newborn. *British Medical Journal* 1950; **2**: 1419–1422.

22 Spears, R.S., Yeh, A., Fisher, D.M. and Zwass, M.S. The 'educated hand'. Can anesthesiologists assess changes in neonatal pulmonary compliance manually? *Anesthesiology* 1991; **75**: 693–6.

23 Froese, A.B. and Rose, D.K. A detailed analysis of T-piece systems. In: Steward, D.J. (ed.). *Aspects of Paediatric Anaesthesia.* Amsterdam: Excerpta Medica, 1982; 101–36.

24 Lindahl, S.G.E., Hulse, M.J. and Hatch, D.J. Ventilation and gas exchange during anaesthesia and surgery in spontaneously breathing infants and children. *British Journal of Anaesthesia* 1984; **56**: 121–9.

25 Hatch, D.J., Yates, A.P. and Lindahl, S.G.E. Flow requirements and rebreathing during mechanically controlled ventilation in a T-piece (Mapleson E) system. *British Journal of Anaesthesia* 1987; **59**: 1533–40.

26 Badgewell, J.M., Heavner, J.E., May, W.S., Goldthorn, J.F. and Lerman, J. End-tidal PCO_2 monitoring in infants and children ventilated with either a partial rebreathing or a non-rebreathing circuit. *Anesthesiology* 1987; **66**: 405–10.

27 Miller, D.M. Early detection of rebreathing in afferent and efferent breathing systems using capnography. *British Journal of Anaesthesia* 1990; **64**: 251–5.

28 Bain, J.A. and Spoerel, W.E. A streamlined anaesthetic system. *Canadian Anaesthetists Society Journal* 1972; **19**: 426–35.

29 Humphrey, D. A new anaesthetic system combining Mapleson A, D and E principles. *Anaesthesia* 1983; **38**: 361–72.

30 Orlikowski, C.E.P., Ewart, M.C. and Bingham, R.M. The Humphrey ADE system: evaluation in paediatric use. *British Journal of Anaesthesia* 1991; **66**: 253–7.

31 Cotter, S.M., Petros, A.J., Doré, C.J., Barber, N.D. and White, D.C. Low-flow anaesthesia. Practice, cost implications and acceptability. *Anaesthesia* 1991; **46**: 1009–12.

32 Baum, J.A. and Aitkenhead, A.R. Low-flow anaesthesia. *Anaesthesia* 1995; **50**: 37–44.

33 Baxter, A.D. Low and minimal flow inhalational anaesthesia. *Canadian Journal of Anaesthesia* 1997; **44**: 643–53.

34 Perkins, R. and Meakin, G. Economics of low-flow anaesthesia in children. *Anaesthesia* 1996; **51**: 1089–92.

35 Rasch, D.K., Bunegin, L., Ledbetter, J. and Kaminskas, D. Comparison of circle absorber and Jackson Rees systems for paediatric anaesthesia. *Canadian Journal of Anaesthesia* 1988; **35**: 25–30.

36 Conterato, J.P., Sten, G.E., Lindahl, G.E., Meyer, D.M. and Bires, J.A. Assessment of spontaneous ventilation in anesthetized children with the use of a pediatric circle or a Jackson–Rees system. *Anesthesia and Analgesia* 1989; **69**: 484–90.

37 Fröhlich, D., Schwall, B., Funk, W. and Hobbhan, J. Laryngeal mask airway and uncuffed tubes are equally effective for low-flow or closed system anaesthesia in children. *British Journal of Anaesthesia* 1997; **79**: 289–92.

38 Logan, M. Breathing systems: effect of fresh gas flow rate on enflurane consumption. *British Journal of Anaesthesia* 1994; **73**: 775–8.

39 Frink, E.J., Green, W.B., Brown, E.A., *et al.* Compound A concentrations during sevoflurane anaesthesia in children. *Anesthesiology* 1996; **84**: 566–71.

40 Mazze, R.I. and Jamison, R.L. Low flow (1 l/min) sevoflurane: is it safe? *Anesthesiology* 1997; **86**: 1225–7.

40a Peters, J.W.B., Bezstarosti-van Eeden, J., Erdmann, W. and Meursing, A.E.E. Safety and efficacy of semi-closed circle ventilation in small infants. *Paediatric Anaesthesia* 1998; **8**: 299–304.

41 Mushin, W.W., Mapleson, W.W. and Lunn, J.N. Problems of automatic ventilation in infants and young children. *British Journal of Anaesthesia* 1962; **43**: 514–22.

42 Newton, N.I., Hillman, K.M. and Varley, J.G. Automatic ventilation with the Ayre's T-piece. *Anaesthesia* 1981; **36**: 22–36.

43 Hatch, D.J., Chakrabarti, M.K., Whitwam, J.G., Bingham, R.M. and Mackersie, A.M. Comparison of two ventilators used with the T-piece in anaesthesia. *British Journal of Anaesthesia* 1990; **65**: 262–7.

44 Barrie, J.R., Meakin, G., Campbell, I.T., Beatty, P.C.W. and Healy, T.E.J. Efficiency of the Carden 'Ventmasta' in A and D modes during controlled ventilation in children. *British Journal of Anaesthesia* 1994; **73**: 453–7.

45 Badgewell, J.M., Swan, J. and Foster, A.C. Volume controlled ventilation is made possible in infants by using compliant breathing circuits with large compression volume. *Anesthesia and Analgesia* 1996; **82**: 719–23.

46 Stevenson, G.W., Tobin, M.J., Horn, B.J., *et al.* The effect of circuit compliance on delivered ventilation with use of an adult circle system for time cycled volume controlled ventilation using an infant lung model. *Paediatric Anaesthesia* 1998; **8**: 139–44.

47 Ohmeda 7900 Anaesthesia Ventilator Operation and Maintenance Manual. Hatfield: Datex-Ohmeda, 1997.

48 Haskins, S.C. and Pratz, J.D. Effects of small and large face masks and translaryngeal and tracheostomy intubation on ventilation, upper-airway dead space, and arterial blood gases. *American Journal of Veterinary Research* 1986; **47**: 945–8.

49 Bagshaw, O.N.T., Southee, R. and Ruiz, K. A comparison of the nasal mask and the nasopharyngeal air way in paediatric chair dental anaesthesia. *Anaesthesia* 1997; **52**: 786–96.

50 Bailie, R., Barnett, M.B. and Fraser, J.F. The Brain laryngeal mask – a comparative study with the nasal mask in paediatric dental outpatients. *Anaesthesia* 1991; **46**: 358–60.

51 Brain, A.I.J. The development of the Laryngeal Mask – a brief history of the invention, early clinical work from which the Laryngeal Mask evolved. *European Journal of Anaesthesiology* 1991; **4**: 5–17.

52 Brimacombe, J.A., Brain, A.I.J. and Berry, A.M. (eds). *The Laryngeal Mask Airway Instruction Manual.* 3rd edn. Maidenhead: Intavent Research, 1996.

53 Eckenhoff, J.E. Some anatomic considerations of the infant larynx influencing endotracheal anesthesia. *Anesthesiology* 1951; **12**: 401–10.

54 Schwartz, R.E., Stayer, S.A. and Pasqueariello, C.A. Tracheal tube leak test –is there inter-observer agreement? *Canadian Journal of Anaesthesia* 1993; **40**: 1049–52.

55 Van den Berg, A.A. and Mphanza, T. Choice of tracheal tube size for children: finger size or age related formula? *Anaesthesia* 1997; **52**: 695–703.

56 Keep, P.J. and Manford, M.L.M. Endotracheal tube size for children. *Anaesthesia* 1974; **29**: 181–5.

57 Knine, H.H., Corddry, D.H., Kettrick, R.G., *et al.* Comparison of cuffed and uncuffed endotracheal tubes in young children during general anesthesia. *Anesthesiology* 1997; **7**: 295–300.

58 Deakers, T.W., Reynolds, G., Stretton, M. and Newth, C.J. Cuffed endotracheal tubes in pediatric intensive care. *Journal of Pediatrics.* 1994; **125**: 57–62.

59 Advanced Life Support Group. *Advanced Paediatric Life Support – The Practical Approach.* London: BMJ, 1997.

60 Pullerits, J. Routine and special pediatric airway equipment. *International Anesthesiology Clinics* 1992; **30**: 109–30.

61 Ring, W.H., Adair, J.C. and Elwyn, R.A. A new pediatric endotracheal tube. *Anesthesia and Analgesia* 1974; **54**: 273–4.

62 Cole, F. A new endotracheal tube for infants. *Anesthesiology* 1945; **6**: 87.

63 Gupta, K. and Harry, R. Cutting paediatric tracheal tubes – a potential cause of morbidity. *British Journal of Anaesthesia* 1997; **78**: 627–8.

64 Freeman, J.A., Doyle, E., Ng Tee Im and Morton, N.S. An audit of percutaneous central venous catheters in paediatric patients *Paediatric Anaesthesia* 1993; **3**: 129–38.

65 Gajraj, N.M., Pennant, J.H. and Watcha, M.F. Eutectic Mixture of Local Anesthetics (EMLA) cream. *Anesthesia and Analgesia* 1994; **78**: 574–83.

66 Teillol-Foo, W.L.M. and Kassab, J.Y. Topical glyceryl trinitrate and eutectic mixture of local anaesthetics in children. A randomised controlled trial on choice of site and ease of venous cannulation. *Anaesthesia* 1991; **46**: 881–4.

67 Jakobson, B. and Nilsson, A. Methemoglobinaemia associated with a prilocaine–lidocaine cream and trimetoprim–sulphamethoxazole. A case report. *Acta Anesthesiology Scandanavica* 1985; **29**: 453–5.

68 Nilsson, A., Engberg, G., Henneberg, S., Danielson, K. and de Verdier, C.H. Inverse relationship between age-dependent erythrocyte activity of methaemoglobin reductase and prilocaine-induced methaemoglobinaemia during infancy. *British Journal of Anaesthesia* 1990; **64**: 72–6.

69 Lawson, R.A., Smart, N.G., Gudgeon, A.C. and Morton, N.S. Evaluation of an amethocaine gel preparation for percutaneous analgesia before venous cannulation in children. *British Journal of Anaesthesia* 1995; **75**: 282–5.

70 Murdoch, L. and Bingham, R. Venous cannulation in infants and small children. *British Journal of Hospital Medicine* 1990; **44**: 405–7.

71 Joshi, H. and Joshi, A. Baby in arms: a good position for peripheral venous cannulation. *Indian Pediatrics* 1993; **30**: 1051–3.

72 Patel, N., Smith, C.E., Pinchak, A.C. and Hancock, D.E. Evaluation of different methods of securing intravenous catheters: measurement of forces during simulated accidental pullout. *Canadian Journal of Anaesthesia* 1995; **42**: 504–10.

73 Livesley, J. and Richardson, S. Securing methods for peripheral cannulae. *Nursing Standard* 1993; **7**: 31–4.

74 Garland, J.S., Dunne, W.M., Havens, P., *et al.* Peripheral intravenous catheter complications in critically ill children: a prospective study. *Pediatrics* 1992; **89**: 1145–50.

75 Fullilove, S. and Fixsen, J. Major limb deformities as complications of vascular access in neonates. *Paediatric Anaesthesia* 1997; **7**: 247–50.

76 Thiagarajan, R.R., Ramamoorthy, C., Gettmann, T. and Bratton, S.L. Survey of the use of peripherally inserted central venous catheters in children. *Pediatrics* 1997; **99**: E4.

77 Chameides, L. and Hazinski, M.F. (eds). *Textbook of Pediatric Advanced Life Support.* American Academy of Pediatrics, American Heart Association, 1994.

78 Forrest, E.T.S., Silk, J.M. and Mackersie, A. An audit of percutaneous central venous catheters in paediatric patients. *Paediatric Anaesthesia* 1993; **3**: 147–52.

79 Alderson, P.J., Burrows, F.A., Stemp, L.I. and Holtby, H.M. Use of ultrasound to evaluate internal jugular vein anatomy and to facilitate central venous cannulation in paediatric patients. *British Journal of Anaesthesia* 1993; **70**: 145–8.

80 Lumb, P.D. Complications of central venous catheters. *Critical Care Medicine* 1993; **21**: 1105–6.

81 Neubauer, A.-P. Percutaneous central iv access in the neonate: experience with 535 silastic catheters. *Acta Paediatrica Scandinavica* 1995; **84**: 756–60.

82 Tweddle, D.A., Windebank, K.P., Brett, A.M., Leese, D.C. and Gowing, R. Central venous catheter use in UKCCSG oncology centres. *Archives of Disease in Childhood* 1997; **77**: 58–9.

83 Hollyoak, M.A., Ong, T.H. and Leditschke, J.F. Critical appraisal of surgical venous access in children. *Pediatric Surgery* 1997; **12**: 177–82.

84 Venkataraman, S.T., Thompson, A.E. and Orr, R.A. Femoral vascular catheterization in critically ill infants and children. *Clinical Pediatrics* 1997; **36**: 311–19.

85 Lavandosky, G., Gomez, R. and Montes, J. Potentially lethal misplacement of femoral central venous catheters. *Critical Care Medicine* 1996; **24**: 893–6.

86 Oriot, D. and Defawe, G. Percutaneous catheterization of the axillary vein in neonates. *Critical Care Medicine* 1988; **16**: 285–6.

87 Mason, D.G. and Weir, P.M. Axillary vein cannulation in neonates. *Critical Care Medicine* 1991; **19**: 303.

88 Richmond, C.E. and Bingham, R.M. Paediatric cardiopulmonary resuscitation. *Paediatric Anaesthesia* 1995; **5**: 11–27.

89 Fiser, D.H. Intraosseous infusion. *New England Journal of Medicine* 1990; **322**: 1579–81.

90 Stewart, F.C. and Kain, Z.N. Intraosseous infusion: elective use in pediatric anesthesia. *Anesthesia and Analgesia* 1992; **75**: 626–9.

91 Schwartz, R.E., Pasquariello, C.A., Stayer, S.A. and Stewart, F.C. Elective use in pediatric anesthesia of intraosseous infusion: proceed only with extreme caution. *Anesthesia and Analgesia* 1993; **76**: 918–19.

92 Ben-Arush, M. and Berant, M. Retention of drugs in venous access port chamber: a note of caution. *British Medical Journal* 1996; **312**: 496–7.

93 Hack, W.W.M., Vos, A., van der Lei, J. and Okken, A. Incidence and duration of total occlusion of the radial artery in newborn infants after catheter removal. *European Journal of Pediatrics* 1990; **149**: 275–7.

94 Taylor, L.M., Troutman, R., Feliciano, P., Menashe, V., Sunderland, C. and Porter, J.M. Late complications after femoral artery catheterization in children less than five years of age. *Journal of Vascular Surgery* 1990; **11**: 297–304.

95 Cantwell, G.P., Holzman, B.H. and Caceres, M.J. Percutaneous catheterization of the axillary artery in the pediatric patient. *Critical Care Medicine* 1990; **18**: 880–1.

96 Wass, C.T., Lanier, W.L., Hofer, R.E., Schithauer, B.W. and Andrews, A.G. Temperature changes 10°C alter functional neurologic outcome and histopathology in a canine model of complete cerebral ischemia. *Anesthesiology* 1995; **83**: 325–35.

97 Sessler, D.I. Mild perioperative hypothermia. *New England Journal of Medicine* 1997; **336**: 1730–7.

98 Imrie, M.M. and Hall, G.M. Body temperature and anaesthesia. *British Journal of Anaesthesia* 1990; **64**: 346–54.

99 Desborough, J. Body temperature control and anaesthesia. *British Journal of Hospital Medicine* 1997; **57**: 440–2.

100 Bissonnette, B. Temperature monitoring in pediatric anesthesia. *International Anesthesiology Clinics* 1992; **30**: 63–76.

101 Sessler, D.I. and Moayeri, B.A. Skin surface warming: heat flux and central temperature. *Anesthesiology* 1990; **73**: 218–24.

102 Lyon, A.J., Pikaar, M.E., Badger, P. and McIntosh, N. Temperature control in very low birthweight infants during first five days of life. *Archives of Disease in Childhood Fetal & Neonatal Edition* 1997; **76**: F47–50.

103 Plattner, O., Semsroth, M., Sessler, D.I., Papousek, A., Klases, C. and Wagner, O. Lack of nonshivering thermogenesis in infants anesthetized with fentanyl and propofol. *Anesthesiology* 1997; **86**: 772–7.

104 Sessler, D.I., McGuire, J. and Sessler, A.M. Perioperative thermal insulation. *Anesthesiology* 1992; **74**: 875–9.

105 Russell, S.H. and Freeman, J.W. Prevention of hypothermia during orthoptic liver transplantation: comparison of three different intraoperative warming methods. *British Journal of Anaesthesia* 1995; **74**: 415–18.

106 Kurtz, A., Kurtz, M., Poeschl, G., Faryniak, B., Redi, G. and Hackl, W. Forced-air warming maintains intraoperative normothermia better than circulating water mattresses. *Anesthesia and Analgesia* 1993; **77**: 89–95.

107 Hedley, R.M. and Allt-Graham, J. Heat and moisture exchangers and breathing filters. *British Journal of Anaesthesia* 1994; **73**: 227–36.

108 Runti, G., Bertuzzi, C. and Scarpa, R. Value of HME antibacterial filters in neonatal and pediatric anesthesia. Comparison with traditional heating humidifiers *Cahiers d'Anesthesiologie* 1994; **42**: 153–7.

109 Snowdon, S.L. Hygiene standards for breathing systems? *British Journal of Anaesthesia* 1994; **72**: 143–4.

110 Presson, R.G., Bezruczko, A.P., Alexander, P., Hillier, S.C. and McNiece, W.L. Evaluation of a new fluid warmer at low to moderate flow rates. *Anesthesiology* 1993; **78**: 974–80.

111 Sadler, R, Lord, W.D. and Blakey, A. A quantitative study of maternal anxiety when accompanying their child during the induction of anaesthesia. Abstract Presented at Association of Paediatric Anaesthetists Annual Meeting, Leeds, UK; March 1998.

112 Tan, C.H. and Onsiong, M.K. Pain on injection of Propofol. *Anaesthesia* 1998; **53**: s468–76.

113 Wodey, E., Pladys, P., Copin, C., *et al*. Comparative hemodynamic depression of sevoflurane versus halothane in infants. *Anesthesiology* 1997; **87**: 795–800.

114 Sigston, P.E., Jenkins, A.M.C., Jackson, E.A., Sury, M.J., MacKersie, A.M. and Hatch, D.J. Rapid inhalation induction in children: 8% sevoflurane compared with 5% halothane. *British Journal of Anaesthesia* 1997; **78**: 362–5.

115 Laycock, G.J.A. and McNicol, L.R. Hypoxaemia during induction of anaesthesia – an audit of children who underwent general anaesthesia for routine elective surgery. *Anaesthesia* 1988; **43**: 981–4.

116 Kong, A.S., Brennan, L., Bingham, R., *et al*. An audit of induction of anaesthesia in neonates and small infants using pulse oximetry. *Anaesthesia* 1992; **47**: 896–9.

117 Logan, A.St.C., Ashford, P. and Gosling, A.J. Arterial oxygen saturation during induction of anaesthesia and laryngeal mask insertion in children: prospective evaluation of two techniques. *British Journal of Anaesthesia* 1994; **73**: 718–19P.

118 Kinouchi, K., Tanigami, H., Tashiro, C., *et al*. Duration of apnea in anesthetized infants and children required for deaturation of hemoglobin to 95%. *Anesthesiology* 1992; **77**: 1105–7.

119 Thurlow, J.A. and Madden, A.P. Sevoflurane for intubation of an infant with croup. *British Journal of Anaesthesia* 1998; **80**: 699–700.

120 Wang, C.Y., Chui, C.L. and Delilkan, A.E. Sevoflurane for difficult intubation in children. *British Journal of Anaesthesia* 1998; **80**: 408.

121 Vessey, J.A., Bogetz, M.S., Dunleavy, M.F., *et al*. Memories of being anaesthetised as a child. *Anesthesiology* 1994; **81**: A1384.

122 Kotiniemi, L.H. and Ryhanen, P.T. Behavioural changes and children's memories after intravenous, inhalation and rectal induction of anaesthesia. *Paediatric Anaesthesia* 1996; **6**: 201–7.

123 McGraw, T. and Kendrick, A. Oral midazolam premedication and postoperative behaviour in children. *Paediatric Anaesthesia* 1998; **8**: 117–21.

124 Hoerauf, K., Funk, W., Harth, M. and Hobbhahn, B.J. Occupational exposure to sevoflurane, halothane and nitrous oxide during paediatric anaesthesia. *Anaesthesia* 1997; **52**: 215–19.

125 Bricker, S.J.W., McLuckie, A. and Nightingale, D.A. Gastric aspirates after trauma in children. *Anaesthesia* 1989; **44**: 721–4.

126 Wetzel, R.C. Gastro-oesophageal reflux: theory over experience? *Paediatric Anaesthesia* 1998; **8**: 101–4.

127 Salem, M.R., Wong, A.Y. and Fizzoti, G.F. Efficacy of cricoid pressure in preventing aspiration of gastric contents in paediatric patitents. *British Journal of Anaesthesia* 1972; **44**: 401–4.

128 Motoyama, E.K. Anesthesia and the upper airway. *International Anesthesiology Clinics* 1992; **30**: 17–19.

129 Haynes, S.R. and Morton, N.S. The laryngeal mask airway: a review of its use in paediatric anaesthesia. *Paediatric Anaesthesia* 1993; **3**: 65–73.

130 Rowbottom, S.J. and Simpson, D.L. The laryngeal mask airway in children: a fibreoptic assessment of positioning. *Anaesthesia* 1991; **46**: 489–91.

131 Mason, D.G. and Bingham, R.M. The Laryngeal mask airway in children. *Anaesthesia* 1990; **45**: 760–3.

132 Johnston, D.F., Wrigley, S.R., Robb, P.J. and Jones, H.E. The Laryngeal mask airway in paediatric anaesthesia. *Anaesthesia* 1990; **45**: 924–7.

133 McNicol, L.R. Insertion of the laryngeal mask airway in children. *Anaesthesia* 1991; **37**: 509–13.

134 Allsop, E., Innes, P., Jackson, M. and Cunliffe, M. Dose of propofol required to insert the laryngeal mask airway in children. *Paediatric Anaesthesia* 1995; **6**: 47–51.

135 Selby, I.R. and Morris, P. Intermittent positive ventilation through a laryngeal mask in children: does it cause gastric dilatation? *Paediatric Anaesthesia* 1997; **7**: 305–8.

136 Gursoy, F., Algren, J. and Shjonsby, B. Positive pressure ventilation with the LMA in children. *Anesthesia and Analgesia* 1996; **82**: 33–8.

137 Brimacombe, J. The laryngeal mask airway for neonatal resuscitation. *Pediatrics* 1994; **93**: 874.

138 Kitching, A.J., Walpole, A.R. and Blogg, C.E. Removal of the laryngeal mask airway in children: anaesthetized compared with awake. *British Journal of Anesthesia* 1996; **76**: 874–6.

139 Laffon, M., Plaud, B., Duousset, A.M., Ben Haj'Hmida, R. and Ecoffey, C. Removal of laryngeal mask airway: airway complications in children, anaesthetised versus awake. *Paediatric Anaesthesia*. 1994; **4**: 35–7.

140 Parry, M., Glaisyer, H.R. and Bailey, P.M. Letter. *British Journal of Anaesthesia* 1997; **78**: 337–44.

141 Liu, L.M., DeCook, T.H., Goudsouzian, N.G., Ryan, J.F. and Liu, P.L. Dose response to intramuscular succinylcholine in children. *Anesthesiology* 1981; **55**: 599–602.

142 Reynolds, L.M., Lau, M., Brown, R., Luks, A. and Fischer, D. Intramuscular rocuronium in infants and children – dose ranging and tracheal intubating conditions. *Anesthesiology* 1997; **87**: 1096–105.

143 O'Brien, K., Kumar, R. and Morton, N.S. Sevoflurane compared with halothane for tracheal intubation in children. *British Journal of Anaesthesia* 1998; **80**: 452–5.

144 Inomata, S., Yamashita, S., Toyooka, H., *et al*. Anaesthetic induction time for tracheal intubation using sevoflurane or halothane in children. *Anaesthesia* 1998; **53**: 440–5.

145 Olsson, G.L. and Hallen, B. Laryngospasm during anaesthesia. A computer-aided incidence study in 136,929 patients. *Acta Anaesthesiologica Scandinavica* 1984; **28**: 567–75.

146 Lyons, B., Frizelle, H., Kirkby, F., *et al*. The effect of passive smoking on the incidence of airway complications in children undergoing general anaesthesia. *Anaesthesia* 1996; **51**: 324–6.

147 Lakshmipathy, N., Bokesch, P.M., Cowen, D.E., *et al*. Environmental tobacco smoke: a risk factor for pediatric laryngospasm. *Anesthesia and Analgesia* 1996; **82**: 724–7.

148 Tiret, L., Nivoche, Y., Hatton, F., Desmonts, J.M. and Vourc'h, G. Complications related to anaesthesia in infants and children. *British Journal of Anaesthesia* 1988; **61**: 263–9.

CHAPTER 7

Monitoring in paediatric anaesthesia

GUNNAR OLSSON

INTRODUCTION

The purpose of anaesthesia is to provide optimal conditions for surgery and other procedures. Major morbidity and mortality resulting from anaesthesia are not acceptable. Anaesthesia involves drugs and techniques that affect vital organ function and mistakes can rapidly lead to disaster. Well-trained anaesthetists who continuously monitor their patients with their own hands and senses can never be replaced by electronic monitoring equipment. However, modern bioengineers have developed better and more practical monitoring devices to aid anaesthetists in their essential task of guiding the patient safely through the procedure. The development of new and sophisticated monitoring equipment also has financial implications and inevitably prompts a reassessment of what exactly is meant by 'a reasonable standard of care'.[1]

Mortality and major morbidity in anaesthesia have been, and will probably continue to be, caused partly by ignorance and negligence. Avoiding complications during anaesthesia primarily involves careful preoperative history taking and evaluation and then, after optimizing a sick patient's condition, selecting the proper anaesthetic technique.[2] Complications may be expected and unavoidable in high-risk patients. Unexpected major complications can be caused by equipment failure, dosage errors, erroneous intubation, etc. With rapidly reacting electronic monitoring equipment, important diagnoses such as hypoxia and apnoea will be revealed promptly and early action may be taken. One may compare the times for response to a fresh gas disconnection when patients were only monitored with electrocardiography (ECG) and blood pressure (i.e. the mid-1980s) with the immediate response by modern alarms for capnography, apnoea and pulse oximetry. It is not at all easy to conduct controlled studies on the decrease in major complications attributable to modern monitoring equipment, and there are few scientific studies proving a beneficial effect of monitoring on decreasing morbidity and mortality.[3] However, it seems reasonable to infer that early diagnosis would lead to less serious hypoxic events.

From a technical standpoint, the monitoring of physiological parameters is not the same in infants as in adults, owing to their size. There are also physiological factors that make different monitoring demands. Pathophysiological changes such as hypoxia, hypercarbia, hypovolaemia and hypothermia can appear very rapidly in children because they have a low functional residual capacity (FRC), a high minute ventilation and cardiac output, a high rate of metabolism and a large body surface relative to body weight. The time taken for SpO_2 to fall below 95% during apnoea is inversely correlated with age[4] and this is further augmented if the child has symptomatic upper respiratory infection.[5] Fast response and continuity are therefore important characteristics of paediatric monitoring devices. Minimal invasiveness is also desirable. Accuracy and specificity can be reasonably well compensated for by the combined use of many indirect but continuous monitoring variables. The newborn CNS is fortunately more resistant to damage caused by hypoxia than the adult, but this is no excuse for reduced vigilance.

In many countries standards for monitoring during anaesthesia have been published by the national anaesthetic society.[6–10] Standards are different in different countries and they change frequently with the development of technology.[1] Compliance with set standards also varies.[11,12]

In recommending guidelines for monitoring the patient during anaesthesia it must first be emphasized, as already stated, that the presence of well-educated anaesthetic staff during the entire procedure is a prerequisite for giving general anaesthesia to a child and the incidence of cardiac arrest during anaesthesia has been shown to vary inversely with the availability of fully trained anaesthetists.[13] The organization of anaesthetic work is different in different coutries. In many countries anaesthetic nurses are employed after proper training to supervise anaesthetics and sometimes even to induce anaesthesia. For every anaesthetic, however, a specialist anaesthetist or consultant responsible for the anaesthetic should be immediately available.

Palpation of pulse, auscultation of heart and breath sounds, observation of chest movement, the colour of the patient and movements of the breathing bag are basic parameters that the anaesthetist automatically checks almost continuously. Routine monitoring devices include ECG, blood pressure, pulse oximetry and capnography if the the child is intubated or where ventilation is managed by laryngeal mask. During longer procedures temperature measurement should be used more often than in adults because of the increased risk of hypothermia in patients with a relatively large body surface.

Monitoring the anaesthetic delivery system must always include the inspired oxygen fraction, and FiO_2 monitors are now usually included in the anaesthetic machine. There should be alarms for low inspiratory oxygen and apnoea, low expiratory volumes or interruption in ventilation. There should also be alarms for low SpO_2 (oxygen saturation of haemoglobin measured by pulse oximetry). Monitoring should start before induction and go on as long into the postoperative period as there is a risk of compromise of vital functions.

A sudden failure of one component in an electronic device may lead to its complete failure and therefore costly back-up facilities must be available.[14] Electronic equipment is becoming more and more complicated and the major importance of basic bedside clinical monitoring cannot be overstated.

RESPIRATORY FUNCTION

Auscultation of the chest with a stethoscope is of the utmost importance in monitoring both ventilation and heart sounds in the child during anaesthesia. It must, however, be emphasized that in the newborn this method is inadequate for confirming the position of a tracheal tube. Incorrect positioning of the tube in the oesophagus can easily be misinterpreted by auscultation and observation of chest movements. Wherever the stethoscope is placed on the chest it is just a few centimetres from the tube, whether in the trachea or in the oesophagus. A direct view of the tube entering the larynx, verified with end-tidal partial pressure of carbon dioxide ($PeCO_2$), is the best way to ensure correct intubation.

A pneumotachometer and a pressure transducer can easily measure flow, volume and pressure relations. Monitoring ventilation in infants is, however, hampered by factors such as shallow and rapid respiration, lack of patient co-operation, use of uncuffed, leaking tubes, a relatively high airway humidity and problems with increasing apparatus dead space. Measurements of lung mechanics have therefore seldom been used continuously during paediatric anaesthesia.[15] During anaesthesia with mechanical ventilation a high compressible volume compared to tidal volume makes the interpretation of delivered values of tidal and minute ventilation less reliable. Electronic devices for monitoring tidal volume and pressure–volume curves are available[16] but can only be used routinely in the operating room in conjunction with a sophisticated ventilator. If the anaesthetic circuit includes a circle with an absorber a mechanical spirometer can be used. Expired volumes can be measured with a Wright respirometer, although this is inaccurate for low volumes.[17] A model adapted for infants has been available since the late 1980s[18] and recently an electronic version was tested, including alarms for airway pressure, minute volume and apnoea.[19] The volume alarm can detect fresh gas failure and breathing system disconnection within 15 s. When using the T-piece, as opposed to an anaesthetic circuit including absorber and circle, the continuous fresh gas flow makes accurate measurement of tidal volume and minute volume difficult. This is, however, not necessary in a simple critical incident monitoring device, as long as changes in volume can be rapidly detected.

Respiratory strength can be monitored before extubation. Negative inspiratory pressure is measured during transient airway occlusion; this pressure is proportional to phrenic nerve output.[20]

Anaesthetists often emphasize the importance of feeling the compliance of the lungs when compressing the anaesthetic bag. The limitations of the 'educated hand' have, however, been highlighted in a study where clamping of the tracheal tube was hard even for qualified anaesthetists to detect.[21,22] Total respiratory system compliance can be measured with an occlusion technique using a Fleisch pneumotachograph and a low-pressure-range transducer, although this procedure can be unreliable.[23]

Trend monitoring is essential. An increase in blood pressure indicating a stress response will make it easier to interpret, for example, minor changes in $PeCO_2$ due to pneumothorax. Trend monitoring of respiratory rate and heart rate can be as valuable as Po_2 in detecting central apnoea. The heart rate of the neonate responds to hypoxia by slowing, in contrast to the adult. Preterm and ex-preterm infants are at risk of life-threatening apnoea after general anaesthesia and should be closely monitored for 24 h after anaesthesia up to a postconceptional age of 44 weeks.[24]

BLOOD GASES

Although less invasive forms of monitoring are preferable the use of an arterial line cannot be entirely eliminated from paediatric anaesthesia and critical care. Percutaneous cannulation is preferable, as is the selection of a peripheral rather than a central artery. Most commonly the radial artery is chosen but in neonates the posterial tibial or the dorsalis pedis artery may be safer for preventing retrograde flow of air or particles entering the cerebral circulation. The hand and the connector must be kept in plain view at all times. They should never be covered. A leaking arterial catheter can rapidly lead to hypovolaemic shock before the blood loss is noticed under a blanket. The arterial partial pressure of oxygen (PaO_2) is accurate, but only reflects oxygenation at the moment when the sample was drawn. Arterial pH and base excess will give important information on metabolic status. Metabolic acidosis is an important warning sign and causative factors such as inadequate circulation, hypoglycaemia, hyperkalaemia and loss of base must be identified and treated.

Capillary sampling is a simple alternative to arterial sampling. Capillary blood gases accurately reflect arterial pH and carbon dioxide tension ($PaCO_2$) in paediatric patients if the peripheral circulation and temperature are normal.[25]

Recently, intravascular catheters for continuous monitoring of blood gases have become available.[26,27] Their role in the clinical situation during anaesthesia is not yet established and controlled studies demonstrating an improvement in outcome with the use of these monitors have not yet been published.[28] Recent reports conclude that one system (Paratrend 7) is practical, reliable and clinically accurate in infants with cyanotic heart disease.[29] The size of the sensor limits its use intra-arterially in children but placement in a peripheral vein has been shown to be accurate and can give valuable information on metabolic status.[30] Differences between $PeCO_2$ and venous carbon dioxide tension ($PvCO_2$) can be of value when the accuracy of $PeCO_2$ devices is in doubt from sampling error, alterations in the ventilation–perfusion ratio or increases in dead space and/or shunt fractions.

PULSE OXIMETRY

Pulse oximetry is a simple and non-invasive method for the continuous evaluation of the oxygen saturation of haemoglobin (SaO_2). Its ability to respond rapidly to changes in SaO_2 makes it extremely useful in monitoring infants and children. The different absorption of energy from emitted light at 660 nm (red) and 940 nm (infrared) by oxyhaemoglobin and deoxyhaemoglobin is used for calculation of saturation.[31] Pulse oximeters are usually calibrated against *in vitro* arterial blood samples tested in a co-oximeter, a multi-wavelength spectrophotometer which measures oxygenated haemoglobin.[32]

A good correlation between arterial SaO_2 and SpO_2 has been demonstrated in children. In view of the shape of the oxyhaemoglobin dissociation curve, the oxygen content of the blood in hypoxaemic infants is more sensitively expressed in terms of haemoglobin saturation than PO_2. However, in many clinical situations the accuracy of displayed values decreases.[33] In hypoxic infants SpO_2 sometimes fails to detect severe hypoxia and a large, variable and unpredictable error of pulse oximetry at low saturations has been demonstrated.[34] For routine monitoring during anaesthesia in non-cardiac patients this is of minor concern because all desaturations below 90% should be avoided.

Pulse oximetry is dependent on pulsatile flow and if vascular resistance is increased as a result of hypovolaemia, low cardiac output or infusion of vasoactive drugs SpO_2 is less reliable.[35,36] Lower readings are obtained in patients with reduced systemic vascular resistence, e.g. in patients with sepsis.[37] At low temperatures peripheral circulation is decreased

and in one study in small infants almost half of the SpO_2 readings were outside reference standards in both directions when peripheral temperatures fell below 27°C.[38]

During anaesthesia artefacts due to movement are less frequent, although malfunction due to electromagnetic interference is often seen during surgical cautery.

In the postoperative ward and the intensive care setting, however, movements frequently disturb the SpO_2 monitor, falsely indicating desaturation. Thirty per cent of the readings of the SpO_2 signal can be uninterpretable.[39,40] Examination of the waveform or comparing heart rate obtained from the ECG will identify most artefacts. Manufacturers tend to incorporate computer algorithms for detecting movement artefacts in modern pulse oximeters.[41]

Pulse oximeters can give measurements differing from true SaO_2 because of differing calibration algorithms. Thus, different alarm limits should be set depending on which instrument is used. This is of particular importance in avoiding hyperoxia in preterm neonates.[42]

SaO_2 can be calculated from blood gas measurement of PO_2, pH and PCO_2. This is a less reliable measurement if the 2,3-diphosphoglycerate (2,3-DPG) concentration is outside the normal range or if abnormal haemoglobins are present.[43]

FiO_2 should always be measured in the inspiratory limb of the system as close to the patient as possible. There is a delay in the response of SpO_2 after a fresh gas supply failure, and delay can also be due to a compromised peripheral circulation. During epidural anaesthesia response times of SpO_2 are shorter.[44]

Carbon monoxide binds strongly to haemoglobin and this will not be detected by SpO_2, since at the red wavelength used by the pulse oximeter, the absorption of light by carboxyhaemoglobin and oxyhaemoglobin is almost identical.[45] Smoking can produce levels of carboxyhaemoglobin as high as 10%. Children are seldom heavy smokers, but when carbon monoxide poisoning is suspected SpO_2 should not be relied on.

Methaemoglobin formation can be induced by various drugs, including the application of EMLA cream (eutectic mixture of local anaesthetic) in excess (prilocaine) in infants and neonates or in infants receiving sulphonamides. In particular, a combination of drugs can lead to substantial formation of methaemoglobin. This causes an underestimation at SaO_2 above 70% and an overestimation below 70%.[43]

Some pulse oximetry probes may develop sharp edges when applied to a finger so that injury, especially to the eye, may occur during a restless awakening.[46]

Neonates

There are some special considerations when monitoring SpO_2 in neonates and infants. In the immediate postpartum period the neonate is relatively desaturated, partly because of a R–L shunt through the ductus arteriosus. In some neonates and infants with persistent pulmonary hypertension this can also occur outside the immediate postpartum period. In these cases the pulse oximetry sensor should be placed on the right hand and not on the foot where postductal unsaturated blood will give a falsely low value.[47] If the ductus arteriosus is closed it is often convenient in the preterm baby to tape the probe to the instep, ankle or wrist.[48]

It has been shown that fetal haemoglobin does not influence the accuracy of *in vivo* pulse oximetry readings SaO_2 in the clinical range.[49] At low saturations, a high concentration of HbF will lead to underestimation of the saturation.[43]

Hyperoxia must be avoided in the preterm baby. Retinopathy of the premature (ROP) and possible pulmonary toxicity are serious adverse effects of high oxygen administration. In preterm neonates in the neonatal intensive care unit (NICU) FiO_2 is usually set to give a PaO_2 between 6.5 and 9.5 kPa. This is less easy to accomplish during anaesthesia. It is not known whether shorter periods of high PaO_2 during surgery in preterm babies increase the frequency of ROP. The relationship between blood oxygen content, tension or duration of hyperoxia and ROP remains undefined. In the NICU setting transcutaneous PaO_2 is recommended wherever possible in very small babies in order to minimize the risk of ROP.[50]

Reflection pulse oximetry

In reflection pulse oximetry the light-detecting and transmitting sensors do not need to have tissue in between them and thus the probe can be placed directly on the skin in such areas as the forehead. However, the accuracy of reflection pulse oximetry may sometimes be insufficient.[51,52]

Intravascular SaO_2 and SvO_2

Recently, paediatric-size oximetry catheters have become available. Two flexible fibreoptic bundles are included in the catheter and measurements use the reflection oximetry method. The small size (5.5 Fr) makes pressure tracings damped and oxygen saturation measurements have been demonstrated to show systematic deviation as well as scattering.[53] Mixed venous saturation (catheter in pulmonary artery) can give valuable information on oxygen consumption and circulatory status. The mixed venous saturation of oxygen (SvO_2) gives a measure of the balance between oxygen delivery and consumption and SvO_2 monitoring serves particularly as a surveillance and early warning system,[54] helping to guide therapy in situations such as hypovolaemia, increased O_2 consumption (e.g. pain, fever, shivering, seizures) and decreasing myocardial performance.[55] Pulmonary artery catheters are not commonplace during paediatric surgery, and the incidence of complications when they are used in children is higher than in adults. Central venous oxygen content is a more easy available measure, although even in adults the accuracy of these measurements has been questioned.[56–58]

Transcutaneous PO_2

Monitoring of hyperoxaemia is best performed by continuously measuring partial pressure; this technique has been widely used in neonatal intensive care,[59] but has not gained popularity in paediatric anaesthesia. It requires site preparation, an airtight seal, and frequent calibration. Response time varies and a periodic change of site is required to prevent skin damage.[60] Moreover, pressure readings vary according to whether the baby is asleep, active, feeding, etc.[61] Transutaneous partial pressure of oxygen ($PtcO_2$) significantly underestimates PaO_2 in patients with bronchopulmonary dysplasia (BPD).[48]

MONITORING CARBON DIOXIDE

The human body has a large storage capacity for CO_2, the concentration of which is dependent on its formation in the body and alveolar ventilation, and affected by several factors during anaesthesia and surgery.[62,63] CO_2 is best measured by $PaCO_2$ in an arterial blood sample. Arterial catheters are, however, invasive and usually only used during major surgical procedures.

Capnography

Infants and children are especially vulnerable to ventilatory complications during anaesthesia.[64–66] Anaesthetic agents depress ventilation in children and neonates, and both laryngeal irritability and a tendency to airway closure are more pronounced in children than in adults.[67] The combination of pulse oximetry and capnography is the most effective means of detecting such complications and thereby reducing anaesthetic mortality and morbidity. CO_2 absorbs infrared light within a narrow wavelength (4.3 μm) sent through a chamber with the gas to be measured and the absorption is dependent on its concentration.[68] The capnogram is the graphic display of the CO_2 concentration versus time or volume. In the clinical setting time capnography is usually used. The inspiratory segment is called phase 0. Phase I is the first part of expiration when dead space gas without CO_2 is exhaled. Phase II is S-shaped and represents a mixture of dead space and alveolar gas. Phase III is the alveolar plateau representing alveolar gas and $PeCO_2$ is the value obtained in the end of this phase. The angle (α-angle) between the steep rise (phase II) and the alveolar plateau (phase III) can give information on ventilation/perfusion mismatch or airway obstruction.[69] Capnography has limited value during rebreathing. The displayed value is normally the highest value during expiration but the real time for the start of inspiration is not integrated into the system, so the instrument goes on measuring inspiratory CO_2 if there is rebreathing. This can

be seen on the capnogram as a less steep downwards slope during inspiration (β-angle). In pregnant and obese patients a terminal upswing after the alveolar plateau can be seen (phase IV).

As well as measuring alveolar ventilation, potentially life-threatening events such as malignant hyperthermia, circuit disconnection and leak, equipment failure, accidental extubation, bronchial intubation or kinked tube can be detected rapidly.[70,71] Inadvertent oesophageal intubation is detected more rapidly by capnography than by pulse oximetry.[72] Capnographs using infrared absorption as the method of measurement are of two types. Mainstream capnographs use a cuvette in the breathing system. Cuvettes with low dead space (2 ml) are available and the cuvette should be placed as near to the tracheal tube as possible. They usually give good readings even in the neonate. In preterm neonates with body weight less than 2 kg the increase of dead space of 2 ml will lead to a small increase in PCO_2. In sidestream capnography, gas is sampled from near the patient and sucked through tubing to the apparatus where the measurement is performed. With long tubing there will be a considerable delay, and the sampling flow rate can make it unreliable in the smallest infants. Because alveolar ventilation is a smaller fraction of the fresh gas flow in infants than in adults, discrepancies between the true end-tidal gas concentration and the sampled end-tidal gas concentration may be clinically significant. Devices for sidestream sampling are available in many different sizes and in neonates and infants significant rebreathing can occur if a size inappropriate to the body weight of the infant is chosen. This is especially important if the breathing is spontaneous. $PeCO_2$ measurements obtained from the proximal (machine) end of the tracheal tube have been shown to be inaccurate in predicting $PaCO_2$ measurements in children weighing less than 8 kg. If gas is sampled from the distal (patient) end of the tracheal tube more accurate measurements can be obtained in neonates.[73] If a 19G sampling catheter is inserted in an tracheal tube of size 3 or 3.5 mm the decrease in cross-sectional area of the tube will not significantly affect measurement or give rise to any complications.[74] A recognizable plateau of the $PeCO_2$ curve during expiration should be seen on the display. If mainstream or distal sampling sidestream $PeCO_2$ is used a good correlation with $PaCO_2$ is seen in sick neonates, even in the absence of a flat alveolar plateau.[75]

High respiratory frequency and low tidal volumes decrease accuracy. During manual ventilation tidal volumes can easily be varied and the shape of the curve can visually indicate satisfactory readings. A short interruption of fresh gas flow during reading will also increase the accuracy.[76] The total delay time with gas sampling at 150 ml min^{-1}, 1 m of sampling tubing and a 19G tracheal sampling catheter can be less than 1 s. Longer delay times than the respiratory cycle which can be seen in infants may give inaccurate[77] or distorted recordings.[78] In general, $PeCO_2$ underestimates $PaCO_2$ and prolonged expiration with or without hyperinflation will not improve the estimation.[79]

When using the laryngeal mask airway (LMA) in adults accurate measurements of $PeCO_2$ have been obtained.[80] In children, however, when using the LMA during spontaneous ventilation correlation between $PaCO_2$ and $PeCO_2$ is often poor. $PeCO_2$ meaurements will in this situation give lower values than $PaCO_2$ and during spontaneous ventilation, and hypoventilation may be missed.[81] However, when the LMA is used during mechanical ventilation in children above 10 kg body weight $PeCO_2$ is an accurate indicator of $PaCO_2$.[82] Gas should be withdrawn at the distal end of the LMA[83] and not at the elbow of the connecting system.

During conscious and deep sedation monitoring of PCO_2 is important. Sedative drugs can lead to respiratory depression that is not detected early by pulse oximetry in patients with supplemental oxygen. $PeCO_2$ can be sampled by a nasal cannula and accurate values can be obtained, even in children.[84] Accuracy will, however, be affected if there is mouth breathing, airway obstruction, oxygen delivery through the ipsilateral nasal cannula or cyanotic heart disease.[85]

In general, in patients with significant lung pathology $PeCO_2$ is a less accurate measure of $PaCO_2$. With pulmonary ventilation/perfusion mismatch, lung pathology or R–L shunting, $PeCO_2$ will underestimate $PaCO_2$ and overestimate alveolar ventilation.[86,87] In children with cyanotic congenital heart disease and severe pulmonary disease calculation of physiological dead space and alveolar ventilation should be based on direct measurements of $PaCO_2$. In children with venous congestion of the lungs a higher $PeCO_2$ reading may be obtained, possibly resulting from an increased pulmonary blood volume, causing an alveolar CO_2 tension closer to the venous than arterial value.

A decreasing pulmonary blood flow and unchanged ventilation will lead to decreasing $PeCO_2$. A sudden decrease in $PeCO_2$ could be an early sign of sudden cardiac arrest. $PeCO_2$ will indicate the effectiveness of the cardiopulmonary resuscitation (CPR) and there is a positive relation between $PeCO_2$ and survival after CPR.[88–91]

$PeCO_2$ measurements are especially useful in patients undergoing craniotomy in the sitting position, where a sudden fall is usually indicative of an air embolus.[92]

End-tidal CO_2 is also an important adjunct in the detection of malignant hyperthermia.

Colorimetric end-tidal CO_2 detector

When capnography is not always readily available, e.g. in accident and emergency departments, a portable, disposable CO_2 detector can be used for confirming tracheal tube position.[93] The device changes colour when pH decreases owing to expired CO_2. This simple monitor can also be of value during cardiopulmonary resuscitation.[94] Continuous use of the device in small children and infants is not recommended because it increases dead space considerably. During transportation, when there is an increased risk of extubation, a simple device for detecting CO_2 can be of value.[95] However, hypoventilation due to patient deterioration, airway problems or unintentional hyperventilation may occur in this situation and a portable capnograph giving more exact measurement of $PeCO_2$ is preferable. Compact models introduced recently by several manufacturers are particularly appropriate in these circumstances.[96]

TRANSCUTANEOUS PCO_2

In the intensive care setting, where neonates often have severe lung disease, transcutaneous carbon dioxide tension ($PtcCO_2$) gives an accurate estimation of $PaCO_2$. Acidosis negatively affects the correlation between $PtcCO_2$ and $PaCO_2$.[97] $PtcCO_2$ is, however, often not practical to use for monitoring during anaesthesia. A long stabilization and calibration time is needed and it is necessary to change the sensor site every 2–4 h to avoid skin burns.[74]

ANAESTHETIC GASES

Overdose of inhaled anaesthetic agents is an important cause of anaesthetic-related cardiac arrest.[13,98] Varying accuracy of delivered gas concentrations by even modern vaporizers can lead to clinically significant errors in delivered inhalation dose.[99] Major complications from overdosage will hopefully be less common when measurement of anaesthetic gas concentration during anaesthesia is applied more widely. Gas is drawn from a sidestream connector, usually near the proximal end of the tracheal tube. End-tidal and inspiratory concentrations of the anaesthetic gas are displayed. Both inspiratory and expiratory concentrations of oxygen and nitrous oxide are also usually measured. Depending on gas flow and anaesthetic circuit configuration the same errors as with $PeCO_2$ must be anticipated in infants and smaller children (below 8–12 kg body weight). According to current recommendations in many countries monitoring of vapour concentration is desirable,[12] particularly when low gas flows are used.

Gas analysis can be performed in different ways: monochromatic or polychromatic infrared spectrometry, mass spectrometry and raman scattering spectrometry. In infrared spectrometry infrared light is sent through the sample gas and energy is absorbed in proportion to the concentration of the gas to be measured. The device cannot distinguish between agents and the correct calibration setting must be used. The setting of a wrong agent can give a reading of only one-fifth of the true concentration, which would easily lead to overdosage.[100] Older monochromatic devices are calibrated for halothane, methoxyflurane,

enflurane and isoflurane, but not for sevoflurane and desflurane. It has been claimed that sevoflurane can be measured using the setting for methoxyflurane,[101,102] but great care must be taken if the manufacturers' recommendations are not followed. Alcohol in a patient's blood may provide another source of erroneous readings.[103]

In polychromatic infrared spectrometry multiple long wavelength infrared light is used and this enables identification of the anaesthetic agent and even measurement of several agents at the same time. It is advantageous if a vapour monitor can identify other gases such as trifluoromethane from breakdown of isoflurane in low-flow circle systems[104] or other chemicals that can contaminate the system.[105]

Mass spectrometers are large, heavy and expensive. Where they are used it is usually in a time-share option. Up to 16 operating rooms or intensive care beds are connected to the device, often with 25-m long collecting catheters. This will give some time delay and if many rooms are connected each patient is only monitored for a small portion of the time. Multiple gases can be measured simultaneously and the measurements are usually correct. Recently, a new portable mass spectrometer has come on the market.[106] It is smaller, weighs only 34 kg and offers a comparable level of accuracy.

In raman scattering spectrometry a laser is sent though a gas sample. The light is scattered when it hits gas molecules. This gives a shift of frequency that can be measured and used to identify different gases and their concentrations. Water vapour does not interfere with results and absolute values can be measured accurately. Multiple gases can be analysed simultaneously.[107]

CIRCULATORY FUNCTION

The importance of observing the patient directly and monitoring heart sounds with a stethoscope must first be emphasized. In neonates and infants oesophageal stethoscopes are often used. The cardiodepressive effect of a high alveolar concentration of halothane is readily detected by the change in heart sound. Early detection of hypovolaemia and shock during anaesthesia in infants and children requires careful observation of clinical signs (capillary refill, skin mottling, peripheral temperature, pulse rate, etc.) since blood pressure may be relatively well maintained at first. Hypoxia, vagal stimulation and commonly administered drugs such as neostigmine lead to the rapid onset of bradycardia, which is more significant in young children since they depend primarily on heart rate for cardiac output. However, recent studies with echocardiography have demonstrated an important role for variation of stroke volume even in neonates and infants.[108,109] Serious arrhythmias during anaesthesia are less common in children, except when deep halothane anaesthesia is combined with elevated PCO_2.

MONITORING

Electrocardiogram

In paediatric anaesthesia the ECG is mainly used for measuring heart rate and identifying arrhythmias. Neonates and infants react to hypoxia with bradycardia. As cardiac output in infants is more dependent on changes in heart rate than in stroke volume, early detection of bradycardia for early intervention is important. A combination of halothane anaesthesia, hypercapnia and adrenaline administration (e.g. by the surgeon for reducing bleeding) may induce arrhythmias and ECG can detect this early. Arrhythmias after succinylcholine administration are common and could be serious in the presence of coexisting muscle disease or serum potassium abnormalities. Evaluating changes in ECG such as depression of the ST-segment due to ischaemia is of less importance in children than in adults during anaesthesia. This is partly due to the rareness of coronary artery disease but also to differences in QRS-axis and R- and T-wave shape. In newborns the right ventricle is dominant.[110] T-waves are usually increased in children and infants and the ECG can easily count both the QRS-complex and the T-wave when calculating heart rate, which will result in doubled frequency.

A normal ECG does not give information on circulation and pulseless electrical activity can occur.[111] In patients where surface electrodes cannot be applied or for special arrhythmia monitoring oesophageal electrodes may be used.[112] Although monitoring of heart rate with ECG does not give good information about circulatory function it is a very easy and reliable measurement and in acute severely ill infants where pulse oximetry and non-invasive blood pressure (NIBP) monitoring may not give satisfactory readings ECG can be valuable. The most significant risk in ECG monitoring during surgery is that of inducing burns on the patient because of faulty ground isolation.[113] The risk is greater if the electrodes are small as in paediatric anaesthesia or if oesophageal electrodes are used.

Blood pressure

Anaesthetics often decrease the systemic vascular resistance and have a negative effect on myocardial contractility. These effects are more pronouced in infants and children than in adults and thus blood pressure is decreased more by anaesthetics in children. Blood pressure is usually monitored non-invasively (NIBP).

Non-invasive oscillometry

Oscillometric measurements have been shown to correlate well with intra-arterial measurements[114] as well as with manual auscultatory method.[115] A pump inflates a cuff and a pressure sensor records the oscillations in pressure that the pulse wave generates when pressure is decreased to the systolic pressure. These oscillations increase and reach a maximum approximately at mean arterial pressure and decrease at diastolic pressure. It is important to use the correct cuff size in children; if the cuff is too small a reading that is too high may be obtained and with a too large cuff readings will be too low. The error with too large a cuff is less than with one which is too small. The cuff should almost encircle the arm. The cuff can also be placed on the thigh, which gives higher readings[116] or, in older children and adolescents, on a finger using a neonatal cuff.[117] Devices using the oscillometric methods are now the most widely produced by most monitoring equipment manufacturers.

Other non-invasive methods

With a cuff and a sphygmomanometer any device that identifies blood flow distal to the cuff can be used for blood pressure monitoring. The radial artery is not always easily palpable and devices with a microphone to detect Korotkoff sounds or a Doppler sensor to detect flow are available.[118] The correlation with true systolic, diastolic and mean pressures is much better with the oscillometric technique than with determination of Korotkoff sounds. Pulse oximetry can also be used for detection of flow when deflating a cuff. The readings are best taken when the oximeter loses its display during inflation. The pulse oximeter can otherwise shift to pulse search mode.[119]

A pulse monitor based on the principle of a finger plethysmograph which tranforms a change in volume into a change in pressure has been shown to measure blood pressure accurately in paediatric patients.[120] As with other non-invasive methods, plethysmography is of limited value in patients with severe peripheral vasoconstriction, low cardiac output or low systolic blood pressure.

Invasive methods

At low blood pressures, when accuracy is needed most, NIBP monitors are poor indicators of true blood pressure. An intra-arterial catheter and transducer are useful in situations when hypotension can be expected, including open heart surgery, induced hypotension and other major surgery where blood loss may be sudden and massive. Continuous arterial flushing with heparinized saline in neonates can add a substantial amount of fluid and flow rates of even less than 1 ml h^{-1} should be used. Newborns often have a catheter inserted in the umbilical artery and a good correlation has been demonstrated between umbilical arterial and peripheral arterial pressures.[121] Injecting as little as 0.2 ml of air through an umbilical artery catheter can occlude blood flow to the lower extremities for several hours.

More information can be obtained from the arterial blood pressure tracing than merely the systolic, mean and diastolic pressures. A damped tracing is usually caused by an air bubble in the line or by myocardial dysfunction.

Pulmonary artery catheters with options for thermodilution are available but seldom used in paediatric anaesthesia.[122] Even in adult cardiac anaesthesia pulmonary artery catheters are not included in standard monitoring.[12] It may be valuable to monitor pulmonary artery pressure in cases where postoperative pulmonary hypertension is likely to occur. This is, however, a very invasive technique associated with considerable risk of complications and is not often used outside cardiac surgery. Pulmonary hypertension can be evaluated with less invasive methods such as echocardiography.

MONITORING CARDIAC OUTPUT

Fick's method of measuring cardiac output is the gold standard. Measuring oxygen uptake from inhaled air and sampling arterial and central venous blood for saturation by co-oximetry provide the most accurate value of cardiac output. This is not practical in the operating room but with analysis of inspiratory and end-expiratory gas concentrations some devices, known as metabolic monitors, display uptake of oxygen and carbon dioxide production. Using a fibreoptic pulmonary artery catheter for measuring mixed venous saturation and routine pulse oximetry, cardiac output can be relatively easily and almost continuously monitored during anaesthesia. Although there are several sources of error with the different measurements a good correlation has been demonstrated with this method compared with thermodilution.[123]

Dye dilution with indocyanine can be used in children,[124] although it is not very practical in the operating room setting. The thermodilution method has been considered by some as the standard for cardiac output measurements, even in children.[125] In adults thermodilution measurements have an error range of approximately 15%. The error is probably higher in children, owing to a smaller injectate and a lower flow. Rapid injection of cold saline may slow the heart rate,[126] and repeated measurements of cardiac output may cause overhydration in infants because 3–10 ml of fluid is required for each determination. Catheters as small as size 3.5F are available.

Thoracic electrical bioimpedance

This is a non-invasive continuous technique to monitor cardiac output and has been shown to give accurate measurement in neonates. However, there are often difficulties in obtaining electrical signals, and the technique is limited to patients with a heart rate below 180 beats min^{-1} and is not applicable during arrhythmias or left-to-right intracardiac shunts.[127] The current recommendation is to limit the use of this technique to children over 2 years old.

Doppler ultrasound

Non-invasive techniques also include pulsed or continuous wave Doppler ultrasound technology.[128] Whilst some have found excellent agreement with cardiac output measurement during cardiac catheterization in children when Doppler and the Fick method were employed, others have shown that the pulsed Doppler method of cardiac output determination is not sufficiently accurate to serve as a guide to therapy for critically ill children.[125] For assessment of trends in cardiac output transoesophageal Doppler is easy to use and rapid to place, and has been found to be reliable, providing clinically acceptable information concerning changes in cardiac index.[129] Left-to-right flow through the ductus arteriosus is included in the measurements. In this situation changes in cardiac output may reflect changes in ductus shunting and not in effective systemic flow.

Transoesophageal echocardiography

When probes for transoesophageal use in neonates became available during the late 1980s the use of intraoperative echocardiography added important information during cardiac surgery.[130] Four-millimetre transoesophageal probes are now available.[131] Transoesophageal echocardiography (TOE) for monitoring surgical repair perioperatively in paediatric cardiac surgery is now a reliable diagnostic tool,[132–136] although the equipment, including probes, is quite expensive. Cardiac output can be measured with TOE, not only by Doppler technique but also by the two-dimensional method, in which end-systolic and end-diastolic volumes are measured and the differ-

ence between these is multiplied by heart rate to reflect cardiac output.[137] There may be significant interobserver and interwindow variability and it has been suggested that the assessment of ventricular function in the operating room should be viewed as a qualitative rather than quantitative measurement.[138] More derived haemodynamic information can be obtained from echocardiography,[139] including information on preload, contractility, etc., and the TOE technique is used more and more also in paediatric anaesthesia.[109,140] Biplane probes are now used in neonates as small as 2.2 kg, not only during cardiac surgery but also for monitoring neurosurgical and orthopaedic procedures or whenever additional cardiac monitoring is required.[141]

Venous air embolism during neurosurgery in the sitting position can be detected early by TOE, minimizing the risk of circulatory impairment and paradoxical air embolism if air reaches the systemic circulation through intracardiac and transpulmonary passages. In one study microbubbles were found in the right atrium in all patients operated on in the sitting position.[142]

There are few complications to TOE, although the probe can cause airway obstruction, even in older children. Other complications include bronchospasm, hypoxia, arrhythmia, minor pharyngeal bleeding and pressure necrosis in the oesophagus owing to long-standing pressure from a probe in the flexed position.[143]

Technical development in this area is advancing quickly and TOE may possibly be incorporated in routine monitoring during major surgery in infants and children in the foreseeable future.

MONITORING INTRAVASCULAR BLOOD VOLUME

Infants and children have a large extracellular fluid volume (ECV), a high rate of metabolism and a large surface area relative to body weight. These factors make the child vulnerable to hypovolaemia during anaesthesia. There are no practical methods of measuring blood volume and ECV perioperatively. Lost blood and fluids must be precisely monitored and given volumes of blood and fluids recorded. During major surgery a record should be kept of blood and fluid balance that should be updated every 15 min, or more often if losses are rapid. A rising heart rate is often the first sign of hypovolaemia. Infants lose their baroresponses with approximately 0.5 MAC halothane. Therefore, a heart rate within the normal range does not necessarily indicate normal blood flow. Decrease in blood pressure is a much later symptom than decreased peripheral circulation, with pale skin, decreased peripheral skin temperature and decreased capillary fill, which is easily checked by compression of the nail beds. The arterial blood pressure is often within normal limits despite 10% volume depletion. Mechanical ventilation is more likely to cause variations in arterial blood pressure if the child is hypovolaemic. Urinary output is valuable, although not useful in situations of rapid losses.

When major blood loss is expected more invasive arterial monitoring is indicated, and may show the dicrotic notch to be in a lower position on the wave form. Central venous pressure (CVP) should be measured continuously when blood loss is expected. The rapidity with which the CVP falls in young children with blood loss is impressive. Complications of central venous catheters (CVC) include thrombosis, infection and even perforation of the heart.[144] Thus, there must be a clear indication for using them in children. If there is a pulmonary artery catheter in use pulmonary capillary wedge pressure can be monitored. However, TOE, which is much less invasive, can give valuable information on left ventricular preload. When major blood loss is expected, as in scoliosis surgery, a moderate degree of controlled hypotension is often used.[145] Intraoperative autologous transfusion can be used in infants during surgery where expected blood loss is large, such as surgery for craniosynostosis.[146]

Mixed venous saturation can be used as an index of overall tissue oxygenation. If O_2 delivery decreases because of hypovolaemia, mixed venous PO_2 will also decrease. Cold stress will, however, increase oxygen consumption and lead to the same effect. This is also true for changes in circulatory distribution and shifts of the oxyhaemoglobin dissociation curve.

Tissue pH is extremely sensitive to changes in intravascular volume and blood flow, and gastric intramucosal pH can be a useful technique for haemodynamic monitoring in children.[147]

MONITORING TEMPERATURE

With the exception of ketamine, general anaesthetics impair the thermoregulatory response to the large thermal stresses to which patients are subject during anaesthesia and surgery.[148] Thermal losses from large open surgical fields, in combination with loss of protective measures during anaesthesia, may lead to hypothermia. Heat production will decrease owing to a low metabolic rate during anaesthesia. Shivering, which is poorly developed in the newborn, is extremely energy and oxygen consuming and should be avoided in the recovery period.

Neonates and young infants are at especially high risk of developing hypothermia during anaesthesia if adequate warming facilities are not used. The relatively large body surface is the most important reason but also the surgical wound area is often relatively large. In particular, the large head with a high cutaneous blood flow increases the risk. Covering the head is advisable during major surgery with a large wound surface. Hypothermic children are slow to awaken and recover from anaesthesia because anaesthetic solubility is greater at low temperatures. There is also increased risk of hypoxaemia and hypercapnoea.

Cold intravenous fluids, irrigating fluids and skin preparation fluids should be avoided, and anaesthetic gases should be warm and humid. Plastic and reflective wraps can be used to decrease heat loss. The relative humidity inside wraps reaches 100% and thus effectively prevents evaporative heat loss.[149] Heating with forced air has recently been found superior to heating by circulating water blankets.[150] Humidification and warming inspired gases are very important for decreasing heat loss. Radiant heaters are used in the recovery period. The temperature of all external heat sources must be carefully monitored to avoid thermal damage to the patient. Even when they are used, the temperature in the operating room must also be carefully monitored. Prior to the introduction of the more efficient forced-air devices, ambient temperature had to be kept as high as was tolerable for the surgical staff, and for neonates a temperature of 26°C was often required. Neonates with a body temperature below 35–36°C are preferably kept anaesthetized postoperatively and allowed to warm up in an incubator with mechanical ventilation.

Temperature monitoring is also important for detecting hyperthermia, although malignant hyperthermia is uncommon. Hyperthermia is less well tolerated than hypothermia and human proteins begin to denature at 42°C.

During deliberate hypothermia temperature is usually monitored in different areas. Measuring both core and peripheral skin temperature gives important information about the thermal status. During normal anaesthesia it is usually only core temperature that is measured. Core temperature can be monitored in the rectum, oesophagus, urinary bladder or tympanic membrane.[151] When using the oesophageal approach the probe must be placed in the lower part of the oesophagus, below the main airways, in order not to be influenced by the temperature of inspired gases. This will be at the level of maximum heart sounds. Oesophageal probes are used only if the child is intubated. The tympanic membrane has not been adopted in most centres, since inserting the probe too far can perforate the eardrum. Rectal temperature is the most commonly used technique. Rectal temperatures should not be measured in patients with inflammatory processes in the bowel or with absolute neutropenia. In infants weighing less than 3 kg the rectum can be perforated with the temperature probe or thermometer. If a pulmonary artery catheter for thermodilution is used the true core temperature is monitored in the blood. Incorrect positioning of the probe results in unreliable axillary temperature readings.

Electric probes are usually used for measuring temperature. These are thermistors that change their resistance according to temperature. Thermocouples are composed of two metals and when the temperature changes a current is induced between the metals. Infrared emission detection thermometry is another useful and reliable method.[152] Liquid crystal temperature sensors can be used for measuring skin temperature.[153]

MONITORING NEUROMUSCULAR BLOCK

Although neuromuscular monitoring is not widely used in paediatric anaesthesia some form of monitoring is advisable, especially in neonates when non-depolarizing agents are used. Neonates do not respond to head-lift or hand-squeeze tests, making clinical judgement less valuable.

Simple non-expensive stimulators are available that can stimulate in different modes. The train-of-four (TOF, 2 Hz for 2 s, repeated every 10–20 s) method is the one most often used. Other stimulation modes include single twitch, tetanus, post-tetanic count and double-burst stimulation.[154,155] During tetanic stimulation neonates demonstrate a fade of twitch at low frequencies[156] and the fourth twitch is normally lower in neonates.[157] Infants have longer elimination half-lives of non-depolarizing muscle relaxants and repeat doses should be administered at longer intervals.[158]

Recording is most easily carried out by direct observation of thumb movement during TOF stimulation or by feeling the mechanical force in the thumb. If just one twitch is seen the patient is adequately relaxed for surgery. This approximately equates to five twitches on the post-tetanic count. Visual or tactile assessments of thumb movements only give a rough estimation and, especially for determining residual muscular block towards the end of anaesthesia, more sophisticated measuring methods, such as mechanomyography, electromyography (EMG) or accelography, are preferable.[159] Observing the twitches directly usually suggests a less profound block with the same total amount of drug and more precise monitoring enhances better timing of neuromuscular relaxant administration.[160] When the TOF ratio (ratio of the fourth/first response) exceeds 70% muscular function is generally believed to be restored, although a ratio of 80% has been suggested. Mechanomyography is considered by many to be the gold standard.[161] The arm is mounted rigidly and a pressure transducer on the thumb measures the force of the contraction of the adductor pollicis muscle. It is, however, cumbersome and time consuming to set up and is not commonly used in routine practice. The electrical activity in the adductor pollicis muscle after stimulation of the ulnar nerve can be measured with cutaneous electrodes (EMG) and standard equipment for this is available. The EMG response of adductor digiti minimi can also be monitored,[162] but correct electrode placement is important.[163] Still easier and more practical is accelomyography. The acceleration of the thumb after nerve stimulation is measured with a piezoelectric transducer applied to a freely movable thumb. It has been shown that accelography underestimates neuromuscular block in children compared with mechanomyography, so that the two methods should not be used interchangeably in research studies.[164] This is probably of minor importance in the clinical setting.[165] Accelography monitors are available on the market and are reliable clinical monitors in daily anaesthesia practice.[166]

Stimulation of a motor nerve is performed supramaximally, i.e. all nerve fibres should be depolarized. This is painful and should not be used in children before induction.[167] Neuromuscular monitoring has also been advocated in the intensive care unit.[168] If stimulation is used in this setting sedation and analgesia must be taken into consideration.

Higher dose requirements for children than for adults, as well as technical complications with intravenous lines, increase the indication for monitoring when modern, shorter acting, non-depolarizing muscle relaxants such as mivacurium or atracurium are used by continuous infusion.[169]

Neuromuscular monitoring consists of nerve stimulation and recording. The ulnar nerve at the wrist or at the elbow is easily stimulated. In infants the posterior tibial nerve at the ankle can be stimulated if the ulnar nerve is inaccessible and the responses of the flexor hallucis brevis muscle can be studied by accelography. The acceleration transducer can be applied to the big toe and this will give similar results to those that arise from stimulating the ulnar nerve.[170] The temporal branch of the facial nerve can also be stimulated. The orbicularis oculi muscle reacts to non-depolarizing muscle relaxants in the same way as the diaphragm and laryngeal muscles, and visual assessment of this muscle will give a good indication of the time for intubation. It relaxes earlier than the adductor pollicis.[171]

Neuromuscular monitoring is perhaps most valuable during emergence from anaesthesia,[20,172,173] when it must be decided whether the patient's muscular strength is sufficient to support protective reflexes and ventilation. Although spontaneous recovery from neuromuscular block is more rapid in children (1–10 years old) than in adults,[174] reversal is usually performed and monitoring is valuable in assessing the timing of this.[175]

CNS MONITORING

Surgery close to the CNS, such as spinal surgery and intracranial surgery, can have neurological sequelae. Indeed, this is often unavoidable, e.g. during brain tumour or CNS-malformation surgery. Neurophysiological monitoring can give early warning and reduce neurological sequelae.[176] This is of special importance during surgery for scoliosis.[177,178] Cardiac surgery and surgery on arteries supplying the CNS involve a risk of inducing cerebral hypoxia and neurological dysfunction owing to decreased blood flow or embolization.[179,180] When using CNS monitoring during paediatric cardiac surgery a very high incidence of changes in brain perfusion or metabolism has been demonstrated.[181] Austin *et al.* demonstrated that interventions based on neurophysiological monitoring decreased the incidence of postoperative neurological sequelae and reduced the length of hospital stay.[181] Neurophysiological monitoring techniques based on electroencephalograms (EEG) and evoked potentials were considered cost-effective.

The EEG can detect ischaemia during surgery. However, it is a cumbersome technique and to be worthwhile it has been proposed that an EEG technician focusing entirely on the neurophysiological monitoring is indispensable.[182] Children below the age of 2 years have an EEG pattern that is not yet mature and is very hard to interpret. Automatic processing of the EEG may make it useful during anaesthesia[183] and with the cerebral function analysing monitor (CFAM) it has been shown to be possible to measure depth of anaesthesia during isoflurane inhalation.[184] Conventional EEG analysis has a low specificity, monitoring is complex and more specific methods have been developed.[185] With compressed spectral assay (CSA), spectral edge frequency (SEF)[186] computer algorithms speed up the interpreting of the EEG. During cerebral ischaemia, hypoxia, hypothermia and general anaesthesia low frequencies increase in the EEG. These delta frequencies have been assessed and used for monitoring in areas such as paediatric cardiac surgery [augmented delta quotient (ADQ)], which is easier and faster than CSA.[187]

Recently, it has been demonstrated that the bispectral index will give an accurate estimation of anaesthetic depth.[188]

EEG changes after sensory stimulation can give more information. This is performed by stimulation of skin or peripheral nerves [somatosensory evoked potentials (SEP)], through auditory clicking sounds delivered by earphones [auditory evoked potentials (AEP)][189] or though visual stimulation (VEP). EEG is then measured from the cortex using scalp electrodes. Brainstem auditory evoked potentials (BAEP) are measured with skin electrodes over, for example, the mastoids and, as with cortical EEG, are difficult to interpret in children below 2 years of age.[190] In children, anaesthesia depresses scalp EEG more than spinal EEG and therefore electrodes over the cervical spine are preferable for recording cervical spine SEP.[176] The use of AEP with an index derived from shifts in both frequency and amplitude has recently been proposed as a reliable indicator of potential awareness during anaesthesia.[191]

Techniques based on blood flow and oxygenation

With transcranial Doppler ultrasonography (TCD) real-time measures of intracranial perfusion are possible even without an open fontanelle. This technique has been used in children with hydrocephalus during shunt operations[192] and a wide range of perfusion abnormalities can be detected with it during paediatric cardiac surgery.[179,181]

Cerebral oxygenation can now be monitored non-invasively and continuously with percutaneous reflectance near-infrared spectrophotometry (NIRS).[179,181,193]

MONITORING DURING SEDATION

During conscious sedation the patient is arousable and can answer when spoken to. Protective reflexes are maintained. This type of sedation is often used by non-anaesthetists. The most important thing to monitor is that the child remains conscious. Thus, talking to the child to confirm consciousness is the most approriate measure. Pulse oximetry is very easy to use and should also be recommended.

During deep sedation the patient is not readily arousable; protective reflexes and patency of airways may be lost. Deep sedation should be supervised by an anaesthetist. Often a higher degree of monitoring is needed than during general anaesthesia. Monitoring standards should be set[194,195] and a monitoring protocol should be used.[196] Patient selection, fasting, recovery facilities, discharge criteria, etc., should be taken into consideration, as during anaesthesia. Children with underlying medical conditions and those who are very young are at increased risk of adverse events during sedation.[197] A significant morbidity and mortality has been directly attributed to sedation in children.[196] Drug overdose and inadequate monitoring are common causative factors. Monitoring during deep sedation should include pulse oximetry, ECG, respiratory rate, blood pressure and capnography. Respiratory depression resulting from opioid administration in a spontaneously breathing child can often be detected earlier by $PeCO_2$ than by SaO_2.[198] The patient is not readily available inside the tube of the magnetic resonance imaging (MRI) machine. The anaesthetist is often in another room and there may be a considerable delay in acting on deteriorations in vital parameters. In the MRI environment electrical cables and metal-containing equipment cannot be used.[199] All types of commonly used monitoring devices designed for use in the MRI environment are now available, such as ECG, SpO_2, NIBP and $PeCO_2$.

MONITORING DURING RECOVERY

In the postoperative period there can still be residual effects of anaesthetic drugs. Opioids and neuromuscular blocking agents, in particular, can induce respiratory depression. In the operating theatre the anaesthetist is beside the patient all the time but in the recovery room this fundamental clinical monitoring must be delegated to suitably trained non-medical staff. Thus, there is a high demand for monitoring devices until the patient has safely recovered. However, during transportation to the recovery room, which happens very soon after emergence from anaesthesia, there is a considerable risk for respiratory depression. This is especially true when the transportation is long, e.g. from the X-ray department.

When standards for clinical and electronic monitoring are discussed the motivation of the personnel in the recovery unit must be considered, as recently demonstrated;[200] the incidence of low SaO_2 in the recovery room decreased when personnel were aware that they were being studied.

Monitoring of ex-premature infants has been mentioned previously, but full-term neonates also have an increased risk of apnoea and periodic breathing.[201]

When spinal opioids are given to infants and small children there is a risk of late respiratory depression and monitoring should continue for 18–24 h after the administration of the drug.[202,203]

REFERENCES

1 Winter, A. and Spence, A.A. An international consensus on monitoring? *British Journal of Anaesthesia* 1990; **64**: 263–6.

2 Olsson, G.L. Complications during anaesthesia and outcome of paediatric intensive care. A computerized study. Thesis. Stockholm: Karolinska Institute, 1987.

3 Orkin, F.K. Practice standards: the Midas touch or the emperor's new clothes? *Anesthesiology* 1989; **70**: 567–71.

4 Xue, F.S., Luo, L.K., Tong, S.Y., Liao, X., Deng, X.M. and An, G. Study of the safe threshold of apneic period in children during anesthesia induction. *Journal of Clinical Anesthesiology* 1996; **8**: 568–74.

5 Kinouchi, K., Tanigami, H., Tashiro, C., Nishimura, M., Fukumitsu, K. and Takauchi, Y. Duration of apnea in anesthetized infants and children required for desaturation of hemoglobin to 95%. *Anesthesiology* 1992; **77**: 1105–7.

6 Recommendations for Standards of Monitoring During Anaesthesia and Recovery. London: Association of Anaesthetists of Great Britain and Ireland, 1994.

7 Guidelines to the practice of anaesthesia as recommended by the Canadian Anaesthetist's Society. Members Guide 1993.

8 Guide de l'exercise de l'anestésie. Publication de la corporation de médicins du Québec, 1992: 6.

9 American Society of Anesthesiologists. Standards for basic anesthetic monitoring. In: *ASA Directory of Members*. Park Ridge, IL: American Society of Anesthesiologists, 1994: 735–6.

10 Samlade riktlinjer (Assembled Guidelines). KalmarSund Tryck: Swedish Society of Anaesthesia and Intensive Care, 1997.

11 Cockroft, S. Use of monitoring devices during anesthesia for cardiac surgery: a survey of practices at public hospitals within the United Kingdom and Ireland. *Journal of Cardiothoracic and Vascular Anesthesia* 1994; **8**: 382–5.

12 Feneck, R.O. Standards of monitoring. *Journal of Cardiothoracic and Vascular Anaesthesia* 1994; **8**: 379–81.

13 Olsson, G.L. and Hallén, B. Cardiac arrest during anaesthesia. A computer-aided study in 250,543 anaesthetics. *Acta Anesthesiologica Scandinavica* 1988; **32**: 653–64.

14 Girgis, Y. and Bromme, U. Monitoring failure and awareness hazard during prolonged surgery. *Anaesthesia* 1997; **52**: 504–5.

15 Miyasaka, K. Respiratory monitoring of the infant in anaesthesia and intensive care. *Canadian Journal of Anaesthesia* 1990; **37**: Scxxiv–xxviii.

16 Berman, L.S., Banner, M.J., Blanch, P.B. and Widner, L.R. A new pediatric respiratory monitor that accurately measures imposed work of breathing: a validation study. *Journal of Clinical Monitoring* 1995; **11**: 14–17.

17 Bushman, J.A. Effects of different flow patterns on the Wright spirometer. *British Journal of Anaesthesia* 1979; **51**: 895–8.

18 Hatch, D.J. and Williams, G.M.E. The Haloscale 'Infanta' Wright respirometer. *In vitro* and *in vivo* assessment. *British Journal of Anaesthesia* 1988; **60**: 232–8.

19 Hatch, D.J. and Jackson, E.A. A new critical incident monitor for use with the paediatric T-piece. *In vitro* evaluation and clinical experience with the Magtrak Infanta Electronic Respirometer. *Anaesthesia* 1996; **51**: 839–42.

20 Withington, D.E., Davis, G.M., Vallinis, P., Del Sonno, P. and Bevan, J.C. Respiratory function in children during recovery from neuromuscular blockade. *Paediatric Anaesthesia* 1998; **8**: 41–7.

21 Spears, R.S., Yeh, A., Fischer, D.M. and Zwass, M.S. The 'educated hand'. Can anesthesiologists assess changes in neonatal pulmonary compliance manually? *Anesthesiology* 1991; **75**: 693–6.

22 Tan, S.S., Sury, M.J. and Hatch, D.J. The 'educated hand' in paediatric anaesthesia – does it exist? *Paediatric Anaesthesia* 1993; **3**: 291–5.

23 Stocks, J., Nothen, U., Sutherland, P., Hatch, D. and Helms, P. Improved accuracy of the occlusion technique for assessing total respiratory compliance in infants. *Pediatric Pulmonology* 1987; **3**: 71–7.

24 Malviya, S., Swartz, J. and Lerman, J. Are all preterm infants younger than 60 weeks postconceptual age at risk for postanesthetic apnea? *Anesthesiology* 1993; **78**: 1076–81.

25 Harrison, A.M., Lynch, J.M., Dean, J.M. and White, M.K. Comparison of simultaneously obtained arterial and

capillary blood gases in paediatric intensive care unit patients. *Critical Care Medicine* 1997; **25**: 1904–8.

26 Abraham, E., Gallagher, T.J. and Fink, S. Clinical evaluation of a multiparameter intra-arterial blood gas sensor. *Intensive Care Medicine* 1996; **22**: 507–13.

27 Weiss, I.K., Fink, S., Edmunds, S., Harrison, R. and Donnelly, K. Continuous arterial gas monitoring: initial experience with the Paratrend 7 in children. *Intensive Care Medicine* 1996; **22**: 1414–17.

28 Venkatesh, B. and Hendry, S.P. Continuous intra-arterial blood gas monitoring. *Intensive Care Medicine* 1996; **22**: 818–28.

29 Hatherhill, M., Tibby, S.M., Durward, A., Rajah, V. and Murdoch, I.A. Continuous intra-arterial blood-gas monitoring in infants and children with cyanotic heart disease. *British Journal of Anaesthesia* 1997; **79**: 665–7.

30 Tobias, J.D., Meyer, D.J., Jr and Helikson, M.A. Monitoring of pH and PC2 in children using the Paratrend 7 in a peripheral vein. *Canadian Journal of Anaesthesia* 1998; **45**: 81–3.

31 Gravenstein, D., Lampotang, S., Huda, W. and Sultan, A. Basic principles of optical radiation and some common applications in anesthesia. *Journal of Clinical Monitoring* 1996; **12**: 445–54.

32 Moyle, J.T.B. Uses and abuses of pulse oximetry. *Archive of Diseases in Childhood* 1996; **74**: 77–80.

33 Webb, R.K., Ralston, A.C. and Runciman, W.B. Potential errors in pulse oximetry. II. Effects of changes in saturation and signal quality. *Anaesthesia* 1991; **46**: 207–12.

34 Fanconi, S. Reliability of pulse oximetry in hypoxic infants. *Journal of Pediatrics* 1988; **112**: 424–7.

35 Clayton, D.G., Webb, R.K., Ralston, A.C., Duthie, D. and Runciman, W.B. A comparison of the perfromance of 20 pulse oximeters under conditions of poor perfusion. *Anaesthesia* 1991; **46**: 3–10.

36 Ralston, A.C., Webb, R.K. and Runciman, W.B. Potential errors in pulse oximetry. I. Pulse oximeter evaluation. *Anaesthesia* 1991; **46**: 202–6.

37 Secker, C. and Spiers, P. Accuracy of pulse oximetry in patients with low systemic vascular resistance. *Anaesthesia* 1997; **52**: 127–30.

38 Iyer, P., McDougall, P., Loughnan, P., Mee, R.B., Al-Tawil, K. and Carlin, J. Accuracy of pulse oximetry in hypothermic neonates and infants undergoing cardiac surgery. *Critical Care Medicine* 1996; **24**: 507–11.

39 Spraque, D., Richardson, M.S., Baish, J.W. and Kemp, J.S. A new system to record reliable pulse oximeter data from the Nellcor-200 and its applications in studies of variability in infant oxygenation. *Journal of Clinical Monitoring* 1996; **12**: 17–25.

40 Poets, C.F. and Stebbens, V.A. Detection of movement artifact in recorded pulse oximeter saturation. *European Journal of Pediatrics* 1997; **156**: 808–11.

41 Plummer, J.L., Ilsley, A.H., Fronsko, R.R. and Owen, H. Identification of movement artefacts by the Nellcor N-200 and N-3000 pulse oximeters. *Journal of Clinical Monitoring* 1997; **13**: 109–13.

42 Grieve, S.H., McIntosh, N. and Laing, I.A. Comparison of two different pulse oximeters in monitoring preterm infants. *Critical Care Medicine* 1997; **25**: 2051–4.

43 Nijland, R., Jongsma, H.W., Nijhuis, J.G., Oeseburg, B. and Zijlstra, W.G. Notes on the apparent discordance of pulse oximetry and multi-wavelength haemoglobin

photometry. *Acta Anaesthesiologica Scandinavica* 1995; **39** Suppl. 107: 49–52.

44 Xue, F.S., Liao, X., Tong, S.Y., Liu, O.H., An, G. and Luo, L.K. Effect of epidural block on the lag time of pulse oximeter response. *Anaesthesia* 1996; **51**: 1102–5.

45 Bazeman, W.P., Myers, R.A. and Barish, R.A. Confirmation of the pulse oximetry gap in carbon monoxide poisoning. *Annals of Emergency Medicine* 1997; **30**: 608–11.

46 Ball, D.R. A Pulse oximetry probe hazard. Anesth Analg 1995; **80**: 1251.

47 Dimich, I., Singh, P.P., Adell, A., Hendler, M., Sonnenklar, N. and Jhaveri, M. Evaluation of oxygen saturation monitoring by pulse oximetry in neonates in the delivery system. *Canadian Journal of Anaesthesia* 1991; **38**: 985–8.

48 Block, F.E., Jr, Fuhrman, T.M., Cordero, L., *et al.* Technology evaluation report: obtaining pulse oximeter signals when the usual probe cannot be used. *International Journal of Clinical Monitoring Computing* 1997; **14**: 23–8.

49 Durand, M. and Ramanathan, R. Pulse oximetry for continuous oxygen monitoring in sick new-born infants. *Journal of Pediatrics* 1986; **109**: 1052–6.

50 Whyte, R.K., Jangaard, K.A. and Dooley, K.C. From oxygen content to pulse oximetry: completing the picture in the newborn. *Acta Anaesthesiologica Scandinavica* 1995; **39** Suppl. 107: 95–100.

51 Lindberg, L.G., Lennmarken, C. and Vegfors, M. Pulse oximetry – clinical implications and recent technical development. *Acta Anaesthesiologica Scandinavica* 1995; **39**: 279–87.

52 Jorgensen, J.S., Schmid, E.R., Konig, V., Faisst, K., Huch, A. and Huch, R. Limitations of forehead pulse oximetry. *Journal of Clinical Monitoring* 1995; **11**: 253–6.

53 Schranz, D., Schmitt, S., Oelert, H., *et al.* Continuous monitoring of mixed venous oxygen saturation in infants after cardiac surgery. *Intensive Care Medicine* 1989; **15**: 228–32.

54 Sanders, C.L. Making clinical decisions using SvO_2 in PICU patients. *Dimensions in Critical Care Nursing* 1997; **16**: 257–64.

55 Oxhöj, H. Oximetry catheters in diagnostic heart catheterization. *Cardiology* 1995; **86**: 384–7.

56 Faber, T. Central venous versus mixed venous oxygen content. *Acta Anaesthesiologica Scandinavica* 1995; **39** Suppl. 107: 33–6.

57 Martin, C., Auffray, J.P., Badetti, C., Perrin, G., Papazian, L. and Gouin, F. Monitoring of central venous oxygen saturation versus mixed venous oxygen concentration in critically ill patients. *Intensive Care Medicine* 1992; **18**: 101–4.

58 Cohendy, R., Périès, C., Lefrant, J.Y., Doucot, P.Y., Saissi, G. and Eledjam, J.J. Continuous monitoring of the central venous oxygen saturation in surgical patients: comparison to the monitoring of the mixed venous saturation. *Acta Anesthesiologica Scandinavica* 1996; **40**: 956.

59 Huch, A. Transcutaneous blood gas monitoring. *Acta Anaesthesiologica Scandinavica* 1995; **39** Suppl. 107: 87–90.

60 Fanconi, S., Doherty, P., Edmonds, J.F., Barker, G.A. and Bohn, D.J. Pulse oximetry in pediatric intensive care: comparison with measured saturations and transcuta-

neous oxygen tensions. *Journal of Pediatrics* 1985; **107**: 362–6.

61 Mok, J.Y.Q., McLaughlin, F.J., Pintar, M., Hak, H., Amaro-Galvez, R. and Levison, H. Transcutaneous monitoring of oxygenation: what is normal? *Journal of Pediatrics* 1986; **108**: 365–71.

62 Lindahl, S.G., Yates, A.P. and Hatch, D.J. Respiratory depression in children at different end tidal halothane concentrations. *Anaesthesia* 1987; **42**: 1267–75.

63 Lindahl, S.G.E., Offord, K.P., Johannesson, G.P., Meyer, D.M. and Hatch, D.J. Carbon dioxide elimination in anaesthetized children. *Canadian Journal of Anaesthesia* 1989; **36**: 113–19.

64 Badgwell, J.M., McLeod, M.E., Lerman, J. and Creighton, R.E. End-tidal PCO_2 measurements sampled at the distal and proximal ends of the tracheal tube in infants and children. *Anesthesia and Analgesia* 1987; **66**: 959–64.

65 Olsson, G.L. and Hallén, B. Laryngospsm during anaesthesia. A computer-aided incidence study in 136,929 patients. *Acta Anaesthesiologica Scandinavica* 1984; **28**: 567–75.

66 Olsson, G.L. Bronchospasm during anaesthesia. A computer-aided incidence study in 136,929 patients. *Acta Anaesthesiologica Scandinavica* 1987; **31**: 244–52.

67 Olsson, G.L., Hallén, B. and Hambraeus-Jonzon, K. Aspiration during anaesthesia: a computer-aided study of 185,358 anaesthetics. *Acta Anaesthesiologica Scandinavica* 1986; **30**: 84–92.

68 Hatch, D. and Fletcher, M. Anaesthesia and the ventilatory system in infants and young children. *British Journal of Anaesthesia* 1992; **68**: 389–410.

69 Mogue, L.R. and Rantala, B. Knowing your equipment. Capnometers. *Journal of Clinical Monitoring* 1988; **4**: 115–21.

70 Bhavani-Shankar, K., Kumar, A.Y., Moseley, H.S.L. and Ahyee-Hallsworth, R. Terminology and the current limitations of time capnography: a brief review. *Journal of Clinical Monitoring* 1995; **11**: 175–82.

71 Coté, C.J., Liu, L.M.P., Szyfelbein, S.K., *et al.* Intraoperative events diagnosed by expired carbon dioxide monitoring in children. *Canadian Journal of Anaesthesia* 1986; **33**: 315–20.

72 Dubreuil, M. Capnography in pediatric anaesthesia: pitfalls and applications. [In French.] *Cahiers d'Anesthesiologie* 1995; **43**: 61–5.

73 Guggenberger, H., Lenz, G. and Federle, R. Early detection of inadvertent oesophageal intubation: pulse oximetry vs. capnography. *Acta Anaesthesiologica Scandinavica* 1989; **33**: 112–15.

74 McEvedy, B.A.B., McLeod, M.E., Mulrea, M., Kirpalani, H. and Lerman, J. End-tidal, trancutaneous and arterial PCO_2 measurements in critically ill neonates: a comparative study. *Anesthesiology* 1988; **69**: 112–16.

75 McEvedy, B.A.B., McLeod, M.E., Kirpalani, H. and Lerman, J. End-tidal carbon dioxide measurements in critically ill neonates: a comparison of side stream and mainstream capnometers. *Canadian Journal of Anaesthesia* 1990; **37**: 322–6.

76 Bisonette, B. and Lerman, J. Single breath end-tidal CO_2 estimates of arterial PCO_2 in infants and children. *Canadian Journal of Anaesthesia* 1989; **36**: 110–12.

77 Schena, J., Thompson, J. and Crone, R.K. Mechanical influences on the capnogram. *Critical Care Medicine* 1984; **12**: 672–4.

78 Pascucci, R.C., Schena, J.A. and Thompson, J.E. Comparison of a sidestream and mainstream capnometer in infants. *Critical Care Medicine* 1989; **17**: 560–2.

79 Tavernier, B., Rey, D., Thevenin, D., Triboulet, J.-P. and Scherpereel, P. Can prolonged expiration manoevres improve the prediction of arterial PCO_2 from end-tidal PCO_2? *British Journal of Anaesthesia* 1997; **78**: 536–40.

80 Hicks, I.R., Soni, N.C. and Shephard, J.N. Comparison of end-tidal and arterial cabon dioxide measurements during anaesthesia with the laryngeal mask airway. *British Journal of Anaesthesia* 1993; **71**: 734–5.

81 Spahr-Schopfer, I.A., Bissonnette, B. and Hartly, E.J. Capnometry and paediatric laryngeal mask airway. *Canadian Journal of Anaesthesia* 1993; **40**: 1038–43.

82 Chhibber, A.K., Kolano, J.W. and Roberts, W.A. Relationship between end-tidal and arterial carbon dioxide with laryngeal mask airways and endothracheal tubes in children. *Anesthesia and Analgesia* 1996; **82**: 247–50.

83 Newell, S. and Brimacombe, J. A modified tracheal tube mount for sampling gases from the distal shaft of the laryngeal mask airway. *Journal of Clinical Anaesthesia* 1995; **7**: 444–5.

84 Tobias, J.D., Flanagan, J.F.K., Wheeler, T.J., Garret, J.S. and Burney, C. Noninvasive monitoring of end-tidal CO_2 via nasal cannulas in spontaneous breathing children during the perioperative period. *Critical Care Medicine* 1994; **22**: 1805–8.

85 Friesen, R.H. and Alswang, M. End-tidal PCO_2 monitoring via nasal cannulae in pediatric patients: accuracy and sources of error. *Journal of Clinical Monitoring* 1996; **12**: 155–9.

86 Lindahl, S.G.E., Yates, A.P. and Hatch, D. Relationship between invasive and noninvasive measurements of gas exchange in anesthetized infants and children. *Anesthesiology* 1987; **66**: 168–75.

87 Lazzell, V.A. and Burrows, F.A. Stability of the intraoperative arterial to end-tidal carbon dioxide partial pressure difference in children with congenital heart disease. *Canadian Journal of Anaesthesia* 1991; **38**: 859–65.

88 Kalenda, Z. The capnogram as a guide to the efficacy of cardiac massage. *Resuscitation* 1978; **6**: 259–63.

89 Falk, J.L., Rackow, E.C. and Weil, M.H. End-tidal carbon dioxide concentration during cardiopulmonary resuscitation. *New England Journal of Medicine* 1988; **318**: 607–11.

90 Sanders, A.B., Kern, K.B., Otto, C.W., Milander, M.M. and Ewy, G.A. End-tidal carbon dioxide monitoring during cardiopulmonary resuscitation. *Journal of the American Medical Association* 1989; **262**: 1347–51.

91 Callaham, M. and Barton, C. Prediction of outcome of cardiopulmonary resuscitation from end-tidal carbon dioxide concentration. *Critical Care Medicine* 1990; **18**: 358–62.

92 Simo Moyo, J., Adnet, P. and Wambo, M. Detection of gas embolism in neurosurgery by capnography. Apropos of 32 patients surgically treated in the seated position. [In French.] *Cahiers d'Anesthesiologie* 1995; **43**: 77–9.

93 Bhende, M.S. and Thompson, A.E. Evaluation of an end-tidal CO_2 detector during pediatric cardiopulmonary resuscitation. *Pediatrics* 1995; **95**: 395–9.

94 Bhende, M.S., Karasic, D.G. and Menegazzi, J.J. Evaluation of an end-tidal CO_2 detector during cardiopulmon-

ary resuscitation in a canine model for pediatric cardiac arrest. *Pediatric Emergency Care* 1995; **11**: 365–8.

95 Higgins, D., Forrest, E.T.S. and LLoyd-Thomas, A. Colorimetric end-tidal CO₂ monitoring during transfer of intubated children. *Intensive Care Medicine* 1991; **17**: 63–4.

96 Tobias, J.D., Lynch, A. and Garrett, J. Alterations of end-tidal carbon dioxide during the intrahospital transport of children. *Pediatric Emergency Care* 1966; **12**: 249–51.

97 Hand, I.L., Shepard, E.K., Krauss, A.N. and Auld, P.A.M. Discrepancies between transcutaneous and end-tidal carbon dioxide monitoring in the critically ill neonate with respiratory distess syndrome. *Critical Care Medicine.* 1989; **17**: 556–9.

98 Keenan, R. and Boyan, C. Cardiac arrest due to anesthesia. *Journal of the American Medical Association* 1985; **253**: 2373–7.

99 Swedlow, D.B. Respiratory gas monitoring. In: Saidman, L.J. and Smith, N.T. (eds). *Monitoring in Anesthesia.* Boston, MA: Butterworth-Heineman, 1993: 27–50.

100 Guyton, D.C. and Gravenstein, N. Infrared analysis of volatile anesthetics: impact of monitor agent setting, volatile mixtures, and alcohol. *Journal of Clinical Monitoring* 1990; **6**: 203–6.

101 Shirley, P.J. Safety issues and volatile agent analysers. *British Journal of Anaesthesia* 1997; **78**: 107–8.

102 Gyermek, L. Can the old vapor monitors measure new vapor anesthetics. *Journal of Clinical Anesthesiology* 1997; **9**: 171–2.

103 Foley, M.A., Wood, P.R., Peel, W.J., Jones, G.M. and Lawler, P.G. The effect of exhaled alcohol on the performance of the Datex Capnomac *Anaesthesia* 1990; **45**: 232–4.

104 Woehlck, H.J., Dunning, M.B., Kulier, A.H., Sasse, F.J., Nitipataikom, K. and Henry, D.W. The response of anesthetic agent monitors to trifluoromethane warns of the presence of carbon monoxide from anesthetic breakdown. *Journal of Clinical Monitoring* 1997; **13**: 149–55.

105 Strachan, A.N. and Richmond, M.N. Ether in an isoflurane vaporizer and the use of vapour analysers in safe anaesthesia. *British Journal of Anaesthesia* 1997; **78**: 107–8.

106 Delaney, P.A., Barnas, G.M. and Mackenzie, C.F. Response time studies of a new, portable mass spectrometer. *Journal of Clinical Monitoring* 1997; **13**: 181–9.

107 Westenscow, D.R., Smith, K., Coleman, D., Gregonis, D.E. and Van Wagenen, R.A. Clinical evaluation of a raman scattering multiple gas analyzer for the operating room. *Anesthesiology* 1989; **70**: 350–5.

108 Winberg, P. and Lundell, B.P.W. Left ventricular stroke volume and output in health term infants. *American Journal of Perinatology* 1990; **7**: 223–6.

109 McAuliffe, G., Bisonnette, B., Cavalle-Garrido, T. and Boutin, C. Heart rate and cardiac output after atropine in anaesthetised infants and children. *Canadian Journal of Anaesthesia* 1997; **44**: 154–9.

110 Park, M.K. and Guntheroth, W.G. *How to Read Pediatric ECGs.* Chicago, IL: Year Book Medical Publishers, 1987.

111 Audenaert, S.M. Atropine, halothane and pulseless electrical activity. *Anesthesia and Analgesia* 1995; **80**: 634–5.

112 Reid, M., Shaw, P. and Taylor, R.H. Oesophageal ECG in a child for burns surgery. *Paediatric Anaesthesia* 1997; **7**: 73–6.

113 Perrino, A.C., Feldman, J.M. and Barash, P.G. Non-invasive cardiovascular monitoring. In: Saidman, L.J. and Smith, N.T. (eds). *Monitoring in Anesthesia.* Boston, MA: Butterworth-Heineman, 1993: 101–45.

114 Park, M.K. and Menard, S.M. Accuracy of blood pressure measurements by the Dinamap monitor in infants and children. *Pediatrics* 1987; **79**: 907–14.

115 Ling, J., Ohara, Y., Orime, Y., Noon, G.P. and Takatani, S. Clinical evaluation of the oscillometeric blood pressure monitor in adults and children based on the 1992 AAMI SP-10 standards. *Journal of Clinical Monitoring* 1995; **11**: 123–30.

116 Goldthorp, S.L., Cameron, A. and Ashbury, A.J. Dinamap arm and thigh arterial pressure measurements. *Anaesthesia* 1986; **41**: 1032–5.

117 Lyew, M.A. and Jamieson, J.W. Blood pressure measurements using oscillometric finger cuffs in children and young adults. A comparison with arm cuffs during general anaesthesia. *Anaesthesia* 1994; **49**: 895–9.

118 Reder, R.F., Dimich, I., Cohen, M.L. and Steinfeld, L. Evaluating indirect blood pressure measurement techniques: a comparison of three systems in infants and children. *Pediatrics* 1978; **62**: 326–9.

119 Wallace, C.T., Baker, J.D., Alpert, C.C., Tankersley, S.J., Conroy, J.M. and Kerns, R.E. Comparison of blood pressure measurement by doppler and by pulse oximetry techniques. *Anesthesia and Analgesia* 1987; **66**: 1018–19.

120 Wong, D.T. and Volgyesi, G.A. Systolic arterial pressure determination by a new pulse monitor technique. *Canadian Journal of Anaesthesia* 1992; **39**: 596–9.

121 Butt, W.W. and Whyte, H. Blood pressure monitoring in neonates: comparison of umbilical and peripheral artery catheter measurements. *Journal of Pediatrics* 1984; **105**: 630–2.

122 Purday, J.P. Monitoring during paediatric cardiac anaesthesia. *Canadian Journal of Anaesthesia* 1994; **41**: 818–44.

123 Wipperman, C.F., Huth, R.G., Schmidt, F.X., Thul, J., Betancor, M. and Schranz, D. Continuous measurement of cardiac output by the Fick principle in infants and children. *Intensive Care Medicine* 1996; **22**: 467–71.

124 Fanconi, S. and Burger, R. Measurement of cardiac output in children. *Intensive Care World* 1992; **9**: 8–12.

125 Notterman, D.A., Castello, F.V., Steinberg, C., Greenwald, B., O'Loughlin, J.E. and Gold, J.P. A comparison of thermodilution and pulsed Doppler cardiac output in critically ill children. *Journal of Pediatrics* 1989; **115**: 554–60.

126 Harris, A.P., Miller, C.F., Beattie, C., *et al.* The slowing of sinus rhythm during thermodilution cardiac output determination and the effect of altering injectate temperature. *Anesthesiology* 1985; **63**: 540–1.

127 Tibballs, J. A comparative study of cardiac output in neonates supported by mechanical ventilation: measurement with thoracic electrical bioimpedance and pulsed Doppler ultrasound. *Journal of Pediatrics* 1989; **114**: 632–5.

128 Alverson, D.C., Eldridge, M.W., Johnson, J.D., Aldrich, M., Angelus, P. and Berman, W. Noninvasive measurement of cardiac output in healthy preterm and term

newborn infants. *American Journal of Perinatology* 1984; **1**: 148–51.

129 Murdoch, I.A., Marsh, M.J., Tibby, S.M. and McLuckie, A. Continuous haemodynamic monitoring in children: use of transoesophageal Doppler. *Acta Paediatrica Scandinavica* 1995; **84**: 761–4.

130 Muhiudeen, I.A., Roberson, D.A., Sivlerman, N.H., Haas, G., Turley, K. and Cahalan, M.K. Intraoperative echocardiography in infants and children with congenital shunt lesions: transesophageal versus epicardial echocardiography. *Journal of the American College of Cardiology* 1990; **16**: 1687–95.

131 Lam, J., Neirotti, R.A., Hardjowijono, R., Blom-Muilwijk, C.M., Schuller, J.L. and Visser, C.A. Transesophageal echocardiography with the use of a four-millimeter probe. *Journal of the American Society of Echocardiography* 1997; **10**: 499–504.

132 Stevenson, J.G. Role of intraoperative transoesophageal echocardiography during repair of congenital cardiac defects. *Acta Paediatrica Scandinavica* 1995; Suppl. 410: 23–33.

133 Xu, J., Shiota, T., Ge, S., Rice, M.J., Cobanoglu, A. and Sahn, D.J. Intraoperative transesophageal echocardiography using high-resolution biplane 7.5 MHz probes with continuous-wave Doppler capability in infants and children with tetralogy of Fallot. *American Journal of Cardiology* 1996; **77**: 539–42.

134 Shiota, T., Omoto, R., Cobanoglu, A., *et al.* Usefulness of transesophageal imaging of flow convergence region in the operating room for evaluating isloated patent ductus arteriosus. *American Journal of Cardiology* 1997; **80**: 1108–12.

135 Singh, G.K., Shiota, T., Cobanoglu, A., Droukas, P., Rice, M.J. and Sahn, D.J. Diagnostic accuracy and role of intraoperative biplane transesophgeal echocardiography in pediatric patients with left ventricle outflow tract lesions. *Journal of the American Society of Echocardiography* 1998; **11**: 47–56.

136 Kantoch, M.J., Frost, G.F. and Robertson, M.A. Use of transoesophageal echocardiography in radiofrequency ablation in children and adolescents. *Canadian Journal of Cardiology* 1998; **14**: 519–23.

137 Smith, M.D., MacPhail, B., Harrison, M.R., Lenhoff, S.J. and De-Maria, A.N. Value and limitations of transoesophageal echocradiography in determination of left ventricular volumes and ejection fraction. *Journal of the American College of Cardiology* 1992; **19**: 1213–22.

138 Bailey, J.M., Shanewise, J.S., Kikura, M. and Sharma, S. A comparison of transesophageal and transthoracic echocardiographic assessment of left ventricular function in pediatric patients with congenital heart disease. *Journal of Cardiothoracic and Vascular Anaesthesia* 1995; **9**: 665–9.

139 Huemer, G. and Zimpfer, M. Intraoperative echocardiography. *Acta Anaesthesiologica Scandinavica* 1996; **40** Suppl. 109: 194–7.

140 Gueugniaud, P.Y., Muchada, R., Moussa, M., Haro, D. and Petit, P. Continuous oesophageal aortic blood flow echo-Doppler measurement during general anaesthesia in infants. *Canadian Journal of Anaesthesia* 1997; **44**: 745–50.

141 Lavoie, J. Oesophageal aortic echo-Doppler and TEE. *Canadian Journal of Anaesthesia* 1998; **45**: 93–4.

142 Mammamoto, T., Hayashi, Y., Ohnishi, Y. and Kuro, M. Incidence of venous and paradoxical air embolism in neurosurgical patients in the sitting position. Detection by transoesophageal echocardiography. *Acta Anaesthesiologica Scandinavica* 1998; **42**: 643–7.

143 Zestos, M.M., Chehade, M. and Mossad, E. A transesophageal echocardiography probe causes airway obstruction in an older child. *Journal of Cardiothoracic and Vascular Anesthesia* 1998; **12**: 65–6.

144 Welch, R.H., Gravenstein, N. and Blackshear, R.H. Multilumen central venous catheters in children: relative potential to perforate vessels. An *in vitro* study. *Journal of Clinical Monitoring* 1997; **13**: 75–9.

145 Fievez, E., Schultze-Balin, C., Herbaux, B., Dalmas, S. and Scherpereel, P. A study of blood loss during surgery for scoliosis. Posterior approach in 319 adolescents. [In French.] *Cahiers d'Anesthesiologie* 1995; **43**: 425–33.

146 Jimenez, D.F. and Barone, C.M. Intraoperative autologous blood transfusion in the surgical correction of craniosynostosis. *Neurosurgery* 1996; **39**: 1075–9.

147 Reinoso-Barbero, F., Calvo, C., Ruza, F., López-Herce, J., Bueno, M. and Garcia, S. Reference values of gastric intramucosal pH in children. *Paediatric Anaesthesia* 1998; **8**: 135–8.

148 Imrie, M.M. and Hall, G.M. Body temperature and anaesthesia. *British Journal of Anaesthesia* 1990; **64**: 346–54.

149 Deacock, S. and Holdcroft, A. Heat retention using passive systems during anaesthesia: comparison of two plastic wraps, one with reflective properties. *British Journal of Anaesthesia* 1997; **79**: 766–9.

150 Kurz, A., Kurz, M., Poeschl, G., Faryniak, B., Redl, G. and Hackl, W. Forced-air warming maintains intraoperative normothermia better than circulating-water mattresses. *Anesthesia and Analgesia* 1993; **77**: 89–95.

151 Bissonnette, B., Sessler, D.I. and LaFlamme, P. Intraoperative monitoring sites in infants and children and the effect of inspired gas warming on esophageal temperature. *Anesthesia and Analgesia* 1989; **69**: 192–6.

152 Harasawa, K., Kemmotsu, O., Mayumi, T. and Kawano, Y. Comparison of tympanic, esophageal, and blood temperatures during mild hypothermic cardiopulmonary bypass: a study using an infrared emission detection tympanic thermometer. *Journal of Clinical Monitoring* 1997; **13**: 19–24.

153 Burgess, G. III, Cooper, J. and Marino, R. Continuous monitoring of skin temperature using a liquid-crystal thermometer during anesthesia. *Southern Medical Journal* 1978; **71**: 516–18.

154 Donati, F. Monitoring of neuromuscular blockade. In: Saidman, L.J. and Smith, N.T. (eds). *Monitoring in Anesthesia*. Boston, MA: Butterworth-Heineman, 1993: 157–68.

155 Ridley, S.A. and Hatch, D.J. Post-tetanic count and profound muscular blockade with atracurium infusion in paediatric patients. *British Journal of Anaesthesia* 1988; **60**: 31–5.

156 Fischer, D.M., O'Keefe, C., Stsanski, D. *et al.* Pharmacokinetics and pharmacodynamics of d-tubocurarine in infants, children, and adults. *Anesthesiology* 1982; **57**: 203–8.

157 Goudsouzian, N. Maturation of neuromuscular transmission in the infant. *British Journal of Anaesthesia* 1980; **52**: 205–13.

158 Goudsouzian, N., Crone, R. and Todres, I.D. Recovery from pancuronium blockade in the neonatal intensive care unit. *British Journal of Anaesthesia* 1981; **53**: 1303–9.

159 Ansermino, J.M., Sanderson, P.M., Bevan, J.C. and Bevan, D.R. Accelomyography improves dectection of residual neuromuscular block in children. *Canadian Journal of Anaesthesia* 1996; **43**: 589–94.

160 Martin, R., Bourdua, I., Therialut, S., Tetrault, J.P. and Pilote, M. Neuromuscular monitoring: does it make a difference? *Canadian Journal of Anaesthesia* 1996; **43**: 585–8.

161 Engbaek, J., Roed, J., Hangaard, N. and Viby-Mogensen, J. The agreement between adductor pollicis mechanomyogram and first dorsal interosseous electromyogram: a pharmacodynamic study of rocuronium and vecuronium. *Acta Anaesthesiologica Scandinavica* 1994; **38**: 869–78.

162 Woolf, R.L., Crawford, M.W. and Choo, S.M. Dose–response of rocuronium bromide in children anesthetized with propofol: a comparison with succinylcholine. *Anesthesiology* 1997; **87**: 1368–72.

163 Kirkegaard-Nielsen, H., Helbo-Hansen, H.S., Lindholm, P., Stougaard Petersen, H.H., Krogh Severinsen, I. and Brauner Smidt, M. New equipment for neuromuscular transmission monitoring: a comparison of the TOF-GUARD with the Myograph 2000. *Journal of Clinical Monitoring* 1998; **14**: 19–27.

164 McCluskey, A., Meakin, G., Hopkinson, J.M. and Baker, R.D. A comparison of acceleromyography and mechanomyography for determination of the dose–response curve of rocuronium in children. *Anaesthesia* 1997; **52**: 345–9.

165 Kalli, I. Effect of surface electrode positioning on the compound action potential evoked by ulnar nerve stimulation in anaesthetized infants and children. *British Journal of Anaesthesia* 1992; **62**: 188–93.

166 Dahaba, A.A., Rehak, P.H. and List, W.F. Assessment of accelography with TOF-Guard: a comparison with electromyelography. *European Journal of Anaesthesiology* 1997; **14**: 623–9.

167 Stoddart, P.A. and Mather, S.J. Onset of neuromuscular blockade and intubating conditions one minute after the administration of rocuronium in children. *Paediatric Anaesthesia* 1998; **8**: 37–40.

168 Hodges, U.M. Vecuronium infusion requirements in paediatric patients in intensive care units: the use of accelomyography. *British Journal of Anaesthesia* 1996; **76**: 23–8.

169 Goudsouzian, N.G. Mivacurium in infants and children. *Paediatric Anaesthesia* 1997; **7**: 183–90.

170 Kitajima, T., Ishii, K. and Ogata, H. Assessment of neuromuscular block in the thumb and the great toe using accelography in infants. *Anaesthesia* 1996; **51**: 341–3.

171 Plaud, B., Laffon, M., Ecoffey, C. and Meistelman, C. Monitoring orbicularis oculi predicts good intubation conditions after vecuronium in children. *Canadian Journal of Anaesthesia* 1997; **44**: 712–16.

172 Hunter, J.M. Is it always necessary to antagonize residual neuromuscular block? Do children differ from adults? *British Journal of Anaesthesia* 1996; **77**: 707–9.

173 Mortensen, C.R., Berg, H., El-Mahdy, A. and Viby-Mogensen, J. Peroperative monitoring of neuromuscular transmission using acceleromyography prevents residual neuromuscular block following pancuronium. *Acta Anaesthesiologica Scandinavica* 1995; **39**: 797–801.

174 Bevan, D.R., Doanti, F. and Kopman, A.F. Reversal of neuromuscular block. *Anesthesiology* 1992; **77**: 785–805.

175 Abdulatif, M., Al-Ghamdi, A., Al-Sanabary, M. and Abdel-Gaffar, M.E. Edrophonium antagonism of intense mivacurium-induced neuromuscular block in children. *British Journal of Anaesthesia* 1996; **76**: 239–44.

176 Harper, C.M. and Nelson, K.R. Intraoperative electrophysiological monitoring in children. *Journal of Clinical Neurophysiology* 1992; **9**: 342–56.

177 Loughnan, B.A. and Fennely, M.E. Editorial. Spinal cord monitoring. *Anaesthesia* 1995; **59**: 101–2.

178 Agarwal, R., Roitman, K.J. and Stokes, M. Improvement of intraoperative somatosensory evoked potentials by ketamine. *Paediatric Anaesthesia* 1998; **8**: 263–6.

179 Edmonds, H.L., Jr, Rodriguez, R.A., Audenaert, S.M., Austin, E.H. III, Pollock, S.B., Jr and Ganzel, B.L. The role of neuromonitoring in cardiovascular surgery. *Journal of Cardiothoracic and Vascular Surgery* 1996; **10**: 15–23.

180 Ferry, P.C. Neurologic sequelae of open-heart surgery in children. *American Journal of Disease in Childhood* 1990; **144**: 369–73.

181 Austin, E.H. III, Edmonds, H.L., Jr, Auden, S.M., *et al.* Benefit of neurophysiologic monitoring for pediatric cardiac surgery. *Journal of Thoracic and Cardiovascular Surgery* 1997; **114**: 707–15.

182 Burgess, R.C. Technology and equipment review. Intraoperative monitoring equipment. *Journal of Clinical Neurophysiology* 1993; **10**: 526–33.

183 Maynard, D.E. and Jenkinson, J.L. The cerebral function analysing monitor. *Anaesthesia* 1984; **39**: 678–90.

184 Lloyd-Thomas, A.R., Cole, P.V. and Prior, P.F. Quantitative EEG and brainstem auditory evoked potentials: comparison of isoflurane with halothane using the cerebral function analysing monitor. *British Journal of Anaesthesia* 1990; **65**: 306–12.

185 Thomsen, C.E. and Prior, P.F. Quantitative EEG in assessment of anaesthetic depth; comparative study of methodology. *British Journal of Anaesthesia* 1996; **77**: 172–80.

186 Young, W.L., Silverberg, P.A., Ornstein, E., *et al.* A computer system for study of the EEG during carotid endarterectomy. *Journal of Clinical Monitoring* 1985; **1**: 100–1.

187 Burrows, F.A., Volgyesi, G.A. and James, P.D. Clinical evaluation of the augmented delta quotient monitor for intraoperative electroencephalographic monitoring of children during surgery and cardiopulmonary bypass for repair of congenital cardiac defects. *British Journal of Anaesthesia* 1989; **63**: 565–73.

188 Struys, M., Versichelen, L., Mortier, E., *et al.* Comparison of spontaneous frontal EMG, EEG power spectrum and bispectral index to monitor propofol drug effect and emergence. *Acta Anaesthesiologica Scandinavica* 1998; **42**: 628–36.

189 Rodriguez, R.A., Audenaert, S.M., Austin, E.H. III and Edmonds, H.L., Jr. Auditory evoked responses in children during hypothermic cardiopulmonary bypass. *Clinical Neurophysiology* 1995; **12**: 168–76.

190 O'Kelly, S.W., Smith, D.C. and Pilkington, S.N. The auditory evoked potential and paediatric anaesthesia. *British Journal of Anaesthesia* 1995; **75**: 428–30.

191 Mantzaridis, H. and Kenny, G.N.C. Auditory evoked potential index: a quantitative measure of changes in auditory evoked potentials during general anaesthesia. *Anaesthesia* 1997; **52**: 1030–6.

192 Iacopino, D.G., Zaccone, C., Molina, D., Todaro, C., Tomasello, F. and Cardia, E. Intraoperative monitoring of cerebral blood flow during ventricular shunting in hydrocephalic pediatric patients. *Childs Nervous System* 1995; **11**: 483–6.

193 Murkin, J.M. Monitoring cerebral oxygenation. *Canadian Journal of Anaesthesia*. 1994; **41**: 1027–32.

194 Committee on Drugs. Guidelines for monitoring and management of pediatric patients during and after sedation for diagnostic and therapeutic procedures. *Pediatrics* 1992; **89**: 1110–15.

195 Morton, N.S. and Oomen, G.J. Development of a sedation and monitoring protocol for safe sedation of children. *Paediatric Anaesthesia* 1988; **8**: 65–8.

196 Coté, C.J., Alderfer, R.J., Notterman, D.A., *et al*. Sedation disasters: adverse drug reports in *Pediatrics* FDA, USP and others. *Anesthesiology* 1995; **83**: A1182.

197 Malviya, S., Voepel-Lewis, T. and Tait, A.R. Adverse events and risk factors associated with sedation of children by nonanesthesiologists. *Anesthesia and Analgesia* 1997; **85**: 1207–13.

198 Hart, L.S., Berns, S.D., Houck, C.S. and Boenning, D.A. The value of end-tidal CO_2 monitoring when comparing three methods of conscious sedation for children undergoing painful procedures in the emergency department. *Pediatric Emergency Care* 1997; **13**: 189–93.

199 Selldén, H., de Chateau, P., Ekman, G., Linder, B., Saaf, J. and Wahlund, L.O. Circulatory monitoring of children during anaesthesia in low-field magnetic resonance imaging. *Acta Anaesthesiologica Scandinavica* 1990; **34**: 41–3.

200 Rheineck-Leyssius, A.T., Kalkman, C.J. and Trouwborst, A. Influence of motivation of care providers on the incidence of postoperative hypoxaemia in the recovery room. *British Journal of Anaesthesia* 1996; **77**: 453–7.

201 Bell, C., Dubose, R., Seashore, J., *et al*. Infant apnea detection after herniorrhaphy. *Journal of Clinical Monitoring* 1995; **7**: 219–33.

202 Karl, H.W., Tyler, D.C. and Krane, E.J. Respiratory depression after low-dose caudal morphine. *Canadian Journal of Anaesthesia* 1996; **43**: 1065–7.

203 Vila, R., Miguel, E., Montferrer, N., *et al*. Respiratory depression following epidural morphine in an infant of three months of age. *Paediatric Anaesthesia* 1997; **7**: 61–4.

CHAPTER 8

Fluid balance: all aspects

LUCINDA HUSKISSON

This chapter aims to cover the basics of fluid balance. It is loosely divided into four sections. The first outlines fluid physiology. The use of crystalloid maintenance fluids is dealt with in the second. The third section deals with colloids and touches on the crystalloid:colloid debate for volume replacement. The final part covers the use of blood and its components in paediatric anaesthesia.

FLUID PHYSIOLOGY

TOTAL BODY WATER AND FLUID BALANCE

Total body water varies with degree of adiposity (90% of muscle weight is water vs 10% of fat), disease state and age. Ninety-four per cent of the body weight of a 12-week fetus is water and this falls to 80% by 32 weeks' gestation and 78% by term. There is a further reduction of about 5% in the first week of life, followed by a gradual fall to adult levels of 50–60% by 18 months of age.[1]

Body water is conventionally divided into three compartments: intracellular, extracellular and transcellular. In adults 60% of water is intracellular, 10% transcellular and 30% extracellular, of which 7.5% is intravascular. Although it is well recognized that disease states may affect the distribution of water in the body, it is less well known that age will also influence it. Extracellular water decreases from 60% in a 20-week fetus to 45% at term and falls a further 5% in the first 5 days of life.[1] Adult levels are reached by the end of the second year of life.

THE STARLING EQUATION

The extracellular compartment is further subdivided into the interstitial and intravascular spaces, with the interstitial space being three and a half times larger than the intravascular.[2] Fluid flux between the two was first described by Starling, who noted that the rate of fluid movement into or out of a capillary was related to the net hydrostatic pressure minus the net osmotic pressure.[3] The Starling equation:[4]

$$J_v = K_{fc}[(P_c - P_t) - \delta_c(\pi_c - \pi_t)],$$

where J_v = rate of fluid movement into/out of

capillary; K_{fc} = capillary filtration coefficient; P_c = capillary hydrostatic pressure; P_t = tissue fluid hydrostatic pressure; δ_c = reflection coefficient; π_c = capillary colloid osmotic pressure; π_t = tissue colloid osmotic pressure, has been further modified to incorporate coefficients which represent the permeabilty of the capillary membrane to small solutes (K_{fc}) and the reflection coefficient which describes the membrane's ability to prevent large molecules such as plasma proteins from crossing it: the Starling coefficient (sc).[5] If sc is 1, then a fluid can realize its full osmotic pressure; if sc for a membrane is 0 then fluids will pass freely across it and no pressure will be exerted. The coefficients vary between different organs of the body and are altered by disease. Burns, sepsis and cardiopulmonary bypass, in particular, reduce sc, resulting in capillaries which are increasingly 'leaky'. This has two effects: it allows water to leak out causing tissue oedema and it allows osmotically active particles to escape into the interstitial space. If sc then increases again, these particles will remain in the interstitial space, increasing its osmotic pressure and altering the balance of the Starling equation until they can be removed by the lymphatic system.

Most of the components of the Starling equation can be measured only with difficulty in the laboratory but the intravascular osmotic pressure and the capillary hydrostatic pressure can be measured clinically.[6,7] Guyton *et al.* describe certain 'oedema protection factors', such as increased lymphatic flow, which prevent the accumulation of oedema until the capillary hydrostatic pressure has increased by more than 15 mmHg.[8] This is supported clinically by the observation that in the absence of pulmonary capillary damage, the left atrial pressure (equivalent to hydrostatic pressure) must be increased to 15–20 mmHg before pulmonary oedema is seen.

One of the main differences between the fluid balance of adults and infants is the relatively large water turnover in the infant. The water contained within the extracellular space of a 70 kg man is about 14 l. Just under 3 l day^{-1} is lost in urine, faeces, sweat and during respiration (20%). In a 7 kg infant, the extracellular space contains about 1.6 l and obligatory losses are around 0.7 l day^{-1} (44%).[2] Any relatively small increase in losses will therefore have a much greater effect on a small child and this explains why diarrhoea remains such an important cause of infant mortality world-wide.

MAINTENANCE CRYSTALLOID REQUIREMENTS

MAINTENANCE WATER REQUIREMENTS

Although there are numerous formulae for calculating maintenance fluid requirements, it is important to stress that these are all guidelines only. They may be used as a starting point but the individual child's response to the fluid given must be monitored and appropriate adjustments made to the regimen.

The formulae available for calculating fluid requirement have as their basis body surface area (BSA), calorie requirement and the weight of the child.

Body surface area

Various nomograms are published which calculate BSA from height and weight. In older children the calculation of BSA is relatively easy and accurate because it is possible to obtain an accurate height. Measurements of the length of a neonate or small infant are not as reliable and errors of up to 20% in BSA are well recognized in babies less than 3 kg.[9] Because the height/length measurement is inaccurate, most centres now use a formula based on weight alone to calculate fluid requirement and the use of BSA has fallen from favour.[10]

Calorie requirements

The metabolism of 1 calorie requires 1 ml of water because, although 0.2 ml of water is produced, a further 1.2 ml is consumed. Therefore, 100 calories will require 100 ml of water for metabolism and knowing the calorie requirement of a child will also reveal the water requirement.[11] In 1911 Howland calculated the calorie requirement of an infant from 3–10 kg to be 100 cal kg^{-1}, with older children needing 75 and adults 35 cal kg^{-1}. The extra calories metabolized by the younger children he attributed to proportionally larger surface area and growth.[12] In infants of less than 10 kg body weight, 50 cal kg^{-1} will be needed for basal metabolic requirements and the rest for growth. Children of less than 20 kg body weight need 1000 calories for the first 10 kg but only 50 cal kg^{-1} for the next 10 kg because of slower growth rate, and larger children and adults need only three times the calories of a neonate (1500 calories for the first 20 kg and 20 cal kg^{-1} thereafter).[11]

Normal maintenance fluid requirements calculated by weight

Whatever mechanism is used to calculate fluid requirements, it must be simple and foolproof because small miscalculations can result in significant errors in fluids administered. It has already been said that 100 calories requires 100 ml of water. A 25 kg child, therefore, requires 100 ml kg^{-1} for the first 10 kg (1000 ml), 50 ml kg^{-1} for the next 10 kg (500 ml) and 20 ml kg^{-1} thereafter (100 ml), making a total of 1600 ml per day or 66 ml h^{-1}. This can be simplified by assuming that there are 25 h in a day. The child then needs 4 ml kg^{-1} h^{-1} for the first 10 kg (40 ml), 2 ml kg^{-1} h^{-1} for the next 10 kg (20 ml) and 1 ml kg^{-1} h^{-1} thereafter (5 ml), giving an hourly total of 65 ml, which can be computed at the bedside without a calculator.

Neonates have greater fluid requirements than infants. As a general rule, most neonatal units allow 60 ml kg^{-1} for the first day, increasing by 30 ml kg^{-1} day^{-1} to 150 ml kg^{-1} for a term neonate and 180 ml^{-1} kg^{-1} day^{-1} for a preterm. This requirement will be affected by

Table 8.1 Normal maintenance fluid requirements

Weight (kg)	Maintenance fluid requirement (cumulative values) (ml kg^{-1} day^{-1})
< 10	100
11–20	50
> 20	20

environment (overhead heaters increase water loss compared with incubators), by whether the baby is ventilated (when there will be a humidifier in the circuit) and by the general state of the neonate. A premature baby with a patent ductus arteriosus may close the duct in response to fluid restriction and this may avoid the need for more aggressive management.

Dextrose requirements

In the UK, intravenous dextrose infusions are usually supplied as 4%, 5%, 10% and 20% strengths. In addition, 50% dextrose is available for management of hypoglycaemia. Most infants and children require 4% or 5% dextrose. A recent study from Germany, however, suggests that when these infusions are given peroperatively, children may become hyperglycaemic with dextrose concentrations as low as 2.5% although these were administered at large volumes equivalent to 200 ml kg^{-1} day^{-1}.[13] Neonates have poor glycogen stores and require higher glucose infusions to maintain their blood glucose levels. The majority of neonates, therefore, are traditionally managed using infusions of 10% dextrose which can be given through a peripheral cannula. Sick neonates on the intensive care unit, particularly in the presence of sepsis, may require higher infusions than this. Such patients may also need fluid restriction and it is not uncommon for small septic babies to need 20% infusions of dextrose. A neonate who cannot be fed enterally for more than a couple of days will require parenteral hyperalimentation rather than simple dextrose saline solutions. Hyperglycaemia can develop in response to stress. Both hypoglycaemia and hyperglycaemia can occur and blood sugar levels should be regularly monitored.

Electrolyte requirements

Electrolyte requirements vary with prematurity, losses and disease states. There is some debate as to whether a neonate needs sodium on the first day of life. Some units use a dextrose solution without added electrolytes, whilst others add sodium, potassium and calcium, particularly for premature infants. Preterm breast milk contains higher concentrations of sodium, calcium and phosphorus for the first 2–

4 weeks of lactation, and meets the preterm infant's increased requirements for these elements. Preterm formulae with similar electrolyte composition are also available. As a guide for prescribing, most children require 2–3 mmol kg^{-1} of sodium and 2 mmol kg^{-1} of potassium. This means that a 10 kg infant who needs 1000 ml of fluid per day will also need around 30 mmol of sodium. In the UK, fluids are available as dextrose (4% or 10%) and 0.18% saline (i.e. containing 30 mmol l^{-1}). For most patients, a ready-made bag of fluid will provide their electrolyte needs. In some instances, additional sodium will be required. This can be added to a standard bag using a strong sodium (30%; 5000 mmol l^{-1}) solution, or Normal saline (0.9%; 150 mmol l^{-1}) or half Normal saline (0.45%; 75 mmol l^{-1}) can be used in its place.

The amount of sodium administered to neonates in the immediate postoperative period needs to be monitored. Krummel *et al.* studied 20 surgical newborns and found that hypernatraemia occurred in 64% of term babies and 67% of preterms. In all cases this appeared to be due predominantly to an administered sodium load of more than 400% of the estimated maintenance requirements. This was compounded by a slightly reduced ability to excrete sodium and a short period of postoperative sodium retention.[14]

SPECIAL REQUIREMENTS

Gastrointestinal losses

Gastrointestinal surgery is relatively common in small infants. Ileus may also occur in a sick child; therefore, gastrointestinal losses are of importance. Nasogastric aspirates should be replaced volume for volume with normal saline containing 10 mmol potassium chloride per 500 ml. This sodium load allows the patient's kidneys to correct the hydrogen deficit incurred by the loss of gastric secretions. Stoma losses may also need to be replaced. High stomas in particular may be associated with significant sodium losses leading to as much a 6-fold increase in sodium requirements. Losses of more than 40 ml kg^{-1} day^{-1} are likely to require parenteral replacement using the same solution of normal saline with 10 mmol potass-

ium per 500 ml. Usually, 0.5 ml is replaced for every 1 ml lost but, depending on the volume of losses and the site of the stoma, anything from one-third to three-quarter replacement may be required. Children who have ileus, either from gastrointestinal surgery and pathology or secondary to another cause, can secrete large amounts of fluid within the gut and peritoneal cavity. Babies with abdominal distension due to Hirschsprung's disease (colonic aganglionosis) may be intravascularly depleted in the presence of steady weight or even weight gain and such patients may need intravascular volume replacement despite normal indices.

Pyloric stenosis

Hypertrophic pyloric stenosis is a common condition with an incidence of about 1 : 200. All babies with this condition vomit and will require preoperative intravenous fluids. About 50% of patients will have a significant derangement of their electrolytes and acid : base status as a result of vomiting. The most useful electrolyte to gauge the seriousness of the metabolic upset is chloride, which can be used to calculate the chloride deficit and this must often be specifically requested as it is no longer performed routinely in most hospitals. While the serum chloride remains low, the infant will be alkalotic.[15] The vomiting of HCl, together with the kidney's attempts to conserve sodium, results in a metabolic alkalosis and a depletion of total body potassium. Because potassium is an intracellular ion, the serum potassium is a poor guide to potassium requirements and will usually be within the normal range.

To correct the metabolic alkalosis, the infant must be given sufficient sodium and potassium so that the kidneys can conserve hydrogen ions and correct the acid : base status. Chloride is also given as the anion to both sodium and potassium. Most babies with mild derangement (sodium bicarbonate < 35 mmol) will be corrected within 24 h using a solution of 5% dextrose plus 0.45% saline with 15 mmol of potassium chloride per 500 ml bag at 150–180 ml kg^{-1} day^{-1}. In extreme cases, normal saline (or 4.5% albumin which contains 150 mmol NaCl l^{-1}) may be required and 2–3 days of parenteral fluids may be needed preoperatively. It is also important to remember that any gastric distension results in more gastric juices being secreted and lost. A wide-bore nasogastric tube should be left on free drainage with regular aspirations and any nasogastric losses should be replaced millilitre for millilitre with normal saline with added potassium (10 mmol in 500 ml).

Posterior urethral valves

Posterior urethral valves cause a congenital obstruction of the male posterior urethra and affected infants may also have a degree of renal dysplasia. Nowadays, the condition is increasingly diagnosed antenatally and most other children present within the first month of life. The initial management of a neonate with valves is to catheterize the patient and then confirm the diagnosis by cystogram and/or cystoscopy. Surgery consists of valve ablation via the cystoscope. A significant number of these children will have renal impairment which may be long-term, and almost all have a diuresis in response to catheterization and relief of the obstruction. Urine output must be closely monitored in these patients and their fluid intake will be based on their creatinine and their output. Most of these babies are well enough to receive oral feeds but will also require parenteral supplementary fluids to keep up with urinary losses. This diuretic phase can last for between 24 h and a couple of weeks, again emphasizing that strict criteria cannot be laid down for neonatal fluid infusions.

Congenital diaphragmatic hernia

The fluid handling of a neonate with congenital diaphragmatic hernia merits special mention. There appears to be only a narrow path between hypovolaemia and fluid overload, either of which may have catastrophic effects resulting in a worsening spiral of acidosis and hypoxia. Rowe *et al.* studied the urine output and osmolarity of both urine and serum in 22 infants with diaphragmatic hernia vs 12 control infants undergoing laparotomy for some other reason. They found that although all controls responded appropriately, 64% of the diaphragmatic hernia group inappropriately retained fluid in the first 16 h after surgery and one-third still had an inappropriate urine output

24 h after surgery.[16] Fluid management of these children involves strict crystalloid restrictions (30 ml kg^{-1} day^{-1} for the first 24 h) and colloid boluses to maintain normovolaemia. Close monitoring of urine output and serum and urine osmolarity will help in the management.

Phototherapy

Neonatal 'physiological' jaundice is relatively common and is worsened by dehydration. Some neonates with a rising unconjugated hyperbilirubinaemia can be managed simply by liberalizing their fluids. This may need to be via a nasogastric tube or parenterally as the jaundice tends to make the baby sleepy and therefore less able to feed, which compounds the problem. If phototherapy is required, environmental water loss is increased significantly and an extra 25 ml kg^{-1} day^{-1} should be added to the fluids to compensate.

Effects of surgery

In 1968 Reid showed in adult patients that fluid accumulation occurred in the early postoperative phase and that this occurred entirely within the extravascular space. There was no change in the intravascular volume even when large fluid increases were seen extravascularly.[17] Seven years earlier, Shires *et al.* had studied fluid shifts peroperatively and noted an acute contraction of the functional extracellular fluid which, in the absence of blood loss, they presumed to be due to internal redistribution. They noted that the magnitude of the internal redistribution was related to the degree of surgical trauma and particularly to the duration and degree of retraction. They concluded that this was a major stimulus to the fluid and sodium retention seen postoperatively.[18] Certainly, after major abdominal surgery there is a fall in the serum sodium and evidence of fluid retention with periorbital and dependent oedema, which can be reduced by restricting fluids for the first 24–48 h following surgery. Following minor procedures patients are allowed their full maintenance fluids, but after any major surgery their intake is reduced to 50% of requirements for the first postoperative day, and if additional fluid is required it may be better to be given as colloid.

Sepsis

Hyponatraemia in sepsis is well recognized and is associated with a worse prognosis. Hannon and Boston looked at fluid and ion redistribution in an animal model of sepsis and found significant shifts of sodium, chloride and water into cells compared with sham controls.[19] They found this trend to be exacerbated by infusing 5% dextrose compared with normal saline with fluid shifts occurring when the volume infused was less than the estimated fluid requirement. They suggested that the hyponatraemia and plasma hypo-osmolality were caused by a combination of intracellular shift of sodium and water, and a dilution of the extracellular space, probably caused by physiological antidiuretic hormone (ADH) secretion. Their conclusion was that, in the presence of sepsis, 4% dextrose + 0.18% sodium chloride is inappropriate, potentially dangerous and should be avoided.

Burns (see also Chapter 15)

Significant burns cause large fluid losses and burns patients require large volumes of fluid resuscitation. In addition to normal maintenance fluids, such patients need resuscitation fluid administered as Normal saline, Ringer's solution or Gelofusine® given over at least the first 36 h after injury. The 36 h are divided into six periods: three of 4 h, two of 6 h and one of 12 h. The timing starts from the moment of injury so that the first infusion is inevitably delayed. During each period the child needs an average of 0.5 ml kg^{-1} per % burn. The precise volume given is adjusted on the basis of urine output, urine and plasma osmolality, perfusion and the calculated plasma deficit. This can be calculated from the formula:

$$\text{plasma deficit} = \text{blood volume} - \left(\text{blood volume} \times \frac{\text{normal haematocrit}}{\text{observed haematocrit}}\right)$$

Deep burns result in red cell destruction and the usual blood requirement is of 1% of normal blood volume per 1% burn for deep burns of more than 10% surface area. Because the haematocrit is a useful guide to the plasma deficit, blood is usually best administered during the last 12 h of fluid resuscitation.[20]

Clinical assessment of dehydration

Although thirst appears with the loss of approximately 2% of total body water, the state of the peripheral circulation is the most sensitive guide to more serious levels of clinical dehydration in children. Core–peripheral temperature difference becomes clinically detectable and mucous membranes dry at around 5% loss of total body water. With 10% dehydration the peripheries are cold and capillary refill, normally complete within 2 s, is delayed. Pulse and respiratory rates increase, consciousness may be clouded, and in the neonate the fontanelle is sunken. Blood pressure may fall, although because of the increased cardiac output caused by the tachycardia this is not an early or reliable sign. Urine output is decreased. At 15% dehydration capillary refill may be incomplete even after 10 s, the mouth is parched and the eyes are sunken. The pulse is rapid and thready and blood pressure low. The child is stuporose and oliguric, and may show signs of respiratory distress. Losses in excess of 20% may be fatal.

COLLOIDS

THE CRYSTALLOID VERSUS COLLOID DEBATE

The superiority of colloid over crystalloid for volume replacement remains controversial.[21,22] Whilst crystalloids are generally more popular in the USA, colloids are preferred in Europe.[23] The debate centres on which fluid space needs replenishing and the importance or otherwise of colloid osmotic pressure.

Colloids theoretically remain within the intravascular space, therefore expanding the intravascular volume more efficiently, producing the same increase in cardiac output for a smaller volume of fluid. The proponents of crystalloid argue that the whole extracellular fluid space is reduced in hypovolaemia because of fluid movement from the interstitial compartment and crystalloids enter this space more reliably and rapidly.[24] Certainly, two to three times the volume of crystalloid must be infused to produce an equivalent effect on intravascular volume. This increase in volume carries with it a risk of tissue oedema. The crystalloid school maintains that this is not harmful, although it has been associated with hypoxia and delayed healing of bowel anastomoses.[25,26]

Those who use colloid emphasize the importance of maintaining the colloid osmotic pressure above 10 mmHg or above capillary hydrostatic pressure because lower levels are associated with a poor prognosis. Colloids can maintain the water-retaining capacity of blood by replenishing the oncotic strength.[27,28] In patients with capillary leak, however, the colloids may leak out of the capillaries, increasing the oncotic pressure of the interstitial space, which is detrimental.[29]

In 1989, Velanovich compared the mortality data from several published clinical trials using meta-analysis to compare crystalloid and colloid. He suggested that in trauma there was a 12.3% difference in mortality in favour of crystalloid, whilst pooled data from studies using nontrauma data found a difference of 7.8% in favour of colloid.[30]

In the UK colloids are generally preferred to crystalloid for volume replacement, with human albumin solution being the colloid of choice.[31] Few studies have compared crystalloid with colloid in paediatric patients and colloids remain the resuscitation fluid of choice in this age group. A recent review of 30 previously published studies of albumin has suggested a higher mortality in the patients receiving albumin. In some of these studies, the albumin group received colloid in addition to cystalloid as an extra volume and in others, the albumin group included patients given the older plasma protein fraction, which is no longer used because of impurities such as bradykinins. This paper suggests that controlled trials are necessary to compare crystalloid and colloid.[32]

THE NEED FOR VOLUME REPLACEMENT

One of the difficulties in assessing hypovolaemia in paediatric patients is that they are able to compensate for large volume losses with minimal signs. A normal blood pressure may be encountered in the presence of loss of up to 25% of the circulating blood volume. Although tachycardia is often seen in hypovolaemia, the unwary may be caught out by a bradycardic neonate. Two of the more reliable signs of hypovolaemia are poor tissue perfusion (capillary refill time) and core–peripheral temperature difference.[33,34] Invasive monitoring of patients may also be difficult: the smallest Swan–Ganz catheter, for example, is inappropriately large for a premature infant. Frequent blood sampling to monitor acid–base status, haematocrit and electrolytes can result in significant volumes of blood loss requiring transfusion.

CRYSTALLOIDS FOR VOLUME REPLACEMENT

Because dextrose is immediately metabolized, fluids containing only dextrose are equivalent to free water. This can equilibrate rapidly between all three fluid compartments so that only 7.5 ml out of each 100 ml infused will remain in the intravascular space, making it inappropriate for volume replacement. Isotonic crystalloids such as normal saline and Hartmann's solution are appropriate as resuscitation fluids but, as has been mentioned before, only about one-third of the volume will remain in the intravascular space, with the rest equilibrating through the extracellular compartment.

Hypertonic saline solutions have been used successfully to maintain the circulation by infusing small volumes of 7.5% saline.[35,36] They are untried in paediatrics and may be inappropriate in the neonate whose sodium handling is immature.[14,37]

COLLOIDS FOR VOLUME REPLACEMENT

The colloids available for volume replacement may be natural, including blood, fresh-frozen plasma (FFP) and albumin, or synthetic, such as dextrans, hydroxyethyl starches and the gelatins. Blood will be discussed in detail later in the chapter.

Injury and surgery can both cause coagulopathy and because of this there has been a tendency for FFP to be used for simple volume replacement, particularly in neonatology where there is a risk of spontaneous intracranial haemorrhage. FFP is derived from whole blood and frozen within 6 h of harvest and is not pasteurized. The National Institute of Health consensus conference in 1985 laid down strict criteria for the use of FFP.[38] These include cases of specific depletion of clotting factors, immunodeficiencies, rapid reversal of warfarin, treatment of thrombotic thrombocytopenic purpura and following transfusion of more than one blood volume within a few hours. The conclusion of the conference was that FFP conferred no benefits as a volume expander and the potential risk of blood-borne infection outweighed any potential advantages outside their criteria.[39] FFP showed no benefits over albumin when compared with albumin solutions for volume replacement in ventilated neonates on a neonatal intensive care unit. In particular, there was no difference in incidence of intracranial haemorrhage.

Dextrans are carbohydrate-based plasma expanders. They are associated with coagulopathies and with a high incidence of allergic reactions. These effects can be minimized by pretreating the patient with hapten dextran (molecular weight 1000).[40] Having fallen from favour because of their adverse effects, they have recently been used increasingly in adult orthopaedics where their use is associated with a reduction in venous thrombosis. Since this is an uncommon problem in paediatric surgical patients, this benefit does not outweigh their disadvantages.

Before looking at albumin, the hydroxyethyl starches and the gelatins, it is worth considering the properties of the ideal colloid solution: it would produce a guaranteed plasma expansion for a reproducible period even if the reflection coefficient of the Starling equation (sc) was less than 1; it would be completely eliminated from the body even in the presence of renal failure; it would have no adverse effects and would be free from the risk of blood-borne infection; finally, it would be freely available at low cost, be acceptable to all religious groups and have a long shelf-life with no special storage requirements.

PLASMA SUBSTITUTES VERSUS PLASMA EXPANDERS

Albumin and the gelatins are plasma substitutes, whereas the hydroxyethyl starches are true plasma expanders; that is, they produce an increase in plasma volume greater than the volume infused by drawing in fluid from the interstitial space.[41] Although this may be of benefit, particularly on intensive care, there is an increased risk of fluid overload and significant haemodilution if used by unwary prescribers.

PHARMACOLOGY OF NATURAL AND SYNTHETIC COLLOIDS

Human albumin solution is derived from donated blood by a process of fractionation and/or plasmaphoresis. It is then stabilized by agents such as caprylates before pasteurization. Albumin is available either as a 4.5% (iso-oncotic) solution or as concentrated 'salt-poor' 10 or 20% solutions.[42] It is monodisperse (all of the molecules within a solution are the same size) and both its weight average (Mw) and number average (Mñ) molecular weights are the same (Table 8.2):

$$Mw = \frac{the\ sum\ of\ each\ molecules\ weight}{(weight\ of\ total\ mixture)(weight\ of\ the\ molecule)}$$

$$M\tilde{n} = \frac{mass\ of\ the\ sample\ in\ grams}{total\ number\ of\ chains}$$

Although only half of the body's albumin is intravascular and it represents about half of the plasma protein fraction, it contributes 80% of the intravascular osmotic pressure in healthy states. On intensive care, when 'acute-phase proteins' may be raised, its contribution is lower. Albumin persists in the body for about 20 days, although its duration of action as a plasma substitute varies from less than 2 h to 1 day.[43]

The new-generation gelatins are derived from bovine collagen by hydrolysis. The gel thus formed is further modified by succinylation (forming the modified fluid or succinylated

Table 8.2 Molecular weights of three colloids

	Albumin	Hespan®	Gelofusine®
Mw	69 000	450 000	30 000
Mñ	69 000	69 000	22 600
Mw/Mñ	1	6.43	1.33

gelatins such as Gelofusine; B. Braun Medical) or by urea linkage resulting in the polygeline or urea-linked gelatins (e.g. Haemaccel®; Behring).[44]

In common with all the synthetic colloids, the gelatins are polydisperse, which results in two molecular weights, as defined above. The weight average molecular weight (Mw) determines the viscosity, whilst the number average molecular weight (Mñ) gives an indication of the osmotic potential of the fluid. The values are given in Table 8.2. Although their weight average molecular weight is less than that of albumin, the gelatins can sustain a useful osmotic pressure. Webb *et al.* studied the *in vitro* colloid osmotic pressure of various fluids across membranes which allowed molecules of either 10 000 or 50 000 molecular weight to cross.[45] Although a urea-linked gelatin was less effective than albumin, the succinylated gelatin–Gelofusine exerted a greater pressure, with the implication that in situations of capillary leak Gelofusine may be a more useful fluid than albumin, which leaks out rapidly.

Reports from the adult literature suggest that, overall, the succinylated are preferable to the urea-linked gelatins. In addition to adverse effects, which will be discussed later, the urea-linked gelatins contain significant amounts of calcium, whilst the succinylated gelatins contain only trace amounts, which means that they can be given through the same giving set as blood.[46]

The gelatins have a duration of action of between 2 and 6 h. They persist in the body for about a week and are renally excreted, although some of the larger molecules may be broken down by proteases.

The hydroxyethyl starches have a structure similar to glycogen and are derived from amylopectin and stabilized by hydroxyethylation with ethylene oxide.[47,48] The number of hydroxyethyl groups substituted reflects the resistance of the molecule to degradation.[49] Hetastarch (e.g. Hespan®; du Pont) has seven hydroxyethyl groups per 10 glucose units. In solution it contains molecules with a wide range of molecular weights and there is a huge discrepancy between the number average and weight average molecular weights. Pentastarch has five substitutions per 10 glucose units and has no molecules greater than 1 (10^6 molecular weight. This gives it the advantage of a similar efficacy but shorter half-life within the body.[50] Hetastarch persists for a long time both intravascularly (reported duration of effect is up to 24 h) and in the body, where survival has been reported for up to 60 days.[47,51] The larger molecules are taken up by the reticuloendothelial system, whilst the smaller molecules and some of the intermediate molecules, having been broken down by amylase, are renally excreted.[52]

ADVERSE EFFECTS OF COLLOIDS

Unfortunately, adverse effects have been recorded with all available colloids, both synthetic and natural. The most important are allergic reactions and effects on haemostasis.

Table 8.3 Basic characteristics of three colloids

	Albumin	Hespan®	Gelofusine®
Sodium (mmol l^{-1})	130–160	154	154
Potassium (mmol l^{-1})	< 2	–	< 0.4
Citrate (mmol l^{-1})	4–10	–	–
mOsmol l^{-1}	300	310	279
Oncotic pressure[a]	0.36	0.58	0.37
% Colloid	4.5	6	4
Volume expansion (%)	100	100–172	≈ 80
Duration of expansion	4–24	12–24	3–6
Excretion	Metabolized	Amylase and renal excretion	Renal excretion and ? proteases

[a]Ratio of oncotic pressure exerted across a membrane with a permeability of 50 000 versus 10 000 Daltons.[44]

Anaphylactoid reactions are classified as mild/moderate (such as fever, rash, nausea) or severe with life-threatening smooth muscle spasm or cardiorespiratory arrest.[53]

The pathogenesis is unclear.[54] Although antibodies have been identified in the serum of patients who have received both hetastarch and gelatins, their presence does not correlate with allergy. Complement has been implicated in the reactions to both synthetic colloids,[55] but histamine release is likely to be the most important factor in reactions to the gelatins. Lorenz et al. found that they could significantly reduce reactions to a urea-linked gelatin by pretreating the patients with H_1 and H_2 blockers.[56] Reactions are twice as common with the urea-linked than with the succinylated gelatins (0.1% vs 0.05%, respectively), possibly because of the release of di-isocyanate during manufacture of the urea-linked compounds. The gelatins should probably be avoided in patients with severe atopy or such patients should be pretreated with histamine blockade.

Allergy has been reported with albumin solutions. This has usually been attributed to impurities such as bradykinins in the solutions. The stabilizing agents may also initiate allergy in susceptible patients.[53]

Although serious when they occur, immediate life-threatening reactions to hydroxyethyl starch, albumin and the succinylated gelatins are rare, with an incidence of between 1 : 5000 and 1 : 10 000 infusions.[57] This is likely to be less common in the paediatric population, which has a reduced incidence of allergic reactions.

The effects of these fluids on coagulation have been well studied in animal models and the adult literature. Coagulation effects of albumin are usually attributed to dilution alone, although fibrinogen levels may drop more than expected with a greater prolongation of the prothrombin time.[58] This may result from the albumin load switching off hepatic synthesis of clotting factors, in addition to the well-recognized inhibition of synthesis of albumin itself.[59,60]

Hetastarch has more profound effects on coagulation. In addition to haemodilutional effects, in moderate doses it causes a prolongation of the partial thromboplastin time.[61] Although these effects are trivial in doses less than 20 ml kg^{-1}, profound effects have been recorded, particularly in patients undergoing neurosurgical procedures.[62–65] This effect on the partial thromboplastin time is due to a reduction in factor VIII levels.[66,67]

Succinylated gelatins have not been studied to the same extent as the other two fluids, but they do not appear to have any effect on coagulation in the quantities used in normal clinical practice.[68]

Recent work compared the coagulation effects of Hespan, albumin and Gelofusine in 60 children undergoing abdominal surgery. In all three groups there was a small effect on the laboratory assessment of haemostasis, presumably due to haemodilution. The Hespan group showed a prolongation of the partial thromboplastin time at 24 h which was significantly greater than baseline and than in the other two groups. This was beyond the normal range for the hospital laboratory and occurred at moderate doses of no more than 20 ml kg^{-1}. This corresponded to a significant fall in factor VIII levels but was not associated with any clinical adverse effect.[69]

EFFICACY OF COLLOIDS

An effective plasma substitute will restore the circulating blood volume and allow perfusion of vital organs following infusion. There have been many adult studies comparing the efficacy of hydroxyethyl starches, albumin and the new-generation gelatins. In the early 1970s, Metcalfe et al. found that hetastarch gave immediate volume expansion.[70] Other workers found that hetastarch had a greater effect than either albumin or gelatin on circulating volume.[71,72] In addition, oxygen transport has been found to be equal following infusion of either albumin or hetastarch.[73] Edwards et al. studied the haemodynamic and oxygen transport effects of succinylated gelatin in critically ill patients on intensive care and demonstrated significant increases in oxygen delivery with improved mean arterial pressure and stroke volume.[74]

The efficacy of Hespan, albumin and Gelofusine in the postoperative period following paediatric open heart surgery has been compared.[69] Albumin and Gelofusine were found to be equally efficacious. Hespan resulted in a greater increase in arterial pressure, supporting the thesis that it is a plasma expander.

VOLUME OF COLLOID REQUIRED

On an intensive care unit with monitoring lines, colloid can be infused in small boluses which are repeated based on filling pressures. In most paediatric situations such monitoring is not available. Colloid is infused as boluses of 10–20 ml kg^{-1} body weight. Paediatric patients often require significantly larger volumes than adult patients. An infant weighing 7 kg with intussusception may need 40–50 ml kg^{-1} of colloid for resuscitation. This would be the equivalent of a 70 kg male receiving 3.5 l of colloid which would result in significant haemodilution.

BLOOD AND BLOOD PRODUCTS

USE OF BLOOD

In 1994, the Royal College of Physicians of Edinburgh convened a consensus conference of haematologists, clinicians, health-care professionals and epidemiologists to consider various factors related to red cell transfusion, including patient information, transfusion guidelines, autologous transfusion, the use of erythropoietin and artificial oxygen carriers. In summary, because red cell transfusion is part of a patient's overall treatment, information regarding a proposed transfusion should be given as part of the explanation of overall management. In emergency situations, however, this may not be possible and transfusion should be given except in positions where there is a clearly expressed objection (see *Jehovah's Witnesses*).

There are no universal clinical guidelines to assist in red cell transfusion and clinicians show wide variations in clinical practice over the decision whether to transfuse in any particular situation.[75] In particular, there is no agreement as to the lowest acceptable haemoglobin. Most of the studies assessing this have been per-

formed in adults where ischaemic heart disease is common and symptoms relating to this dictate the need for red cell transfusion. Although historically most clinicians recommend perioperative transfusion for a haemoglobin level less than 10 g dl^{-1}, in the absence of ischaemic heart disease, a haemoglobin level as low as 6 g dl^{-1} will be tolerated by most adults.[76] In paediatrics, most information relates to ventilator- or oxygen-dependent neonates, where there is some evidence that oxygen requirements are less if the haemoglobin is maintained above 10 g dl^{-1}.[77]

The American College of Physicians' guidelines for transfusion for transient anaemia from acute blood loss in adults suggest that crystalloid should be used for volume replacement initially. Since normovolaemic anaemia is generally well tolerated, asymptomatic patients should not be transfused regardless of haemoglobin levels. If symptoms develop (syncope, dyspnoea, postural hypotension, angina or transient ischaemic attacks) blood should be transfused unit by unit until the patient is again asymptomatic. Although these guidelines do not give a lower safe haemoglobin, 7 g dl^{-1} has been suggested as a lower safety margin.[78]

One of the problems in neonatal surgery is that the circulating blood volume is small. A neonate weighing 1 kg has a blood volume of about 80 ml, so that 10 ml of blood loss is more than 10% of the circulating blood volume. For this reason, blood should be cross-matched preoperatively for any procedure more invasive than a pyloromyotomy or a herniotomy.

RISKS OF TRANSFUSION

Infection

The most widely recognized risk of transfusion is blood-borne infection. All blood and plasma donations are screened for antibodies to human immunodeficiency virus (HIV)-1 and HIV-2, hepatitis C, hepatitis B surface antigen and syphilis. Despite such screening programmes and strict exclusion criteria for donors, the quoted risk of acquired infection is 1 : 13 000 for hepatitis C, 1 : 20 000 for hepatitis B and 1 : 3 000 000 for HIV.[79]

Recent Department of Health guidelines have suggested that blood transfusions may be associated with a risk of transmitting Creutz-feldt-Jakob disease and that all transfusions should be filtered to remove leucocytes, which are the vectors for the virus.

There is some evidence to suggest that red cell transfusion is associated with impaired resistance to infection. Jensen *et al.* studied postoperative infection rates and natural killer cell function in patients undergoing elective colorectal surgery. They found a significantly increased risk of infection in the group that received whole blood transfusions when compared with no blood or filtered blood. In addition, the patients receiving whole blood had significantly impaired natural killer cell function up to 30 days postsurgery.[80]

Immunosuppression

The reduction in natural killer cell function, together with increased suppressor lymphocyte activity, may have further detrimental effects. Preliminary studies have suggested that adult patients receiving whole blood transfusions have an increased risk of developing tumours within 10 years of their transfusion, although the causal link has not been proven.[81] That transfusion produces immunosuppression is certain and this does have some beneficial effects in reducing the rate of allograft rejection after renal transplant and in decreasing the rate of Crohn's recurrence.[82]

Effects on immunosuppression are thought to be leucocyte related. Whilst whole blood has been shown to reduce the T-helper : T-suppressor ratio, filtered blood or reconstituted blood (SAG-m) does not have the same effect.[83]

AUTOLOGOUS BLOOD TRANSFUSION

Autologous blood transfusion includes preoperative staged donations, acute normovolaemic haemodilution and perioperative red cell salvage. Autologous blood transfusions in children have been used more extensively in the USA and Japan than in the UK. The problems associated with their use are largely logistic. Blood collected by staged donation must be used within 35 days or frozen for storage. Predeposits need to be of volumes greater than 150 ml because of volume reduction during freezing and the blood must be collected through a large-bore needle to prevent haemolysis. For these reasons it is impractical in children weighing less than 15 kg. Children weighing between 20 and 50 kg are bled into a 250 ml paediatric blood pack, whilst older children are bled into an adult unit of 450 ml. Parental consent must be obtained and the procedure must be fully explained to the child. No child should be forced to undergo donation. It is only reasonable to proceed if there is a reasonable expectation that a blood transfusion will be required. The child should receive iron supplementation and there should be a gap of at least 4 days between the last donation and surgery.

Perioperative cell salvage has been used extensively in adult vascular and liver surgery and it has been used successfully in orthopaedics. It is contraindicated in operations where the blood loss is potentially contaminated by either blood or tumour cells. The general surgical procedures most commonly associated with significant peroperative blood loss are gastrointestinal and tumour resections rendering cell salvage unsuitable. The procedure requires expensive equipment which is not universally available.

The risks of autologous transfusion include dilutional coagulopathy, bacterial contamination of stored blood, cytokine release during storage and improper storage. There is also a tendency to overtransfuse because of the availablity of the blood.[78]

COST OF TRANSFUSIONS

Although paediatric units of packed cells are expensive, leucocyte-depleted filtered blood costs almost twice as much. The cost of a unit of autologous blood is approximately double that of an allogeneic unit.

PLATELETS

Platelet counts of less than 50 000 require platelet transfusion prior to surgical intervention. A count of less than 15 000 puts the child at risk of spontaneous haemorrhage and any such patient should also be transfused. A low platelet count is a contraindication to epidural or spinal anaesthesia. The other indication for platelets is a child who has undergone a circulating volume transfusion of red cells. In babies and infants, a transfusion of 5–10 ml kg^{-1} is usually sufficient, whilst unit transfusions are appropriate in older patients.

FRESH-FROZEN PLASMA AND CRYOPRECIPITATE

FFP contains 1 unit of factor activity per millilitre of plasma. A decision to use FFP or cryoprecipitate should be based on a combination of clinical and laboratory findings. An INT of less than 1.4 or a partial thromboplastin time of less than 60 s is unlikely to cause significant bleeding problems and correction is not required. Laboratory values greater than these levels or significant bleeding will require correction. An empiric dose of 5–10 ml kg^{-1} is usually adequate or the dose can be calculated by body weight, plasma volume and desired increment of clotting factors.

Cryoprecipitate is a poor source of factors II, V, IX, X, XI and XII but contains factors VIII : C, VIIIvWF, XIII, fibrinogen and fibronectin. Indications for its use include haemophilia A, von Willebrand disease, fibrinogen deficiency, massive transfusion and uraemic platelet dysfunction. Its advantage over FFP is that it is concentrated and one bag (of 15–20 ml) is the dose per 10 kg body weight.

SPECIAL SITUATIONS

Jehovah's witnesses

The Royal College of Surgeons of England have produced a code of practice for the surgical management of Jehovah's Witnesses. This acknowledges that the children of Jehovah's Witnesses requiring blood transfusion present a most difficult management problem.[84] There are some mitigating factors, however. Either parent may sign a consent form permitting a transfusion. Most operations on children do not require or involve blood transfusion, but it is unethical to let a child die for want of a blood transfusion. The surgeon and anaesthetist must, however, respect the beliefs of the family and should make every effort to avoid the perioperative use of blood or blood products. For children under 13 years of age who require or may require a transfusion but whose parents refuse to give consent, legal advice should be sought. Such children will normally be made a temporary ward of court. This subject is covered more fully in Chapter 2.

Sickle cell disease

Traditionally, patients with sickle cell disease have been routinely transfused before elective surgery. There has, however, been little consensus as to whether simple correction of the anaemia is sufficient or whether the level of HbS should be reduced to less than 30%. Vichinsky *et al.* compared a conservative regimen (transfusing to a haemoglobin level of around 10 g dl^{-1}) with an aggressive regimen (haemaglobin of around 10 g dl^{-1} and an HbS level of less than 30%). They found the conservative regimen to be as effective in preventing perioperative complications and this group had half as many transfusion-associated complications.[85] Similarly, immediately preoperative transfusion to a haematocrit of more than 36% was as efficacious as two-volume exchanges beginning 2 weeks prior to surgery, with less disruption to the family.[86] Patients with HbSS disease should receive transfusions to correct their anaemia. They should be given adequate perioperative hydration with crystalloid. Postoperatively, they should receive adequate analgesia in addition to oxygen and physiotherapy to prevent atelectasis. For more information, see Chapter 1.

CONCLUSION

Fluid management in paediatrics is an art as well as a science; clinicians need to monitor the response to therapy and change the regimen appropriately. This chapter contains guidelines and suggestions for safe fluid administration but cannot replace clinical experience.

REFERENCES

1 Rowe, M.I. A dynamic approach to fluid and electrolyte management of the newborn. *Zeitschrift für Kinderchirurgie* 1985; **40**: 270–7.
2 Lippold, O.C.J. and Winton, F.R. The distribution of body fluids. In: Lippold, O.C.J. and Winton, F.R. (eds). *Human Physiology*. Edinburgh: Churchill Livingstone, 1979: 118–21.
3 Starling, E.H. On the absorption of fluids from the connective tissue spaces. *Journal of Physiology* 1896; **19**: 312–26.
4 Bush, G.H. Intravenous fluid therapy in paediatrics. *Annals RCS* 1971; **49**: 92–101.
5 Bevan, D.R. Colloid osmotic pressure. *Anaesthesia* 1980; **35**: 263–70.
6 Morissette, M.P. Colloid osmotic pressure: its measurement and clinical value. *Canadian Medical Association Journal* 1977; **116**: 897–900.
7 Barclay, S.A. Colloid osmotic pressure: its measurement and role in clinical cardiovascular medicine. PhD Thesis, University of London, 1988.
8 Guyton, A.C., Granger, H.J. and Taylor, A.E. Interstitial fluid pressure. *Physiology Review* 1971; **51**: 527–63.
9 Boyd, E. *Growth of Surface Area of the Human Body*. Institute of Child Welfare, Monograph Series 10. Minneapolis, MN: University of Minnesota Press, 1935.
10 Oliver, W.J., Graham, B.D. and Wilson, J.L. Lack of scientific validity of body surface as a basis for parenteral fluid dosage. *Journal of the American Medical Association* 1958; **167**: 1211–18.
11 Siker, D. Pediatric fluids and electrolytes. In: Gregory, G.A. (ed.). *Pediatric Anaesthesia*. 2nd edn. New York: Churchill Livingstone, 1989: 581–617.
12 Howland, J. The fundamental requirements of an infant's nutrition. *American Journal of Diseases of Childhood* 1911; **2**: 49.
13 Fosel, T.H., Uth M, Wilhelm W, Gruness Z. Comparison of two solutions with different glucose concentrations for infusion therapy during laparotomies in infants. *Infusionstherapie und Transfusionsmedizin* 1996; **23**: 80–4.
14 Krummel, T.M., Lloyd, D.A. and Rowe, M.I. The postoperative response of the term and preterm newborn infant to sodium administration. *Journal of Pediatric Surgery* 1985; **20**: 803–9.
15 Goh, D.W., Hall, S.K., Gomall, P., Buick, R.G., Green, A. and Corkery, J.J. Plasma chloride and alkalaemia in pyloric stenosis. *British Journal of Surgery* 1990; **77** 922–3.
16 Rowe, M.I., Smith, S.D. and Cheu, H. inappropriate fluid response in congenital diaphragmatic hernia: first report of a frequent occurrence. *Journal of Pediatric Surgery* 1988; **23**: 1147–53.
17 Reid, D.J. Intracellular and extracellular fluid volume during surgery. *British Journal of Surgery* 1968; **55**: 594–6.
18 Shires, T., Williams, J. and Brown, F. Acute changes in extracellular fluids associated with major surgical procedures. *Annals of Surgery* 1961; **154**: 803–10.
19 Hannon, R.J. and Boston, V.E. Hyponatraemia and intracellular water in sepsis: an experimental comparison of the effect of fluid replacement with either 0.9% Normal saline or 5% dextrose. *Journal of Pediatric Surgery* 1990; **25**: 422–5.
20 Muir, I.F.K. and Barclay, T.L. Treatment of burn shock. In: *Burns and Their Treatment*. London: Lloyd-Luke, 1962.
21 Laks, H., O'Connor, N.E., Anderson, W., *et al* Crystalloid versus colloid hemodilution in man. *Surgery, Gynecology and Obstetrics* 1976; **142**: 506–12.
22 Poole, G.V., Meredith, J.W., Pennell, T. *et al*. Comparisons of colloids and crystalloids in resuscitation from hemorrhagic shock. *Surgery, Gynecology and Obstetrics* 1982; **154**: 577–86.
23 Shoemaker, W.C. Hemodynamic and oxygen transport effects of crystalloids and colloids in critically ill patients. *Current Studies in Hematology and Blood Transfusion* 1986; **53**: 155–76.
24 Ross, A.D. and Angaran, D.M. Colloids versus crystalloids – a continuing controversy. *Drug Intelligence and Clinical Pharmacology* 1986; **18**: 202–12.
25 Hunt, T.K., Rabkin, J. and von Smitten, K. Effects of edema and anemia on wound healing and infection. *Current Studies in Hematology and Blood Transfusion* 1986; **53**: 101–11.
26 Chan, S.T.F., Kapadia, C.R., Johnson, A.W., *et al*. Extracellular fluid volume expansion and third space sequestration at the site of small bowel anastomoses. *British Journal of Surgery* 1983; **70**: 36–9.
27 Falk, J.L., Rackow, E.C., Astiz, M., *et al*. Fluid resuscitation in shock. *Journal of Cardiothoracic Anesthesia* 1988; **2** Suppl.: 33–8.
28 Weil, M.H., Henning, R.J., Morisette, M.P., *et al*. Relationship between colloid osmotic pressure and pulmonary artery wedge pressure in patients with acute cardiorespiratory failure. *American Journal of Medicine* 1978; **64**: 643–50.
29 Viriglio, R.W., Rice, C.L., Smith, D.E., *et al*. Crystalloid versus colloid resuscitation: is one better? A randomized clinical study. *Surgery* 1979; **85**: 129–39.
30 Velanovich, V. Crystalloid versus colloid fluid resuscitation; a meta-analysis of mortality. *Surgery* 1989; **105**: 65–71.
31 Huskisson, L.J. Intravenous volume replacement – which fluid and why. *Archives of Disease in Childhood* 1992; **67**: 649–53.
32 Cochrane Injuries Group Albumin Reviewers. Human albumin administration in critically ill patients; systemic review of randomised controlled trials. *British Medical Journal* 1998; **317**: 235–40.
33 APLS, Advanced Life Support Group. London: BMA Publishing 1997.
34 Ryan, C.A. and Soder, C.M. Relationship between core/peripheral temperature gradient and central hemodynamics in children after open heart surgery. *Critical Care Medicine* 1989; **17**: 638–40.
35 de Felippe, J., Timoner, J., Velasco, I.T., *et al*. Treatment of refractory hypovolaemic shock by 7.5% sodium chloride injections. *Lancet* 1980; **ii**: 1002–4.
36 Vincent, J.-L. Fluids for resuscitation. *British Journal of Anaesthesia* 1991; **67**: 185–93.
37 Wilkins, B.H. Renal function in sick very low birthweight infants: 3. Sodium, potassium and water excretion. *Archives of Disease in Childhood* 1992; **67**: 1154–61.

38 National Institute of Health Consensus Conference. Fresh frozen plasma. Indications and risks. *Journal of the American Medical Association* 1985; **253**: 551–3.

39 Messmer, K. Chapter 2. In: Lowe, K.C. (ed.). *Blood Substitutes, Preparation, Physiology and Medical Application.* Hemel Hempstead: Ellis Horwood Series in Biomedicine, 1988.

40 Ring, J. Anaphylactoid reactions to plasma substitutes. *International Anesthesiology Clinics* 1985; **23**: 67–95.

41 Quon, C.Y. Clinical pharmacokinetics and pharmacodynamics of colloidal plasma volume expanders. *Journal of Cardiothoracic Anesthesia* 1988; **2**: 13–23.

42 McClelland, D.B.L. Human albumin solutions. *British Medical Journal* 1990; **300**: 35–7.

43 Lewis, R.T. Albumin: role and discriminative use in surgery. *Canadian Journal of Surgery* 1980; **23**: 322–8.

44 Saddler, J.M. and Horsey, P.J. The new generation gelatins. *Anaesthesia* 1987; **42**: 998–1004.

45 Webb, A.R., Barclay, S.A. and Bennett, E.D. *In vitro* colloid osmotic pressure of commonly used plasma expanders and substitutes: a study of the diffusibility of colloid molecules. *Intensive Care Medicine* 1989; **15**: 116–20.

46 Edwards, M.P., Clark, D.J., Mark, J.S. *et al.* Compound sodium lactate (Hartmann's solution). Caution: risk of clotting. *Anaesthesia* 1986; **41**: 1053–4.

47 Hulse, J.D. and Yacobi, A. Hetastarch: an overview of the colloid and its metabolism. *Drug Intelligence and Clinical Pharmacology* 1983; **17**: 334–41.

48 Mishler, J.M. Synthetic plasma volume expanders – their pharmacology, safety and clinical efficacy. *Clinics in Hematology* 1984; **13**: 75–92.

49 Klotz, U. and Kroemer, H. Clinical pharmacological considerations in the use of plasma expanders. *Clinical pharmacokinetics* 1987; **12**: 123–35.

50 Waxman, K., Holness, R., Tominaga, G., *et al.* Hemodynamics and oxygen transport effects of pentastarch in burn resuscitation. *Annals of Surgery* 1989; **209**: 341–5.

51 Thompson, W., Fukushima, T. and Rutherford, R.B. Intravascular persistence, tissue storage and excretion of hydroxyethyl starch. *Surgery, Gynecology and Obstetrics* 1970; **131**: 965–72.

52 Lawrence, D.A. and Schell, R.F. Influence of hydroxyethyl starch on humoral and cell-mediated immune response in mice. *Transfusion* 1985; **25**: 223–9.

53 Ring, J. and Messmer, K. Incidence and severity of anaphylactoid reactions to colloid volume substitutes. *Lancet* 1977; **i**: 466–9.

54 Adelmann-Grill, B. and Schoning, B. Lack of evidence for immunological reactions to gelatin. *Developmental Biological Standards* 1981; **48**: 235–40.

55 Watkins, J., Wild, G., Appleyard, T.N., *et al.* Complement activation by polystarch and gelatin volume expanders. *Lancet* 1990; **335**: 233.

56 Lorenz, W., Duda, D., Dick, W., *et al.* Incidence and clinical importance of perioperative histamine release: randomised study of volume loading and antihistamines after induction of anaesthesia. *Lancet* 1994; **343**: 933–40.

57 Watkins, J. Allergic and pseudoallergic reactions to colloid plasma substitutes: which colloid? *Care of the Critically Ill* 1991; **7**: 213–17.

58 Johnson, S.D., Lucas, C.E., Gerrick, S.J., *et al.* Altered coagulation after albumin supplements for treatment of oligaemic shock. *Archives of Surgery* 1979; **114**: 379–83.

59 Tullis, J.L. Albumin 1. Background and use. *Journal of the American Medical Association* 1977; **237**: 355–9.

60 Strauss, R.G. Volume replacement and coagulation: a comparative review. *Journal of Cardiothoracic Anesthesia* 1988; **2**: 24–32.

61 Macintyre, E., Mackie, I.J., Ho, D., *et al.* The haemostatic effects of hydroxyethyl starch used as a volume expander. *Intensive Care Medicine* 1985; **11**: 300–3.

62 Diehl, J.T., Lester, J.L. III and Cosgrove, D.M. Clinical comparison of hetastarch and albumin in postoperative cardiac patients. *Annals of Thoracic Surgery* 1982; **34**: 674–9.

63 Falk, J.L., Rackow, E.C., Astiz, M., *et al.* Effects of hetastarch and albumin on coagulation in patients with septic shock. *Journal of Clinical Pharmacology* 1988; **28**: 412–15.

64 Cully, M.C., Larson, C.P. and Silverberg, G.D. Hetastarch coagulopathy in a neurosurgical patient. *Anaesthesiology* 1987; **66**: 706–7.

65 Lockwood, D.N.J., Bullen, C. and Machin, S.J. A severe coagulopathy following volume replacement with hydroxyethyl starch in a Jehovah's Witness. *Anaesthesia* 1988; **43**: 391–3.

66 Stump, D.C., Strauss, R.G. and Henriksen, R.A. Effects of hydroxyethyl starch on blood coagulation, particularly Factor VIII. *Transfusion* 1985; **25**: 349–54.

67 Alexander, B., Odake, K., Lawlor, D., *et al.* Coagulation, hemostasis and plasma expanders: a quarter century enigma. *Federation Proceedings* 1975; **34**: 1429–40.

68 Fujii, K., Kaneko, K., Iwahori, Y., *et al.* The influence of Gelofusine on the blood coagulating function. *Japanese Gelofusine Symposium* 1967.

69 Huskisson, L.J. Evaluation of synthetic colloids in paediatric surgical practice. MS Thesis, 1994. University of London.

70 Metcalfe, W., Papadopoulos, A., Tufaro, R., *et al.* A clinical physiologic study of hydroxyethyl starch. *Surgery, Gynecology and Obstetrics* 1970; **131**: 255–67.

71 Kilian, J., Spilker, D. and Borst, R. The effect of 6% HES, 4.5% Dextran and 5.5% Oxypol Gel on blood volume and circulation in human volunteers. *Anaesthesist* 1975; **24**: 193–7.

72 Lamke, L.-O. and Liljedahl, S.-O. Plasma volume changes after infusion of various plasma expanders. *Resuscitation* 1976; **5**: 93–102.

73 Lazrove, S., Waxman, K., Shippy, C., *et al.* Hemodynamic, blood volume and oxygen transport responses to albumin and HES infusions in critically ill postoperative patients. *Critical Care Medicine* 1980; **8**: 302–6.

74 Edwards, J.D., Nightingale, P., Wilkins, R.G., *et al.* Hemodynamic and oxygen transport response to modified fluid gelatin in critically ill patients. *Critical Care Medicine* 1989; **17**: 996–8.

75 Sudhindran, S. Perioperative blood transfusion: a plea for guidelines. *Annals of the Royal College of Surgeons of England* 1997; **79**: 299–302.

76 Spence, R.K., Carson, J.A., Poses, R., *et al.* Elective surgery without transfusion: influence of preoperative hemoglobin level and blood loss on mortality. *American Journal of Surgery* 1990; **159**: 320–4.

77 James, L., Greenough, A. and Naik, S. The effect of blood transfusion on oxygenation in premature venti-

lated neonates. *European Journal of Pediatrics* 1997; **156**: 139–41.

78 Welch, H.G., Meechan, K.R. and Greenought, L.T. Prudent strategies for elective red blood cell transfusion. *Annals of Internal Medicine* 1992; **116**: 393–402.

79 Contreras, M. and Chapman, C.E. Autologous transfusion and reducing allogenic blood exposure. *Archives of Disease in Childhood* 1994; **71**: 105–7.

80 Jensen, L.S., Anderson, A.J., Christiansen, P.M., *et al.* Postoperative infection and natural killer cell function following blood transfusion in patients undergoing elective colorectal surgery. *British Journal of Surgery* 1992; **79**: 513–16.

81 Nielsen, H.J. Detrimental effects of perioperative blood transfusion. *British Journal of Surgery* 1995; **82**: 582–7.

82 Blumberg, N., Agarwal, M.M. and Chuang, C. Relation between recurrence of cancer of the colon and blood transfusion. *British Medical Journal* 1985; **290**: 1037–9.

83 Kaplan, J., Sarnaik, S., Gitlin, J., *et al.* Diminished helper/suppressor lymphocyte ratios and natural killer activity in recipients of repeated blood transfusions. *Blood* 1984; **64**: 308–10.

84 The Royal College of Surgeons of England. Code of practice for the surgical management of Jehovah's Witnesses, 1996.

85 Vichinsky, E.P., Haberkern, C.M., Neuayr, L., *et al.* A comparison of conservative and aggressive transfusion regimens in the perioperative management of sickle cell disease. *New England Journal of Medicine* 1995; **333**: 206–13.

86 Janik, J. and Seeler, R.A. Perioperative management of children with sickle hemoglobinopathy. *Journal of Pediatric Surgery* 1980; **15**: 117–20.

CHAPTER 9

Regional anaesthesia

ANDREA MESSERI

INTRODUCTION

Regional anaesthesia has become an essential component of modern paediatric anaesthetic practice, even though it was in the past considered unsuitable for children. The major advance in paediatric anaesthesia and post-operative pain management during the 1990s has probably been the widespread application of regional anaesthesia, both as a supplement to light general anaesthesia intraoperatively and for postoperative use.

Key factors in encouraging widespread use and acceptance of regional techniques have been (1) the favourable outcome observed in children undergoing combined general anaesthesia and epidural analgesia for urology and thoracic surgery, (2) the routine practice of caudal or peripheral nerve blocks to provide smooth painless emergence for subumbilical procedures, and (3) the efficacy of chronic implanted epidural catheters for pain relief in oncology patients.

HISTORY

Before attempting to define the role of paediatric regional anaesthesia it is worth putting the subject in a historical perspective and examining the factors that have influenced its development over the years. Regional anaesthesia has had a chequered history during its first 100 years. Twenty-four years passed between the isolation of cocaine by Albert Niemann in 1860[1] and the bold step taken by Karl Koller when he used the drug for topical anaesthesia of the eye in 1884.[2] Then, a flurry of excited exploration took place at the turn of the century, when in the manner of an academic gold-rush, pioneers staked out injections for every conceivable nerve in the anatomical atlas. These techniques were also used in children. Of the six cases of spinal anaesthesia with cocaine, described in the classic paper by August Bier in 1899,[3] the third case was a 14-year-old boy who required treatment for tuberculous ankylosis of his left knee, and the fourth was an 11-year-old boy with a tuberculous ischium. In 1901 Bainbridge reported his experience of spinal anaesthesia in children between the ages of 3 months and 6 years.[4]

During the first decade of the twentieth century the method gained in popularity and a number of reports from Gray, based on larger clinical series, attested to the usefulness and safety of spinal anaesthesia in children.[5] Further support was produced by Farr, who reported a reduction in morbidity and mortality with the use of this technique.[6] An early publication by Campbell on caudals in children appeared in 1933, describing such an anaesthetic method for paediatric urological surgery,[7] but then enthusiasm waxed and waned. The advent of curare seemed to deal a mortal blow to regional anaesthesia, for the muscle relaxants suddenly gave general anaesthesia a flexibility and a gentleness that had never been known before, while regional anaesthesia became outmoded and outmanoeuvred.

Only the stubborn dedication of a few enthusiasts kept paediatric regional techniques alive. Ruston introduced a modern technique combining regional and general anaesthesia and he used continuous lumbar anaesthesia in children in 1957.[8] Spiegel published the first paper dealing exclusively with caudal anaesthesia in children, suggesting a formula to calculate the proper dose of the local anaesthetic using as a parameter the distance between C7 and the sacral hiatus.[9] Fortuna in 1967 demonstrated that caudal anaesthesia in children was a simple, safe and reliable technique which can be utilized for a wide range of surgical operations including emergency surgery.[10] Virtually all techniques in use until the end of the 1970s were an imitation of what was known and described for adults. During the later part of the 1980s other significant developments occurred as the successful use of epidural anaesthesia was described.[11,12] The more 'perfect' anatomy of children compared with that of adults greatly facilitated the performance of neural blockades: because of anatomical and physiological peculiarities, infants and children proved to be ideal for the application of regional anaesthesia techniques. In addition, the renewed interest in pain and its control in infants and children has guided the research towards such techniques as neural blocks. These techniques provide an effective attenuation of stress responses to surgery and a quality of postoperative analgesia that can be achieved by systemic opioids only at the cost of greater side-effects.[13] Therefore, during the 1990s, we have observed a widespread application of regional anaesthesia, both as a supplement to light general anaesthesia intraoperatively and for postoperative use. Recently, new techniques have been described, appropriate paediatric equipment has been made available and pharmacokinetic data have been obtained even for small infants. As we approach the next millennium, the circle of development has been completed by the links back to the pioneering era of Bier, Baimbridge and Gray.

GENERAL CONSIDERATIONS

GENERAL ANAESTHESIA

Children are far from being a homogeneous group, varying as they do from tiny preterm neonates to quite large adolescents. The psychological approach to each patient must, of course, vary enormously. A premature infant can be given a spinal or a caudal anaesthetic and remain awake with the simple aid of a comforter.[14,15] As children grow and become emotionally dependent on their parents the whole approach changes if unnecessary distress is to be avoided. In most cases, general anaesthesia is induced before proceeding to the regional block. Is block placement in an anaesthetized or heavily sedated child a reasonable and safe technique? There are no data available to support or reject the hypothesis that it is acceptable to place blocks in anaesthetized children apart from the subjective opinion that 'this is how it is always done in paediatric patients'[16] and the fact that no one could cite an incident or a case report in which a child was injured using this technique. It is now commonly accepted that is impractical, if not impossible, to place central or peripheral blocks safely in a terrified, awake, moving and crying child.[17] Obviously, there are benefits and limitations when combining regional techniques with general anaesthesia and these aspects have long been discussed (Table 9.1).[18] In the author's experience, with the use of laryngeal mask airway, in fit children, and with the increasing practice of peripheral nerve blocks, there may not be the need for an assistant. There are limited circumstances in which a block can be performed as a sole anaesthetic technique: for inguinal hernia repair in premature and former premature infants, in certain emergency situations, such as a patient with full stomach, in children at risk of malignant hyperthermia or with neuromuscular or chronic pulmonary disease, or in older or co-operative children who wish to remain awake.

ANATOMY AND PHYSIOLOGY

In view of the anatomical and physiological changes that occur as a child grows, important differences in the performance and in the effects produced by neural blockades must be kept in mind before inducing a regional block. First of all, there are some differences between neonates and adults in the anatomy of the vertebral column and in the spinal cord meninges; these affect the placement of central neural blocks. The normal curves of the spine do not become fixed until after puberty. At birth the vertebral column forms a single, long shallow curve extending from the first cervical to the fifth lumbar segment. The spinous processes are more parallel to each other than in adults and consequently the epidural approaches are facilitated at all levels. The end of both the spinal cord and the dural sac is located further down than in adults (Figure 9.1). The tip of the spinal

cord is at L3 at birth and reaches L1–L2 at 1 year of age. The dural sac is found at S3–S4.[19] Therefore, accidental dural puncture is also possible when performing a caudal block. In early life, the ossification of the sacral vertebrae is not completed and the sacrum consists of five distinct vertebrae. The vertebral bodies are separated by intervertebral discs and, posteriorly, the ligamentum flavum still persists.[20] As the ossification proceeds, fusion occurs between the sacral segments, beginning with the two lowest, about the age of 18 years, and extends cephalad until the process is completed between 25 and 30 years of age. The practical implication of these anatomical differences is that a sacral intervertebral epidural approach is always possible in children.[21] The contents of the epidural space in infants differ from those of adults. Instead of having mature, densely packed fat lobules divided by fibrous strands, they have spongy, gelatinous lobules with distinct spaces, permitting the wide longitudinal spread of injected solutions and the upward progression of the epidural catheters.[22] Liga-

Table 9.1 Advantages and disadvantages of paediatric regional anaesthesia

Advantages	Disadvantages
Analgesia without physiological alterations	Light general anaesthesia is required
Total amount of general anaesthesia is decreased	Need for an extra pair of hands
Wake-up times are decreased	Special training
More rapid and pain-free recovery	Risks and complications of general and regional anaesthesia

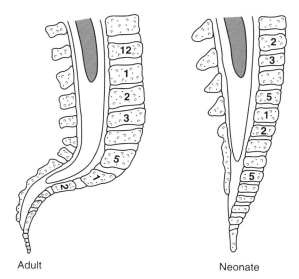

Adult · Neonate

Figure 9.1 Diagram of the anatomical differences of the lumbosacral region between adults and children. In adults the spinal cord ends at the level of the first lumbar vertebra, whereas in children it reaches the level of the third lumbar vertebra. Dural sac is found at S1–S2 in adults, but in children as low as S4. In children the ligamentum flavum, at the sacral level, is not yet ossified and the sacral angle is less prominent.

ments and fascia are thinner in children and easier to penetrate compared with those of adults. In infants myelination is incomplete; therefore, diffusion and penetration of local anaesthetic can occur easily, and satisfactory blocks can be achieved with lower concentrations of drug than would be required in adults. However, incomplete myelination results in slower rates of nerve conduction and this must be evaluated when the effectiveness of a block is being assessed. There are also important differences in the anatomical landmarks. On average, the intercristal line passes through the spinous process of the fourth lumbar vertebra in adults, and crosses the fifth lumbar vertebra in children and the L5–S1 interspace in neonates[23] (Figure 9.2).

The first important physiological difference between adults and children is that even very high central blocks (spinal and epidural) cause little or no change in blood pressure or heart rate up to the age of about 6 years.[24,25] The adaptation to the hydrostatic pressure changes

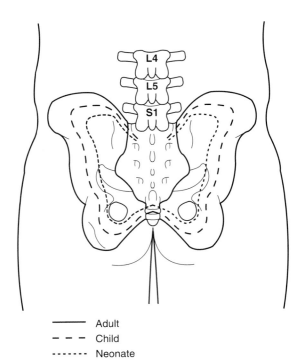

	Adult
- - -	Child
......	Neonate

Figure 9.2 Anatomical landmarks: age-related differences. The intercristal line crosses the fourth lumbar vertebra in adults, the fifth in children, and the L5–S1 interspace in small infants and neonates.

brought about by posture and height are very underdeveloped because such adaptation is unnecessary in small individuals. Hypotension requiring treatment is rare.[26] However, spinal anaesthesia is of much shorter duration in babies than in older children or adults, presumably because they have a different pattern of cerebrospinal fluid (CSF) formation and circulation. Stress responses to surgery are quantitatively and qualitatively different from those of the adult as the hormonal and metabolic changes are of shorter duration despite a greater magnitude of change for a given degree of surgical trauma.[27] The practical implication of this is that it is important to maintain continuous neural blockades for only 24–36 h to modulate the stress response to major surgery.

SAFETY ADVICE

With the introduction of any treatment to a new population safety concerns are prominent and the following safety rules represent some practical guidelines for using regional anaesthesia techniques in infants and children: selection of appropriate equipment; careful and meticulous technique; selection of the appropriate block; and appropriate dosage.

APPROPRIATE EQUIPMENT

The minimum equipment requirements for performing a regional block are a needle and a syringe. Depending on the block, a catheter for reinjections and a nerve stimulator may be required. All resuscitation drugs and all equipment required for coping with possible complications should be available prior to performing a neural blockade.

In a prospective multicentre study, performed by the French-Language Society of Pediatric Anesthesiologists (ADARPEF), regarding the complications of regional anaesthesia in children,[28] half of all complications reported were ascribed to wrong equipment. Although the correct equipment remains a matter of some debate, and more details would be helpful to confirm or reject the assertion of this epidemiological study, it is important to stress some points. Several different types of needle can be used for peripheral and central blocks. Sterile, disposable needles should be used. It is advisable to limit oneself to a few selected needles in order to become familiar with them and to become accustomed to their feel when different anatomical structures are pierced. In practice, the choice of the material could be as follows.

Peripheral nerve blocks

Peripheral nerve blocks should be performed using a straight, short bevelled needle.

Spinal

Depending on the age of the patient, spinal anaesthesia can be performed with a 22G short or long spinal needle; 25G–27G are useful as well. Thinner needles are available and their use has been recommended in order to reduce the incidence of a postdural headache, especially in adults. These needles are rather difficult to control and require careful use, but the incidence of postspinal headache is reduced with their use, even in children.[29] Comparisons between 25 and 29G Quincke spinal needles have been reported in paediatric day-case surgery.[30] The puncture characteristics favour the 25G needle.

Epidural

Epidural anaesthesia is best performed with Tuohy needles. The size used depends on the age and the weight of the patient: 22G up to 1 year, 20G from 1 to 5–6 years, and 19–18G in children older than 7 years.

Caudal

Caudal anaesthesia can be performed with specially designed caudal needles, Tuohy needles, Crawford needles, intravenous cannulae or normal syringe needles according to preference. Three available needles (21G and 23G standard bevelled intramuscular needles and 22G short bevelled 'regional block' needles) have been compared to determine whether complication and success rates were influenced by either needle size or type.[31] The study showed that

there was no clear short-term benefit to be gained from any one of the needles. Theoretically, needles without a stylet could cause an epidermal tumour carrying superficial cells into the epidural space. The author has routinely used standard intravenous cannulae to perform caudal anaesthesia in more than 15 000 patients over a 20-year period, without observing any epidermal tumours. Dalens and Broadman recommend the use of stylleted needles in performing caudal blocks as well.[17,32]

Epidural catheter

Technical problems with catheters are common in paediatric practice. Many groups have commented on difficulties with 23 and 24G catheters, such as with threading, kinking[33] and, most commonly, with high infusion pressures and leakage.[34] These occur because of the extremely small diameter that is required of these catheters in order to allow them to pass through the Tuohy needles used in paediatric units, e.g. 23G catheters passing through 19G needles. The obvious way round this is to use 18G needles; however, the length of these, although suitable for adults, is unsuitable for infants where the tip of the needle may enter the ligaments for a distance of less than 1 cm. Shorter 18G Tuohy needle have recently become available for use in infants. A possible alternative is to use a technique that allows an inclination of the needle. For example, a lumbosacral or sacral epidural approach allows a cephalad inclination of the needle in such a manner that the effective depth of the epidural space available for the bevel of the needle is increased, in comparison with the 90° approach. The inclination of the needle also makes the insertion of the epidural catheter easier (Figure 9.3).

Nerve stimulator

A nerve stimulator allows localization of a nerve by electrical stimulation of its motor component and is particularly useful when the patient is already anaesthetized, which generally is the case when regional anaesthesia is performed in children. Not all peripheral blocks require the use of a neurostimulator. However, often in children, anatomical land-

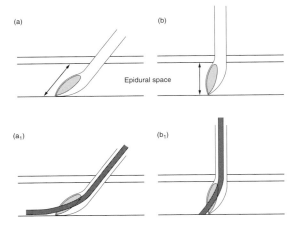

Figure 9.3 Importance of the inclination of the needle in approaching the epidural space in children. With an upward inclination of the Tuohy needle (a) the effective depth of the epidural space available for the bevel of the needle is increased. If the Tuohy needle encounters the dura, it is the round part of the tip that makes contact. This is in contrast with the 90° approach (b), in which the sharp part of the tip contacts the dura first. In addition, the inclination of the Tuohy needle is favourable for an upward threading of the catheter (a₁), whereas a perpendicular approach could cause the tip of the catheter to impact the dura with consequent possible migration into the subdural space (b₁).

marks are poorly developed and are difficult to identify, fascial sheets are thinner and identifying loss of resistance can be impossible. Therefore, on these occasions the use of a nerve stimulator is essential. Most anaesthetists prefer to use insulated needles which deliver maximum current density at the tip of the needle. Unsheathed, non-insulated, short-bevelled needles can be successfully used as well.[35]

CAREFUL AND METICULOUS TECHNIQUE

Regional blockade in children is usually performed under general anaesthesia, masking the perception of pain or paresthesiae and increasing the risk of inflicting unintentional neurological damage. The hazard of injury may diminish provided that:

- appropriate needles are selected (see above);

- slow insertion is combined with a careful detection technique for the epidural space;
- since the spinal cord terminates at the level of the third lumbar vertebra at term, spinal or low epidural approaches (lumbosacral, sacral, caudal) are preferred, and extreme caution is exercised in both the thoracic and lumbar regions. It must be remembered that peripheral blocks are often a simple and safe alternative;
- the procedure is abandoned if injury to neural tissue is suspected;
- there is close follow-up of the presumed injured patient, early neurological assessment and prompt referral to a neurosurgical unit for timely diagnosis and surgery if required.

Loss of resistance technique

Detection of the loss of resistance technique (LORT) is frequently used to locate the epidural space. A similar technique is also used to detect the perineural or the aponeurotic spaces. LORT can be use with a small volume of a gas, air or medical CO_2,[36] or fluid, normal saline or the local anaesthetic solution. Air to locate the epidural space has been suggested as a possible cause of neurological damage[37] and saline recommended as the safest option in children.[38] However, a critical look at the case histories reported by Flandin-Blety and Barrier showed some examples of serious neurological complications ascribed, probably incorrectly, to air used to locate the epidural space. A recent large epidemiological study of the complications of paediatric regional anaesthesia demonstrated that the method for identifying the epidural space (air or saline) was not correlated with any of the reported complications.[28] Therefore, before accepting the restrictive recommendation of not using air for the LORT, it is important to stress some points: air is a simple method and 'what is simple is usually safer'. There is no evidence that saline reduces the risks to patients. Using fluid carries the risk of injecting the wrong drug and, more importantly, accidental dural puncture is difficult to detect owing to low CSF pressure in small babies; saline certainly further dilutes the local anaesthetic concentrations and increases the volume of injection, thus resulting in less effective sensory block with a higher upper limit.[39] Obviously, when using air to identify the epidural space, venous air embolism is a possibility.[40] However, Scott commented on the same recommendation regarding air and LORT in adults: 'Nothing in medicine is completely safe, and trying to avoid a small problem often leads to a bigger one. My advice to those physicians who use the loss of resistance to air technique is not to change, provided their success rate in locating the epidural space is acceptable. As in many areas of medical practice, there is no substitute for good training and common sense.'[41] With careful use of the LORT, no air or only a tiny amount of air is injected into the epidural space. The pressure of the anaesthetist's thumb on the plunge of the detection syringe must be applied by quick, intermittent (not continuous as when saline is used) movements. As soon as 'a change' in resistance (rather than 'loss') is encountered, noted by the lack of the elastic recoil of the plunge, any pressure on the plunger should be stopped, thus avoiding any subsequent injection of air into the epidural space. An aspiration test must be performed immediately and, as a result, the introduced air (if any) is drawn out. The present author uses air but does not inject it for the LORT.[39] In conclusion, the accuracy of the technique plays a crucial role in determining a successful and uneventful epidural block.

Regarding the technique of injection, Dalens and Saint-Maurice recommended five safety rules for all regional block procedures:[42]

- Rule 1: Aspiration prior to each injection.
- Rule 2: Evaluation of the effects of a test dose containing adrenaline is made except in the area of an end artery.
- Rule 3: Slow rate of injection over about 90 s.
- Rule 4: Repeated intermittent aspirations during the course of an injection.
- Rule 5: Stop injection if any abnormal signs or symptoms occur.

These rules represent highly recommendable safety advice, but rule 2 deserves some comment.

Test dosing is an imperfect marker for intravascular injection. Several cases of intravascular injection were apparently preceded by uneventful test doses.[43] Problems related to the low predictive value of test dosing have been outlined recently.[44] These findings support the view that dosing of local anaesthetics for major

conduction blockade should be fractionated and continuous electrocardiographic (ECG) monitoring should be used to detect signs in addition to tachycardia, including bradycardia, changes in QRS morphology and ventricular ectopy.[45]

Localization of a nerve or a spinal/epidural space may sometimes be difficult and, if the first attempt fails, the procedure should be restarted from the beginning after verifying the patient's position and confirming the anatomical landmarks. After three failed attempts, the technique should be abandoned and an alternative technique, such as another block or opioid analgesia, should be used.

SELECTION OF THE APPROPRIATE BLOCK

In selecting the block an appropriate balance has to be found between successful analgesia and unwanted side-effects; it must be remembered that adequate analgesia may be achieved for relatively minor operations using simpler techniques such as wound infiltration and there is no block that is suitable for all operations.

Peripheral nerve blocks are especially useful for children undergoing minor procedures as outpatients, since these blocks provide analgesia with rapid emergence and a lower incidence of nausea than comparable analgesia produced by systemic opioids.[46]

Caudal anaesthesia is a safe, easily learned technique which has a versatile role providing intraoperative and postoperative analgesia for surgical procedures on the lower abdomen and lower limbs. It remains the most frequently utilized regional block in children. However, other approaches may provide effective postoperative analgesia whilst avoiding the possible adverse effects associated with central blocks or by decreasing the dose of local anaesthetic. For example, ilioinguinal/iliohypogastric nerve blocks are effective for perioperative pain management of patients undergoing inguinal hernia repair.

Thoracic epidural puncture in anaesthetized children should be restricted to patients with severe illness undergoing extensive thoracoabdominal surgery, and to practitioners who have gained considerable expertise in both adult thoracic epidural and paediatric lumbar epidural techniques.[46]

The primary rationale for epidural analgesia is to provide excellent analgesia with acceptable side-effects. In order to accomplish this, the key factor is proper patient selection. For instance, the likelihood of urinary retention from lumbar or caudal epidural infusions is sufficiently high to limit the procedure primarily to patients who require bladder catheters for reasons related to the length or complexity of surgery.

With short-term use the risk of infection from postoperative epidural infusions is quite rare. A recent study[47] found no postoperative epidural infections among 1620 infusions; another large series report found similar results.[48] However, the incidence of epidural catheter tip contamination is increased with the caudal route of insertion when compared with lumbar catheter placement.[49] Skin infection,[50] subcutaneous abscess[51] and epidural abscess[52] resulting from epidural catheter placement have occasionally been described. All cases were successfully treated using catheter removal, incision and drainage with culture and antimicrobial therapy when signs of systemic infection were present. As a preventive measure, a strict aseptic technique has to be emphasized: daily inspection of the catheter entry wound while the catheter is in place and for 72 h after catheter removal, and prompt catheter removal if infection is suspected.

APPROPRIATE DOSAGE

The sites of systemic local anaesthetic toxicity are the central nervous and cardiovascular systems and are manifest when the blood levels of these agents exceed safe concentrations. This may occur by unintended intravenous or intraosseous administration or by accumulation of excessive amounts of drug administered either by repeated bolus dosing or by continuous infusion.[53–55] This situation is more likely to remain undetected in children until a large volume of local anaesthetic is injected because most children are under general anaesthesia and subjective symptoms of a test dose are lost. Intravascular injection is more likely as small veins collapse easily on attempted aspiration. Toxicity in the central nervous system (CNS) manifests itself in convulsions and in the cardiovascular system by malignant ventricular dysrhythmias resistant to therapy or by sudden

cardiovascular collapse. Plasma concentrations of lignocaine from 10 μg ml^{-1} and bupivacaine 3–5 μg ml^{-1} in adults may be expected to produce these effects. There are too many factors influencing the onset of systemic toxicity to focus on absolute levels. Subtoxic levels producing a range of cardiovascular and CNS symptoms may be used as indicators of impending major toxicity but would be masked by general anaesthesia or sedation in children. Hence, signs of irritability, restlessness, or hypertension and tachycardia could be misinterpreted as pain in these patients[13] (see also Chapter 12).

Safe doses of local anaesthetic both as initial boluses and as continuous infusions depend upon meagre kinetic data. Safe administrations guidelines for single doses of bupivacaine and lignocaine have been developed[53] on the basis of pharmacokinetic studies of infants and children receiving wound infiltration, peripheral nerve blocks, or epidural and interpleural analgesia[56–61] (see *Pharmacology* section). Eyres reviewed local anaesthetic pharmacokinetics in infancy and concluded that 'paediatric anaesthetists should stop thinking in ml kg^{-1} but work instead in mg kg^{-1}'.[62] This conclusion seems to be appropriate in order to use a safe dosage of local anaesthetic.

Regarding the treatment of toxicity, it is worth mentioning the words of Fortuna, one of the pioneers of regional anaesthesia in children: 'no vein, no block!' (Fontuna, A., personal communication). In practice, it may be deemed negligent not to have access to a reliable open vein during administration of significant doses of local anaesthetic and minimal monitoring should include pulse oximetry and ECG monitoring to assist in the interpretation of electrical changes. During neuroaxial blockade, if signs of toxicity occur, there is universal agreement that the first step is the maintenance or institution of adequate ventilation.[63] This inhibits or delays the development of acidosis, which promotes further toxicity.[64,65] Following accidental intravenous injection, CNS toxicity is often limited in time and respiratory support may be adequate treatment. If more than ventilatory support is required for cardiovascular resuscitation a number of drugs has been suggested, although intravenous phenytoin may be the treatment of choice.[66–70] According to Eyres, it must be remembered that 'local anaesthetic toxicity is transient and all resuscitation resources should be utilized including extracorporeal support, where available and if indicated'.[62]

PHARMACOLOGY

In spite of their low therapeutic index local anaesthetics are good drugs. They are safe and effective and are being used in an expanding variety of clinical applications.

Pharmacological, pharmacokinetic and pharmacodynamic knowledge underpins the rational selection of safe and effective drug dosage for paediatric patients.

The amide local anaesthetics have been most frequently used and studied and as ester-type local anaesthetic agents are now used much less frequently this classification has more historical than pharmacological importance.

Hydrolysis by plasma pseudocholinesterase accounts for a majority of the metabolism of the ester-type agents. A metabolite resulting from the hydrolysis of procaine-like compounds is para-aminobenzoic acid. This metabolite has been implicated in allergic reactions which can occur following the administration of these ester-type drugs. As plasma pseudocolinesterases do not reach adult levels until about 6 months of life it would seem prudent to use reduced doses of the ester local anaesthetics in this age group.[71,72] However, there is no evidence that reduced metabolism of the ester local anaesthetic agents has clinical significance.

It is generally accepted that the amide-type local anaesthetics are metabolized principally by the liver, with the exception of prilocaine. One metabolite of prilocaine is responsible for methaemoglobinaemia. This problem is more likely to occur in the first 3 months of life, when reductive enzyme activity is lower.[73,74]

The clearance of lignocaine, which has an intermediate hepatic extraction ratio, depends on both hepatic perfusion and enzyme activity, while that of bupivacaine and mepivacaine, with low hepatic extraction ratios, depends on enzyme activity.

Mepivacaine is mainly metabolized by hydroxylation. Hydroxylation of mepivacaine is considerably slower in newborns than in adults and renal excretion is the primary mode of clearance.[75]

For a long time, protein binding was considered to be the principal factor regulating the free fraction of local anaesthetics, on which depends the toxicity. The affinity of a local anaesthetic for proteins concerns not only plasma protein but also tissue protein.

The major protein complex to which these drugs bind has been identified as α_1-acid glycoprotein (AAG). The plasma concentration of this glycoprotein is lower in neonates and infants than in older children and adults.[76,77] Neonates and infants are, thus, more vulnerable regarding the development of toxic free plasma concentration and the use of lower doses of local anaesthetics in this age group has been advocated.[53] Recently, concern has arisen about the importance of protein binding, especially after bolus injection.[78]

Following single epidural injection in adults maximum concentrations were generally reached in 10–30 min, with only marginal differences between agents. After 2.5–3 mg kg^{-1} caudal bupivacaine in infants under 6 months t_{max} was 28 ± 13 min, peak plasma concentrations were 0.97 ± 0.42 μg ml^{-1}, clearance was 7.1 ± 3.2 ml min^{-1} kg^{-1}, the volume of distribution (VD) at steady state was 3.9 ± 2 l kg^{-1} and $t_{1/2\beta}$ was 7.7 ± 2.4 h.[56]

Using a group of children aged 3–192 months, receiving bupivacaine for intercostal nerve block, it was found that the half-life of elimination was very similar to that reported for adults. The total body clearance, however, was twice that reported for adults (16.0 and 6.7 ml min^{-1} kg^{-1}, respectively).[61,79] Prolonged continuous paravertebral infusion of bupivacaine 0.25 mg kg^{-1} h^{-1} in 22 infants with a median age of 1.5 weeks resulted in a serum bupivacaine concentration > 3 μg ml^{-1} in three cases after 48 h.[80,81]

Owing to the relationship $t_{1/2} = VD \times \ln 2/ CL$, any increase in VD will raise the $t_{1/2}$. Despite an augmented clearance neonates have an increase in VD owing to their total body water and consequently a longer $t_{1/2}$.

Weston and Bourchier demonstrated that very-low-birth-weight infants have a markedly different pharmacokinetic profile.[82] After a single dose of 2 mg kg^{-1} of bupivacaine by the intrapleural route in this infant population, the half-life was longer, the clearance lower and volume of distribution greater than in term infants. Although the drug did not reach toxic levels at this dose ($< 4 \mu$g ml^{-1}), caution should be observed when redosing as the accumulation of the drug may be unpredictable. It is possible that a once-only dose might be sufficient for adequate analgesia. Multiple redosing in very-low-birth-weight infants might therefore only be safe if blood level analysis is rapidly available. Luz *et al.* measured bupivacaine plasma concentrations during 5 h of continuous epidural anaesthesia in infants.[83] They found higher plasma concentrations in infants up to 4 months than in older infants and after 5 h there is a tendency to accumulation, although within safe limits. They suggest that continuous administration for more than 5 h might cause an additional increase in bupivacaine plasma concentrations. If analgesia is not sufficient the dose should not be increased, as this could lead to toxicity in this age group.

Concern over the cardiotoxicity of bupivacaine has led to development of two alternative compounds, ropivacaine, which has recently been licensed, and levobupivacaine, which is currently undergoing clinical evaluation. Ropivacaine is the *N-n*-propyl homologue of mepivacaine and bupivacaine, but differs from these agents in that the single *S*-isomer has been developed for clinical use. In a preliminary report 0.2% caudal ropivacaine for minor surgical procedures in children provided adequate analgesia with minimal motor block.[84] A comparison between 2 mg kg^{-1} 0.2% caudal ropivacaine and 2.5 mg kg^{-1} of 0.25% bupivacaine demonstrated that the two drugs shared a similar clinical profile after low abdominal procedures in children.[85] A pilot sudy with 0.2% epidural ropivacaine 0.2–0.4 mg kg^{-1} h^{-1} (0.1–0.2 ml kg^{-1} h^{-1}) after abdominal and thoracic surgery in children showed that this dose regimen with ropivacaine as sole agent was ineffective. The use of epidural ropivacaine (0.2%) with regular diclofenac resulted in excellent analgesia, minimal motor block and no other epidural opioid-related complications.[86] (See also p. 324 for treatment of local anaesthetic toxicity.)

CENTRAL BLOCKS

SINGLE-SHOT CAUDAL ANAESTHESIA

In the caudal block the anaesthetic agent is injected through the sacral hiatus, puncturing the sacrococcygeal membrane, into the epidural space.

Technical guidelines

The approach to the sacral hiatus is made with the child in the lateral position with the upper leg flexed at the hip. Awake caudal anaesthesia in newborns is better performed in genupectoral position. After cleansing the skin over the sacrum, the anatomical landmarks are carefully identified. The sacral hiatus is identified by palpating the crista sacralis media moving in a caudad direction until a triangular depression is felt. This triangular depression lies directly over the sacrococcygeal membrane and is recognized by the prominent sacral cornua superiorly at its apex. The most common mistake in the performance of this block is to insert the needle too low. Marking the sacral cornua and the spinous process of the fifth sacral vertebra (where the crista sacralis media ends) allows a triangle to be drawn and the needle should be inserted at the higher apex of the triangle. The needle should be neither too long (the dural sac is very close) nor too thin (lack of blood or CSF reflux). A good example could be a 25-mm metallic needle 21G with a stylet. The author uses a standard intravenous cannula (20–22G) according to the child's age. The technique is very similar to venous cannulation: the needle is inserted at an angle of 90° to the skin and, after penetrating the sacrococcygeal membrane, depressed in a caudal direction through an angle of approximately 55–60° (Figure 9.4). At this point the metal stylet is withdrawn slightly (as in the venous cannulation) and the plastic cannula is advanced cephalad in the epidural space. Easy advancement of the cannula is indicative of successful placement in the epidural space. The blunt cannula tip reduces the chance of accidental dural puncture, subarachnoid injection and injury to underlying structures. The advancement along the canal should be no more than necessary, remembering that the

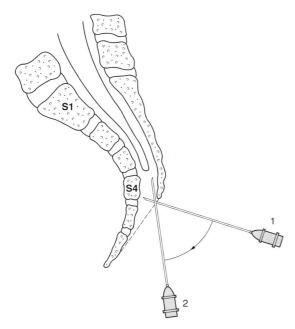

Figure 9.4 Diagram of the best fit angle for needle insertion into the caudal space. The needle is inserted at an angle of 90° to the skin (position 1), and then depressed in a caudal direction from position 1 to position 2.

shortest distance to the dural sac ranges from 19 to 34 mm in adults,[87] much less in small infants (Figure 9.5). The needle is then withdrawn completely and after ascertaining, by aspiration, that the catheter is not in the subarachnoid space or in a blood vessel, the chosen local anaesthetic is injected. No resistance must be encountered during the injection and since the level of analgesia is not affected by the rate of injection, it seems prudent to adopt a slow rate of injection (1 ml 10 s^{-1}).[88]

The duration and the extent of the caudal block are determined by the patient's age, the drug concentration, the drug volume and the presence or absence of additives to local anaesthetic solutions. Bupivacaine is the most commonly used agent in caudal epidural anaesthesia, but lignocaine and mepivacaine have been used extensively as well. Many dose regimens have been proposed and they tend to fall into two groups.[9,89,90] Firstly, there are regimens in which the recommended dose will guarantee a successful block over a given area. The extent or height of the block is not a pri-

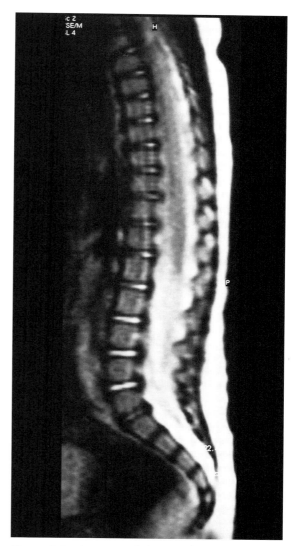

Figure 9.5 Anatomy of the sacral extradural space shown by magnetic resonance imaging.

mary concern. The emphasis is on a satisfactory clinical outcome. This is the case with Armitage's formula, where 0.5 ml kg^{-1}, 1 ml kg^{-1} or 1.25 ml kg^{-1} is administered to obtain a lumbosacral, thoracolumbar or midthoracic block, respectively.[91] When this calculation gives a volume less than 20 ml, 0.25% bupivacaine is used. For volumes greater than 20 ml, one part of saline is added to three parts of drug, giving a concentration of 0.19%. Secondly, there are regimens based on statistical studies which show graphical correlations between various indices such as weight, age, extent of block and mass of drug used. This approach is illustrated in Figure 9.6, which shows two nomograms compiled by Busoni and Andreuccetti for single-shot caudal anaesthesia.[92] Knowing the child's age or weight, the anaesthetist can read off the volume of drug required to produce anaesthesia at various dermatomal levels. Wolf *et al.* studied the optimal effective bupivacaine concentration for infants and children between the ages of 6 months and 10 years undergoing elective superficial lower abdominal or genital surgery.[81] They demonstrated that 0.0625% bupivacaine was ineffective for caudal epidural anaesthesia and that 0.125% bupivacaine with 1 : 200 000 adrenaline provided equipotent caudal epidural anaesthesia with less motor blockade than 0.25% bupivacaine. Various additives to local anaesthetic solutions have been used to prolong the duration of caudal analgesia provided by a single injection. The duration of action of adrenaline-added solutions is controversial in paediatric patients[25,93,94] as it has been implicated in several cases of neurological deficit associated with spinal cord ischaemia and hypoxic irritability.[95] Although there is very little convincing evidence to support this sugges-

tion, the optimal dose and associated risks are not well defined in neonates and infants. There is no doubt about the efficacy of opioids introduced into the caudal epidural space for providing prolonged postoperative analgesia (see below). Several studies have demonstrated that 1–2 μg kg^{-1} of clonidine in addition to the caudal analgesic mixture more than doubled the analgesic time, without affecting vital parameters.[94–98] In the author's experience 1 μg kg^{-1} clonidine added to 10 mg kg^{-1} caudal mepivacaine showed an increase in the postoperative analgesia and sedation time in comparison to a control group. Ketamine 0.5 mg kg^{-1} added to bupivacane 0.25% 1 ml kg^{-1} provided a longer duration of post-operative analgesia than clonidine 2 μg kg^{-1} or adrenaline 5 μg ml^{-1} for orchidopexy.[98] In practice, the use of caudal opioids should be reserved for major surgery when patients will receive a period of postoperative high-dependency care. The use of clonidine and ketamine offers the potential to prolong the duration of single-shot caudal analgesia greatly with minimal risk of side-effects. There is a need for dose-finding studies with these compounds to provide a more complete picture of the benefits and incidence of side-effects when these drugs are added to local anaesthetic solutions for caudal epidural use.

Indications

Single-shot caudal anaesthesia is the technique of choice for operations to T9, lasting for around 60–90 min. The majority of ambulatory surgical procedures below the diaphragm, including surgery involving lower extremities, hip, pelvis, urogenital and perianal regions, can be performed with such a technique. It alleviates pain after bone marrow harvesting.[99]

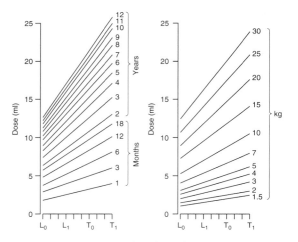

Figure 9.6 Diagrams for the relationship between dose, the spread of analgesia and age (left); and dose, the spread of analgesia and weight (right), useful in selecting the mean dosage of local anaesthetic in caudal blocks. The ordinates represent dose in millilitres. The abscissae represent the upper level of the block in dermatomes. (From Busoni and Andreuccetti[92] with permission.)

Advantages

Clinical experience with paediatric caudal block is quite extensive and reports of large series have been published.[26,92,100] Caudal anaesthesia combines the advantages of a simple and safe technique with a high success rate. It has a wide range of indication in paediatric practice.

Disadvantages

Persistent paresthesia and weakness in the lower extremities have proved distressing to some patients. In practice, lowering the concentrations of the local anaesthetic minimizes these problems.

CONTINUOUS CAUDAL ANAESTHESIA

The main disadvantage of single-shot caudal anaesthesia is the short duration of action. A catheter can be introduced into the epidural space via the sacral hiatus (Figure 9.7) and used to administer repeated doses or continuous infusions through the caudal needle (Tuohy, Crawford, intravenous cannula). Ideally, the tip of the catheter should lie in close proximity to the dermatomes that need to be blocked. Bosenberg and others took advantage of the difference in epidural fat between infants and adults to thread caudal catheters in the thoracic region.[101] This technique was used successfully for surgical correction of biliary atresia and to reduce the postoperative ventilatory requirements of a group of poor-risk infants undergoing repair of tracheo-oesophageal fistulae.[102] Initial reports claimed a very high success rate with caudally placed thoracic catheters and some authors proposed using this technique in older children and suggested that it was unnecessary to confirm the catheter position by X-ray.[103] However, more recent data have shown that in children older than 1 year the progression of the catheter is made difficult by the lumbosacral curvature that appears as a consequence of standing and walking, making this technique unreliable, with an unacceptable failure rate.[104] A segmental approach to the thoracic epidural space requires a highly experienced anaesthetist and, even in neonates and infants, catheter misplacement has been described. Bleeding must be regarded as a possible hazard and epidurographic control is suggested.[105]

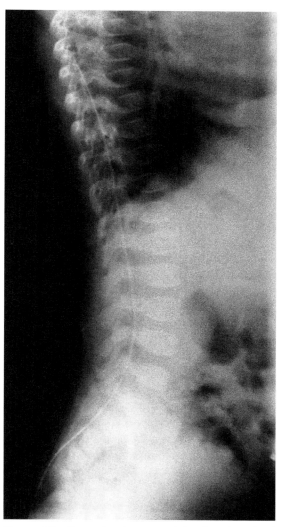

Figure 9.7 X-ray showing a caudally placed epidural catheter reaching the thoracic level.

SACRAL INTERVERTEBRAL, LUMBAR AND THORACIC EPIDURAL BLOCKADES

Although caudal epidural anaesthesia has been used successfully for upper abdominal or thoracic surgical procedures, it is evident that the volume of local anaesthetic required to achieve thoracic levels reliably by the caudal route is excessive. In addition, because of the possibility of faecal contamination, the safety of leaving an indwelling caudal catheter in place has not been adequately addressed. Sacral intervertebral, lumbar and thoracic epidural blockades are effective alternatives and well-established techniques in paediatric practice.

GRIP OF THE NEEDLE

It is important to be fully trained in the different ways of advancing the needle when performing sacral, lumbar or thoracic epidural blocks in children of different sizes. The back of the patient, the hand of the anaesthetist and the needle are a system in which variations relate to changes in the patient's body size. In adults and older children, the firmness of the grip on the needle is of greatest importance and Bromage's grip is probably ideal (Figure 9.8). In infants and newborns, the size of the anaesthetist's hand becomes relevant and is very large compared to the child's back. In this case sensitivity is more important than firmness of the grip. As the fingertips are the most sensitive, this will increase with the number of the fingertips used in performing the different techniques. The grip illustrated in Figure 9.9 is less firm, but allows the needle to be held between the first and second fingers, with the other three fingers maintaining contact with the child's back. The fingertips are used exclusively, so that maximum sensitivity is obtained. Even the slightest respiratory movements can be

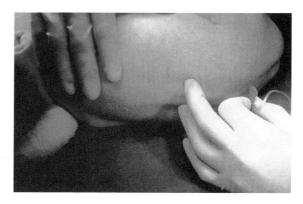

Figure 9.9 Grip of the needle for the epidural approach in neonates and small infants. The first two fingers of the left hand hold the wings of the needle and the other three fingers maintain the contact with the child's back (spider-like grip).

detected and the needle can be delicately advanced into the epidural space. Maximum flexibility can be achieved if extension tubing is used between the needle and the loss-of-resistance syringe.

SACRAL INTERVERTEBRAL EPIDURAL BLOCK

In 1986 Busoni and Sarti described this approach to the epidural space through the sacral interspaces.[21]

Technical guidelines

With the child in a lateral decubitus position, a line is drawn between the posterior superior iliac spines. This line crosses the second vertebral arch and, immediately below it, in the midline, the S2–S3 interspace is located by palpation (Figure 9.10). The needle is inserted in this interspace and the epidural space is identified with the LORT. Saint-Maurice uses this technique approaching the epidural space with a technique similar to that used for caudals; he relies only on feeling the 'give', which is clearly evident as the needle penetrates the ligamentum flavum and enters the epidural space (Saint-Maurice, C., personal communication). Although other sacral intervertebral spaces could be used safely, S2–S3 is frequently chosen because it is large and easy to identify.

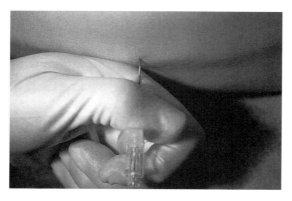

Figure 9.8 Bromage's grip for performing lumbar epidural in adult. This grip is also useful in older children.

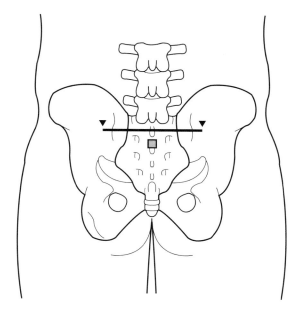

■ S$_2$S$_3$ Interspace

▼ Pasterior superior
iliac spine

Figure 9.10 Anatomical landmarks for sacral intervertebral epidural block. A line joining the posterior superior iliac spines crosses the vertebral body of the second sacral vertebra. The needle is inserted immediately below it in the midline (S2–S3 interspace).

The spread of local anaesthetic is similar to that of caudal anaesthetic. Therefore, it is possible to use the same nomograms to calculate the desired level of anaesthesia. The Tuohy needle is inserted perpendicular to the skin and as the needle passes between the two rudimentary spinous processes, upward or downward inclination of the needle can be used (Figure 9.11).

Indications

An upward inclination is mainly used for single-shot procedures as an alternative to a caudal block. If a catheter is to be inserted, a downward needle inclination is useful to keep the catheter in a safe space, since nervous structures are located higher in the spinal canal and a subdural migration of the catheter is unlikely (Figure 9.12); it is easy to tape the catheter to the child's back or it is possible to tunnel the

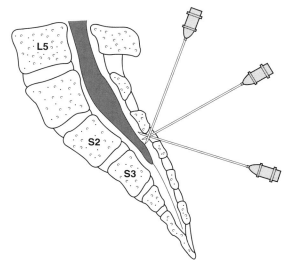

Figure 9.11 At the sacral level, owing to the rudimentary spinous processes, the Tuohy needle can be inserted using any inclination. A classical perpendicular approach, a cephalad or even a downward inclination of the needle can be used.

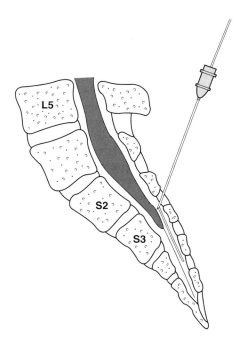

Figure 9.12 Sacral intervertebral epidural block with a downward catheter insertion. (From Messeri *et al.*[106] with permission.)

catheter under the skin. This unusual downward insertion of an epidural catheter is useful for postoperative analgesia after surgical correction of bladder exstrophy to eliminate discomfort caused by Bryant's traction.[106]

Advantages

Sacral intervertebral epidural block offers several advantages compared both with the lumbar epidural and with the caudal block: flexion of the lumbar spine is not required to facilitate the passage of the needle; any inclination of the Tuohy needle is possible; if a catheter is inserted, there is less danger of infection due to soiling than with caudal; traumatic injuries of the spinal cord and spinal arteries are unlikely compared with the lumbar approach; when training inexperienced anaesthetists, it is safer to use this technique than the more difficult and potentially more dangerous higher epidural blocks.

Disadvantages

Accidental dural puncture is possible as in children the dural sac ends at S3 and occasionally as low as S4.

SACROLUMBAR EPIDURAL APPROACH

The L5–S1 interspace is the largest in the vertebral column. In adults the spinous process of the fifth lumbar vertebra projects caudally in such a manner as to preclude entry into the epidural space from a skin area directly over it. In 1940 Taylor described the lateral approach to the L5–S1 interspace. Since the sacral vertebral angle is less prominent in children than in adults and the spinous process of the first sacral vertebra is rudimentary, Taylor's description, originally applied to adults, has been modified so that the space is approached in the midline, but the cephalad inclination of the needle has been retained.[107] With this modification the effective depth of the epidural space available for the bevel of the needle is increased and the insertion of an epidural catheter is facilitated.

Indications

This technique has proved to be useful and safe for abdominal urological procedures in infants and children for both intraoperative and postoperative pain control.

LUMBAR EPIDURAL BLOCK

Lumbar epidural spaces can be approached in children in the same way as in adults, although the distance from the skin to the epidural space is short and the ligaments are soft.

Skin dura distance

Prediction of the depth of the epidural space, with awareness of its variability, may increase the success and safety of the epidural procedure. Several formulae have been proposed to calculate the distance from the skin to the lumbar epidural space. The distance at L2–L3 is about 10 mm at birth and increases linearly with age according to the following equation: distance (mm) = (age in years × 2) + 10.[108] The age in years is a non-continuous number (i.e. no differences can be made between 12-month-old and a 23-month-old baby) and the body size could be quite different in various parts of the world, even at the same age in years. High correlation was reported between the depth of the lumbar puncture and body surface area.[109] However, body surface area is rarely used in clinical practice and body weight has been proposed as a more suitable parameter. The following clinically useful formula was derived: distance at L3–L4 (mm) = (body weight + 10) × 0.8.[110] Others found that the depth of the epidural space in older infants and children was correlated with age and weight, with a regression equation of depth (cm) = 1 + 0.15 × age (years) and depth (cm) = 0.8 + 0.05 × weight (kg), respectively.[111] The hypothesis that the distance is 1 mm kg^{-1} body weight is a simple and useful guideline for children aged between 6 months and 10 years.[112]

The criteria for the selection of the local anaesthetic solutions depend on the general condition and age of the patient, the need for motor block, the duration of postoperative analgesia required and the concomitant use of other analgesics. As with caudals, several formulae have been proposed to calculate the desired level of anaesthesia. The author has found that the mathematical model suggested by Romiti et al. according to an equation based on weight, age and desired level of anaesthesia fits well for paediatric requirements (Table 9.2).[113]

Advantages

Lumbar epidural anaesthesia provides analgesia with haemodynamic stability in children.[114–116] In a series of term newborns and former preterm infants undergoing primarily abdomi-

Table 9.2 Mathematical model of the relationship between volume of anaesthetic (ml), level of analgesia required and age and body weight useful in selecting the dosage of local anaesthetic in lumbar epidural block

Age (years)	Body weight (kg)	T12	T10	T7	T5	Age (years)	Body weight (kg)	T12	T10	T7	T5
12	60	16.3	17.8	19.8	21.1	6	30	10.8	11.8	13.1	14.0
	55	16.0	17.5	19.5	20.8		25	10.5	11.4	12.7	13.6
	50	25.8	17.2	19.2	20.4		20	10.1	11.0	12.3	13.1
	45	25.5	16.9	18.9	20.1		15	9.6	10.5	11.7	12.5
	40	25.2	16.6	18.5	19.7	5	25	9.7	10.6	11.8	12.5
	35	14.9	16.3	18.1	19.3		20	9.3	10.2	11.4	12.1
	30	14.5	15.9	17.7	18.8		15	8.9	9.7	10.8	11.5
11	55	15.5	16.9	18.8	20.0	4	20	8.5	9.3	10.3	11.0
	50	15.5	16.9	18.5	19.7		15	8.1	8.8	9.8	10.5
	45	15.0	16.3	18.2	19.4		10	7.6	8.3	9.2	9.8
	40	14.7	16.0	17.9	19.0	3	20	7.5	8.2	9.1	9.7
	35	14.4	15.7	17.5	18.6		15	7.2	7.8	8.7	9.3
	30	14.0	15.3	17.0	18.1		10	6.7	7.3	8.1	8.7
	25	13.6	14.8	16.5	17.6	2	15	6.0	6.6	7.3	7.8
10	50	14.6	15.9	17.8	18.9		10	5.6	6.1	6.8	7.3
	45	14.4	15.7	17.5	18.6	1.5	15	5.3	5.8	6.5	6.9
	40	14.1	15.4	17.1	18.2		10	5.0	5.4	6.0	6.4
	35	13.8	15.0	16.8	17.8	(months)					
	25	13.4	14.7	16.3	17.4	12	10.5	4.2	4.6	5.1	5.4
	20	13.0	14.2	15.9	16.9		8.5	4.1	4.4	4.9	5.3
9	45	13.7	15.0	16.7	17.0	9	10.0	3.7	4.0	4.5	4.8
	40	13.5	14.7	16.4	17.4		8.0	3.6	3.9	4.3	4.6
	35	13.2	14.4	16.0	17.0	6	8.0	3.0	3.3	3.6	3.9
	30	12.8	14.0	15.6	16.6		6.0	2.9	3.1	3.5	3.7
	25	12.5	13.6	15.2	16.1	3	6.5	2.2	2.4	2.7	2.8
	20	12.0	13.1	14.6	15.6		5.5	2.1	2.3	2.5	2.7
8	40	12.8	14.0	15.6	16.6		4.5	2.0	2.2	2.5	2.6
	35	12.5	13.7	15.2	16.2	1	5.0	1.3	1.4	1.5	1.6
	30	12.2	13.3	14.9	15.8		3.5	1.1	1.3	1.4	1.5
	25	11.8	12.9	14.4	15.3	< 1	4.0	0.92	1.00	1.12	1.19
	20	11.4	12.5	13.9	14.8		3.5	0.90	0.98	1.09	1.18
7	35	11.8	12.9	14.4	15.3		2.5	0.85	0.93	1.03	1.10
	30	11.5	12.6	14.0	14.9						
	25	11.2	12.2	13.6	14.5						
	20	10.2	11.8	13.1	14.0						

Modified from Romiti et al.[113]
Model: $Y = aX^B W^T T^S E$ (E)$Y = 0.817X^{0.430}W^{0.163}T^{0.524}$, where X = age; W = weight; T = number of analgesic dermatomes; E = estimated local anaesthetic dose (ml).

nal procedures, a combined lumbar epidural light general anaesthesia technique allowed extubation of all infants, maintainance of excellent haemodynamic and respiratory stability with very low pain scores in the post-operative period.[117] A successful epidural block reduces intraoperative anaesthetic requirements, attenuates the stress responses and assures good-quality postoperative pain relief.[118]

Disadvantages

Continuous lumbar extradural block is generally a safe technique; however, the smaller the child or the higher the dose of local anaesthetic and opioid, if any, administered, the greater the chance of complications.The amount of monitoring required is a direct function of the complexity of the technique employed and this varies from institution to institution.

THORACIC EPIDURAL BLOCK

Meignier first showed that thoracic epidural analgesia permitted a group of infants and children with severe pulmonary disease to undergo major thoracoabdominal procedures with excellent recovery of pulmonary function.[119] For the approach to the thoracic interspace the LORT can be used; a two-handed grip and the Macintosh balloon is a possible alternative (Figure 9.13). However, with the Macintosh balloon, unless the tip of the needle is well inside the thick ligamentum flavum, the air tends to spread into the softer surrounding tissues and the balloon will not remain inflated. The spinous processes of the dorsal vertebrae are long, triangular on transverse section, directed obliquely downward and terminate in a tubercular extremity. The angulation of the epidural needle should, therefore, be at its greatest in the midthoracic region. Above and below this level, the angulation decreases until, at the lower thoracic interspaces, the needle is inserted perpendicular to the child's back (Figure 9.14). Dosages and concentrations of the local anaesthetic solutions are calculated as follows:[120] for children less than 10 kg, 1% mepivacaine or 0.25% bupivacaine and the volume (ml) given is one-third of the body weight (kg); for children more than 10 kg, 1.5% mepivacaine or 0.5% bupivacaine and

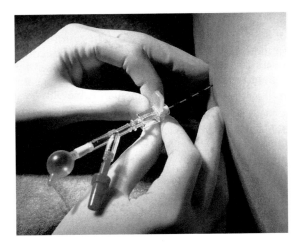

Figure 9.13 Macintosh balloon for the identification of the epidural space at the thoracic level. As the needle enters the epidural space the balloon will deflate.

the volume (ml) is one-quarter of the body weight (kg). With this regimen, analgesia spreads from T2 to T12. Top-up dosages are on average half the first dose.

Indications

Indications for this block must be carefully considered. It is reserved for seriously ill

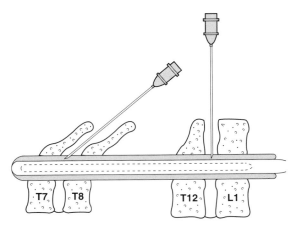

Figure 9.14 Thoracic epidural approach. The spinous processes of the thoracic vertebrae are directed obliquely downward in the midthoracic region; above and below this level the angulation of the spinous processes is less pronounced. At the lower thoracic interspaces the needle is inserted perpendicular to the child's back.

children undergoing major thoracoabdominal procedures.

Advantages

Thoracic epidural block overcomes the problems of the caudal and lumbar routes by anaesthetizing the specific segments that innervate the operative site.

Disadvantages

This block is technically more difficult and potentially more dangerous than the alternative. It should be performed only by expert hands.

SPINAL

Although spinal anaesthesia was the first regional technique described for use in children, only sporadic reports appeared in the literature until Abaijian *et al.* reintroduced it as a safe alternative to general anaesthesia in high-risk infants.[15] Spinals have also been used in older children and adolescents.[121,122] The doses of local anaesthetic and the duration of the block have not yet been well established in this age group.

Technical guidelines

The subarachnoid space can be approached at any interspace below L3, although L5–S1 has been reported to be the safest approach.[123] In awake newborns and small infants, spinal puncture should be made with the baby placed in the lateral or sitting position with the head reasonably extended to prevent oxygen desaturation from airway obstruction.[124] An assistant should firmly restrain the patient, because it is easy to dislodge the needle during the procedure. The needle is inserted in the midline and advanced at right angles to the skin. The characteristic click that is often felt when the needle pierces the ligmantum flavum and the dura is less distinct in the preterm infant than in older children. It is not uncommon to obtain a bloody or a dry tap during the performance of spinal puncture, especially in premature infants. These events are caused by improper needle placement: bloody tap might occur if the needle is not advanced exactly in the midline and dry

tap might be related to an excessive advancement of the needle. If blood is aspirated or there is failure to detect the free return of CSF during the procedure, it is advisable to move to another interspace after checking the accuracy of the technique. Isobaric bupivacaine can be used according to the body weight: $0.6–0.8$ mg kg^{-1} is a generally accepted dosage. In practice, using 0.5% bupivacaine 0.4, 0.5, 0.6 ml will adequately anaesthetize babies with weights of 1.5–2.4, 2.5–3.4 and 3.5–4.4 kg, respectively. Although hyperbaric 5% lignocaine has been used in children, it cannot be recommended because of the risk of neurotoxicity.[125,126]

Indications

Spinal anaesthesia is mainly used for children under the age of 1 year, especially for high-risk ex-premature infants, as an alternative to general anaesthesia for lower abdominal and lower extremity surgery.[15,127,128] Spinal anaesthesia can be used in emergency procedures, such as repair of testicular torsion, in unsedated and co-operative older children.

Advantages

No other technique can provide such extensive anaesthesia with so small a dose of local anaesthetic,[129] which is particularly useful in newborns and infants, who are at greater risk from local anaesthetic toxicity. Spinal anaesthesia has a more rapid onset time and stronger anaesthetic and muscle relaxant effects than any other central block.

Unlike older children and adults, neonates tolerate high thoracic spinal anaesthesia with minimal changes in heart rate, arterial blood pressure and respiratory activity. A prospective study showed that in ex-premature infants, postoperative bradycardia and oxygen desaturation were accentuated after general anaesthesia but not after spinal anaesthesia.[130] The effect of decreased sympathetic activity could be offset by arterial baroreflex-mediated vagal withdrawal.[131]

Disadvantages

The main risk of spinal anaesthesia in babies is a high block with ventilatory depression and apnoea.[132] The risk is greater when a high lumbar approach and large doses are used or if the baby's legs are raised after a block with hyperbaric solution.[123] The duration of spinal anaesthesia in infants is shorter than in older children or in adults and no postoperative analgesia can be achieved. Attempts to prolong the duration of spinal anaesthesia by the addition of adrenaline have been unsuccessful.[133]

EPIDURAL AND SPINAL OPIOIDS

Caudal/epidural opioids

The aim of epidural opioid administration is to achieve long-lasting, profound analgesia without undesiderable systemic side-effects (e.g. respiratory depression) and to avoid motor, sensory and autonomic blockade. Several studies have provided evidence of the long-lasting analgesia which is produced in children after the administration of 30–50 μg kg^{-1} epidural morphine.[134-136] Following the administration of caudal morphine, the plasma morphine concentration is much lower than that required for analgesia after systemic administration, suggesting that the effect of epidural opioids on analgesia is due to an action on spinal cord opioid receptors as opposed to an effect after systemic absorption. In clinical practice, for postoperative epidural analgesia the combination of opioid and very diluted local anesthetics is more commonly used than opioids alone, since this combination produces synergistic analgesic effects, perhaps because nociceptive pathways are interrupted at different sites with the two drugs: axonal membranes with the local anaesthetic and opioid receptors with the narcotic.[137] After orchidopexy, patients receiving morphine 0.05 mg kg^{-1} combined with 0.75 ml kg^{-1} of 0.125% bupivacaine did not require further analgesics, while over 50% of those receiving bupivacaine alone required opioid analgesia.[138] As in adults, the use of the more lipophilic agent requires continuous administration, because of the short duration of postoperative analgesia obtained. Since lipophilic opioids provide intense analgesia in the areas of administration without extensive spread, it is advisable to place the catheter tip near the dermatomal level of the surgical site. Infusions of 0.0625–0.1% bupivacaine with the addition of fentanyl 1–2 μg ml^{-1} at rates of 0.15–0.3 ml kg^{-1} h^{-1} have been employed.[139] Continuous epidural infusion of bupivacaine/-fentanyl mixture (fentanyl 2 μg ml^{-1} and bupivacaine 1 mg ml^{-1} infused at a rate of 0.25 ml kg^{-1} h^{-1}) was found to be superior to intermittent epidural morphine (30 μg kg^{-1} every 8 h) for postoperative pain management in children.[140]

Pruritus, urinary retention, sedation, nausea, vomiting and hypoventilation are the side-effects reported following epidural opioids, but the overall incidence of these effects in children is not known. A small reduction in ventilation, without significant increases in arterial and expired carbon dioxide tension, has been detected after 0.05–0.075 mg kg^{-1} of caudal or lumbar morphine.[141,142]

Early respiratory depression occurring in the first 2 h following epidural narcotic injection is the result of vascular uptake and redistribution (i.e. the same mechanism that follows intramuscular injection). Delayed hypoventilation, occurring up to 24 h following epidural injection, is the consequence of rostral spread of the narcotic in CSF to the respiratory centres located in the floor of the fourth ventricle. A series of 138 children given caudal morphine reported an incidence of 11 cases of clinically detected hypoventilation (8%).[143] Seven of these 11 children received parenteral opioids in addition to epidural morphine: the concurrent systemic use of opioids or any other sedative drug is a known risk factor at any age.[144] Eight cases were below 3 months of age. Pharmacokinetic and pharmacodynamic reasons for increased sensitivity to opioids of children up to 4 months is well known: children in this age group, given even small doses of opioids by any route, will have an increased incidence of hypoventilation. In children older than 4 months, the risk of hypoventilation is similar to that seen in adults. In a large, multicentre Swedish survey the incidence of 'depression requiring naloxone' was 0.25–0.4%.[145] In a survey of 74 American institutions, the incidence of 'respiratory insufficiency' was 1.9–2.3%.[145] In a prospective study of 1085 patients in a single institution, the incidence of 'respiratory depression' was 0.9%.[146] These data suggest that, after analgesic doses of epidural morphine the occurrence of clinically significant hypoventilation is rare. The duration of the at-risk period is unknown, possibly up to 12 h, even 24 h. Respiratory rate alone is an inadequate and a late indicator of the ventilatory status in postoperative patients receiving epidural narcotics.[147]

In patients breathing air and with no concurrent pulmonary or cardiovascular disease a pulse oximeter is an useful and sensitive postoperative monitor for ventilatory depression after epidural opioid administration:[148] in children breathing air an SpO_2 value (oxygen saturation of haemoglobin measured by pulse oximetry) of less than 94% should be considered a sign that hypoventilation has occurred. Oversedation and somnolence are always associated with hypoventilation: the detection of these symptoms, presumably resulting from carbon dioxide narcosis or to a spread of the drug in CSF to receptors in the thalamus, limbic system and cortex, can give a warning of the onset of respiratory depression.[149]

In a high-dependency unit postoperative monitoring by experienced nursing staff and continuous pulse oximetry recording should be mandatory up to 24 h after surgery. No other sedative or opioid drug should be administered by any route. Monitoring should include regular assessment of level of consciousness and a sedation score.[150] If hypoventilation is detected, intravenous naloxone (0.01–0.1 mg kg^{-1}) will promptly restore adequate spontaneous ventilation, but repeated doses are sometimes necessary: this drug should be kept at the bedside. The administration of opioids in the epidural space, alone or in combination with local anaesthetics, should be limited to major orthopaedic and abdominal surgery, excluding day-case surgery.[151]

Spinal opioids

Intrathecal opioids are used less commonly in children than are epidural opioids, probably because epidural techniques are much more common than spinal blocks in children. Nevertheless, 3.75–10 μg kg^{-1} spinal morphine has been successfully used to treat postoperative pain following thoracic or upper abdominal procedures.[152]

In conclusion, central neuroaxis opioids are increasing in popularity for use in children; the duration of analgesia increases in a dose-related manner, as does the incidence of side-effects. Late respiratory depression can occur; neonates and small infants receiving similar weight-related doses to older children are more likely to develop side-effects and must be closely monitored.

PERIPHERAL NERVE BLOCKS

NERVE BLOCKS OF THE LOWER LIMB

Femoral nerve and lateral cutaneous nerve of thigh blocks

It has been demonstrated by means of anatomical dissections that the femoral nerve[153] and the lateral cutaneous nerve of the thigh[154] run in canals which can be relatively easily located using two basic principles: (1) loss of resistance or a 'pop' can be felt when a short bevelled needle is passed through fascia or aponeurosis; and (2) it is difficult to inject when the needle tip is in muscle or dense fibrofatty tissue.[155]

Technical guidelines

The femoral nerve can be located below the inguinal ligament just lateral to the pulsations of the femoral artery by feeling two losses of resistance or 'pops' as the needle passes through fascia lata and then fascia iliaca. A line drawn between the anterior superior iliac spine and pubic tubercle indicates the position of the inguinal ligament. The needle is inserted 0.5–1 cm below the inguinal ligament, 0.5–1 cm lateral to the pulsation of the femoral artery, and advanced until loss of resistance is twice appreciated (Figure 9.15). If it is then easy to inject one can be confident of being in the canal with the femoral nerve. If it is not easy to inject the needle may have entered the nerve or the muscle deep to the nerve. The two fascial layers are sometimes fused and the apparent second loss of resistance may occur when the needle enters muscle. The correct space can usually be found by slowly withdrawing the needle until it is easy to inject. The femoral nerve is adequately blocked by 0.3 ml kg^{-1} of local anaesthetic

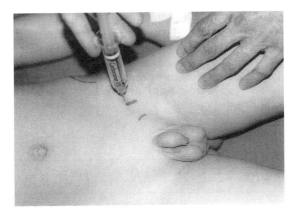

Figure 9.15 Anatomical landmarks of femoral block. The needle is inserted 0.5–1 cm below the inguinal ligament, 0.5–1 cm lateral to the pulsation of the femoral artery. Anterior superior iliac spine, femoral artery and pubic tubercles are marked.

solutions. After penetration of the femoral canal, a catheter can be introduced thorough a standard Tuohy needle and advanced cephalad for 5–8 cm. Continuous femoral nerve blockade with an infusion of 0.3 ml kg^{-1} h^{-1} of 0.125% bupivacaine is a simple and safe method of pain relief in children with, for example, femoral fractures.[156]

The best place to block the lateral cutaneous nerve of the thigh is immediately medial to the anterior superior iliac spine. As the needle is advanced a loss of resistance is felt as the external oblique aponeurosis is penetrated. The needle is advanced with a syringe attached and gentle pressure applied to the plunger. It is difficult to inject while passing through the internal oblique muscle. As the needle enters the nerve canal it suddenly becomes easy to inject. Two to three millilitres of local anaesthetic will fill the canal and provide a good block.

Indications

These nerve blocks are particularly useful in children for muscle biopsies and for donor areas for skin harvesting in burns. In patients with femoral shaft fractures both blocks provide analgesia and relieve muscle spasm.

Advantages

The accurate location of the nerves makes it possible to block the nerve with a relatively low dose of local anaesthetic, avoiding large volumes necessary when a fan-wise injection is used.

Disadvantages

Injury to adjacent blood vessels and nerve damage are possible, although minor, complications of these techniques. It is important to stress that nothing should be injected if there is undue resistance.

Fascia iliaca compartment block

The fascia iliaca compartment block has been described as an alternative to the 'three-in-one' nerve block for analgesia in the lower limbs in children. The femoral, obturator and lateral cutaneous nerves are blocked using a single injection into the fascia iliaca compartment.[157]

Technical guidelines

The technique involves injection of local anaesthetic into the fascia iliaca compartment, which is a potential space between the iliacus muscle and the fascia iliaca which covers it. The anatomical landmarks consist of the anterior superior iliac spine, the pubic tubercle and the inguinal ligament. With the patient supine, a needle is inserted perpendicular to the skin 0.5 cm below the junction of the lateral third and the medial two-thirds of the inguinal ligament (Figure 9.16). The loss of resistance is appreciated twice, when the needle passes through the fascia lata and then the fascia iliaca. The anaesthetic solution is injected at this level and, at the same time, firm compression is applied immediately caudad to the needle to favour the upward spread of the anaesthetic. Dalens *et al.*[157] used a 50 : 50 mixture of 1% lignocaine and 0.5% bupivacaine with 1 : 200 000 adrenaline, with the volume calculated on weight basis: 0.7 ml kg^{-1} for less than 20 kg, 15 ml for 20–30 kg, 20 ml for 30–40 kg, 25 ml for 40–50 kg and 27.5 ml for more than 50 kg. However, 2 mg kg^{-1} of 0.25% bupivacaine can also be used successfully.

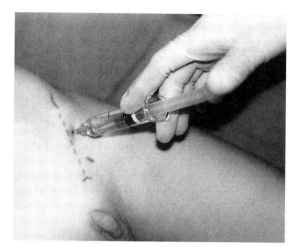

Figure 9.16 Anatomical landmarks of fascia iliaca compartment block. The needle is inserted 0.5 cm below the junction of the lateral third and medial two-thirds of the inguinal ligament.

Indications

Fascia iliaca compartment block is used in hip surgery, femoral osteotomies, femoral fractures, knee arthroscopy and muscle biopsies in the thigh.

Advantages

This block does not require the use of a nerve stimulator or the production of paraesthesiae and is performed away from blood vessels and nerves so that the chance of inadvertent nerve injury or intravascular injection is remote. The technique has been shown to have a higher success rate (95%) than the 'three-in-one' block (20%) in children.

Disadvantages

The block requires almost the maximal dose of local anaesthetic, but absorption is low from this compartment, especially when adrenaline is added to the solution, and toxic levels of bupivacaine are not reached.[158]

Sciatic nerve blocks and saphenous nerve block

The sciatic nerve is a mixed nerve which supplies sensory innervation to the foot, ankle, posterior

and lateral parts of the leg, including the periosteum of the tibia.

Technical guidelines

Many approaches have been described to block the sciatic nerve. According to Dalens the safest, and easiest, proximal approach is the lateral.[159] The child is placed in the dorsal decubitus position with the limb in a neutral position or slightly internally rotated (if possible). The landmark is the skin projection of the greater trochanter of the femur on the lateral aspect of the thigh. The puncture site is marked 0.5–1 cm below the greater trochanter and the needle is inserted horizontally, in the direction of the lower border of the femur under which runs the sciatic nerve, until twitches are elicited in the leg or foot (Figure 9.17).

An alternative technique is to block the division of the sciatic nerve (tibial and common peroneal nerve) within the popliteal fossa.[160] The use of a neurostimulator makes blockade of the tibial nerve and common peroneal nerve reliable and prevents any tempt-

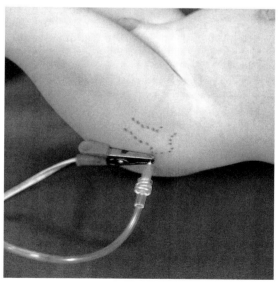

Figure 9.17 Anatomical landmarks of lateral approach to the sciatic nerve. The needle is inserted 0.5–1 cm below the skin projection of the great trochanter of the femur on the lateral aspect of the thigh and advanced in the direction of the lower border of the femur until twitches are elicited in the leg or foot.

ation to place the needle too deep, where it may damage the popliteal vessels. The patient is turned to the lateral or semiprone position with the leg to be blocked uppermost. The needle is inserted lateral to the pulsations of the popliteal artery midway between the intercondylar line and the apex of the popliteal fossa (Figure 9.18). A 'pop' is felt as the needle passes through the popliteal membrane. The tibial nerve is found about 0.5 cm deeper and the position is confirmed by flexor muscle twitching when the nerve is stimulated. The common peroneal nerve is found immediately beneath the popliteal membrane and is located by the nerve stimulator causing twitching of the peroneal muscles and dorsiflexion and eversion of the foot. Then, 0.5 ml kg^{-1} 0.5% bupivacaine is injected and successful blockade is manifest by fading of the muscle twitch until it disappears after 1 or 2 min.

The saphenous nerve (terminal branch of the femoral nerve) can be blocked with subcutaneous infiltration on the medial aspect of the leg just below the knee.

Indications

Sciatic nerve blocks are recommended for surgery on the foot (especially club foot) and for pain relief in patients with traumatic lesions

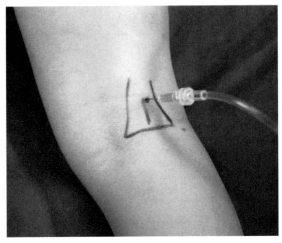

Figure 9.18 Anatomical landmarks of tibial nerve block. The needle is inserted lateral to the midline axis of the popliteal space about midway between the intercondylar line and the apex lateral to the palpable popliteal artery.

of the leg (fractured tibia) and foot. Block of the tibial and common peroneal nerve has been used in children for postoperative analgesia, as a diagnostic block, and as an adjunct to the physiotherapy management of severe equinus deformity after brain injury.

Advantages

Local analgesic blockade of the tibial nerve, common peroneal nerve and saphenous nerve provides good analgesia following surgery below the knee. It is an alternative to blocking the sciatic nerve in the thigh and to blocking the nerves at the ankle. Its advantages are that the nerves are more superficial and the depth can be located by feeling the penetration of the popliteal membrane.

Disadvantages

Tibial fracure and tibial osteotomy should be considered contraindications for nerve block in the popliteal fossa because of subsequent inability to recognize a compartment syndrome.

NERVE BLOCKS FOR EXTERNAL GENITALIA AND ABDOMINAL SURGERY

Penile block

The dorsal nerves of the penis are a terminal branch of the pudendal nerve. Arising in the pudendal canal they run forward along the ramus of the ischium and then along the margin of the inferior ramus of the pubis. They pass through the gap between the perineal membrane and the inferior pubic ligament to enter the subpubic space (where they can be blocked with a subpubic approach). The nerves lie on the dorsal surface of the corpora cavernosa as they pass forward on the dorsum of the penis and supply the glans and most of the shaft of the penis (Figure 9.19).

Technical guidelines

Several techniques for dorsal penile nerve blockade have been described which depend on the level at which the nerves are approached, the inclination of the needle and the choice of a single or double injection. The technique of blocking the nerves at the level of the base of the

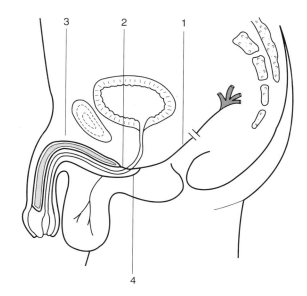

Figure 9.19 Gross anatomy of the pudendal nerve and its divisions. 1: pudendal nerve; 2: dorsal nerve of the penis; 3: subpubic space; 4: perineal nerve.

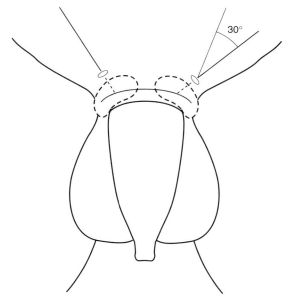

Figure 9.20 Bilateral subcutaneous injection for penile block.

penis by injecting the anaesthetic in the space between Buck's fascia and the corpora cavernosa is dangerous and may lead to injury of penile vessels.[161] Dalens *et al.* have described the subpubic approach to the penile nerves.[162] Two puncture sites are marked below the symphysis pubis, 0.5–1 cm lateral to the midline. The needle is inserted almost perpendicular to the skin, pointing slightly medially and caudally, until it crosses Scarpa's fascia with a perceptible 'give' and enters the subpubic space. The first half of the local anaesthetic is injected. The procedure is then repeated at the other puncture site to achieve complete anaesthesia of the penis, foreskin and glans.

An alternative technique has been performed by Broadman *et al.*, injecting the solution around the shaft of the penis near the base, producing a subcutaneous ring; most of the volume is administered dorsally in the midline.[163]

The author uses a subcutaneous injection 0.5–1 cm bilaterally to the symphysis pubis until a swelling of the penile base is achieved (Figure 9.20). Recommended volumes of local anaesthetic vary from 1.0 to 5 ml in children up to 12 years old depending on age. Adrenaline should never be used with dorsal nerve blocks

because spasm in the dorsal arteries could lead to ischaemia, with dire consequences.

Topical analgesia with lignocaine has been used to produce pain relief after circumcision,[164] although a dorsal nerve block may prove more effective.[165] EMLA cream (eutectic mixture of local anaesthetics) has been shown to be efficacious and safe for the prevention of pain from circumcision in neonates.[166]

Indications

This block is recommended for superficial surgery of the penis (circumcision, phimosis) and for postoperative analgesia of hypospadias repair, provided that the base of the penis has not been included in the surgery.

Advantages

It is easy to perform, safe and reliable. The procedure does not require special skill and complications are unlikely.

Disadvantages

Possible complications are haematoma formation and ischaemia. Haematoma formation is unlikely unless the dorsal vessels or the corporus cavernosum are punctured.

Ilioinguinal and iliohypogastric nerve block

At the level of the anterior superior iliac spine these two branches of the lumbar plexus run immediately below the external oblique fascia where they can easily be approached percutaneously (here the ilioinguinal and iliohypogastric nerves lie between the external oblique and internal oblique muscles).

Technical guidelines

Two finger breadths of the child 1 cm above, medial to the anterior superior iliac spine, a needle is inserted at an angle of 30° to the skin and directed parallel to the inguinal ligament (Figure 9.21). When the needle tip pierces the aponeurosis of the external oblique muscle a loss of resistance or a 'pop' is felt. At this point, after aspiration, 80% of the solution is injected; the remaining 20% is injected subcutaneously in lines radiating inferiorly and medially from the injection point to block the missed cutaneous nerve fibres. The most common local anaesthetic solution administered is 0.25–0.5% bupivacaine 2 mg kg^{-1}; 1–2% mepivacaine or the equivalent can also be used. In children weighing less than 15 kg rapid absorption with high plasma levels can occur; it is therefore prudent

to use a dose of bupivacaine not exceeding 1.25 mg kg^{-1}, especially if repeated or bilateral blocks are required.[167]

Indications

Ilioinguinal and iliohypogastric nerve block are commonly used for inguinal hernia repair, hydrocele, orchidopexy and varicocele.

Advantages

If this block is performed before surgery, it decreases the requirement for a deep level of general anaesthesia and provides similar duration and quality of postoperative analgesia for orchidopexy and inguinal hernia repair as a caudal block.[168]

Disadvantages

This block by itself does not provide sufficient anaesthesia for surgery and is primarly used to provide postoperative analgesia. It does not abolish the visceral pain produced by traction on the spermatic cord structures or on the peritoneum. Some surgeons feel that locally infiltrated anaesthetic solutions obscure the anatomical landmarks necessary for surgery. If this is the case, the block can be successfully performed, intraoperatively, under direct vision, by the surgeon.[169] If the injection is performed too deeply, under the fascia covering iliacus muscle, femoral nerve block can occur.[170] Perforation of visceral organs might occasionally happen, but no serious complications have been reported.

Rectus sheath block and paraumbilical block

Although only recently described for use in children, these blocks provide analgesia for surgical procedures in the umbilical area.[171,172] Continuous rectus sheath block has been used for postoperative analgesia after Nissen fundoplication in an infant with bronchopulmonary dysplasia.[173]

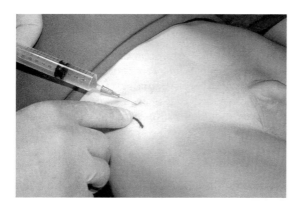

Figure 9.21 Iliohypogastric and ilioinguinal nerve block. The needle should be inserted about 1 cm above the anterior superior iliac spine (marked), at an angle of about 30° to the skin, directed parallel to the inguinal ligament.

NERVE BLOCKS OF THE UPPER LIMB

The upper extremity is supplied by the brachial plexus, which is formed from the union of C4–

C5 to T1–T2 spinal nerves. This plexus is located in the interscalene space, enclosed in a continuous sheath derived from the deep cervical fascia: thus, a single injection within this envelope allows complete plexus block. This space is divided in two by a transverse barrier at the level of the coracoid process of the scapula: therefore, supraclavicular and axillary approaches to the brachial plexus are not equivalent.

Supraclavicular brachial plexus blocks

Owing to the close relationships of the brachial plexus with vital structures of the head and neck, supraclavicular blocks have been little used or even contraindicated in children.

Parascalene approach

Dalens *et al.* have described in children a new approach to the brachial plexus within the interscalene space, the parascalene approach, which avoids major structures.[174]

Technical guidelines

The patient is placed in the dorsal decubitus position, the head turned away from the side to be blocked, after placement of roll under the shoulders and neck to stretch and superficialize the plexus nerves. The landmarks are the midpoint of the clavicle and Chassaignac's tubercle (transverse process of C6) at the posterior border of the sternocleidomastoid muscle, on the circular line passing over the cricoid cartilage. The puncture site is marked at the union of the lower third with the upper two-thirds of the line joining the two landmarks. The needle is inserted perpendicular to the skin, i.e. strictly anteroposteriorly, until twitches are elicited in the forearm or hand (not the shoulder) (Figure 9.22). With this insertion route, the needle cannot threaten the greater

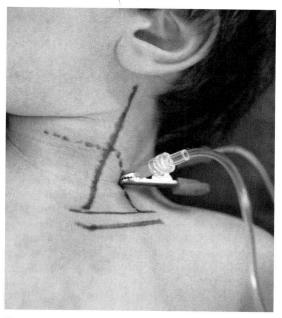

Figure 9.22 Anatomical landmarks of parascalene block. The puncture site is marked at the union of the upper two-thirds and lower one-third of the line joining the midpoint of the clavicle and Chassaignac's tubercle.

vessels of the neck or the apical pleura. The recommended volume of local anesthetic solution (Table 9.3) is then injected at a slow rate. Anaesthesia distributes rapidly to distal branches of the cervical plexus and upper branches of the brachial plexus, whereas the lower branches of the brachial plexus (supplying the wrist and hand) are blocked later, and sometimes incompletely.

Indications

Parascalene block is recommended for surgery of the shoulder, arm and elbow (especially

Table 9.3 Suggested local anaesthetic volumes for brachial plexus block

Brachial plexus block	Body weight (kg)							
	< 10	15	20	25	30	40	50	60
Parascalene approach	1 ml kg^{-1}	12.5 ml	15 ml	17.5 ml	20 ml	22.5 ml	25 ml	27.5 ml
Axillary block	0.5 ml kg^{-1}	7.5 ml	10 ml	10 ml	12.5 ml	15 ml	17.5 ml	20 ml

supracondylar fractures) but is less appropriate than axillary blocks for surgery of the forearm and hand.

AXILLARY BRACHIAL PLEXUS BLOCK

For paediatric patients axillary block is the most common and the safest technique.

Technical guidelines

Since solutions spread easily along nerve paths, high axillary approaches are unnecessary and are better avoided. The patient is positioned supine with the arm abducted to 90° and with the elbow flexed. The axillary artery is identified by palpation in the axillary fossa with the index finger of the left hand. The artery is identified by palpating the tissues overlying the humerus at the juction of pectoralis major and coracobrachialis muscles. With the index finger placed over the artery, a short-bevel needle, with an extension set, is inserted with the right hand immediately above the finger at an angle of 30° to the skin and directed parallel to, and just above, the artery. The needle is then slowly advanced until it starts to pulsate, which is the sign that the needle is placed correctly (Figure 9.23). If the artery is penetrated, the needle is withdrawn until blood is no longer aspirated. The anaesthetic solution is then slowly injected

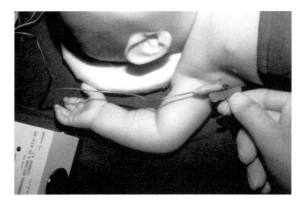

Figure 9.23 Axillary brachiac plexus block. The arterial pulse is palpated in the axilla. The needle is directed parallel to, and just above, the artery. The needle should be seen to pulsate distinctly and the position can be confirmed with a nerve stimulator if required.

according to recommended volumes (Table 9.3). A reinjection catheter can easily be introduced for providing long-lasting postoperative pain relief when necessary. In neonates, 5 mg kg^{-1} of 0.75–2% lignocaine has been used; 0.5 ml kg^{-1} of 1% mepivacaine or 0.25% bupivacaine usually produces adequate analgesia in infants and children.

Indications

The axillary block is indicated for surgery involving the arm and hand. It has recently been used successfully for venous catheterization in low- and very-low-birthweight infants.[175]

Advantages

The axillary block is an easy, effective and safe technique. The use of a nerve stimulator can be avoided.

Disadvantages

Upper arm procedures and surgery to the clavicle cannot be performed with this block. Intravascular injection, haematoma formation and vascular damage can occasionally occur.

NEURAL BLOCKADES FOR THORAX AND UPPER ABDOMEN

Thoracotomy is a painful procedure which causes marked impairment of pulmonary function. Neural blockade has been advocated by many authors to reduce or negate the need for parenteral opioids after thoracotomy. Techniques described include epidural blockade (see specific paragraph) and intercostal nerve block either via injection of multiple intercostal spaces, or by insertion of a catheter to provide continuous blockade of intercostal nerves. These catheters may be placed in the interpleural space (interpleural block), alongside the nerve (subcostal catheter techniques) or in the extrapleural space (extrapleural intercostal nerve block). Evidence suggests that all three of these techniques may have the same sites of spread to multiple levels, both along adjacent intercostal spaces extrapleurally and via the paravertebral space.[176]

Interpleural block

The interpleural block should only be used during thoracotomy, since the percutaneous technique has a substantial risk of pneumothorax in a child who does not have a chest drain. A catheter is inserted under direct vision during the surgical procedure between the visceral and parietal pleurae, and a continuous infusion of local anaesthetic is started. Although regimens using high-volume, low-concentration infusion have been reported as safe,[177,178] the high dose of local anaesthetic required for effective interpleural block has raised concerns about toxicity.

Intercostal nerve block

Subcostal catheter techniques

Individual intercostal nerve block at several levels performed during surgery has a relatively short duration of action, but placement of single or multiple catheters alongside the nerve in the subcostal groove provides effective analgesia with spread to multiple levels in the extrapleural space.[179] However, if inserted percutaneuously, these catheters can be technically difficult to feed onwards and may risk neural or vascular damage.

Continuous extrapleural intercostal nerve block

This technique, recently described by Downs and Cooper in children, consists of the placement of a catheter extrapleurally in the paravertebral gutter under direct vision at surgery.[180] This approach overcomes the problems of the subcostal techniques and obviates the need for more than one catheter. However, with continuous extrapleural intercostal nerve block the optimal route, bolus and infusion dosage need to be established in neonates, infants and children. These techniques may not be appropriate when there is potential for markedly increased uptake of local anaesthetics, such as with pulmonary angiomas or pleural inflammation.[54]

Paravertebral block

Lönnqvist described the use of paravertebral block in children and the gross and radiological anatomy for its successful and safe execution.[181–184]

Technical guidelines

With the child in a lateral decubitus position the skin of the back is punctured 1–2 cm lateral to the spinous process of T7–T9. The Tuohy needle is advanced until contact is made with the transverse process and then 'walked off' its superior border through the costotransverse ligament until the paravertebral space is located with the LORT. A catheter is then introduced for 2–3 cm and a bolus dose of 0.5 ml kg^{-1} 0.25% bupivacaine is injected.

The risk of pneumothorax and damage to blood vessels makes this technique less popular than the epidural approach.

BLOCKS FOR CLEFT LIP AND PALATE REPAIR

Infraorbital nerve block

The infraorbital nerve runs forward in the infraorbital groove and canal. It enters the face through the infraorbital foramen and supplies sensory innervation to the skin and mucous membrane of the upper lip and lower eyelid, to the skin between them and to the side of the nose. Bosenberg performed an anatomical surface study in neonates to determine the landmarks that can be useful for the transcutaneous approach to this nerve and its clinical application.[185]

Technical guidelines

The infraorbital nerve lies halfway between the midpoint of the palpebral fissure and the angle of the mouth, approximately 7.5 mm from the alar base. The needle is introduced at this point perpendicular to the skin and advanced until bony resistance is felt. The needle is then slowly withdrawn and 0.5% bupivacaine 0.5–0.75 ml with adrenaline 1 : 200 000 is injected. If resistance to injection is noted, the position of the needle tip should be adjusted.

In older children the author prefers the transoral approach to the nerve. The needle is inserted through the superior buccal sulcus, at the second upper premolar tooth level, and directed upwards to the infraorbital foramen, which is being palpated with the other hand. The needle tip can be felt as it approaches the foramen and a swelling is observed as the local anaesthetic (1–2 ml 0.5% bupivacaine, 2% mepivacaine or their equivalent) is injected.

Indications

Bilateral block of the nerve can be used for all surgical procedures on the upper lip. It is especially useful for cleft lip repair.

Advantages

A very small amount of local anaesthetic produces satisfactory intraoperative and post-operative analgesia, whereas profound general anaesthesia with opioids can cause respiratory depression.

Disadvantages

No problems have been reported with the use of this block.

Nasopalatine and palatine nerve block

Anaesthesia of the nasopalatine and palatine nerve will provide palatal hard and soft tissue anaesthesia.

Technical guidelines

The nasopalatine nerve is blocked with an injection performed into the incisive papilla just behind the maxillary central incisors (Figure 9.24a). Because the soft tissue is sparse in this area only a few drops of local anaesthetic can be injected. The palatine nerve emerges into the palate through the greater palatine foramen and passes forwards in a groove parallel to the molar teeth. The foramen is located between the second and third maxillary molars about 0.5 cm from the teeth, towards the midline. The foramen is approached from the opposite side with the needle at a right angle to the palatal bone (Figure 9.24b). Here, a few drops of local anaesthetic can also be injected.

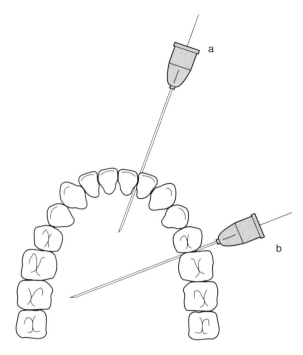

Figure 9.24 (a) Nasopalatine nerve block. The needle is inserted into the incisive papilla behind the maxillary central incisors. (b) Palatine nerve block. The needle is inserted from the opposite side, keeping it as near to a right angle as possible with the curvature of the palate.

Indication

Cleft palate repair.

Advantages

The technique is relatively simple. This area is usually infiltrated with vasoconstrictors for surgical purposes; a local anaesthetic solution with adrenaline will anaesthetize and at the same time provide a bloodless surgical field.

WOUND INFILTRATION

Small superficial wounds can be infiltrated with local anaesthetics at the end of surgery for providing pain relief. The technique has mainly been used after inguinal hernia repair,[186,187] pyloromyotomy[188] and craniotomy.[189] A concentration of 0.5 ml kg^{-1} of 0.125–0.25% bupivacaine can be safely used.

The administration, usually in the subcutaneous space, by infiltration or irrigation,[190,191] seems to be safe.[192] No toxic effects have been observed or any significant increase in wound infection reported; however, a dose–response study has not been published.

In paediatric patients there are no reports regarding wound infiltration for major surgical procedures. The short duration of local anaesthetic is a major problem; irrigation of all the parts of the surgical wound with a continuous infusion seems to be technically difficult, particularly because of the age of the patients. Ropivacaine, a new aminoamide local anaesthetic, could be utilized in the future for incisional use because of its long-lasting effects and minimal cardiovascular toxicity.

ACKNOWLEDGEMENTS

I dedicate this chapter to Paolo Busoni, teacher and good friend, who realized early on the importance of using regional anaesthesia techniques in children. A special thanks to all my colleagues for their encouragement and help, especially to Marco Calamandrei for his invaluable work on pharmacology and illustrations.

REFERENCES

1 Niemann, A. Uber eine neue organische. Base in den Cocablattern. Inaug. Diss. Gottingen, 1860.

2 Koller, C. On the use of cocaine for producing anaesthesia on the eye. *Lancet* 1884; **ii**: 990.

3 Bier, A. Versuche uber cocainisirung des ruckenmarkes. *Deutsches Zeitschrift der Chirurgie* 1899; **51**: 361–9.

4 Bainbridge, W.S. A report of 12 operations on infants and young children using spinal anesthesia. *Archives of Pediatrics* 1901; **18**: 510–20.

5 Gray, H.T. A study of spinal anaesthesia in children and infants from a series of 200 cases. *Lancet* 1909; **ii**: 913–17.

6 Farr, R.E. Local anesthesia in infancy and childhood. *Archives of Pediatrics* 1920; **37**: 381.

7 Campbell, M.F. Caudal anesthesia in children. *American Journal of Urology* 1933; **30**: 245–9.

8 Ruston, F.G. Epidural anaesthesia in infants and children. *Canadian Anaesthetists' Society Journal* 1954; **1**: 37–44.

9 Spiegel, P. Caudal anesthesia in children: a preliminary report. *Anesthesia and Analgesia* 1962; **41**: 218–21.

10 Fortuna, A. Caudal analgesia: a simple and safe technique in paediatric surgery. *British Journal of Anaesthesia* 1967; **39**: 165–70.

11 Dalens, B. Regional anesthesia in children. *Anesthesia and Analgesia* 1989; **68**: 654–72.

12 Yaster, M. and Maxwell L.G. Pediatric regional anesthesia. *Anesthesiology* 1989; **70**: 324–38.

13 Wolf, A.R., Eyres, R.L., Laussen, P.C., *et al.* Effect of extradural analgesia on stress responses to abdominal surgery in infants. *British Journal of Anaesthesia* 1993; **70**: 654–60.

14 Arthur, D.S. Caudal anaesthesia in neonates and infants. *Anaesthesia* 1980; **35**: 1136–7.

15 Abajian, J.C., Melish, R.W.P., Browne, A.F., Lambert, D.H. and Mazuzan, J.E. Spinal anesthesia for surgery in high risk-infant. *Anesthesia and Analgesia* 1984; **63**: 359–62.

16 Bromage, P.R. Masked mischief. *Regional Anesthesia* 1996; **21** (6S): 62–3.

17 Broadman, L.M. Where should advocacy for pediatric patients end and concern for patient safety begin? *Regional Anesthesia* 1997; **22**: 205–8.

18 Bosenberg, A.T. and Ivani, G. Regional anaesthesia – children are different. *Paediatric Anaesthesia* 1998; **8**: 447–50

19 Busoni, P. Anatomy. In: Saint-Maurice, C. and Schulte Steinberg, O.H. (eds). *Regional Anaesthesia in Children*. Fribourg: Mediglobe, 1990: 16–25.

20 Pick, P.T. and Howden, R.*Gray's Anatomy. Descriptive and Surgical*. Philadelphia, PA: Running Press, 1974: 49–50.

21 Busoni, P. and Sarti, A. Sacral intervertebral epidural block. *Anesthesiology* 1987; **67**: 993–5.

22 Brown, T.C.K. and Schulte-Steinberg, O.H. Neural blockade for pediatric surgery. In: Cousins, M.L. and Bridenbaugh, P.O. (eds). *Neural Blockade in Clinical Anesthesia and Management of Pain*. Philadelphia, PA: Lippincott, 1988: 662.

23 Busoni, P. and Messeri, A. Spinal anesthesia in children: surface anatomy. *Anesthesia and Analgesia* 1989; **68**: 418–19.

24 Dohi, S., Naito, H. and Takahashi, T. Age related changes in blood pressure and duration of motor block in spinal anesthesia. *Anesthesiology* 1979; **50**: 319–23.

25 Murat, I., Delleur, M.M., Estève, C., Egu, J.F., Raynaud, P. and Saint-Maurice, C. Continuous epidural anaesthesia in children. Clinical and haemodynamic implications. *British Journal of Anaesthesia* 1987; **59**: 1441–5.

26 Broadman, L.M., Hannallah, R.S., Norden, R.S. and McGill, W.A. 'Kiddie caudals': experience with 1154 consecutive cases without complications. *Anesthesia and Analgesia* 1987; **66**: S18.

27 Anand, K.J.S. and Hickey, P.R. Pain and its effects in the human neonate and fetus. *New England Journal of Medicine* 1987; **317**: 1321–9.

28 Giaufrè, E., Dalens, B. and Gombert, A. Epidemiology and morbidity of regional anesthesia on children: a one year prospective survey of the French-Language Society of Pediatric Anesthesiologists. *Anesthesia and Analgesia* 1996; **83**: 904–12.

29 Kokki, H. Postdural puncture headache is not an age-related symptom in children: a prospective open randomized parallel group study comparing a 22-G

Quicke with a 22-G Whitacre needle. *Paediatric Anaesthesia* 1999; **9**: in press.

30 Kokki, H. and Hendolin, H. Comparison of 25G and 29G Quincke spinal needles in paediatric day case surgery. A prospective randomized study of the puncture characteristics, success rate and postoperative complaints. *Paediatric Anaesthesia* 1996; **6**: 115–19.

31 Newman, P.J., Bushnell, T.G. and Radford, P. The effect of needle size and type in paediatric caudal analgesia. *Paediatric Anaesthesia* 1996; **6**: 459–61.

32 Dalens, B. and Hasnaoui, A. Caudal anesthesia in pediatric surgery: success rate and adverse effects in 750 consecutive patients. *Anesthesia and Analgesia* 1989; **68**: 83–9.

33 Wood, C.E., Goreski, G.V., Kuwahara, B. and Neil, S.C. Complications of continuous epidural infusions for postoperative analgesia in children. *Canadian Journal of Anaesthesia* 1994; **41**: 613–20.

34 Wilson, P.T.J. and Lloyd-Thomas, A.R. An audit of extradural analgesia in children. *Anaesthesia* 1993; **48**: 718–23.

35 Bosenberg, A.T. Lower limb nerve blocks in children using unsheathed needles and a nerve stimulator. *Anaesthesia* 1995; **50**: 206–10.

36 Dalens, B. and Chrysostome, Y. Intervertebral epidural anaesthesia in paediatric surgery: success rate and adverse effects in 650 consecutive procedures. *Paediatric Anaesthesia* 1991; **1**: 107–17.

37 Flandin-Blety, C. and Barrrier, G. Accident following extradural analgesia in children. *Paediatric Anaesthesia* 1995; **5**: 41–5.

38 Goldman, L. Complications in regional anaesthesia. *Paediatric Anaesthesia* 1995; **5**: 3–9.

39 Busoni, P. and Messeri, A. Loss of resistance technique to air for identifying the epidural space in infants and children. Use an appropriate technique! *Paediatric Anaesthesia* 1995; **5**: 347–8.

40 Naulty, J.S., Ostheimer, G.W., Datta, S., Knapp, R. and Weiss, J.B. Incidence of venous air embolism during epidural catheter insertion. *Anesthesiology* 1982; **57**: 410–2.

41 Scott, D.B. Identification of the epidural space: loss of resistance to air or saline? *Regional Anesthesia* 1997; **22**: 1–2.

42 Dalens, B. and Saint-Maurice, C. Practical considerations and recommended monitoring for regional anesthesia. In: Dalens, B. (ed.). *Regional Anesthesia in Infants, Children and Adolescent*. Baltimore, MD: William & Wilkins, 1985: 133–60.

43 Desparmet, J., Mateo, J., Ecoffey, C. and Mazoit, J.X. Efficacy of an epidural test dose in children anesthetized with halothane. *Anesthesiology* 1990; **72**: 249–51.

44 Toledano, A., Roizen, M.F. and Foss, J. When is testing the test dose the wrong thing to do? *Anesthesia and Analgesia* 1995; **80**: 861–3.

45 Berde, C. Regional anesthesia in children: what have we learned? *Anesthesia and Analgesia* 1996; **83**: 897–900.

46 Berde, C.B. Epidural analgesia in children. *Canadian Journal of Anaesthesia* 1994; **41**: 555–60.

47 Strafford, M.A., Wilder, R.T. and Berde, C.B. Risk of infection from epidural analgesia in children: a review of 1620 cases. *Anesthesia and Analgesia* 1995; **80**: 234–8.

48 Strong, W.E. Epidural abscess associated with epidural catheterization: a rare event? Report of two cases with markedly delayed presentation. *Anesthesiology* 1991; **74**: 943–6.

49 McNeely, J.K., Trentadue, N.C., Rusy, L.M. and Farber, N.E. Culture of bacteria from lumbar and caudal epidural catheters used for postoperative analgesia in children. *Regional Anesthesia* 1997; **22**: 428–31.

50 Meunier, J.F., Norwood, P., Dartayet, B., Dubousset, A.M. and Ecoffey, C. Skin abscess with lumbar epidural catheterization in infants: is it dangerous? Report of two cases. *Anesthesia and Analgesia* 1997; **84**: 1248–9.

51 Emmanuel, E.R. Post-sacral extradural catheter abscess in a child. *British Journal of Anaesthesia* 1994; **73**: 548–9.

52 Larsson, B.A., Lundeberg, S. and Olsson, G.L. Epidural abscess in a one-year-old boy after continuous epidural analgesia. *Anesthesia and Analgesia* 1997; **84**: 1245–7.

53 Berde, C.B. Convulsions associated with pediatric regional anesthesia. *Anesthesia and Analgesia* 1992; **75**: 164–6.

54 Agarwal, R., Gutlove, D.P. and Lockhart, C.H. Seizures occurring in pediatric patients receiving continuous infusion of bupivacaine. *Anesthesia and Analgesia* 1992; **75**: 284–6.

55 McCloskey, J.J., Haun, S.E. and Deshpande, J.K. Bupivacaine toxicity secondary to continuous caudal epidural in children. *Anesthesia and Analgesia* 1992; **75**: 287–90.

56 Mazoit, J.X., Denson, D.D. and Samii, K. Pharmacokinetics of bupivacaine following caudal anesthesia in infants. *Anesthesiology* 1988; **68**: 387–91.

57 Ecoffey, C., Desparmet, J., Maury, M., Berdeaux, A., Giudicelli, J.F. and Saint-Maurice, C. Bupivacaine in children: pharmacokinetics following caudal anesthesia. *Anesthesiology* 1985; **63**: 447–8.

58 Eyres, R.L., Bishop, W., Oppenheim, R.C. and Brown, T.C.K. Plasma bupivacaine concentrations in children during caudal epidural analgesia. *Anaesthesia and Intensive Care* 1983; **11**: 20–2.

59 Eyres, R.L., Hastings, C., Brown, T.C.K. and Oppenheim, R.C. Plasma bupivacaine concentrations following lumbar epidural anaesthesia in children. *Anaesthesia and Intensive Care* 1986; **14**: 131–4.

60 Mobley, K.A., Wandless, J.G. and Fell, D. Serum bupivacaine concentrations following wound infiltration in children undergoing inguinal herniotomy. *Anaesthesia* 1991; **46**: 500–1.

61 Rothstein, P., Arthur, G.R., Feldman, H.S., Kopf, G.S. and Covino, B.G. Bupivacaine for intercostal nerve blocks in children. *Anesthesia and Analgesia* 1986; **65**: 625–9.

62 Eyres, R.L. Local anaesthetic agents in infancy. *Paediatric Anaesthesia* 1995; **5**: 213–8.

63 Moore, D.C. Administer oxygen first in the treatment of local anesthetic-induced convulsions. *Anesthesiology* 1980; **53**: 346–7.

64 Moore, D.C., Crawford, R.D. and Scurlock, J.E. Severe hypoxia and acidosis following local anesthetic-induced convulsions. *Anesthesiology* 1980; **53**: 259–60.

65 Rosen, M.A., Thigpen, J.W., Shnider, S.M., Fouk, S.E., Levinson, G. and Koike, M. Bupivacaine-induced cardiotoxicity in hypoxic and acidotic sheep. *Anesthesia and Analgesia* 1985; **64**: 1089–96.

66 Moore, D.C. and Scurlock, J.E. Possible role of epinephrine in prevention or correction of myocardial

depression associated with bupivacaine. *Anesthesia and Analgesia* 1983; **62**: 450–3.

67 Solomon, D., Bunegin, L. and Albin, M. The effect of magnesium sulfate administration on cerebral and cardiac toxicity of bupivacaine in dogs. *Anesthesiology* 1990; **72**: 341–6.

68 Kasten, G.V. and Martin, S.T. Bupivacaine cardiovascular toxicity: comparison of treatment with bretylium and lidocaine. *Anesthesia and Analgesia* 1985; **64**: 491–5.

69 Haasio, J. and Rosemberg, P.H. Treatment of bupivacaine-induced cardiac arrhythmias in hypoxic and hypercarbic pigs with amiodarone and bretylium. *Regional Anesthesia* 1990; **15**: 174–9.

70 Maxwell, L.G., Martin, L.D. and Yaster, M. Bupivacaine-induced cardiac toxicity in neonates: successful treatment with intravenous phenytoin. *Anesthesiology* 1994; **80**: 682–6.

71 DiFazio, C.A. Metabolism of local anaesthetics in the fetus, newborn and adult. *British Journal of Anaesthesia* 1979; **51**: 29–36.

72 Zsigmond, E.X. and Downs, J.R. Plasma cholinesterase activity in newborns and infants. *Canadian Journal of Anaesthesia* 1982; **18**: 278–85.

73 Nilsson, A., Engberg, G., Henneberg, S., Danielson, K. and De Verdier, C.H. Inverse relationships between age-dependent erythrocyte activity of methaemoglobin reductase and prilocaine-induced methaemoglobinemia during infancy. *British Journal of Anaesthesia* 1990; **64**: 72–6.

74 Engberg, G., Danielson, K., Hennemberg, S. and Nilsson, A. Plasma concentrations of prilocaine and lidocaine and methaemoglobin formation in infants after epicutaneous application of a 5% lidocaine–prilocaine cream (EMLA). *Acta Anaesthesiologica Scandinavica* 1987; **31**: 624–8.

75 Meffin, G., Long, G.J. and Thomas, J. Clearance and metabolism of mepivacaine in the human neonates. *Clinics in Pharmacology and Therapy* 1973; **14**: 218–25.

76 Tucker, G.T., Boyes, R.N., Bridenbugh, P.O. and Moore, D.C. Binding of anilide-type local anesthetics in human plasma: relationship between binding, physicochemical properties and anesthetic activity. *Anesthesiology* 1970; **33**: 287–303.

77 Lönnqvist, P.A. Alpha-1-acid glycoprotein levels in infants during cardiopulmonary bypass and deep hypothermic cardiac arrest. *Perfusion* 1991; **6**: 261–4.

78 Anderson, B.J, McKee, A.D. and Holfort, N.H.G. Size, myths and the clinical pharmacokinetics of analgesia in paediatric patients. *Clinical Pharmacokinetics* 1997; **33**: 313–27.

79 Tucker, G.T. and Mather, L.E. Pharmacokinetics of local anaesthetics. *British Journal of Anaesthesia* 1975; **47**: 213–24.

80 Cheung, S.L.W., Booker, P.D., Franks, R. and Pozzi, M. Serum concentrations of bupivacaine during prolonged continuous paravertebral infusion in young infants. *British Journal of Anaesthesia* 1997; **79**: 9–13.

81 Wolf, A.R., Valley, R.D., Fear, D.W., Roy, W.L. and Lerman, J. Bupivacaine for caudal analgesia in infants and children: the optimum effective concentration. *Anesthesiology* 1988; **69**: 102–6.

82 Weston, P.J. and Bourchier, D. The pharmacokinetics of bupivacaine following interpleural nerve block in infants of very low birthweight. *Paediatric Anaesthesia* 1995; **5**: 219–22.

83 Luz, G., Innerhofer, P., Bachmann, B., Frischut, B., Menardi, G. and Benzer, A. Bupivacaine plasma concentrations during continuous epidural anesthesia in infants and children. *Anesthesia and Analgesia* 1996; **82**: 231–4.

84 Ivani, G., Mereto, N., Lampugnani, E., *et al*. Ropivacaine in paediatric surgery: preliminary results. *Paediatric Anaesthesia* 1998; **8**: 127–9.

85 Ivani, G., Mazzarello, G., Lampugnani, E., *et al*. Ropivacaine in paediatric regional anaesthesia: a comparison with bupivacaine. *British Journal of Anaesthesia* 1998; **81**: 247–8.

86 Moriarty, A. Use of ropivacaine in postoperative infusions. *Paediatric Anaesthesia* 1997; **7**: 478.

87 Crighton, I.M., Barry, B.P. and Hobbs, G.J. A study of the caudal space using magnetic resonance imaging. *British Journal of Anaesthesia* 1997; **78**: 391–5.

88 Blanco, D., Mazo, V., Ortiz, M., Fernandez-Llamazares, J. and Vidal, F. Spread of local anesthetic into the epidural caudal space for two rates of injection in children. *Regional Anesthesia* 1996; **21**: 442–5.

89 Schulte Steinberg, O. and Rahlfs, V.W.Caudal anaesthesia in children and spread of 1% lignocaine.*British Journal of Anaesthesia* 1970; **42**: 1093–7.

90 Takasaki, M., Dohl, S. and Kawabata, Y. Dosage of lidocaine for caudal anesthesia in infants and children. *Anesthesiology* 1977; **47**: 527–31.

91 Armitage, E.N. Caudal block in children. *Anaesthesia* 1979; 34: 396–400.

92 Busoni, P. and Andreuccetti, T. The spread of caudal anaesthesia in children: a mathematical model. *Anaesthesia and Intensive* Care 1986; **14**: 140–4.

93 Warner, M.A., Kunkel, S.E., Offord, K.O., Atchison, S.R. and Dawson, B. The effects of age, epinephrine, and operative site on duration of caudal analgesia in pediatric patients. *Anesthesia and Analgesia* 1987; **66**: 995–8.

94 Jamali, S., Monin, S., Begon, C., Dubousset, A.M. and Ecoffey, C. Clonidine in pediatric caudal anesthesia. *Anesthesia and Analgesia* 1994; **78**: 663–6.

95 Naadkari, A.V. and Tondare, A.S. Localized clonic convulsions after spinal anesthesia with lidocaine and epinephrine. *Anesthesia and Analgesia* 1982; **61**: 945–7.

96 Lee, J.J. and Rubin, A.P. Comparison of a bupivacaine–clonidine mixture for caudal analgesia in children. *British Journal of Anaesthesia* 1994; **72**: 258–62.

97 Ivani, G., Mattioli, G., Rega, M., Conio, A., Jasonni, V. and De Negri, P. Clonidine-mepivacaine mixture vs plain mepivacaine in paediatric surgery. *Paediatric Anaesthesia* 1996; **6**: 111–14.

98 Cook, B., Grubb, D.J. and Aldridge, L.A. Comparison of the effects of adrenaline, clonidine and ketamine on the duration of caudal analgesia produced by bupivacaine in children. *British Journal of Anaesthesia* 1995; **75**: 698–701.

99 Tesno, B., Jones, M.B., Yu, L. and Wall, D.A. Use of caudal block for pain control after bone marrow harvest in children. *American Journal of Pediatric Hematology/Oncology* 1994; **16**: 305–8.

100 Gunther, J. Caudal anesthesia in children. A survey. *Anesthesiology* 1991; **75**: A936.

101 Bosenberg, A.T., Bland, B.A.R., Schulte-Steinberg, O. and Downing, J.W. Thoracic epidural anaesthesia via caudal route in infants. *Anesthesiology* 1988; **69**: 265–9.

102 Bosenberg, A.T., Hadley, G.P. and Wiersma, R. Oeso-phageal atresia: caudothoracic epidural anaesthesia reduces the need for postoperative ventilatory support. *Paediatric Surgery International* 1992; **7**: 289–91.

103 Gunter, J.B. and Eng, C. Thoracic epidural anesthesia via the caudal approach in children. *Anesthesiology* 1992; **76**: 935–8.

104 Blank, J.W., Houck, C.S., McClain, B.C and Berde, C.B. Cephalad advancement of epidural catheters: radio-graphic correlation. *Anesthesiology* 1994; **58**: A1345.

105 Van Niekerk, J., Bax-Vermeire, B.M.J., Geurts, J.W.M. and Kramer, P.P.C. Epidurography in premature infants. *Anaesthesia* 1990; **45**: 722–5.

106 Messeri, A., Romiti, M., Andreuccetti, T. and Busoni, P. Continuous epidural block for pain control in bladder exstrophy: report of a case and description of technique. *Paediatric Anaesthesia* 1995; **5**: 229–32.

107 Busoni, P., Messeri, A. and Sarti, A. The lumbosacral epidural block: a modified Taylor approach for abdom-inal urologic surgery in children. *Anaesthesia and Intensive Care* 1991; **19**: 325–8.

108 Busoni, P. Anatomy. In: Saint-Maurice, C. and Sculte-Steinberg, O. (eds). *Regional Anaesthesia in Children.* Norwalk, CT: Appleton & Lange, 1990: 16–25.

109 Bonadio, W.A., Smith, D.S., Metrou, M. and Dewitz, B. Estimating lumbar puncture depth in children. *New England Journal of Medicine* 1988; **319**: 952–3.

110 Uemura, A. and Yamashita, M. A formula for determin-ing the distance from the skin to the lumbar epidural space in infants and children. *Paediatric Anaesthesia* 1992; **2**: 305–7.

111 Hasan, M.A., Howard, R.F. and Lloyd-Thomas, A.R. Depth of epidural space in children. *Anaesthesia* 1994; **49**: 1085–7.

112 Bosenberg, A.T. and Gouws, E. Skin–epidural distance in children. *Anaesthesia* 1995; **50**: 895–7.

113 Romiti, M., Casadio, C., Calamandrei, M. and Busoni, P. L'anestesia epidurale lombare in pediatria. *Anestesia e Rianimazione* 1987; **28**: 259–62.

114 Desparmet, J., Meistelman, C., Barre, J. and Saint-Maurice, C. Continuous epidural infusion of bupivacaine for postoperative pain relief in children. *Anesthesiology* 1987; **67**: 108–10.

115 Ecoffey, C., Dubousset, A.M. and Samii, K. Lumbar and thoracic epidural anesthesia for urologic and upper abdominal surgery in infants and children. *Anesthesiol-ogy* 1986; **65**: 87–90.

116 Murat, I., Delleur, M.M., Levy, J., Esteve, C. and Saint-Maurice, C. Continuous epidural anaesthesia for major abdominal surgery in young children. *European Journal of Anaesthesiology* 1987; **4**: 327–35.

117 Murrel, D., Gibson, P.R. and Cohen, R.C. Continuous epidural analgesia in newborn infants undergoing major surgery. *Journal of Pediatric Surgery* 1993; **28**: 548–53.

118 Wolf, A.R., Eyres, R.L., Laussen, P.C., Edwards, J., Rowe, P. and Simon, L. Effect of extradural analgesia on sress responses to abdominal surgery in infants. *British Journal of Anaesthesia* 1993; **70**: 654–60.

119 Meignier, M., Souron, R. and Le Neel, J.C. Post-operative dorsal epidural analgesia in the child with respiratory disabilities. *Anesthesiology* 1983; **59**: 473–6.

120 Busoni, P. Single shot thoracic epidural block. In: Saint-Maurice, C. and Schulte-Steinberg, O. (eds). *Regional Anaesthesia in Children.* Norwalk, CT: Medi Globe, 1990: 110.

121 Kokki, H. and Hendolin. H. Comparison of spinal anaesthesia with epidural anaesthesia in paediatric surgery. *Acta Anaesthesiologica Scandinavica.* 1995; **39**: 896–900.

122 Hirabayashi, Y., Shimizu, R., Saitoh, K. and Fukuda, H. Spread of subarachnoid hyperbaric amethocaine in adolescents. *British Journal of Anaesthesia* 1995; **74**: 41–5.

123 Busoni, P. and Messeri, A. Spinal anesthesia in infants: could a L5–S1 approach be safer? *Anesthesiology* 1991; **75**: 168–9.

124 Gleason, C.A., Martin, R. and Anderson, J.V. Optimal position for a spinal tap in preterm infants. *Pediatrics* 1983; **71**: 31–5.

125 Hampl, K.F., Schneider, M.C., Gut, J., Drasner, K. and Drewe, J.Transient radicular irritation after 2% or 5% lidocaine for hyperbaric spinal anesthesia. *Anesthesiol-ogy* 1995; **83**: A811.

126 Drasner, K. Lidocaine spinal anesthesia. A vanishing therapeutic index? *Anesthesiology* 1977; **87**: 469–72.

127 Harnik, E.V., Hoy, G.R., Potolicchio, S., Stewart, D.R. and Siegelman, R.E. Spinal anesthesia in premature infants recovering from respiratory distress syndrome. *Anesthesiology* 1986; **64**: 95–99.

128 Welborn, L.G., Rice, L.J. and Hannallah, R.S. Post-operative apnea in former preterm infants: prospective comparison of spinal and general anesthesia. *Anesthe-siology* 1990; **72**: 838–42.

129 Saint-Maurice, C. Spinal block. In: Saint-Maurice, C. and Steinberg, O. (eds). *Regional Anaesthesia in Children.* Norwalk, CT: Appleton & Lange, 1990: 119–25.

130 Krane, E.J., Haberkern, C.M. and Jacobson, L.E. Post-operative apnea, bradycardia, and oxygen desaturation in formerly premature infants: prospective comparison of spinal and general anesthesia. *Anesthesia and Analgesia* 1995; **80**: 7–13.

131 Oberlander, T.F., Berde, C.B., Lam, K.H., Rappaport, L.A. and Saul, J.P. Infants tolerate spinal anesthesia with minimal overall autonomic changes: analysis of heart variability in former premature infants undergoing hernia repair. *Anesthesia and Analgesia* 1995; **80**: 20–7.

132 Wright, T.E., Orr, R.J., Haberkern, C.M. and Walbergh, E.J. Complications during spinal anesthesia in infants. High spinal blockade. *Anesthesiology* 1990; **73**: 1290–1.

133 Beauvoir, C. Spinal anaesthesia in newborns: total and free bupivacaine plasma concentration. *Paediatric Anaesthesia* 1996; **6**: 195–9.

134 Tyler, C. and Krane, E. Epidural opioids in children. *Journal of Pediatric Surgery* 1989; **24**: 469–73.

135 Krane, E.J., Tyler, D.C. and Jacobson, L.E. The dose response of caudal morphine in children. *Anesthesiology* 1989; **71**: 48–52.

136 Taylor, G. and Boswell, M. Continuous epidural infusion of low doses morphine for postoperative analgesia in children. *Anesthesiology* 1991; **75**: A937.

137 Kaneko, M., Saito, Y. and Kirihara, J. Synergistic antinoceptive interaction after epidural co-administra-tion of morphine and lidocaine in rats. *Anesthesiology* 1994; **80**: 137–50.

138 Wolf, A.R., Hughes, D. and Wade, A. Postoperative analgesia after paediatric orchidopexy: evaluation of a bupivacaine–morphine mixture. *British Journal of Anaesthesia* 1990; **64**: 430–5.

139 Berde, C.B., Sethna, N.F. and Yemen, T.A. Continuous bupivacaine–fentanyl infusions in children following ureteral reimplantation. *Anesthesiology* 1990; **73**: A1128.

140 Kart, T., Walther-Larsen, S., Svejborg, T.F., Feilberg, V., Eriksen, K. and Rasmussen, M. Comparison of continuous epidural infusion of fentanyl and bupivacaine with intermittent epidural administration of morphine for postoperative pain management in children. *Acta Anaesthesiologica Scandinavica* 1997; **41**: 461–5.

141 Rosen, K.R. and Rosen, D.A. Caudal epidural morphine for control of pain following open heart surgery in children. *Anesthesiology* 1989; **70**: 418–21.

142 Attia, J., Ecoffey, C. and Sandouk, P. Epidural morphine in children. Pharmacokinetics and CO_2 sensitivity. *Anesthesiology* 1986; **65**: 590–4.

143 Valley, R.D. and Bailey, A.G. Caudal morphine for postoperative analgesia in infants and children: a report of 138 cases. *Anesthesia and Analgesia* 1991; **72**: 120–4.

144 Gustafsson, L.L., Schildt, B. and Jacobsen, K.J. Adverse effects of extradural and intrathecal opiates: report of a nationwide survey in Sweden. *British Journal of Anaesthesia* 1982; **54**: 479–85.

145 Mott, J.M. and Eisele, J.H. A survey of monitoring practices following spinal opiate administration. *Anesthesia and Analgesia* 1986; **65**: S1.

146 Stenseth, R., Sellevold, O. and Breivik, H. Epidural morphine for postoperative pain: experience with 1085 patients. *Acta Anaesthesiologica Scandinavica* 1985; **29**: 148–55.

147 Kluger, M.T., Owen, H. and Watson, D. Oxyhaemoglobin saturation following elective abdominal surgery in patients receiving continuous intravenous infusion or intramuscular morphine analgesia. *Anaesthesia* 1992; **47**: 256–60.

148 Hutton, P. and Clutton-Brock, T. The benefits and pitfalls of pulseoximetry. *British Medical Journal* 1993; **307**: 457–8.

149 Morton, N.S. Development of a monitoring protocol for the safe use of opioids in children. *Paediatric Anaesthesia* 1993; **3**: 179–84.

150 Lloyd-Thomas, A.R. and Howard, R. Postoperative pain control in children. *British Medical Journal* 1992; **304**: 1174–5.

151 Cook, B. and Doyle, E. The use of additives to local anaesthetic solutions for caudal epidural blockade. *Paediatric Anaesthesia* 1996; **6**: 353–9.

152 Krechel, S.W., Helikson, M.A. and Kittle, D. and Eggers, G.W.N. Intrathecal morphine for postoperative pain control in children: a comparison with nalbuphine patient controlled analgesia. *Paediatric Anaesthesia* 1995; **5**: 177–83.

153 Khoo, S.T. and Brown, T.C.K. Femoral nerve block – the anatomical basis for a single injection technique. *Anaesthesia and Intensive Care* 1983; **11**: 40–3.

154 Brown, T.C.K. and Dickens, D.R.V. Another approach to the lateral cutaneous nerve of thigh. *Anaesthesia and Intensive Care* 1986; **14**: 126–8.

155 Brown, T.C.K. Leg blocks in children. *Paediatric Anaesthesia* 1996; **6**: 245.

156 Johnson, C.M. Continuous femoral nerve blockade for analgesia in children with femoral fractures. *Anaesthesia and Intensive Care* 1994; **22**: 281–3.

157 Dalens, B., Vanneuville, G. and Tanguy, A. Comparison of the fascia iliaca compartment block with the 3-in-1 block in children. *Anaesthesia and Analgesia* 1989; **69**: 705–13.

158 Doyle, E., Morton, N.S. and McNicol, L.R. Plasma bupivacaine levels after fascia iliaca compartment block with and without adrenaline. *Paediatric Anaesthesia* 1997; **7**: 121–4.

159 Dalens, B., Tanguy, A. and Vanneuville, G. Sciatic nerve blocks in children: comparison of the posterior, anterior, and lateral approaches in 180 pediatric patients. *Anesthesia and Analgesia* 1990; **70**: 131–7.

160 Kempthorne, P.M. and Brown, T.C.K. Nerve blocks around the knee in children. *Anaesthesia and Intensive Care* 1984; **12**: 14–17.

161 Sara, C.A. and Lowry, C.J. A complication of circumcision and dorsal nerve block of the penis. *Anaesthesia and Intensive Care* 1984; **13**: 79–85.

162 Dalens, B., Vanneuville, G. and Dechelotte, P. Penile block via the subpubic space in 100 children. *Anaesthesia and Analgesia* 1989; **69**: 41–5.

163 Broadman, L.M., Hannallah, R., Belman, A.B., Elder, P.T., Ruttimann, U. and Epstein, B.S. Post circumcision analgesia – a prospective evaluation of subcutaneous ring block of the penis. *Anesthesiology* 1987; **67**: 399–402.

164 Tree-Trakarn, T., Pirayavaraporn, S. and Lertakyamanee, J. Topical analgesia for relief of postcircumcision pain. *Anesthesiology* 1987; **67**: 395–9.

165 Lee, J.J. and Forrester, P. EMLA for postoperative analgesia for day case circumcision in children. A comparison with dorsal nerve of penis block. *Anaesthesia* 1992; **47**: 1081–3.

166 Taddio, A., Stevens, B., Craig, K., *et al.* Efficacy and safety of lidocaine–prilocaine cream for pain during circumcision. *New England Journal of Medicine* 1997; **336**: 1197–201.

167 Smith, T., Moratin, P. and Wulf, H. Smaller children have greater bupivacaine plasma concentrations after ilioinguinal block. *British Journal of Anaesthesia* 1996; **76**: 452–5.

168 Hannallah, R.S., Broadman, L.M. and Belman, A.B. Comparison of caudal and ilioinguinal/iliohypogastric nerve block for control of post-orchiopexy pain in pediatric ambulatory surgery. *Anesthesiology* 1987; **66**: 832–4.

169 Trotter, C., Martin, P., Youngson, G. and Johnston, G. A comparison between ilioinguinal–iliohypogastric nerve block performed by anaesthetist or surgeon for postoperative analgesia following groin surgery in children. *Paediatric Anaesthesia* 1995; **5**: 363–7.

170 Derrick, J.L. and Aun, C.S.T. Transient femoral nerve palsy after ilioinguinal block. *Anaesthesia and Intensive Care* 1996; **24**: 115.

171 Ferguson, S., Thomas, V. and Lewis, I. The rectus sheath block in paediatric anaesthesia: new indications for an old technique? *Paediatric Anaesthesia* 1996; **6**: 463–6.

172 Courreges, P., Poddevin, F. and Lecoutre, D. Paraumbilical block: a new concept for regional anaesthesia in children. *Paediatric Anaesthesia* 1997; **7**: 211–14.

173 Cornish, P., Anderson, B. and Chambers, C. Continuous rectus sheath block analgesia for an infant with bronchopulmonary dysplasia. *Paediatric Anaesthesia* 1993; **3**: 191–2.

174 Dalens, B., Vanneuville, G. and Tanguy, A. A new approach to the brachial plexus in children: comparison with the supraclavicular approach. *Anesthesia and Analgesia* 1987; **66**: 1264–8.

175 Messeri, A., Calamandrei, M., Agostino, M.R. and Busoni, P. The use of brachial plexus block for central venous catheterization in low and very low birthweight infants. *Anesthesiology* 1998; **88**: 837.

176 McKenzie, A.G. and Mathe, S. Interpleural local anaesthesia: anatomical basis for mechanism of action. *British Journal of Anaesthesia* 1996; **76**: 297–9.

177 Giaufrè, E., Bruguerolle, B., Rastello, C., Coquet, M. and Lorec, A.M. New regimen for interpleural block. *Paediatric Anaesthesia* 1995; **5**: 125–8.

178 Stayer, S.A., Pasquariello, C.A., Schwartz, R.E., Balsara, R.K. and Lear, B.R. The safety of continuous pleural lignocaine after thoracotomy in children and adolescent. *Paediatric Anaesthesia* 1995; **5**: 307–10.

179 Cooper, M.G. and Seaton, H.L. Intra-operative placement of intercostal catheter for post thoracotomy pain relief in a child. *Paediatric Anaesthesia* 1992; **2**: 165–7.

180 Downs, C.S. and Cooper, M.G. Continuous extrapleural intercostal nerve block for post thoracotomy analgesia in children. *Anaesthesia and Intensive Care* 1997; **25**: 390–7.

181 Lönnqvist, P.A. Continuous paravertebral block in children – initial experience. *Anaesthesia* 1992; **47**: 607–9.

182 Lönnqvist, P.A. and Hesser, U. Location of the paravertebral space in children and adolescents in relation to surface anatomy assed by computer tomography. *Paediatric Anaesthesia* 1992; **2**: 285–9.

183 Lönnqvist, P.A. and Hesser, U. Radiological and clinical distribution of thoracic paravertebral blockade in infants and children. *Paediatric Anaesthesia* 1993; **3**: 83–7.

184 Lönnqvist, P.A. and Hesser, U. Depth from the skin to the paravertebral space in infants and children. *Paediatric Anaesthesia* 1994; **4**: 99–100.

185 Bosenberg, A.T. and Kimble, F.W. Infraorbital nerve block in neonates for cleft lip repair: anatomical study and clinical application. *British Journal of Anaesthesia* 1995; **74**: 506–8.

186 Reid, M.F., Harris, R., Phillips, P.D., Barker, I., Pereira, N.H. and Bennett, N.R. Day case herniotomy in children. A comparison of ilioinguinal nerve block and wound infiltration for postoperative analgesia. *Anaesthesia* 1987; **42**: 658–61.

187 Fell, D., Derrington, M.C., Taylor, E. and Wandless, J.G. Paediatric postoperative analgesia. A comparison between caudal block and wound infiltration of local anesthetic. *Anaesthesia* 1988; **43**: 107–10

188 McNicol, L.R., Martin, C.S., Smart, N.G. and Logan, R.W. Perioperative bupivacaine for pyloromyotomy pain. *Lancet* 1990; **6**: 54–5.

189 Hartley, E.J., Bissonette, B. and St Louis, P. Scalp infiltration with bupivacaine in pediatric brain surgery. *Anesthesia and Analgesia* 1991; **73**: 29–32.

190 Casey, W.F., Rice, L.J., Hannallah, R.S., Broadman, L.M., Norden, J.M. and Guzzetta, P. A comparison between bupivacaine instillation versus ilioinguinal/iliohypogastric nerve block for postoperative analgesia following inguinal herniorrhaphy in children. *Anesthesiology* 1990; **72**: 637–9.

191 Shenfeld, O., Eldar, I., Lotan, G., Avigad, I. and Goldwasser, B. Intraoperative irrigation with bupivacaine for analgesia after orchiopexy and herniorrhaphy in children. *Journal of Urology* 1995; **153**: 185–7.

192 Mobley, K.A., Wandless, J.G. and Fell, D. Serum bupivacaine concentrations following wound infiltration in children undergoing inguinal herniotomy. *Anaesthesia* 1991; **46**: 500–1.

CHAPTER 10

The immediate recovery period

MEHERNOOR WATCHA

INTRODUCTION

Most surgical procedures in children are now performed on an ambulatory or day-case basis where rapid recovery is essential to ensure safe discharge of the child on the day of surgery. When this practice was first introduced, anaesthetists considered it prudent to limit cases managed on an outpatient basis to brief procedures that did not involve major body cavities, were associated with minimal blood loss or were for patients rated to have an American Society of Anesthesiologists physical status I or II.[1] With the advent of short-acting anaesthetic agents, minimally invasive surgery and increased financial pressures to limit hospitalization costs, many patients who would previously have been admitted to the hospital are now discharged home shortly after the procedure. In addition, ambulatory surgery is now performed on chronically ill children, as they and their families benefit from the reduced disruption of their normal schedules, and a decreased risk of nosocomial infections with hospital-acquired resistant organisms. This trend towards performing more complex operations in sicker children on a day-case basis has challenged anaesthetists to make thorough evaluations and decisions about the discharge readiness of such children in order to limit postanaesthetic complications.[2]

In this chapter the factors associated with increased postoperative complications are reviewed. However, it is obvious that the actions that anaesthetists can take to reduce these complications are not limited to those in the post-anaesthetic care unit (PACU), but include all aspects of anaesthetic care, extending from the preoperative evaluation to the time when the patient is ready to resume normal daily activities.

PHASES OF RECOVERY FROM ANAESTHESIA

Recovery from ambulatory surgery occurs in three phases: early, intermediate and late.[3] Early or phase-1 recovery occurs in the PACU where close observation is essential until the patient demonstrates return to consciousness, the ability to maintain a patent airway and normal oxygen saturation in room air. During this phase the patient is recumbent and the nurse : patient ratio is usually 1 : 1. In the intermediate phase (phase-2 recovery) the patient continues to recover sitting up in a chair or often on the parent's lap. This phase ends when the child achieves preset 'home readiness' discharge criteria that are discussed in more detail below. During phase-2 recovery, parents or other family members help in patient care under the supervision of a nurse, and the nurse : patient ratio is lower than during phase-1 recovery. Nursing routines of frequent cardio-respiratory monitoring are justified during phase-1 recovery, but may be limited during phase-2 recovery as the taking of these measurements often upsets the child. The third or final phase occurs at home where a normal playful level of activity gradually returns and those caring for the child can resume their daily routine. In adults this phase is completed when the patient has achieved 'street fitness'.

In recent years, the distinction between inpatient and outpatient surgery has been blurred in a number of facilities that keep selected patients overnight for the management of pain, persistent nausea and vomiting and for observation for bleeding.[2] These facilities are variously termed 23-h admission, extended observation, short-stay recovery or day surgery admission units. Parents may provide much of the care in these areas, with one or two nurses available for supervision of care.

INCIDENCE OF COMPLICATIONS

The overall mortality and morbidity associated with anaesthesia in paediatric patients have been reported in a few large studies from Canada and France and also in the Closed Claims Studies from the USA and Australia.[4-7] In general, the complication rates are higher for the paediatric patient population than in adults, with the neonatal and infant subgroups having the highest rates. In one study the overall major complication rate for paediatric inpatients was reported to be 7 per 10 000, but the rate in infants was much higher (43 per 10 000 vs 5 per 10 000 for older children).[5] The intraoperative complication rates for older children (over 2 years of age) and adults are similar (9/10 000 children vs 10.6/10 000 adults). In contrast, the postoperative complication rates are much higher in children, with major life-threatening events occurring in about 4% of children vs 0.5% of adults (Tables 10.1–10.3).[4,8,9]

These differences are even more marked when the rates for minor complications are compared. In the Canadian study, approximately 21% of children had minor complications in the first 3 postoperative days, compared with 9.4% of adults (Table 10.3).[4,8,9] The most common

Table 10.1 Incidence of perioperative complication rates (%) in children and adults[8,9]

	Neonates	Infants	1–5 years	6–10 years	11+ years	Adults
Intraoperative events	15.0%	7.3%	7.1%	12.2%	9.7%	10.6%
PACU event	16.6%	7.23%	12.2%	14.9%	15.2%	5.9%
Any postoperative event						
Minor event	13.6%	10.3%	20.3%	31.5%	32.4%	9.4%
Major event	23.8%	7.5%	3.3%	3.4%	3.3%	0.5%
Any event	48.9%	25.9%	37.5%	50.5%	51.3%	31.6%

Table 10.2 Phase 1 and 2 recovery event rates per 10 000 anaesthetics

	Neonates	Infants	1–5 years	6–10 years	11+ years	Adults
Respiratory events:						
Airway obstruction	28	161	444	260	184	0.6
Laryngospasm	28	43	187	177	165	N/a
Other respiratory	1163	248	105	78	103	9.6
PONV	0	83	410	855	935	555
Cardiac events:						
Blood pressure	1385	12	10	15	32	219
Arrhythmia	0	12	8	15	9	57.3 (other)
Cardiac arrest	55	4	2	1	0	*
Surgical complication	28	63	131	167	76	30.9

*Incidence of myocardial infaction was 13.7 per 10 000 anaesthetics.

Table 10.3 Event rates during first 3 days per 10 000 anaesthetics[8,9]

	Neonates	Infants	1–5 years	6–10 years	11+ years	Adults
PONV	481	489	2011	3424	3209	555
Respiratory events:						
Sore throat	N/a	N/a	43	145	316	139
Croup	74	108	133	47	28	N/a
Other respiratory	2519	592	196	142	178	9.6
Headache	N/a	N/a	41	116	292	44
Muscle pains	N/a	N/a	33	63	128	33.9
Cardiac events	630	117	30	49	44	71*
Surgical complications	37	259	180	214	152	N/a

*Incidence of myocardial infarction was 13.7 per 10 000 anaesthetics.

problems in neonates were respiratory and cardiovascular, while older children were more likely to develop nausea and vomiting, sore throat, headache and muscle pains. The true incidence of the minor complications of sore throat and muscle pains may be higher in the younger child who is unable to express these symptoms. The data from the Canadian studies include inpatients and outpatients. It is likely that the incidence of the minor complications will be higher in the outpatient population. Patel and Hannallah compared the incidence of unanticipated admission to hospital after outpatient surgery during two periods (Table 10.4), and noted that the major cause for unanticipated admission remained postoperative emesis.[10]

Postanaesthetic complications may occur during any of the three phases of recovery, but

Table 10.4 Reasons for unplanned admissions to the hospital after outpatient surgery[10]

	1983–1986	1988–1991
Number of outpatient surgical patients	10 000	15 245
Admission rates	90 per 10 000	30 per 10 000
Protracted vomiting	33%	39%
Complicated surgery	17%	9%
Bleeding	3%	9%
Croup	9%	11%
Excessive drowsiness	2%	4%
Social reasons	7%	11%
Respiratory monitoring	N/a	4%
Other	22%	13%

the serious problems occur most often during phase 1. These include hypoxaemia during transport from the operating room to the PACU, bleeding, airway obstruction, croup, pain, emergence delirium, hypothermia, nausea and vomiting. In phase 2 the major problems relate to bleeding, nausea and vomiting, pain, dizziness and excessive drowsiness. In phase 3 problems reported include pain, nausea and vomiting, bleeding and behavioural changes.

RESPIRATORY COMPLICATIONS

Children may develop hypoxaemia following upper airway obstruction, laryngospasm, apnoea and postintubation croup. Upper airway obstruction is a very common postoperative respiratory complication in this patient population, particularly following otolaryngological airway surgery (e.g. adenotonsillectomy).[11–14] During transport from the operating room to the PACU, oxygen saturation values have been reported to decrease from a mean of $97.6 \pm 0.2\%$ to $93 \pm 0.5\%$ if the child is breathing room air.[11] In both adults and children, the incidence of postoperative hypoxaemia during transport did not correlate significantly with anaesthetic agent, age or duration of anaesthesia.[11,13] In the initial report by Motoyama and Glazener, oxygen saturation levels increased with awakening.[11] However, others have shown that the incidence of hypoxaemia did not correlate with the level of consciousness or Aldrete's recovery score.[11,13,15]

The anaesthetist must be very aware of the breathing pattern of the child during transport from the operating room to the PACU and should administer oxygen or monitor oxygen saturation continuously during this phase. The combination of airway obstruction and residual volatile agents may further depress respiratory drive, increasing blood carbon dioxide tension and setting off a vicious cycle of hypoxaemia, hypercarbia, further depression of respiration and ultimately cardiac dysrhythmias and cardiac arrest.[6] Airway manipulation with the jaw thrust manoeuvre, neck extension and mouth

opening may not always be enough to correct the problem. At times, it may be necessary to insert a nasopharyngeal airway, and maintain positive pressure with a bag and face mask. If all measures to maintain ventilation fail, urgent tracheal intubation is essential and the anaesthetist should consider the risks and benefits of administering a dose of a rapidly acting muscle relaxant to facilitate intubation.

The duration of oxygen therapy should be determined by the oxygen saturation values in the PACU and not by the anaesthetic regimen.[16] Although there are some reports of decreased critical respiratory events when total intravenous anaesthesia has been used in adults, these findings were not confirmed in children.[17,18] The presence of secretions in the oropharynx may be responsible for these airway-related complications and the ability to handle secretions may improve as the patient becomes more awake. However, the timing of tracheal extubation has not been shown to alter the incidence of hypoxaemia. In randomized studies the incidence of low oxygen saturation did not decrease when the trachea was extubated with the child fully awake compared with tracheal extubation with the child still deeply anaesthetized. Some of these studies may be criticized for having a low power to detect differences between the two groups.[19,20] The skills of the recovery room personnel and the availability of anaesthetists to respond to airway-related emergencies in the PACU may be more important factors in the outcome than the decision on the timing of tracheal extubation.

Anaesthetists should anticipate increased perioperative respiratory problems in children with: (1) a recent upper respiratory tract infection, particularly if tracheal intubation is required; (2) a history of prematurity; (3) chronic, obstructive sleep apnoea; (4) passive exposure to tobacco smoke; or (5) postintubation croup.

UPPER RESPIRATORY INFECTIONS

The incidence of airway-related complications of hypoxaemia, laryngospasm and bronchospasm increase 11-fold if the child has had a recent upper respiratory infection (URI).[21] Both major and minor desaturation events occur more frequently in children with

URI.[22,23] In a case–control study, Schreiner *et al.* noted that the 123 patients who developed laryngopasm were at least twice [95% confidence interval (CI) 1.2–3.5] as likely to have an active URI as a control group of 492 patients ($p = 0.01$).[24] Tracheal intubation is associated with increased bronchospasm in the presence of a recent URI, leading some to recommend the preferential use of a laryngeal mask airway in these children.[22,25] Airway irritability after URI continues for 3–6 weeks, a time when most patients are asymptomatic, and one should anticipate perioperative respiratory problems in this patient population.[26]

EX-PREMATURE INFANTS AND APNOEA

Similarly, anaesthetists should anticipate problems with apnoea during recovery from general anaesthesia in babies previously requiring admission to a premature baby (neonatal) intensive care unit (NICU). Apnoea may be central, obstructive or mixed and is defined as cessation of breathing for 15 s or for less than 15 s if associated with pallor, cyanosis or bradycardia. Briefer pauses without bradycardia are termed periodic breathing, which is normal in some neonates. The probability of apnoea in the former premature baby is inversely proportional to the gestational and postconceptional age. At greatest risk are infants with a history of apnoea, and/or anaemia and a postconceptional age less than 46 weeks. A recent combined analysis used the original data on 255 patients enrolled in eight prospective studies of postoperative apnoea in this patient population.[27] The authors determined that the probability of apnoea was increased (1) with a low gestational and postconceptional age; (2) if the baby had a history of continuing apnoea at home; and (3) with anaemia (hematocrit < 30%). Small-for-gestational age babies seemed to be better protected from postoperative apnoea than appropriate and large-for-gestational age babies.[27] These authors concluded that the data 'do not allow prediction with confidence up to what age the precaution of admitting patients for monitoring should continue to be taken for infants with anaemia.' The data were insufficient to allow recommendations regarding how long infants should be observed in recovery. However, in the subgroup of patients free from anaemia and from apnoea in the recovery room, the risk of subsequent apnoea was greater than 5% (with 95% statistical confidence) until the postconceptional age was ≥ 48 weeks for babies born at 35 weeks (Table 10.5). Risks of apnoea were at least 1% until the postconceptional age was 56 weeks for babies born at a gestational age of 32 weeks, and the postconceptional age was 54 weeks for babies born at 34 weeks' gestation. The authors also stated that there was 'additional uncertainty in the results due to the dramatically different rates of detected apnoea in different institutions, which appear to be related to the use of different monitoring devices. Given the limitations of this combined analysis, each physician and institution must decide what is an acceptable risk for postoperative apnoea.'

Although some have suggested that regional anaesthesia or the administration of caffeine 10 mg kg^{-1} or doxapram (1–1.5 mg kg^{-1}) may control this complication, there are reports of apnoea following pure regional anaesthesia techniques.[28] The more conservative approach would involve admitting all children below 56 weeks' postconceptional age, for a minimum of 12–24 h for observation for apnoea regardless of the type of anaesthetic used, particularly if the haematocrit is below 30%.

CHRONIC OBSTRUCTIVE SLEEP APNOEA

Children with chronic obstructive sleep apnoea constitute another group with a predilection to hypoxaemia and postoperative apnoea.[29,30] A significant incidence of postoperative respiratory distress, need for oxygen and intensive monitoring has been reported in children below 3 years of age who have undergone tonsillect-

Table 10.5 Risks of postoperative apnoea in the graduate of the neonatal intensive care unit[27]

Gestational age	Postconceptual age	Risk of apnoea
≤35 weeks	≥48 weeks	5%
≤32 weeks	≥50 weeks	5%
≤35 weeks	≥54 weeks	1%
≤32 weeks	≥56 weeks	1%

omy, particularly if the child has difficulty breathing during sleep, loud snoring with apnoea and restless sleep.[29] The risks increase further in patients with prematurity, cerebral palsy and coexisting medical conditions such as congenital heart disease, seizures,[29,31–33] neuromuscular disorders and chromosomal abnormalities (e.g. Down's syndrome).[32] In one study the risk of respiratory complications was increased three-fold if the child had a URI within 4 weeks of surgery.[29] Chest X-rays, electrocardiograms (ECG) and polysomnograms have not been shown to be useful in predicting which patients can be safely managed on an ambulatory basis.[31] Although shorter acting anaesthetic agents, opioids and non-sedating antiemetics may be associated with a more rapid awakening, postoperative hypoxaemia may still occur, and it has been shown that the Aldrete score (a measure of awakening in the PACU) does not correlate with the incidence of hypoxaemia.[15] The frequency of these complications has led the Paediatric Otolaryngology Committee of the American Academy of Otolaryngology – Head and Neck Surgery to issue guidelines recommending close observation of children below 3 years and those with other risk factors.

TOBACCO SMOKE

Children who have been passively exposed to tobacco smoke at home have an increased risk of perioperative airway-related complications.[34,35] In a retrospective, cohort study of 310 patients, the risk of laryngospasm severe enough to require succinylcholine was 10 times greater in children with environmental tobacco exposure (9.4% vs 0.9%).[34] In a prospective study, high urinary cotinine (a metabolic derivative of tobacco) levels were associated with a threefold increased risk of perioperative respiratory complications and unanticipated admission to an ICU or other monitored bed.[36]

POSTINTUBATION CROUP

Children may also present with airway obstruction in the PACU if they develop postintubation croup. The risk may be increased in patients with URI, perhaps because the ciliated columnar epithelium of the mucosa at the narrowest part of the child's airway (the cricoid ring) is more adherent to the underlying structures than the more resilient squamous epithelium of the supraglottic structures. Mild oedema of the mucosa at the cricoid ring may result in clinically important increases in resistance to air flow.[37] The incidence of postintubation croup has decreased since the late 1970s with the advent of polyvinyl tracheal tubes that meet the international standards of decreased tissue reactivity. Anaesthetists are also routinely using smaller tubes than before and are willing to replace a tracheal tube with a smaller one if there is no air leak around the tube with airway pressures of 30 cmH_2O.[38,39] The wider use of steroids during adenotonsillectomy surgery, one of the most common paediatric operations, may be an additional factor in the decrease in postintubation croup.[40–43]

For many years it was believed that children below 8 years of age were more prone to develop postextubation stridor if cuffed tracheal tubes were used. The reasons cited for avoiding cuffed tubes were: (1) a good seal could be achieved with an appropriately sized uncuffed tube as the narrowest portion of the child's airway was at the cricoid ring; (2) addition of a cuff necessitated the use of a smaller tube and increased the work of breathing; and (3) a cuff increased the chances of trauma and swelling of the mucosa at the cricoid ring.[44] However, in one study conducted in a paediatric ICU, the overall incidence of postextubation stridor was 14.9%, with no significant differences between patients who had cuffed or uncuffed tracheal tubes, even after controlling for patient age, duration of intubation, trauma, leak around tracheal tubes before extubation, and paediatric risk of mortality score. There was also no difference in the number of patients who required reintubation of the trachea for severe postextubation stridor.[45] This study led Khine *et al.* to examine the incidence of croup with cuffed and uncuffed tubes in a study of 488 children undergoing anaesthesia.[44] Different formulae were used to determine the size of cuffed and uncuffed tubes [Cuffed tube size in mm internal diameter = (age/4) + 3; Uncuffed tube size in mm internal diameter = (age/4) + 4]. Cuffed tracheal tubes permitted the use of low fresh gas flows, decreased contamination of ambient air by anaesthetic gases and decreased the need for repeated laryngoscopy and tube changes (1.2% vs 23%). Cuffed tubes did not increase the incidence or severity of croup as the number that required therapy or unanticipated admission for management of this complication did not differ between the two groups.[44]

If a child develops croup in the PACU, humidified mist should be administered. If symptoms persist or progress, 0.5 ml of 2.25% racemic adrenaline should be nebulized with 3–5 ml normal saline. Children should be observed for a minimum of 2 h after racemic adrenaline therapy to ensure that a rebound phenomenon does not occur. If multiple doses of racemic adrenaline are required, the child should be admitted to hospital. A few may require tracheal reintubation with a smaller tube than used initially. This subgroup may benefit from the use of steroids (dexamethasone 0.25 mg kg^{-1} i.v., then 0.1 mg kg^{-1} 6-hourly).

EMERGENCE DELIRIUM

Some children emerge from anaesthesia disoriented, screaming, thrashing around and difficult to control. A number of factors is associated with increased emergence delirium, including the young age of the child, increased preoperative anxiety, postoperative pain, hypoxaemia and the use of ketamine, midazolam, anticholinergic medications or sevoflurane. Rapid awakening has been stated to be a major factor in emergence delirium. This problem is not new, as it was noted around 1970 during the era of cyclopropane use, when it was speculated that delirium was a specific pharmacological action of the anaesthetic agent.[46]

Depending on the surgical procedure and anaesthetic technique used, the incidence of this complication has been reported to vary between 12 and 50%, with the higher incidence noted in preschool non-verbal children who had received desflurane. However, in this study, no preoperative sedatives or intraoperative analgesics were used.[47,48] The incidence of emergence delirium with sevoflurane was lower in comparative studies but still higher than with halothane.[48,49] Rapid awakening also occurs

with propofol and remifentanil, but the incidence of emergence delirium has not been well documented with these drugs.[50] However, propofol does not have any analgesic effect and the analgesic effect of remifentanil is short lived. It is not surprising that patients receiving these drugs without supplemental analgesia had higher pain scores in the PACU.[50]

Pain-related behaviour may be interpreted as emergence delirium in some cases as it is often very difficult to gauge what is upsetting a preschool child. While pain may be a major factor in the uncontrollable child that cannot be readily consoled in the PACU, other factors may also be responsible for this behaviour. The child may be upset by the presence of an intravenous infusion line, surgical dressing or awakening in a strange environment without the presence of familiar faces, rather than by pain alone. It is more humane if the person caring for the child assumes that pain is a major cause of this behaviour and treats it with opioids. However, there are data to indicate that this behaviour also occurs in some patients free from pain.[51] In a study of children undergoing hernia surgery, Auno and colleagues excluded patients with preoperative agitation, an inadequate caudal epidural block or other reason to believe the child had postoperative pain. However, they noted a higher incidence of emergence delirium in the preschool children receiving sevoflurane rather than halothane, and higher in younger than in older children receiving either sevoflurane or halothane for maintenance of anaesthesia. The benefits of rapid emergence need to be re-examined, as it has not been accompanied by an earlier discharge from hospital.[47,49,51] The comments of Bastron and Moyers are interesting as they stated in 1967 that 'Perhaps we have gone too far in our efforts to have patients wide awake at the conclusion of operations.'[46]

PERIOPERATIVE TEMPERATURE CONTROL

Perioperative hypothermia is a common problem because of the inhibition of thermoregulatory mechanisms during both regional and general anaesthesia.[52,53] In infants but not in adults, non-shivering thermogenesis is an important thermoregulatory defence mechanism mediated by the β_3-adrenergic receptors in the brown adipose tissue, which has an uncoupling protein that permits direct transformation of substrate to heat.[54] Non-shivering thermogenesis does not occur in adults or children under anaesthesia, regardless of the anaesthetic drug: propofol, opioids or inhalation agents.[53–56] During general anaesthesia, the threshold for vasoconstriction of the arteriovenous shunts located in the fingers and toes is decreased, resulting in a redistribution of body heat from the core to the periphery, and a consequent inadvertent perioperative hypothermia in the typical cold operating room environment is common.[54–57] Regional anaesthesia also impairs the central control of thermal regulation, as the regulatory system judges the skin temperature in the blocked area to be abnormally high and increases blood flow to that area. Unless special precautions are taken during the intraoperative period, even the patient who has received only a regional block may arrive in the PACU with a decreased body temperature. Since most patients also receive some form of sedation during regional anaesthesia, the potential for hypothermia is increased. This is perhaps an even greater risk in paediatric patients who have regional blocks placed after induction of anaesthesia.

There is now convincing evidence that the typical 2°C reduction in temperature during surgery predisposes to numerous complications, including increased coagulopathy, cardiac events in adults, prolonged hospitalization and surgical wound infections.[53,58,59] Mild hypothermia decreases the metabolism of drugs such as muscle relaxants and propofol and, in adults, prolongs recovery.[59] However, in infants, mild hypothermia *per se* neither impairs respiratory function nor prolongs postanaesthetic recovery following peripheral surgery.[60]

Fortunately, effective methods are available for preventing hypothermia. These include increasing environmental temperature, heating intravenous fluids and reducing heat loss by covering the patient with one to three layers of blankets, impervious drapes or plastic bags.[52,53,57,60] In infants (but not adults) active or passive humidification of airway gases is an important mechanism of intraoperative heat conservation.[55,57]

Once heat loss has occurred, active heating is the best method of re-establishing normal body temperature. This should preferably be performed while the patient is still in the operating room and the introduction of forced air warming devices into clinical practice has made this easier. Some patients have stated that they were more distressed by uncontrollable shivering in the PACU than by incisional pain. It is a common practice to administer meperidine or clonidine to diminish shivering, but patients must be warmed actively. While the younger paediatric patient does not shiver in the PACU as often as his or her adult counterpart, hypothermia is still possible. Many children receive both a general anaesthetic and a regional nerve block, both of which impair central and peripheral thermoregulation. Most paediatric anaesthetists are aware of the importance of keeping neonates warm and paediatric surgeons are accustomed to working in a much warmer environment than those dealing with adult patients. Despite these measures some children arrive hypothermic in the PACU and active warming by overhead radiant heaters, forced air warmers and warmed blankets should be performed in these children.

POSTOPERATIVE NAUSEA AND VOMITING

Nausea, vomiting and retching are common postoperative complications that are viewed as minor complications by some physicians, while patients have reported that these sequelae are sometimes more debilitating than the consequences of the operation itself.[61,62] Postoperative nausea and vomiting (PONV) not only cause patient discomfort, but when severe may be associated with tension and bleeding on suture lines, muscular fatigue and tracheal aspiration of vomitus. More commonly, PONV can lead to prolonged times to discharge from ambulatory surgery centres, increased resource utilization and unanticipated hospital admission.[63,64] The overall incidence in many large studies is 10% in the PACU, 30% in the first 24 h, with recurrent emesis in 0.1% and unanticipated hospital admission in 1 in 3000. However, rates of 40–80% have been reported in some high-risk groups.[61] Some factors affecting PONV are not under the direct control of the anaesthetist. These include the age and gender of the patient, the nature, site and duration of the operation. Higher rates of PONV are seen in children aged 11–14 years, particularly if they are very nervous, in post-menarchal females, in those with a previous history of PONV or motion sickness and after strabismus, adenotonsillectomy, orchiopexy, middle ear, otoplasty, cardiac catheterization and dental rehabilitation procedures.

The multifactorial nature of PONV makes it difficult to sort out the effects of an individual drug on the incidence of this complication.[64] The quality of clinical trials on PONV varies considerably, making it difficult to determine the clinical usefulness of the data, even if the differences in the incidence of PONV in a study achieve statistical significance. Quantitative systematic reviews and meta-analyses help resolve questions arising from conflicting results in two or more studies and will increase the statistical power of the conclusions compared with studies with small numbers.[65] While statistical significance has been achieved in many studies, the clinical importance of the proposed strategy often remains unclear unless the numbers-needed-to-treat (NNT) are calculated. This method determines how many patients need to be treated with the proposed strategy to avoid the complication in one patient who would have otherwise developed the problem if the alternative strategy was used. If the NNT are low, then the proposed strategy has both clinical importance and statistical significance.

Factors that affect PONV and are under the control of the anaesthetist include: preanaesthetic sedation, anaesthetic drugs used for induction and maintenance, nitrous oxide (N_2O), neostigmine, non-steroidal anti-inflammatory drugs (NSAID), nursing protocols and antiemetic prophylaxis.

PREANAESTHETIC SEDATION

Prior to the advent of benzodiazepines, it was routine to administer opioids for preinduction sedation. However, the administration of opioids by any route (oral transmucosal, nasal, orogastric, intramuscular or intravenous) is associated with increased emesis.[66] The concomitant use of atropine or scopolamine, but not glycopyrrolate, would ameliorate the increased PONV.[61] The oral transmucosal administration of fentanyl in a sucrose candy matrix (Fentanyl Oralet) has been useful in sedating children undergoing painful procedures outside the operating rooms.[66,67] However, the associated increased incidence of preinduction emesis has been a major drawback to its more widespread use as a routine preanaesthetic sedative.[66] In contrast, premedication with oral benzodiazepines (midazolam) has become more popular as the route of administration is more acceptable, side-effects of respiratory depression are less likely and this practice may be associated with decreased emesis.[68,69] However, some patients have paradoxical reactions with agitation after midazolam. Clonidine, an α_2 antagonist, has also been used orally for effective preoperative sedation, and is associated with decreased PONV.[70]

ANAESTHETIC DRUGS USED FOR INDUCTION AND MAINTENANCE

Induction with the older inhalation agents ether and cyclopropane was associated with increased PONV, but there seems to be little difference among halothane, isoflurane, sevoflurane or desflurane with regard to PONV.[61] Intravenous induction with ketamine and etomidate is associated with increased emesis, while induction with propofol is associated with decreased PONV.[62,71] This beneficial effect of propofol is more prominent when it is used for both induction and maintenance of anaesthesia, and seems to be limited to the early (0–6 h) postoperative period. Tramer *et al.* performed a quantitative systematic review of 84 studies of 6069 patients who received propofol.[72] They concluded that it would require nine patients to be induced with propofol to prevent PONV in one (NNT = 9). However, if propofol was used for both the induction and maintenance of anaesthesia, the NNT would be 6. If studies were limited to those with a 20–60% PONV rate in the comparator group, the NNT to prevent early nausea was 4.7 (95% CI 3.8–6.3), vomiting

4.9 (4–6.1) and any emetic event 4.9 (3.7–7.1). Thus, of five patients in this population treated with propofol for maintenance of anaesthesia, one will not vomit or be nauseated in the immediate postoperative period who would otherwise have vomited or been nauseated. The authors claimed that the difference between propofol and control may have reached statistical significance in other situations but was of doubtful clinical relevance.[72] However, this conclusion is based on an arbitrary definition that any strategy where the NNT exceed 5 is of limited clinical value.

While there are some reports of the use of low-dose propofol in the PACU for managing established PONV, this antiemetic action is short lived and its mechanism is unknown.[73–75] The high cost of propofol and the need to waste residual drug make its routine use in all ambulatory surgery prohibitively expensive in some countries. However, it should be considered as part of the intraoperative management of patients with previous PONV undergoing operations with a high risk for this complication.[62]

NITROUS OXIDE

While volunteers breathing nitrous oxide in oxygen develop nausea and vomiting, it has been more difficult to prove there is increased PONV when nitrous oxide is part of the anaesthetic technique, perhaps because the studies had limited power. More recently, three separate meta-analyses concluded that omission of nitrous oxide reduced the incidence of PONV.[76–78] Part of the earlier confusion may be related to different effects of nitrous oxide on nausea and emesis. Tramer *et al.* used meta-analysis to show that omitting nitrous oxide has no effect on early or late nausea, but decreased both early and late vomiting. This decrease was noted only if the baseline incidence was high.[76] Although there was a significant reduction in emesis when a nitrous oxide free regimen was used, it would require anaesthetists to treat 13 patients with this regimen to prevent both early and late vomiting in one (95% CI 9–30). In studies with a baseline risk higher than the mean of all reports, the NNT to prevent both early and late vomiting with a nitrous oxide-free anaesthetic was 5 (95% CI 4–10). When the

baseline risk was lower than the mean, omitting nitrous oxide did not improve outcome. However, the nitrous oxide-free regimen was not without risks. For every 46 patients treated with this method, one would develop intraoperative awareness, limiting the value of this technique.[76]

NEOSTIGMINE

Routine antagonism of residual neuromuscular blockade has been a standard practice because of concerns about postextubation airway complications. However, anticholinesterases such as neostigmine have muscarinic actions on the gastrointestinal system. With the introduction of short- and intermediate-acting muscle relaxants, the routine use of antagonists has been questioned and some suggest that spontaneous recovery of neuromuscular blockade (NMB) is preferable in order to minimize the incidence of PONV secondary to reversal agents.[73,79] There are conflicting reports regarding the effect of neostigmine on PONV, with significant differences noted in some studies but not others.[80–82] Perhaps these differences relate to the concomitant use of atropine or glycopyrrolate with neostigmine. In one study, children who received neostigmine 0.07 mg kg^{-1} i.v. and glycopyrrolate 0.01 mg kg^{-1} following mivacurium infusions had more vomiting in the PACU than children who received placebo or edrophonium 1 mg kg^{-1} i.v. with atropine 0.01 mg kg^{-1} i.v.[79] The effect of neostigmine on PONV is limited to the early PACU phase of recovery and avoidance of this drug may not have much clinical significance on 24-h PONV.

NON-STEROIDAL ANTI-INFLAMMATORY DRUGS

Postoperative pain management is important in decreasing PONV, as both pain and the use of opioids increase PONV. Even a single dose of morphine is associated with increased PONV.[83] Regional nerve blocks and wound infiltration with local anaesthetics may decrease postoperative opioid analgesic requirements and so decrease PONV. With the advent of potent NSAIDs such as ketorolac and propacetamol, it is possible to control mild-to-moderate post-operative pain without using opioids.[84] However, the incidence of increased bleeding after tonsillectomy procedures and the relatively high price of ketorolac have led to a decline in the use of this drug in these patients.[85] This is discussed below in more detail.

NURSING PROTOCOLS

Protocols that have been shown to increase PONV include rapid mobilization of children who have received opioids and the insistence that children drink before they are discharged from the ambulatory surgery centre.[86] Gentle handling and the avoidance of rapid positional changes are essential in children who have received opioids. In a major study, Schreiner *et al.* randomized 989 patients to one of two groups: (1) where patients were required to drink clear liquids without vomiting prior to discharge from the hospital, or (2) where children were allowed but not required to drink before discharge. There were no differences in the incidence of emesis in the operating room, during phase-1 recovery or after discharge. However, during phase-2 recovery the incidence of emesis in the group permitted but not required to drink was significantly lower (14% vs 23%, $p < 0.001$) and the times to discharge were significantly shorter (84 ± 40 min vs 101 ± 58 min, $p < 0.001$). The current practice is not to insist that a child drinks before discharge.

ANTIEMETIC PROPHYLAXIS

Routine antiemetic prophylaxis for all patients is not appropriate as less than 30% experience PONV. However, patients at high risk of this complication should receive antiemetic prophylaxis.[87] The complex act of emesis is controlled by the emetic centre situated in the lateral reticular formation of the brainstem, which receives stimuli from the pharynx, gastrointestinal tract and mediastinum, the higher cortical centres (including the visual centre and the vestibular portion of the eighth cranial nerve) and the chemoreceptor trigger zone (CTZ) in the area postrema. The blood–brain barrier is absent in the CTZ and chemical stimuli from both blood and cerebrospinal fluid can activate the CTZ. This area is rich in dopamine, opioid, 5-hydroxytryptamine (5-HT_3, serotonin), histaminic and muscarinic cholinergic receptors, and their blockade may be an important mechanism of action of the currently used antiemetic drugs.[61,73]

There is a vast body of literature comparing the efficacy of antiemetic drugs for both prophylaxis and treatment of established PONV. Many of these studies can be criticized for comparisons with placebo, for being underpowered or for not standardizing the perioperative management.[64] Drugs used include phenothiazines, butyrophenones, antihistaminics, anticholinergics, benzamides and antiserotonin agents.[88] In a quantitative systematic review of drugs used for prophylaxis of PONV after strabismus surgery in children, Tramer *et al.* concluded that droperidol and metoclopramide were both better than placebo in preventing this complication.[89] However, if droperidol 75 μg kg^{-1} i.v. was administered to 100 children, it would prevent vomiting in 25, while 25 would still vomit and the remaining 50 children would not have vomited anyway. Sixteen of the 100 may have minor adverse reactions and less than one child in 100 may have an extrapyramidal reaction. Metoclopramide 0.15 and 0.25 mg kg^{-1} was significantly better than control only for early vomiting.[89]

A new class of drugs, the 5-HT_3 receptor antagonists, has recently been introduced for the management of PONV. These drugs are reported to be more effective and free from the side-effects of the older antiemetics, but more expensive. The large body of literature regarding the use of ondansetron (53 trials of 13 580 patients) has been summarized in meta-analyses.[90] When the subgroup of paediatric patients in this meta-analysis was examined separately, the efficacy of ondansetron was clearly demonstrated, with only five patients being required to be treated to prevent emesis during the first 6 h in one, and three to prevent late emesis (0–48 h).[89] These methods can be applied to comparisons of ondansetron with droperidol and metoclopramide. It is clear that for both children and adults ondansetron is superior to metoclopramide in the prophylaxis of PONV.[91–93] However, there are differences in the relative efficacy of ondansetron and droperidol in children and adults. In adults the efficacy of ondansetron (4 mg) is not superior to droperidol (0.625–1.25 mg), while in children, ondansetron (0.1 mg kg^{-1}) is a better prophylactic antiemetic than droperidol (75 μg kg^{-1}).[94,95] In a study that included both adult and paediatric patients, prophylactic prochlorperazine (0.2 mg kg^{-1} i.m.) and ondansetron 0.06 mg kg^{-1} i.v. were similarly efficacious in reducing nausea with vomiting after tympanoplasty, while prochlorperazine 0.1 mg kg^{-1} i.v. was less efficacious.[96]

Although the efficacy of 5-HT$_3$ antagonists seems to be greater than that of droperidol in children, their high costs have led some to question the practice of routine prophylaxis with antiserotonin or with any antiemetic drug. These investigators have suggested that if prophylaxis is deemed necessary, cheaper drugs should be used (e.g. droperidol, prochlorperazine or dimenhydrinate) and ondansetron be reserved for treating established postoperative PONV.[97]

Many anaesthetists base their choice of antiemetics on personal experience and prejudice, suggesting that there is no single solution to the problem. Since PONV is multifactorial in origin, a multipronged approach is probably required. Antiemetic drug combinations have been avoided until recently because of concerns about enhanced CNS drug toxicity (delayed emergence, drowsiness and extrapyramidal reactions). In any case, the debate on the relative merits of one antiemetic against another has now been sidelined by the emergence of data to suggest that combinations with steroids and/or other antiemetics are more effective than any one individual antiemetic.[98–102]

ANAESTHETIC PLAN FOR PATIENT WITH PREVIOUS SEVERE POSTOPERATIVE NAUSEA AND VOMITING

Based on current knowledge of factors affecting PONV, the anaesthetic plan for a patient with previous severe PONV should include: (1) preanaesthetic sedation with oral midazolam; (2) intravenous induction and maintenance with propofol; (3) avoidance of nitrous oxide and antagonists of neuromuscular blocking agents; (4) minimization of opioid usage by administering ketorolac, local anaesthetics and nerve blocks, but vigorous pain therapy in the PACU; (5) atropine, if opioids or neuromuscular antagonists are used; (6) liberal intravenous fluids to replace fluid deficits, discharge home without insisting the patient drink; and (7) a combination of antiemetics given prophylactically at the end of surgery along with steroids. A good case can be made for a combination of ondansetron, steroids and droperidol or perphenazine to prevent PONV in this patient. It should be the aim of anaesthetists to make emetic sequelae as unacceptable as pain in the postoperative period.

POSTOPERATIVE PAIN AND DISCOMFORT

Postoperative pain and discomfort are very common problems following surgery in children and are discussed in detail elsewhere in this book. However, the principles of postoperative pain management will be reiterated here, as both pain and drugs used in its management are associated with side-effects. During the 1990s it has become well recognized that even premature infants feel pain, and that there are serious adverse effects from poor management of postoperative pain. Part of the problem has been the limited ability to asses pain in non-verbal children. Various observational pain scales, such as the Children's Hospital of Eastern Ontario Pain Scale (CHEOPS) and the Objective Pain Scales, have been used along with patient reports based on the Visual Analogue Score, 'Faces' scale, or other scales. These tools need modification for age, culture and cognitive ability of the child. It is beyond the scope of this chapter to discuss these in more detail here, except to state that these tools are used in pain management decisions. Postoperative pain management starts in the operating room and should perhaps start before stimuli from the surgical site arrive in the dorsal horn of the spinal cord and set up a 'wind-up' phenomenon. Although there are many animal studies demonstrating the superiority of pre-emptive analgesia, these have been difficult to duplicate clinically. More recently, authorities have been recommending a multimodal approach where local anaesthetics, anti-inflammatory drugs and opioids have been used. These approaches are discussed in more detail elsewhere in the book.

SURGICAL COMPLICATIONS: BLEEDING

Bleeding remains a major cause for readmission after ambulatory surgery. This is particularly true for tonsillectomy patients, where a 1–2% rate in the first 24 h has been noted in many studies. Secondary haemorrhage after this operation can occur 3–7 days later and is not under the control of the anaesthetist. This has led to much debate about the time at which patients can be safely discharged after the operation.[29,30,103] In a study of the times to first bleed after adenotonsillectomy, Carithers noted in 1987 that 19% of patients could be released 4 h postoperatively with an 8.1% chance of subsequent complications. Of the remaining patients, 85.9% could be released 8 h after surgery or 98.2% could be released 10 h after surgery, all with a less than 10% chance of subsequent complications.[104] This study supports keeping tonsilloadenoidectomy patients for at least 8 h and possibly for 10 h after surgery to minimize the risk of complications after discharge. In most institutions a minimum stay of 4–6 h has been advocated for this operation. However, children below 3 years of age are more likely to develop airway obstruction and it is routine practice to admit these patients.

As described above, pain management in these children is a major challenge as the procedure is associated with considerable postoperative pain and yet the opioid drugs commonly used to treat it are associated with a potential for life-threatening respiratory depression. When ketorolac was first introduced, it achieved considerable popularity when it was shown to be as effective as morphine 0.1 mg kg^{-1}, but without the associated increased respiratory depression or vomiting.[84] Early reports failed to show any increased bleeding.[105–107] However, when the reoperation

rate of larger groups of patients undergoing tonsillectomy was examined retrospectively, an increased incidence of bleeding was noted in the ketorolac group.[108,109] In one retrospective study, 58 of 311 patients who underwent tonsillectomy received intraoperative ketorolac with an overall postoperative bleeding rate of 17%, compared with 4.4% in 253 patients who received traditional opioid analgesics.[108] In double-blind studies an increased difficulty in establishing haemostasis was noted in patients receiving ketorolac.[110] In a similar patient population, Gunter *et al.* demonstrated that subjects receiving ketorolac had more major bleeding that required intervention (5/49 vs 0/47, $p < 0.05$) and more bleeding episodes (0.22 per subject vs 0.04, $p < 0.05$) than children receiving morphine.[85] The risk of bleeding is limited to the first 24 h after a single dose of ketorolac. The increased risk of bleeding after ketorolac seems to be limited to the tonsillectomy patient population.[109,111–113] The study by Rusy *et al.* showed that rectal acetaminophen 30 mg kg^{-1} was as effective an analgesic as ketorolac but free from the increased bleeding, and this has currently become the practice in the USA.[110]

Other surgical complications relate to the site and type of surgery. The presence of tight dressings and splints may cause discomfort and have the potential to result in compartment syndromes after orthopaedic procedures. It is imperative that the surgeon examine the child before discharge to ensure that the wound site is satisfactory.

DISCHARGE CRITERIA

Children should be discharged from the ambulatory surgery unit when they have stable vital signs, can maintain a patent airway, cough, gag and swallow reflexes have returned, and the child is free from cardiorespiratory distress, excessive bleeding, pain and vomiting. Scoring systems have been described for discharge from the PACU by Steward and by Aldrete.[29,30,114,115] Numeric values are assigned to various attributes and the sum of these values provides the score. In the modified Aldrete scoring system, a score of 0, 1 or 2 is assigned to motor activity, respiration, blood pressure, consciousness and colour, respectively. There have been suggestions that oxygen saturation values in room air replace colour as an attribute. In the Steward scale a similar score of 0, 1 or 2 is applied to evaluations of the level of consciousness, airway and patient movement. Both of these scales apply to phase-1 recovery, with the patient achieving higher scores when he or she becomes more awake. A modified Aldrete score of 9 or more indicated that the patient is ready for discharge from phase-1 PACU. However, the maximum Steward score can only be 6.

Clinical discharge criteria have also been described for discharge readiness from phase-2 recovery.[116,117] Simple checklists are used to confirm that the patient has stable vital signs, and has returned to an alert, orientated state, with intact coughing, swallowing reflexes, the ability to walk and freedom from surgical bleeding, respiratory distress, nausea, vomiting and dizziness. A postanaesthetic discharge scoring system (PADS) was developed and validated by Chung *et al.* to measure home readiness (Table 10.6).[118] In the initial description of the PADS, the ability to accept oral intake and void were required prior to discharge. However, with the demonstration that insisting on oral intake prior to discharge increases in-hospital emesis, the PADS score has been modified to remove both voiding and oral intake as criteria for discharge readiness.[118] The PADS score has not been validated in children, but similar criteria are used in most hospitals in the USA. The discharge criteria should also take into account the capabilities of

the person who will be caring for the child, the presence of other medical problems and the distance that the family has to travel to obtain medical assistance. It is more important to individualize the times of discharge rather than insist on minimum stays.

POSTDISCHARGE PROBLEMS

A good day-surgery programme presupposes well-established lines of communication in the event of postdischarge problems. Postdischarge follow-up is essential and written instructions to the family on how to manage problems are important. In a study of 551 children in Finland, the incidence of postdischarge symptoms was highest on the day of the operation, with only 79 (14%) children being free of symptoms.[119] The incidence of pain was 56%, with the most problems noted after tonsillectomy (mild pain in 38% and severe in 25%; pain lasted for 7 days or longer in 33%).[119] The authors concluded that pain management and the instructions given in hospital for the treatment of postdischarge pain needed to be improved. Only 78% of all children reported to have pain on the day of the operation received analgesics, and this decreased to 60% on the next day and later to 58%.[119] These authors also studied the incidence of behavioural changes following discharge.[120] Problematical changes were most common in the 1.0–2.9 year olds and the incidence decreased significantly from 46% on the day of the operation

Table 10.6   Postanaesthetic discharge score (PADS)

	0	1	2
Change in vital signs	≤40% preoperative value	20–40% of preoperative value	Within 20% of preoperative value
Ambulation and mental status	Not ambulating/dizzy	Ambulates well	Steady gait/not dizzy
Nausea and vomiting	Severe	Moderate	None or mild
Pain	Severe	Moderate	None or mild
Surgical bleeding	Severe	Moderate	None or mild

Patients may be discharged if the PADS is 9 or higher.

to 9% 4 weeks later. Pain on the day of the operation predicted the occurrence of behavioural problems up to the 4th week, 2–4 weeks longer than the duration of pain itself, emphasizing the importance of effective prevention of postoperative pain.[118,120]

CONCLUSIONS

Fortunately, the incidence of postanaesthetic complications is low as children recover quickly from surgery. Most families rate their overall experience of day surgery as excellent. While newer drugs have been introduced to speed recovery, their overall costs usually exceed those of the older group of drugs, but the new drugs have not been shown to decrease times to discharge readiness. Clinical research has concentrated more on the immediate recovery phase while the child is still in hospital and not on the effects of the new drugs after discharge. Research should focus on determining what modifications to the anaesthetic technique help patients and their families recover and return to their preoperative routines faster. The foremost concern is to ensure the provision of satisfactory care as judged by the parent. The anaesthetist should ensure that the management of pain, emergence delirium, respiratory complications, temperature control and emesis are optimal.

REFERENCES

1 Hannallah, R.S. Selection of patients for paediatric ambulatory surgery [Review]. *Canadian Journal of Anaesthesia* 1991; **38**: 887–90.

2 Patel, R.I., Leith, P. and Hannallah, R.S. Evaluation of the difficult pediatric patient. *Anesthesiology Clinics of North America* 1996; **14**: 753–66.

3 Herbert, M., Healy, T.E., Bourke, J.B., Fletcher, I.R. and Rose, J.M. Profile of recovery after general anaesthesia. *British Medical Journal (Clinical Research Ed.)* 1994; **1983**: 1539–42.

4 Cohen, M.M., Cameron, C.B. and Duncan, P.G. Pediatric anesthesia morbidity and mortality in the perioperative period. *Anesthesia and Analgesia* 1990; **70**: 160–7.

5 Tiret, L., Nivoche, Y., Hatton, F., Desmonts, J.M. and Vourc'h, G. Complications related to anaesthesia in infants and children. A prospective survey of 40240 anaesthetics. *British Journal of Anaesthesia* 1988; **61**: 263–9.

6 Morray, J.P., Geiduschek, J.M., Caplan, R.A., Posner, K.L., Gild, W.M. and Cheney, F.W. A comparison of pediatric and adult anesthesia closed malpractice claims. *Anesthesiology* 1993; **78**: 461–7.

7 Van der Walt, J.H., Sweeney, D.B., Runciman, W.B. and Webb, R.K. The Australian Incident Monitoring Study. Paediatric incidents in anaesthesia: an analysis of 2000 incident reports. *Anaesthesia and Intensive Care* 1993; **21**: 655–8.

8 Cohen, M.M., Duncan, P.G., Pope, W.D., *et al.* The Canadian four-centre study of anaesthetic outcomes: II. Can outcomes be used to assess the quality of anaesthesia care? *Canadian Journal of Anaesthesia* 1992; **39**: 430–9.

9 Cohen, M.M., Duncan, P.G., Tweed, W.A., *et al.* The Canadian four-centre study of anaesthetic outcomes: I. Description of methods and populations. *Canadian Journal of Anaesthesia* 1992; **39**: 420–9.

10 Patel, R.I. and Hannallah, R.S. Anesthetic complications following pediatric ambulatory surgery: a 3-year study. *Anesthesiology* 1988; **69**: 1009–12.

11 Motoyama, E.K. and Glazener, C.H. Hypoxemia after general anesthesia in children. *Anesthesia and Analgesia* 1986; **65**: 267–72.

12 Rose, D.K., Cohen, M.M., Wigglesworth, D.F. and DeBoer, D.P. Critical respiratory events in the postanesthesia care unit. Patient, surgical, and anesthetic factors. *Anesthesiology* 1994; **81**: 410–18.

13 Tyler, I.L., Tantisira, B., Winter, P.M. and Motoyama, E.K. Continuous monitoring of arterial oxygen saturation with pulse oximetry during transfer to the recovery room. *Anesthesia and Analgesia* 1985; **64**: 1108–12.

14 Xue, F.S., Huang, Y.G., Tong, S.Y., *et al.* A comparative study of early postoperative hypoxemia in infants, children, and adults undergoing elective plastic surgery. *Anesthesia and Analgesia* 1996; **83**: 709–15.

15 Soliman, I.E., Patel, R.I., Ehrenpreis, M.B. and Hannallah, R.S. Recovery scores do not correlate with postoperative hypoxemia in children. *Anesthesia and Analgesia* 1988; **67**: 53–6.

16 Gift, A.G., Stanik, J., Karpenick, J., Whitmore, K. and Bolgiano, C.S. Oxygen saturation in postoperative patients at low risk for hypoxemia: is oxygen therapy needed? *Anesthesia and Analgesia* 1995; **80**: 368–72.

17 Georgiou, L.G., Vourlioti, A.N., Kremastinou, F.I., Stefanou, P.S., Tsiotou, A.G. and Kokkinou, M.D. Influence of anaesthetic technique on early postoperative hypoxemia. *Acta Anaesthesiologica Scandinavica* 1996; **40**: 75–80.

18 Watcha, M.F., RamirezRuiz, M., Schweiger, C., Jones, M.B., Lagueruela, R.G. and White, P.F. Postoperative oxygen saturation following propofol nitrous oxide versus halothane nitrous oxide anaesthesia in children. *Paediatric Anaesthesia* 1994; **4**: 383–9.

19 Patel, R.I., Hannallah, R.S., Norden, J., Casey, W.F. and Verghese, S.T. Emergence airway complications in children: a comparison of tracheal extubation in awake and deeply anesthetized patients. *Anesthesia and Analgesia* 1991; **73**: 266–70.

20 Pounder, D.R., Blackstock, D. and Steward, D.J. Tracheal extubation in children: halothane versus isoflurane, anesthetized versus awake. *Anesthesiology* 1991; **74**: 653–5.

21 Cohen, M.M. and Cameron, C.B. Should you cancel the operation when a child has an upper respiratory tract infection? *Anesthesia and Analgesia* 1991; **72**: 282–288.

22 Rolf, N. and Cote, C.J. Frequency and severity of desaturation events during general anesthesia in children with and without upper respiratory infections. *Journal of Clinical Anesthesia* 1992; **4**: 200–3.

23 DeSoto, H., Patel, R.I., Soliman, I.E. and Hannallah, R.S. Changes in oxygen saturation following general anesthesia in children with upper respiratory infection signs and symptoms undergoing otolaryngological procedures. *Anesthesiology* 1988; **68**: 276–9.

24 Schreiner, M.S., O'Hara, I., Markakis, D.A. and Politis, G.D. Do children who experience laryngospasm have an increased risk of upper respiratory tract infection? *Anesthesiology* 1996; **85**: 475–80.

25 Tait, A.R., Pandit, U.A., Voepel-Lewis, T., Munro, H.M. and Malviya, S. Use of the laryngeal mask airway in children with upper respiratory tract infections: a comparison with endotracheal intubation. *Anesthesia and Analgesia* 1998; **86**: 706–11.

26 Aquilina, A.T., Hall, W.J., Douglas, R.G.J. and Utell, M.J. Airway reactivity in subjects with viral upper respiratory tract infections: the effects of exercise and cold air. *American Review of Respiratory Disease* 1980; **122**: 3–10.

27 Cote, C.J., Zaslavsky, A., Downes, J.J., et al. Post-operative apnea in former preterm infants after inguinal herniorrhaphy. A combined analysis. *Anesthesiology* 1995; **82**: 809–22.

28 Watcha, M.F., Thach, B.T. and Gunter, J.B. Postoperative apnea after caudal anesthesia in an ex-premature infant. *Anesthesiology* 1989; **71**: 613–15.

29 Gerber, M.E., O'Connor, D.M., Adler, E. and Myer, C.M. Selected risk factors in pediatric adenotonsillectomy. *Archives of Otolaryngology – Head and Neck Surgery* 1996; **122**: 811–14.

30 Guida, R.A. and Mattucci, K.F. Tonsillectomy and adenoidectomy: an inpatient or outpatient procedure? *Laryngoscope* 1990; **100**: 491–3.

31 Biavati, M.J., Manning, S.C. and Phillips, D.L. Predictive factors for respiratory complications after tonsillectomy and adenoidectomy in children. *Archives of Otolaryngology – Head and Neck Surgery* 1997; **123**: 517–21.

32 McGowan, F.X., Kenna, M.A., Fleming, J.A. and O'Connor, T. Adenotonsillectomy for upper airway obstruction carries increased risk in children with a history of prematurity. *Pediatric Pulmonology* 1992; **13**: 222–6.

33 Randall, D.A. and Hoffer, M.E. Complications of tonsillectomy and adenoidectomy [Review]. *Otolaryngology – Head and Neck Surgery* 1998; **118**: 61–8.

34 Lakshmipathy, N., Bokesch, P.M., Cowen, D.E., Lisman, S.R. and Schmid, C.H. Environmental tobacco smoke: a risk factor for pediatric laryngospasm. *Anesthesia and Analgesia* 1996; **82**: 724–7.

35 Lyons, B., Frizelle, H., Kirby, F. and Casey, W. The effect of passive smoking on the incidence of airway complications in children undergoing general anaesthesia. *Anaesthesia* 1996; **51**: 324–6.

36 Skolnick, E.T. and Vomvolakis, M.A. Exposure to environmental tobacco smoke and clinical outcome in children receiving general anesthesia (Abstract). *Anesthesiology* 1996; **85**: A1066.

37 Shemie, S. Steroids for anything that swells: dexamethasone and postextubation airway obstruction [Editorial; Comment]. *Critical Care Medicine* 1996; **24**: 1613–14.

38 Koka, B.V., Jeon, I.S., Andre, J.M., MacKay, I. and Smith, R.M. Postintubation croup in children. *Anesthesia and Analgesia* 1977; **56**: 501–5.

39 Litman, R.S. and Keon, T.P. Postintubation croup in children [Letter]. *Anesthesiology* 1991; **75**: 1122–3.

40 Postma, D.S., Prazma, J., Woods, C.I., Sidman, J. and Pillsbury, H.C. Use of steroids and a long-acting vasoconstrictor in the treatment of postintubation croup. A ferret model. *Archives of Otolaryngology – Head and Neck Surgery* 1987; **113**: 844–9.

41 Splinter, W.M. and Roberts, D.J. Dexamethasone decreases vomiting by children after tonsillectomy. *Anesthesia and Analgesia* 1996; **83**: 913–16.

42 Tom, L.W., Templeton, J.J., Thompson, M.E. and Marsh, R.R. Dexamethasone in adenotonsillectomy. *International Journal of Pediatric Otorhinolaryngology* 1996; **37**: 115–20.

43 April, M.M., Callan, N.D., Nowak, D.M. and Hausdorff, M.A. The effect of intravenous dexamethasone in pediatric adenotonsillectomy. *Archives of Otolaryngology – Head and Neck Surgery* 1996; **122**: 117–20.

44 Khine, H.H., Corddry, D.H., Kettrick, R.G., et al. Comparison of cuffed and uncuffed endotracheal tubes in young children during general anesthesia. *Anesthesiology* 1997; **86**: 627–31.

45 Deakers, T.W., Reynolds, G., Stretton, M. and Newth, C.J. Cuffed endotracheal tubes in pediatric intensive care. *Journal of Pediatrics* 1994; **125**: 57–62.

46 Bastron, R.D. and Moyers, J. Emergence delirium. *Journal of the American Medical Association* 1967; **200**: 883.

47 Davis, P.J., Cohen, I.T., McGowan, F.X.J. and Latta, K. Recovery characteristics of desflurane versus halothane for maintenance of anesthesia in pediatric ambulatory patients. *Anesthesiology* 1994; **80**: 298–302.

48 Lerman, J., Davis, P.J., Welborn, L.G., et al. Induction, recovery, and safety characteristics of sevoflurane in children undergoing ambulatory surgery. A comparison with halothane. *Anesthesiology* 1996; **84**: 1332–40.

49 Welborn, L.G., Hannallah, R.S., Norden, J.M., Ruttimann, U.E. and Callan, C.M. Comparison of emergence and recovery characteristics of sevoflurane, desflurane, and halothane in pediatric ambulatory patients. *Anesthesia and Analgesia* 1996; **83**: 917–20.

50 Davis, P.J., Lerman, J., Suresh, S., et al. A randomized multicenter study of remifentanil compared with alfentanil, isoflurane, or propofol in anesthetized pediatric patients undergoing elective strabismus surgery. *Anesthesia and Analgesia* 1997; **84**: 982–9.

51 Aono, J., Ueda, W., Mamiya, K., Takimoto, E. and Manabe, M. Greater incidence of delirium during recovery from sevoflurane anesthesia in preschool boys. *Anesthesiology* 1997; **87**: 1298–300.

52 Sessler, D.I. Perioperative thermoregulation and heat balance [Review]. *Annals of the New York Academy of Sciences* 1997; **813**: 757–77.

53 Sessler, D.I. Mild perioperative hypothermia [Review]. *New England Journal of Medicine* 1997; **336**: 1730–7.

54 Plattner, O., Semsroth, M., Sessler, D.I., Papousek, A., Klasen, C. and Wagner, O. Lack of nonshivering thermogenesis in infants anesthetized with fentanyl and propofol. *Anesthesiology* 1997; **86**: 772–7.

55 Bissonnette, B. and Sessler, D.I. The thermoregulatory threshold in infants and children anesthetized with isoflurane and caudal bupivacaine. *Anesthesiology* 1990; **73**: 1114–18.

56 Lindahl, S.G. Sensing cold and producing heat [Editorial; Comment]. *Anesthesiology* 1997; **86**: 758–9.

57 Sessler, D.I. Perianesthetic thermoregulation and heat balance in humans [Review]. *FASEB Journal* 1993; **7**: 638–44.

58 Kurz, A., Sessler, D.I. and Lenhardt, R. Perioperative normothermia to reduce the incidence of surgical-wound infection and shorten hospitalization. Study of Wound Infection and Temperature Group. *New England.Journal.of Medicine* 1996; **334**: 1209–15.

59 Lenhardt, R., Marker, E., Goll, V., *et al.* Mild intraoperative hypothermia prolongs postanesthetic recovery. *Anesthesiology* 1997; **87**: 1318–23.

60 Bissonnette, B. and Sessler, D.I. Mild hypothermia does not impair postanesthetic recovery in infants and children. *Anesthesia and Analgesia* 1993; **76**: 168–72.

61 Watcha, M.F. and White, P.F. Postoperative nausea and vomiting. Its etiology, treatment, and prevention [Review]. *Anesthesiology* 1992; **77**: 162–84.

62 Watcha, M.F. and White, P.F. Post-operative nausea and vomiting: do they matter? *European Journal of Anaesthesiology* 1995; **10** Suppl.: 18–23.

63 Korttila, K., Clergue, F., Leeser, J., *et al.* Intravenous dolasetron and ondansetron in prevention of postoperative nausea and vomiting: a multicenter, double-blind, placebo-controlled study. *Acta Anaesthesiologica Scandinavica* 1997; **41**: 914–22.

64 Korttila, K. The study of postoperative nausea and vomiting [Review]. *British Journal of Anaesthesia* 1992; **69** Suppl.: 23S.

65 Tramer, M.R. What can systematic reviews teach us in anaesthesia? *Acta Anaesthesiologica Scandinavica* 1997; **111**: 235–6.

66 Epstein, R.H., Mendel, H.G., Witkowski, T.A., *et al.* The safety and efficacy of oral transmucosal fentanyl citrate for preoperative sedation in young children. *Anesthesia and Analgesia* 1996; **83**: 1200–5.

67 Schecter, N.L., Weisman, S.J., Rosenblum, M., Bernstein, B. and Conrad, P.L. The use of oral tranmucosal fentanyl citrate for painful procedures in children. *Pediatrics* 1995; **95**: 335–9.

68 Khalil, S.N., Berry, J.M., Howard, G., *et al.* The antiemetic effect of lorazepam after outpatient strabismus surgery in children. *Anesthesiology* 1992; **77**: 915–19.

69 Splinter, W.M., MacNeill, H.B., Menard, E.A., *et al.* Midazolam reduces vomiting after tonsillectomy in children. *Canadian Journal of Anaesthesia* 1995; **42**: 201–3.

70 Mikawa, K., Nishina, K., Maekawa, N., *et al.* Oral clonidine reduces vomiting after strabismus surgery. *Canadian Journal of Anaesthesia* 1995; **42**: 977–81.

71 Watcha, M.F. and White, P.F. New antiemetic drugs [Review]. *International Anesthesiology Clinics* 1995; **33**: 1–200.

72 Tramer, M., Moore, A. and McQuay, H. Propofol anaesthesia and postoperative nausea and vomiting: quantitative systematic review of randomized controlled studies. *British Journal of Anaesthesia* 1997; **78**: 247–55.

73 Appadu, B.L. and Lambert, D.G. Interaction of i.v. anaesthetic agents with 5-HT$_3$ receptors. *British Journal of Anaesthesia* 1996; **76**: 271–3.

74 Appadu, B.L., Strange, P.G. and Lambert, D.G. Does propofol interact with D$_2$ dopamine receptors? *Anesthesia and Analgesia* 1994; **79**: 1191–2.

75 Borgeat, A., Wilder-Smith, O.H. and Suter, P.M. The nonhypnotic therapeutic applications of propofol [Review]. *Anesthesiology* 1994; **80**: 642–56.

76 Tramer, M., Moore, A. and McQuay, H. Omitting nitrous oxide in general anaesthesia: meta-analysis of intraoperative awareness and postoperative emesis in randomized controlled trials. *British Journal of Anaesthesia* 1996; **76**: 186–93.

77 Divatia, J.V., Vaidya, J.S., Badwe, R.A. and Hawaldar, R.W. Omission of nitrous oxide during anesthesia reduces the incidence of postoperative nausea and vomiting. A meta-analysis. *Anesthesiology* 1996; **85**: 1055–62.

78 Hartung, J. Twenty-four of twenty-seven studies show a greater incidence of emesis associated with nitrous oxide than with alternative anesthetics. *Anesthesia and Analgesia* 1996; **83**: 114–16.

79 Watcha, M.F., Safavi, F.Z., McCulloch, D.A., Tan, T.S. and White, P.F. Effect of antagonism of mivacurium-induced neuromuscular block on postoperative emesis in children. *Anesthesia and Analgesia* 1995; **80**: 713–17.

80 Boeke, A.J., de Lange, J.J., van Druenen, B. and Langemeijer, J.J. Effect of antagonizing residual neuromuscular block by neostigmine and atropine on postoperative vomiting. *British Journal of Anaesthesia* 1994; **72**: 654–6.

81 Hovorka, J., Korttila, K., Nelskyla, K., *et al.* Reversal of neuromuscular blockade with neostigmine has no effect on the incidence or severity of postoperative nausea and vomiting. *Anesthesia and Analgesia* 1997; **85**: 1359–61.

82 Ding, Y., Fredman, B. and White, P.F. Use of mivacurium during laparoscopic surgery: effect of reversal drugs on postoperative recovery. *Anesthesia and Analgesia* 1994; **78**: 450–4.

83 Weinstein, M.S., Nicolson, S.C. and Schreiner, M.S. A single dose of morphine sulfate increases the incidence of vomiting after outpatient inguinal surgery in children. *Anesthesiology* 1994; **81**: 572–7.

84 Watcha, M.F., Jones, M.B., Lagueruela, R.G., Schweiger, C. and White, P.F. Comparison of ketorolac and morphine as adjuvants during pediatric surgery. *Anesthesiology* 1992; **76**: 368–72.

85 Gunter, J.B., Varughese, A.M., Harrington, J.F., *et al.* Recovery and complications after tonsillectomy in children: a comparison of ketorolac and morphine. *Anesthesia and Analgesia* 1995; **81**: 1136–41.

86 Schreiner, M.S., Nicolson, S.C., Martin, T. and Whitney, L. Should children drink before discharge from day surgery? *Anesthesiology* 1992; **76**: 528–33.

87 Watcha, M.F. and Smith, I. Cost-effectiveness analysis of antiemetic therapy for ambulatory surgery. *Journal of Clinical Anesthesia* 1994; **6**: 370–7.

88 Baines, D. Postoperative nausea and vomiting in children [Review]. *Paediatric Anaesthesia* 1996; **6**: 7–14.

89 Tramer, M., Moore, A. and McQuay, H. Prevention of vomiting after paediatric strabismus surgery: a systematic review using the numbers-needed-to-treat method [Review]. *British Journal of Anaesthesia* 1995; **75**: 556–61.

90 Tramer, M.R., Reynolds, D.J., Moore, R.A. and McQuay, H.J. Efficacy, dose–response, and safety of ondansetron in prevention of postoperative nausea and vomiting: a quantitative systematic review of randomized placebo-controlled trials. *Anesthesiology* 1997; **87**: 1277–89.

91 Shende, D. and Mandal, N.G. Efficacy of ondansetron and metoclopramide for preventing postoperative emesis following strabismus surgery in children. *Anaesthesia* 1997; **52**: 496–500.

92 Rose, J.B., Martin, T.M., Corddry, D.H., Zagnoev, M. and Kettrick, R.G. Ondansetron reduces the incidence and severity of poststrabismus repair vomiting in children. *Anesthesia and Analgesia* 1994; **79**: 486–9.

93 Raphael, J.H. and Norton, A.C. Antiemetic efficacy of prophylactic ondansetron in laparoscopic surgery: randomized, double-blind comparison with metoclopramide. *British Journal of Anaesthesia* 1993; **71**: 845–8.

94 Davis, P.J., McGowan, F.X.J., Landsman, I., Maloney, K. and Hoffmann, P. Effect of antiemetic therapy on recovery and hospital discharge time. A double-blind assessment of ondansetron, droperidol, and placebo in pediatric patients undergoing ambulatory surgery. *Anesthesiology* 1995; **83**: 956–60.

95 Fortney, J.T., Gan, T.J., Graczyk, S., *et al.* A comparison of the efficacy, safety and patient satisfaction of ondansetron versus droperidol as antiemetics for elective outpatient surgical procedures. *Anesthesia and Analgesia* 1998; **86**: 731–8.

96 van den Berg, A.A. A comparison of ondansetron and prochlorperazine for the prevention of nausea and vomiting after tympanoplasty. *Canadian Journal.of Anaesthesia* 1996; **43**: 939–45.

97 Tramer, M.R., Moore, R.A., Reynolds, D.J. and McQuay, H.J. A quantitative systematic review of ondansetron in treatment of established postoperative nausea and vomiting. *British Medical Journal* 1997; **314**: 1088–92.

98 Koivuranta, M., Jokela, R., Kiviluoma, K. and Alahuhta, S. The anti-emetic efficacy of a combination of ondansetron and droperidol. *Anaesthesia* 1997; **52**: 863–8.

99 McKenzie, R., Uy, N.T., Riley, T.J. and Hamilton, D.L. Droperidol/ondansetron combination controls nausea and vomiting after tubal banding [published erratum appears in *Anesth Analg* 1997 Mar; 84(3): 704]. *Anesthesia and Analgesia* 1996; **83**: 1218–22.

100 Steinbrook, R.A., Freiberger, D., Gosnell, J.L. and Brooks, D.C. Prophylactic antiemetics for laparoscopic cholecystectomy: ondansetron versus droperidol plus metoclopramide. *Anesthesia and Analgesia* 1996; **83**: 1081–3.

101 Wrench, I.J., Ward, J.E., Walder, A.D. and Hobbs, G.J. The prevention of postoperative nausea and vomiting using a combination of ondansetron and droperidol. *Anaesthesia* 1996; **51**: 776–8.

102 Pueyo, F.J., Carrascosa, F., Lopez, L., Iribarren, M.J., Garcia-Pedrajas, F. and Saez, A. Combination of ondansetron and droperidol in the prophylaxis of postoperative nausea and vomiting. *Anesthesia and Analgesia* 1996; **83**: 117–22.

103 Mitchell, R.B., Pereira, K.D., Friedman, N.R. and Lazar, R.H. Outpatient adenotonsillectomy. Is it safe in children younger than 3 years? *Archives of Otolaryngology – Head and Neck Surgery* 1997; **123**: 681–3.

104 Carithers, J.S., Gebhart, D.E. and Williams, J.A. Postoperative risks of pediatric tonsilloadenoidectomy. *Laryngoscope* 1987; **97**: 422–9.

105 Forrest, J.B., Heitlinger, E.L. and Revell, S. Ketorolac for postoperative pain management in children [Review]. *Drug Safety* 1997; **16**: 309–29.

106 Sutters, K.A., Levine, J.D., Dibble, S., Savedra, M. and Miaskowski, C. Analgesic efficacy and safety of single-dose intramuscular ketorolac for postoperative pain management in children following tonsillectomy. *Pain* 1995; **61**: 145–53.

107 Buck, M.L. Clinical experience with ketorolac in children. *Annals of Pharmacotherapy* 1994; **28**: 1009–13.

108 Judkins, J.H., Dray, T.G. and Hubbell, R.N. Intraoperative ketorolac and posttonsillectomy bleeding. *Archives of Otolaryngology – Head and Neck Surgery* 1996; **122**: 937–40.

109 Gallagher, J.E., Blauth, J. and Fornadley, J.A. Perioperative ketorolac tromethamine and postoperative hemorrhage in cases of tonsillectomy and adenoidectomy. *Laryngoscope* 1995; **105**: 606–9.

110 Rusy, L.M., Houck, C.S., Sullivan, L.J., *et al.* A double-blind evaluation of ketorolac tromethamine versus acetaminophen in pediatric tonsillectomy: analgesia and bleeding. *Anesthesia and Analgesia* 1995; **80**: 226–9.

111 Bailey, R., Sinha, C. and Burgess, L.P. Ketorolac tromethamine and hemorrhage in tonsillectomy: a prospective, randomized, double-blind study. *Laryngoscope* 1997; **107**: 166–9.

112 Splinter, W.M., Rhine, E.J., Roberts, D.W., Reid, C.W. and MacNeill, H.B. Preoperative ketorolac increases bleeding after tonsillectomy in children. *Canadian Journal of Anaesthesia* 1996; **43**: 560–3.

113 Hall, S.C. Tonsillectomies, ketorolac, and the march of progress [Editorial; Comment]. *Canadian Journal of Anaesthesia* 1996; **43**: 544–8.

114 Aldrete, J.A. and Kroulik, D. A postanesthetic recovery score. *Anesthesia and Analgesia* 1970; **49**: 924–34.

115 Steward, D.J. A simplified scoring system for the postoperative recovery room. *Canadian Anaesthetists Society Journal* 1975; **22**: 111–13.

116 Korttila, K. Recovery from outpatient anaesthesia. Factors affecting outcome. [Review]. *Anaesthesia* 1995; **50** Suppl.: 8.

117 Korttila, K. Full recovery after different anesthesia techniques for short diagnostic procedures. *Acta Anaesthesiologica Belgica* 1984; **35** Suppl.: 411.

118 Chung, F., Chan, V.W. and Ong, D. A post-anesthetic discharge scoring system for home readiness after ambulatory surgery. *Journal of Clinical Anesthesia* 1995; **7**: 500–6.

119 Kotiniemi, L.H., Ryhanen, P.T., Valanne, J., Jokela, R., Mustonen, A. and Poukkula, E. Postoperative symptoms at home following day-case surgery in children: a multicentre survey of 551 children. *Anaesthesia* 1997; **52**: 963–9.

120 Kotiniemi, L.H., Ryhanen, P.T. and Moilanen, I.K. Behavioural changes in children following day-case surgery: a 4-week follow-up of 551 children. *Anaesthesia* 1997; **52**: 970–6.

CHAPTER 11

Immediate postoperative intensive care

ROBERT EYRES

INTRODUCTION

The postoperative management of acute neo-natal surgical conditions can usually be planned in advance. Babies with moderate to large gastroschisis or exomphalos, for example, will remain electively intubated and ventilated post-operatively because of abdominal distension, whilst neonates with tracheo-oesophageal fistula may often be extubated immediately following surgery with judicious pain management provided by thoracic epidural[1] or low-dose morphine (5 μg kg^{-1} h^{-1}). The introduction of postoperative recovery areas where children can be carefully observed and treated in the first few hours after surgery has greatly reduced the need for unexpected admission to the intensive care unit (ICU), although these will always occur. Decisions to admit a child to the ICU are sometimes a matter of fine judgement, and may be influence by organizational factors such as the level of staffing and ability to monitor children closely in the general wards.

Occasionally, infants and young children who require large doses of narcotic analgesics for pain management may be at risk of respiratory failure and may have to be managed in the ICU. Immediate problems of recovery are fully discussed in Chapter 10. The purpose of this chapter is to describe the main reasons why children may require intensive care following surgery, to outline the main indications for admission to ICU and to give a brief summary of initial ICU management.

PATHOPHYSIOLOGICAL FACTORS PREDISPOSING CHILDREN TO INTENSIVE CARE ADMISSION

RESPIRATORY

Cohen et al.,[2] in a survey of 29 220 procedures, noted that the most common adverse effects in patients aged less than 12 months were related to the respiratory system. This was most obvious in the neonatal age group, with an event (laryngospasm, apnoea or aspiration, etc.) noted in 25% of patients. Respiratory complications are the most common events in the under-5 year olds, whereas above 6 years of age nausea and vomiting are more common.

Glazener and Motoyama[3] studied 65 ASA I patients aged 1 month to 17 years in the immediate postoperative period and found that the oxygen saturation changed from 97.5 ± 0.2% (mean ± SEM) preoperatively to 93.3 ± 0.54% (range 100–84%) postoperatively, which improved with time after anaesthesia and arousal. Tomkins et al. confirmed this pattern of desaturation in a study in infants[4] where 24% of patients recorded saturations of less than 90% in room air. These cases of desaturation occurred in the first 10 min of the postoperative period. No correlation was found between these events and the use of opioids. Indeed, ventilation may be impaired in the presence of severe pain. Cass and Howard described an infant in whom premature cessation of epidural analgesia after thoracotomy led

to respiratory failure, which was rapidly corrected when the epidural infusion was restarted.[5] Tyler et al. showed that older infants and children receiving opioids postoperatively suffered less episodic hypoventilation and desaturation than did adults.[6]

Several factors in small children, and particularly infants and ex-preterm patients, predispose to the adverse respiratory events in the immediate postoperative period (Table 11.1).

Functional residual capacity

The functional residual capacity (FRC) is determined by the outward force of the thorax balanced by the elastic recoil of the lungs at rest. In the neonate the thorax is easily deformable and provides little outward force. The elasticity of the lung is only slightly less than that in adults and the relaxed FRC in the neonate would fall well below closing volume, which would result in airway closure, atelectasis and a V/Q mismatch causing a decrease in arterial O_2 saturation. In the awake neonate a number of mechanisms exists to defend the dynamic FRC to approximately 40% of total lung capacity: (1) laryngeal braking:[7] partial adduction of the vocal cords during expiration retards expiratory flow and in effect is a form of physiological positive end-expiratory pressure (PEEP). During rapid eye movement (REM) sleep this activity is less pronounced and end-expiratory volume falls;[8] (2) infants terminate expiration before the lung volume reaches resting FRC;[9] and (3) inspiratory muscle activity continues during the phase of expiration altering the stiffness of the chest wall[10] and maintaining a higher FRC.

During a normal respiratory cycle adults breathe down to a relaxed FRC at end-expiration without the use of these dynamic mechanisms. Because of the relatively stiff chest wall the FRC remains above closing volume. This change from dynamically maintained to a relaxed end-expiratory volume in the infant occurs between 6 months and 1 year of age.[11] In spite of these dynamic mechanisms newborns maintain an FRC that is only 40% of total lung capacity, which renders them more susceptible to airway closure and subsequent atelectasis. During REM sleep some of these dynamic mechanisms become inoperative and FRC is

Table 11.1 Reasons why infants are at risk of respiratory events in the postoperative period

- Infants have a low FRC
- Anaesthesia reduces FRC further, causing airway closure and atelectasis
- Respiratory control in newborns is immature and subject to periodic breathing
- Subanaesthetic concentrations of anaesthetic agents alter ventilatory control
- Infants are prone to airway obstruction and this is exacerbated by anaesthesia

reduced by up to 31% compared with FRC in quiet sleep. This reduction during the REM state may render the infant more vulnerable to hypoxia in this period.

General anaesthesia, with or without muscle relaxants, decreases the FRC in adults,[12] causing atelectasis and a decreased compliance, and these changes remain for prolonged periods. Motoyama *et al.*[13] demonstrated in infants under 1 year of age that when anaesthetized with halothane/N_2O relaxant there was a decrease in FRC to 38.5% of predicted values with a marked increase in alveolar to arterial oxygen gradient. This decrease in FRC in this age group is greater than seen in 1–8 year olds (58.7% of predicted value). Halothane anaesthesia at 0.75 MAC produced ventilatory depression in infants less than 1 year old, which is significantly greater than seen in older age groups.[14] This depression of respiration is due to a thoracic paradox as a consequence of preferential depression of the inspiratory intercostal activity with relative sparing of diaphragmatic activity. This intercostal activity is essential in stabilizing the compliant infant rib cage during the respiratory cycle.

Respiratory control

In the healthy human control of ventilation is the function of chemoreceptors in the medulla and the periphery (carotid body, aortic arch). Although both receptor areas respond to arterial carbon dioxide and oxygen tensions ($PaCO_2$ and PaO_2), the primary role of the peripheral chemoreceptors is to respond to changes in arterial PaO_2. A decrease in PaO_2 to below 60 mmHg results in an increase in ventilation at all ages except for preterm infants and possibly newborns. In preterm infants there is a biphasic response to both high and low oxygen partial pressures.[15] The preterm infant responds to hypoxia by an immediate and brief increase followed by a sustained decrease in respiratory minute volume. Conversely, when breathing 100% oxygen there is an immediate and brief decrease followed by sustained increase in minute ventilation. The response to hypoxia matures by about the third week of life,[14] changing to a more adult pattern of a sustained increase in ventilation. This suggests that hypoxaemia in the newborn depresses the

respiratory centre, leading to hypoventilation, periodic breathing and apnoea.

Preterm infants also demonstrate an altered response to carbon dioxide. Preterm infants suffering from periodic breathing chronically hypoventilate and show a significant shift in the CO_2 response curves to the right, with a 22% decrease in slope.[16] The major defect in this response was at the site of the central chemoreceptors. This decrease in sensitivity to CO_2 decreases with decreasing gestational age. Even at a postconceptional age of 37 weeks, a relatively mature infant in clinical terms, the response to CO_2 is blunted for the first few days.[17]

Apnoea and periodic breathing are not uncommon in the newborn but the frequency of the events will depend on the definition used. Apnoea is usually defined as the cessation of respiration for a period of greater than 15 s. Normal full-term infants occasionally have apnoeic spells of 10, 11 or 12 s and until the age of 6 months the majority will have a small amount of periodic breathing during sleep.[18] Apnoeic episodes occur frequently in preterm newborns and although these events are not often observed in full-term neonates their prevalence increases with decreasing gestational age, suggesting that prematurity is a major risk factor for apnoea.

Subanaesthetic concentrations of anaesthetic agents alter ventilatory control. Depending on anaesthetic management practice, the conscious state of patients in the postoperative environment will vary from awake and alert to completely obtunded, according to the influence of residual anaesthetic agents and their kinetics. All anaesthetic agents depress respiration in a dose-dependent manner. One of the primary effects of the opioids via the μ-receptor is the depression of respiration at brainstem level. Volatile anaesthetic agents decrease ventilation and the ventilatory response to carbon dioxide in a dose-related fashion. Trace concentrations of halothane (0.1 MAC) decrease the ventilatory response to hypoxia to less than one-third of control values by impairing the reflex mediated by the peripheral chemoreceptors.[19,20] A 50–80% decreased response was found with the equivalent concentrations (0.1 MAC) of enflurane and isoflurane,[21,22] but more recently it was thought that the peripheral chemoreceptors are more resistant to the effect of isoflurane.[23] This level of anaesthesia (0.1 MAC) is expected in awake patients recovering from anaesthesia from volatile agents, and implies that hypoxia due to other causes will not result in reflex increase in ventilation.

Patency of the human infant upper airway

Upper airway obstruction is not uncommon in the newborn and infants, as a number of anatomical and physiological factors combines to predispose this age group to partial or complete obstruction. From birth to approximately 6 months of age newborn infants are obligatory nose breathers, but the resistance in the nose only contributes approximately 42% of the total airway resistance in the infant,[24] compared with 63% in adults.[25] This may increase significantly with infection, secretions or anatomical abnormalities (choanal narrowing). A small decrease in cross-sectional area caused by the placement of a size 5 French gauge nasogastric tube in the dominant nostril will increase the resistance to airflow by 138%.[26] Pharyngeal obstruction can be both anatomical and physiological. Flexion of the neck in the infant causes oropharyngeal closure, which can be opposed by the application of positive transmural pressure to the pharynx. Neck extension increases the airway diameter.[27] It has been suggested that spontaneous neck flexion causing airway obstruction is an important factor in the pathogenesis of apnoea in preterm infants.[28] In the pharynx there is interaction between airway pressure and the airway muscle tension. Negative and positive airway pressures potentially influence the internal configuration of the airway, while muscles surrounding the upper airway increase or decrease tension concurrently in phase with respiration. Negative transmural pressure in the upper airway has a constricting effect from the vocal cords to the choanae. The most compliant area is the oropharynx and the least compliant is the larynx. In small preterm infants the hypopharynx at the level of the epiglottic folds is nearly as compliant as the oropharynx.[27] Lowering the pharyngeal pressure causes inward movement of the anterior, posterior and lateral pharyngeal walls until occlusion

occurs. Once the airway is closed additional tension in the airway muscles or pressure in the pharynx is needed to restore patency, suggesting adhesive forces between the airway mucosa maintain closure. Tension in the genioglossus muscle is pivotal in maintaining this upper airway patency during the inspiratory phase, but in newborn kittens it has been demonstrated that tension in this muscle is selectively depressed during halothane anaesthesia. Anaesthesia with halothane results in greater airway obstruction in kittens than in adult cats because of the selective depression of the genioglossus in this younger age group.[29]

The larynx acts as a valve controlling airflow but is also an important sensory organ protecting the lower airways from foreign substances. In the neonate laryngeal stimulation may result in prolonged apnoea and respiratory arrest. In healthy full-term infants and preterm infants while sleeping, the response to stimulation of the larynx with small amounts of fluid insufficient in volume to cause airway obstruction per se results in brief or prolonged apnoea and cough. Prolonged apnoea is more common in preterm than full-term infants. This is in contrast to more mature responses of cough or swallowing when small volumes of fluid are deposited in the pharynx.[30]

CARDIOVASCULAR

In their respective studies, both Cohen et al.[2] and Fogliani et al.[31] noted that in the recovery room the profile of adverse events experienced by children differed considerably from that of adults: children were less likely to experience problems with dysrhythmias or hypotension but were more likely to experience problems related to the respiratory system.

Cardiac function in the newborn and infant has fewer reserves than later in life and cardiac failure is frequently related to disorders in other systems such as fluid over load, pulmonary disease or sepsis.

Approximately 30% of the mass of the newborn myocardium is contractile (compared with 60% in the adult), with the contractile sarcomeres being arranged more in random fashion than in parallel sequences. Optimal sarcomere length (2–2.2 u) and arrangement in the infant occur at higher filling pressures than in the adult, and cardiac output is best when peripheral resistance is low. If sarcomere length exceeds 2.2 u, contractility is suboptimal and the heart begins to fail. Heart failure may begin as predominantly left- or right-sided, but because the ventricles are more interdependent in infancy, both sides are rapidly involved. Thus, classic signs of right heart failure, including an enlarging liver [ascites, pleural effusions and peripheral oedema (a very late sign in children)] , and those of left heart failure (cardiac enlargement, pulmonary oedema with dyspnoea and tachpnoea) all tend to be seen in infants with heart failure.

While clinical signs of heart failure, including the characteristic diastolic gallop rhythm, together with chest X-ray and electrocardiographic (ECG) changes, remain very important, non-invasive assessments using echocardiography and Doppler are crucial (see Chapter 13). These techniques not only provide accurate diagnosis and functional assessments, but can also be used to monitor progress in the treatment of cardiac failure closely.

Postoperative bradycardia in children is likely to be due to medications, such as anticholinesterases or fentanyl, or associated with the more obvious situation of severe hypoxia. Tachycardia is most likely to be due to pain and anxiety, antimuscarinics or hypovolaemia. Young children usually compensate well for volume depletion and hypotension is a relatively late feature of hypovolaemia unless large fluid losses are incurred in a short space of time. In the recovery room it is important to exclude and treat ongoing bleeding of surgical origin.

The intensive care environment allows close monitoring of all parameters and usually involves invasive monitoring of arterial, central venous and possibly pulmonary artery pressures. Advanced support of all organ systems is provided as necessary and close monitoring of fluid intake and output, as well as core and peripheral temperatures, is mandatory.

SPECIFIC INDICATIONS FOR ADMISSION FROM THEATRE/ RECOVERY AREA TO INTENSIVE CARE

Over a 3-year period in a large specialized Children's Hospital (Royal Children's Hospital, Melbourne), 61 patients were transferred from the general theatre recovery area (excluding cardiac surgery) to the general ICU (excluding the neonatal ICU). Of this number, 51 were unexpected admissions. In most instances the transfer to intensive care is following initial therapy in the recovery area with admission to intensive care overnight for ongoing observation and support. In keeping with Cohen's survey on postoperative morbidity,[2] 65% of the problems experienced were respiratory, 20% related to the cardiovascular system and approximately 10% were central nervous system (CNS) problems. Airway problems include bleeding with associated obstruction following adenotonsillectomy, pre-existing deformity or disease (subglottic stenosis, cleft palate, Pierre–Robin), respiratory care following extensive craniofacial surgery, unexpected apnoea following anaesthesia and observation following severe laryngospasm. Planned admission for obvious potential problems is desirable even if the problem is not realized and the admission cancelled postoperatively. Patients with severe obstructive sleep apnoea (OSA), surgery for subglottic stenosis and surgery for severe restrictive kyphoscoliosis fall into this particular category.

The main indications for postoperative intensive care are listed in Table 11.2.

RESPIRATORY

Respiratory failure

Respiratory failure may be defined as an elevated $PaCO_2$ greater than 8 kPa (60 mmHg) or the failure of arterial oxygenation with a PaO_2 less than 9 kPa (70 mmHg) with an inspiratory oxygen fraction (FiO_2) greater than 0.6. In practice, the clinical

Table 11.2 Indications for admission to the intensive care unit following anaesthesia

Respiratory	
For ventilation	Respiratory failure
	Phrenic nerve paralysis
	Neonate following major procedures,
	e.g. gastroschisis, diaphragmatic hernia
	Increased intracranial pressure
Tracheal tube care	Tracheomalacia or bronchomalacia
	Postcricoid split
	Following tracheostomy
	Tumours of mediastinum and airway
Airway care	Foreign body
	Craniofacial procedures
	Severe postextubation croup
	Airway trauma
Pulmonary disorders	Aspiration
	Post-tonsillectomy for obstructive sleep apnoea
	Postoperative apnoea in infants
Cardiovascular	
Postcardiac arrest	Postcardiac surgery
	Underlying cardiac disease
Cardiovascular instability	
Central nervous system	
Following surgery for head injury	
Following major surgery on patients with neurological disorders	Myasthenia gravis
	Muscular dystrophy
Miscellaneous	
Severe metabolic derangements	Hypothermia
	Difficult pain management

diagnosis of respiratory failure may be more important than blood gas results alone. These may include increasing respiratory and pulse rate, use of the accessory muscles of respiration, increasing rib retraction and obvious exhaustion. The phrenic nerves are vulnerable to damage during cardiac surgery, and phrenic nerve palsy should be considered when infants fail to wean from ventilatory support in the presence of normal cardiovascular function. Respiratory support may also be initiated for less well-defined reasons, such as to decrease the work of breathing,[32,33] to overcome the work imposed by a tracheal tube[34] or to improve the left ventricular performance in situations of cardiac failure.[35,36] This last reason is an important one, which is not always recognized.

Tracheal tube care

Admission to intensive care is necessary for the routine care of any tracheal tube left *in situ* to prevent complications. Patients with unstable airways, such as tracheomalacia or bronchomalacia, may require intubation for prolonged periods of weeks to months. Following surgery for subglottic stenosis, such as cricoid split, a tracheal tube may be required for shorter periods. Intubation for mediastinal tumours, such as lymphomas, does not ensure stability as these tumours may compress the heart and great vessels as well as the airway, and may rapidly increase in size.

Airway care

One critical function performed by intensive care is observation in the postoperative period after surgical manipulation or trauma to the airway, such as may occur during removal of a foreign body from the bronchus, bleeding or partial obstruction of the airway following tonsillectomy, cleft palate repair or extensive craniofacial surgery. Postextubation croup, developing oedema or structural instability may compromise airway patency, which is only manifest with the passage of time. There are no defined guidelines for intervention in circumstances of airway obstruction that are mild or moderate, as management will depend on operator experience and unit practice.

POSTEXTUBATION STRIDOR

Postextubation stridor is not a common occurrence in paediatric anaesthesia. In 1977 the overall incidence was quoted as approximately 1%[37], but Litman in 1991,[38] using more defined criteria, cited an incidence of only 0.1% and attributed this difference to a change in practice and equipment. The relative size of the sub-glottic region in the infant predisposes this age group to extubation croup. The cricoid cartilage is the only circumferential ring in the trachea and intubation with a tracheal tube or endo-scope is capable of causing ischaemia of the mucosal lining with subsequent mucosal oedema after extubation. Resistance (R) to air flow in a tube varies inversely according to the fourth power of changes in the lumen radius (r), so that very small changes in r have a large influence on R.

A circumferential swelling of 1 mm in a small orifice of 4 mm in diameter, the diameter of the internal lumen of the cricoid will reduce the lumen by up to 70%, giving rise to stridor. Other factors in children that may predispose them to postextubation croup, apart from an oversized tube, may include unrecognized infec-tion, difficult or traumatic intubation, and frequent or excessive movement of a tracheal tube *in situ*. Patient factors include a past history of croup and Down's syndrome. Cohen's study on perioperative morbidity[2] found an incidence of postextubation croup of 0.87% in 22 760 patients, with the peak incidence in the 1–5-year-old group. This observation may suggest that in the newborn more care is taken, more experienced personnel are involved, or there are other unknown patient factors. In patients with Down's syn-drome, following a moderately prolonged anaesthetic and recovery,[39] the frequency of postextubation stridor was 38.4% compared with an overall incidence of 2.8%. Management of postextubation stridor consists of reviewing the cause or predisposing conditions. The possibility of foreign-body or other obstruction should be considered, especially if procedures have been performed on the head or neck. Routine laryngoscopy is not advised, but observation of the patient is essential to assess the degree of obstruction and any trend towards resolution or deterioration. Steroids and/or racemic adrenaline have been suggested in viral croup[40,41] and postextubation croup. Dexamethasone 0.25 mg kg^{-1} i.v. and/or neb-ulized 1% racemic adrenaline should be tried for moderate to severe postextubation croup.

Reintubation to relieve the airway obstruction in this situation is rarely required.

Pulmonary disorders

Aspiration syndrome

Unlike in obstetric practice, if acid aspiration syndrome is seen in children it is not associated with a significant mortality. In a retrospective study of 50 000 paediatric anaesthetics an approximate incidence of 1 : 1000 of this syn-drome was noted,[42] but because of the subtle course of mild aspiration in children this figure may be understated. Approximately 80% of the incidents occurred during induction and passive regurgitation was more common (50%) than active vomiting (40%). Among the different paediatric age groups aspiration was most common in children aged 6–11 years. Even in the more overt cases morbidity is slight in paediatrics; in the above series there was no mortality attributable to aspiration. Despite the best management aspiration will occur and may go unrecognized. Silent aspiration around cuffed tracheal tubes in adults was found to be 0–38.5%;[43] a higher incidence was noted in children with uncuffed tubes.[44] More recently, an increased risk of aspiration has been reported with the use of the laryngeal mask airway (LMA). It has been postulated that inflation of the cuff of the LMA in the pharynx causes distension and reduces the lower oesophageal sphincter tone, reducing the barrier pressure and leading to an increased risk of reflux.[45]

The damage caused by the inhalation of gastric contents can be divided into direct primary and secondary injury. Until recently, the emphasis of therapeutic manoeuvres has been directed towards the direct damage caused by strong acid and particulate matter which results in a combination of pneumonitis and obstruction. Contributory factors to morbidity include the agent used for anaesthesia[46] and excessive oxygen concentrations used in therapy.[47] Therapy has been directed towards strict adherence to fasting time, prophylactic treatment of patients at risk with antacids, H_2 receptor antagonists and/or the use of dopa-mine antagonists. If aspiration is recognized then effective suction or bronchoscopy for removal of particulate matter, if appropriate, is followed by supportive treatment of the pneumonitis with oxygen therapy, intubation and PEEP, or in the most severe cases intermittent positive pressure ventilation. Routine prophylactic antibiotics and steroids are not recommended presently. Of more interest is the secondary injury provoked by acid aspiration. Evidence is emerging that the pneumonitis seen with the acid aspiration syndrome is immunologically based.[48] Using animal studies it has been shown the neutrophils are the primary mediators of secondary lung and systemic organ injury. Acid aspiration into one lung causes injury of the contralateral lung as well as injury in the small intestine. Recombinant human soluble complement receptor I (sCR1) used in experimental treatment of this syndrome showed an 85% reduction in injury.[49]

Obstructive sleep apnoea

Patients in the recovery phase of an anaesthetic with a diagnosis of OSA are at risk of airway compromise. In the paediatric age group these patients are most often in recovery following adenotonsillectomy, as this procedure is an important indication for the treatment of OSA. The diagnosis and treatment of this condition may not be easy.[50,51] Often patients on an ENT list are given a diagnosis of OSA but do not meet the accepted criteria. Characteristically, the sleep-related apnoeas can be classified as obstructive, central or mixed. Obstruction is both anatomical and physiological. The physiological basis for the obstructive component of the syndrome lies in the decrease in tone of the pharyngeal dilator muscles with a resultant loss of patency of the pharyngeal airway during sleep (especially REM sleep) and anaesthesia. Importantly, during recovery, even trace levels of anaesthetics may have an effect.[52] The central component consists of an impaired ventilatory response to carbon dioxide in these patients, which is also further compromised by other respiratory depressants in the perioperative period. Immediately postoperatively, patients having an adenotonsillectomy for OSA may be significantly worse than before, as the obstruction caused by enlarged tonsils and adenoids is often only partially relieved after their removal and obstruction is further exacerbated by postoperative oedema, residual anaesthetic agents and narcotic analgesics. McColley et al.[53] noted that the incidence of respiratory compromise

needing intervention in children aged under 3 years was 52%, but in the short term the operation appeared effective in most patients. Preoperatively and postoperatively, these patients need to be assessed to determine whether they will be nursed and observed in a high-dependency unit or a normal ward. Monitoring with pulse oximetry is the minimal requirement. Analgesia presents a problem as adenotonsillectomy pain is often not relieved adequately by non-steroidal anti-inflammatory drugs and these patients are sensitive to the respiratory depressant effect of the opioids. Careful titration is advised to identify the minimal effective dose. A recent report of respiratory arrest in three adults 2–3 days postoperatively on a narcotic infusion highlights the risk involved.[54] Only very rarely following postoperative extubation of these patients will severe obstruction occur necessitating reintubation and admission to an ICU for respiratory care for a period of 24–48 h before attempted re-extubation. (See also Chapter 11.)

Postoperative apnoea in infants

Previously in this chapter, mention has been made of the influence of anaesthesia on the respiratory system of infants and in particular the preterm, which increases the risk of apnoea in the postoperative period. Ex-preterm infants at risk of postoperative apnoea, especially if on intravenous opioid infusion, must be admitted to and be nursed in a high-dependency area or an ICU. (See also Chapters 1 and 10.)

Apnoea is defined as the absence of air movement at the mouth or nose for 15 s or longer, but less than 15 s if bradycardia (heart rate below 100 beats min^{-1}) or desaturation (oxygen saturation less than 90%) occurs. Apnoea so defined for this section refers to idiopathic apnoea not overtly related to hypoxia, hypercapnia, drugs, hypothermia, hypoglycaemia, electrolytic disturbances or neurological disease.

Steward[55] alerted anaesthetists to the risk of respiratory complications, particularly apnoea following anaesthesia in ex-preterm infants. Since that time a number of investigators, including Wellborn et al.[56] and Kurth et al.[57], have provided information to evaluate the problem. Combined analysis by Coté et al.[58] and a review by Sims and Johnson[59] contribute to the following information.

- Postoperative apnoea is particularly likely in the preterm infant if the postconceptional age is 44 weeks or less.
- There are no reports of healthy former preterm infants aged over 52 weeks postconceptional age developing apnoea more than 2 h after minor surgery.
- No studies have reported the onset of apnoea occurring later than the first 12 h after surgery.
- Full-term infants may develop postoperative apnoea but are at a much lower risk. A lower age limit of 44 weeks postconceptional age takes into consideration the oldest reported case of apnoea in a term infant.

No doubt, in the future, reports will emerge of events occurring outside these time frames and the goalposts will have to be moved slightly. Each practitioner will have to consider each individual case and be guided by good clinical judgement. Other factors also influence the management process. Wellborn *et al.*[60,61] reported anaemia to increase the frequency of apnoea in preterm infants, but others have not confirmed this. Neurological disease makes postoperative apnoea more likely at an older postconceptional age and may also increase theincidence. The most common surgical procedure performed on these particular infants is inguinal herniorrhaphy. Wellborn *et al.*[62] found that the incidence of apnoea was zero using spinal anaesthesia, compared with a cohort given general anaesthesia, where the incidence approximated 30%. This safety margin for spinal anaesthesia may decrease if any inhalational or intravenous adjunct is administered.[63]

Both aminophylline 5 mg kg^{-1} and caffeine 5–10 mg kg^{-1} intravenously have been effective therapy for the treatment of apnoea of prematurity and, depending on availability, either is recommended for postoperative use. Any term or preterm infant perceived to be at risk of postoperative apnoea, regardless of anaesthetic management, must be monitored for apnoea for at least 12 h postoperatively in an appropriate environment.

CARDIOVASCULAR

Postoperative admissions to the ICU for cardiovascular reasons include:

1 all patients who have undergone cardiac surgery, even though nowadays many have a 'fast-track' pathway postoperatively;
2 any patient with underlying cardiac disease, such as cardiomyopathy or pulmonary hypertension, or who may have a previous history of a cardiac problem. Any patient with previously treated cardiac failure who develops sepsis, fluid shifts or dysrhythmias is at risk from sudden decompensation;
3 following cardiac arrest in the operating theatre from any cause it is mandatory to admit the patient to the ICU for therapy or observation. Causes of cardiac arrest in the operating theatre environment include respiratory obstruction, anaphylaxis, hypovolaemia and direct trauma during thoracic operations or hypertensive crisis. Ventilation of the lungs following cardiac arrest may reduce the risk of neurological damage;
4 any patient who has cardiovascular instability postoperatively, especially if a low cardiac output does not respond to a fluid challenge or if severe dysrhythmias require treatment;
5 unexpected admission to intensive care for cardiovascular instability after cardiac catheterization. These patients may be unstable preoperatively, have severe cardiac disease including pulmonary hypertension and may spend up to 4 h undergoing cardiac catheterization. During the procedure respiration may be compromised as a result of sedation or anaesthesia, and blood loss may be significant. Patients may become hypothermic because of inadequate heating facilities, and suffer multiple arrhythmias or even cardiac tamponade as a result of myocardial perforation. On admission to intensive care this last group of patients often needs more than observation and support.

NEUROLOGICAL

Head injuries in children remain a significant cause of morbidity and mortality, and those who require surgery should normally be admitted to the ICU postoperatively. In addition, if children with neurological disorders such as myasthenia gravis (described in Chapter 1) require surgery for any reason they may also need postoperative intensive care.

INITIAL INTENSIVE CARE MANAGEMENT

RESPIRATORY

Modes of respiratory support

Constant positive airway pressure (CPAP) refers to the maintenance of positive airway pressure throughout the respiratory cycle with no positive pressure breaths provided. This form of therapy may be used during the gradual initiation of or weaning from respiratory support. CPAP may be provided by a tracheal tube, nasopharyngeal CPAP, nasal prongs or a facemask

Tracheal CPAP is the most reliable method and provides control of the airway, but incurs all disadvantages of an indwelling tracheal tube. Nasopharyngeal CPAP is provided by withdrawing or inserting the tracheal tube into the nose or pharynx and is frequently used for neonates and small infants for obligatory nose breathers. The constancy of a given pressure is not as reliable as for tracheal CPAP but is usually very effective. Nasal prongs provide CPAP similar to nasopharyngeal application but are more prone to obstruction.[64] A facemask with a good seal fitted over the nose and mouth with pressure applied can be used to provide CPAP in co-operative individuals only, but not for long periods because of pressure sores.

All of the above methods of CPAP application may increase the work of breathing, all are capable of causing gastric distension with air and all increase the risk of aspiration. The effect of CPAP is to increase FRC or to maintain airway patency in patients with unstable airways, e.g. tracheomalacia or bronchomalacia.

Modes and methods of intermittent positive pressure ventilation (IPPV) are dealt with elsewhere (Chapter 11).

Weaning from respiratory support

The indications for initiation of weaning are the converse of those indications for interventional therapy. Rigid guidelines do not exist for the weaning process, but the following apply: the underlying disease process should show signs of improvement; the patient should be able to sustain spontaneous ventilation; the patient should be able to maintain adequate gas exchange; and close observation during the weaning process with the ability to reverse any incremental changes made as necessary. The weaning process should be initiated and expedited as soon as clinical indications exist, as discharge from intensive care at the earliest possible time is important for both clinical and economical reasons.

CARDIOVASCULAR

Volume expansion is the first manoeuvre in any hypotensive and hypoperfused child.

It is difficult to calculate or measure fluid deficits during an operative procedure. Suitable solutions include blood, albumin-containing solutions or other colloids and crystalloids. Because of the possible transmission of disease [e.g. hepatitis, acquired immunodeficiency syndrome (AIDS), unrecognized micro-organisms], blood transfusion has been rationalized to a situation of 'only if necessary'. Administration of blood will depend on the haematocrit limits tolerated by the patients. Children being relatively free of degenerative diseases do not have obstructive vascular lesions in the CNS and coronary vessels' resulting in uninterrupted blood flow and the ability to compensate for a decrease in haematocrit. Experience in managing patients with reduced haematocrits has been gained from Jehovah's Witnesses and the use of haemodilution techniques during cardiopulmonary bypass. Berry[65] calls this informed approach to the risk factors involved a judgement issue, and has given guidelines for acceptable haematocrits according to age (Table 11.3).

Berry qualifies these limits in that they are arbitrary and subject to change with more experience. If an underlying condition exists involving either the respiratory or cardiovascular system with limits to physiological change with the surgical challenge then the levels may need to be higher. Albumin 5% or the more recently introduced 4% is preferred for newborns as a volume expander, especially in situations such as gastroschisis where the loss of protein-rich fluid perioperatively may

Table 11.3 Normal and acceptable haematocrits in paediatric patients

Age group	Normal HCT		Acceptable HCT
	Mean	Range	
Premature	45	40–45	35
Newborn	54	45–65	30–35
3 months	36	30–42	25
1 year	38	34–42	20–25
6 years	38	35–43	20–25

approach 50% of the estimated circulating blood volume. Albumin-containing solutions have a longer half-life in the circulation compared with colloids. The preparation of human protein solutions presently is said to eliminate known infectious micro-organisms and particles. Colloids such as a haemaccel and dextrans are suitable alternatives to the more expensive albumin, especially in the older child. The latter two still suffer from a significant incidence of sensitivity reactions. As crystalloids rapidly equilibrate with extracellular fluid volume when used for blood replacement a volume three times the estimated blood loss should be infused. Hartmanns solution is not isotonic (256 mmol l^{-1}), so excessive volumes should not be used. Dextrose solutions effectively are metabolized to free water and may also result in hyperglycaemia, possibly augmenting brain damage in neurosurgical patients.[66]

Because of a relatively non-compliant ventricle in the newborn, central venous pressure measurement is difficult to interpret as a means of estimating volume state, and in the newborn and preterm infants, blood pressure is a better guide to adequacy of fluid replacement. Titrating aliquots of 20–30 ml kg^{-1} and appreciating the changes in haemodynamic status are appropriate therapy. From experience in renal patients it has been demonstrated that on administration of warm crystalloid over a 1-h period without any ongoing fluid loss, 100 ml kg^{-1} is well tolerated. In infants during treatment of fluid deficit it is always prudent to treat in excess of the estimated loss.

Treatment of heart failure includes respiratory support, which removes the work of breathing, ensures adequate oxygenation and is valuable cardiac support.

Ventricular function can be enhanced by modifying preload, afterload and contractility, and by the treatment of dysrhythmia. Preload is increased by a fluid challenge or decreased by fluid restriction, diuretics or the removal of fluid from body cavities. Afterload reduction is achieved with peripheral and pulmonary vasodilatation using drugs such as enoximone (a phosphodiesterase inhibitor which is also a positive inotropic agent), nitroglycerine or nitroprusside intravenously, or an angiotensin-converting enzyme inhibitor, such as captopril, orally. Inhaled nitric oxide (5–40 parts per million) is the current treatment for pulmonary hypertension. The use of various inotropic agents is discussed on p. 359, but includes drugs such as dopamine, dobutamine, isoprenaline and adrenaline. Improvements in cardiac output are seen with increasing pulse rate and blood pressure, a rise in peripheral temperature so that the gradient between core and periphery is less than 2°C, good urine output (more than 1 ml kg^{-1} h^{-1}), normal pulmonary gas exchange and acid–base status.

REFERENCES

1 Bosenberg, A.T., Bland, B.A.R., Schulte-Steinberg, O., *et al.* Thoracic epidural anesthesia via caudal route in children. *Anesthesiology* 1988; **69**: 265–9.

2 Cohen, M.M., Cameron, C.B. and Duncan, P.G. Pediatric anesthesia morbidity and mortality in the perioperative period. *Anesthesia and Analgesia* 1990; **70**: 160–7.

3 Glazener, C.H. and Motoyama, E.K. Hypoxemia after general anesthesia in children. *Anesthesiology* 1984; **61**: A416.

4 Tomkins, D.P., Gaukroger, P.B. and Bentley, M.W. Hypoxia in children following general anaesthesia. *Anaesthesia and Intensive Care* 1988; **16**: 177–81.

5 Cass, L.J. and Howard, R.F. Respiratory complications due to inadequate analgesia following thoracotomy in a neonate. *Anaesthesia* 1994; **49**: 879–80.

6 Tyler, D.C., Woodham, M., Stocks, J., *et al.* Oxygen saturation in children in the postoperative period. *Anesthesia and Analgesia* 1995; **80**: 14–19.

7 Hardcastle, W.J. The physiology of the larynx. In: *Physiology of Speech Production*. London: Academic, 1976; **4**: 63–4.

8 Henderson-Smart, D.J. and Read, D.J.C. Reduced lung volume during behavioural active sleep in the newborn. *Journal of Applied Physiology* 1979; **46**: 1081–1085.

9 Kosch, P.C. and Stark, A.R. Determination and homeostasis of the FRC in infants. *Physiologist* 1979; **22**: 71.

10 Mortola, J.P., Milic-Emili, J., Noworaj, A., *et al.* Muscle pressure and flow during expiration in infants. *American Review of Respiratory Diseases* 1983; **129**: 49–54.

11 Colin, A.A., Wohl, M.E.B., Mead, J., *et al.* Transition from dynamically maintained to relaxed end expiratory volume in human infants. *Journal of Applied Physiology* 1989; **67**: 2107–11.

12 Westbrook, P.R., Stubbs, S.E., Sessler, A.D., *et al.* Effects of anaesthesia and muscle paralysis on respiratory mechanics in normal man. *Journal of Applied Physiology* 1973; **34**: 81–6.

13 Motoyama, E.K., Brinkmeyer, S.D., Mutich, R.L., *et al.* Reduced FRC in anesthetized infants: effect of low PEEP [Abstract]. *Anesthesiology* 1982; **57** (3): A418.

14 Benameur, M., Goldman, M.D., Ecoffey, C., *et al.* Ventilation and thoraco-abdominal asynchrony during halothane anaesthesia in infants. *Journal of Applied Physiology* 1993; **74**: 1591–6.

15 Rigatto, H., Brady, J.P. and Torre Verduzco, R. Chemoreceptor reflexes in preterm infants I: the effect of gestational and post-natal age on the ventilatory response to inhalation of 100% and 15% oxygen. *Pediatrics* 1975; **55**: 604–13.

16 Rigatto, H. and Brady, J.P. Periodic breathing and apnoea in preterm infants I: evidence for hypoventilation, possibly due to central respiratory depression. *Paediatrics* 1972; **50**: 202–17.

17 Rigatto, H., Brady, J.P. and Torre Verduzco, R. Chemoreceptor reflexes in preterm infants II: the effects of gestation and post-natal age on the ventilatory response to inhaled carbon dioxide. *Pediatrics* 1975; **55**: 614–20.

18 Kelly, D.H., Stellwagen, L.M., Kaitz, E., *et al.* Apnea and periodic breathing in normal full term infants during the first twelve months. *Pediatric Pulmonology* 1985; **1**: 215–19.

19 Knill, R.L. and Gelb, A.W. Ventilatory response to hypoxia and hypercapnia during halothane sedation and anesthesia in man. *Anesthesiology* 1978; **49**: 244–51.

20 Dahan, A., Van den Elsen, M.J.L.J., Berkenbosch, A., *et al.* Effects of sub-anesthetic halothane on the ventilatory responses to hypercapnia and acute hypoxemia in healthy volunteers. *Anesthesiology* 1994; **80**: 727–38.

21 Knill, R.L., Manninen, P.H. and Clement, J.L. Ventilation and chemoreflexes during enflurane sedation and anaesthesia in man. *Canadian Anaesthetists Society Journal* 1979; **26**: 353–60.

22 Knill, R.L. and Kieraszewiczht-Dodgsen, B.G. Chemoregulation of ventilation during isoflurane sedation and anaesthesia in humans. *Canadian Anaesthetists Society Journal* 1983; **30**: 607–14.

23 Rowbotham, J.L. Do low dose inhalational agents alter ventilatory control? [Editorial]. *Anesthesiology* 1994; **80**: 723–6.

24 Polgar, G. and Kong, G.P. The nasal resistance of newborn infants. *Journal of Pediatrics* 1965; **67**: 557–67.

25 Butler, J. The work of breathing through the nose. *Clinical Science* 1960; **19**: 55.

26 Stocks, J. Effect of nasogastric tubes on nasal resistance during infancy. *Archives of Disease in Childhood* 1980; **55**: 17–21.

27 Reed, W.R., Roberts, J.L. and Thach, B.T. Factors influencing regional patency and configuration of the human infant upper airway. *Journal of Applied Physiology* 1985; **58**: 635–43.

28 Thach, B.T. and Stark, A.R. Spontaneous neck flexion and airway obstruction during apneic spells in preterm infants. *Journal of Pediatrics* 1979; **94**: 275–81.

29 Ochiai, R., Guthrie, R.D. and Motoyama, E.K. Differential sensitivity to halothane anesthesia of the genioglossus, intercostals and diaphragm in kittens. *Anesthesia and Analgesia* 1992; **74**: 338–44.

30 Pickens, D.L., Schefft, G.L. and Thach, B.T. Pharyngeal fluid clearance and aspiration preventative mechanisms in sleeping infants. *Journal of Applied Physiology* 1989; **66**: 1164–71.

31 Fogliani, J., Didier, G., Domenget, J.F., *et al.* Clinical surveillance of wakening from anaesthesia following 1006 regular operations. *Canadian Journal of Anaesthesia* 1982; **30**: 1003–18.

32 Burzstein, S., Taitelman, U., DeMyttenaere, S., *et al.* Reduced oxygen consumption in catabolic states with mechanical ventilation. *Critical Care Medicine* 1978; **6**: 162–4.

33 Field, S., Kelly, S.M. and Macklem, P.T. The oxygen cost of breathing in patients with cardiorespiratory disease. *American Review of Respiratory Disease* 1982; **126**: 9–13.

34 Fiastro, J.F., Habib, M.P. and Quan, S.F. Pressure support compensation for inspiratory work due to endotracheal tubes and demand CPAP. *Chest* 1988; **93**: 499–505.

35 Buda, A.J., Pinsky, M.R., Ingels, N.B., *et al.* Effects of intrathoracic pressure on left ventricular performance. *New England Journal of Medicine* 1979; **301**: 453–9.

36 Pinsky, M.R. and Summer, W.R. Cardiac augmentation biphasic high intrathoracic pressure support. *Chest* 1983; **84**: 370–5.

37 Koka, B.V., Jeon, I.S., Andre, J.M., *et al.* Post-intubation croup in children. *Anesthesia and Analgesia* 1977; **56**: 501–5.

38 Litman, R.S. and Keon, T.P. Post-intubation croup in children. *Anesthesiology* 1991; **75**: **6**: 1122–3.

39 Sherry, K.M. Post-extubation stridor in downs syndrome. *British Journal of Anaesthesia* 1983; **55**: 53–4.

40 Freezer, N., Butt, W. and Phelan, P. Steroids in croup: do they increase the incidence of successful extubation? *Anaesthesia and Intensive Care* 1990; **18**: 224–8.

41 Kuusela, A. and Vesikari, T. A randomised double blind placebo controlled trial of dexamethasone and racemic epinephrine in the treatment of croup. *Acta Paediatrica Scandinavia* 1988; **77**: 99–104.

42 Borland, L.M. Induction of anaesthesia and endotracheal intubation. In: Motoyama, E.K. and Davis, P.J. (eds). *Smith's Anaesthesia for Infants and Children*, 6th edn. New York: Mosby, 1996; 304.

43 Bernhardt WN, Cottrell JE, Sivakumaran C., *et al.* Adjustment of intracuff pressure to prevent aspiration. *Anesthesiology* 1979; **50**: 363–6.

44 Browning, D.H. and Graves, S.A. Incidence of aspiration with tracheal tubes in children. *Journal of Pediatrics* 1983; **102**: 582–4.

45 Rabey, P.G., Murphy, P.J., Langton, J.A., *et al.* Effect of the laryngeal mask airway on lower oesophageal sphincter pressure in patients during general anaesthesia. *British Journal of Anaesthesia* 1992; **69**: 346–8.

46 Nader-Djalal, N., Knight, P.R., Bacon, M.F., *et al.* Alterations in the course of acid induced lung injury in rats after general anesthesia; volatile anesthetics versus ketamine. *Anesthesia and Analgesia* 1998; **86**: 141–6.

47 Nader-Djalal, N., Knight, P.R., Davidson, B.A., *et al.* Hyperoxia exacerbates microvascular lung injury following aspiration. *Chest* 1997; **112**: 1607–14.

48 Nishizawa, H., Yamada, H., Miyazaki, H., *et al.* Soluble complement receptor type I inhibited the systemic organ injury caused by acid instillation into a lung. *Anesthesiology* 1996; **85**: 1120–8.

49 Weiser, M.R., Pechett, T., Williams, J.P., *et al.* Experimental murine acid aspiration injury is mediated by neutrophils and the alternative complement pathway. *Journal of Applied Physiology* 1997; **83**: 1090–5.

50 Aboussouan, L.S., Golish, J.A., Dinner, D.S., *et al.* Limitations and promise in the diagnosis and treatment of obstructive sleep apnoea. *Respiratory Medicine* 1997; **91**: 181–91.

51 Strohl, K.P., Cherniack, N.S. and Gothe, B. Physiologic basis of therapy for sleep apnea. *American Review of Respiratory Diseases* 1986; **134**: 791–802.

52 Hwang, J., St John, W.N. and Bartlett, D. Respiratory related hypoglossal nerve activity: influence of anaesthetics. *Journal of Applied Physiology* 1983; **55**: 785–92.

53 McColley, S.A., April, M.M., Carroll, J.L., *et al.* Respiratory compromise after adenotonsillectomy in children with obstructive sleep apnoea. *Archives of Otolaryngology, Head and Neck Surgery* 1992; **118**: 940–3.

54 Ostermeier, A.M., Roizen, M.F., Hautkappe, M., *et al.*Three sudden postoperative respiratory arrests associated with epidural opioids in patients with sleep apnea. *Anesthesia and Analgesia* 1997; **85**: 452–60.

55 Steward, D.J. Preterm infants are more prone to complications following minor surgery than are term infants. *Anesthesiology* 1982; **56**: 304–6.

56 Wellborn, L.G., Ramirez, N., Oh, T.H., *et al.* Post-anesthetic apnea and periodic breathing in infants. *Anesthesiology* 1986; **65**: 658–61.

57 Kurth, C.D., Spitzer, A.R., Broennle, A.M., *et al.* Postoperative apnea in preterm infants. *Anesthesiology* 1987; **66**: 483–8.

58 Coté, C.J., Zaslavsky, A., Downes, J.J., *et al.* Postoperative apnea in former preterm infants after inguinal herniorrhaphy. *Anesthesiology* 1995; **82**: 809–822.

59 Sims, C. and Johnson, C.M. Postoperative apnoea in infants (Review). *Anaesthesia and Intensive Care* 1994; **22**: 40–5.

60 Wellborn, L.G., Desotto, H., Hannallah, R.S., *et al.* The use of caffeine in the control of post-anesthetic apnea in former preterm infants. *Anesthesiology* 1988; **68**: 796–8.

61 Wellborn, H.G., Hannallah, R.S., Luban, N.L.G., *et al.* Anemia and postoperative apnea in former preterm infants. *Anesthesiology* 1991; **74**: 1003–6.

62 Wellborn, L.G., Rice, L.J., Hannallah, R.S., *et al.* Postoperative apnea in former preterm infants: prospective comparison of spinal and general anesthesia. *Anesthesiology* 1990; **72**: 838–42.

63 Sartorelli, K.H., Abajian, J.C., Kreutz, J.M., *et al.* Improved outcome utilising spinal anesthesia in high risk neonate. *Journal of Pediatric Surgery* 1992; **27**: 1022–5.

64 Kattwinkel, J., Fleming, D., Cha, C.C., *et al.* A device for administration of continuous positive airway pressure by nasal route. *Pediatrics* 1973; **52**: 131–4.

65 Berry, F. Fluid and electrolyte therapy in pediatrics. Annual Refresher Course Lectures, American Society of Anesthesiologists, 1997; **166**: 1–7.

66 Lanier, W.L., Strangland, K.G. and Scheithaur, B.W. Effects of dextrose infusion and head position on neurological outcome after complete cerebral ischaemia in primates: examination of a model. *Anesthesiology* 1987; **66**: 39–48.

CHAPTER 12

Pain management in children

RICHARD HOWARD AND ADRIAN LLOYD-THOMAS

INTRODUCTION

The undertreatment of children who were in pain following injury or operations[1,2] and medical illnesses[3] has been recognized. Inadequate treatment of neonates and premature babies was widespread.[4,5] However, the 1990s have seen physicians change wholly their perceptions of neonatal pain[6] and modern analgesic techniques have been refined for use in children.[7] These advances have been based on an increased understanding of the neurophysiology of pain,[8,9] combined with the concurrent development of clinical pain services,[10] as well as sophisticated analgesia delivery devices and monitoring protocols.[11] In view of the advances in fetal surgery consideration is now being given to pain perception by the fetus.[12–15]

THE NEUROBIOLOGY OF PAIN

The conscious perception of pain following injury or operations is reliant on the transmission of action potentials via the dorsal horn by nociceptive neurons.[16] Our understanding of the nociceptive system has been enhanced by the development of experimental models of postoperative pain transmission.[17,18] Action potentials arise from mechanical and heat stimuli, or from direct chemical activation (bradykinin, hydrogen ions, serotonin, histamine, prostaglandins, leukotrienes and thromboxanes).[19] The absence of full myelination in the neonatal and infant nervous system, including the poorly myelinated thalamocortical radiation, was thought to be an indicator of non-function.[20] It is, however, a reflection of immaturity, not an indication of lack of function. This has been shown by observation of responses to noxious stimuli, including movement,[21] cardiovascular variables,[22–24] facial expression[25–27] and crying.[28–30]

Nociceptive information from the periphery enters the dorsal horn to synapse with two types of secondary nociceptive neuron, the nociceptive specific neuron (NSN) and the wide dynamic range neuron (WDR). These neurons are themselves influenced by the convergence of multiple neural transmissions, including (1) nociceptive and non-nociceptive afferents (which may be excitatory or inhibitory), (2) local dorsal horn interneurons (also excitatory or inhibitory), and (3) descending inhibitory inputs from supraspinal sites.[31] The net result of these dorsal horn influences is the modulation of onward transmission in the spinothalamic tracts.

The neurophysiology of the immature nociceptive system is different. Experimental data suggest that the receptive field for each individual WDR neuron may be much larger in the immature nervous system of neonates and infants.[8] This implies that the younger patient cannot localize pain as accurately as the adult, and the corresponding perception of nociceptive sensation may be more widespread. In the newborn, non-nociceptive stimuli, carried by non-nociceptive fibres (Aβ), can give rise to the expression of c-fos in the dorsal horn. C-fos is an immediate early gene induced by noxious stimuli.[32] This suggests that neonatal low threshold fibres can activate laminae which are predominantly nociceptive in the adult (high threshold).[33] It may be that innocuous stimuli result in 'pain' perception in the very young. This may be further enhanced if hyperalgesia develops (see below).

The descending inhibitory pathways are less well developed, allowing unattenuated nociceptive input to the spinal cord.[34] Experimental data suggest that there may be differences in the proportion of subclasses of opioid receptors in neonates,[35] which may contribute to a reduced ability to modulate nociceptive transmission.[36]

The nervous system is plastic and the release of algogenic substances and transmitters[37,38] leads to sensitization of both peripheral nociceptors[39–42] and the dorsal horn.[43–46] Cell membrane damage in the periphery results in the production of prostaglandins via arachidonic acid, whilst repetitive C-fibre activity in the dorsal horn causes intracellular Ca^{2+} release which then also results in arachidonic acid production from membranes. In turn, by production of a stimulatory guanine nucleotide regulator protein (Gs),[39] the neuron becomes sensitized. Nitric oxide may be implicated in the facilitation of dorsal horn transmission.[47] C-fos expression by nociceptive afferent traffic[48] may be one factor in long-term structural and functional changes[49] consequent on unchecked afferent input. C-fos expression is reduced by opioids,[50] α_2 agonists and NMDA receptor antagonists.[46]

The clinical manifestation of these physiological mechanisms is the development of primary and secondary hyperalgesia, in which hypersensitivity gives rise to the sensation of pain consequent on non-nociceptive stimuli. Experimental data show that repetitive C-fibre activation results in (1) facilitation of the flexor motor neural responses, (2) expansion of receptive fields, and (3) a fall in the threshold of dorsal horn neurons.[31] In addition, Aβ (low-threshold) mechanoreceptors may gain access to nociceptive neurons by a presynaptic link in the dorsal horn, resulting in the development of allodynia.[51]

The ability of local anaesthesia,[52] N-methyl-d-aspartate (NMDA) antagonists[44,53,54] and opioids[55] to ameliorate the development of secondary hyperalgesia has given rise to the concept of pre-emptive treatment to stop this adaptation of thresholds according to input.[56] Combination therapy may have a further physiological basis, in that opioid receptors appear not to function in isolation, but also rely in part on other receptors such as NMDA to elicit their effects.[57] There are few data to suggest that these mechanisms are not fully functional in the neonate or infant, but in the experimental model receptor populations are different,[34] descending inhibitory pathways are less developed and NMDA-mediated effects are more marked in the immature nervous system.[8,57–59] This indicates that careful attention to pain control should be a part of all children's management.

PAIN MEMORY

Pain is a subjective experience. Given that memories of neonatal and early infant life are few, does pain perception matter? Older children (15–16 years) are able to recall with accuracy the extent and intensity of pain experiences.[60] Surgery before the age of 5 years may influence impulsivity and activity,[61] whilst painful experiences in very low birthweight infants may result in significantly higher somatosization scores.[62] Moreover, pain behaviour at immunization is adversely affected by prior noxious experience (circumcision) without any analgesia.[63,64] As well as these psychological changes, physical consequences of early noxious stimuli may be manifest in the dense cutaneous innervation seen in experimental models of early injury.[65]

PAIN ASSESSMENT

The difficulty of pain assessment in children has been part of the constraint on adequate analgesic therapy.[66] Substantial research has gone into the development of scores for behavioural observation[67–73] and self-report scales (Table 12.1). The fact that there are a multiplicity of scales suggests that there are numerous drawbacks and no ideal measure. In general, however, difficulties arise because of the cognitive development of children which renders certain assessment criteria invalid in the wide range of ages to be studied. Pain verbalization changes with age;[74] the specificity of respiratory and cardiovascular responses is low[75] (in particular, measures of oxygenation will be influenced by underlying pulmonary or cardiac pathology, whilst cry cannot be estimated in intubated patients receiving respiratory support); facial expression changes with age;[76] and postoperative behaviour may be blunted, leading to underestimation of pain.[77] Despite these shortcomings, it must be remembered that these parameters are a significant constituent of most behavioural observation scales, so caution is required in their use. If these tools are used with care and their limitations are realized, they can assist objective assessment.[78] In any research process, a careful choice of validated scale is essential, taking account of the setting in which the investigation is to be performed, the age of the subjects to be studied

and their underlying pathology. Comparisons between studies may be very difficult when different pain measurement tools are employed. Nevertheless, it is possible to make some suggestions: for neonates use CRIES (crying requires increased oxygen administration, increased vital signs, expression, sleeplessness),[72] for infants use OPS[71] and after the age of 5 years self-report scales with visual aids will provide a range of scores tailored to the age and understanding of the patient to be studied. If self-report is impractical, CHEOPS (Children's Hospital of Eastern Ontario pain score) can be employed.[78–80]

Although scales have their place in objective pain measurement, they should be employed as a part of the complex psychosocial processes involved in pain assessment. For everyday clinical work, assessment by an experienced nurse,[81] backed up by simple sedation and pain scales,[10,11] will afford sufficiently accurate measurements to direct therapy safely and effectively.[82]

PAIN CONTROL TEAMS

Physicians and nurses with special responsibility for postoperative pain control were first suggested by Ready *et al.*[83] and their introduction was supported by the Intercollegiate Report of 1990.[84] Clinical nurse specialists have a central role in pain control teams.[7] They are there to advise on patient management, to support ward nurses in their clinical pain decisions, to educate ward staff in all techniques of analgesia thereby ensuring patient safety and to facilitate prospective clinical audit.[7] A pain service should provide agreed protocols which are followed by all clinicians; the protocols should cover analgesic techniques, patient observations, control of side-effects and response to critical incidents (e.g. respiratory depression).

Patient observations should be undertaken hourly and should encompass assessment by pain and sedation scales, respiratory rate and volume of medication infused (Table 12.2).

Table 12.1 Summary of published neonatal pain assessment tools

Assessment tool	Applicability/notes	Pros	Cons
NFCS[42] (Neonatal Facial Coding System)	Yes/Tested in healthy neonates	Behavioural	Training required. 9-item descriptive tool
NIPS[21] (Neonatal Infant Pain Scale)	Yes/Validated in intensive care; 6-item (3-point) score	Behavioural. Can be used in premature neonates	Unsuitable for the very sick or paralysed
MNIPS[80] (Modified NIPS)	Yes/Not validated in equivalent settings to NIPS	Behavioural. Crying (from NIPS) is replaced by hand/finger tone	
PIPP[81] (Premature Infant Pain Profile)[a]	Yes/For intensive care and postoperative use		Possible too complex for routine clinical use. 7-item (4 points in each) score
LIDS[82] (Liverpool Infant Distress Scores)	Yes/Designed for postoperative pain	Observational	For scientific evaluation of different treatments. Complex 8-item (6 points in each) score
SBES[83] (Short Bedside Evaluation Score)	Yes/behavioural. Intended for acute pain. Preterm and term babies evaluated after heel lancing	Easy 5-item score	
OPS[84] (Objective Pain Scale)	Probably/For postoperative pain. Validated in older age groups, appearing robust	5 items of score appropriate to neonates	Requires blood pressure (BP) measurement
CRIES[87] [a] (see p. 319)	Yes/Used in postoperative intensive care setting	Some nurses preferred it to OPS. 5-item simple score	Unusable if unable to cry. Requires BP. O_2 measurements may mislead in those with cardiorespiratory disease
POPS[88] (Post-Operative Pain Scale)[a]	Probably/Described for use in children < 1 year old	Behavioural	10-item score, where a high value = comfort
DSVNI[90] (Distress Scale for Ventilated Newborn Infants)[a]	Yes/For use in ventilated neonates to guide analgesia	Routine observations: many physiological parameters only if monitoring is already *in situ*	7-item score
NACS[92] (Neurological and Adaptive Capacity Score)	Yes/Assesses pain, discomfort and neurobehaviour	Sensitive to drug effects, and straightforward. Useful in intensive care	Too long to remember (20 items, 3 points in each) score where a high value is normal.

[a]The possibility of intrathoracic shunts may complicate the assessment.

MULTIMODAL ANALGESIA

The increased understanding of pain transmission has underlined a need to use a wide spectrum of analgesic medications simultaneously for optimal patient management: this is the concept of 'balanced analgesia'.[85] A balanced technique of analgesia uses drugs that modify nociceptive transmission at different points in the pain pathway. Using single agents increases the incidence of unwanted effects as doses are raised to try and produce effective analgesia.[86] By approaching the pain pathway at different points, analgesia can be produced using minimal doses of drugs, thereby reducing side-effects.

Balanced analgesia not only implies the use of medication, but will also use the skills of nurses and parents in distraction techniques and other forms of comfort therapy. Furthermore, in babies, the administration of agents such as sucrose can have profound analgesic effects.[87,88]

PHARMACOLOGY OF ANALGESIC AGENTS

PARACETAMOL

This cornerstone of paediatric analgesia has been in use since the early twentieth century. Its mechanism of action remains uncertain, but seems to exert its analgesic and antipyretic effects centrally by inhibiting cyclo-oxygenase.[89] There is also a debate on the correct dosage for analgesia in children.[90] At present, by both the oral and rectal route, the maximum recommended dose of paracetamol is $90 \text{ mg kg}^{-1} \text{ day}^{-1}$, and less for a newborn.[82,91] Newborns form the reactive product responsible for liver damage by the glucuronide process even with a low level of cytochrome P450 system, but the rate constant for the sulphonation metabolic pathway is greater in the newborn than in adults and is the most important route of metabolism[92] The slower and more erratic absorption of paracetamol given by the

Table 12.2 Examples of pain and sedation scales

		Action (instructions in bold for Pain Service only)
Pain		
P1	Pain free	
P2	Comfortable except on moving	NCA: give bolus
		PCA: encourage bolus (10 min before activity)
P3	Uncomfortable	NCA: give bolus
		PCA: encourage bolus (10 min before activity).
		Contact Pain Service
		Epidural: increase rate
P4	Distressed but can be comforted	NCA: contact Pain Service
		PCA: give bolus or increase background infusion
		Encourage bolus, increase background infusion
		or shorten lockout interval
		Epidural: give bolus and/or increase rate
P5	Distressed	Contact Pain Service
Sedation		
S1	Awake	
S2	Drowsy	
S3	Asleep, but moves spontaneously	
S4	Asleep, responds to stimulation	Stop infusion until returns to level 3
S5	Hard to rouse	Stop infusion
		Call Pain Service

rectal route has led to recommendations for a longer dosing interval and larger dose (Table 12.3).[82,92,93] However, even this may still be conservative, as rectal loading doses of 35–45 mg kg^{-1} are required to achieve antipyretic plasma levels of 10–20 mg l^{-1} which are usually equated with the levels required for analgesia.[94–96]

However, even higher plasma levels (25 mg l^{-1}) are required to achieve satisfactory analgesia in 60% of children undergoing adenotonsillectomy.[96] In order to realize plasma levels of 25 mg l^{-1}, Anderson and Holford used a pharmacokinetic model to suggest rectal-loading doses of 70 mg kg^{-1} with maintenance doses of 50 mg kg^{-1} every 8 h. It should be noted that doses of 150 mg kg^{-1} day^{-1} are associated with reversible liver toxicity and these high doses need to be further investigated before they can possibly be recommended.[97] More conservatively, the same authors suggest that a rectal loading dose of 50 mg kg^{-1} and maintenance doses of 30 mg kg^{-1} every 6 h thereafter are needed to achieve reliable antipyretic plasma levels. The suggestion that larger doses of paracetamol are needed when using rectal administration in children is further supported by Lyn and co-workers,[98] who found that even in preterm neonates 20 mg kg^{-1} of rectal paracetamol resulted in low plasma levels. Although further research is needed to identify the optimum rectal dose and dosing interval, the doses of paracetamol suggested in Table 12.3 can be regarded as safe, but it may be necessary to increase these recommendations in the light of further research.

Rectal administration of paracetamol is chosen in children who are unable to take the medication orally. The advent of propacetamol, an intravenous preparation of a prodrug that hydrolyses to paracetamol, with a peak effect in 20 min, makes an injectable form of paracetamol a reality.[99] Intravenous propacetamol 1 g yields 0.5 g of paracetamol. Propacetamol (30 mg kg^{-1}) is an effective analgesic after orthopaedic surgery in children[100] and may have 'stronger' analgesic effect than equivalent doses of oral paracetamol. Studies in adults show a morphine-sparing effect.[101]

The traditional combination of paracetamol and codeine phosphate as an analgesic for acute pain must not be forgotten. Moore et al.,[102] in a meta-analysis of randomized trials identified that codeine added to paracetamol produces worthwhile additional pain relief, even in single oral doses. In children, codeine doses of 1 mg kg^{-1} on an 8-h basis can be combined with paracetamol.[103] Codeine is metabolized to morphine, which may be the mechanism of its

Table 12.3 Suggested doses of paracetamol and NSAIDs

	Loading dose (mg kg^{-1})	Maintenance dose (mg kg^{-1})	Dose interval (h)	Maximum daily dose (mg kg^{-1} 24 h^{-1})
Paracetamol				
Oral				
Antipyretic	20	10	4–6	Neonates 60 Infants 90
Analgesic	20	15–20	4–6	Children 90
Rectal				
Neonates	20	15		Neonates 60
Antipyretic	30	15	6–8	Infants 90
Analgesic	30	20	6–8	Children 90
Ibuprofen				
Oral	5	4–10	6–8	20
Diclofenac				
Oral		1[a]	8–12	3 mg kg^{-1}
Rectal		1[a]	8–12	150 mg day^{-1} (maximum)

The data follow the guidelines issued by the Working Party of the Royal College of Paediatrics and Child Health.[82]
[a]From 1 year.

analgesic action.[104] The minimal incidence of nausea and vomiting with codeine makes this medication useful in day-care surgery.

NON-STEROIDAL ANTI-INFLAMMATORY DRUGS

Prostaglandins sensitize and activate peripheral nociceptors to tissue agents such as bradykinin, released as a result of trauma.[105] Arachidonic acid is converted to prostaglandins by cyclo-oxygenase, an enzyme which is inhibited by non-steroidal anti-inflammatory drugs (NSAIDs). Peripheral analgesia occurs by reducing prostaglandin production, thereby ameliorating the development of primary hyperalgesia. NSAIDs also provide direct spinal analgesia by a similar mechanism,[106] namely, preventing the conversion of arachidonic acid to prostaglandins. Arachidonic acid is released in the dorsal horn following repetitive C-fibre impulses, as a result of peripheral nociceptor activity. In addition, unrelated to prostaglandins, NSAIDs inhibit the release of mediators of inflammation from neutrophils and macrophages.[107]

The inhibition of cyclo-oxygenase, however, is also responsible for unwanted NSAID effects; for example, reduced platelet aggregation, gastrointestinal haemorrhage and renal insufficiency. These side-effects are most commonly seen in adults with pre-existing disorders. Such pre-existing pathology is much less common in children, but if present, indicates that NSAIDs should be used with caution or withheld altogether. The syndrome of nasal polyposis, asthma and aspirin hypersensitivity (with which there may be NSAID cross-sensitivity) is very rare in children but is an absolute contra-indication to their use. Reversible airways obstruction, however, is increasingly common and there is often concern that NSAIDs may worsen asthma. A sensible approach is to avoid NSAIDs in those children receiving active asthma management (regular inhaled β-agonists with regular inhaled steroids or regular inhaled cromoglycate, oral steroid mediation, hospitalization for parental asthma therapy). Those having occasional therapy may receive NSAIDs used with caution, and parents must be advised to stop therapy if there is any deterioration in the child's symptoms.

Few data exist on the pharmacokinetics of NSAIDs in infants, although from the age of 3 months they are probably the same as in adults.[108] NSAIDs should be avoided in neonates in whom inhibition of renal prostaglandins, which cause vasodilatation, may reduce renal perfusion, thereby causing oliguria and fluid retention.

Two NSAIDs are useful in paediatric postoperative analgesia (Table 12.4), but in the UK only the suspension of ibuprofen is licensed for pain relief in children over the age of 6 months. Concern over antiplatelet activity in the perioperative period, particularly for adenotonsillectomy, can be avoided by administration at the end of surgery. The slow onset of NSAID analgesia (even intravenous ketorolac)[109] indicates that they are better used as prophylactic medication, given regularly for a fixed period, rather than as acute analgesics, a role to which opioids or local anaesthetic blocks are better suited. A suitable dose of diclofenac is 1–3 mg kg^{-1} day^{-1} in divided doses, e.g. every 8 h. The regular administration of NSAIDs may help to reduce morphine consumption; moreover, some data in adults suggest that ketoprofen (an NSAID) may reduce susceptibility to morphine-induced respiratory de-

Table 12.4 NSAID dosage and preparations

Dose	Preparations	Frequency
Ibuprofen 5 mg kg^{-1} dose^{-1}	*Oral suspension* 20 mg ml^{-1} *Tablets* 200 mg 400 mg 600 mg	6–8 hourly
Diclofenac 1 mg kg^{-1} dose^{-1}	*Tablets* 25 mg 50 mg *Dispersible tabs* 50 mg *Suppositories* 12.5 mg 25 mg 50 mg 100 mg	8 hourly

pression.[110] Paracetamol and NSAIDs are vital supplemental analgesics when using local anaesthesia in paediatric pain control. The combination of local anaesthesia with general anaesthesia is a common, effective and safe approach to pain management in children.[111]

LOCAL ANAESTHETICS

The ability of neonates and infants to metabolize local anaesthetic drugs is of concern when using these agents in very young patients. Indeed, there have been several reports of toxicity from local anaesthetics,[112,113] especially when they are given by continuous infusion,[114–117] although high doses of local anaesthetics were used in some of these reports (see also p. 258).

METABOLISM AND CLEARANCE

Amide local anaesthetics undergo dealkylation, hydroxylation and conjugation. There are few studies on the hepatic handling of local anaesthetic drugs in neonates, although some data suggest a limitation of capacity in comparison with older children.[118] The extensive data available for narcotics are much needed for local anaesthetic agents.

The metabolic half-life of local anaesthetics ($t_{1/2\beta}$) is longer in neonates and infants than in adults; however, the clearance of bupivacaine is higher;[119] moreover, the volume of distribution is much larger.[119,121,122] The prolonged half-life seen in neonates and infants may in part be due to this larger volume of distribution, as $t_{1/2\beta} = 0.693 \times$ volume of distribution (VD)/clearance (CL).[118]

Plasma levels seen following local anaesthetic injections may also be influenced by the age of the recipient. Potentially toxic levels were recorded in some infants of 10–15 kg body weight who received an ilioinguinal–iliohypogastric nerve block, even though the dose administered (1.25 mg kg^{-1} of 0.5% bupivacaine) was both conservative and carefully calculated according to patient weight.[123] The comparator group in this study (15–30 kg) did not have high plasma levels.[123] This effect, which requires confirmation by other groups, may be due to (1) an increased cardiac output with more rapid absorption, (2) decreased tissue binding of local anaesthetic, or (3) delayed metabolism in the younger patients. Absolute plasma levels are not the only factor in the manifestation of toxicity to local anaesthetics (vide below), but these data support the general principle of using cautious doses of all local anaesthetics in young patients.

Our present understanding suggests that carefully administered 'single-shot' blocks are likely to be safe, but accumulation is a significant hazard in neonates and infants receiving continuous local anaesthetic infusions. Careful titration of dose to effect is mandatory when infusions are employed.[124,125]

TOXICITY

The toxicity of a local anaesthetic drug is dependent on (1) the rate of rise of plasma local anaesthetic concentration, (2) protein binding of local anaesthetic agent, and hence free drug concentration, (3) concurrent use of central nervous system depressants, and (4) immaturity of the blood–brain barrier.[118] Local anaesthetics bind to plasma proteins. In particular, they bind to α_1-acid glycoprotein (AAG) and albumin,[126] with the majority of the drug being bound to the former. Lerman and co-workers showed that AAG levels were present in low concentrations in the neonate and infant of less than 3–6 months of age. As a consequence, the free fraction of lignocaine was inversely proportional to the AAG level.[126] Moreover, the degree of protein binding is determined by the plasma pH; acidosis causes an increase in the free fraction of drug in plasma.[118] The combination of acidosis and low protein binding may lead to high plasma-free local anaesthetic levels with a consequent risk of central nervous system (CNS) or cardiovascular (CVS) toxicity. Surgical 'stress' may also influence AAG levels, causing an increase which may be protective, although even maximally elevated AAG levels will be less than those seen in adults; however, any increase is unpredictable and will not be seen in the very sick patient who is most at risk of toxicity.[127] It is clear that these drugs need to be used with care in the very young, and dosage recommendations will be presented during consideration of the individual blocks.

TREATMENT OF TOXICITY

Toxicity from local anaesthetic drugs may result in CNS or CVS symptoms and signs. Somnolence, heaviness of the head and impaired postural ability are early signs of CNS toxicity, which can then progress to perioral paraesthesiae, tinnitus, visual disturbance, dysarthria and eventually convulsions.[128] Regional anaesthesia is most often performed in the anaesthetized child,[129,130] which renders these symptoms and signs useless. Indeed, cardiac arrhythmia or CVS collapse may be the first sign of local anaesthetic toxicity in a child. Extrasystoles, broadening of the QRS complex, ventricular tachycardia and fibrillation may all occur, especially with the longer acting agents.[113,131]

Basic life support is the first step in the management of local anaesthetic toxicity; this should include the correction of any acidosis. CNS toxicity (convulsions) can be treated with diazepam or midazolam, although concern has been expressed over the displacement of local anaesthetic from plasma proteins by competition from benzodiazepines.[118] Short-acting neuromuscular blockade, with ventilatory support, may help to reduce the acidaemia consequent on convulsive activity.[132]

By contrast, CVS toxicity is more difficult to treat. There are four potential mechanisms of cardiotoxicity and a wide range of therapeutic options is described, including lignocaine, adrenaline, bretylium and amiodarone.[118] In an experimental study, a combination of clonidine and dobutamine was shown to be effective in correcting bupivacaine-induced cardiotoxicity.[133] More recently, intravenous phenytoin 5 mg kg^{-1} repeated at 5-min intervals to a maximum of 15 mg kg^{-1} has been effective in aborting bupivacaine-induced ventricular tachydysrrhythmias in two neonates and is now thought to be the treatment of choice.[113]

Careful attention to technique and careful use of minimal doses should ensure the lowest risk of toxicity from long-acting local anaesthetics. Ropivacaine[133] and laevo-bupivacaine may be less prone to cause CVS toxicity and further data are required on the side-effect profile of these drugs in young patients.

OPIOID ANALGESICS

Many opioids have been used in children, but the extensive experience with morphine means that it remains the drug of choice for postoperative analgesia in most children following major surgery.

MORPHINE PHARMACOKINETICS

The metabolism and pharmacokinetics of all opioids, apart from remifentanil, alter with age. The developmental aspects of morphine metabolism have been the subject of excellent reviews.[134–137] In essence, glucuronidation is the main metabolic pathway for morphine even in very premature neonates. The ability to glucuronidate is diminished by immature liver enzymes (cytochrome P450). As a result, plasma ratios of M3G : morphine and M6G : morphine are reduced in neonates and young infants, when compared with older children or adults. The ratio of metabolites (M6G : M3G) increases with decreasing birth weight.[138] Morphine half-life is prolonged in the very young (preterm: 9 ± 3.4, term: 6.5 ± 2.8 and infants: 2 ± 1.8 h); the volume of distribution is increased and the clearance is reduced.[135] Surgery and critical illness will further distort the pharmacokinetic picture in these babies.[139,140] Birth weight, gestational age and postnatal age influence the ability of the liver to glucuronidate. However, all studies have shown wide variance between subjects, such that a mature, healthy term neonate of 2 weeks of age may have morphine metabolism, clearance and half-life figures similar to an adult, whilst another infant of 6 weeks of age may still have immature metabolism and a long half-life.

Protein binding is also reduced in infancy and the neonatal period,[138,141,142] with as little as 18–22% of morphine being bound in early life compared with 20–35% in adulthood.[142] This may lead to more free drug being available in plasma to bind to opioid receptors. The percentage protein binding varies from opioid to opioid. Alfentanil and fentanyl are bound to a much greater extent than morphine (79% and 70% respectively, in term neonates).[143] Although increasing prematurity is usually associated with less protein binding, Wilson *et al.*[143] found that preterm infants had more fentanyl bound than term infants (77% vs 70%), but the general rule was adhered to by alfentanil (79% vs 65%). It should be remembered that plasma pH may play a role in determining protein binding for basic drugs such as fentanyl (pK_a 8.43).

GENERAL PRINCIPLES OF POSTOPERATIVE PAIN MANAGEMENT

A considerable amount of information is now available regarding children's pain and its treatment which must be assimilated and adapted for clinical use. In most circumstances it is the paediatric anaesthetist on whom the responsibility for postoperative pain management devolves. Nursing staff in the postoperative recovery room and in ward areas play an important role in the assessment and delivery of analgesia but they can only be effective if they are given adequate support. The plan of postoperative analgesia should be part of the anaesthetic management plan, and preferably supported by a written protocol. In order that the quality of care is maintained, audit of outcomes should be undertaken and protocols amended from time to time. Protocols may be specific for a surgical procedure, patient category or a technique of analgesia such as patient-controlled analgesia (PCA) or epidural infusion. All personnel involved should be aware of the protocol, and it should be available for consultation at the bedside or nearby. A record of postoperative analgesia should be kept, which might include the protocol, prescription and details of patient observations or outcomes such as pain score, sedation score and cardiorespiratory parameters (Table 12.2).

The side-effects of a technique should be anticipated and promptly treated; if this is to be done by nursing staff the correct prescriptions and procedures to be followed must be available. As successful pain management requires a considerable amount of organization it is most easily accomplished within the framework of an acute pain service or team (see above). The team can function as facilitator, resource and monitor of good pain management.

The aim of postoperative pain therapy is to provide subjective comfort while enhancing the restoration of normal function.[144] Treatment using drugs from several therapeutic groups is generally indicated as part of a multimodal approach, typically paracetamol and an NSAID, local anaesthesia with or without an opioid, α-agonist or NMDA receptor antagonist.

The choice of postoperative analgesia is influenced by the technique of anaesthesia used, the complexity and duration of surgery, the expected severity of pain, and the expected duration of postoperative gastrointestinal inactivity. Patient-related factors must also be considered, including the age, physical status, developmental level and any individual special needs. The availability of equipment and facilities for postoperative care are also important.

MILD AND MODERATE POSTOPERATIVE PAIN

Many procedures performed on children are now planned on an outpatient basis. This is economic and minimizes disruption for patients and their families. One of the prerequisites of discharge on the day of surgery is that the child should be fully recovered from anaesthesia, free from pain and not suffering from potentially dangerous or incapacitating side-effects.[144] Any persistent pain should be amenable to treatment at home and parents should be given clear instructions and prescriptions or, preferably, suitable analgesics to take with them. There is evidence that parents tend to undertreat postoperative pain at home and they should be advised to administer simple analgesics on a regular basis.[145] Certain procedures, particularly circumcision, tonsillectomy and strabismus surgery, are associated with significant pain on the operative and subsequent days.[146,147] Local anaesthesia, NSAIDs and paracetamol do not potentiate general anaesthetics or cause nausea and vomiting and so are very suitable for this type of surgery.

Local anaesthesia

Local anaesthetic drugs reversibly block pain impulse conduction, often with little or no effect on other physiological systems. In particular, the sedative and depressant effects of general anaesthetic drugs are not potentiated when local anaesthetics are used correctly and this gives them an enormous advantage, particularly in very young patients and for day care. A disadvantage is that usually these agents must be injected and therefore given initially under general anaesthesia and cannot be repeated after surgery. Bupivacaine is currently the most widely used local anaesthetic in paediatric practice, because its long duration of action is particularly useful. Unfortunately, both neuro-toxicity and cardiotoxicity have been described with this agent and so care should be taken that recommended dosages are not exceeded.[128,148] The newer drug, ropivacaine, which is structurally similar, has many of the therapeutic properties of bupivacaine with lower reported toxicity. Ropivacaine appears to be suitable for paediatric use and initial reports are encouraging with significantly less motor block.[149] The purified optical isomer of bupivacaine, l-bupivacaine, is also interesting, with a higher therapeutic ratio than the mixture of both isomers. Local anaesthetics can be incorporated into timed-release delivery systems such as liposomes and polymers. This raises the possibility of a very long duration of action from a single injection, although no preparation for clinical use is available at present.[150]

Topical preparations of local anaesthetics have become very popular for short or minor procedures such as venepuncture, lumbar puncture and various biopsies including renal biopsy.[151,152] Commercially available preparations are EMLA, a eutectic (lowest melting point) mixture of lignocaine and prilocaine, and Ametop, an aqueous suspension of amethocaine. EMLA has also been used for post-circumcision pain, and for its anti-inflammatory and analgesic effect in burned patients.[153–155]

Subcutaneous infiltration of the incision with local anaesthetic at the end of surgery can provide significant analgesia in the early postoperative period.[156–158] The technique is useful when other forms of local analgesia have not been used. It is simple to perform and relatively non-invasive. Plasma concentrations of local anaesthetic are low and well below toxic levels.[159] It may be an underutilized technique as it can easily be forgotten at the end of a procedure. Infiltration of the tonsillar bed with bupivacaine has been described and this reduces early postoperative pain after tonsillectomy.[160]

Specific nerve blocks and caudal analgesia

A large number of blocks of individual and groups of nerves has now been described in children, as discussed in detail in Chapter 9. They are most often performed just after induction of anaesthesia and they generally make an important contribution to postoperative analgesia, particularly in the early phase.[161,162]

Some of the most frequently used blocks for moderately painful procedures and in day surgery are shown in Table 12.5. Combining a perioperative local block with an NSAID and paracetamol will reduce and may frequently obviate the need for opioids in some common paediatric procedures, e.g. inguinal hernia, umbilical hernia or orchidopexy.[163–165]

Table 12.5 Commonly performed nerve blocks

Local block	Nerves anaesthetized	Surgical procedures
Inguinal	Ilioinguinal nerve and iliohypogastric nerve	Inguinal hernia repair Orchidopexy
Penile	Dorsal nerves of penis	Circumcision Hypospadias repair
Axillary	Brachial plexus	Arm and hand surgery
Femoral	Femoral nerve	Surgery to femur and thigh
Caudal	Volume dependent	Surgery below umbilicus

Caudal block is suitable for most surgery below the level of the umbilicus (10th thoracic dermatome). The number of dermatomes blocked by this technique depends on the volume of local anaesthetic injected and various formulae have been suggested in order to calculate the correct dosage.[166–168] A single injection of bupivacaine will last for 4–6 h, by which time oral medication should be tolerated after most minor surgery. Leg weakness can occur after caudal block, femoral nerve blocks and occasionally after inguinal blocks. This side-effect should be noted, although it should not delay discharge in the younger patient and should be less frequent in the future with newer drugs such as ropivacaine.

Paracetamol is a very safe mild analgesic and antipyretic and is probably the most widely used in paediatrics. It can be used in all ages and is available in convenient oral, rectal and, in some countries, parenteral formulations (see above). It does not have a significant anti-inflammatory effect and can be used logically and effectively in conjunction with the NSAIDs, local anaesthetics and opioids. Traditionally, it has often been combined with the low-potency opioid codeine, with good effect.[172,173] A suggested oral absorption of paracetamol is excellent and complete within 60 min. It is available as a suspension and in tablet formulation. Oral dosage is 20 mg kg^{-1} loading dose and 15 mg kg^{-1} maintenance every 4–6 h with a daily maximum of 90 mg kg^{-1} (reduced to 60 mg kg^{-1} in neonates).

Rectal administration results in slow and somewhat erratic absorption and so should be used in higher dosage and less frequently. Suppositories are generally available in doses of 60 mg, 120 mg, 240 mg, 500 mg and 1 g. A loading dose of 30 mg kg^{-1} is recommended, with maintenance doses of 20 mg kg^{-1}, daily maxima as above and a dosing interval of at least 6 h. These doses should probably be reduced in neonates to 20 mg kg^{-1} and 15 mg kg^{-1}, respectively. Propacetamol (see above), the parenteral form of paracetamol, is a prodrug which is metabolized to paracetamol.[170] It is a potentially useful agent which, at the time of writing, has only limited availability in some countries.[101]

NSAIDs, currently ibuprofen and diclofenac, are the most commonly recommended for use in children (Table 12.4). Many others have been used in various situations, including indomethacin, ketorolac, ketoprofen and flubiprofen. Aspirin should not be used in children under 12 years old, owing to the known association with Reye's syndrome.[171,174]

The NSAIDs are effective for mild to moderate postoperative pain and unlike paracetamol and opioids also have marked anti-inflammatory properties. The NSAIDs produce significant postoperative analgesia and are also known to have an opioid-sparing effect.[109] The incidence of postoperative nausea and vomiting (PONV) is lower with NSAIDs than with opioids and a number of convenient formulations of this group of drugs is available. Suppositories are particularly useful, especially if given early after induction of anaesthesia. Potent NSAIDs are effective alone for pain after minor procedures, particularly ENT surgery, dental procedures and some minor orthopaedics. NSAIDs should not be combined with each other, but logically they can be used in combination with local anaesthesia, paracetamol and the opioids.[173,174]

Although this group of drugs is regarded as generally very safe for short-term use, they should be used with caution in patients with severe asthma or renal impairment and they are not generally prescribed for neonates (see above).

PAIN AFTER MAJOR SURGERY

Opioids

Opioids, despite their potentially serious side-effects, are the mainstay in the management of severe postoperative pain and considerable experience has now been gained in their safe use, even in the very young. The maximum analgesia that can be obtained varies from drug to drug; the moderate-potency codeine and high-potency morphine are the most widely used in paediatric practice, although codeine must not be given intravenously.[175] Codeine is often used for pain associated with head injury and after neurosurgery as it causes minimal interference with physical signs of increasing intracranial pressure.[176]

Opioids are effective by all routes, although major differences in bioavailability are apparent. Parenteral administration is generally required postoperatively and has the most predictable effects. Intravenous and subcutaneous infusion can be recommended but intramuscular injection, although effective, is no longer employed routinely. Whatever the route, the principal side-effects of opioids are nausea and vomiting, sedation, respiratory depression, pruritus and constipation. Pruritus is not usually troublesome in short-term postoperative use, unless the epidural or intrathecal route is employed. Constipation normally only occurs after several days' treatment. Tolerance, addiction and dependence can also occur with opioids but are rare in the postoperative situation.

Oral and sublingual

Generally speaking, the oral bioavailability of opioids is low, with the exception of codeine, which is largely metabolized to morphine by whichever route it is given.[177] Several oral preparations of morphine are available which are commonly used for certain chronic painful conditions and in palliative care. Buprenorphine, a partial agonist, is available in a sublingual presentation which can be useful in older children.[178–180] Buprenorphine has a high affinity for the opioid receptor and can be difficult to reverse with naloxone.[181]

Parenteral administration

Morphine is the drug of choice for postoperative infusion in children. It is given as a continuous infusion with or without the modification of extra bolus injections when required. Children older than 5 years can use PCA devices to self-administer morphine, although some modifications may be required to equipment and programming. Younger children may benefit from nurse-controlled analgesia (NCA), nurse-administered boluses as a supplement to a continuous infusion. Both intravenous and subcutaneous routes are satisfactory for infusion. Dosages and typical preparations are:

- continuous infusion: morphine sulphate 10–30 μg kg^{-1} h^{-1} as required;
- intravenous preparation: morphine 1 mg kg^{-1} in 50 ml 5% dextrose rate 0.5–1.5 ml h^{-1};

- subcutaneous preparation: morphine 1 mg kg^{-1} in 20 ml 5% dextrose rate 0.2–0.6 ml h^{-1}.

Nurse-controlled analgesia

NCA is a modified morphine infusion using PCA technology. It is suitable for all children who are either too young or unable to use PCA. A continuous infusion of morphine in the range 10–20 μg kg^{-1} h^{-1} is given together with the option for nursing staff to administer extra boluses of 10–20 μg kg^{-1} two or three times an hour. NCA can be used either intravenously or subcutaneously using the preparations described above. NCA programming is shown in Table 12.6. When NCA is employed it is important to emphasize that extra boluses are to be given by the primary nurse alone. Parents, and if possible the patients themselves should be consulted about the timing and need for analgesia in NCA.

Patient-controlled analgesia

PCA can be used for the majority of children above the age of 5 years. Sometimes even younger patients are able to understand the concept and operate the equipment. Although standard handsets are usually satisfactory, a number has been designed especially for children. Preoperative instruction is always profitable and frequent reminders can be necessary, particularly in the early postoperative phase. Despite the temptation to do otherwise, it is essential for safety in this technique that all concerned understand that only the patient should operate the handset. A small background infusion is beneficial in children, improving the quality of analgesia and duration of night-time sleep, and reduces the incidence of PONV.[182,183] When compared with intermittent injection or simple infusion the total dose of morphine received is generally larger, quality of analgesia is improved and side-effects are slightly increased.[184,185] Although PCA is generally safe, serious respiration depression has been reported, equipment malfunction can also occur and the use of antireflux and antisyphon valves is recommended.[186] PCA can be either intravenous or subcutaneous. Recommended programming is shown in Table 12.6.

Table 12.6 PCA and NCA programming

	Loading dose (μg kg^{-1})	Back-ground infusion (μg kg^{-1})	Bolus dose (μg kg^{-1})	Lockout min.
NCA	50 or 100	< 20	10 or 20	20 or 30
PCA	50 or 100	0 or 4	10 or 20	5 or 10

OPIOID SIDE-EFFECTS AND MONITORING

Nausea and vomiting (PONV), sedation and respiratory depression are all seen with opioid use. When these drugs are continuously infused the potential for side-effects is obviously increased. Frequent assessments by experienced nursing staff will identify complications early and allow appropriate treatment to be instigated. Ideally, as well as basic cardiorespiratory parameters and pain score, sedation, nausea and vomiting and possibly oxygen saturation in air should be recorded.[187] Antiemetics should be prescribed and naloxone (4 μg kg^{-1}) administered if an emergency situation arises, for example if a preselected minimum respiratory rate is reached.

The location for nursing patients with epidural and morphine infusions is controversial and local preferences should prevail. However, if the patients are undergoing regular assessments of pain and sedation using simple 5-point scales and are under the overall care of a pain service, the nursing on the ordinary postoperative surgical ward should be safe.

LOCAL ANAESTHESIA FOLLOWING MAJOR SURGERY

Maximum doses of local anaesthetics are quickly reached when large areas of the body must be covered. Although they are effective, wound infiltration and field blocks are limited by the potential for local anaesthetic toxicity. Infusions of local anaesthetics through catheters are popular but must also take account of maximum dosages and the rate of absorption from the site of infusion. For these reasons central nerve blocks are the most favoured techniques after major surgery. Other approaches have their advocates: for example,

continuous paravertebral block has been used for abdominal surgery in children, with satisfactory results.[188,189] Intrapleural block has also been described and it has even been used in low birth-weight infants, although there has been some concern about potential rapid absorption and subsequent toxic plasma levels of local anaesthetic from this area.[190,191]

EPIDURAL ANALGESIA

The epidural space is very accessible in children and thoracic, lumbar, trans-sacral and caudal techniques have been described. Single injections into the epidural space have the advantage of allowing extensive analgesia with a low dose of local anaesthetic relative to more superficial nerve blocks. Their effect in the postoperative period has been extended by the addition of other drugs, such as opioids, clonidine and ketamine, with reasonable success after moderately painful surgery. The use of a catheter in the epidural space is common and it can be left safely *in situ* for some time.

The caudal epidural has an important place in paediatric practice, being easy to learn, simple to perform, versatile and very safe.[192] Traditionally, it has been used for perineal and urological surgery, but the technique can be used for most surgery below the level of the umbilicus and especially for major surgery in the lower abdominal, perineal and genital areas, such as bladder exstrophy, epispadias and genitoplasty. The number of segments blocked depends on the volume of solution injected and is discussed above and in Chapter 9. Caudal catheters for use following major surgery have been described and it is possible to thread a catheter as far as thoracic dermatomes in neonates and small infants, allowing postoperative analgesia for thoracotomy or upper abdominal surgery.[193] This technique is particularly suitable when direct lumbar or thoracic approaches are found to be technically too difficult.

THORACIC, LUMBAR AND TRANS-SACRAL EPIDURALS

'Single-shot' and continuous epidural blocks have been described in children, and several large series have been reported, with continuous lumbar epidural block now being employed routinely in most major centres around the world.[194-196]

Insertion technique

Although fundamentally similar to that used in adult practice, the following points should be remembered, which will help in the postoperative period.

1 Asepsis: a strict aseptic technique should be observed and the catheter should be securely fixed such that the insertion site can be easily observed in the postoperative period. The potential for contamination is high in infants, particularly if the catheter is in the nappy area. If redness, swelling or pus is observed, the catheter should be removed and micro-biological culture performed.[197]

2 Loss of resistance technique: the skin–epidural distance is short; indeed, it may be less than 0.5 cm in a newborn baby. The ligamentum flavum is softer and may not easily be detected, so a technique using continuous pressure on the syringe plunger should be employed. Saline rather than air has been particularly recommended in children, both to reduce the likelihood of inadvertent air embolus and to prevent air pockets from impeding even spread of the local anaesthetic, although this remains controversial (see Chapter 9).[198,199]

3 Length of catheter in the epidural space: catheters are easily dislodged in children even when securely fixed, at least 3 or 4 cm left in the space will reduce the incidence of this complication.

4 Site of epidural: although it is most convenient to access the epidural space close to the dermatomes to be blocked, the relatively short and straight spine in children, particu-

larly those weighing less than 10 kg, will allow a catheter to be threaded to the required level.

Bupivacaine or its equivalent is the drug of choice, and a suitable regime is:

- initial dose, lumbar or sacral level: bupivacaine 0.25%, 0.75 ml kg^{-1}, maximum 15 ml;
- thoracic: bupivacaine 0.25%, 0.5 ml kg^{-1}, maximum 10 ml.

Further incremental doses can be given as required. For postoperative use more dilute solutions are suitable as minimal motor block is required. Analgesia is improved and tachyphylaxis avoided by combination with an opioid; diamorphine, morphine and fentanyl have been used successfully. There is some evidence that ropivacaine might be effective alone as it can be used in higher concentration without motor block and has a better therapeutic ratio.[149] A regime for bupivacaine/morphine is:

- preparation: bupivacaine 0.125% + morphine sulphate (preservative free) 0.001%;
- infusion rate: neonates, 0.1–0.2 ml kg^{-1} h^{-1}; older children, 0.1–0.4 ml kg^{-1} h^{-1}.

The infusion can be continued for 2 or 3 days as required, reducing the rate daily provided that analgesia is satisfactory.

Side-effects

The principal side-effects are attributable to the opioid, being itching, nausea and vomiting, urinary retention and rarely respiratory depression, although more serious complications have been described, including permanent neurological deficit.[200] It is common to prescribe antiemetics, antipruritics and naloxone to be given if necessary. The technique is subject to a relatively high technical failure rate which discourages its use except where strong indications are present (Table 12.7) and a risk–benefit analysis should be considered for individual patients.[201,202]

Monitoring

The principal requirement is for skilled nursing and the availability of an anaesthetist familiar with the management of continuous epidurals. In most instances the nurse : patient ratio

Table 12.7 Indications for continuous postoperative epidural analgesia

Major/extensive surgery
Thoracic surgery
Surgery leading to respiratory compromise
Pre-existing significant respiratory disease
Poor previous experience of opioid analgesia

should be 2 : 1 or better. Minimum levels of monitoring should include hourly observations of pulse, respiration, blood pressure, level of sedation and analgesia score (Table 12.2).

MANAGEMENT OF PROCEDURAL PAIN

Increasingly, children undergo medical procedures in hospital which can be painful, distressing or both. Very often no protocols or guidelines exist for the management of such procedures and the outcome is a negative experience for all concerned. The management of painful procedures without anaesthesia is a difficult problem to which no simple solution exists. Although anaesthesia may seem to be clearly indicated for operative procedures, there is a large number of other diagnostic and therapeutic procedures which are performed regularly for which the optimal management is less obvious.[203] In a comparison of cognitive–behavioural management and general anaesthesia for bone marrow aspiration, neither the children nor their parents found one method to be clearly preferable and there were advantages and disadvantages to both.[204] Clearly, short procedures such as venepuncture or vaccination should not warrant invasive or complex techniques to make them tolerable; however, if they are badly managed, there may be significant consequences for the child and their subsequent management.[205,206] Techniques for the management of procedural pain may be classified as primarily either psychological or pharmacological. Most successful treatments are likely to involve a combination of both.

Psychological approaches include preparation, coping strategies and behaviour therapy.[207] Preparation usually consists of the provision of information about the procedure itself and the process surrounding it. It may also include sensory information, for example, about noises, smells or other accompanying sensations. Equipment may be shown and actually handled, play or rehearsal of the procedure might be possible, and videos and other visual material can be used.

Coping strategies may take the form of breathing exercises, self-hypnosis and distraction therapy. The presence of a key individual or favourite toy may be helpful for some children.

Behavioural therapy includes desensitization and reinforcement-type exercises. Desensitization is the gradual introduction of an anxiety-provoking stimulus; it is probably unsuited to routine clinical use, but may be helpful in certain situations. Non-pharmacological physical interventions, such as transcutaneous electrical nerve stimulation (TENS), acupuncture, aromatherapy and massage, may also be useful.

Pharmacological aids may be as simple as the application of a topical local anaesthetic or may extend to analgesic–sedative combinations of several drugs. When selecting suitable drugs or drug combinations, it is important to consider that in some situations general anaesthesia may be safer and, therefore, more appropriate.

Benzodiazepines, particularly midazolam which can be given orally, intranasally or intravenously, are commonly employed. Analgesic supplementation either using local anaesthetic infiltration or systemic analgesics may also be necessary. Entonox has a useful role in the management of procedural pain and has been used in dentistry and accident departments, and for painful dressing changes and removal of chest drains.[208,209]

REFERENCES

1 Mather, L. and Mackie, J. The incidence of postoperative pain in children. *Pain* 1983; **15**: 271–82.
2 Purcell-Jones, G., Dormon, F. and Sumner, E. The use of opioids in neonates. A retrospective study of 933 cases. *Anaesthesia* 1987; **42**: 1316–20.
3 Grundy, R., Howard, R.F. and Evans, J. Practical management of pain in sickling disorders. *Archives of Disease in Childhood* 1993; **69**: 256–9.
4 Anand, K.J.S. and Aynsley-Green, A. Metabolic and endocrine effects of surgical ligation of patent ductus arteriosus: are there implications for further improve-

ment of post-operative outcome? *Modern Problems in Paediatrics* 1985; **23**: 143–57.

5 Purcell-Jones, G., Dorman, F. and Sumner, E. Paediatraic anaesthetists perception of neonatal and infant pain. *Pain* 1988; **33**: 181–7.

6 de Lima, J., Lloyd-Thomas, A.R., Howard, R.F., *et al.* Anaesthetists perceptions of and prescribing for infant and neonatal pain. *British Medical Journal* 1996; **313**: 787.

7 Lloyd-Thomas, A.R., Howard, R.F. and Llewellyn, N.E. The management of acute and post-operative pain in infancy and childhood. In: Aynsley-Green, A., Ward Platt, M.P. and Lloyd-Thomas, A.R. (eds). *Clinical Paediatrics: Stress and Pain in Infancy and Childhood.* London: Balliere Tindall, 1995: 579–99.

8 Fitzgerald, M. Neurobiology of fetal and neonatal pain. In: Wall, P.D. and Melzack, R. (eds). *Textbook of Pain.* London: Churchill Livingstone, 1994: 153–63.

9 Aynsley-Green, A., Lloyd-Thomas, A.R. and Ward Platt, M.P. In: Aynsley-Green, A., Ward Platt, M.P. and Lloyd-Thomas, A.R (eds). *Clinical Paediatrics: Stress and Pain in Infancy and Childhood.* London: Balliere Tindall, 1995: ix–xi.

10 Lloyd-Thomas, A.R. and Howard, R.F. A pain service for children. *Paediatric Anaesthesia* 1994; **4**: 3–15.

11 Morton, N.S. Development of a monitoring protocol for the safe use of opioids in children. *Paediatric Anaesthesia* 1993; **3**: 179–84.

12 Derbyshire, S.W.G. and Fureda, I.A. 'Foetal Pain' is a misnomer. *British Medical Journal* 1996; **313**: 795.

13 Glover, B. and Fisk, N. We don't know; better to err on the safe side from mid-gestation. *British Medical Journal* 1996; **313**: 796.

14 Szawarski, Z. Probably no pain in the absence of 'self'. *British Medical Journal* 1996; **313**: 796.

15 Lloyd-Thomas, A.R. and Fitzgerald, M. Reflex responses do not necessarily signify pain. *British Medical Journal* 1996; **313**: 797–8.

16 Bonica, J.J. Anatomic and physiologic basis of nociception and pain. In: Bonica, J.J. (ed.). *The Managment of Pain.* Malvern: Lea & Fibinger, 1990: 28–94.

17 Abram, S.E. Necessity for an animal model of post-operative pain (Editorial). *Anesthesiology* 1997; **86**: 1015–17.

18 Zahn, P.K., Gysbers, D. and Brennan, T.J. Effect of systemic and intrathecal morphine in a rat model of postoperative pain. *Anesthesiology* 1997; **86**: 1066–77.

19 Dray, A. Inflammatory mediators of pain. *British Journal of Anaesthesia* 1995; **75**: 125–31.

20 Tilney, F. and Rossett, J. The value of brain lipoids as an index of brain development. *Bulletin of the Neurological Institute of New York* 1938; **1**: 28–71.

21 Pozanski, E.P. Children's reactions to pain: a psychiatrist's perspective. *Clinical Pediatrics* 1976; **15**: 1114–19.

22 Holve, D.S., Bromberger, B.J., Groverman, H.D., *et al.* Regional anesthesia during newborn circumcision: effect on pain response. *Clinical Pediatrics* 1983; **22**: 813–18.

23 Williamson, P.S. and Williamson, M.L. Physiologic stress reduction by a local anesthetic during newborn circumcision. *Pediatrics* 1983; **71**: 36–40.

24 Field, T. and Goldson, E. Pacifying effects of non-nutritive sucking on term and preterm neonates during heelstick procedures. *Pediatrics* 1984; **74**: 1012–15.

25 Eckman, P. and Oster, H. Facial expressions of emotion. *Annual Review of Psychology* 1979; **30**: 527–54.

26 Izard, C.E., Huebner, R.R., Risser, D., *et al.* The young infant's ability to produce discrete emotional expressions. *Developments in Psychology* 1980; **16**: 132–40.

27 Izard, C.E., Hembree, E.A. and Huebner, R.R. Infants emotional expressions to acute pain: developmental change and stability of individual differences. *Developments in Psychology* 1987; **23**: 105–13.

28 Wasz-Hockert, O., Lind, J. and Vuorenkoski, V. The infant cry: a spectographic and auditory analysis. *Clinics in Developmental Medicine* 1968; **2**: 9–42.

29 Levin, J.D. and Gordon, N.C. Pain in pre-lingual children and its evaluation by pain induced vocalisation. *Pain* 1982; **14**: 85–93.

30 Porter, F.L., Miller, R.H. and Marshall, R.E. Neonatal pain cries, effect of circumcision on acoustic features and percieved urgency. *Child Development* 1986; **57**: 790–802.

31 Dahl, J.B. Neuronal plasticity and pre-emptive analgesia: implications for the management of postoperative pain. *Danish Medical Bulletin* 1994; **41**: 434–42.

32 Yi, D.K. and Barr, G.A. The induction of fos-like immunoreactivity by noxious thermal, mechanical and chemical stimuli in the lumbar spinal cord of infant rats. *Pain* 1995; **60**: 257–65.

33 Jennings, E. and Fitzgerald, M. C-fos can be induced in the neonatal rat spinal cord by both noxious and innocuous stimulation. *Pain* 1996; **68**: 301–6.

34 Kar, S. and Quirion, R. Neuropeptide receptors in developing and adult rat spinal cord: an *in vitro* quantitative autoradiography study of calcitonin gene-related peptide, neurokinins, β-opioid, lanin, omatostatin, neurotension and vasoactive intestinal polypeptide receptors. *Journal of Comparative Neurology* 1995; **354**: 253–81.

35 Leslie, R.M., Tso, S. and Harlbutt, D.E. Differential appearance of opiate receptor subtypes in neonatal rat brain. *Life Sciences* 1982; **31**: 1393–6.

36 Andrews, K. and Fitzgerald, M. The cutaneous withdrawal reflex in human neonates: sensitization, receptive fields, and the effects of contralateral stimulation. *Pain* 1994; **56**: 95–101.

37 Levine, J.D., Codderre, T.J. and Basbaum, A.I. The peripheral nervous system and the inflammatory process. In: Dubner, R., Gebhart, G.F. and Bond, M.R. (eds). *Proceedings of the V World Congress on Pain.* Amsterdam: Elsevier, 1988: 33–43.

38 Handwerker, H.O. and Reeh, P.W. Chemosensitivity and sensitisation by chemical agents. In: Willis, W. (ed.). *Hyperalgesia and Allodynia.* New York: Raven Press, 1992: 107–15.

39 Taiwo, Y.O. and Levine, J.D. Contribution of guanine neucleotide regulatory proteins to prostaglandin hyperalgesia in the rat. *Brain Research* 1989; **492**: 396–9.

40 Pitchford, S. and Levine, J.D. Prostaglandin sensitive nociceptors in cell culture. *Neuroscience Letters* 1991; **131**: 105–8.

41 Treede, R.D., Meyer, R.A., Raja, S.N., *et al.* Peripheral and central mechanisms of cutaneous hyperalgesia. *Progress in Neurobiology* 1992; **38**: 397–421.

42 Taiwo, Y.O. and Levine, J.D. Mediation of serotonin hyperalgesia by the cyclic AMP seond messenger system. *Neuroscience* 1992; **48**: 479–83.

43 Woolf, C.J. Recent advances in the pathophysiology of acute pain. *British Journal of Anaesthesia* 1989; **63**: 139–46.

44 Dickenson, A.H. Recent advances in the physiology and pharmacology of pain: plasticity and its implications for clinical analgesia. *Journal of Psychopharmacology* 1991; **5**: 342–51.

45 Woolf, C.J. The dorsal horn: state dependent sensory processing and the generation of pain. In: Wall, P.D. and Melzack, R. (eds). *The Textbook of Pain*. London: Churchill Livingstone, 1994: 101–12.

46 Munglani, R., Fleming, B.G. and Hunt, S.P. Remembrance of times past: the significance of c-*fos* in pain (Editorial). *British Journal of Anaesthesia* 1996; **76**: 1–4.

47 Anbar, M. and Gratt, B.M. Role of nitric oxide in the physiopathology of pain. *Journal of Pain and Symptom Management* 1997; **14**: 225–54.

48 Bullitt, E. Somatotropy of spinal nociceptive processing. *Journal of Comparative Neurology* 1991; **312**: 279–90.

49 Morgan, J.I. and Curran, T. Stimulus–transcription coupling in the nervous system: involvement of the inducible oncogenes foa and jun. *Annual Review of Neuroscience* 1991; **14**: 421–51.

50 Sun, W.Z., Shyn, B.C. and Shieh, J.Y. Nitrous-oxide or halothane or both fail to supress c-fos expression in rat spinal cord dorsal horn neurones after subcutaneous formalin. *British Journal of Anaesthesia* 1996; **76**: 99–105.

51 Cervero, F. and Laird, J.M.A. Mechanisms of touch-evoked pain (allodynia): a new model (Review). *Pain* 1996; **68**: 13–23.

52 LaMotte, R.H., Shain, C.N., Simone, D.A., *et al.* Neurogenic hyperalgesia: psychophysical studies of underlying mechanisms. *Journal of Neurophysiology* 1991; **66**: 190–211.

53 Ma, Q.P. and Woolf, C.J. Noxious stimuli induce an *N*-methyl d-aspartate receptor dependent hypersensitivity of the flexion withdrawal to touch: implications for the treatment of mechanical allodynia. *Pain* 1995; **61**: 383–90.

54 Woolf, C.J. Somatic pain – pathogenesis and prevention. *British Journal of Anaesthesia* 1995; **75**: 169–76.

55 Dickenson, A.H. and Sullivan, A.F. Subcutaneous formalin induced activity of dorsal horn neurones in the rat: differential response to an intrathecal opiate administered pre or post-formalin. *Pain* 1987; **30**: 349–60.

56 Wall, P.D. The prevention of postoperative pain. *Pain* 1988; **33**: 289–90.

57 Marsh, D.F., Hatch, D.J. and Fitzgerald, M. Opioid systems and the newborn. *British Journal of Anaesthesia* 1997; **79**: 787–95.

58 Fitzgerald, M. and Anand, K.J.S. Developmental neuroanatomy and neurophysiology of pain. In: Schechter, N.L., Berde, C.B. and Yaster, M. (eds). *Pain in Infants, Children and Adolescents*. Baltimore, MD: Williams and Wilkins, 1993: 11–31.

59 Fitzgerald, M. Pain in infancy – some unanswered questions. *Pain Review* 1995; **2**: 77–91.

60 Zonneveld, L.N.L., McGrath, P.J., Reid, G.J., *et al.* Accuracy of children's pain memories. *Pain* 1997; **71**: 297–302.

61 Stevenson, J. Long-term sequelae of acute stress in early life. In: Aynsley-Green, A., Ward Platt, M.P. and Lloyd-Thomas, A.R. (eds) *Clinical Paediatrics: Stress and Pain in Infancy and Childhood*. London: Balliere Tindall, 1995: 619–31.

62 Grunau, R.V.E., Whitfield, M.F., Petrie, J.H., *et al.* Early pain experience, child and family factors, as precursors of somatization: a prospective study of extremely premature and fullterm children. *Pain* 1994; **56**: 353–9.

63 Taddio, A., Goldbach, M., Ipp, M., *et al.* Effects of neonatal circumcision on pain responses during vaccination in boys. *Lancet* 1995; **345**: 291–2.

64 Taddio, A., Katz, J., Illersich, A.L., *et al.* Effect of neonatal circumcision on pain response during subsequent routine vaccination. *Lancet* 1997; **349**: 599–603.

65 Reynolds, M.L. and Fitzgerald, M. Longtem sensory hyper-innervation following neonatal skin wounds. *Journal of Comparative Neurology* 1995; **358**: 487–98.

66 Hester, N.O. Assessment of acute pain. In: Aynsley-Green, A., Ward Platt, M.P. and Lloyd-Thomas, A.R. (eds). *Clinical Paediatrics: Stress and Pain in Infancy and Childhood*. London: Balliere Tindall, 1995: 561–77.

67 Grunau, R.V.E. and Craig, K.D. Pain expression in neonates: facial action and cry. *Pain* 1987; **28**: 395–410.

68 Lawrence, J., Alcock, D., McGrath, P., *et al.* The development of a tool to assess neonatal pain. *Neonatal Network* 1993; **12**: 59–65.

69 Horgan, M. and Choonara, I. Measuring pain in neonates: an objective score. *Paediatric Nursing* 1996; **8**: 24–7.

70 Hannallah, R.S., Broadman, L.M., Belman, A.B., *et al.* Comparison of caudal and ilioinguinal/iliohypogastric nerve blocks for control of post-orchidopexy pain in pediatric ambulatory surgery. *Anesthesiology* 1987; **66**: 832–4.

71 Broadman, L.M., Rice, L.J. and Hannallah, R.S. Testing the validity of an objective pain scale for infants and children (Abstract). *Anesthesiology* 1988; **69**: A770.

72 Krechel, S.W. and Bildner, J. CRIES: a new neonatal postoperative pain measurement score. Initial testing of validity and reliability. *Paediatric Anaesthesia* 1995; **5**: 53–61.

73 Sparshott, M.M. The development of a clinical distress scale for ventilated newborn infants: identification of pain and distress based on validated behavioural scores. *Journal of Neonatal Nursing* 1996; April: 5–11.

74 Hester, N.O., Foster, R.L. and Bayer, J.E. Clinical judgement in assessing childrens' pain. In: Watt-Watson, J.H. and Donovan, M.I. (eds). *Pain Management: Nursing Perspective*. St. Louis, MO: Mosby-Yearbook, 1992: 236–94.

75 McGrath, P.A. An assessment of children's pain: a review of behavioral, physiological and direct scaling techniques. *Pain* 1987; **31**: 147–76.

76 Craig, K.D. The facial expression of pain: better than a thousand words? *American Pain Society Journal* 1992; **1**: 153–62.

77 Beyer, J.E., McGrath, P.J. and Berde, C.B. Discordance between self-report and behavioural pain measures in children aged 3–7 years after surgery. *Journal of Pain Symptom Management* 1990; **5**: 350–6.

78 Tyler, D.C., Tu, A., Douthit, J., *et al.* Toward validation of pain measurement tools for children: a pilot study. *Pain* 1993; **52**: 301–9.

79 McGrath, P.J., Johnson, G., Goodman, J.T., Schillinger, J., Dunn, J. and Chapman, J. CHEOPS: a behavioural scale for rating postoperative pain in children. In: Fields, H.L., Dubner, R. and Cervero, F. (eds). *Advances in Pain Research and Therapy*. New York: Raven Press, 1985: 395–402.

80 Morton, N.S. Pain assessment in children (Review). *Paediatric Anaesthesia* 1997; **7**: 267–72.

81 Manne, S.L., Jacobsen, P.B. and Redd, W.H. Assessment of acute pediatric pain: do child self-report, parent ratings, and nurse ratings measure the same phenomenon? *Pain* 1992; **48**: 45–52.

82 Southall, D.P. (ed.). *Prevention and Control of Pain in Children: A Manual for Healthcare Professionals. Report of the Working Party of the Royal College of Paediatrics and Child Health*. London: British Medical Journal Publications, 1997.

83 Ready, L.B., Oden, R., Chadwick, H.S., *et al*. Development of an anesthesiology-based postoperative pain management service. *Anesthesiology* 1988; **68**: 100–6.

84 *Report of the Working Party on Pain after Surgery. Commission on the Provision of Surgical Services*. London: Royal College of Surgeons of England and College of Anaesthetists, 1990: 1–36.

85 Kehlet, H. Postoperative pain relief – what is the issue? *British Journal of Anaesthesia* 1994; **72**: 375–8.

86 Kehlet, H. Surgical stress – the role of pain and analgesia. *British Journal of Anaesthesia* 1989; **63**: 189–95.

87 Blass, E.M. and Hoffmeyer, L.B. Sucrose as an analgesic for newborn infants. *Pediatrics* 1991; **87**: 215–18.

88 Johnston, C.C., Stremler, R.L., Stevens, B.J., *et al*. Effectiveness of oral sucrose and simulated rocking on pain response in preterm neonates. *Pain* 1997; **72**: 193–9.

89 Flower, R.J. and Vane, J.R. Inhibition of prostaglandin synthetase in brain explains the anti-pyretic action of paracetamol. *Nature* 1972; **240**: 410–11.

90 Gaudreault, P., Guay, J., Nicol, O., *et al*. Pharmacokinetics and clinical efficacy of intrarectal solutions of acetaminophen. *Canadian Journal of Anaesthesia* 1988; **35**: 149–52.

91 Temple, A.R. Pediatric dosing of acetominophen. *Pediatric Pharmacology* 1983; **3**: 321–7.

92 Hopkins, C.S., Underhill, S. and Booker, P.D. Pharmacokinetics of paracetamol after cardiac surgery. *Archives of Disease inChildhood* 1990; **65**: 971–6.

93 Anderson, B.J., Woolard, G.A. and Holford, N.H.G. Pharmacokinetics of rectal paracetamol after major surgery in children. *Paediatric Anaesthesia* 1995; **5**: 237–42.

94 Montgomery, C.J., McCormack, J.P., Reichert, C.C., *et al*. Plasma concentrations after high-dose (45 mg.kg^{-1}) rectal acetaminophen in children. *Canadian Journal of Anaesthesia* 1995; **42**: 982–6.

95 Birmingham, P.K., Tobin, M.J., Henthorn, T.K., *et al*. Twenty-four-hour pharmacokinetics of rectal acetaminophen in children. *Anesthesiology* 1997; **87**: 244–52.

96 Anderson, B., Kanagasundarum, S. and Woolard, G. Analgesic efficacy of paracetamol in children undergoing tonsillectomy as a pain model. *Anaesthesia and Intensive Care* 1996; **24**: 669–73.

97 Anderson, B.J. and Holford, H.N.G. Rectal paracetamol dosing regimens: determination by computer simulation. *Paediatric Anaesthesia* 1997; **7**: 451–5.

98 Lyn, Y.C., Sussman, H.H. and Benitz, W.E. Plasma concentration after rectal adminstration of acetaminophen in pre-term neonates. *Paediatric Anaesthesia* 1997; **7**: 457–59.

99 Bannwarth, B., Netter, P., Lapicque, F., *et al*. Plasma and cerebrospinal fluid concentration of paracetamol after a single intravenous dose of propacetamol. *British Journal of Clinical Pharmacology* 1992; **34**: 79–81.

100 Granry, J.C., Rod, B., Monrigal, J.P., *et al*. The analgesic efficacy of an injectable pro-drug of acetaminophen in children after orthopaedic surgery. *Paediatric Anaesthesia* 1997; **7**: 445–9.

101 Delbos, A. and Boccard, E. The morphine-sparing effect of propacetamol in orthopedic postoperative pain. *Journal of Pain Symptom Management* 1995; **10**: 279–86.

102 Moore, A., Collins, S., Carroll, D., *et al*. Paracetamol with and without codeine in acute pain: a quantitative systematic review. *Pain* 1997; **70**: 193–201.

103 Houck, C.S., Troshynski, T. and Berde, C.B. Treatment of pain in children. In: Wall, P.D. and Melzack, R. (eds). *Textbook of Pain*. London: Churchill Livingstone, 1994: 1419–34.

104 Quiding, H., Osson, G.L., Boreus, L.O., *et al*. Infants and young children metabolise codeine to morphine. A study after single and repeated rectal administration. *British Journal of Clinical Pharmacology* 1992; **33**: 45–9.

105 Sunshine, A. and Olson, N.Z. Nonnarcotic analgesics. In: Wall, P.D and Melzack, R. (eds). *Textbook of Pain*. London: Churchill Livingstone, 1994: 923–42.

106 Malmberg, A.B. and Yaksh, T.L. Hyper-algesia mediated by spinal glutomate or substance receptor blocked by spinal cyclooxygenase inhibition. *Science* 1992; **257**: 1277–80.

107 Abramson, S. Therapy with and mechanisms of nonsteroidal anti-inflammatory drugs. *Curent Opinion in Rheumatology* 1991; **3**: 336–40.

108 Kauffman, R.E. and Nelson, M.V. Effect of age on ibuprofen pharmacokinetics and anti-pyretic response. *Journal of Pediatrics* 1992; **121**: 969–73.

109 Maunuksela, E.-L., Kokki, H. and Bullingham, R.E.S. Comparison of intravenous ketorolac with morphine for postoperative pain in children. *Clinical Pharmacology and Therapeutics* 1992; **52**: 436–43.

110 Moren, J., Francois, T., Blanloeil, Y., *et al*. The effects of nonsteroidal antiinflammatory drugs (ketoprofen) on morphine respiratory depression: a double-blind, randomized study in volunteers. *Anesthesia and Analgesia* 1997; **85**: 400–5.

111 Giaufre, E., Dalens, B. and Gombert, a. Epidemiology and morbidity of regional anesthesia in children: a one-year prospective survey of the French-Language Society of Pediatric Anesthesiologists. *Anesthesia and Analgesia* 1996; **83**: 904–12.

112 Ved, S.A., Pinosky, M. and Nicodemus, H. Ventricular tachycardia and brief cardiovascular collapse in two infants after caudal anesthesia using a bupivacaine-epinephrine solution. *Anesthesiology* 1993; **79**: 1121–3.

113 Maxwell, L.G, Martin, L.D. and Yaster, M. Bupivacaine-induced cardiac toxicity in neonates: successful treatment with intravenous phenytoin. *Anesthesiology* 1994; **80**: 682–6.

114 Agarwal, R., Gutlove, D.P. and Lockhart, C.H. Seizures occuring in pediatric patients receiving continuous

infusion of bupivacaine. *Anesthesia and Analgesia* 1992; **75**: 284–6.

115 McCloskey, J.J., Haun, S.E. and Deshpande, J.K. Bupivacaine toxicity secondary to continuous caudal epidural infusion in children. *Anesthesia and Analgesia* 1992; **75**: 287–90.

116 Berde, C.B. Convulsions associated with pediatric regional anesthesia. *Anesthesia and Analgesia* 1992; **75**: 164–6.

117 Larsson, B.A., Olsson, G.L. and Lonnqvist, P.A. Plasma concentrations of bupivacaine in young infants after continuous epidural infusion. *Paediatric Anaesthesia* 1994; **4**: 159–162.

118 Eyres, R.L. Local anaesthetic agents in infancy. *Paediatric Anaesthesia* 1995; **5**: 213–18.

119 Desparmet, J., Meistelman, C., Barre, J., *et al.* Continuous epidural infusion of bupivacaine for postoperative pain relief in children. *Anesthesiology* 1987; **67**: 108–10.

120 Mazoit, J.X., Denson, D.D. and Samii, K. Pharmacokinetics of bupivacaine following caudal anesthesia in infants. *Anesthesiology* 1988; **68**: 387–91.

121 Bricker, R.W., Telford, R.J. and Booker, P.D. Pharmacokinetics of bupivacaine following intraoperative intercostal nerve block in neonates and infants less than 6 months. *Anesthesiology* 1989; **70**: 942–7.

122 Weston, P.J. and Bourchier, D. The pharmacokinetics of bupivacaine following interpleural nerve block in infants of very low birthweight. *Paediatric Anaesthesia* 1995; **5**: 219–22.

123 Smith, T., Moratin, P. and Wulf, H. Smaller children have greater bupivacaine plasma concentrations after ilioinguinal block. *British Journal of Anaesthesia* 1996; **76**: 452–5.

124 Cheung, S.L.W., Booker, P.D., Franks, R., *et al.* Serum concentrations of bupivacaine during prolonged continuous paravertebral infusion in young infants. *British Journal of Anaesthesia* 1997; **79**: 9–13.

125 Peutrell, J.M., Holder, K. and Gregory, M. Plasma bupivacaine concentrations associated with continuous extradural infusions in babies. *British Journal of Anaesthesia* 1997; **78**: 160–2.

126 Lerman, J., Strong, H.A., LeDez, K.M., *et al.* Effects of age on the serum concentration of 1-acid glycoprotein and the binding of lidocaine in pediatric patients. *Clinical Pharmacology and Therapeutics* 1989; **46**: 219–25.

127 Booker, P.D., Taylor, C. and Saba, G. Perioperative changes in α_1-acid glycoprotein centrations n infants undergoing major surgery. *British Journal of Anaesthesia* 1996; **76**: 365–8.

128 Peutrell, J.M. and Hughes, D.G. A grand-mal convulsion in a child in association with a continuous epidural infusion of bupivacaine. *Anaesthesia* 1995; **50**: 563–4.

129 Berde, C.B. Regional anesthesia in children: what have we learned? *Anesthesia and Analgesia* 1996; **83**: 897–900.

130 De la Coussaye, J.E., Brugada, J. and Allessia, M.A. Electrophysiological and arrythmogenic effects of bupivacaine. *Anesthesiology* 1992; **77**: 132–41.

131 Dalens, B. *Regional Anesthesia in Infants, Children and Adolescents.* London: Williams and Wilkins, Waverley Europe, 1995.

132 De la Coussaye, J.E., Bassoul, B., Brugada, J., *et al.* Reversal of electrophysiological and haemodynamic effects induced by high doses of bupivacaine by the combination of clonidine and dobutamine in anesthetised dogs. *Anesthesia and Analgesia* 1992; **74**: 703–11.

133 McClure, J.H. Ropivacaine. *British Journal of Anaesthesia* 1996; **76**: 300–7.

134 Hartley, R. and Levene, M.I. Opioid pharmacology in the newborn. In: Aynsley-Green, A., Ward Platt, M.P. and Lloyd-Thomas, A.R. (eds). *Clinical Paediatrics: Stress and Pain in Infancy and Childhood.* London: Balliere Tindall, 1995: 467–93.

135 Kart, T., Christrup, L.L. and Rasmussen, M. Recommended use of morphine in neonates, infants and children based on a literature review: Part 1 – Pharmacokinetics (Review). *Paediatric Anaesthesia* 1997; **7**: 5–11.

136 Kart, T., Christrup, L.L. and Rasmussen, M. Recommended use of morphine in neonates, infants and children based on a literature review: Part 2 – Clinical use (Review). *Paediatric Anaesthesia* 1997; **7**: 93–101.

137 McRorie, T.I., Lynn, A.M., Nespeca, M.K., *et al.* The maturation of morphine clearance and metabolism. *American Journal of Disease in Childhood* 1992; **146**: 972–6.

138 Dahlstrom, B., Bolme, P., Feychting, H., *et al.* Morphine kinetics in children. *Clinical Pharmacology and Therapeutics* 1979; **26**: 354–65.

139 Dagan, O., Klein, J., Bohn, D., *et al.* Morphine pharmacokinetics in children following cardiac surgery: effects of disease and inotropic support. *Journal of Cardiothoracic and Vascular Anesthesia* 1993; **7**: 396–8.

140 Morselli, P.L., Franco-Morselli, R. and Borsi, L. Clinical pharmacokinetics in newborns and infants: age related differences and therapeutic implications. *Clinical Pharmacokinetics* 1980; **5**: 485–527.

141 Bhat, R., Chari, G., Gulati, A., *et al.* Pharmacokinetics of a single dose of morphine in preterm infants during the first week of life. *Journal of Pediatrics* 1990; **117**: 477–481.

142 Glare, P.A. and Walsh, T.D. Clinical pharmacokinetics of morphine. *Therapeutic Drug Monitoring* 1991; **13**: 1–23.

143 Wilson, A.S., Stiller, R.L., Davis, P.J., *et al.* Fentanyl and alfentanil plasma protein binding in preterm and term neonates. *Anesthesia and Analgesia* 1997; **84**: 315–18.

144 Sikich, N., Carr, A.S. and Lerman, J. Parental perceptions, expectations and preferences for the postanaesthetic recovery of children. *Paediatric Anaesthesia* 1997; **7**: 139–42.

145 Finley, G.A., McGrath, P.J., Forward, S.P., McNeill, G. and Fitzgerald, P. Parents' management of children's pain following 'minor' surgery. *Pain* 1996; **64**: 83–7.

146 Tan, S.G.M., May, H.A. and Cunliffe, M. An audit of pain and vomiting in paediatric day case surgery. *Paediatric Anaesthesia* 1994; **4**: 105–9.

147 Knight, J.C. Postoperatve pain in children after day case surgery. *Paediatric Anaesthesia* 1994; **4**: 45–51.

148 Berde, C.B. Convulsions associated with pediatric regional anesthesia. *Anaesthesia and Analgesia* 1992; **75**: 164–6.

149 Moriarty, A. Use of ropivacaine in postoperative infusions. *Paediatric Anaesthesia* 1998; **7**: 478–9.

150 Kuzma, P., Kline, J., Mark, D., *et al.* Progress in the development of ultra-long-acting local anesthetics. *Regional Anesthesia* 1998; **22**: 543–51.

151 Halperin, D., Koren, G., Attas, D. *et al.* Topical skin anesthesia for venous, subcutaneous drug reservoir and lumbar punctures in children. *Pediatrics* 1989; **84**: 281–4.

152 Ogborn, M.R. The use of a eutectic mixture of local anesthetic in pediatric renal biopsy. *Pediatric Nephrology* 1992; **6**: 276–7.

153 MacKinlay, G.A. Save the prepuce. Painless separation of preputial adhesions in the outpatient clinic. *British Medical Journal* 1988; **297**: 590–1.

154 Lee, J.J. and Forrester, P. EMLA for postoperative analgesia for day case circumcision in children: a comparison with dorsal nerve of penis block. *Anaesthesia* 1992; **47**: 1081–3.

155 Pedersen, J.L., Callesen, T., Moiniche, S. and Kehlet, H. Analgesic and anti-inflammatory effects of lignocaine–prilocaine (EMLA) cream in human burn injury. *British Journal of Anaesthesia* 1996; **76**: 806–10.

156 Schindler, M., Swann, M. and Crawford, M. A comparison of postoperative analgesia provided by wound infiltration or caudal analgesia. *Anaesthesia and Intensive Care* 1991; **19**: 46–9.

157 Casey, W.F., Rice, L.J., Hannallah, R.S., Broadman, L., Norden, J.M. and Guzzetta, P. A comparison between bupivacaine instillation versus ilioinguinal/iliohypogastric nerve block for postoperative analgesia following inguinal herniorraphy in children. *Anesthesiology* 1990; **72**: 637–9.

158 Wright, J.E. Controlled trial of wound infiltration with bupivacaine for postoperative pain relief after appendicectomy in children. *British Journal of Surgery* 1993; **80**: 110–11.

159 Mobley, K.A., Wandless, J.G., Fell, D. and McBurney, A. Serum bupivacaine concentrations following wound infiltration in children undergoing inguinal herniotomy. *Anaesthesia* 1991; **46**: 500–1.

160 Wong, A.K., Braude, B.M., Macdonald, R.M. and Fear, D.W. Post-tonsillectomy infiltration with bupivacaine reduces immediate postoperative pain in children. *Canadian Journal of Anaesthesia* 1995; **42**: 770–4.

161 Watt, I. and Ledingham, I.McA. Mortality amongst multiple trauma patients admitted to an intensive therapy unit. *Anaesthesia* 1984; **39**: 973–81.

162 Broadman, L.M. Regional anaesthesia in paediatric practice. *Canadian Journal of Anaesthesia Suppl.* 1987; **34**: 43–8.

163 Moores, M.A., Wandless, J.G. and Fell, D. Paediatric postoperative analgesia. A comparison of rectal diclofenac with caudal bupivacaine after inguinal herniotomy. *Anaesthesia* 1990; **45**: 156–8.

164 Mannion, D., Armstrong, C., O'Leary, G. and Casey, W. Paediatric post orchidopexy analgesia – effect of diclofenac combined with ilioinguinal/iliohypogastric nerve block. *Paediatric Anaesthesia* 1994; **4**: 327–30.

165 Maunuksela, E.-L., Ryhanen, P. and Janhunen, L. Efficacy of rectal Ibuprofen in controlling postoperative pain in children. *Canadian Journal of Anaesthesia* 1992; **39**: 226–30.

166 Armitage, E.N. Caudal block in children. *Anaesthesia* 1979; **34**: 396–401.

167 Shulte Steinberg, O. and Rahlfs, V.W. Caudal anaesthesia in children and spread of 1% lignocaine. *British Journal of Anaesthesia* 1970; **42**: 1093–7.

168 Takasaki, M., Dohl, S. and Kawabata, Y., *et al.* Dosage of lidocaine for caudal anesthesia in infants and children. *Anesthesiology* 1977; **47**: 527–29.

169 Moore, A., Collins, S., Carroll, D. and McQuay, H. Paracetamol with and without codeine in acute pain: a quantitative systematic review. *Pain* 1997; **70**: 193–201.

170 Granry, J.C., Boccard, E., Hermann, P., Gendron, A. and Saint-Maurice, C. Pharmacokinetics and antipyretic effects of an injectable pro-drug of paracetamol (propacetamol) in children. *Paediatric Anaesthesia* 1992; **2**: 291–5.

171 Porter, J.D.H., Robinson, P.H., Glasgow, J.F.T., Banks, J.H. and Hall, S.M. Trends in the incidence of Reye's syndrome and the use of aspirin. *Archives of Disease in Childhood* 1990; **65**: 826–9.

172 Hurwitz, E., Barrett, M. and Bregman, D. Public health service study of Reye's syndrome and medications. *Journal of the American Medical Association* 1987; **257**: 1905–11.

173 McQuay, H.J., Carroll, D. and Watts, P.G. Codeine 20 mg increases pain relief from ibuprofen 400 mg after molar surgery. A rapid-dosing comparison of ibuprofen and ibuprofen–codeine combination. *Pain* 1989; **37**: 7–13.

174 *Guidelines for the Use of Nonsteriodal Anti-inflammatory Drugs in the Perioperative Period.* London: Royal College of Anaesthetists, 1998.

175 Shanahan, E.C., Marshall, A.G. and Garrett, C.P.O. Adverse reactions to intravenous codeine phosphate in children. A report of three cases. *Anaesthesia* 1983; **38**: 40–3.

176 Goldsack, C., Scuplak, S.M. and Smith, M. A double-blind comparison of codeine and morphine for post-operative analgesia following intracranial surgery. *Anaesthesia* 1996; **51**: 1029–32.

177 Quiding, H., Olsson, G.L., Boreus, L.O. and Bondesson, U. Infants and young children metabolise codeine to morphine. A study after single and repeated rectal administration. *British Journal of Clinical Pharmacology* 1992; **33**: 45–9.

178 Maunuksela, E.-L., Korpela, R. and Olkkola, K.T. Double-blind, multiple-dose comparison of buprenorphine and morphine in postoperative pain of children. *British Journal of Anaesthesia* 1988; **60**: 48–55.

179 Maunuksela, E.-L., Korpela, R. and Olkkola, K.T. Comparison of buprenorphine with morphine in the treatment of postoperative pain in children. *Anesthesia and Analgesia* 1988; **67**: 233–9.

180 Olkkola, K.T., Leijala, M.A. and Maunuksela, E.-L. Paediatric ventilatory effects of morphine and buprenorphine revisited. *Paediatric Anaesthesia* 1995; **5**: 303–5.

181 Zanette, G., Manani, G., Giusti, F., Pittoni, G. and Ori, C. Respiratory depression following administration of low dose buprenorphine as a postoperative analgesic after fentanyl balanced anaesthesia. *Paediatric Anaesthesia* 1996; **6**: 419–22.

182 Doyle, E., Robinson, D. and Morton, N.S. Comparison of patient controlled analgesia with and without a background infusion after lower abdominal surgery in children. *British Journal of Anaesthesia* 1993; **71**: 670–3.

183 Doyle, E., Harper, I. and Morton, N.S. Patient-controlled analgesia with low dose background infusions after lower abdominal surgery in children. *British Journal of Anaesthesia* 1993; **71**: 818–22.

184 Bray, R.J., Woodhams, A.M., Vallis, C.J., Kelly, P.J. and Ward-Platt, M.P. A double-blind comparison of morphine infusion and patient controlled analgesia in children. *Paediatric Anaesthesia* 1996; **6**: 121–7.

185 Bray, R.J., Woodhams, A.M., Vallis, C.J. and Kelly, P.J. Morphine consumption and respiratory depression in children receiving postoperative analgesia from continuous morphine infusion or patient controlled analgesia. *Paediatric Anaesthesia* 1996; **6**: 129–34.

186 Southern, D.A. and Read, M.S. Overdosage of opiate from patient controlled analgesia devices. *British Medical Journal* 1994; **309**: 1002.

187 Morton, N.S. Development of a monitoring protocol for the safe use of opioids in children. *Paediatric Anaesthesia* 1993; **3**: 179–84.

188 Lonnqvist, P.A., MacKenzie, J., Soni, A.K. and Conacher, I.D. Paravertebral blockade. Failure rate and complications. *Anaesthesia* 1995; **50**: 813–15.

189 Lonnqvist, P.A. and Hesser, U. Depth from the skin to the thoracic paravertebral space in infants and children. *Paediatric Anaesthesia* 1994; **4**: 99–100.

190 McIlvaine, W.B., Knox, R.F., Fennessey, P.V. and Goldstein, M. Continuous infusion of bupivacaine *via* intrapleural catheter for analgesia after thoracotomy in children. *Anesthesiology* 1988; **69**: 261–4.

191 Weston, P.J. and Bourchier, D. The pharmacokinetics of bupivacaine following interpleural nerve block in infants of very low birthweight. *Paediatric Anaesthesia* 1995; **5**: 219–22.

192 Dalens, B. and Hasanaoui, A. Caudal anesthesia in pediatric surgery: success rate and adverse events in 750 consecutive patients. *Anesthesia and Analgesia* 1989; **68**: 83–9.

193 Bosenberg, A.T., Bland, B.A.R., Schulte-Steinberg, O. and Downing, J.W. Thoracic epidural anesthesia *via* caudal route in infants. *Anesthesiology* 1988; **69**: 265–9.

194 Dalens, B. and Chrysostome, Y. Intervertebral epidural anaesthesia in paediatric surgery: success rate and adverse effects in 650 consecutive procedures. *Paediatric Anaesthesia* 1991; **1**: 107–17.

195 Dalens, B., Tanguy, A. and Haberer, J.P. Lumbar epidural anesthesia for operative and post-operative pain relief in infants and young children. *Anesthesia and Analgesia* 1986; **65**: 1069–73.

196 Ecoffey, C., Dubousset, A.-M. and Samii, K. Lumbar and thoracic epidural anesthesia for urologic and upper abdominal surgery in infants and children. *Anesthesiology* 1986; **65**: 87–90.

197 Strafford, M.A., Wilder, R.T. and Berde, C.B. The risk of infection from epidural analgesia in children: a review of 1620 cases. *Anesthesia and Analgesia* 1995; **80**: 234–8.

198 Dalens, B., Bazin, J.E. and Haberer, J.P. Epidural bubbles as a cause of incomplete analgesia during epidural anesthesia. *Anesthesia and Analgesia* 1987; **66**: 679–83.

199 Sethna, N.F. and Berde, C.B. Venous air embolism during identification of the epidural space in children (Editorial). *Anesthesia and Analgesia* 1993; **76**: 925–7.

200 Flandin-Blety, C. and Barrier, G. Accidents following extradural analgesia in children. The results of a retrospective study. *Paediatric Anaesthesia* 1995; **5**: 41–6.

201 Berde, C.B. Epidural analgesia in children. *Canadian Journal of Anaesthesia* 1994; **41**: 555–60.

202 Wood, C.E., Goresky, G.V., Klassen, K.A., Kuwahara, B. and Neil, S.G. Complications of continuous epidural infusions for postoperative analgesia in children. *Canadian Journal of Anaesthesia* 1994; **41**: 613–20.

203 Berde, C. Pediatric oncology procedures: to sleep or perchance to dream? (Editorial). *Pain* 1995; **62**: 1–2.

204 Jay, S., Elliott, C.H., Fitzgibbons, I., Woody, P. and Siegel, S. A comparative study of cognitive behavior therapy versus general anesthesia for painful medical procedures in children. *Pain* 1995; **62**: 3–9.

205 Taddio, A., Goldbach, M., Ipp, M., Stevens, B. and Koren, G. Effects of neonatal circumcision on pain responses during vaccination in boys. *Lancet* 1995; **345**: 291–2.

206 Brown, R.E. and Fanurik, D. Editorial 'It'll only hurt for a little while'. Managing procedural pain in children. *Paediatric Anaesthesia* 1996; **6**: 249–50.

207 Hamilton, A. and Zeltzer, L. Psychological approaches to procedural pain. In: Aynsley-Green, A., Ward Platt, M.P. and Lloyd-Thomas, A.R. (eds). *Clinical Paediatrics: Stress and Pain in Infancy and Childhood*. London: Balliere Tindall, 1995; 601–18.

208 Warren, V.N., Crawford, A.N. and Young ,T.M. The use of Entonox as a sedation agent for children who have refused operative dentistry. *Journal of Dentistry* 1983; **11**: 306–12.

209 Griffin, G.C., Campbell, V.D. and Jones, R. Nitrous oxide–oxygen sedation for minor surgery. *Journal of the American Medical Association* 1981; **245**: 2411–13.

CHAPTER 13

Anaesthesia for patients with cardiac disease

EDWARD SUMNER

INTRODUCTION

Anaesthesia for infants with cardiac disease, whether for palliative or corrective cardiac surgery or for associated or intercurrent disease, requires a full knowledge of the pathophysiological background of the particular disease. The anaesthetist is an invaluable member of the team involved in the treatment of the patient from hospital admission to recovery.

Over the past few years the trend has been for the correction of many lesions in the early weeks of life.[1] Although most cardiac surgery for infants is performed in specialized centres, many anaesthetists will encounter the increasing number of children with corrected, palliated or uncorrected cardiac lesions who present for non-cardiac surgery.

In children, cardiothoracic surgery is undertaken mainly for congenital heart disease, which has a fairly constant world-wide incidence of 8 : 1000 live births.[2] No specific causes are found in most cases, but congenital rubella infection and fetal alcohol syndrome are well-documented causes of congenital heart disease. Some 30–40% of children with trisomy 21 (Down's syndrome) have heart disease and very many chromosomal abnormalities are associated with different cardiac lesions. The risk of recurrence of structural heart disease rises to 3–5% if there is an affected sibling and the incidence is even higher if one parent is affected.[3] Many autosomal dominant and recessive syndromes include cardiac malformations and there is a high incidence of other associated abnormalities, particularly midline defects, such as cleft lip and palate or gut atresias. Approximately 15–20% of babies with tracheo-oesophageal fistula have a cardiac defect, commonly a ventricular septal defect (VSD)[4] (Table 13.1).

Modern antenatal echocardiography identifies most forms of congenital heart disease with accuracy by 16 weeks of gestation, which allows earlier treatment of affected babies, but it is not universally available.[5] If left untreated, more than 20% of infants would die from cardiac

Table 13.1   More common forms of congenital heart disease with medical and surgical management

Incidence	Disease (%)	Treatment
Patent ductus arteriosus (PDA)	10–15	Newborn: trial of indomethacin, ligation or clipping Older: ligation Transcatheter umbrella/coil occlusion
Ventricular septal defect (ASD)	1–20	Closure on bypass
Atrial septal defect (ASD) (secundum)	5–15	Closure on bypass/transcatheter device closure
Atrial septal defect (ASD) (primum)	1–3	Closure on bypass
Atrioventricular septal defect (AVSD)		Closure on bypass
Total anomalous pulmonary venous drainage (TAPVD)	1–2	Immediate repair on bypass
Pulmonary stenosis (PS) (valvular)	5–10	Treatment of choice: balloon pulmonary valvuloplasty Newborn: valvotomy; inflow occlusion Older: valvotomy on bypass
Coarctation of aorta	2–5	Subclavian angioplasty or resection
Aortic arch anomalies	0.5–10	
Persistent truncus arteriosus	1–2	Correction with conduit right ventricle to pulmonary artery (RV–PA)
Aortic stenosis (all types)	3–5	Newborn: valvotomy/vavuloplasty; inflow occlusion Older: Konno/valvuloplasty on bypass
Tetralogy of Fallot	5–10	Modified Blalock–Taussig shunt Early correction
Pulmonary atresia +VSD	1	Blalock shunt/later closure VSD, RV–PA homograft
Tricuspid atresia (TA)	1–3	Blalock shunt; Fontan later
Transposition of great arteries (TGA)	5–15	Balloon atrial septostomy; arterial switch on bypass. Older: Senning on bypass
Corrected TGA (CTGA)	<1	
Univentricular heart (UVH)	1–2	Banding of pulmonary artery/palliative arterial switch; later Fontan
Ebstein's anomaly	<1	Tricuspid valve replacement; ASD closure on bypass
Hypoplastic left heart syndrome	1–2	No intervention/staged palliation (Norwood–Glenn–Fontan)

diseases in the first year of life, half of these within the first month.[6]

PATHOPHYSIOLOGY

Anderson has advocated a sequential segmental approach to naming and classification of congenital heart disease.[7] This system depends on the atrial arrangement (situs), the atrioventricular (A-V) junction connections (type of connection) and the morphology of the A-V valves (mode of connection). The topology of the ventricular mass and the relations of the ventricular chambers within it are determined. The ventriculoatrial (V-A) junctions are analysed in terms of type and mode of connection, in conjunction with a list of associated cardiac malformations. This system, useful for cardiologists and surgeons, permits an unambiguous description of all cardiac defects. However, anaesthetists are more concerned with pathophysiology and applied physiology and pharmacology and a functional approach may be more useful in clinical practice[8] (Table 13.2).

FUNCTIONAL GROUPING OF LESIONS

Four basic functional groups of patients can be identified, each of which poses distinct anaesthetic problems.

1 Patients with increased pulmonary blood flow, including patent ductus arteriosus (PDA), septal defects, aorto-pulmonary (A-P) windows, truncus arteriosus and total anomalous pulmonary venous drainage (TAPVD). Inhalational induction is normal, but respiratory failure may occur because of reduced pulmonary compliance and the increased work of breathing. Untreated cases die early in cardiac failure or develop pulmonary vascular disease and eventually Eisenmenger's syndrome (reversal of shunt). A fall in systemic vascular resistance may

Table 13.2 Haemodynamic characteristics of various congenital cardiac lesions (Reproduced with kind permission of Professor Carol Lake and Appleton and Lange.)

Increased pulmonary blood-flow lesions
Atrial septal defect
Ventricular septal defect
Patent ductus anteriosus
Endocardial cushion defect (atrioventricular canal abnormality)
Anomalous origin of coronary arteries
Transposition of the great arteries
Anomalous pulmonary venous drainage
Truncus arteriosus
Single ventricle

Decreased pulmonary blood-flow lesions
Tetralogy of Fallot
Pulmonary atresia
Tricuspid atresia
Ebstein's anomaly
Transposition of the great arteries
Single ventricle

Obstructive lesions
Aortic stenosis
Pulmonary stenosis
Coarctation of the aorta
Asymmetric septal hypertrophy

cause reversal of the shunt, severe cyanosis and even death.

2 Patients with reduced pulmonary blood flow, often with severe cyanosis and polycythaemia including Fallot's tetralogy, pulmonary stenosis or atresia and tricuspid atresia. Inhalational induction is very slow. Systemic hypotension causes increased right-to-left shunting and infundibular spasm causes catastrophic hypoxia and subsequent acidosis. Severe lesions of this type are dependent on patency of the ductus arteriosus and benefit from preoperative prostaglandin therapy. Cyanosis occurs with a reduction in pulmonary blood flow (anatomical) or with intracardiac mixing (right–left shunt).

3 Patients with transposition of the great vessels which may be complicated by PDA and VSD, have a combination of cyanosis

and increased pulmonary blood flow. An arterial 'switch' operation is performed in the early days of life for 'simple' transposition before the pulmonary vascular resistance (PVR) falls and the left ventricle can no longer support the systemic vascular resistance. With VSD or PDA the operation can be delayed, but not so long that pulmonary vascular disease develops. The alternative is to perform an atrial direction of flow during the first year of life (Senning operation). A Rashkind's balloon septostomy is always required soon after diagnosis to increase mixing at atrial level, but even with good mixing at atrial level by 2 years of age the mortality without correction approaches 50%. Survival is impossible without intracardiac mixing.

4 Patients in whom left ventricular outflow obstruction causes low cardiac output, myocardial ischaemia and eventually myocardial fibrosis with aortic stenosis, subvalvular or valvular and aortic arch problems such as coarctation of the aorta. Patients presenting with symptoms early in life often have very poor cardiac function and may require considerable preoperative support: mechanical ventilation, prostaglandins, inotropes, vasodilators, renal dialysis, etc. However, surgery should not be delayed for too long.

FETAL AND TRANSITIONAL CIRCULATION

The fetal channels, ductus arteriosus (DA) and foramen ovale are important in considerations of abnormal haemodynamics. In fetal life the DA is large, so it allows equal pressures in the aorta and pulmonary artery. The blood flow to the lungs therefore depends on the relative resistances of the lungs and placenta. As the lungs are not expanded and have a high PVR they take only 10% of the cardiac output. The vascular bed of the placenta has a low resistance and takes at least 50% of the total cardiac output. In all, 60% of the oxygenated blood from the placenta crosses from right to left

through the foramen ovale to the aorta, coronaries and developing brain. The rest of the blood passes via the ductus venosus through the liver to the short inferior vena cava and is ejected by the right ventricle to the pulmonary artery, DA and hence to the lower part of the body. Fetal arterial oxygen tension (PaO_2) in the upper part of the body is approximately 4 kPa (60% saturated) and in the lower part 3 kPa (38% saturated).

After the first breath and clamping of the umbilical cord, cessation of umbilical blood flow causes a fall in right atrial pressure. Increasing pulmonary blood flow allows the left atrial pressure to rise and when this is at a sustained level, greater than right atrial pressure, the foramen ovale closes. It is initially only held closed by the difference in pressure between the two atria and it is potentially patent in 30% of normal adults. PVR falls further under the influence of increasing PaO_2 and rising pH [falling arterial carbon dioxide tension ($PaCO_2$)], together with release of bradykinin from inactive precursors triggered by a fall in temperature and pH of umbilical venous blood at birth.[9]

The media of the ductus contains spirally arranged dense smooth muscle which begins to contract from the pulmonary artery end under the influence of increasing PaO_2. Physiological closure is completed within 24 h but permanent closure, requiring fibrosis, takes at least 3 weeks. Isolated ductal tissue of the fetal lamb is relaxed by prostaglandins E_1 and E_2, which are the agents assumed to maintain patency during fetal life. The increased PaO_2 in the newborn period inhibits prostaglandin E_2 synthesis which, when coupled with the activation of cytochrome P450 metabolism in mitochondria of periductal tissue, causes contraction of the smooth muscle of the ductus via the EP 4 and other receptors.[10] Persistent patency beyond the age of 4 months may be caused by a defect in the media of the ductus arteriosus. Prostaglandins are not stored but are synthesized from arachidonic acid and released in response to stimuli such as hypoxia. Synthesis is blocked by prostaglandin synthetase inhibitors such as corticosteroids, aspirin or indomethacin.[11]

The premature ductus is less sensitive to the factors which cause closure; many more remain open in this age group. This is partly because of exposure to low PaO_2 and also attributable to factors such as fluid overload at a time when the oxygen mechanism for closure of the ductus is not fully developed. If the PVR is less than systemic there will be a left-to-right shunt through a PDA causing heart failure, pulmonary oedema and increased work of breathing so that the duct may require urgent medical or surgical attention. The presence of a PDA in a baby dependent on mechanical ventilation may contribute to the appearance of bronchopulmonary dysplasia and thus be an indication to close the ductus.

It is possible to monitor the effects of a closing ductus using echocardiography because the size of the left atrium decreases with the reduction in the left-to-right shunt. Indomethacin is given orally for three 6-hourly doses of 0.2 mg kg^{-1}, but PVR is increased, an effect intensified by hypoxia and more marked in the preterm than the mature baby. This rise in PVR may outweigh the advantage of the 'medical' closure of the ductus.[12]

Prostaglandin E$_1$ or E$_2$ is used therapeutically in doses of 0.05–0.1 μg kg^{-1} min^{-1} by intravenous infusions to maintain ductal patency in babies with severe cyanotic congenital heart disease with very low pulmonary blood flow.[13] Such duct-dependent lesions include severe tetralogy of Fallot and pulmonary atresia with intact septum. Opening of the duct increases pulmonary blood flow and oxygenation, allowing stabilization of the infant and subsequent surgery in more favourable circumstances. Prostaglandin E$_1$ is also useful in patients with reduced systemic blood flow, such as in coarctation of the aorta. Prostaglandin therapy has undoubtedly made a major contribution to the reduction in mortality and morbidity in these lesions. High doses of prostaglandin E$_1$ cause apnoea and facilities for respiratory support should always be readily available when treatment is started.

PULMONARY VASCULATURE

Changes in the PVR are of the greatest importance in congenital heart disease as they easily affect the successful outcome of any corrective surgery. Normally, PVR is low, falling from systemic levels to adult levels within the first few weeks of life. At birth the media of the peripheral pulmonary arterioles contains abundant smooth muscle which regresses gradually, during which time the pulmonary vascular bed is very reactive.[14] Vasoconstrictive reaction to hypoxia, hypercarbia and acidosis by an adrenergic mechanism may cause fetal channels to reopen with a right-to-left shunt and critical hypoxaemia. Transmembrane influx of Ca^{2+} may be involved in pulmonary vasoconstriction and intravenous $CaCl_2$ bolus injection almost always increases PVR.[15]

Irreversible fixed pulmonary vascular disease is often the limiting factor in operability of congenital heart disease and even minor changes may preclude the formation of a Fontan-type of univentricular circulation.

Abnormalities such as VSD, PDA, atrioventricular septal defects, transposition of the great arteries (TGA) and truncus arteriosus cause a high pulmonary artery pressure and an initially high pulmonary blood flow with subsequent development of pulmonary vascular disease. Initially, the small vessels become muscularized very rapidly, possibly within days of birth, first on the arterial and then the venous side, and subsequently the intra-acinar vessels, which normally develop during late fetal life and form mainly after birth, fail to do so.[16] The larger the lesion, for example VSD, the greater the flow of blood from the high pressure left side to the right and the greater the pulmonary blood flow. This causes a fixed increase in PVR as well as the potential for a reversible component by constriction of the abundant smooth muscle, at least in the earlier stages of pulmonary vascular disease.

Dependent shunts occur when ventricular pressures are equal and flow is determined by the relative resistances, whereas an obligatory shunt occurs from a high-pressure chamber to a lower. For example, with atrioventricular septal defect blood shunts from the left ventricle to right atrium, causing a continuous shunt. Most infants with large left-to-right shunts have a low PVR and high flow with hyperaemic lungs with actual or incipient pulmonary oedema, reduced pulmonary compliance, increased work of breathing causing tachypnoea and possible cardiorespiratory failure.

Pulmonary vascular disease is a serious risk if the pulmonary artery (PA) pressure is greater than half systemic pressure with a pulmonary: systemic flow ratio greater than 3 : 1. Resistance usually rises after the first year of life, but the Eisenmenger syndrome does not appear until after the age of 10–20 years. Cyanosis, causing pulmonary vasoconstriction and polycythaemia, which increases resistance to blood flow, complicates pulmonary vascular disease and greatly accelerates its course. Down's syndrome children develop pulmonary vascular disease earlier than other children with similar cardiac lesions.

The diagnosis of pulmonary hypertension in infancy is crucial. Preoperative assessment of PVR is made using cardiac catheter data to obtain the ratio of pulmonary to systemic resistance ($R_p : R_s$), which is normally 0.2. The use of ratios has the advantage that assumptions made in the calculation of both resistances cancel each other out. Absolute values of pulmonary blood flow (Q_p) are difficult to obtain (Figure 13.1).

With difficult or advanced cases a lung biopsy is taken and a progressive series of obliterative structural changes in the peripheral pulmonary arteries is classified into six grades from medial hypertrophy to acute arterial necrosis.[17] Grades IV or more are irreversible, but grades III and IV increase the risk of correcting the abnormality – death from low cardiac output and right ventricular failure or the persistence of pulmonary hypertension. Even those in whom the PA pressure falls to normal postoperatively may show an abnormal increase in PA pressure on exercise, indicating a permanent reduction in the overall capacity of the pulmonary vascular bed.

Calculation of pulmonary vascular resistance

$$Q_p = \frac{\text{oxygen uptake}}{\text{pulmonary A-V O}_2 \text{ difference}} \qquad Q_s = \frac{\text{oxygen uptake}}{\text{systemic A-V O}_2 \text{ difference}}$$

$$\therefore \frac{Q_p}{Q_s} = \frac{\text{systemic A-V O}_2 \text{ difference}}{\text{pulmonary A-V O}_2 \text{ difference}} \quad \text{because } R_p = \frac{P_p}{Q_p} \text{ and } R_s = \frac{P_s}{Q_s}$$

$$R_p/R_s = \frac{P_p}{P_s} \times \frac{Q_s}{Q_p} = \frac{P_p}{P_s} \times \frac{\text{pulmonary A-V O}_2 \text{ difference}}{\text{systemic A-V O}_2 \text{ difference}}$$

Q_p = pulmonary blood flow; Q_s = aortic blood flow; R_p = pulmonary resistance; R_s = systemic resistance; P_p = pressure drop across pulmonary vascular bed; P_s = systemic pressure difference.

Figure 13.1 Calculation of pulmonary vascular resistance.

Fall in peripheral resistance when PVR is severe, associated, for example, with induction of anaesthesia or prolonged diuretic therapy, is poorly tolerated and sudden reversal of the shunt may occur. Factors associated with anaesthesia which cause changes in systemic and pulmonary circulations are listed in Table 13.3.

LOW PULMONARY BLOOD FLOW

A dependent right-to-left shunt occurs when venous and systemic circulations communicate and the resistance of the right ventricular outflow is variable, for example, in tetralogy of Fallot. An obligatory right-to-left shunt occurs when the normal pulmonary pathway is obstructed and blood shunts to the left side at a more proximal level, for example, in pulmonary stenosis or atresia. In TGA the obligatory shunt is of systemic venous blood to systemic arterial circulation and pulmonary to pulmonary.

Cyanotic patients make a number of adaptations to compensate for reduced oxygen delivery to the tissues. The oxygen dissociation curve is shifted to the right to allow improved unloading of oxygen to the tissues, a shift caused by a mild persistent metabolic acidosis and a rise in level of 2,3-diphosphoglycerate in red cells.

There is enlargement of the systemic venous bed, doubling of blood volume with collateral formation which in the digits is manifest as clubbing. The oxygen-carrying capacity of the blood is increased by a rising haemoglobin level, sometimes exceeding 20 g dl^{-1}.

Progress of cyanotic disease, for example pulmonary atresia, is easily monitored from haemoglobin levels and a rising level may be an indication for further palliative surgery or even total correction. As the haematocrit rises there is an increase in blood viscosity, impairing perfusion of vital organs such as the kidneys. At levels above 70% there is sludging of cells in peripheral vessels and a danger of thromboembolism, especially in the cerebral circulation, and particularly if the child becomes dehydrated. Preoperative starvation, diuretic therapy and sudden diarrhoea are all common contributory factors to such a catastrophe. Exchange transfusion with plasma may be necessary to reduce the haematocrit.

A further compensatory mechanism counteracting the tendency to thrombosis is a coagulo-

Table 13.3 Anaesthetic implications of cardiac pathophysiology (Reproduced with kind permission of Professor Carol Lake and Appleton and Lange.)

Perianaesthetic factors influencing cardiovascular flow and resistance

Flow (cardiac output)
Systemic and pulmonary circulations

Increase	Volume loading
	Chronotropic agents
	Inotropic agents
	Vasodilators (with adequate volume)
	Inhalation anaesthetics
	β-Adrenergic antagonists
Decrease	Inhalation anaesthetics
	Hypovolaemia
	Vasodilators (with inadequate volume)
	Arrhythmias
	Ischaemia
	Calcium slow-channel blocking agents
	High mean airway pressure (with inadequate volume)

Resistance
Systemic circulation

Increase	Sympathetic stimulation
	α-Adrenergic agonists
Decrease	Anaesthetics[a]
	Vasodilators
	α-Adrenergic antagonists
	β-Adrenergic agonists
	Calcium slow-channel blocking agents

Pulmonary circulation

Increase	Hypoxia
	Hypercarbia
	Acidosis
	High mean airway pressure
	Sympathetic stimulation
	α-Adrenergic agonists
	Hypervolaemia
	Anaesthetics[a]
Decrease	Oxygen
	Hypocarbia
	Alkalosis
	Prostaglandin E_1/prostacyclin
	α-Adrenergic antagonists
	Vasodilators
	Anaesthetics[a]
	Nitric oxide

[a]Effects of non-inhalational agents may be unpredictable.

pathy with reduced prothrombin and poor platelet function, which often causes bleeding problems after surgery performed on cardiopulmonary bypass (CBP). Blood products such as platelets, fresh-frozen plasma and cryoprecipitate should be available.

Cyanotic attacks, which are sometimes very severe (hypercyanotic), occur in tetralogy of Fallot if systemic resistance is reduced or right ventricular outflow trace resistance rises. They can occur during crying or feeding but are commonly associated with cardiac catheterization or the prebypass phase of surgery, particularly at induction of anaesthesia. The squatting which is so characteristic of the Fallot is an attempt to minimize right-to-left shunting by increasing peripheral resistance. Attacks can be controlled with β-blockade (e.g. propranolol), which is usually discontinued before surgery because of its myocardial depressant effect after bypass. Hypercyanotic attacks require urgent treatment, including sedation with morphine (0.2 mg kg^{-1}), oxygen, sodium bicarbonate (1 mmol kg^{-1}), propranolol (0.2 mg kg^{-1}) and an infusion of noradrenaline. Noradrenaline (dose range 0.01–0.5 μg kg^{-1} min^{-1}, 30 μg kg^{-1} in 50 ml 5% dextrose at 5 ml h^{-1} i.v. = 0.05 μg kg^{-1} min^{-1}) is the drug of first choice for attacks occurring during surgery. Surgery becomes more urgent since the combination of systemic hypotension, hypoxaemia and acidosis may be rapidly fatal. Care should be taken not to overventilate these children, as intermittent positive pressure ventilation (IPPV) with distending pressure will further reduce pulmonary blood flow. Vigorous manual hyperventilation of a hypercyanotic child should be resisted.

PREOPERATIVE ASSESSMENT OF MURMURS

Diastolic, pansystolic and continuous murmurs are organic murmurs, indicate underlying structural heart disease and require preoperative consultation.[18] A high index of suspicion for an organic heart murmur should be present if a history is positive for:

- prematurity;
- small for gestational age/failure to thrive;
- associated congenital anomalies;
- recurrent respiratory tract infections.

The healthy asymptomatic child may, on occasion, present with an undiagnosed heart murmur and identification of the ejection systolic murmur which signifies organic heart disease may fall to the anaesthesiologist. The murmurs of idiopathic hypertrophic subaortic stenosis (IHSS), atrial septal defect (ASD), bicuspid aortic valve and coarctation of the aorta are four organic murmurs which occasionally masquerade as innocent systolic ejection murmurs. Distinction between the innocent and pathological murmurs in children has been extensively reviewed by Rosenthal.[19] Auscultation of the heart in both the supine and sitting position may be useful, since outflow murmurs will be louder in the supine position. This is because in the supine position, the end-diastolic volume is larger, the stroke volume greater and the murmur louder compared with the sitting position. Murmurs arising from the right heart will increase in intensity during inspiration. Those arising from the left heart will be louder in expiration.

Still's murmur is the most common innocent murmur of childhood and is characterized by a vibratory musical quality best heard between the apex and left lower sternal border. The most important differential diagnosis to exclude, in the presence of such a murmur, is that of IHSS. The absence of a positive family history and the absence of a rapid carotid upstroke argue against a diagnosis of IHSS. Murmurs which increase in intensity in the sitting position should alert the anaesthesiologist to the possibility of IHSS. A valsalva manoeuvre performed by asking the child to place his or her thumb in their mouth and then blowing hard against it will also cause the intensity of the murmur of IHSS to increase. Table 13.4 shows an algorithm for the preoperative management of children older than 1 year with a murmur.[20]

A systolic murmur best heard over the second left intercostal space may indicate the presence of an ASD. An ASD may also be associated with a widely split second heart sound and/or a hyperdynamic cardiac impulse at the xiphoid. A supraclavicular arterial bruit and any murmur heard at the right upper sternal border may

Table 13.4 Algorithm for preoperative management for children older than 1 year[20]

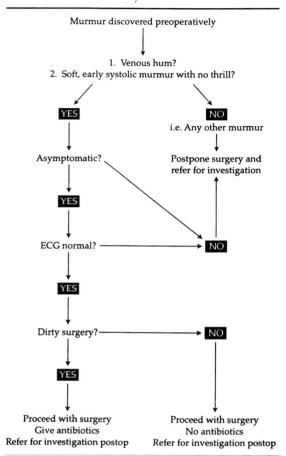

indicate organic heart disease, namely a bicuspid aortic valve which requires antimicrobial prophylaxis (see appendices).[21] A supraclavicular murmur may indicate a benign arterial bruit or a coarctation of the aorta, a diagnosis which is suggested by diminished or delayed femoral pulses compared with the radial pulses.

CONGESTIVE HEART FAILURE

Heart failure is associated with large left-to-right shunts, mitral or aortic valve disease, total anomolous pulmonary venous connection (TAPVC) or valve atresia and is often precipitated by a chest infection or anaemia. Early signs include hepatomegaly since the infant liver is so distensible, tachypnoea and tachycardia with a gallop rhythm. Peripheral oedema occurs late. Wheezing heard on chest auscultation in a baby is often a sign of increased lung interstitial water, rather than asthma, as there is very little bronchial musculature in infants. Digoxin and diuretics (frusemide up to 1 mg kg^{-1} 8-hourly or spironolactone) with potassium supplements (1 mmol kg^{-1} b.d.) are standard treatment. Prolonged therapy with diuretics often leads to hypovolaemia in infancy as well as reduction in total body potassium, manifest by a metabolic alkalosis. Hypomagnesaemia is usually present, in addition, and is poorly reflected in serum levels. Digoxin therapy is usually stopped preoperatively as toxicity postbypass is possible and at that stage stronger inotropic agents such as dopamine may be indicated.

MYOCARDIAL FUNCTION

Animal work shows that the fetal myocardium develops much less active tension during isometric contraction than the adult and is much more sensitive to the depressant effect of inhalational anaesthetic agents. Newborn myocardium contains only 30% contractile mass, whereas the adult contains 60%, causing the stroke volume of the infant to be relatively fixed. Increases in cardiac output come almost entirely from increases in cardiac rate and bradycardia causes a severe fall in cardiac output. Infants have a lower blood pressure than that found later in life; average systolic blood pressure is 80 mmHg.

CARDIAC INVESTIGATION

A good history and proper physical examination remain the basis of diagnosis in paediatric cardiology, but in addition, chest X-ray, electrocardiography (ECG), echocardiography and cardiac catheterization are often necessary.

From the chest X-ray an evaluation of cardiac size, shape, position and pulmonary vascularity can be made as well as lung fields generally. Cardiothoracic ratio is 0.6 in infancy and the thymus may mimic cardiac enlargement. Classically, the heart is egg-shaped in TGA and boot-shaped in Fallot's tetralogy, but a normal configuration does not necessarily rule out a specific defect. Pulmonary hyperaemia and underperfusion are easily seen, as are all stages of pulmonary oedema.

There are distinct differences between an adult ECG and an ECG in the very young, where there is dominance of the right ventricle and right-axis deviation, so that a left-axis configuration is always abnormal. The adult pattern is seen by 3 years of age. Information on enlargement of chambers, cardiac malpositioning and rhythm abnormalities is also provided by the ECG. Table 13.5 gives normal cardiovascular values for children.

Modern echocardiography from the chest or via the oesophagus has revolutionized cardiac diagnosis and frequently information gained from this non-invasive technique is of superior quality.[22] Serial studies provide accurate data of changes in cardiac output and ventricular function.

M-mode echo records motion of the heart, from which it is possible to measure the thickness of the chamber walls and left ventricular function. If the ECG is recorded at the same time, measurement of systolic time intervals can be made. Left ventricular function is assessed from the shortening fraction (above 0.3 in infants) and left ventricular systolic time intervals. The time between onset of the ECG Q-wave and aortic valve opening is the pre-ejection period (PEP) and the ejection time (ET) is the time during which the aortic valve is open. The PEP:ET ratio should be less than 0.3. The echo shows the velocity of fibre shortening (less than 1 circumference s^{-1}) of the walls and septum.[23] Serial echo investigations are of great importance postoperatively to assess ventricular function and are particularly important after the arterial switch operation for TGA, where the coronary arteries are reimplanted and after the Senning operation for atrial correction of TGA, where the systemic

Table 13.5 Normal cardiovascular values for children

	% Saturated O_2	Pressure (mmHg)		
		Systolic	Diastolic	Mean
Superior vena cava	65–75			2–6
Inferior vena cava	75–80			2–6
Coronary sinus	30–40			2–6
Right atrium	75	a = 5–10	v = 4–10	2–6
Right ventricle	75	15–30	0–5	
Neonate		65–80	0–5	
Pulmonary artery	75	15–30	5–10	10–20
Neonate		65–80	35–50	40–70
Pulmonary artery wedge	96	a = 3–7	v = 5–15	5–12
Pulmonary vein	96–100	a = 6–12	v = 8–15	5–10
Left atrium	96–100	a = 6–12	v = 8–15	5–10
Left ventricle	96–100	80–130	0–10	
Aorta	96–100	80–130	60–90	70–80

	Age		
	<2 years	>2 years	Adult
LV end-diastolic volume (ml m^{-2})	42 ± 10	73 ± 10	70 ± 20
LV end-systolic volume (ml m^{-2})	13.4	27 ± 7	24
LV stroke volume (ml m^{-2})	28.6	44 ± 5	45 ± 13
LV ejection fraction	0.68 ± 0.05	0.63 ± 0.05	0.67 ± 0.08
LV mass (g m^{-2})	92 ± 16	86 ± 11	96 ± 11
RV end-diastolic volume (ml m^{-2})	53 ± 3	75 ± 2	
Left atrial maximum volume (ml m^{-2})	26 ± 5	38 ± 8	34 ± 10

Cardiac index	3–5 l min^{-1} m^{-2}
Systemic arteriolar resistance	10–15 Wood units (mmHg l^{-1} min^{-1} m^{-2})
Pulmonary arteriolar resistance	8–10 Wood units (neonate) and 1–3 units after 6–8 weeks (mmHg l^{-1} min^{-1} m^{-2})
Normal aortic valve area	2 cm^2 m^{-2} (adult, 3–4 cm^2)
Normal pulmonary valve area	2 cm^2 m^{-2} (adult, 2–4 cm^2)
Adult mitral valve	5 cm^2
Adult tricuspid valve	10 cm^2

right ventricular function may not be optimal. Two-dimensional echocardiography allows an accurate diagnosis of the connections of all chambers and great vessels. Pericardial effusions are easily seen and the dimensions of septal defects can be estimated and shunts seen using bubble injections into the venous circulation. Doppler echocardiography detects changes in the velocity of blood flow so that shunts and obstructions as well as cardiac output can be measured.[24]

Cardiac catheterization is required less often, but is necessary to obtain pressures, quantitative flows to calculate shunts and also for the calculation of systemic and pulmonary resistances. For VSD, nowadays, catheterization is rarely necessary to assess PVR as sufficient information is obtained from clinical and echo Doppler examinations.

An increasing number of therapeutic manoeuvres is now performed: balloon atrial septostomy; transluminal angioplasty of aortic coarctation; balloon valvuloplasty of aortic and pulmonary valves; angioplasty of stenotic pulmonary arteries and occlusion of collaterals.[25] PDA and some ASDs may be occluded with suitable devices and abnormal electrical pathways ablated electrophysiologically.

It is possible to perform cardiac catheterization for straightforward cases under sedation, together with local anaesthesia (lignocaine up to 3 mg kg^{-1}), and this is still the practice in some centres (Table 13.6).

In addition, diazepam 0.2 mg kg^{-1} may be given via the catheter as necessary. Full monitoring includes ECG, blood pressure and pulse oximetry. Blood up to 10 ml kg^{-1} is replaced by dextrose and serial haematocrits, blood sugar (BM sticks) and blood gas estimations are made.

General anaesthesia is used for most patients, especially those who are sick or undergoing interventional cardiology, and for the assessment of pulmonary vascular disease, severe rhythm problems, severe failure and cardiac failure from obstructive lesions. For digital subtraction imaging, a completely still patient is required.

Either ketamine 2 mg kg^{-1} i.v. or inhalation of sevoflurane may be used for induction of anaesthesia, as for cardiac surgery.

Anaesthesia always includes a relaxant technique with controlled ventilation and a fixed inspired oxygen concentration, usually 30% to simplify the calculation of shunts. The anaesthetist must be prepared to deal with periods of low cardiac output and dysrhythmia. Monitoring of arterial pressure is therefore usually direct, although access to the central venous circulation is via the catheter.

Angiography with its contrast load may be poorly tolerated in sick infants as the circulation has to cope with a biphasic insult, first from a hyperosmolar fluid load and then from an osmotic diuresis. Protection against hypother-

Table 13.6 Sedation protocol for cardiac investigations

Age	Weight	Drug	Dose	Route	Comments
Tetralogy of Fallot		Morphine	250 μg kg^{-1}	i.m.	30 min precatheter
For all other patients					
Newbornes up to 1 month + infants	<5 kg	Inj. Peth. Co.	0.05 ml kg^{-1}	i.m.	30 min precatheter
Older children	All weights	Trimeprazine	2 mg kg^{-1} **Max dose**: 100 mg	p.o.	3 h precatheter
Followed by:	≥ 5 kg to 15 kg	Inj. Peth. Co.	0.1 ml kg^{-1} **Max dose**: 1.5 ml	i.m.	30 min precatheter Smaller babies in poor condition should have a reduced dose
Or:	≥ 15 kg	Morphine	202 μg kg^{-1} **Max dose**: 10 mg	i.m.	30 min precatheter
		Hyoscine	100 μg kg^{-1} **Max dose**: 500 μg	i.m.	Sick children (e.g. transplant assessments) may need reduced doses

Sedation the night before catheter: triclolos 30 mg kg^{-1} p.o. nocte.
Children >2.5 years who are just under 15 kg body weight are usually best sedated with morphine and hyoscine rather than Inj. Peth. Co.
Most children require the full dose of sedation.
Timing is very important because of patient preparation time and the duration of the investigation.
Supplementary sedation to be given only by a doctor skilled in paediatric resuscitation: diazemuls 200–300 μg kg^{-1} i.v. in increments of 100 μg
NB. EMLA/Ametop should be applied to all children.

mia is necessary. Assessment of pulmonary vascular disease requires a period of 10 min of ventilation with 100% O_2, infusion of prostaglandin starting at 10 ng kg^{-1} min^{-1}, rising to 20 ng kg^{-1} min^{-1}, and inhalation of nitric oxide starting at 5 ppm and rising to 10 ppm to assess the reversible component of the resistance.[26] All three agents may be necessary before a response is seen. A hypercyanotic attack in a child with tetralogy of Fallot is not uncommon during cardiac catheterization.

ANAESTHETIC MANAGEMENT

The general principles of anaesthesia for cardiac surgery in children do not differ greatly from those in adults, but there are specific differences related to the diversity of lesions in childhood. The immaturity of all organ systems and smaller blood volumes mean that sudden major haemorrhage is more likely to be catastrophic. Adequate depth of anaesthesia with intense analgesia is necessary to obtund a major stress response with biochemical changes such as hyperglycaemia, peripheral vasoconstriction, increasing chance of dysrhythmia and increasing right ventricular outflow obstruction in, for example, tetralogy of Fallot. Systemic embolism is a potential danger in children with right-to-left shunts such as TGA and ASD. Great care must be taken to avoid injection of air or particulate matter and cerebral, coronary and renal arteries are at particular risk from embolization. Stopcocks are an important source of air so the line should be aspirated with the syringe before injection and the last millilitre from the syringe should not be used; injection with a needle into a rubber bung is an alternative.

ANTIBIOTICS

The prevention of bacterial endocarditis is a major concern in children and antibiotic prophylaxis is routine to cover all heart surgery as transient bacteraemia is a risk at any stage of the procedure. Routine cover may consist of genta-

Table 13.7 Antibiotic prophylaxis for cardiac surgery

Age	Drug	Dose	Comments
All cases except for reoperations and patients allergic to penicillins			
0–4 weeks	Amikacin	10 mg kg^{-1} stat dose	
> 4 weeks	Amikacin	10 mg kg^{-1} 12 hourly	
0–4weeks	Flucloxacillin	25 mg kg^{-1} 8 hourly	Repeat 25 mg kg^{-1} stable off bypass
>4 weeks	Flucloxacillin	25 mg kg^{-1} 6 hourly	Repeat 25 mg kg^{-1} when stable off bypass
Reoperations during same hospital admission or patients allergic to penicillins			
0–4 weeks	Amikacin	10 mg kg^{-1} stat dose	
5–8 weeks	Amikacin	10 mg kg^{-1} 12 hourly	
8 weeks	Amikacin	10 mg kg^{-1} 12 hourly	
0–4 weeks	Teicoplanin	16 mg kg^{-1} stat dose	
5–8 weeks	Teicoplanin	15 mg kg^{-1} stat dose	
>8 weeks	Teicoplanin	10 mg kg^{-1} 12 hourly	

Duration of prophylactic cover should be 24 h. First dose: on induction of anaesthesia; bypass cases – additional flucloxacillin dose off bypass. Subsequent doses: to complete 24 h cover from induction.
Antibiotic levels are not indicated as prophylaxis is for 24 h only.
Preterm infants and special situations, e.g. renal failure, long standing and complex cases. Discuss regime with consultant microbiologist.
Teicoplanin administration: patients > 8 weeks, intravenous bolus; neonates = 8 weeks, 30-min infusion.

micin or amikacin plus flucloxacillin given on induction of anaesthesia and an additional dose of flucloxacillin after bypass (see Table 13.7). Flucloxacillin given intravenously postbypass may cause hypotension. For those with penicillin allergy teicoplanin is substituted for flucloxacillin. Antibiotic prophylaxis for patients with corrected or uncorrected cardiac lesions, especially after implantation of prosthetic material, follows the recommendations of the American Heart Association (1997)[27] (see Appendix 4).

ASSESSMENT AND PREMEDICATION

Heart surgery is a tremendously anxious time for parents and patients. All aspects of anaesthesia and surgery should be discussed fully, including the known risks such as postoperative cardiac, renal and neurological problems, which should be quantified where possible. The patients have often been in hospital on previous occasions and anxiety may be intense. The preoperative visit also allows the anaesthetist to define the lesion and to find out what the surgeon intends to do, as well as assessing the clinical condition, the degree of cyanosis, the exercise tolerance, the ability to feed, etc. The presence of any other congenital abnormalities should be noted.

It is usual for the parents to be shown the postoperative intensive care unit (ICU) on the day prior to surgery so that the shock of seeing their own child postoperatively should be lessened. Some small sick babies will already be receiving full intensive care and indeed a period of mechanical ventilation, fully monitored with prostaglandin and inotropic agents, may be beneficial as myocardial glycogen stores may be replenished and poor renal function improved.

A checklist for preoperative investigations with the results is useful and should include haemoglobin, haematocrit, electrolytes, clotting studies and platelet count, a recent chest X-ray and the current status of drug therapy such as digoxin, diuretics or β-blockers. Any dental infection should be treated preoperatively together with the appropriate antibiotic cover.

Children are given clear fluids up to 2 h preoperatively. Children with polycythaemia should not be starved for too long and if the time of surgery is unpredictable then fluids should be given intravenously.

Many centres have established care pathways for specific lesions in an attempt to increase efficiency and safety and to allow fast tracking for patients with simpler lesions such as ASD, pulmonary stenosis or partial atrioventricular septal defect, with the result that morbidity is reduced and cost-effectiveness improved.

Establishment of a rapport with the parents and the child is essential, but the use of an anxiolytic drug preoperatively is usually beneficial. A local anaesthetic cream such as EMLA (eutectic mixture of local anaesthetics) or Ametop is used routinely. Even for very small babies, such as those for the arterial switch operation, sedative premedication such as triclofos (chloral hydrate 30–50 mg kg^{-1} orally 40 min preoperatively) is of benefit (Table 13.8).

Table 13.8 Premedication for cardiac surgery[a]

Age	Weight	Drug	Dose	Comments
<4 weeks		Atropine		
Between 4 weeks and 6 kg		Triclofos	50–75 mg kg^{-1}	
	6–15 kg	Triclofos	50–75 mg kg^{-1}	
	>15 kg	Midazolam syrup	500 μg–1 mg	Max. dose: 15 mg
		Temazepam	500 μg–1 mg	Max. dose: 20 mg
				Use tablets not elixir

[a]Closed heart operations and bypass surgery.

ANAESTHETIC AGENTS

There is no anaesthetic agent or opioid which does not affect cardiovascular function and if the myocardium is poor, the effects may be profound, especially with cyanotic patients.

Halothane, which is still commonly used for inhalational induction of anaesthesia in children, is a myocardial depressant and may also cause the loss of sinus rhythm. In all patients it is contraindicated except in low doses until full monitoring has been established, and in patients with obstructive lesions only minute doses may be given. Laishley *et al.* and Hensley *et al.* found that induction with halothane, nitrous oxide and oxygen actually increased oxygen saturation in children with cyanotic congenital heart disease. This was particularly so in those with the potential for variable pulmonary outflow tract obstruction, and was possibly caused by a decrease in cardiac output but a maintenance of pulmonary blood flow.[28,29] Isoflurane is claimed to have a less depressive cardiac effect than halothane but it decreases systemic resistance, which is unwise in patients with balanced shunts. However, it has been shown in children by Murray *et al.* that halothane and isoflurane both decrease mean blood pressure from an awake level; both decrease cardiac index at 1.25 minimum alveolar concentration (MAC) with a significant decrease in ejection fractions.[30] Sevoflurane may have a similar effect.[31] Large right-to-left shunts may affect the speed of inhalational induction and the more insoluble the agent the greater will be the slowing, i.e. greater with sevoflurane than halothane.[32,33] After a fluid load the ejection fraction decreased significantly with halothane but increased with isoflurane. This response to fluid may show that a greater cardiovascular reserve exists during isoflurane anaesthesia than with halothane. Isoflurane is a small-vessel coronary dilator and this type of vasodilator may cause myocardial ischaemia by diverting flow from areas of borderline perfusion towards areas that are already well perfused. This 'coronary steal' may be deleterious in children whose coronary flow is already prejudiced.[34]

Sevoflurane causes a dose-dependent reduction in blood pressure but constricts peripheral veins, which may make venepuncture more difficult, although cardiac output is well maintained.[35]

Thiopentone decreases cardiac output by at least 30%, reducing sympathetic tone and availability of calcium to cardiac muscle fibres, effects which are related to dose and speed of injection.

Ketamine, which produces rapid hypnosis and profound analgesia without respiratory or cardiovascular depression, has regained popularity as an induction agent for paediatric cardiac anaesthesia. It produces a non-dose-related increase in heart rate and cardiac index, and increases in systemic and pulmonary artery pressures.[36] There is a potential for increasing PVR, although this effect and any effect on balanced shunts is trivial if the airway is secured and controlled ventilation started.[37] Clinical practice has also confirmed ketamine's safety in this respect. Ketamine has a direct negative inotropic action on myocardial muscle, but inhibition of neuronal catecholamine uptake overcomes this. If noradrenaline stores have been depleted ketamine has no positive inotropic effect and there may be a profound fall in blood pressure if given to patients on long-term catecholamine therapy. It is also an *N*-methyl-D-aspartate (NMDA) receptor antagonist which may possibly have a beneficial effect in babies undergoing deep hypothermic circulatory arrest.[38] Tachycardia, increased cardiac output and increased myocardial oxygen consumption may be undesirable in children with severe valvar stenoses.[39]

INDUCTION AND MONITORING: OPEN HEART SURGERY

Before induction of anaesthesia it is wise to have 8.4% sodium bicarbonate, 1 : 10 000 adrenaline and 10% calcium chloride readily available for possible use. Whichever agents are chosen for induction, minimal quantities to provide a smooth induction should be used and respiratory obstruction or depression avoided. The airway should be rapidly secured and mechanical ventilation commenced. Rapid, smooth and safe induction is achieved by either sevoflurane in oxygen and nitrous oxide, which have minimal cardiovascular effects for a brief period, or ketamine 2 mg kg^{-1} i.v. A local anaesthetic cream allows early painless venous access, whichever agent is chosen and this is a priority. Intravenous induction agents should be given with care as any bubbles of air will gain access to the brain with a right-to-left shunt and in these cases the induction agent crosses to the left side affecting the brain and myocardium immediately, so all intravenous injections should be slow.

Thiopentone, which is suitable for use in fitter patients, should be used with the greatest of care in patients with fixed cardiac output, for example in those with with aortic stenosis or constrictive pericarditis.

Pancuronium (0.1 mg kg^{-1}) continues to be the muscle relaxant of choice given by bolus, and although it occasionally causes a troublesome tachycardia, this can usually be offset by the bradycardia seen with intravenous fentanyl. Other short-acting relaxants can be given by continuous infusion.

Most infants undergoing cardiac surgery require some postoperative respiratory support so that a firm nasal fixation of the tracheal tube is preferred. The tube should be of a sufficient size to allow a small air leak through the cricoid at 25 cmH$_2$O inflation pressure and at least 3 cm of tube should lie in the trachea. The tip should lie in the mid-trachea and on the chest X-ray be seen between the clavicles.

The process of inducing anaesthesia is a time of potential instability and clinical signs should be carefully observed: mottling of the skin and cooling of the hands and feet mean a falling cardiac output. Clinical observation is reinforced by the use of the precordial stethoscope, non-invasive blood pressure (NIBP), ECG and pulse oximetry at this stage.

VASCULAR ACCESS LINES

It is now common practice, in addition to the largest possible cannula in a peripheral vein, to stitch in place a multilumen catheter in a central vein, usually the right internal jugular vein. An alternative is to use multiple single cannulae, either in the same central vein or in different ones. At least three separate lumens are required, one for continuous monitoring of central venous pressure (CVP), one for infusion of drugs such as inotropic and/or vasodilating agents and one or more for the infusion of crystalloids and colloids, which occasionally may need to be very rapid. A fluid warmer (Hotline, for example) is used routinely. Other sites for central vein catheterization, for example, left superior vena cava (SVC), femorals or subclavians, are probably less satisfactory, although the left internal jugular vein can be used if there is dextrocardia, a persistent left SVC or if a Glenn procedure is being performed. Insertion should be with aseptic precautions, but it is wise not to cover the whole child as clinical monitoring signs are lost. Great care should be taken not to introduce air into the circulation. CVP readings in infancy may not be reliable because the venous system has a great capacity as the liver is so distensible. Considerable volumes of fluid may be given with no rise in CVP at all, although the liver has enlarged enormously. Right atrial pressure does not necessarily correspond with severity of congestive cardiac failure in small infants.

Direct monitoring of arterial pressure is via a 24–20G Teflon cannula inserted percutaneously into a radial artery, although the femoral or axillary routes last longer postoperatively.[40] Complications of monitoring lines are few in children.

In infants the technique of transfixation is likely to be more successful than a direct puncture technique. The cannula is connected to a short extension with a three-way stopcock to allow frequent sampling and is continuously flushed with heparinized saline (1 U ml^{-1}) using an intraflow type of device (3 ml h^{-1}), except in very small babies when a syringe pump set to 1 ml h^{-1} is used.

This stage of anaesthesia should not be prolonged; 15–20 min should be sufficient or the child will tend to become vasoconstricted and acidotic. In addition, a nasogastric tube (postoperative ileus), a silastic urinary catheter, peripheral temperature, nasopharyngeal temperature reflecting cerebral temperature) and oesophageal temperature probes (reflecting cardiac temperature) are inserted. In patients at risk from postoperative pulmonary hypertensive crisis a 20 or 22G catheter may be coiled up in the right atrium via the right internal jugular vein to be passed on into the pulmonary artery by the surgeon before completing the operation. A Swan–Ganz catheter is rarely used intraoperatively.

Other monitoring includes end-tidal CO_2 which is higher than arterial CO_2 when pulmonary blood flow is reduced. Cerebral function monitors are not routinely used as they provide only limited, global information, although they would show any residual cerebral activity prior to circulatory arrest.

MAINTENANCE OF ANAESTHESIA

The patient is transferred to the operating table on a heated mattress (at this stage switched off) and connected to a mechanical ventilator. A small bridge is used to lift the chest forward for median sternotomy. The chest movement is checked and ventilator adjustments made after blood gas analysis to give a $PaCO_2$ of 5 kPa. It should be remembered that patients with left-to-right shunts have non-compliant lungs, whilst those with right-to-left shunts have compliant lungs; overventilation of these will further reduce pulmonary blood flow. When monitoring lines have been connected, anaesthesia is supplemented with, for example, fentanyl, which can be given as boluses or by continuous infusion. It is advisable, in the absence of surgical stimulation to give an initial small dose of fentanyl, for example: 1–2 μg kg^{-1}, but followed by 10–20 μg kg^{-1}, repeated as necessary before skin incision and sternotomy, and together with a full dose of relaxant before bypass.[41] These fentanyl dosages provide unique cardiovascular stability.[42] The ultra-short-acting opioid remifentanil is now being used for open heart surgery, by continuous infusion in both adults and children in doses of 0.5–1 μg kg^{-1} h^{-1}. Other forms of analgesia are provided before the infusion is finally terminated. Supplementation with midazolam 0.2–0.4 mg kg^{-1} will reduce the risk of awareness.

Inspired oxygen concentration is adjusted to give a reasonable PaO_2, depending on the lesion, but 100% should be used if cardiac output falls – the balance is best made up with nitrous oxide. During opening of the chest, particularly by sternotomy, low doses of inhala-

tional agents such as halothane or isoflurane will control the hypertension and may actually be beneficial to the myocardium;[28] a systolic pressure of 90–100 mmHg is satisfactory. Serial blood gas analyses should be made as a tendency to an increase in acidosis is common and should be corrected if the base excess is greater than 5 mmol l^{-1} (weight/5 × 1/2 base deficit = ml 8.4% HCO_3).

Patients on long-term diuretic therapy are often found to have metabolic alkalosis and low total body potassium. This is associated with dysrhythmia, and diluted increments of 0.5–1 mmol K$^+$ are given slowly to keep serum levels above 4 mmol l^{-1}.

Rapid transfusion may be necessary at any time, e.g. during aortic cannulation, so equipment to pressurize the infusion should be available. Bleeding from sternotomy in older children with cyanotic disease may be enormous and in repeat operations there is a danger that one of the cardiac chambers will be entered inadvertently. Surgical manipulation always interferes with cardiac output, especially when putting in venous purse strings and 'snuggers' for the venous tourniquets. It is now usual to begin bypass with one cannula in the right atrial appendage, which causes minimal disruption to cardiac function, and to put the second into the IVC as soon as bypass is established. A bolus injection of $CaCl_2$ is a powerful inotropic stimulus but it should be remembered that severe bradycardia and even asystole may occur if K$^+$ is low or if myocardial oxygenation is very borderline. A very small dose of 1 : 100 000 adrenaline may be better to improve cardiac output if the systemic blood pressure does not return to a reasonable level after surgical manipulations have stopped.

A control level of activated clotting time (ACT) is measured prior to heparinization and should be in the region of 90–140 s (Hemochron R automatic ACT device). Heparin 300 U kg^{-1} is given intravenously before aortic cannulation and the ACT should be greater than 400 s before and during bypass. Further heparin is required if the ACT falls below that level, but in practice with heparin given to the bypass prime and hypothermic conditions, further heparin is seldom needed. However, ACT continues to be used because a few patients have a decreased response[43] and inadequate anticoagulation may result in damaging low-grade fibrinolysis.

Aprotinin (Trasylol), a proteinase inhibitor, is frequently used in children where excessive bleeding, is expected as in redo surgery. Its mechanism of action has not been fully defined but has a protective effect on platelet function and antifibrinolytic activity via a direct inhibition of plasmin and the kinin–kallikrein system.[44] Studies have shown a large reduction in bleeding after cardiac and other major surgery. A usual dosage regime is a test dose of 1–2 ml, then a slow intravenous bolus of 1 ml kg^{-1} and the same to the pump prime, and thereafter a continuous infusion of 1 ml kg^{-1} h^{-1} until bleeding stops postoperatively. Kaolin is used as the clotting time activator in these cases.[45]

CARDIOPULMONARY BYPASS

A further full dose of relaxant and analgesic is given a few minutes before bypass to allow time for the drugs to fix at the end-plate and to achieve complete muscular paralysis. It is a disaster if respiratory movements start during deep hypothermic circulatory arrest; if air is sucked into the heart with an ASD, air embolism is a very real possibility. There is no agreement on how to manage the lungs during bypass, but ventilation continues until there is full flow from the bypass and the venous drainage blood looks well oxygenated, after which the lungs may be left to collapse or maintained with 3–5 cmH$_2$O distending pressure with oxygen or oxygen and air. Lung damage is more likely to occur from the vascular side and blood from the left side must be vented continuously. Left-to-right shunts through a PDA or Blalock shunt must be controlled immediately after the start of bypass.

Mean perfusion pressures of 30–60 mmHg on bypass at full flow (2.4 l m^{-2} min^{-1}) are considered suitable. Vasoconstrictors are rarely necessary as progressive cooling usually causes a rise in peripheral resistance. To combat a rise in perfusion pressure, isoflurane, nitroglycerine (2–10 μg kg^{-1} min^{-1}) or sodium nitroprusside (2–10 μg kg^{-1} min^{-1}) may be given into the pump.

At low temperatures cerebral metabolism and oxygen consumption are greatly reduced; at 18–20°C they are only 17% of basal requirements.[46] Periods of circulatory arrest up to 30–45 min may be used safely at this temperature. Deep hypothermic circulatory arrest is used routinely for periods in open heart surgery for small babies where the usual venous cannulae would obstruct a delicate repair.[47] This allows even the most complex surgery to be carried out with dramatic decrease in mortality and morbidity.

The venous cannulae are removed after circulatory arrest and replaced prior to recommencement of bypass. Catecholamine levels are enormously elevated after deep hypothermic circulatory arrest, contributing to extreme vasoconstriction; surface cooling (see below) causes even higher levels.[48] Lactate and pyruvate levels are surprisingly low even after long periods of arrest and myocardial protection is maximized by preventing the heart being rewarmed by surrounding tissues using ice slush in the pericardium.

Alternatively, low flow can be maintained where possible with the venous cannulae left *in situ* with levels of flow as low as 0.5 l m^{-2} min^{-1} (approx. 50 ml kg^{-1} min^{-1}) in which case only moderate hypothermia is required (22–25°C).[49] Uniform cooling before arrest is very important and requires all temperatures to read 17–18°C with at least 12 min of bypass. Methylprednisolone 30 mg kg^{-1} to stabilize membranes is given before arrest and moderate haemodilution to a haematocrit of 20 is used to promote peripheral blood flow.

Potassium supplementation is always required on CPB, as K$^+$ is very frequently low and losses into the cells, urine and bypass continue; 1 mmol kg^{-1} can be given slowly into the pump prime during bypass. Serum Mg^{2+} is also low and further reduced by CPB which is not well reflected in serum levels. Mg^{2+} may prevent coronary vessel spasm, reduce the incidence of dysrhythmia, reduce systemic vascular resistance and improve cardiac output.[50] It may help to prevent deleterious effects of reperfusion.[51]

SURFACE COOLING

The technique of surface cooling before beginning surgery has largely been abandoned in favour of a very short prebypass period and core cooling on bypass. It was claimed that the technique produced more even cooling, particularly of the peripheral muscular bed to prevent readjustment of temperatures and possible rewarming after arrest. A measure of cerebral protection would be achieved if cardiac output fell or cardiac arrest occurred during sternotomy.[52,53] No metabolic differences have been found between surface cooling and core cooling. Icebags are packed around the baby over the major arteries after anaesthesia, but care is taken to avoid the precordium, kidneys or limb extremities. Peripheral vasodilatation is promoted by adequate anaesthesia (isoflurane) and as the temperature falls, CO_2 production is diminished so 2.5–5% CO_2 is added to the inspired gases to maintain $PaCO_2$ over 6 kPa. This improves cerebral perfusion. Very frequent blood gas (corrected for temperature) and K^+ analyses are essential and severe acidosis is corrected. Cardiac stability is easily achieved during cooling if K^+ supplements are given (0.5–1 mmol) as K^+ levels fall with movement into the cells. Crystalloid 10–20 ml kg^{-1} i.v. helps to maintain peripheral blood flow. Active cooling is discontinued when the nasopharyngeal temperature is 26°C. A 2°C afterdrop is to be expected and surgery then proceeds.

CARDIOPLEGIA

It is routine to infuse cold cardioplegic solution into the root of the aorta after aortic cross-clamping to cause diastolic arrest and cool the myocardium.[54] The cardioplegic solution (e.g. Ringer's solution containing KCl 1.193 g, procaine 272.8 mg and magnesium chloride 3.253 g l^{-1}; St Thomas' solution), is infused at 150 mmHg pressure at a dose of 20–30 ml kg^{-1} bodyweight to preserve myocardial function. A half-dose is repeated at intervals of 30 min of aortic cross-clamping to prevent electrical activity. As the aorta is clamped the solution is aspirated by the discard suction from the right atrium and usually none enters the perfusate.

There is no agreement as to which regimen of cardioplegia, temperature and delivery pressure damages the myocardium the least and results in minimal reperfusion injury. Minimally diluted tepid blood cardioplegia, which has a greater buffering activity and O_2-carrying capacity, may give the best postoperative ventricular function.[55] After cross-clamping and administration of cardioplegia many surgeons pack the heart in ice slush. There is some anecdotal evidence that procaine may increase the incidence of atrioventricular block in the immediate postbypass period, but this does not seem to be of any clinical significance.

EXTRACORPOREAL CIRCULATION

Extracorporeal circulation is now safe and routine, with flow rates at normothermia of 2.2–2.5 l min^{-1} m^{-2} providing a margin of safety. Although pulsatile flow from the pump may help organ perfusion, particularly in the kidneys, it is not routinely used[56] as there seems to be no proven clinical advantage. The peripheral circulation should be maximal at any temperature and this is related to oxygen consumption (Figure 13.2). The temperature gradient between perfusate and the patient should never exceed 10°C on rewarming. Systemic venous pressure should always be low (< 10 mmHg) or cerebral oedema will occur, so the largest possible venous cannulae should be used as drainage is a passive, syphonic process.[57]

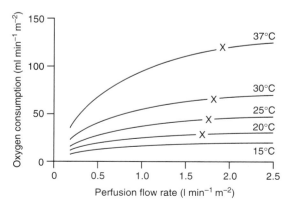

Figure 13.2 Normogram of the relation between oxygen consumption (V_{O_2}) and perfusion flow rate (Q) at various temperatures. (From Kirklin *et al.*, 1985, with permission.[57])

The following formula is used for calculating haematocrit of the prime for cardiopulmonary bypass:

$$Htpm = \frac{(\text{kg body weight} \times f \times 1000)(Htp)}{(\text{kg body weight} \times f \times 1000) + \text{machine BV}},$$

where *Htpm* is the desired total haematocrit (25–30), *Htp* is the *Ht* of the patient and *f* is 0.08 in infants and young children.

Stored blood should ideally be as fresh as possible and requires 3000 units of heparin, 10 ml 8.4% $NaHCO_3$ and 5 ml 10% $CaCl_2$ to be added to each 500 ml of blood. Hartmann's solution is used for dilution. Blood sugar levels are always well maintained on bypass[58] but will require close monitoring afterwards. CPB technology is constantly improving with smaller priming volumes. PaO_2 levels are held between 15 and 25 kPa, but the management of pH and $PaCO_2$ is more controversial and two strategies are in use: alphastat (temperature uncorrected) and pH stat (temperature corrected), the latter requiring the addition of CO_2 to maintain a temperature corrected pH of 7.4. The advantages claimed for alphastat are: the preservation of intracellular neutrality and an improvement in the efficiency of intracellular enzyme function.[59]

Other constituents of the prime include 100 ml 20% albumin to increase the oncotic pressure and 0.5 g kg^{-1} mannitol to promote osmotic diuresis. Approximately 0.5–1 mmol kg^{-1} of potassium is required during bypass; this can be given incrementally after aortic cross-clamping to maintain a serum K^+ of at least 4.5 mmol l^{-1}.

Occasionally in infancy, CBP may produce lung and tissue damage, including severe extravasation of plasma and greatly increased interstitial fluid plus a coagulopathy. Complement activation is assumed to play an important role in the lung damage, possibly with sequestration of polymorphs in the lungs. Many of the deleterious effects of CPB on fluid retention can be reversed by modified ultrafiltration postbypass.[60]

CEREBRAL PROTECTION

The use of deep hypothermia with or without circulatory arrest has dramatically improved the results of infant cardiac surgery, so that for many lesions mortality is approaching zero.[61]

However, neurological problems such as seizures may affect 3–8% of infants, most of which are minor and transitory but may be related to the length of the circulatory arrest (Figure 13.3). It is not always possible to find a cause and apart from a major hypoxic–ischaemic episode, many neurological problems are blamed on thromboembolic episodes of air or particulate matter. Cerebral metabolic changes associated with, for example, hypotension, hypothermia, circulatory arrest and changes in blood sugar, are being investigated and strategies to minimize brain damage devised.[62,63]

Global cerebral blood flow, metabolic rate and oxygen consumption can be investigated clinically by near-infrared spectroscopy or measurement of jugular venous bulb saturations. This requires the placement of a catheter or probe retrogradely in the internal jugular vein. Venous oxygen saturations will peak at a certain temperature, indicating that cerebral metabolism is as low as possible at that level of temperature, i.e. oxygen extraction is minimal. Additional cooling may be required before arresting the circulation if the jugular bulb saturations have not peaked[64] (Figure 13.4).

A pH stat strategy (addition of CO_2) may be beneficial early in bypass to allow cerebral

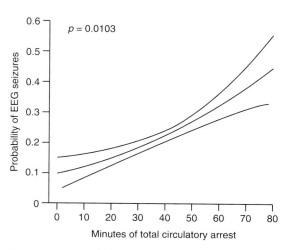

Figure 13.3 Probability of EEG-monitored seizures postoperatively as a function of duration of hypothermic circulatory arrest. (Reproduced by kind permission of J. Newburger and *New England Journal of Medicine*.)

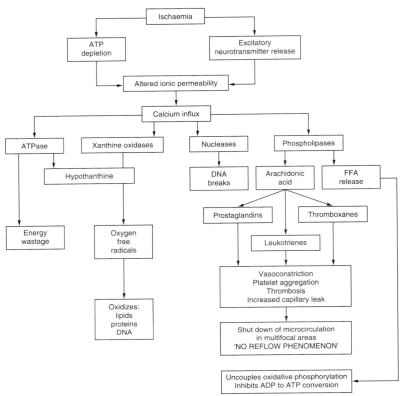

Figure 13.4 Flowchart describing cellular events associated with normothermic arrest.[47] (Reproduced by kind permission of Kern, F.M. *et al.* and Mosby Year Book Publishers.)

vasodilation and thorough cerebral cooling, even of the watershed areas. Alpha stat is then used for the rest of bypass.[65]

Topical cooling of the head with ice packs is used for all children undergoing circulatory arrest; this has been shown to enhance cerebral protection and improves brain recovery after the arrest period.[47]

Experimental evidence using magnetic resonance spectroscopy shows that high-energy phosphates in cerebral cells are depleted after 30–40 min of circulatory arrest at 18°C.[66] It is supposed that the likelihood of cerebral damage will increase the longer the arrest period extends after this time.

Pulsatile bypass flow does improve tissue perfusion and may improve cerebral and other organ function, but is not widely used.[67] Circulatory arrest damages cerebral NMDA receptors, allowing free influx of Ca^{2+} which may destroy the cell. Release of excitatory amino acid neurotransmitters is a sensitive index of cerebral injury. NMDA receptor antagonists such as ketamine may have a protective role. The use of specific cerebroplegia solutions has not reached clinical practice.[68]

Hyperglycaemia may be implicated in worsening neurological outcome after a hypoxic–ischaemic episode.[69,70]

REWARMING

Just before the aortic clamp is released, rewarming starts with a temperature gradient of no more than 10°C between patient and perfusate or perfusate and heat exchange. During rewarming heat is provided mainly by the heat exchanger, but heat also comes from the heating mattress, which is now turned on, and from heated humidified inspired gases. At this stage, to overcome the intense peripheral vasospasm induced by hypothermia, it is common practice to infuse a vasodilator such as nitroprusside or nitroglycerine, although their efficacy has been questioned.

Suction is attached to the aortic needle vent as the cross-clamp is removed. Removal of every trace of air is crucial to avoid cerebral air embolism. The cardiac action should be vigorous and the lungs inflated to drive air out of the pulmonary veins; venous pressure is increased and the heart, especially the left atrial appendage, is massaged. The heart begins to eject at this point and mechanical ventilation is recommended. It is also usual to position the patient in the head-down position so that any ejected air bubbles do not go to the brain. To minimize reperfusion injury after aortic unclamping flow on bypass should be reduced for 1 or 2 min.

Intracardiac lines are placed into pulmonary artery or left atrium at this stage. Monitoring of the left atrial pressure is necessary whenever left ventricular or mitral valve function requires close monitoring and is particularly important in the Fontan operation. Intracardiac lines, if placed with meticulous care, have a very low morbidity.[71] It is wise to leave the chest drains *in situ* and to have a unit of blood cross-matched before these lines are removed in the postoperative period.

After circulatory arrest cerebral metabolism does not immediately return to normal with dysfunctional oxygen utilization, although topical cooling and ultrafiltration speed the process.

POSTBYPASS

Partial bypass is established after deaeration so that the heart can eject and bypass is slowly withdrawn by constriction in the venous drainage line. After venous drainage is stopped the patient is transfused via the aortic cannula to a systolic pressure of 80 mmHg and superior vena caval pressure of 10–12 mmHg, with left atrial pressure no more than 15 mmHg. If arterial pressure remains low with high filling pressures then inotropic support is necessary, as it is essential that the heart is not left with poor myocardial perfusion pressures and poor myocardial oxygen delivery, causing increasing hypoxia and acidosis.

It is acceptable to provide an initial inotropic 'kick' to the myocardium with a small bolus of

1 : 100 000 adrenaline or 10% $CaCl_2$ and, in many cases, this is all that will be necessary. Other patients will require dopamine 5–10 μg kg^{-1} min^{-1}, which is often the first choice, or dobutamine in a similar starting dose for those patients judged to have a labile PVR, but these may be less effective than adrenaline at the time of coming off bypass.[72] It is logical to use both dopamine and dobutamine, the former in a low renal vasodilating dose and the latter in higher dosage for inotropic action without vasoconstriction (Table 13.9).

It should be remembered that the venous system is very compliant and it is dangerously easy to overload a small patient with colloid without any change in CVP. Small babies have a rate-dependent cardiac output, so chronotropic drugs such as isoprenaline may be required. Once all the cardiac cannulae have been removed, colloid is transfused to keep filling pressures within normal limits, using whole blood if the haematocrit is below 40, or colloid (for example, fresh frozen plasma) if the haematocrit is high. Initially, ventilation is with 100% oxygen to ensure complete oxygenation before the first blood gas analysis.

Haemodilution to a haematocrit of 20–25 is routine to optimize flow at low temperatures and will also allow saving of the use of donor blood, but always causes an increase in total body water and occasionally a capillary leak syndrome. This leads to suboptimal myocardial and pulmonary function.[60]

Towards the end of bypass and afterwards, urine flow should be at least 1 ml kg^{-1} h^{-1}. Urine output before bypass and during periods of low flow and hypothermia is of no interest. Suboptimal renal function associated with open heart surgery in the very young is common and mannitol in the prime, low, renal vasodilating doses of dopamine (3–4 μg kg^{-1} min^{-1}) and small doses of frusemide (0.25 mg kg^{-1}) may help to minimize this. Where renal failure existed preoperatively in patients with major lesions (e.g. truncus arteriosus) or in all neonates after CPB it is common practice to insert a peritoneal drain which can also be used as a dialysis catheter. Failure to respond to diuretics is a further indication for early dialysis. Many centres use a modified ultrafiltration after bypass, taking from the aorta and returning to

Table 13.9   Cardiac drugs with dosages

Dopamine 6 mg kg^{-1}in 100 ml 5% dextrose	1 ml h^{-1} = 1 μg kg^{-1} min^{-1}
	dose, 5–10 μg kg^{-1} min^{-1}
Dobutamine 6 mg kg^{-1} in 100 ml 5% dextrose	1 ml h^{-1} = 1 μg kg^{-1} min^{-1}
	dose, 5–10 μg kg^{-1} min^{-1}
Adrenaline 60 μg kg^{-1}in 100 ml 5% dextrose	1 ml h^{-1} = 0.01 μg kg^{-1} min^{-1}
	dose, 0.01–0.5 μg kg^{-1} min^{-1}
Isoprenaline 60 μg kg^{-1}in 100 ml 5% dextrose	1 ml h^{-1} = 0.01 μg kg^{-1} min^{-1}
	dose, 0.01–0.5 μg kg^{-1} min^{-1}
Noradrenaline 60 μg kg^{-1} in 100 ml 5% dextrose	1 ml h^{-1} = 0.01 μg kg^{-1} min^{-1}
	dose, 0.01–0.5 μg kg^{-1} min^{-1}
Dextrose/insulin 2 g dextrose : 1 unit insulin	dose, 0.5 g kg^{-1}
Calcium chloride	10–20 mg kg^{-1}
Sodium nitroprusside 6 mg kg^{-1} in 100 ml 5%dextrose	1 ml h^{-1} = 1 μg kg^{-1} min^{-1}
	dose, 0.5–5 μg kg^{-1} min^{-1}
Enoximine 100 mg in40 ml H$_2$O	dose, 1 mg kg^{-1} slow bolus
	5–10 μg kg^{-1} min^{-1}
	(dedicated line)
Nitroglycerine 6 mg kg^{-1}in 100 ml 5% dextrose	1 ml h^{-1} = 1 μg kg^{-1} min^{-1}
	dose, 0.5–5 μg kg^{-1} min^{-1}

the right atrium, to return the haematocrit towards 40. During the process haemodynamics steadily improve and cerebral function is more rapidly restored to prebypass levels. The mechanism of action is unknown but may include falling PVR with full oxygenated blood returning to the right atrium and possible removal by filtration of vasoactive cytokinins.[73,74]

Protamine is given to reverse heparin in doses up to 6 mg kg^{-1} with ACT control, although very small patients may require greater doses. Heparin levels in the patient coming off bypass are often in excess of those before going on as a result of heparin added to the prime; although ACT is not specific for heparinization, it is useful to know whether the level has returned to the baseline. Protamine causes a degree of hypotension in most patients, occasionally profound, although not to the same degree as in adults. This possibly arises from the release of histamine or other vasoactive substances by the heparin–protamine moiety and is possibly also related to the activation of complement.[75] The reaction may be more severe if myocardial function is suboptimal.[76] Vascular effects of protamine can be minimized by very slow infusion, possibly after a small test dose, into a peripheral rather than central vein or even into the left side of the heart via the LA line,

although this should be done with meticulous care to avoid air embolism. Fresh-frozen plasma, cryoprecipitate and platelet-rich plasma may all be necessary before haemostasis is finally achieved and the ACT has returned to the baseline level.

The insertion of temporary pacemaker wires is routine; these can be for direct ventricular pacing or atrioventricular sequential pacing. Rhythm problems in children are not particularly common, but troublesome dysrhythmias do occur: supraventricular tachycardias, junctional rhythm and atrioventricular block with a fall in cardiac output when the myocardium is under stress or with electrolyte and blood gas abnormalities. Slow dysrhythmias are often easily corrected by small doses of isoprenaline. Fast dysrhythmias with an acute fall in cardiac output may be treated by d.c. shock or adenosine in increments of 50 μg kg^{-1} to a maximum on 250 μg kg^{-1}. It has a half-life of 15 s. If the change in rhythm is less catastrophic it can be treated by digoxin, β-adrenergic blockade or amiodarone 5 mg kg^{-1} by slow intravenous infusion to a maximum of 20 mg kg^{-1} day^{-1}. Amiodarone blocks K$^+$ channels and prolongs refractoriness.[77,78]

When the haemodynamics are stable, pressures in the cardiac chambers can be measured by direct needle puncture, and of particular interest is the right ventricular pressure, for example after repair of VSD or tetralogy of Fallot, or gradients across repaired valves. Many patients, particularly infants in whom vasoconstrictive compensatory mechanisms are very active, benefit from reduction in the left ventricular afterload. Either sodium nitroprusside ($1–2$ μg kg^{-1} min^{-1}) or nitroglycerine ($2–4$ μg kg^{-1} min^{-1}) may be used, although nitroglycerine in low doses specifically dilates venous capacitance vessels, and is particularly indicated in mitral valve regurgitation and coronary artery dysfunction (e.g. after the arterial switch operation for TGA). It also has more effect on pulmonary than on systemic resistance. Measurement of cardiac output is not routinely performed as it has many limitations in the infant patient. Transoesophageal echocardiography (TOE) and/or epicardial echo are more useful tools to assess the cardiac repair and cardiac function at this stage and are used increasingly.[79,80]

In spite of myocardial protection by cooling and cardioplegia, cardiac function may be very poor after bypass, especially in newborns, and catecholamine receptors may have become downregulated.[81,82] TOE has demonstrated dyskinetic ventricles with poor diastolic function, especially after repair of tetralogy of Fallot. Phosphodiesterase inhibitor inodilators such as milrinone or enoximone may dramatically improve cardiac function in these cases. The combination of enoximone and adrenaline is a potent inotropic cocktail.[83]

Occasionally, in spite of maximal inotropic therapy, cardiac function is so poor that bypass support is required and sometimes a period of $1–2$ h on bypass will allow the heart to regain function. If there is a good prospect for cerebral and cardiac survival, a period of several days on extracorporeal membrane oxygenation (ECMO), if available, may prove successful.[84,85]

In many small babies after major surgery on bypass (e.g. arterial switch) cardiac size is greater than preoperatively and when the sternum is closed cardiac output may drop dramatically. In these cases the sternum can be stented open and the wound closed with a Silastic sheet. In most cases the chest can be closed in the ICU in 24–48 h with no increased risk of sepsis.[86]

Respiratory and cardiac support is continued into the postoperative period where indicated. Patients with simple lesions are weaned from the ventilator and extubated after a very short time, but others may require a prolonged weaning period. It is usually beneficial to continue inotropic support until the patient is weaned from the ventilator. Analgesia is with a continuous morphine infusion of 0.5 mg kg^{-1} in 50 ml at 2 ml h^{-1} ($= 20$ μg kg^{-1} h^{-1}), which continues even in the spontaneously breathing patient until after the chest drains have been removed, usually on the first postoperative day.

Older children may benefit from an infusion of propofol started after bypass at 3 mg kg^{-1} h^{-1}, reducing to 2 mg kg^{-1} h^{-1} when they have returned to the ICU. This prevents hypertension and unstable haemodynamics on the transfer from theatre to unit and allows early extubation.

PULMONARY HYPERTENSIVE CRISIS

In conditions of left-to-right shunt and TAPVC the smooth muscle of the media of the pulmonary arterioles does not regress at birth as normally happens. There is an overgrowth of muscle so that these small vessels in the lung peripheries become unusually contractile and allow the PVR to be extremely labile.[87] The vessels constrict with the stimuli of hypoxia and acidosis, probably via an adrenergic mechanism. If the fetal channels, PDA and patent foramen ovale (PFO) are open the increase in PVR causes the reversion to a transitional circulation and critical hypoxaemia, but if these channels are closed, as they are after surgery, then severe right heart failure is followed by left heart failure, since in infancy both ventricles fail in parallel.

The patients at risk from pulmonary hypertensive crises (PHC) are all newborns and those with a previously high pulmonary blood flow from left-to-right shunt; unrestrictive VSD, atrioventricular septal defect, especially Down's syndrome; truncus, TGA and VSD, and TAPVC. Many of these have monitoring of the pulmonary arterial (PA) or right ventricular (RV) pressures postoperatively, especially if pulmonary resistance is known to be raised. Nowadays, these problems occur most commonly in patients with pulmonary venous hypertension, such as the obstructed TAPVC or severe mitral valve lesions.

The PA catheter can be introduced directly by the surgeon, or a catheter may be inserted via the internal jugular vein and allowed to coil in the right atrium (RA). When the repair is complete, the surgeon threads it into the PA. Only by monitoring PA pressures in relation to systemic can the effects of restlessness, tracheal suctioning or weaning from controlled ventilation be seen. The first sign of a PHC may be a rise in CVP.

Increases in PA pressure can be categorized into minor events if PA pressure acutely exceeds 80% of systemic, but without a fall in systemic pressure, and a major crisis if PA pressure exceeds systemic, with a fall in systemic pressure and reduction in SpO_2 and cardiac output (peripheral temperature falls).

Phenoxybenzamine, a long-acting α-adrenergic blocking agent, was used perioperatively (1 mg kg^{-1} every 12 h) to prevent crises, but is not now so favoured. The patient remains on full mechanical ventilation with mild hyperventilation and PaO_2 over 14 kPa; paralysis with pancuronium or vecuronium is an advantage. Morphine infusions, which are routinely used for postoperative analgesia in other patients, may cause pulmonary vasoconstriction and hypotension, whereas fentanyl has no effect on the pulmonary vasculature. A fentanyl infusion of 4–10 μg kg^{-1} h^{-1} plus boluses of up to 25 μg kg^{-1} blunt stress responses associated with tracheal suctioning.[88]

If the pulmonary artery pressure rises to the level of systemic pressure or above, immediate steps must be taken to reverse the PVR; as the patient becomes hypoxic, pulmonary vasoconstriction gets worse and may be very difficult to reverse at this stage. Sedation and hyperventilation by hand with 100% oxygen may be effective and provide the first-line approach.

Drugs previously used in the treatment of sustained pulmonary hypertension, multiple minor events or a crisis, nitroglycerine, tolazoline and prostacyclin, have been superceded by inhaled nitric oxide (NO).[89] NO is released from endothelial cells of blood vessels and other tissues (endothelial relaxing factor) stimulated by the longitudinal shear stress on the cells by pulsatile flow. NO causes a rise in levels of cyclic granosine monophosphate, a vasorelaxant. This is the mechanism of action of the nitrovasodilators. NO is now used as a selective pulmonary vasodilator for all forms of pulmonary hypertension in children and will also reduce the need for ECMO in many babies with persistent pulmonary hypertension of the newborn.[90] Concentrations up to 20 ppm are used at the outset, but this can often be reduced to as little as 3–5 ppm, although occasionally a response is not seen until 80 ppm is used. NO has been used to help weaning from bypass when this failed because of very high pulmonary resistances.[91]

NO is supplied in cylinders and specific amounts are introduced into the ventilator circuit via a flow meter. Concentrations of both NO and nitrogen dioxide (NO_2), formed from oxidation of NO, are continuously analysed. NO_2, which is toxic, should never rise above 5 ppm. Methaemoglobin is formed as NO is inactivated and levels should be checked and should not rise above 5%. If NO is stopped too soon, there is often a rebound in pulmonary resistance and the agent should be continued for several days at a low concentration until the pulmonary endothelial synthesis of NO has been normalized.

REOPERATIONS

Many patients whose cardiac surgery has involved the use of a homograft conduit (truncus arteriosus, pulmonary atresia, Rastelli operation) will eventually require this to be replaced, either because it is non-functional with increasing calcification, or because the conduit inserted in infancy has become inadequate with the growth of the child. The conduit usually lies just beneath the sternum and may even be attached to it. The greatest care is required for the opening of the sternum, and usually the iliac artery is prepared for bypass should one of the cardiac chambers be opened inadvertently. Occasionally, the conduit or right ventricle lies immediately behind the sternum and in these cases femorofemoral bypass is commenced before the sternum is opened. An external defibrillator plate is placed beneath the chest before surgery starts. It is advisable to secure extra venous access for these cases, and to have blood and colloid in readiness, together with pressure infusion devices in case urgent transfusion should become necessary.

Aprotinin (Trasylol) is commonly used to reduce bleeding in redo operations. The second procedure is usually well tolerated and is not necessarily a lengthy procedure.

CLOSED CARDIAC AND PALLIATIVE SURGERY

In any unit which receives the whole range of paediatric cardiac anomalies approximately 40% of the surgical procedures are performed via thoracotomy and usually without bypass. Many patients are cyanotic and/or in severe heart failure and some may require preoperative intensive care with respiratory and cardiac support. Induction of anaesthesia and levels of monitoring are usually the same as for open heart surgery.

A nasogastric tube is inserted, as ileus is very common after thoracotomy. For patients expected to be extubated at the end of the procedure the fentanyl dose should not exceed 5–10 μg kg^{-1} and anaesthesia can be supplemented with small doses of an inhalational agent such as isoflurane or halothane. However, a great many patients are extremely sick and inhalational agents are contraindicated, so that full doses of opioids may be given and postoperative respiratory support via a nasotracheal tube is undertaken.

For many patients a local anaesthetic technique can be used, such as thoracic epidural, with a catheter either inserted at a thoracic level or threaded from the caudal route. Spinal, paravertebral, interpleural and intercostal blocks will also provide intraoperative and postoperative analgesia.

PATENT DUCTUS ARTERIOSUS

Any premature baby is at risk from PDA because the mechanisms which cause the duct to close are also immature; fluid overload in the neonatal period may also cause the ductus to remain open. PDA is also associated with many forms of congenital heart disease, but may be a single, chance finding. It is estimated that 25% of babies weighing below 1500 g and recovering from hyaline membrane disease have a PDA. The greatly increased pulmonary blood flow will contribute to the development of bronchopulmonary dysplasia and any small baby who is ventilator dependent should have a PDA ligated. There may be no murmur so echocardiographic investigation should be routine. These small patients may be fragile, already ventilated and will require very careful monitoring, with the operation sometimes even being performed in the ICU. A relaxant technique with oxygen, nitrous oxide or air and oxygen mixtures with fentanyl up to 10 μg kg^{-1} is an excellent technique for a small baby not expected to breathe spontaneously in the early postoperative period.[41,92] Direct arterial monitoring is not routinely undertaken except in the very frail baby. Oxygen saturation should remain between 90 and 92% to minimize the risk of retinopathy of prematurity.

The surgical approach is via a left thoracotomy and the ductus is either doubly ligated or clipped. Sudden ligation of the ductus may cause a surge in arterial pressure and increase the possibility of intraventricular cerebral haemorrhage in this vulnerable age group. Before the PDA is finally ligated, a trial clamping takes place to demonstrate any serious cardiovascular consequences and there should be two suckers, vascular clamps and blood ready to transfuse in the unlikely event that the ductus is torn during ligation. Transfusion of blood is otherwise rarely necessary.

Most older children have PDA occluded by interventional cardiology with an occlusion device introduced via a cardiac catheter, but occasionally require a surgical approach. These children do not require direct arterial monitoring. During the ligation of a very large and tense ductus a reduction in systemic blood pressure, for example with isoflurane or sodium nitroprusside, makes the surgery safer.

COARCTATION OF THE AORTA

NEONATAL

These babies are often very sick indeed, with severe left ventricular failure and a tight juxtaductal aortic stenosis or a hypoplastic aortic arch and little, if any, collateral flow. Clinical diagnosis is confirmed by echocardiography, which will also find any other cardiac pathology.

Prostaglandin infusion to maintain patency of the ductus is usually beneficial, but respiratory support and an inotrope may also be required preoperatively. It is preferable if all vascular access is achieved in the ICU before the baby is taken to the operating room. The arterial line is preferably in the right arm, as the left subclavian artery is usually clamped during the surgery, which takes place via a left thoracotomy.

The anaesthetic technique which provides the greatest stability for these very sick patients is relaxant, oxygen/air and fentanyl (10–20 μg kg^{-1}); inhalation agents such as halothane are contraindicated. Total body potassium is frequently very low and contributes to cardiac instability. The time of greatest risk is at unclamping of the aorta when hypotension reduces myocardial perfusion. The aorta can be repeatedly clamped to increase coronary perfusion pressure and, with transfusion of 10–20% blood volume, the clamp can eventually be completely removed. The peripheral vasculature is often reactive, so an infusion of sodium nitroprusside may be necessary later to maintain the blood pressure between 80 and 100 mmHg in the postoperative period. Respiratory support should continue postoperatively, although recovery is usually rapid if the repair is satisfactory and other lesions, for example VSD, are not present.

OLDER CHILDREN

The patients are not usually unfit, but may be hypertensive with large collateral flow through the intercostal arteries. Without mild induced hypotension the thoracotomy may bleed profusely. Mild hypotension without tachycardia is easily achieved with a combination of 0.5–1 mg kg^{-1} labetalol i.v. and isoflurane. Severe hypertension after application of the aortic clamps, indicating poor collateral circulation, is an indication for further induced hypotension, for example with sodium nitroprusside. Satisfactory cerebral, renal and spinal cord perfusion during the repair is ensured if the distal aortic pressure is kept above a mean of 45–50 mmHg. The clamping time should never exceed 20–25 min. In more problematic cases a heparin-bonded shunt or some form of left heart bypass should be used. Sodium nitroprusside infusion is usually required postoperatively to maintain the blood pressure between 90 and 100 mmHg and, although the patients are extubated before returning to the unit, they require full analgesia and sedation.

BLALOCK–TAUSSIG SHUNTS

Anastomosis of a subclavian artery to the PA of the same side (classical Blalock) will improve pulmonary blood flow and oxygenation. It is frequently required in babies with pulmonary or tricuspid atresia or severe tetralogy of Fallot if the diameter of the main pulmonary artery is less than 30% of the aorta. For tetralogy patients there is controversy as to whether a shunt or a total correction is the better approach for a small baby with symptoms. Not only does the shunt increase peripheral oxygen saturation and prevent damaging hypercyanotic attacks, but the increased flow into the pulmonary artery will also stimulate its growth to a degree, hopefully allowing patients with pulmonary atresia to be fully corrected at a later stage. The shunt most commonly performed is the modified Blalock using 4–6-mm Gore-Tex tube, usually on the side opposite the aortic arch. Direct anastomosis from aorta to pulmonary artery (Waterston's shunt) is not now performed because of the difficulty in judging its size and the increased risk of pulmonary vascular disease which would make subsequent corrective surgery, for example, total cavopulmonary connection procedure for tricuspid atresia, impossible.

The patients are always cyanotic, often with a high haematocrit and excessive mechanical ventilation, will further reduce pulmonary blood flow.

Arterial monitoring should be from the side opposite to the thoracotomy or in a femoral artery and one or two lines are inserted into an internal jugular vein. Great care must be taken not to damage the subclavian artery on the side of the shunt during the insertion of these neck lines. Transfusion during the procedure is with plasma to replace blood loss. An anaesthetic technique with relaxant, oxygen, nitrous oxide or oxygen, air and fentanyl is satisfactory and hand ventilation helps the surgeon during the delicate anastamoses in the mediastinum. Heparin 1 mg kg^{-1} i.v. is given after the Gore-Tex has been sutured to the subclavian artery, before it is joined to the pulmonary artery. Increasing acidosis is a common finding and 1 mmol kg^{-1} sodium bicarbonate is invariably necessary during the procedure. After the shunt is completed peripheral oxygenation and graft patency depends on a normal perfusion pressure, and an infusion of, for example, dopamine 6 μg kg^{-1} min^{-1} may be necessary to achieve this. A short period of intubation postoperatively is invariably beneficial, particularly if the shunt is large and pulmonary compliance falls. If large aortopulmonary collaterals have developed these may need to be ligated to optimize flow into the main pulmonary artery, or a focalization procedure undertaken for the same purpose.

PULMONARY ARTERY BANDING

Banding the main pulmonary artery in patients with a large left-to-right shunt not amenable to early corrective surgery causes equalization of pressures in both ventricles, reducing the volume of the shunt. Pulmonary engorgement is diminished, compliance improves and the work of the left ventricle is reduced, as is the risk of permanent pulmonary vascular disease. Full arterial and venous monitoring is used and respiratory support is invariably required postoperatively since the patients have failed to thrive and have unremitting cardiac failure. The surgical approach is via a left thoracotomy and the band is tightened around the PA until the distal PA pressure is at least half the systemic. Systemic pressure usually rises as PA pressure falls. If the band is too tight the shunt becomes right-to-left with profound desaturation, bradycardia and a fall in cardiac output. Pulse oximetry is most useful in warning of over-banding[93] and the final PaO_2 should be at least 7 kPa (80% saturation).

BLALOCK–HANLON SEPTECTOMY

This operation, performed via a right thoracotomy, is designed to remove a section of atrial septum to equalize the two atrial pressures. In the past the procedure allowed greater mixing of atrial blood in patients with TGA to increase peripheral oxygen saturation. Nowadays it is required only for complicated TGA, where the Rashkind has failed, or in other complex conditions not amenable to corrective surgery where decompression of the left atrium gives considerable palliation, for example mitral atresia. Problems include the potential for severe haemorrhage and periods of very low cardiac output after the pulmonary veins have been snared. Full monitoring and postoperative ventilation are required. Some surgeons prefer the more controlled situation offered by CBP.

VASCULAR RING

The vascular ring around the trachea and oesophagus is commonly based on a double aortic arch with many variations, less frequently by a pulmonary artery sling, with the left PA arising from the right. The patients often present with stridor and the diagnosis is confirmed by a barium swallow, which shows indentation of the oesophagus, and also by echocardiography.[94] The effect on the trachea is variable, ranging from mild tracheomalacia to severe tracheal stenosis. Vascular ring is a cause of respiratory arrest and sudden infant death. The operation via a left thoracotomy divides the PDA and one limb of the double aortic arch, freeing the oesophagus and trachea. Anaesthesia is little more complicated than for a simple PDA, but care should be taken with intubation to have the tip of the tracheal tube at least in the mid-trachea and hand ventilation allows early warning of tracheal obstruction during the dissection. Most patients may be extubated at the end of the procedure and nursed in a humidified headbox.

Pre-existing stridor may be intensified because of tracheal oedema; this may respond to dexamethasone 0.25 mg kg^{-1} i.v. A small group of patients with severe stridor and secretion retention may require nasotracheal intubation and continuous positive airway pressure for several days. Tracheomalacia responds to the distending pressure, which may be continued in the infant with one nasal prong after extubation.

PHRENIC NERVE PALSY

Infants rely solely on function of the diaphragm to breathe. The phrenic nerves are vulnerable during cardiac surgery and are frequently damaged by diathermy, cold injury or traction. A phrenic palsy should be suspected if a small baby fails to wean from the ventilator when cardiac output and pulmonary compliance are normal. The plain chest X-ray may show an elevated hemidiaphragm: two vertebral spaces above the contralateral side are diagnostic, but the diagnosis should also be confirmed by echocardiography or fluoroscopy; occasionally both sides are affected. Often, recovery can be expected between 3 and 6 weeks from the injury. However, the period of respiratory

support will be greatly reduced if surgical plication of the diaphragm is undertaken to prevent the damaging respiratory effects of paradoxical movement. Plication will not prejudice normal diaphragmatic function if the nerve regenerates at a future time.

FLUID BALANCE

Accurate control of fluid balance is crucial to the success of cardiac surgery. In the prebypass period, maintenance fluids of 5–10 ml kg^{-1} h^{-1} may be given as compound sodium lactate (Hartmann's) or lactated Ringer's solutions. These fluids are not strictly necessary in small babies where sufficient volume of crystalloid is maintained by flushing and diluted drugs, but are of greater importance in patients with a high haematocrit or if surface cooling is used. Blood loss is replaced by colloid.

In the postoperative period, severe fluid restriction is used and postbypass patients should be given 20 ml m^{-2} h^{-1} of 5 or 10% dextrose for the day of surgery (day 1); 30 ml m^{-2} h^{-1} on day 2, and 40 ml m^{-2} h^{-1} on day 3; 1 g KCl (13 mmol) can be put into 500 ml of 5% dextrose to maintain serum K$^+$ around 4 mmol l^{-1}.

Nasogastric feeds usually begin on day 2 or 3, starting with half-strength milk, but the total fluid intake should not be exceeded. Blood sugar is never low during surgery, but is checked every 2–4 h postoperatively and if low, boluses of 25% dextrose are given. Closed cases are given 3 ml kg^{-1} h^{-1} of 5 or 10% dextrose on day 1; 4 ml kg^{-1} h^{-1} on day 2, and 5 ml kg^{-1} h^{-1} on day 3.

The infusion of colloid matches losses from the chest drains, although extra volumes are often required to maintain reasonable cardiac filling pressures and warm peripheries. Crystalloid input matches urine output, although on days 1 and 2 urine output should always exceed input and regular doses of diuretics may be necessary to achieve this. Continuous infusions of inotropes such as dopamine may require increased concentrations if fluid restriction is to be maintained; the dilutions are in multiples of

6 mg kg^{-1} in 100 ml 5% dextrose for ease of calculation.

NON-CARDIAC SURGERY

Increasing numbers of patients with cardiac disease which has been corrected, palliated or uncorrected, require surgery for non-cardiac reasons. Patients with corrected cardiac disease may have residual lesions or may never be able to respond to stress with a full cardiac output, for example after Mustard or Senning operation for TGA the active atrial component of ventricular filling may be lost. Patients after the Fontan operation whose success depends on normal PVR may poorly tolerate intermittent positive pressure ventilation and anaesthesia, and many patients have a relatively fixed cardiac output. It is wise preoperatively to seek the opinion of a paediatric cardiologist to assess the current clinical status of the patient. It may even be necessary to perform the cardiac surgery before any general surgery is undertaken. Conditions such as corrected transposition and Ebstein's anomaly have a high incidence of dysrhythmias, e.g. supraventricular tachycardia and atrioventricular block.

Assessment must include the general condition of the patient, including associated pulmonary, renal and hepatic abnormalities. Exercise tolerance is the best guide to tolerance of anaesthesia, assessable in infants by whether they are able to feed and suck without breathlessness and whether growth and development has been normal. The presence and degree of cyanosis are noted, as well as the cardiac drugs used, e.g. β-adrenergic blockers cause a relatively fixed cardiac output.

A preoperative echocardiograph gives crucial information on ventricular function and any residual lesions that may be present. It is very useful to have knowledge of the likely functional outcome after the more common cardiac lesions have been corrected, for example, tetralogy of Fallot or the arterial switch for TGA.

All patients having dental or other surgery require antibiotic prophylaxis, and the following anaesthetic considerations should be included.

1 Full and careful monitoring: direct arterial vascular access is required during major surgery for continuous monitoring of pressure and blood sampling. The use of a pulmonary artery catheter may be indicated for patients with raised PVR undergoing major surgery as these patients are particularly at risk from the changes in systemic and PVRs associated with general anaesthesia.
2 Cardiac output is maintained by a choice of suitable technique, which usually includes controlled ventilation with relaxants, since inhalational agents may be too hypotensive. Peripheral vasodilatation or vasoconstriction should not be excessive, particularly with balanced right-to-left and left-to-right shunts. Maintenance should be with light general anaesthesia together with regional anaesthesia wherever possible; ketamine or sevoflurane are very suitable induction agents.
3 Blood volume should be fully maintained with normal intraoperative fluids as well as colloid to cover blood and plasma losses.
4 Heart rate should be stable at a normal or slightly increased rate; judicial use of atropine intravenously may be necessary to achieve this.
5 Pancuronium may cause undesirable tachycardia, so atracurium or vecuronium by bolus or infusion may be more logical.
6 A high inspired oxygen concentration gives a margin of safety for periods of reduced cardiac output or pulmonary congestion and increased right-to-left intrapulmonary shunting.
7 Postoperative monitoring in a high-dependence unit or ICU may be required, as is an increased inspired oxygen concentration, delivered by facemask, nasal cannula or headbox.

SPECIFIC LESIONS

TETRALOGY OF FALLOT

This is the most common form of cyanotic heart disease presenting in the first year of life and involves a perimembranous VSD, right ventricular outflow obstruction (infundibular and valvar stenosis) and overriding of the ventricular septum by the aorta. It usually presents after the neonatal period with cyanosis and/or hypercyanotic attacks. Critical cyanosis as a duct-dependent lesion may present in a neonate, requiring emergency surgery for a Blalock shunt, although the trend in many centres is for a definitive repair at that stage.

Routine anaesthesia for repair of tetralogy includes morphine premedication and readiness to treat a hypercyanotic spell in the prebypass period by volume expansion and/or the use of sodium bicarbonate, noradrenaline and propranolol intravenously if necessary. Surgery consists of VSD closure and relief of the right ventricular outflow obstruction (RVOTO), often with a patch across the pulmonary valve annulus. Operative mortality is low.

TRANSPOSITION OF GREAT ARTERIES

This is the most common form of cyanotic heart disease presenting at birth and may be complicated by other lesions, for example VSD, univentricular heart or absence of one atrioventricular connection. For survival, a high-flow, low-pressure shunt at atrial level is the most efficient at improving SpO_2 and is provided by an urgent balloon septostomy (Rashkind), usually performed under echo control. An arterial switch procedure is performed in the early days of life before PVR falls and the left ventricle involutes to such a degree that it would never be able to function as the systemic ventricle. In the past an atrial switch (Senning or Mustard) procedure was performed, but resulted in significant late mortality and morbidity. The arterial switch involves switching the great vessels surgically and reimplanting the coronary arteries into the neoaorta. The procedure, although complex for a small newborn, carries a low operative risk (< 5%) regardless of the coronary artery pattern.

UNIVENTRICULAR HEART

This finding of only one functioning (usually the left) ventricle is associated with various lesions, especially tricuspid atresia, and precludes a biventricular surgical repair. The clinical picture of failure and/or cyanosis depends on the degree of pulmonary blood flow. Surgical management involves the Fontan procedure or one of its variants, for example, total cavopulmonary connection. These procedures depend for their success on low/normal pulmonary resistance and good ventricular function. After CBP when PVR may be elevated, modified ultrafiltration, dobutamine, nitroglycerine and even nitric oxide may be beneficial. Although surgery is classified as a palliative procedure, many patients are improved, with removal of cyanosis and reduction of volume load of the single ventricle. There is an increasing mortality and morbidity in follow-up.

HYPOPLASTIC LEFT HEART SYNDROME

Hypoplastic left heart syndrome (HLHS) is the most common cardiac cause of death in the first month of life and is a spectrum of disease of left ventricular and aortic hypoplasia and aortic stenosis or atresia. The diagnosis is usually made antenatally and the condition is fatal unless one of two treatment options is taken: heart transplantation or a staged reconstruction (Norwood) of a viable circulation.[95] Management of these babies at all stages is complex, but is undertaken in many centres around the world with some success. The stage-I procedure is the reconstruction of the aortic arch and formation of a central shunt to carry the pulmonary blood flow. Stage II is a bidirectional cavopulmonary connection and stage III is the completion of the cavopulmonary connection (Fontan). The aim is for all stages to be completed by 2 years of age. After stage-I, pulmonary and systemic blood flow depends on the resistances, the aim being for a $Q_p : Q_s$ ratio of 1. The aim of anaesthesia and postoperative care is to maintain the balance of shunts and promote the function of the right ventricle. The babies are usually ventilated with air to keep SpO_2 at 70–80% and useful information is obtained when the shunt is unclamped at the end of bypass: if the perfusion pressure falls by more than 25 mmHg, Q_p is high and steps are taken to increase PVR, by reducing the inspiratory oxygen fraction and increasing CO_2. As the reconstruction is in three stages, all of which require bypass, great care must be taken to preserve sites of arterial and venous access.

Various strategies to increase or decrease pulmonary blood flow may be necessary post-operatively. Calculation of crucial $Q_p : Q_s$ is achieved by using superior vena caval saturation as a mixed venous saturation.[96] Mortality and morbidity of these procedures remains high.

REFERENCES

1 DiDonato, R.M., Jonas, R.A., Lang, P., *et al.* Neonatal repair of tetralogy of Fallot with or without pulmonary atresia. *Journal of Thoracic and Cardiovascular Surgery* 1991; **101**: 126–37.

2 Fyler, D.C. (ed.). *Nadas' Pediatric Cardiology*. Philadelphia, PA: Hanley and Belfus, 1992.

3 Clarke, E.B. Epidemiology of congenital cardiovascular malformations. In: Emmanouilides, G.C., Riemenschneider, T.A., Allen, H.D. and Gutgesell, H.P. (eds). *Moss and Adams Heart Disease in Infants, Children and Adolescents*. Baltimore, MD: Williams and Wilkins, 1989: 60–70.

4 Chittmittrapap, S., Spitz, L., Kiely, E.M. and Brereton, R.J. Oesophageal atresia and associated anomalies. *Archives of Disease in Childhood* 1989; **64**: 364–8.

5 Cullen, S., Sharland, G.K., Allan, L.D. and Sullivan, I.D. Potential impact of population screening for prenatal diagnosis of congenital heart disease. *Archives of Disease in Childhood* 1992; **67**: 775–8.

6 Stark, J. and de Leval, M.R. *Surgery for Congenital Heart Defects*. 2nd edn. Philadelphia, PA: Saunders, 1994.

7 Anderson, R.H. Terminology. In: Anderson, R.H., Macartney, F.J., Shinebourne, E.A. and Tynan, M. (eds). *Paediatric Cardiology*. Edinburgh: Churchill Livingstone, 1987.

8 Sumner, E. and Cullen, S. Congenital heart disease. In: Vickers, M.D. (ed.). *Medicine for Anaesthetists*. Oxford: Blackwell 1999: (in press).

9 Friedman, A.H. and Fahey, J.T. The transistion from fetal to neonatal circulation: normal responses and implications for infants with heart disease. *Seminars in Perinatology* 1993; **17**: 106–21.

10 Nguyen, M., Camenisch, T., Snouwaert, J.N., *et al.* The prostaglandin receptor EP4 triggers remodelling of the cardiovascular system at birth. *Nature* 1997; **390**: 78–81.

11 Hammerman, C. Patent ductus arteriosus. Clinical relevance of prostaglandins and prostaglandin inhibitors in PDA pathology and treatment. *Clinics in Perinatology* 1995; **22**: 457–79.

12 Clyman, R.I. Ductus arteriosus. In: Gluckman, P.D. and Heyman, M. (eds). *Pediatrics and Perinatology*. 2nd edn. London: Arnold, 1996: 755–61.

13 Greeley, W.J., Leslie, J.B. and Reves, J.G. Prostaglandins and the cardiovascular system: a review and update. *Journal of Cardiothoracic Anesthesia* 1987; **1**: 331–49.

14 Rabinovitch, M. Developmental biology of the pulmonary vasculature. In: Polin, R.A. and Fox, W.W. (eds). *Fetal and Neonatal Physiology*. Philadelphia, PA: Saunders, 1998: 913–23.

15 Mathew, R. Development of the pulmonary circulation; metabolic aspects. In: Polin, R.A. and Fox, W.W. (eds). *Fetal and Neonatal Physiology*. Philadelphia, PA: Saunders, 1998: 924–6.

16 Rabinovitch, M. Pathophysiology of pulmonary hypertension. In: Emmanouilides, G.C., *et al.* (eds). *Moss and Adams Heart Disease in Infants, Children and Adolescents*. Baltimore, MD: Williams and Wilkins, 1995: 1659–95.

17 Haworth, S.G. Lung biopsies in congenital heart disease: computer assisted correlations between structural and hemodynamic abnormalities. In: Doyle, E.F., Engle, M.A., Gersony, W.M., Rashkind, W.J. and Talner, N.S. (eds). *Pediatric Cardiology*. New York: Springer, 1986: 942–5.

18 Roy, D.L. Heart sounds and murmurs – innocent or organic? *Medical Clinics of North America* 1989; **73**: 153–62.

19 Rosenthal, A. How to distinguish between innocent and pathologic murmurs in childhood. *Pediatric Clinics of North America* 1984; **31**: 1229–40.

20 McEwen, A.I., Birch, M. and Bingham, R.M. The preoperative management of the child with a heart murmur. *Paediatric Anaesthesia* 1995; **5**: 151–6.

21 Dajani, A.S., Taubert, K.A., Wilson, W., *et al.* Prevention of bacterial endocarditis. *Circulation* 1997; **96**: 358–66.

22 Scott, P.J., Blackburn, M.E., Wharton, G.A., *et al.* Transoesophageal echocardiography in neonates, infants and children: applicability and diagnostic value in everyday practice of a cardiothoracic unit. *British Heart Journal* 1992; **64**: 488–92.

23 Meyer, R.A. Echocardiography. In: Emmanouilides, G.C. *et al.* (eds). *Moss and Adams Heart Disease in Infants, Children and Adolescents*. Baltimore, MD: Williams and Wilkins, 1995: 241–270.

24 Snider, A.R. and Bengur, A.R. Doppler echocardiography. In Emmanouilides, G.C. *et al.* (eds). *Moss and Adams Heart Disease in Infants, Children and Adolescents*. Baltimore, MD: Williams and Wilkins, 1995: 270–93.

25 Gatzoulis, M.A., Rigby, M.L., Shinebourne, E.A. and Redington, A.N. Contemporary results of balloon valvuloplasty and surgical valvotomy for congenital aortic stenosis. *Archives of Disease in Childhood* 1995; **73**: 66–9.

26 Frostell, C.G., Fratacci, M.-D., Wain, J.C., Jones, R. and Zapol, W.M. Inhaled nitric oxide: a selective pulmonary vasodilator reversing hypoxic pulmonary vasoconstriction. *Circulation* 1991; **83**: 2038–47.

27 Dajani, A.S., Taubert, K.A., Wilson, A.F., *et al.* Prevention of bacterial endocarditis; Recommendation of the American Heart Association. *Journal of the American Medical Association* 1997; **227**: 1794–801.

28 Laishley, R.S., Burrows, F.A., Lerman, J. and Lang, P. Effect of anesthetic induction regimes on oxygen saturation in cyanotic congenital heart disease. *Anesthesiology* 1986; **65**: 673–7.

29 Hensley, F.A., Larach, D.R., Martin, D.E., *et al.* The effect of halothane/nitrous oxide/oxygen mask induction on arterial hemoglobin saturation in cyanotic heart disease. *Journal of Cardiothoracic Anesthesia* 1987; **1**: 289–96.

30 Murray, D., Vadewalker, G., Matherne, P. and Mahoney, L. Pulsed Doppler and two-dimensional echocardiography: comparison of halothane and isoflurane on cardiac function in infants and small children. *Anesthesiology* 1987; **67**: 211–17.

31 Mori, N. and Masahiro, S. Sevoflurane in paediatric anaesthesia: effects on respiration and circulation during induction and recovery. *Paediatric Anaesthesia* 1996; **6**: 95–102.

32 Tanner, G.E., Angers, D.G., Barash, P.G., Mulla, A., *et al.* Effect of L-R, mixed L-R and R-L shunts on inhalational induction in children. *Anesthesia and Analgesia* 1985; **64**: 101–7.

33 Sarner, J.B., Levine, M., Davis, P.J., *et al.* Clinical characteristics of sevoflurane in children – a comparison with halothane. *Anesthesiology* 1995; **82**: 38–46.

34 Slogoff, S., Keats, A.S., Dear, W.E., *et al.* Steal-prone coronary anatomy and myocardial ischemia associated with four primary anesthetic agents in humans. *Anesthesia and Analgesia* 1991; **72**: 22–7.

35 Ebert, T.J., Harkin, C.P. and Muzi, M. Cardiovascular responses to sevoflurane: a review. *Anesthesia and Analgesia* 1995; **811** Suppl. 6: S11–22.

36 Greeley, W.J. Comparative effects of halothane and ketamine on systemic arterial oxygen saturation in children with cyanotic heart disease. *Anesthesiology* 1986; **65**: 666–8.

37 Hickey, P.R., Hansen, D.D., Cramolini, G.M., *et al.* Pulmonary and systemic hemodynamic responses to ketamine in infants with normal and elevated pulmonary vascular resistance. *Anesthesiology* 1985; **62**: 287–93.

38 Orser, B.A., Pennefather, P.S. and MacDonald, J.F. Multiple mechanisms of ketamine blockade of N-methyl-d-aspartate receptors. *Anesthesiology* 1997; **86**: 903–17.

39 Spung, J., Schuetz, S.M., Stewart, R.W. and Moravec, C.S. Effects of ketamine on the contractility of failing and nonfailing human heart muscles *in vitro*. *Anesthesiology* 1998; **88**: 1202–10.

40 Moylan, S.L. and Murdoch, L.J. A prospective survey of axillary artery cannulation in paediatric intensive care. *Paediatric Anaesthesia* 1993; **3**: 37–40.

41 Anand, K.J.S., Sippell, W.G. and Aynsley-Green, A. Randomised trial of fentanyl anaesthesia in preterm babies undergoing surgery: effect on the stress response. *Lancet* 1987; **i**: 243–8.

42 Yaster, M. The dose response of fentanyl in neonatal anesthesia. *Anesthesiology* 1987; **66**: 433–5.

43 Gravlee, G.P., Brauer, S.D., Roy, R.C., *et al.* Predicting the pharmacodynamics of heparin: a clinical evaluation. *Journal of of Cardiothoracic Anesthesia* 1987; **1**: 379–87.

44 Levy, J.H., Pifarre, R., Schaff, H.V., *et al.* A multicenter, double-blind, placebo controlled trial of aprotinin for reducing blood loss and the requirement for donor-blood transfusion in patients undergoing repeat coronary artery bypass grafting. *Circulation* 1995; **92**: 2236–44.

45 Wangs, J.S., Lin, C.Y., Hung, W.T. and Karp, R.B. Monitoring of heparin induced anticoagulation with kaolin-activated clotting time in cardiac surgical patients treated with aprotinin. *Anesthesiology* 1992; **77**: 1080–4.

46 Swain, J.A., Mcdonald, T.J., Balaban, R.S., *et al.* Metabolism of the heart and brain during hypothermic cardiopulmonary bypass. *Annals of Thoracic Surgery* 1991; **51**: 105–9.

47 Kern, F.H., Greeley, W.J. and Ungerleider, R.M. Cardiopulmonary bypass. In: Nichols, D.G., *et al.* (eds) *Critical Heart Disease in Infants and Children.* St Louis, MO: Mosby, 1995: 497–529.

48 Firmin, R.K., Bouloux, P., Allen, P., *et al.* Sympathoadrenal function during cardiac operations in infants with the technique of surface cooling, limited cardiopulmonary bypass and circulatory arrest. *Journal of Cardiovascular Surgery* 1985; **90**: 729–35.

49 Swain, J.A., McDonald, T.J., Griffith, P.K., *et al.* Low flow hypothermic cardiopulmonary bypass protects the brain. *Journal of Thoracic and Cardiovascular Surgery* 1991; **102**: 76–84.

50 Birch, R.F.H. and Lake, C.L. Pro: Magnesium is a valuable therapy in the cardiac surgical patient. *Journal of Cardiothoracic and Vascular Anesthesia* 1991; **5**: 518–21.

51 Aglio, L.S., Stanford, G.G., Maddi, R., *et al.* Hypomagnesemia is common following cardiac surgery. *Journal of Cardiothoracic and Vascular Anesthesia* 1991; **5**: 201–8.

52 Barratt-Boyes, B.G., Simpson, M. and Neutze, J.M. Intracardiac surgery in neonates and infants using deep hypothermia with surface cooling and limited cardiopulmonary bypass. *Circulation* 1971; **43** Suppl. 1: 1–25.

53 Jonas, A.R. and Elliott, M.J. (eds) *Cardiopulmonary Bypass in Neonates, Infants and Young Children.* Oxford: Butterworth-Heinemann, 1994.

54 Buckberg, G.D. A proposed solution to the cardioplegia controversy. *Journal of Thoracic and Cardiovascular Surgery* 1979; **77**: 803–15.

55 Hayashida, N., Isomura, T., Sato, T., *et al.* Minimally diluted tepid blood cardioplegia. *Annals of Thoracic Surgery* 1998; **65**: 615–21.

56 Finlayson, D.C. Nonpulsatile flow is preferable to pulsatile flow during cardiolpumonary bypass. *Journal of Cardiothoracic Anesthesia* 1987; **1**: 169–70.

57 Kirklin, J.K., Kirklin, J.W. and Pacifico, A.D. Cardiopulmonary bypass. In: Archiniegas, E. (ed.) *Pediatric Cardiac Surgery.* Chicago, Il: Year Book Medical Publishing, 1985: 67–77.

58 Ratcliffe, J., Elliott, M.J., Wyse, R.K.H., *et al.* Metabolic consequences of three different crystalloid pump priming fluids in children less than 15 kilos undergoing open heart surgery. *Journal of Cardiovascular Surgery* 1985; **26** Suppl.: 86–91.

59 du Plessis, A.J., Jonas, R.A., Wypij, D., *et al.* Perioperative effects of Alpha-stat versus pH-Stat strategies for deep hypothermic cardiopulmonary bypass in infants. *Journal of Thoracic and Cardiovascular Surgery* 1997; **6**: 991–1000.

60 Elliott, M.J. Modified ultrafiltration and open heart surgery in children. *Paediatric Anaesthesia* 1999; **9**: 1–5.

61 Jonas, R.A. Hypothermia, circulatory arrest and the pediatric brain. *Journal of Cardiothoracic and Vascular Anesthesia* 1996; **10**: 66–74.

62 Mault, J.R., Whitaker, E.G., Heinle, J.S., *et al.* Intermittent perfusions during hypothermic circulatory arrest: a new and effective technique for cerebral protection. *Annals of Thoracic Surgery* 1994; **57**: 96–101.

63 Newburger, J.W., Jonas, R.A., Wernovsky, G., *et al.* A comparison of the perioperative neurologic effects of

hypothermic circulatory arrest versus low-flow cardio-pulmonary bypass in infant heart surgery. *New England Journal of Medicine* 1993; **329**: 1057–64.

64 Greeley, W.J. and Kern, F.H. Cerebral blood flow and metabolism during infant cardiac surgery. *Paediatric Anaesthesia* 1994; **4**: 285–99.

65 Kurth, C.D., O'Rourke, M.M., O'Hara, I.B. and Uher, B. Brain cooling efficiency with pH-Stat and alpha-stat cardiopulmonary bypass in newborn pigs. *Circulation* 1997; **96**: 358–63.

66 Swain, J.A., Robbins, R.G., Balaban, R.S., *et al.* The effect of cardiopulmonary bypass on brain and heart metabolism. A P-31 NMR study. *Magnetic Resonance Medicine* 1990; **15**: 446–55.

67 Watanabe, T., Orita, H., Kobayashi, M., *et al.* Brain tissue pH, oxygen tension and carbon dioxide tension in profoundly hypothermic cardiopulmonary bypass. Comparative study of circulatory arrest. non pulsatile low-flow and pulsatile low-flow perfusion. *Journal of Thoracic and Cardiovascular Surgery* 1989; **97**: 369–401.

68 Aoki, M., Jonas, R.A., Nomura, F., *et al.* Effects of cerebroplegic solutions during hypothermic circulatory arrest and short-term recovery. *Journal of Thoracic and Cardiovascular Surgery* 1994; **108**: 291–301.

69 Lanier, J.R., Stangland, K.J., Scheithauer, B.W., *et al.* The effects of dextrose infusion and head position on neurological outcome after complete cerebral ischemia in primates: examination of model. *Anesthesiology* 1987; **66**: 39–48.

70 Anderson, R.V., Siegman, M.G., Balaban, R.S., *et al.* Hyperglycemia exacerbates cerebral intracellular acidosis during hypothermic circulatory arrest and reperfusion. *Annals of Thoracic Surgery* 1992; **54**: 1126–30.

71 Gold, J.P., Jonas, R.A., Lang, P., *et al.* Transthoracic intracardiac monitoring lines in pediatric surgical patients: a 10 year experience. *Annals of Thoracic Surgery* 1986; **42**: 185–91.

72 Booker, P.D., Evans, C. and Franks, R. Comparison of the haemodynamic effects of dopamine and dobutamine in young children undergoing cardiac surgery. *British Journal of Anaesthesia* 1995; **74**: 419–23.

73 Naik, S.K., Knight, A. and Elliott, M.J. A prospective randomized study of a modified technique of ultrafiltration during pediatric open-heart surgery. *Circulation* 1991; **84**: 422–31.

74 Davies, M.J., Nguyen, K., Gaynor, J.W. and Elliott, M.J. Modified ultrafiltration improves left ventricular systolic function in infants after cardiopulmonary bypass. *Journal of Thoracic and Cardiovascular Surgery* 1998; **115**: 361–9.

75 Kirklin, J.K., Westaby, S., Blackstone, E.H., *et al.* Complement and the damaging effects of cardiopulmonary bypass. *Journal of Cardiovascular Surgery* 1983; **86**: 845–57.

76 Del Re, M.R., Ayd, J.D., Schulyheis, L.W., *et al.* Protamine and left ventricular function: a transesophageal echcardiography study. *Anesthesia and Analgesia* 1993; **77**: 1098–103.

77 Wren, C. and Campbell, R.W.F. (eds). *Paediatric Cardiac Dysrhythmias.* Oxford: Oxford University Press, 1996.

78 Vetter, V.L. What every pediatrician needs to know about arrhythmias in children who have had cardiac surgery. *Pediatric Annals* 1991; **20**: 378–85.

79 Ungerleider, R.M., Greeley, W.J. and Kanter, R.J. The learning curve for intraoperative echocardiography during congenital heart surgery. *Annals of Thoracic Surgery* 1992; **54**: 691–6.

80 O'Leary, P.W., Hapler, D.J., Seward, J.B., *et al.* Biplane intaoperative transesophageal echocardiography in congenital heart disease. *Mayo Clinic Proceedings* 1995; **70**: 317–26.

81 Booker, P.D. Myocardial stunning in the neonate. *British Journal of Anaesthesia* 1998; **80**: 371–83.

82 Schranz, D., Droege, A., Broede, A., *et al.* Uncoupling of human cardiac beta adrenoceptors during cardiopulmonary bypass with cardioplegic cardiac arrest. *Circulation* 1993; **87**: 422–6.

83 Innes, P.A., Frazer, R.S., Booker, P.D., *et al.* Comparison of the haemodynamic effects of dobutamine with enoximone after open heart surgery in small children. *British Journal of Anaesthesia* 1994; **72**: 77–81.

84 UK collaborative randomised trial of neonatal extracorporeal membrane oxygenation. UK Collaborative ECMO Trial Group. *Lancet* 1996; **348**: 75–82.

85 Trittenwein, G., Furst, G., Golej, J., *et al.* Extracorporeal membrane oxygenation in neonates. *Acta Anaesthesiologica Scandinavica* 1997; **111**: 143–4.

86 Iyer, R.S., Jacobs, J.P., de Leval, M.R., *et al.* Outcomes after delayed sternal closure in pediatric heart operations: A 10-year experience. *Annals of Thoracic Surgery* 1997; **63**: 489–91.

87 Haworth, S.G. Pulmonary vascular remodelling in neonatal pulmonary hypertension. State of the art. *Chest* 1988; **93**; 133–8S.

88 Hickey, P.R., Hansen, D.D., Wessel, D.L., *et al.* Blunting of stress responses in the pulmonary circulation of infants by fentanyl. *Anesthesia and Analgesia* 1985; **64**: 1137–42.

89 Frostell, C.G., Blomquist, H., Hedenstierna, G., *et al.* Inhaled nitric oxide selectively reverses human hypoxic pulmonary vasoconstriction without causing systemic vasodilatation. *Anesthesiology* 1993; **78**: 427–35.

90 Atz, A.M. and Wessel, D.L. Inhaled nitric oxide in the neonate with cardiac disease. *Seminars in Perinatology* 1997; **21**: 441–55.

91 Bichel, T., Spahr-Schopfer, I., Berner, M., *et al.* Successful weaning from cardiopulmonary bypass after cardiac surgery using inhaled nitric oxide. *Paediatric Anaesthesia* 1997; **7**: 335–9.

92 Robinson, S. and Gregory, G.A. Fentanyl–air–oxygen anesthesia for ligation of paptent ductus arteriosus. *Anesthesia and Analgesia* 1981; **60**: 31–62.

93 Casthely, P.A., Redko, V., Dluzneski, J., *et al.* Pulse oximetry during pulmonary artery banding. *Journal of Cardiothoracic Anesthesia* 1987; **1**: 297–9.

94 Burch, M., Balaji, S., Deanfield, J.E. and Sullivan, I.D. Investigation of vascular compression of the trachea: the complimentary roles of barium swallow and echocardiography. *Archives of Disease in Childhood* 1993; **71**: 171–6.

95 Castaneda, A.R. Hypoplastic left heart syndrome. In: Castaneda, A.R., Jonas, R.A., Mayer, J.E., Jr, and Hanley, F.L. (eds). *Cardiac Surgery of the Neonate and Infant.* Philadelphia, PA: Saunders, 1994.

96 Rossi, A.F., Sommer, R.J., Lotvin, A., *et al.* Usefulness of intermittent monitoring of mixed venous oxygen saturation after Stage 1 palliation for hypoplastic left heart syndrome. *American Journal of Cardiology* 1994; **73**: 1118–23.

CHAPTER 14

Anaesthesia for patients with cardiac disease: outcome following reconstructive congenital cardiac surgery

PETER LAUSSEN

INTRODUCTION

The advances in paediatric cardiology and cardiac surgery in the 1980s and 1990s have resulted in a substantial decrease in mortality, such that most congenital heart lesions are now amenable either to an anatomical or to a physiological repair. Surgical techniques for many cardiac defects have evolved over this period; today's patients may have a different spectrum of complications from those of the past. In addition, complications related to previous palliative surgery such as a systemic to pulmonary artery shunt or pulmonary artery band may influence late outcome, as does the patient age at which complete repair is undertaken.

The trend over recent years has been towards early surgical correction of defects during the neonatal or infancy period to limit the pathophysiological sequelae, including pulmonary hypertension, ventricular dysfunction and chronic hypoxaemia. An important premise has been that any surgical procedure should allow for growth potential. This has been readily achieved with repair of atrial or ventricular septal defects. Complex lesions involving the great vessels or outflow tracts may not have the same growth potential and complications are more likely to occur later.

ANATOMICAL REPAIRS

This type of repair implies that the morphological left ventricle is connected to the aorta and the right ventricle to the pulmonary artery, and the circulation is in series. It can be categorized further as either a simple or a complex reconstruction (Table 14.1).

SIMPLE RECONSTRUCTION

Following correction of lesions such as an atrial septal defect (ASD), ventricular septal defect (VSD) or patent ductus arteriosus (PDA), the heart is structurally normal and correction is for the most part curative without long-term sequelae.

Considerable remodelling of the ventricles and recovery of function is possible after reconstructive surgery. The period over which irreversible ventricular dysfunction develops is variable, and generally if surgical intervention to correct a volume overload is undertaken within the first year of life, residual dysfunction is uncommon.[1] Ventricular outflow tract obstruction may develop over time after some repairs, but it takes longer to develop significant ventricular dysfunction in patients with a chronic pressure load than in those with a chronic volume load.

In response to an unrestricted left-to-right shunt, pulmonary hypertension may develop as pulmonary vascular obstructive disease (PVOD) progresses owing to structural changes in the pulmonary vasculature. The period over which PVOD develops depends on the size of the shunt and the age at surgery. The progression to PVOD is more rapid when both the volume and pressure load to the pulmonary circulation are increased, such as with a large VSD. When pulmonary flow is increased in the absence of elevated PA pressures, as with an ASD, pulmonary hypertension develops more slowly. For the majority of infants with an unrestrictive shunt at the ventricular level, e.g. large VSD, and pulmonary hypertension, repair of the defect within the first year of life is usually associated with regression of the pulmonary vascular changes.

COMPLEX RECONSTRUCTION

The complex nature of some surgical repairs necessary to achieve an anatomical correction may result in significant long-term sequelae. Regular re-evaluation is necessary because, while patients may report that they are progressing well with few symptoms, when tested objectively significant limitations may be evi-

Table 14.1 Broad classification following reconstructive congenital cardiac surgery

Type of repair		Outcome
Anatomical	LV = systemic ventricle	*Simple reconstruction*
	RV = pulmonary ventricle	Structurally normal after repair, e.g. ASD, VSD, PDA
	Circulation in series	Late complications unlikely
	Cyanosis corrected	*Complex reconstruction*
		Baffle, conduit, outflow reconstruction or A-V valve repair
		Late complications likely
Physiological	Circulation in series	*Two ventricles*
	Cyanosis corrected	RV = systemic ventricle
		LV = pulmonary ventricle
		e.g. Senning or Mustard procedure
		Single ventricle
		i.e. Fontan procedure

RV, right ventricle; LV, left ventricle; ASD, atrial septal defect; VSD, ventricular septal defect; PDA, patent ductus arteriosus; A-V, atrioventricular valve.

dent. Patients who have required extensive outflow reconstruction, atrioventricular valve repair and baffle placement are at particular risk for later complications, and while corrected are not cured. In contrast, the development of the arterial switch operation (ASO) to treat transposition of the great arteries has been associated with few problems on intermediate follow-up, and it is possible that this complex repair may be curative in the long term.

Right ventricle outflow reconstruction

Reconstruction of the right ventricle (RV) outflow tract may lead to significant problems that affect RV function and increase the risk of arrhythmias over time. While most of the long-term outcome data pertain to patients following Fallot's tetralogy repair, similar complications and risks are also likely for those who have undergone extensive RV outflow reconstruction, such as placement of a conduit from the right ventricle to the pulmonary artery for correction of pulmonary atresia, truncus arteriosus and the Rastelli procedure for transposition of the great arteries with pulmonary stenosis.

Complete surgical repair of tetralogy of Fallot has been performed since 1954, with recent data reporting 32- and 36-year actuarial survival rates of 86% and 85% respectively.[2,3] Many patients lead relatively normal lives, but RV dysfunction may progress after repair and only be evident on exercise stress testing or echocardiography. A spectrum of problems develop, ranging from a dilated RV with systolic dysfunction to diastolic dysfunction from a poorly compliant RV (Table 14.2). In addition, continued evaluation is necessary because of the increased risk of ventricular dysrhythmias and late sudden death. Factors that may adversely affect long-term survival include older age at initial repair, initial palliative procedures and residual chronic pressure and/or volume load such as from pulmonary insufficiency or stenosis.

Systolic dysfunction secondary to a residual volume load from pulmonary regurgitation after tetralogy repair is a strong predictor of late morbidity and possibly mortality. It is reflected by cardiomegaly on chest X-ray, an increase in RV end-diastolic volume by echocardiography,[4] and on exercise testing as a reduction in anaerobic threshold, maximal exercise performance and endurance.[5] A mechanicoelectrical relationship has also been demonstrated, with these patients more likely to have a prolonged QRS complex and to be at higher risk of ventricular dysrhythmias and possible sudden death.[6]

It is important to distinguish one group of patients who have a non-restrictive physiology or diastolic dysfunction secondary to reduced ventricular compliance. They usually do not have cardiomegaly, they demonstrate good exercise tolerance and the risk of ventricular dysrhythmias is possibly decreased. Although the RV is hypertrophied, function is generally well preserved on echocardiography with minimal pulmonary regurgitation.[7]

Table 14.2 Right ventricular function on long-term follow-up after Fallot's tetralogy repair

Systolic dysfunction	Non-restrictive RV: dilated, volume loaded
	Cardiomegaly
	Significant pulmonary regurgitation
	↑ RVEDV, ↓ RV ejection fraction
	↓ Maximal exercise capacity and endurance
	↑ Risk of ventricular dysrhythmias and possibly sudden death
Diastolic dysfunction	Restrictive RV: poor compliance
	↓ Cardiomegaly
	↑ RVEDP, contractility maintained
	Limited pulmonary regurgitation
	Improved exercise capacity
	Lower risk of ventricular dysrhythmias

RV, right ventricle; RVEDV, right ventricle end-diastolic volume; RVEDP, right ventricle end-diastolic pressure.

The incidence of significant RV outflow obstruction developing over time is low. Residual obstruction contributes to early mortality within the first year after surgery, but is well tolerated in the long term. A gradient more than 40 mmHg across the RV outflow is uncommon and the pressure ratio between the RV and LV is usually less than 0.5. The gradient may become more significant with time, but as the progression is usually slow, RV dysfunction occurs late.

A wide variation in the incidence of ventricular ectopy has been reported in numerous follow-up studies, including up to 15% of patients on routine electrocardiography (ECG) and up to 75% of patients on a Holter monitor.[8] Multiple risk factors, including an older age at repair, residual haemodynamic abnormalities and the duration of follow-up, have all been considered important.[9,10] In common with these factors is probable myocardial injury and fibrosis from chronic pressure and volume overload, and cyanosis.

While ventricular ectopy is common in asymptomatic patients during ambulatory ECG Holter monitoring and exercise stress testing, it is often low grade and has not identified those patients at risk of sudden death. Electrophysiological induction of sustained ventricular tachycardia (VT), especially when monomorphic, is suggestive of the presence of a re-entrant arrhythmic pathway. Although dependent on the stimulation protocol used to induce VT, the presence of monomorphic VT in a symptomatic patient with syncope and palpitations is significant and indicates treatment with radio-frequency ablation, surgical cryoablation, antiarrhythmic drugs or placement of an implantable cardioversion–defibrillator (ICD).[11] The significance in asymptomatic patients is currently unknown.

The risk of ventricular dysrhythmia during anaesthesia is unknown. While preoperative prophylaxis with antiarrhythmic drugs is not recommended, a means for external defibrillation and pacing must be readily available.

Arterial switch operation

One of the major advances in congenital heart surgery over the past 10–15 years has been the development of the arterial switch operation (ASO) to correct transposition of the great arteries (TGA). In experienced centres, the early hospital mortality is less than 3% and actuarial analyses indicate 98% survival at 5–10 years.[12,13] Long-term survival data are not available, as the oldest survivors are only in their teenage years, but based on intermediate-term follow-up data, the risk for reoperation and complications after the arterial switch operation remains small.

Virtually all coronary artery patterns are amenable to the arterial switch operation. While an intramural coronary artery and a single right coronary artery with retropulmonary course of the circumflex may be associated with an increased incidence of early death after surgery, no particular pattern has been associated with late death. A recent report of coronary artery angiography in 366 patients following the ASO (median age at follow-up 7.9 years) revealed coronary artery stenosis or occlusion in 3% of patients.[14] The long-term significance of these coronary artery abnormalities is yet to be determined. Despite the angiographic findings, evaluation with serial ECG, exercise testing and wall-motion abnormalities on echocardiography rarely demonstrate evidence of ischaemia.[15,16]

After repair, the native pulmonary valve becomes the neoaortic valve. A 30% incidence of trivial to mild aortic regurgitation has been reported on intermediate-term follow-up, without significant haemodynamic changes.[17] Severe regurgitation is unusual.

There appears to be a very low incidence of significant rhythm disturbances after the ASO.[18] Supravalvular pulmonary artery stenosis was an early complication, but is now less common with surgical techniques that extensively mobilize, augment and reconstruct the pulmonary arteries. Supravalvular aortic stenosis may develop, but is rare.

Assessment of myocardial performance, using echocardiography, cardiac catheterization and exercise testing following the ASO, has demonstrated function identical to age-matched controls.[19] Based on the currently available clinical, functional and haemodynamic data, a patient who has undergone a previous ASO with no evidence of subsequent problems should be treated as for any patient with a structurally normal heart when presenting for non-cardiac surgery. Life-long antibiotic prophylaxis is not necessary.

PHYSIOLOGICAL REPAIRS

Patients in this category may have undergone either a single- or two-ventricle repair, and are functionally corrected because cyanosis is relieved and the circulation is in series. However, long-term outcome data, complications and functional status indicate that such repairs may only be palliative.

TWO-VENTRICLE REPAIR

Patients who have a morphological right ventricle remaining as the systemic ventricle and the morphological left ventricle as the pulmonary ventricle can be regarded as having a physiological or functional two-ventricle repair. An example is the Mustard or Senning atrial baffle repair for transposition of the great arteries, effectively resulting in a switch at the atrial level. This surgery was performed in the 1960s and 1970s and significant problems may develop as patients get older (Table 14.3). In particular, this group provides some insight into the ability of the right ventricle to function as the systemic ventricle in the long term.

Creation of an intra-atrial baffle redirects systemic venous return through the mitral valve to the LV and pulmonary artery, while pulmonary venous blood is directed through the tricuspid valve to the RV and aorta. The patient is therefore functionally corrected with the RV remaining the systemic ventricle. In the Senning procedure the atrial baffle is fashioned using the

right atrial wall and the interatrial septum, whereas in the Mustard procedure the baffle is constructed from autologous pericardium or synthetic material after most of the atrial septum has been removed. Superiority of either surgical technique outside individual experience has not been convincingly established and long-term risks and complications are similar for both operations.[20]

Actuarial survival figures at 15 years have been quoted up to 85%.[21,22] However, significant long-term functional deterioration is likely with increasing risk of right ventricle failure, sudden death and dysrhythmias.[23,24]

Right ventricular function may deteriorate over time, highlighting the fact that the morphological RV may be incapable of sustained normal function as the systemic ventricle. This is also of concern for a number of other complex repairs in which the RV remains the systemic ventricle, such as in hypoplastic left heart syndrome.

Tricuspid regurgitation (i.e. regurgitation of the systemic A-V valve) may also progress over time, possibly as a result of trauma to the valve at the time of surgery, but it is predominantly related to progressive RV dysfunction. The tricuspid valve is supported by relatively small papillary muscles and, along with the abnormal concave RV septal surface, the annulus of the tricuspid valve enlarges with RV dilation and dysfunction, thereby causing tricuspid regurgitation.

A residual volume load may result from an intra-atrial baffle shunt. Although trivial baffle leaks have been observed on late postoperative angiography in 10–20% of patients, significant leaks requiring surgery are uncommon.

Either the systemic or pulmonary venous pathways may become stenotic over time. Superior vena caval obstruction occurs in 5–10% of patients, but is usually not associated with symptoms because of decompression by the azygous or hemiazygous systems. Inferior vena caval and pulmonary venous obstruction obstruction are both rare.

Dysrhythmias are a common complication observed on postoperative follow-up. In particular, there is progressive loss of sinus rhythm and increase in atrial dysrhythmias over time. The presence of dysrhythmias may be preceded by right ventricular dysfunction, but may also

Table 14.3 Potential long-term complications following the Mustard or Senning repair for transposition of the great arteries

- Right ventricular failure
- Tricuspid regurgitation
- Supraventricular and ventricular dysrhythmias
- Vena cavae obstruction
- Baffle leak and/or obstruction

be an isolated finding and is potentially the major cause of sudden death in these patients. A number of large follow-up series has reported that the probability of a patient remaining in sinus rhythm after an atrial level repair is 50% at 10 years and 40% at 20 years.[25]

The atrial baffle provides a functional repair, although many patients continue to maintain relatively active lives with few subjective symptoms.[26] Objective exercise testing on intermediate and late follow-up, however, may demonstrate limited right ventricular reserve in as many as 50% of patients; exercise duration, peak heart rate response and peak minute oxygen consumption have all been reported to be reduced compared with age-matched controls.[27]

SINGLE-VENTRICLE REPAIR/FONTAN OPERATION

A major advance in the treatment of congenital heart defects has been the development of single-ventricle repairs, connecting the systemic venous return directly to the pulmonary artery, thereby excluding the pulmonary ventricle.[28] Originally described for tricuspid atresia, the repair is now applied to a wide range of complex single-ventricle defects.

There have been numerous modifications to the initial atriopulmonary connection described by Fontan in 1971, which have been accompanied by an improvement in early survival from 75–80% in the 1970s, to over 90% in the current era.[29,30] This has occurred despite extension of this functional repair to younger patients with complex single-ventricle defects and to those with haemodynamic parameters previously considered to be at high risk. However, as the duration of follow-up increases, the continued risk for late failure of the Fontan circulation remains.

By relieving hypoxaemia, single-ventricle repairs are functionally corrective. In the absence of a pulmonary ventricle, success depends on the right-to-left atrial pressure gradient and unobstructed flow across the pulmonary vascular bed. Pulmonary vascular resistance and ventricular compliance are therefore major factors that influence early and late outcome. Intermediate to late follow-up studies have reported an increasing incidence of cardiac

failure or need for reoperation, with a late decline in functional status and 15-year survival between 60% and 73%.[29–32] However, these figures include patients operated on in the earlier surgical years, and with improved surgical techniques and patient selection, subsequent survival figures may improve. Therefore, while single-ventricle repairs have improved the outlook for children with complex congenital defects, the late decline in survival and functional status implies that these repairs are not curative and should be viewed as palliative at this time.

Complications

Venous hypertension can cause recurrent pleuropericardial effusions in the early postoperative period, although the incidence is reduced with placement of a fenestration in the baffle. Chronic elevation of systemic venous pressure can cause ascites and protein-losing enteropathy (PLE), and contributes to the increasing incidence of supraventricular arrhythmias with time after the Fontan operation.

Arrhythmias, in particular atrial flutter, sick sinus syndrome and heart block, have been reported in 20% or more of survivors 10 years following the Fontan procedure. The probability of freedom from atrial flutter has been reported as approximately 40% at 15 years after the Fontan procedure, although these data include patients from different surgical eras.[33] Predisposing factors include surgery involving the atrium with extensive suture lines, disrupted sinoatrial node blood supply and chronic atrial distension. In addition, older age at operation, longer duration of follow-up and type of surgical procedure are associated with an increased incidence of atrial flutter after Fontan operation.

There is an increased incidence of thromboembolism in patients who have undergone the Fontan procedure. However, the routine use of long-term anticoagulation remains controversial. The actual incidence of thromboembolism is difficult to determine because of the heterogeneous patient population. A large retrospective review of 645 patients who underwent the Fontan procedure at Children's Hospital, Boston, USA, over a 15-year period, between 1978 and 1993, described 17 patients (2.6%)

who suffered a stroke following the Fontan procedure, presumed to be secondary to a thromboembolic event.[34] The nature of the Fontan circulation, with increased venous pressure and stasis of flow through the right atrial baffle, atrial dysrhythmias, alterations in humoural coagulation and recent evidence suggesting increased resting venous tone in this population of patients, are all contributing factors.[35]

The role of prophylactic anticoagulant therapy in congenital heart disease in general and the Fontan population in particular is poorly defined. Antiplatelet therapy with aspirin is commonly used in the immediate and early postoperative period, although the benefit of long-term use has not been evaluated. In high-risk patients and those who have had previous thrombus formation, coumadin therapy for an extended period is recommended. A problem with long-term coumadin therapy in children is the need for frequent blood testing to maintain a therapeutic international normalized ratio (INR) and the potential for significant haemorrhagic complications in children prone to relatively minor trauma.

PLE has been reported in 2.5–14% of patients on long-term follow-up.[36,37] Defined as persistent hypoalbuminaemia (< 3.0 mg dl^{-1}) in the absence of liver and renal disease, with associated clinical features including abdominal pain, diarrhoea, oedema and ascites, its onset is associated with early mortality. Haemodynamic cardiac catheter studies have shown increased systemic venous pressure, decreased cardiac index and increased end-diastolic ventricular pressure. Medical management is only partially successful. Minor abnormalities in enzymic liver function are common, with mild elevation in serum transaminases reported in up to approximately 85% of patients.[37]

Clinical evaluation

The majority of patients demonstrate catch-up growth after the modified Fontan operation, and subsequently maintain growth patterns similar to age-matched controls.

Although full peripheral oxygen saturation in room air is expected after the Fontan procedure, saturations in the 90–95% range are common.[37] This may reflect a low cardiac output and low mixed venous oxygen saturation, but other factors include a residual right-to-left shunt across the baffle fenestration, leak from the baffle suture line, decompressing venous collateral vessels and pulmonary atriovenous malformations.

Following a modified Fontan procedure, no murmur or additional heart sounds should be expected on cardiac examination. Nevertheless, ventricular failure and the effects of chronic systemic venous hypertension need to be evaluated. Ventricular function assessed by echocardiography should be normal in the majority of patients. However, it has been reported as mildly to moderately impaired in about 20% of patients. Atrioventricular valve insufficiency, semilunar valve regurgitation, ventricle outflow tract obstruction and the Fontan baffle pathway should all be evaluated by echocardiography prior to surgery. Mild-to-moderate cardiomegaly on chest X-ray may be evident in about 40% of patients. Encouragingly, postoperative cardiac catheterization performed up to 15 years after the Fontan procedure has demonstrated preserved haemodynamics with pulmonary artery pressure around 12 mmHg and pulmonary artery wedge pressure around 7 mmHg, resulting in a transpulmonary gradient of about 5 mmHg.[37]

Functional assessment

Most patients with stable single-ventricle physiology report subjectively that they are able to lead relatively normal lives with moderate exercise tolerance, but deterioration in function and New York Heart Association classification occurs over longer follow-up.[31,32]

Objective evaluation with exercise testing demonstrates the limited cardiorespiratory reserve of many Fontan patients, and the response to exercise testing may be useful for assessing a patient's ability to tolerate the stress of anaesthesia and surgery. Maximal exercise workload is often reduced, and patients fatigue earlier and take longer to recover after stopping exercise compared with controls. Anaerobic threshold and maximal oxygen consumption are significantly reduced, and patients frequently desaturate and demonstrate an increase in arteriovenous oxygen saturation difference because of the suboptimal increase in cardiac index.[38,39] The inability to increase effective pulmonary blood flow and stroke volume during strenuous exercise underscores the importance of the pulmonary vascular bed in determining ventricular filling and the dependence on heart rate to increase cardiac output.

Cardiac catheterization should be considered if a patient has deteriorating symptoms or function. In particular, prior to major surgery or if significant fluid shifts are anticipated, performing a haemodynamic study under fluoroscopy immediately before surgery is often beneficial. Besides being able to assess baseline haemodynamics, a balloon-tipped catheter can be left positioned in the pulmonary artery for intraoperative and postoperative measurement of pulmonary artery pressure and mixed venous oxygen saturation. Pulmonary capillary wedge pressure can be measured to monitor the transpulmonary gradient. However, the pulmonary catheter is often difficult to wedge without direct vision because there is no pulsatile arterial pulmonary flow and the balloon may not readily float out to a lung segment. Positioning the catheter using pressure tracings alone may be difficult and direct vision using fluoroscopy is preferable. An important

consideration, however, is the risk of thrombosis and obstruction to venous return after central venous line placement.

Considerations for anaesthetic management following a successful Fontan procedure are shown in Table 14.4. Ideally, the Fontan baffle, superior vena cava and branch pulmonary artery pressures should be similar in the range of 10–15 mmHg, with pulmonary venous and atrial pressure between 5 and 10 mmHg.

There are few reports in anaesthesia literature about the potential problems posed by this group of patients when presenting for non-cardiac surgery. Significant haemodynamic abnormalities may persist or develop over time, and 'correction' does not necessarily imply 'cure'. Knowledge of long-term outcome data and potential complications are important when planning anaesthesia management. The disparity between subjective or reported symptoms and objective evaluation of function often seen in these patients, highlights the value of exercise testing preoperatively as a potential means by which the response to stress during surgery and anaesthesia can be assessed.

Table 14.4 Management considerations for patients following a single-ventricle repair

	Aim	Management
Right atrium	RAp 10–15 mmHg	→ or ↑ preload
	Unobstructed venous return	Low intrathoracic pressure
Pulmonary circulation	PVR < 2 Wood units m^{-2}	Avoid increases in PVR, e.g. from acidosis, hypoinflation and hyperinflation of the lung, hypothermia and excess sympathetic stimulation
	Mean PAp < 15 mmHg	Early resumption of spontaneous respiration
	Unobstructed pulmonary vessels	
Left atrium	LAp 5–10 mmHg	Maintain sinus rhythm
	Sinus rhythm	
	Competent A-V valve	→ or ↑ rate to increase CO
	Ventricle:	
	normal diastolic function	→ or ↓ afterload
	normal systolic function	
	no outflow obstruction	→ or ↑ contractility
		Inodilators useful because of vasodilation, inotropic and lusiotropic properties

RAp, right atrial pressure; PVR, pulmonary vascular resistance; PAp, pulmonary artery pressure; LAp, left atrial pressure; A-V, atrioventricular; CO, cardiac output.

REFERENCES

1 Graham, T.P., Jr. Ventricular performance in congenital heart disease. *Circulation* 1991; **84**: 2259–74.

2 Murphy, J.G., Gersh, B.J., Mair, D.D., *et al.* Long-term outcome in patients undergoing surgical repair of tetralogy of Fallot. *New England Journal of Medicine* 1993; **329**: 593–9.

3 Nollert, G., Fischlein, T., Bouterwek, S., *et al.* Long-term survival in patients with repair of tetralogy of Fallot: 36-year follow-up of 490 survivors of the first year after surgical repair. *Journal of the American College of Cardiology* 1997; **30**: 1374–83.

4 Bove, E.L., Byrum, C.J., Thomas, F.D., *et al.* The influence of pulmonary insufficiency on ventricular function following repair of tetralogy of Fallot. *Journal of Thoracic and Cardiovascular Surgery* 1983; **85**: 691–6.

5 Carvalho, J.S., Shinebourne, E.A., Busst, C., *et al.* Exercise capacity after complete repair of tetralogy of Fallot: deleterious effects of residual pulmonary regurgitation. *British Heart Journal* 1992; **67**: 470–3.

6 Gatzoulis, M.A., Till, J.A., Somerville, J., *et al.* Mechanoelectrical interaction in tetralogy of Fallot. *Circulation* 1995; **92**: 231–7.

7 Cullen, S., Shore, D. and Reddington, A. Characterization of right ventricular diastolic performance after complete repair of tetralogy of Fallot. *Circulation* 1995; **91**: 1782–9.

8 Deanfield, J.E., McKenna, W.J. and Hallidie-Smith, K.A. Detection of late arrhythmia and conducting disturbances after correction of tetralogy of Fallot. *British Heart Journal* 1980; **44**: 248–53.

9 Chandar, J.S., Wolff, G.S., Garson, A., *et al.* Ventricular arrhythmia in postoperative tetralogy of Fallot. *American Journal of Cardiology* 1990; **65**: 655–61.

10 Deanfield, J.E., McKenna, W.J., Presbitero, P., *et al.* Ventricular arrhythmia in unrepaired and repaired tetralogy of Fallot. Relation to age, timing of repair and haemodynamic status. *British Heart Journal* 1984; **52**: 77–81.

11 Marie, P.Y., Marcon, F., Brunotte, F., *et al.* Right ventricular overload and induced sustained ventricular tachycardia in operatively 'repaired' tetralogy of Fallot. *American Journal of Cardiology* 1992; **69**: 785–9.

12 Kirklin, J.W., Blackstone, E.H., Tchervenkov, C.I., *et al.* Clinical outcomes after the arterial switch operation for transposition. *Circulation* 1992; **86**: 1501–15.

13 Wernovsky, G., Mayer, J.E., Jr, Jonas, R.A., *et al.* Factors influencing early and late outcome of the arterial switch operation for transposition of the great arteries. *Journal of Thoracic and Cardiovascular Surgery* 1995; **109**; 289–302.

14 Tanel, R.E., Wernovsky, G., Landzberg, M.J., *et al.* Coronary artery abnormalities detected at cardiac catheterization following the arterial switch operation for transposition of the great arteries. *American Journal of Cardiology* 1995; **76**: 153–7.

15 Weindling, S.N., Wernovsky, G., Colan, S.D., *et al.* Myocardial perfusion, function and exercise tolerance after the arterial switch operation. *Journal of the American College of Cardiology* 1994; **23**: 424–33.

16 Massin, M., Hovels-Gurich, H., Dabritz, S., *et al.* Results of the Bruce Treadmill test in children after the arterial switch operation for simple transposition of the great arteries. *American Journal of Cardiology* 1998; **81**: 56–60.

17 Jenkins, K.J., Hanley, F.L., Colan, S.D., *et al.* Function of the anatomic pulmonary valve in the systemic circulation. *Circulation* 1991; **84** Suppl. III: 173–9.

18 Rhodes, L.A., Wernovsky, G., Keane, J.F., *et al.*Arrhythmias and intracardiac conduction after the arterial switch operation. *Journal of Thoracic and Cardiovascular Surgery* 1995; **109**: 303–10.

19 Colan, S.D., Boutin, C., Castaneda, A.R., *et al.*Status of the left ventricle after arterial switch operation for transposition of the great arteries: hemodynamic and echocardiographic evaluation. *Journal of Thoracic and Cardiovascular Surgery* 1995; **109**; 311–21.

20 Helbing, W.A., Hansen, B., Ottenkamp, J., *et al.* Long-term results of atrial correction for transposition of the great arteries. Comparison of Mustard and Senning operations. *Journal of Thoracic and Cardiovascular Surgery* 1994; **108**: 363–72.

21 Williams, H.G., Trusler, G.A., Kirklin, J.W., *et al.* Early and late results of a protocol for simple transposition leading to an atrial switch Mustard repair. *Journal of Thoracic and Cardiovascular Surgery* 1988; **95**: 717–26.

22 Merlo, M., de Tommasi, S.M., Brunelli, F., *et al.* Long term results after atrial correction of complete transposition of the great arteries. *Annals of Thoracic Surgery* 1991; **51**: 227–31.

23 Graham, T.P., Jr, Atwood, G.F., Boucek, R.J., Jr, *et al.* Abnormalities of right ventricular function following Mustard's operation for transposition of the great arteries. *Circulation* 1975; **52**: 678–84.

24 Deanfield, J., Camm, J., Maccartney, F. *et al.* Arrhythmia and late mortality after Mustard and Senning operation for transposition of the great arteries. *Journal of Thoracic and Cardiovascular Surgery* 1988; **96**: 569–76.

25 Gelatt, M., Hamilton, R.M., McCrindle, B.W., *et al.* Arrhythmia and mortality after the Mustard procedure: a 30 year single center experience. *Journal of American College of Cardiology* 1997; **29**: 194–201.

26 Sagin-Saylam, G. and Somerville, J. Palliative Mustard operation for transposition of the great arteries: late results after 15–20 years. *Heart* 1996; **75**: 72–7.

27 Ramsay, J.M., Venebales, A.W., Kelly, M.J., *et al.* Right and left ventricular function at rest and with exercise after the Mustard operation for transposition of the great arteries. *British Heart Journal* 1984; **51**: 364–70.

28 Castaneda, A.R. From Glenn to Fontan. A continuing evolution. *Circulation* 1992; **86** Suppl. II: 80–4.

29 Gentles, T.L., Wernovsky, G., Mayer, J.E., Jr, *et al.* Fontan operation in 500 consecutive patients: factors influencing early and late outcome. *Journal of Thoracic and Cardiovascular Surgery* 1997; **114**: 376–91.

30 Cetta, F., Feldt, R.H., O'Leary, P.W., *et al.* Improved early morbidity and mortality after Fontan operation: the Mayo Clinic experience, 1987 to 1992. *Journal of the American College of Cardiology* 1996; **28**: 480–6.

31 Fontan, F., Kirklin, J.W., Fernandez, G., *et al.*The outcome after a 'perfect' Fontan operation. *Circulation* 1990; **81**: 1520–36.

32 Driscoll, D.J., Offord, K.P., Feldt, R.H., *et al.* Five- to fifteen-year follow-up after Fontan operation. *Circulation* 1992; **85**: 469–96.

33 Fishberger, S.B., Wernovsky, G., Gentles, T.L., *et al.* Factors that influence the development of atrial flutter after the Fontan operation. *Journal of Thoracic and Cardiovascular Surgery* 1997; **113**: 80–6.

34 DuPlessis, A.J., Chang, A.C., Wessel, D.L., *et al.* Cerebrovascular accidents following the Fontan procedure. *Pediatric Neurology* 1995; **12**: 230–6.

35 Cromme-Dijkhuis, A.H., Henkens, C.M., Bijleveld, C.M.A., *et al.* Coagulation factor abnormalities as possible thrombotic risk factors after Fontan operations. *Lancet* 1990; **336**: 1087–90.

36 Feldt, R.H., Driscoll, D.J., Offord, K.P., *et al.* Protein-losing enteropathy after the Fontan operation. *Journal of*

Thoracic and Cardiovascular Surgery 1996; **112**: 672–80.

37 Gentles, T.L., Gauvreau, K., Mayer, J.E., Jr, *et al.* Functional outcome after the Fontan operation: factors influencing late morbidity. *Journal of Thoracic and Cardiovascular Surgery* 1997; **114**: 392–403.

38 Gewillig, M.H., Lundstrom, U.R., Bull, C., *et al.* Exercise responses in patients with congenital heart disease after Fontan repair: patterns and determinants of performance. *Journal of the American College of Cardiology* 1990; **15**: 1424–32.

39 Harrison, D.A., Liu, P., Walters, J.E., *et al.* Cardiopulmonary function in adults late after Fontan repair. *Journal of the American College of Cardiology* 1995; **26**: 1016–21.

CHAPTER 15

Anaesthesia for specific areas of surgery

Section 15.1. Anaesthesia for plastic surgery

MICHAEL SURY

INTRODUCTION

This section covers anaesthesia for surgery for cleft lip and palate, the external ear and syndactyly.

CLEFT LIP AND PALATE SURGERY

NATURAL HISTORY

If left uncorrected, a cleft lip can cause social and psychological difficulties, and a cleft palate interferes with feeding and speech because of the escape of liquid and air through the nose.[1,2]

Both cleft lip and cleft palate develop because of defects in palatal growth during the first trimester. The palate grows inwards and fuses in the midline in two parts: the primary palate is anterior to the incisive foramen, forms the alveolus and lip and fuses by 5–6 weeks, and the secondary palate is posterior to the incisive foramen and fuses later at 7–8 weeks. Impairment of growth and fusion result in a variety of complete, incomplete, unilateral and bilateral clefts. Also, although the mucosa of the secondary palate can fuse, the underlying palatal muscles may not, resulting in a dysfunctional submucous cleft palate.

The incidence of all types of cleft lips and palates is between 1 : 300 and 1 : 600,[1] the highest incidence being in China and other far-east countries. There is an hereditary factor, since incidence of the combination of cleft lip and palate increases from 1 : 1000 in the general population to 1 : 25 of children with first-degree relatives who have clefts.

In the past it was assumed that the majority of clefts occur in otherwise normal infants,[3] but in a review of 1000 cases, over 50% had one or more major anomalies, 22% were syndromic and approximately half of the syndromes were unknown and presumed unique[4] (these infants are often labelled dysmorphic). In general, congenital anomalies are more frequent with isolated cleft palate than with the combination of cleft lip/palate. The common and important associated syndromes are listed in Table 15.1.1 and their anaesthetic problems are discussed in Chapter 20.[1,4,5] Most infants with associated syndromes have a degree of mandibular hypoplasia and this can make both airway management and surgical repair difficult. In the extreme form of Pierre–Robin sequence, for example, in which there is an association between micrognathism (small mandible), glossoptosis (posteriorly placed tongue) and cleft palate, an infant can present with an obstructed upper airway and may require a nasopharyngeal airway or occasionally even a tracheostomy.

HISTORICAL AND GENERAL PERSPECTIVE

In 1847, a year after anaesthesia became available, John Snow reported the use of ether and chloroform in 3–6-week-old infants undergoing repair of a cleft lip.[6] The technique was without a protected airway and the anaesthetic was administered intermittently either by drip on to an open mask or on a sponge applied to a nostril. The potential for airway obstruction due to haemorrhage restricted the surgeon to quick, simple surgery and therefore, at least initially, repair of a cleft palate under anaesthesia was considered too hazardous. By 1900, pharyngeal insufflation allowed the continuous administration of vapour but it was the development of intratracheal insufflation in the 1920s

Table 15.1.1 Common syndromes associated with cleft lip and palate[1,4]

Velocardiofacial (Shprintzen) syndrome
Van der Woude syndrome
Stickler syndrome
Pierre–Robin sequence
Fetal alcohol syndrome
Goldenhar syndrome (facio-auriculo-vertebral sequence or hemifacial microsomia)
Treacher Collins syndrome
Nager syndrome
Down's syndrome

which improved airway protection. Under deep anaesthesia a thin catheter was inserted into the trachea and a larger bore tube was placed just outside the glottis for expired gases: both were protected from blood by gauze packing.[7] Later, during the 1930s, airway protection was available for infants by the use of single large-bore tracheal tube, but even then the tube had to be inserted with great skill without muscle relaxants, under deep anaesthesia. Ayre, in 1937, introduced the 'T-piece' for infants undergoing cleft surgery and was impressed by how much better they fared than those in whom rebreathing methods (which were popular then) were used.[8] The addition of an open-ended bag to the T-piece by Jackson-Rees allowed manual control of ventilation and this became an established technique with the advent of muscle relaxants. Since these pioneering days, advances in the understanding of infant anaesthesia, better drugs, training, equipment and monitoring have improved safety and quality.[9,10]

Not only the skill of the surgeon but also both the timing and type of surgery are factors which have been debated over recent years. The surgeon needs to be experienced before consistently good results can be expected and this has encouraged the concentration of services, including anaesthesia, into centres where fewer surgeons can operate on a larger number of cases.[11–13] These centres should also be able to provide the services necessary to deal with not only the associated feeding, speech and hearing problems, but also the multitude of major and minor anomalies found in children with cleft lip/palates.

CLEFT LIP

Repair of cleft lip challenges the surgeon's skill to achieve a pleasing result. Making a symmetrical nose and lip margin demands accuracy in both dissection and suturing, and although operating equipment has improved, surgical accuracy is more difficult in small patients. Understandably, parents want the repair performed as soon as possible and there are potential advantages in neonatal repair in that wound healing and parental bonding may be improved. Nevertheless, many surgeons prefer to operate from approximately 3 months onwards because by this age any major abnormalities and diseases should have become apparent. Anaesthesia itself may have more risk in neonates than in older infants, although there is much debate on this issue.[1,14–16] Postoperatively, neonates also require more intensive and specialized care. Parents virtually always bond with their babies despite the facial appearance.

Anaesthetic management

Airway considerations

If the infant's face is otherwise normal, there should be few problems with either the maintenance of a clear airway or with laryngoscopy. Occasionally, the laryngoscope can become caught in a deep lip cleft, but this problem can be overcome by filling the cleft with a roll of gauze. In bilateral cleft lip the vomer (or central lip prominence) can hinder midline laryngoscopy,[12] but by using a lateral approach technique and a straight blade,[17] laryngoscopy is much easier (Figure 15.1.1). A south-facing preformed oral tracheal tube is satisfactory and must be placed symmetrically over the chin. A

pharyngeal pack is essential to prevent aspiration of any blood.

Analgesia

In neonates, the postoperative analgesia from both local anaesthetic infiltration and rectal paracetamol is usually sufficient, but older infants usually require extra pain relief with codeine phosphate and diclofenac (the author uses diclofenac in babies over 5 kg). Infraorbital nerve blockade may reduce discomfort,[18,19] but care must be taken with structures nearby. Infants should be able to suckle within a few hours after surgery. Older children need more potent opioid analgesia, such as morphine,[20] or infraorbital nerve blockade. Removal of sutures can be achieved without anaesthesia by skilful nurses 10 days after surgery.

CLEFT PALATE

Primary repair

The head is extended and access to the mouth and pharynx is made possible by the use of a

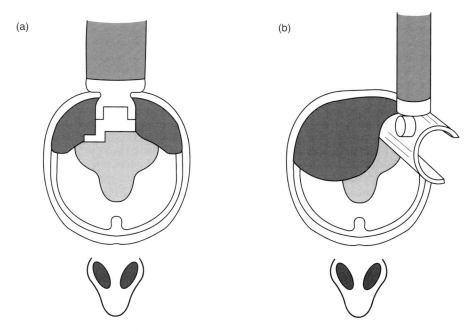

Figure 15.1.1 Oral views of two methods of laryngoscopy. (a) Midline approach: lifting the tongue with a curved blade; (b) lateral approach: sliding past and underneath the tongue with a staight blade.

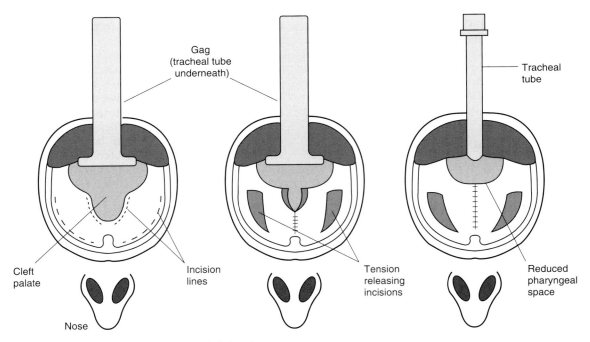

Figure 15.1.2 Oral views of repair of cleft palate.

gag which pushes away the tongue and tracheal tube (Figure 15.1.2). Closure of a cleft palate involves the dissection and mobilization of nasal and buccal mucosae and interposing muscles. Each layer is then sutured and excess tension can be released by making lateral palatal incisions. Damaged blood supply and excess tension are factors responsible for the complications of early wound dehiscence and, later, the development of palatal fistulae.[3,21] Surgery should be complete by 60–90 min, because after 2 or 3 h, excessive pressure from the mouth gag causes tongue ischaemia and oedema which can cause airway obstruction after extubation.[22–24] Although blood should be available for transfusion,[10] appreciable blood loss is unusual. Perioperative antibiotics are recommended, particularly to prevent streptococcal infection.[10]

Closing a cleft palate can affect the airway, by reducing the oropharyngeal space and/or by making the nasopharynx too narrow (Figure 15.1.2). Infants who are unable to mouth-breathe before surgery will be dependent on a patent nasal airway after surgery. Those at particular risk are babies with a small mandible which pushes the tongue against the posterior pharyngeal wall and infants who are too

immature to mouth-breathe if either the nose or nasopharynx is obstructed. For these reasons, cleft palate repair is delayed until well after the neonatal period, usually until 6–9 months.[25]

Secondary cleft palate operations

Speech is affected if the soft palate fails to prevent air escaping through the nose (velopharyngeal incompetence). Once the child is old enough for velopharyngeal incompetence to be demonstrated, revision operations on the soft palate may be attempted. Either a flap is raised from the posterior oropharynx and sutured to the soft palate (Figure 15.1.3) or the mucosa of the posterior pharynx is rearranged to make the nasopharynx smaller. Both operations aim to narrow the nasal airway and thereby prevent velopharyngeal incompetence. The pharyngeal flap operation, however, is associated with severe postoperative respiratory obstruction during sleep, which may persist for several weeks.[26–29] Insertion of a nasopharyngeal airway is likely to damage the flap unless it is placed carefully to one side. In addition, there may be haemorrhage from the pharynx stripped of mucosa, which may only cease after gauze packing and necessitates postoperative tracheal intubation.

Anaesthetic management

Airway considerations at induction

A cleft palate alone should not affect laryngoscopy or the maintenance of a clear airway. However, in infants with a small mandible, such as those with Pierre–Robin sequence, laryngoscopy can be extremely difficult. Restricted neck mobility, as in the Klippel–Feil syndrome, is another well-known factor.[17] Predicting which infants will be difficult is not straightforward, and the grade of laryngoscopy depends on the technique and skill of the anaesthetist.[12,17] In a large survey using a curved blade, difficult laryngoscopy (Cormack and Lehane, grade 3 or 4) occurred in 10% of cases and was associated with either a small mandible or a bilateral cleft lip.[12] The size and position of the tongue are also important, especially if a curved blade is used to lift the tongue in the midline. A straight blade, however, such as the Anderson–Magill, Oxford or the Miller, inserted laterally can slide past or under the tongue and can allow a different and often much easier view of the larynx (Figure 15.1.1). In a survey by the author of infants weighing less than 10 kg, straight-blade laryngoscopy was difficult in those with a maximum mouth opening of less than 2 cm and a short neck, although there were exceptions, as the larynx could not be easily visualized in one infant who had a long neck and ample mouth opening.

Even when conventional laryngoscopy is too difficult, maintaining oxygenation by manual inflation of the lungs via a face mask should be easily achieved, but in infants with severely abnormal facial anatomy safety should be maximized by keeping the infant breathing spontaneously. The laryngeal mask airway is often the best airway tool in these situations. If the mouth opening is severely limited, not only is laryngoscopy difficult but surgery may not be possible. It may be better to abandon the procedure and try again when the infant is larger. If the surgery is possible there are several alternative methods of airway management.

1 A laryngeal mask airway (LMA) can be used throughout surgery, although it is more bulky and is less secure than a tracheal tube.[30,31]
2 Fibreoptic laryngoscopy could be considered, although this is not easy when the pharyngeal space is limited by a small mandible. This problem can sometimes be overcome if a laryngeal mask is used and the fibrescope is inserted through it. A good view of the larynx may be achieved by this method, but passing a tracheal tube over the fibrescope is difficult because of the lack of space inside a small LMA. Even small fibrescopes block the infant trachea and while a tracheal tube is being pushed into the trachea it is difficult to avoid causing a period of hypoxia. It is easier and safer to insert a guide wire into the trachea using the fibrescope so that after the LMA and fibrescope are removed, a tube can be passed over the guide wire into the trachea.[32] The guide wire needs to be stiff enough or it will become dislodged as the tracheal tube is pushed over it.
3 The Bullard laryngoscope is a rigid fibreoptic scope mounted on a curved blade and is reported to be useful in difficult cases.[33]
4 A tracheostomy should be considered, especially if the airway was precarious before anaesthesia.[10]

Tracheal tube types

South-facing preformed plastic tubes are usually satisfactory, although the surgical gag may crush or kink the tube, especially as it becomes warm and soft. Small tubes have thinner walls

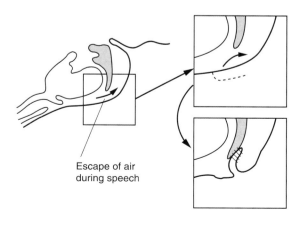

Escape of air during speech

Figure 15.1.3 Sagittal section of pharyngeal flap.

than larger tubes and are particularly susceptible to becoming crushed (the wall thicknesses
of 3.5- and 4.5-mm i.d. plastic tracheal tubes are
0.6–7 and 0.8–9 mm, respectively). Preformed
rubber tubes such as the Oxford are stronger
than plastic but they are no longer in common
use. A reinforced 'armoured' tube will also resist
crushing and kinking but it is difficult to fix at
the correct length: not only can it be pushed
down beyond the carina by the gag but it can
also be dislodged accidentally when the gag is
removed.

Airway considerations at extubation

After extubation the airway may be obstructed
by the combination of a closed palate, a small
mandible pushing the tongue into a small
pharynx, oedema, blood and the residual effects
of anaesthesia (Figure 15.1.4). It is vital that the
infant can lift its tongue forward away from the
posterior pharyngeal wall. The anaesthetist will
need to be able to predict which infants are
likely to be in difficulty and also to manage a
difficult airway at this stage. Anaesthesia should
be tailored to allow maximum control of airway
reflexes at extubation and this usually means
that the infant has to be awake. Opioid
analgesia, if used, must not cause appreciable
postoperative sedation.[10] All infants, particularly those with a small mandible, should be
tested preoperatively to ensure that if the nose is
blocked, they can breathe through their mouth.
For those who cannot mouth-breathe at the end
of surgery, several manoeuvres are possible to
maintain a clear airway. A suture placed

through the tongue and attached to the side of
the mouth can be used to pull the tongue
forward, and is sometimes effective but often
only for a few hours. A nasopharyngeal airway
is safer and provides a clear airway and a port
for nasopharyngeal suctioning; it should not
damage the palate repair if inserted carefully.
Usually, the nasopharyngeal airway is only
required until the following day, by which
time almost all infants have regained their
ability to mouth-breathe. For those who still
rely on the nasal airway, it must remain until the
nasal passage is safe from obstruction from
blood and secretions. A few infants will need
prolonged airway support, probably because of
pharyngeal incoordination as well as a small
pharynx; rarely, a tracheostomy is the safest
course of action.

Analgesia

Local anaesthesia infiltration and paracetamol
provide insufficient postoperative analgesia for
repair of cleft palate. Diclofenac is effective but
opioid analgesia is usually required. The author
prefers intramuscular or rectal codeine phosphate (1.5 mg kg^{-1}) as it is satisfactory for most
infants and causes little postoperative sedation.
Fentanyl (1–2 μg kg^{-1}) provides effective
intraoperative analgesia but a small number of
infants will be too sleepy at extubation. Most
infants can manage either bottle- or breast-
feeding on the following day. It is unnecessary
to splint the arms to prevent the infant
disrupting the sutures.

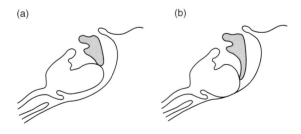

(a)   (b)

(a) Before surgery tongue can lie within cleft palate

(b) After closure of palate tongue may obstruct airway

Figure 15.1.4 Airway obstruction after closure of
cleft palate due to small mandible and posterior
placement of tongue.

EXTERNAL EAR SURGERY

OTOPLASTY

This common and cosmetic operation to correct
prominent ears is usually performed in normal
children and causes postoperative nausea and
vomiting (PONV) which lasts for 1 or 2 days in
up to 85% of cases.[34,35] A major cause of
PONV is the tight packing of the ear contours
by the surgeon after surgery, which stimulates
the vagus and glossopharyngeal nerves. If
packing of the external auditory meatus and

the conchal hollow is avoided PONV is reduced markedly: in one study nausea was reduced from 83% to 7%.[34] Opioid-induced PONV can be avoided by using local anaesthesia, either by infiltration or by nerve block.[35] Regular administration of diclofenac and paracetamol should be sufficient for postoperative pain relief.

RECONSTRUCTION

The external ear can be reconstructed from the costal cartilage.[35] The first-stage operation lasts for 3–4 h, during which the costal cartilage is harvested and carved skilfully into an ear shape which is then inserted into position on the head under a skin flap. Several months later a skin flap is created behind the ear. The surgery is entirely cosmetic and is performed in teenagers in order that an adult-sized ear can be constructed. Many children are normal but others, such as those with Goldenhar's syndrome who have normal intellect, may request surgery. Intraoperative opioid analgesia is required for the harvest of costal cartilage but postoperative pain relief is usually satisfactory with local anaesthesia administered to the costal margin via a catheter. An infusion of 0.25% bupivacaine (0.1 mg kg^{-1} h^{-1}) is effective in most cases, but occasionally the catheter may not be placed perfectly and additional 10 ml bolus doses of local anaesthetic are needed. Regular administration of diclofenac is very helpful and may be more effective than opioids. Surgical dissection on the side of the head causes little pain in comparison with the costal margin. Complications are unusual but include haematoma at the side of the head, which is painful, and pneumothorax.

HAND SURGERY: REPAIR OF SYNDACTYLY

Syndactyly of the hand is most common in children with Apert's syndrome. Surgery is performed at 12–18 months of age, takes 1–2 h and requires a tourniquet. Full-thickness skin grafts may be taken from the groin and, occasionally, pins are inserted into the fingers to

prevent contractures. Despite the associated maxillary hypoplasia and nasal obstruction in these cases, airway control during anaesthesia is usually straightforward, either by tracheal intubation or by laryngeal mask. Venous access, however, may be difficult and the blocked nasal airway may make an inhalational induction awkward until the patient is able to tolerate an oral airway. For intraoperative analgesia, brachial plexus block is extremely effective, reducing the need for opioid supplementation during surgery to less than 10% and making a spontaneous breathing anaesthetic technique easy.[37–40] Using the axillary approach the neurovascular sheath can be cannulated with a 22G intravenous catheter and 0.5 ml kg^{-1} 0.25% bupivacaine injected while applying distal pressure over the sheath.[36] Paracetamol, diclofenac or codeine phosphate is sufficient for postoperative analgesia. Approximately 1 week after surgery the dressings are changed and because this is painful most children will require anaesthesia. Acquired syndactyly is also a feature of certain types of epidermolysis bullosa in which anaesthesia carries risks and management is described on p. 556.

REFERENCES

1 Sommerlad, B.C. Management of cleft lip and palate. *Current Paediatrics* 1994; **4**: 189–95.

2 Habel, A., Sell, D. and Mars, M. Management of cleft lip and palate. *Archives of Diseases of Childhood* 1996; **74**: 360–6.

3 Wilhelmsen, H.R. and Musgrave, R.H. Complications of cleft lip surgery. *Cleft Palate Journal* 1966; **3**: 223–31.

4 Shprintzen, R.J., Siegel-Sadewitz, V.L., Amato, J. and Goldberg, R.B. Anomalies associated with cleft lip, cleft palate, or both. *American Journal of Medical Genetics* 1985; **20**: 585–95.

5 *Smith's Recognisable Patterns of Human Malformation.* 5th edn. Philadelphia, PA: W.B. Saunders, 1997.

6 Jones, R.G. A short history of anaesthesia for hare-lip and cleft palate repair. *British Journal of Anaesthesia* 1971; **43**: 796–802.

7 Magill, I.W. New inventions: an expiratory attachment for endotracheal catheters. *Lancet* 1924; **i**: 1320.

8 Ayres, P. Anaesthesia for hare-lip and palate operation. *British Journal of Surgery* 1937; **25**: 131–2.

9 Jennings, F.O., Delaney, E.J. and Prendiville, J.B. Ether–cyclopropane anaesthesia for the primary repair of cleft

lip and palate (a 20-year experience). *British Journal of Plastic Surgery* 1980; **33**: 301–4.

10 Doyle, E. and Hudson, I. Anaesthesia for primary repair of cleft lip and palate: a review of 244 procedures. *Paediatric Anaethesia* 1992; **2**: 139–45.

11 Huang, M.H., Cohen, S.R., Burstein, F.D. and Simms, C.A. Endoscopic pediatric plastic surgery. *Annals of Plastic Surgery* 1997; **38**: 1–8.

12 Gunawardana, R.H. Difficult laryngoscopy in cleft lip and palate surgery. *British Journal of Anaesthesia* 1996; **76**: 757–9.

13 Clinical Standards Advisory Group. *Cleft Lip and Palate*. London: Department of Health, 1998.

14 Stevens, P., Saunders, P. and Bingham, R. Neonatal cleft lip repair: a retrospective review of anaesthetic complications. *Paediatric Anaesthesia* 1997; **7**: 33–6.

15 Ansermino, J.M. and Sommerlad, B.C. Neonatal cleft lip repair. *Paediatric Anaesthesia* 1998; **8**: 94–5.

16 Freedlander, E., Webster, M.H., Lewis, R.B., Blair, M., Knight, S.L. and Brown, A.I. Neonatal cleft lip repair in Ayrshire; a contribution to the debate. *British Journal of Plastic Surgery* 1990; **43**: 197–202.

17 Hatch, D.J. Airway management in cleft lip and palate surgery. *British Journal of Anaesthesia* 1996; **76**: 755–6.

18 Bosenberg, A.T. and Kimble, F.W. Infraorbital nerve block in neonates for cleft lip repair: anatomical study and clinical implication. *British Journal of Anaesthesia* 1995; **74**: 506–8.

19 Mayer, N.M., Frot, C. and Barrier, G. Anaesthesia for primary repair of cleft lip and palate. *Paediatric Anaesthesia* 1993; **3**: 55.

20 Ward, C.M. and James, I. Survey of 346 patients with unoperated cleft lip and palate in Sri Lanka. *Cleft Palate Journal* 1990; **27**: 11–15.

21 Lees, V.C. and Pigott, R.W. Early postoperative complications in primary cleft lip and palate surgery – how soon may we discharge patients from hospital? *British Journal of Plastic Surgery* 1992; **45**: 232–4.

22 Patane, P.S. and White, S.E. Macroglossia causing airway obstruction following cleft palate repair. *Anesthesiology* 1989; **71**: 995–6.

23 Bell, C., Oh, T.H. and Loeffler, J.R. Massive macroglossia and airway obstruction after cleft palate repair. *Anesthesia and Analgesia* 1988; **67**: 71–4.

24 Lee, J.T. and Kingston, H.G. Airway obstruction due to massive oedema following cleft palate surgery. *Canadian Journal of Anaesthesia* 1985; **32**: 265–7.

25 Hairfield, W.M., Warren, D.W. and Seaton, D.L. Prevalence of mouth breathing in cleft lip and palate. *Cleft Palate Journal* 1988; **25**: 135–8.

26 Orr, W.C., Levine, N.S. and Buchanan, R.T. Effect of cleft palate repair and pharyngeal flap surgery on upper airway obstruction during sleep. *Plastic and Reconstructive Surgery* 1987; **80**: 226–30.

27 Kravath, R.E., Pollack, C.P., Borowiecki, B. and Weittzman, E.D. Obstructive sleep apnea and death associated with surgical correction of velopharyngeal incompetance. *Journal of Pediatrics* 1980; **96**: 645–8.

28 Sirois, M., Caouette-Laberge, L., Laocque, Y. and Egerszegi, P. Sleep apnea following a pharyngeal flap: a feared complication. *Plastic and Reconstructive Surgery* 1994; **93**: 943–7.

29 Xue, F.S., An, S., Tong, S.Y., Liao, X., Liu, J.H. and Luo, L.K. Influence of surgical technique on early postoperative hypoxaemia in children undergoing elective palatoplasty. *British Journal of Anaesthesia* 1998; **80**: 447–51.

30 Chadd, G.D., Crane, D.L., Phillips, R.M. and Tunell, W.P. Extubation and reintubation guided by the laryngeal mask airway in a child with the Pierre–Robin syndrome. *Anesthesiology* 1992; **76**: 640–1.

31 Beveridge, M.E. Laryngeal mask anaesthesia for reair of cleft palate. *Anaesthesia* 1989; **44**: 656–7.

32 Hasan, M.A. and Black, A.E. A new technique for fibreoptic intubation in children. *Anaesthesia* 1994; **49**: 1031–3.

33 Borland, L.M. and Casselbrant, M. The Bullard laryngoscope. A new indirect oral laryngoscope (pediatric version). *Anesthesia and Analgesia* 1990; **70**: 103–4.

34 Ridings, P., Gault, D. and Khan, L. Reduction in postoperative vomiting after surgical correction of prominent ears. *British Journal of Anaesthesia* 1994; **72**: 592–3.

35 Burtles, R. Analgesia for 'bat ear' surgery. *Annals of the Royal College of Surgeons* 1989; **71**: 332.

36 Brent, B. Auricular repair with autogenous rib cartilage grafts: two decades of experience with 600 cases. *Plastic and Reconstructive Surgery* 1992; **90**: 355–74.

37 Tan, T.S.H., Watcha, M.F. and Safavi, F. Cannulation of the axillary brachial sheath in children. *Anesthesia and Analgesia* 1995; **80**: 640–1.

38 Fisher, W.J. and Bingham, R.M. Axillary brachial plexus block for perioperative analgesia in 250 children. *Paediatric Anaesthesia* 1999; (in press).

39 Arthur, D.S. and McNichol, L.R. Local anaesthetic techniques in paediatric surgery. *British Journal of Anaesthesia* 1986; **58**: 760–78.

40 Giaufre, E., Dalens, B. and Gombert, A. Epidemiology and morbidity of regional anesthesia in children: a one-year prospective survey of the French Language Society of Pediatric Anesthesiologists. *Anesthesia and Analgesia* 1996; **83**: 904–12.

Section 15.2. Anaesthesia for general surgery

ANN BLACK

INTRODUCTION

This section covers anaesthesia for genitourinary surgery, renal transplantation, orthopaedics, scoliosis and oncology.

GENITOURINARY SURGERY: ASSESSMENT OF THE CHILD WITH RENAL DISEASE

PHYSIOLOGICAL AND METABOLIC CHANGES

The normal newborn infant has an immature renal system which achieves equivalence to adult function by about 1 year of age. Many children undergoing genitourinary surgery are otherwise healthy and are having procedures such as circumcision or orchidopexy which may be performed on a day-care basis. Some children have associated conditions which have anaesthetic implications (Table 15.2.1).

Significant renal impairment results in multisystem disease. Cardiorespiratory compromise can occur from the effects of hypertension, cardiac failure, severe anaemia, pericarditis, pleural or pericardial effusions and diaphragmatic splinting. The hypertension associated with renal disease may be caused by renal artery stenosis, end-stage renal failure, Wilms' tumour, or it may be secondary to pharmacological treatment, particularly steroid or immunosuppressant therapy. A normocytic normochromic anaemia is physiologically compensated with increases in 2,3-diphosphoglycerate levels and a right shift in the oxyhaemoglobin dissociation curve secondary to metabolic acidosis. Early administration of erythropoietin means that anaemia is less severe and haemoglobin levels of $8–10$ g dl^{-1} are usual. Associated haematological abnormalities may include platelet dysfunction and decreased immunity. Metabolic abnormalities include acidosis, high creatinine and urea levels, hyperkalaemia, hypocalcaemia and hyperphosphataemia. In late stages fragility of the bone due to renal bone disease, secondary hyperparathyroidism and rickets may occur. The pharmacokinetic and pharmacodynamic profiles of many drugs will be altered and concurrent medication must be considered.

DIALYSIS

Patients with end-stage renal failure will be on either peritoneal or haemodialysis. Both treatments are associated with significant fluid and electrolyte shifts. Dialysis should be undertaken $12–36$ h preoperatively in elective cases to allow equilibration of fluid compartments. Preoperative blood tests and a clinical assessment of the child's volume status are required after dialysis and prior to anaesthesia. Haemodialysis involves the use of heparin and platelet dysfunction may occur after treatment. Therefore, a full blood count and clotting must be checked before anaesthesia. The presence of hyperkalae-

Table 15.2.1 Conditions that may need genitourinary surgery: potential anaesthetic implications

Medical condition	Anaesthetic implications
Spina bifida	Latex allergy
Multiple urological procedures	Latex allergy
Prune belly syndrome	Poor respiratory reserve, gastro-oesophageal reflux
Adrenogenital syndrome	Salt and fluid management
Fanconi syndrome, renal tubular acidosis	Salt and fluid management
CHARGE association	Difficult intubation, CHD
Edwards syndrome, trisomy 18	CHD, difficult intubation
Maple syrup urine disease	Glucose and fluid balance
Noonan's syndrome	CHD, difficult intubation
Wilms' tumour	Multiple tumours
Polycystic disease	Lung cysts, pneumothorax

CHD, congenital heart disease.

mia is potentially dangerous. K^+ greater than 5.5 mmol l^{-1} will need consideration of possible causes (drug and dialysis regimen review) and a level above 6.5 mmol l^{-1} requires treatment either with dialysis or with the use of a glucose and insulin infusion or with calcium resonium. Dialysis is associated with an increased risk of blood-borne infection, including hepatitis and human immunodeficiency virus (HIV).

ANAESTHESIA TECHNIQUE

Drugs which wholly or partially rely on renal function for their removal are relatively contra-indicated. In practice, however, there is little to choose between the commonly used intravenous induction agents. Suxamethonium is avoided because of the risk of exacerbating hyperkalae-mia. Atracurium remains the non-depolarizing agent of choice as metabolism is independent of renal function. Mivacurium may also be used, but its effect may be prolonged as plasma cholinesterase activity is decreased by up to 50% in patients with renal failure. Rocuronium and vecuronium both partially rely on renal excretion. Rocuronium has a very rapid onset of action and may be of use if a rapid sequence induction is required. Both drugs have been used successfully in children with diminished renal function, provided neuromuscular func-tion is monitored. Following a single dose of relaxant, effective antagonism of neuromuscular blockade can easily be achieved; accumulation

is likely if infusions are used and these are best avoided.[1] The metabolism of enflurane, sevo-flurane and to a lesser extent halothane pro-duces fluoride ions. The metabolism of sevoflurane is via the cytochrome P450 system and the fluoride ion levels following use are lower in children than in adults. To date there have been no reports of nephrotoxicity[2] (see Chapter 3).

ANALGESIA

The expansion of pain-relief strategies in paediatric practice allows the use of patient- or nurse-controlled morphine infusion techniques, or continuous epidural infusions of bupivacaine alone or with morphine, fentanyl or diamor-phine. These may be achieved via either the lumbar or caudal route. Common compli-cations include nausea, vomiting, pruritus and urinary retention. Metabolites of morphine, morphine-3-glucuronide and morphine-6-glu-curonide, of which the latter is clinically active, are excreted in the urine and can accumulate, so care with dosages and post-operative monitoring of effect are particularly important in this group of patients.

Diclofenac is contraindicated in children with poor renal function, although there are no studies to date that quantify the risk in this group of children. It is wise to be cautious with its use in any condition requiring bilateral renal surgery.

BLADDER SPASMS

Following any operation in which the bladder is opened, postoperative bladder spasms frequently occur and constitute a difficult problem which may significantly prolong the child's hospital stay. Oral oxybutynin, given routinely after surgery, is useful. A lumbar or caudal epidural is useful in treating the spasms but intravenous opioids are not particularly effective. The use of a morphine infusion directly into the bladder, assuming that the bladder is not being continuously drained postoperatively, has been reported to decrease pain and spasm, suggesting that peripheral opioid receptors are present in the bladder mucosa.[3]

RENAL SURGERY

NEPHROBLASTOMA (WILMS' TUMOUR)

Wilms' is the most common tumour of the urinary tract in children (1 : 15 000 live births); in some cases it is congenital but the peak age of occurrence is 3 years. The prognosis is improved if the tumour is small and the child younger than 2 years old and in the earlier stages of the disease. Wilm's is bilateral in 10% of cases and it can occasionally be associated with other syndromal features. Acquired Von Willebrand's disease may also occur. Metastases occur to the lungs, bone, liver, lymph nodes and brain. Preoperative investigations include full blood count, cross-match and clotting screen, liver and renal function tests and chest X-ray. Treatment includes surgery, chemotherapy and radiotherapy. The first step in treatment will often be a biopsy with staging of the tumour and placement of an indwelling venous catheter for chemotherapy. Chemotherapy will decrease tumour size, improving surgical access. Several radiological investigations requiring general anaesthesia may be needed in order to stage the disease. Resection of the mass can be very difficult, particularly when it has extended to, or into, the inferior vena cava (IVC), across the diaphragm or to the retroperitoneal space. Hypertension due to increased renin production may be part of the disease, and this may be

difficult to control preoperatively and may continue into the early postoperative period. Resection requires an extensive upper abdominal laparotomy which may be extended to the thorax. Given that the mass may be large, the abdomen distended and stomach emptying delayed, precautions to prevent regurgitation and potential aspiration of gastric fluid into the lungs must be implemented. Ventilation of the lungs may be compromised by pressure from the mass, abdominal distension or lung metastases.

In addition to routine monitoring, arterial and central venous pressure (CVP) lines are placed. The lower limbs are best avoided as monitoring will be inaccurate and vascular access compromised if the IVC is affected or needs to be clamped during the operative procedure. Surgery, particularly if the disease is bilateral, may involve removal of the kidney, bench dissection and reimplantation. Blood loss with heminephrectomy can be extensive. On rare occasions the tumour may have extended into the right atrium and cardiopulmonary bypass may be necessary. Fluid balance is crucial and blood loss can be major. Precautions to prevent excessive heat loss are important and warming of intravenous fluids is essential. A lumbar epidural using a combination of bupivacaine and opioid will produce good operating conditions and can be continued for the first few postoperative days providing excellent analgesia.

RENAL TRANSPLANTATION

Renal transplantation for end-stage renal failure is an increasingly successful operation and has been extended to include children of 10 kg and above. Donor organs are either from cadaver or live related donors (LRD). Success of the procedure is multifactorial and the results are improved with LRD. Graft thrombosis is the major cause of graft failure and the risk is higher when a young donor kidney is transplanted to a young recipient.[4]

The child's physical condition should be stable before transplantation. This is not usually an emergency operation and cadaveric kidneys stored optimally will maintain good function for up to 48 h. Adequate preparation and psychological support are important. Chronic anaemia is usual and treatment with erythropoietin is beneficial. Preoperative blood transfusion has been shown to improve transplant results. Pretransplant protocols dictate regimens for steroids, immunosuppressants, antibiotics, H_2 receptor antagonists and low-dose heparin. Investigations prior to surgery include full blood count, clotting screen, cross-match of blood, urea, creatinine and electrolyte analysis and a chest X-ray. Important intraoperative issues include management of a major laparotomy and maintenance of adequate intravascular volume to ensure donor kidney perfusion, particularly immediately on reperfusion. Blood is usually given just before the vascular clamps are removed to aid reperfusion and transfusion continued to achieve a normal haemoglobin level. CVP monitoring is essential and intravenous fluids are given to keep the CVP at an adequate level to ensure that the child's volume status is optimal (e.g. 10 cmH₂O). Direct arterial pressure monitoring, sited in the upper limb, is important in young children. However, in older children non-invasive measurements are satisfactory and will avoid potential trauma to the peripheral arteries, which may be required for arteriovenous shunts later in life. For the same reasons care is taken with the choice of intravenous sites. If the radial artery is used the majority will recover patency satisfactorily postoperatively. Lower limb vascular access is not reliable particularly in young children as the anastomosis of the donor vessels is frequently to the aorta and IVC and these vessels may be clamped during vascular surgery.

Acidosis may develop during the period of aortic cross-clamping and potassium toxicity has been reported from the transfusion of cadaver kidney preservation fluid into the circulation. A large kidney may take a significant proportion of the child's cardiac output so that hypotension may occur after the arterial clamps have been removed. Transfusion to a high, normal central venous pressure before the clamps are released will minimize this problem. A large kidney transplanted into a small child requires maximal muscle relaxation during closure; this is easily obtained with atracurium, which does not rely on renal excretion for its elimination. Venous return may be compromised during closure of the abdomen.

A high urine output of at least 2 ml kg⁻¹ h⁻¹ is desirable and this should continue into the postoperative period. Frusemide 1 mg kg⁻¹ i.v. and mannitol 0.5 g kg⁻¹ may be given before the clamps are released and a dopamine infusion of 2–4 μg kg⁻¹ min⁻¹ is also beneficial. Serum and urinary electrolytes and osmolalities as well as haematocrit should be checked regularly and fluid replacement adjusted accordingly.

Opioid analgesia is used taking into account dosages and regimens appropriate to patients with renal failure. Wound infiltration with local anaesthetic is useful and central blockade avoided in view of potential coagulation abnormalities and infection risk from long-standing renal disease and steroid and immunosuppressive use.

Small infants, particularly those weighing less than 20 kg, who are likely to receive a kidney that is large in relation to their body size, may benefit from elective postoperative ventilation. This allows for the physiological effect of the increased intra-abdominal volume and aims to reduce local pressure on the vascular system which could compromise the transplanted kidney. It also allows aggressive management of the intravascular volume without compromising cardiorespiratory function. The potential increase in interstitial lung fluid, decreased functional residual capacity (FRC) and diaphragmatic splinting will all tend to cause a decrease in respiratory function. Management of hypertension includes use of hydralazine, nifedipine or labetalol.

Children who have had a renal transplant may present for surgery unrelated to the transplant.[5] Issues to consider include:

- present status of renal function;
- concurrent medication (antihypertensives, steroid and immunosuppressive regimen and prophylactic antibiotics);
- psychological support for children who must be readmitted on a regular basis;
- avoidance of invasive monitoring if possible;
- maintenance of adequate intravascular volume and avoidance of hypotension;
- potential protracted postoperative course, due to delay in establishing feeding, increased analgesia requirements and a tendency to be slow to mobilize.

The possibility of transplant rejection should be considered in any child who seems generally unwell. Features of potential rejection include fever, oliguria, local graft tenderness or swelling and an increase in serum creatinine greater than 10% of baseline values.

URINARY TRACT SURGERY

Posterior urethral valves result from abnormal development of valve tissue in the male fetal urethra This causes delay in urethral emptying, resulting in back-pressure on the urethra, bladder and ureters, which can result in severe renal damage and a small, hypertrophied bladder. The diagnosis is frequently made antenatally allowing early investigation and management of fluid and acid–base balance, giving the maximum chance for the kidneys to recover and renal function to be in a stable state. Anaesthesia in small babies includes tracheal intubation, although a laryngeal mask airway (LMA) is appropriate in larger infants and a caudal block is usual. Postoperative problems due to large volume, poor quality urine flow resulting in difficulties with post-operative fluid management and sudden electrolyte shift, which were common in the past, are now unusual thanks to careful preoperative care. Drainage of the bladder with either suprapubic or urethral catheter can be achieved on the ward. Early surgery with transurethral resection of the valve tissue or drainage by vesicostomy via a minilaparotomy is under-taken. Later presentation may occur with features of renal insufficiency, increasing vesi-courethral reflux, recurrent infection, dysplasia and failure to thrive. Chronic renal failure may result in 10–15% of children on follow-up.

Pyeloplasty is undertaken for obstruction at the pelviureteric junction. Antenatal scans may diagnose the condition by the presence of hydronephrosis. Renal function is not usually compromised.

For lateral renal incisions the child is positioned on his or her side with the table 'broken' to allow access to the kidney. In babies a flank roll is used. The non-muscle-splitting renal incision will require less analgesia than more extensive incisions. Surgery for reimplantation of the ureters following uretovesical obstruction is a more extensive procedure using a lower abdominal incision. This is associated with considerable pain and bladder spasms; an epidural block and/or opioids may be required. Blood transfusion is most commonly needed in heminephrectomy and in operations on kidneys with a duplex system.

PRUNE BELLY SYNDROME

The prune belly syndrome occurs in 1 : 40 000 births, almost exclusively in males, and may be part of a urethral obstruction malformation complex with megaureter. The condition involves deficiencies in the musculature of the abdominal wall to a varying degree and is associated with cryptorchism, volvulus, pulmonary stenosis, deafness and mental retardation. The skin over the abdomen is classically wrinkled like a prune and the testes are undescended.

Lack of abdominal muscles makes coughing and clearing of respiratory secretions ineffective, which leads to a high incidence of chest infections, especially if there is associated pulmonary hypoplasia. Renal function may be impaired with damage caused by a back-pressure effect of the urine and urinary tract infections.

Surgery is designed to restore function of the urinary tract, promote bladder emptying and preserve renal function. Anaesthesia takes into account the reduced renal function and is managed as if the stomach were full using a rapid sequence induction and cricoid pressure. Controlled ventilation can be maintained without relaxants as the abdomen is very lax. Minor chest infections pose the greatest problem post-operatively and care is therefore taken to avoid oversedation and hypoventilation.[6] For major abdominal surgery a continuous epidural would be suitable.

BLADDER EXSTROPHY

This rare congenital abnormality occurs in less than 1 : 50 000 births. It is often diagnosed antenatally and other abnormalities may be present. Initial closure takes place early in the neonatal period but repeated procedures will be necessary. This is a major abnormality and psychological support is essential for the family. Initial surgery takes into account all the factors important to anaesthesia in neonates. As the repair takes many hours arterial pressure monitoring and intermittent sampling for blood gases, electrolytes and haematocrit are essential. A caudal or lumbar epidural provides excellent conditions and can be retained for up to 2 days postoperatively. Alternatively, intravenous opioids are used. To provide surgical access, pelvic osteotomies may be performed; blood loss will require transfusion and third space losses are high. Postoperatively, plaster of paris splints are applied to promote healing. Usually, the baby is otherwise well and can be extubated at the end of the procedure. Multiple surgical procedures and the use of urinary catheters have caused many patients to develop latex allergy.

BLADDER RECONSTRUCTION

Major surgery to reconstruct the bladder by using segments of bowel is useful in several groups of children, including those with meningomyelocoele and bladder exstrophy. The aim is to establish continence. In the Mitrofanoff operation the newly augmented urinary reservoir is emptied by catheterizing a valved conduit or stoma fashioned from either the relocated appendix or a dilated ureter. Postoperatively, bladder pain and spasms are significant problems.

HYPOSPADIAS

Hypospadias occurs when the external urethral opening is proximal to the tip of the penis. Repair may require either minor or extensive surgery. Meatal advancement and glanduloplasty (MAGPI) is the term used for treatment of distal hypospadias. Minor hypospadias repairs can be carried out on a day-care basis.[7] Anaesthesia involves spontaneous respiration or mechanical ventilation depending on the length of surgery. A caudal block with 0.25% bupivacaine 0.5 ml kg^{-1} is used. The addition of opioids to the caudal, particularly morphine or diamorphine, will delay the need for additional analgesia. The risk of respiratory depression and the requirement to monitor sedation scores and respiratory rate preclude the use of this regimen in day-care patients. The addition of other agents, including adrenaline, ketamine or

clonidine, has been tried with varying success (see Chapter 9).[8,9] A penile block can be used if the hypospadias is distal. The combination of a non-steroidal anti-inflammatory drug (NSAID) with a local block provides very effective postoperative analgesia.[10] Other analgesics, including paracetamol and codeine phosphate, are usually sufficient for postoperative pain management given orally or rectally.

Repeat fistula formation may occur and additional surgery is required. If there is insufficient penile tissue for the repair graft, tissue can be taken from either the buccal or bladder mucosa. This requires a more extensive procedure and adjustments to allow suitable surgical access and use of a site-specific local analgesic regimen. The presence of an erection during hypospasias surgery can make surgery difficult and is best prevented by adequate depth of anaesthesia and an effective caudal blockade.

EPISPADIAS

In epispadias the urethral opening is on the dorsum of the penis rather than at the tip of the glans and this requires extensive surgery which is prolonged and complex. Management is as for a laparotomy and an epidural is very useful for perioperative and postoperative care. Significant blood loss may occur and third space losses are high.

CIRCUMCISION

This is a common procedure required for recurrent infection, phimosis or paraphimosis. In addition, many procedures, performed by non-medical practitioners for social or religious reasons, take place outside the operating theatre without anaesthesia and with little analgesia. There is no consensus as to the best management or most appropriate type of pain relief.[11] Recent work following up a group of infants who underwent circumcision without pain relief has shown that they have a lower pain threshold to later interventions such as immunization.[12]

Children operated on in hospital are usually managed as day patients, with general anaesthesia augmented with analgesia provided by a caudal or penile block with plain bupivacaine. Topical local anaesthetics [lignocaine gel, eutectic mixture of local anaesthetics (EMLA) or

Ametop creams] are all worth considering, particularly in children in whom a local block is contraindicated, such as those with coagulation or anatomical abnormalities. Postoperatively, the use of topical lignocaine gel is very useful, in addition to simple analgesics.

INTERSEX

This may occur in many conditions and may be associated with ambiguous genitalia and difficulties with gender assignment. Surgery may be extensive, repetitive and potentially emotionally traumatic, particularly in older children. Blood loss can be sufficient to require blood transfusion and fluid management may be a problem making close liaison with the metabolic team essential. Use of an epidural for analgesia and perioperative stability is helpful. Congenital adrenal hyperplasia is the most common cause of intersex. Excess androgens are produced owing to a defect in the 21-hydroxylase enzyme required for production of cortisol from progesterone, and this results in masculinization of the female. Severe salt loss from aldosterone deficiency occurs in about 50% of those affected. Preoperative considerations include dependence on exogenous steroids and management of salt and water homeostasis to avoid excessive salt loss and dehydration. Postoperatively, additional steroid cover must be provided and fludrocortisone continued.

SURGERY ON THE TESTIS

Approximately 2% of boys have undescended testes at 2 years of age and will require orchidopexy. In 20% of these the testis is impalpable; it may be high in the inguinal canal, intra-abdominal or absent. Associated potential problems include infertility, local trauma (as the testis is less mobile), torsion and increased risk of malignancy (which is up to 10 times more frequent than in the normally positioned testis). Orchidectomy is very rarely necessary. Anaesthesia for surgery on the testis usually involves spontaneous respiration and provision of a local block, either a caudal or an ilioinguinal block. Although an ilioinguinal block is very effective for this surgery the scrotal incision, if used, may require additional local infiltration as the ilioinguinal and genitofemoral

nerves supply the anterior third of the scrotum but the perineal and posterior femoral nerves supply the rest. Despite a well-functioning local block perioperatively, traction on the testis and vessels can produce a vagally mediated bradycardia best managed by temporarily ceasing surgical stimulation. If the testis is very high a two-stage procedure may be used. Initially, a laparoscopy is undertaken to identify the position of the testis which, if present, is brought down into the inguinal canal at laparotomy; at later surgery the testis is positioned in the scrotum.

Torsion of the testis can occur in the newborn and presents as a bruised scrotum. The testis may be irrevocably damaged and bleeding may be considerable.

In the older child acute torsion of the testis is a surgical emergency and precautions for the management of a child with a potentially full stomach are important. Therefore, anaesthesia is with a rapid sequence induction and tracheal intubation. A local anaesthetic block is useful for postoperative analgesia together with rectal NSAID and paracetamol.

ORTHOPAEDICS

GENERAL PRINCIPLES

Most children undergoing elective orthopaedic procedures are above 1 year of age and otherwise well. Whilst this is so for the majority, orthopaedic conditions do occur in children with syndromes which can be associated with potential anaesthetic problems, the most common group being those with neuromuscular disease (Table 15.2.2).

ANALGESIA

Minor orthopaedic surgery requires the use of simple analgesics. Paracetamol doses in children have recently been revised and an initial dose of 30 mg kg^{-1} (rectally) followed by 15–20 mg kg^{-1} every 6 h is recommended until children are of an appropriate size for adult doses (see Chapter 12). NSAIDs are very useful in children and diclofenac in a total dose of 3 mg

Table 15.2.2 Orthopaedic conditions: associated anaesthetic implications

Medical condition	Anaesthetic implications
Osteognesis imperfecta	Skeletal fragility, scoliosis, temperature control (hyperthermia), care with positioning and moving
Arthrogryposis	Difficult intubation (mandibular hyoplasia), poor lung function, congenital heart disease, difficult vascular access
Meningomyelocoele	Latex allergy, respiratory compromise, renal impairment, scoliosis
Juvenile rheumatoid arthritis (Still's disease)	Difficult intubation, temperomandibular joint fusion, atlanto-axial instability, steroids
Duchenne's muscular dystrophy	Respiratory compromise, scoliosis, cardiomyopathy, arrhythmias, suxamethonium contraindicated
Friedreich's ataxia	Myocardial depression due to fibrosis, scoliosis
Marfans	Congenital heart disease
VATERS	Congenital heart disease, renal impairment

$kg^{-1}\ day^{-1}$ is the most commonly used. Both drugs can be given either orally or as suppositories and the combination of oral analgesics with an oral premedication is useful, particularly in the day-care patient. For the majority of soft-tissue surgery it is sufficient to use simple analgesics and wound infiltration with local anaesthetic or an appropriate nerve block. Procedures such as change of plaster and closed manipulations, whilst non-invasive, can be associated with postoperative pain that requires several doses of analgesia. Pain following major bony surgery may well benefit from the use of a continuous analgesic technique, such as an epidural or intravenous morphine infusion. Preoperative antiemetic administration may be beneficial if opioids are to be used postoperatively. Careful use of postoperative monitoring systems for assessing pain scores and identifying complications (particularly sedation and respiratory depression) allow most pain management techniques to be used safely in these children.

USE OF A TOURNIQUET

Tourniquets are commonly used to improve the surgical exposure during peripheral orthopaedic procedures. Complications are rare but include tissue necrosis or nerve damage. Choice of the widest possible cuff with the lowest acceptable inflation pressure, careful smooth padding of the limb before application of the tourniquet

and avoidance of excessive periods of use will decrease the risk of complications. Tourniquets are avoided if local damage to a nerve is likely, as in patients with multiple exostoses. Tourniquet use in sickle cell disease is controversial. In patients with sickle cell trait no additional risk has been found, although there are reports of increased morbidity when tourniquets are used in patients with homozygous disease, when they are usually avoided.

On release of a single tourniquet it is usual to see a decrease in blood pressure and elevation of end-tidal CO_2, which is thought to be related to the transient acidotic load. This is predictable and can be countered by decreasing the inspired anaesthetic agent, increasing the inspiratory oxygen fraction and administering additional intravenous fluids before the release of the tourniquet. The use of simultaneous bilateral tourniquets in children is potentially hazardous and should be discouraged. If essential they should never be deflated at the same time.

LOWER LIMB SURGERY

Surgery most commonly required in infancy is for correction of talipes and hip surgery for congenital dislocation. Older children most frequently suffer from trauma requiring orthopaedic surgical intervention. Perthes' disease occurs most frequently in boys aged 5–10 years, and results in an osteochondritis of the hip which may require femoral osteotomy, particularly when it occurs in the older child. Slipped femoral epiphysis occurs in a slightly older age group and the epiphysis may need to be manipulated and stabilized by pinning. Children with cerebral palsy or other major neurological impairment may require surgery to prevent joint dislocation or deterioration of function or to aid positioning of the child, in a chair, for example. Multiple soft tissue releases at the hip, knee and feet are used and major hip surgery may be required to prevent dislocation of the femoral head.

Congenital talipes equinovarus

Congenital talipes equinovarus (CTE or club foot) occurs in 1 : 1000 live births and is one of the most common congenital orthopaedic abnormalities requiring surgery in the infant. The majority of children are well, although neuromuscular disorders such as myopathy or congenital myotonic dystrophy may be present and in this small subgroup of patients there may be an increased risk of malignant hyperthermia.[13] If conservative management is not adequate corrective surgery followed by a number of change-of-plaster procedures, associated with manipulation of the foot during anaesthesia, is undertaken in infancy before the child begins to walk. The majority of procedures is managed with the child supine, with the use of an LMA or tracheal intubation depending on the age of the child and the expected duration of surgery. The prone position is sometimes used for posterior release of tissues, making tracheal intubation advisable. A caudal or epidural block provides excellent analgesia which will last for several hours postoperatively, after which opioids such as codeine phosphate 1 mg kg^{-1} every 6 h with NSAIDs will be sufficient. In the severely affected child more extensive bony surgery is required, which may necessitate the use of a postoperative morphine infusion.

Fixation devices

Stabilization of fractures with the use of an external fixator device has been common practice for many years. Increasingly these days complex fixation devices, such as the Illizarov frame, are used to allow lengthening of the limb when there is an inequality between the two sides and also to adjust bone position in all planes if required. These procedures can be prolonged, are sometimes bilateral and often require a series of further procedures with anaesthesia during a course of treatment that lasts for many months. Postoperative pain is significant, in particular immediately after the fixator device has been initially positioned. Diclofenac is not used as it has been shown specifically to inhibit new bone growth in animals, although there are no data in children.

Episiodesis

If limb growth is excessive in one or both limbs surgical destruction of the growing epiphysis is undertaken. This is a relatively minor procedure undertaken with radiological imaging.

HIP SURGERY

Congenital dislocation of the hip

Congenital dislocation of the hip (CDH) is more common in girls, in those born via a breech delivery and in those with a family history of CDH. An arthrogram and application of a spica plaster during anaesthesia may be sufficient to correct the dislocation and this is a short procedure. If exploration of the hip is required it may involve open reduction with or without femoral osteotomy and internal fixation. These major procedures dictate that anaesthesia will include muscle relaxation, tracheal intubation, intermittent positive pressure ventilation (IPPV), perioperative opioid and a caudal or lumbar epidural block with 0.25% bupivacaine 0.75–1.0 ml kg^{-1}. If a lumbar epidural catheter is to be used postoperatively and the child is to be in a spica plaster, practical difficulties arise with monitoring the catheter entry site and allowing both adjustments to the catheter position and removal when required. Some centres use a window cut in the spica posteriorly to allow access, while others rely on intravenous opioids postoperatively so that the catheter, if used, is removed before the spica is applied. For the first surgical intervention blood loss is not usually extensive, although during subsequent surgery blood loss may be a more significant problem. Owing to the support afforded by the spica plaster, postoperative pain is not prolonged.

Later removal of the metalwork from the repaired bone is usually a simple procedure requiring infiltration of the operative site with local anaesthetic, but occasionally excessive bony growth makes removal of metal very difficult.

UPPER LIMB SURGERY

During anaesthesia for hand surgery either use of local infiltration or provision of a brachial plexus block is very successful for analgesia. Other upper limb surgery is less amenable to nerve blockade, and morphine infusions with simple analgesia and local infiltration with bupivacaine are used. Positioning and surgical access for shoulder surgery may dictate the use of tracheal anaesthesia.

CEREBRAL PALSY

Cerebral palsy (CP) is a commonly used term describing a clinical picture with many aetiologies resulting in muscle spasms, contractures and functional problems which may be associated with developmental delay and/or epilepsy. Affected children may require multiple orthopaedic procedures aimed at maintaining or improving their physical function, and helping with management of seating and personal hygiene. The children need careful assessment as the degree of immobility can camouflage serious limitations in cardiovascular and respiratory reserve. A decrease in the requirements for some drugs in this condition has been reported; if the child's physical status is poor even simple sedative premedication can produce respiratory compromise. Some children will require ventilatory support postoperatively and in this high-risk group great care must be taken with opioid use, particularly when planning the postoperative regimen. Simple analgesics and diclofenac are safe and codeine phosphate is usually well tolerated. Postoperative oxygen saturation, respiratory rate and apnoea monitoring are important, particularly if opioids are being given. Children with little muscle bulk and severe CP may be unable to maintain their temperature perioperatively and temperature monitoring is essential. In this group, unpredictable muscle spasms are a common postoperative problem, often exacerbated by the operative stretching of the limb and the fixed position dictated by the presence of a plaster cast. These spasms can be difficult to manage and do not respond to increasing doses of opioids, or to epidural anaesthesia. Many children will be taking baclofen and this should be continued, particularly as sudden withdrawal can exacerbate muscular irritability and epilepsy. Benzodiazepines such as diazepam, 0.2 mg kg^{-1}, given either orally or as a suppository, are the most effective intervention to relieve frequent spasms, if the child can tolerate it.

SCOLIOSIS

Scoliosis in the young is idiopathic in 85% of cases. It can be classified into infantile, juvenile and adolescent types depending on the age at which the majority of change occurs. Adolescent idiopathic scoliosis is the most common type. If the spinal curve is limited or resolving on follow-up, no surgery is required. Known causes of scoliosis include meningomyelocoele, cerebral palsy, poliomyelitis, syringomyelia, neurofibromatosis, Duchenne's muscular dystrophy and Friedreich's ataxia. In these cases the anaesthetic requirements of the specific conditions will need to be carefully assessed. The severity of scoliosis is quantified using measurements defined by Cobb.[14] Surgery is required to stabilize the spine, to prevent further curvature progression or for cosmetic results, and this may involve an anterior and/or posterior approach to the spine.

ASSESSMENT

Full preoperative assessment and explanation is essential for all children undergoing such major surgery and this is best achieved in a preoperative clinic situation when there is sufficient time for discussion with both the child and the parents. The majority of children with idiopathic scoliosis do not have decreased physiological function. They do not require extensive investigations and will tolerate surgery and anaesthesia well. Respiratory compromise is unlikely in idiopathic scoliosis unless the curve is greater than 65°. Children with neuromuscular disease may well have limited cardiorespiratory reserve for any given degree of curvature; they are likely to have a more difficult and protracted postoperative course. Accurate measurements of pulmonary function can be difficult in the young child (under 5 years) or in children with learning difficulties. They are likely to have restrictive lung function with decreased total lung capacity, vital capacity (VC) and FRC. Chest-wall compliance can be severely restricted and this, combined with respiratory muscle weakness, may decrease respiratory reserve and lead to alveolar hypoventilation and potential hypoxaemia and hypercarbia. Major limitation in respiratory function, such as a VC less than 40%, suggests that postoperative respiratory support is more likely to be needed. Whilst there is an increased risk of postoperative morbidity and mortality this should not preclude surgical intervention.[15] A delay in surgery may result in worsening of the scoliosis and a further decrease in respiratory reserve. Postoperative ventilation may be prolonged and occasionally may be long term, particularly in children with advanced neuromuscular disease.[16]

Cardiac function may also be compromised. This can be related to structural abnormalities, particularly mitral valve prolapse, or due to pulmonary hypertension either as a primary pathology or secondary to chronic respiratory disease. Many conditions associated with scoliosis also have associated cardiac involvement: cardiomyopathy, mitral valve abnormalities and dysrhythmias in Duchenne's muscular dystrophy, myocardial failure and dysrhythmias in Friedreich's ataxia, aortic and mitral valve abnormalities in Marfan's syndrome. A preoperative electrocardiogram (ECG) and echocardiogram with review by a paediatric cardiologist are essential in these children. Children with multiple handicaps may benefit from a period of nutritional management preoperatively and those with chronic gastric reflux should have their therapy maximized.

MONITORING SPINAL CORD FUNCTION

The monitoring of gross motor function with the use of a 'wake-up test' is becoming less common, particularly as paediatric patients are sometimes not able to co-operate adequately. It has been mainly superseded by routine operative spinal cord function monitoring using evoked potentials. If a wake-up test is necessary it should be discussed carefully before the operation. When needed, the neuromuscular blocking agent is stopped to allow return of motor function and the anaesthesia titrated to allow co-operation for assessment of function. Use of a propofol and opioid infusion is particularly helpful in this setting. Midazolam may be used after the test to provide amnesia, but even without this patients rarely remember the test being applied.

Many different methods of continuous monitoring of sensory and motor evoked potentials are available and these specialized techniques are constantly evolving.[17–19] The choice and use of anaesthetic agents and changes in physiological conditions can affect these recordings and it is most important that there is close liaison between the anaesthetist and the neurophysiologist throughout the surgical procedure (Table 15.2.3).

Useful data can be recorded once a baseline recording is made and stable anaesthetic levels and conditions are maintained with low inspired concentrations of inhalational agents, 0.5–1% isoflurane, nitrous oxide and an opioid-based anaesthetic or use of a propofol infusion. Recordings can be affected by hypotension and hypothermia, changes in the level of anaesthesia and poor positioning.[20] Clinically important changes in the recording suggest potential compromise of the spinal cord and immediate intervention to reduce stress to the cord may prevent serious damage.

BLOOD LOSS AND FLUID BALANCE

Blood loss is dictated by the duration and complexity of surgery, the underlying pathology and the surgical technique. Special attention to surgical technique helps to minimize blood loss although, particularly with posterior spinal fusion and surgery at multiple levels, this is

Table 15.2.3   Effect of anaesthetic agents on monitoring spinal cord function

Type of monitoring		Effect of anaesthetic agent
Sensory evoked potentials		
Cortical		
Stimulation of posterior tibial nerve, recording from EEG scalp electrodes	Halothane Enflurane Isoflurane	Increase latency, decrease amplitude of recording
	Nitrous oxide	Decreases amplitude
	Fentanyl	Decreases amplitude
	Thiopentone	Little effect
Spinal		
Stimulation of posterior tibial nerve, recording from epidural catheter	Relatively insensitive to anaesthetic agents	
Motor evoked potentials		
Myogenic		
Electrical or magnetic stimulation of scalp, recording from muscle	Volatile agents	Abolish response
	Nitrous oxide	Depresses response
	Fentanyl Ketamine Etomidate Propofol	Minimal effect
Neurogenic		
Electrical or magnetic stimulation, recording from epidural catheter	Isoflurane	Reduces response

See Refs 17–19.

difficult. Increasingly, it is reported that spinal surgery is possible with no allogenic blood use.[21] Other strategies for managing blood loss are mostly appropriate in larger children and include the use of autotransfusion and pre-operatively donated autologous blood where available, and the avoidance of hypertension perioperatively. Blood-saving mechanisms are increasingly being used in many forms of paediatric surgery which involve a potential for large blood loss.[22] Induced hypotension is less frequently used in paediatric practice; although it reduces blood loss and improves surgical conditions the moderate level achieved by balanced anaesthesia and mild hyperventilation may be sufficient. The risk of inadequate perfusion to major organs and the increased risk of spinal-cord damage, along with the difficulty of knowing what perfusion pressure may be required in different age groups, have decreased its use. In older children a degree of hypoten-

sion can be acceptable if monitoring of spinal-cord function is in place. The choice of agent is wide and includes sodium nitroprusside, glyceryl trinitrate, labetalol and nicardipine. Maintenance of intravascular volume is with a combination of crystalloid and colloid. Blood and blood products are given as required based on the results of blood counts and clotting studies. Platelet infusions, cryoprecipitate and fresh-frozen plasma may be required in the more complex cases.

ANAESTHESIA

Premedication can be beneficial and is safe in the majority of children. Precautions to avoid aspiration of gastric contents in children who have chronic reflux problems are advisable. Reinforced tracheal tubes are usually used and changed at the end of the procedure if post-operative IPPV is necessary. Core and peripheral temperature probes and a nasogastric tube are placed. Routine monitoring is initiated and a urinary catheter inserted. Anaesthesia is with fentanyl, and neuromuscular relaxant in addition to low inspired concentrations of isoflurane is usually satisfactory. Owing to the length of surgery and risk of major blood loss, together with the necessity to control arterial blood pressure, venous access must be adequate and central venous and arterial pressure monitoring is required. The positioning of the patient may compromise the accuracy of the CVP recording. Regular perioperative sampling of arterial gases, haematocrit and clotting studies will be required. Temperature-preserving mechanisms are also necessary, including a heating mattress, preferably of the hot-air type, and the use of warmed intravenous fluids. Air or fat embolism may occur via the open venous sinus of the vertebrae. These may be identified by changes in the end-tidal CO_2 or ECG, or other sudden physiological change such as a decrease in blood pressure.

POSITIONING

Positioning requires scrupulous care. An anterior fusion requires the patient to be placed supine for a thoracic or thoracolumbar approach. Use of a double-lumen tube and one-lung anaesthesia may help surgical access in larger children. For posterior spinal fusion the child is positioned prone on specially designed support frames, which allow good surgical access while ensuring that the child is well supported with the abdomen unrestricted to prevent respiratory compromise or the development of venous obstruction. If a combined approach is undertaken the child has to be turned during the procedure.

There is some debate regarding the advantages of combining the anterior and posterior repair in one operation as opposed to separating the procedures by a week or more. The incidence of postoperative complications is higher in children undergoing staged procedures, as is the requirement for blood products.[23]

POSTOPERATIVE MANAGEMENT

Postoperatively, morphine or fentanyl infusions or patient-controlled analgesia (PCA) are used for pain management, in addition to NSAIDs. Successful use of regional techniques has been reported, including the use of epidural opioids for both anterior and posterior fusion.[24] Intrathecal morphine placed once the dura is closed following posterior spinal fusion and epidural catheters placed perioperatively can be tunnelled so that infusions can be used for postoperative analgesia.

Respiratory complications are common but many children can be extubated at the end of the surgery even if their preoperative lung function was diminished. Some children will temporarily require postoperative ventilation and occasionally a child will require tracheostomy and long-term ventilatory support.[15] Postoperative respiratory complications are common. The presence of a chest drain, the effect of pain and difficulties in achieving effective chest physiotherapy make respiratory management an important focus of postoperative care. Other postoperative complications include pneumonia, pneumothorax, pleural effusion, atelectasis, pulmonary embolus, respiratory failure, bleeding, wound infection, neurological damage and urinary complications, including retention and infection.

The possibility of other rare anaesthetic events, such as malignant hyperthermia or latex allergy, should be considered as these conditions occur more frequently in this group of patients.[25]

ONCOLOGY

New methods for management of childhood malignant disease have increased the cure rate and long-term survival in many conditions (see also Chapter 1). Affected children may have multisystem disease and a review of cardiorespiratory, renal, hepatic, haematological and metabolic status is essential, bearing in mind any disease-specific issues. Many will require blood products prior to any procedure. Cachexia and poor nutritional status may be a feature and the need for additional psychological support must be recognized. The therapy already undergone, whether surgery, chemotherapy, radiotherapy or bone marrow

Table 15.2.4 Anaesthetic implications of oncology treatment

Agent	Effect
Chemotherapeutic agents	
Bleomycin	Pulmonary fibrosis
	Additional risk if high inspired oxygen concentration; mucositis
Doxorubicin	Myelosuppression, mucositis, cardiomyopathy: serial ECHO required
Vincristine	Neurotoxicity, parasthesia, ptosis, muscular weakness, convulsions, 2% inappropriate ADH (hyponatraemia, convulsions)
Vinblastine	Myelosuppression
Cyclophosphamide	Myelosuppression, pneumonitis
Methotrexate	Myelosuppression, mucositis
Immunosuppressants	
Azathiaprine	Myelosuppression, decreased requirement for non-depolarizing muscle relaxants, altered liver function.
Cyclosporine	Hypertension, renal impairment
Steroids	Need additional steroid cover, 'steroid facies', potential difficult airway, intubation may be difficult, altered glucose metabolism, hypertension
Radiotherapy	Local fibrosis (airway compromise)

transplant, will have specific anaesthetic implications (Table 15.2.4).

Many children will require repeated general anaesthesia during their treatment, for investigations such as lumbar puncture or bone marrow biopsy and trephine, diagnostic procedures or therapy. Anaesthesia may be required on a frequent, even daily basis as with radiotherapy programmes. Intravenous agents such as ketamine, thiopentone or propofol are very useful. Gas induction with sevoflurane is also popular and, in general, use of a facemask or LMA is sufficient for airway management.

Treatment of children with malignant disease has been revolutionized by the use of indwelling intravenous catheters and implantable intravenous access ports. These are invaluable for giving drugs and chemotherapy, for routine blood sampling, administration of fluids and blood products and occasionally for monitoring. When accessed for anaesthesia a sterile or aseptic non-touch technique is used. Regular flushing of the system with saline followed by heparinized saline $10\ U\ ml^{-1}$ according to local protocols is essential. The system must always be checked before use. If the line is not functioning correctly it is checked to ensure that there is no extravasation and that the position is satisfactory on the chest X-ray. Management of catheter complications is summarized in Table 15.2.5.

COMPLICATIONS

The immunocompromised child has specific needs. Scrupulous care with technique to avoid any risk of infection is essential. Liaison with

Table 15.2.5 Use of indwelling catheters and ports

Complication	Diagnostic features	Management
Thrombosis	Unable to access	Urokinase[a] (can be repeated)
Fibrin sheath	Will flush, will not aspirate	Urokinase; TPA
Vegetation/thrombus	Diagnosed on ECHO	Antibiotics; urokinase; TPA
Infection in line	Blood cultures positive	Antibiotics (if catheter has more than one lumen, each is treated giving antibiotic doses via alternate lumen)

[a]Hickman line: urokinase 5000 U in 1 ml saline; Portacath: urokinase 10 000 units in 2 ml saline.
TPA, tissue plasminogen activator.

the haematology service is important as the need for blood products is high and specific conditions will have specialized needs. Most children will require blood products which are screened for cytomegalovirus (CMV). All children will have prophylactic antibiotics.

Bone marrow transplantation has been used for the treatment of an increasing range of malignant and genetic conditions. Children who have had this treatment are at risk of infection; they may develop graft versus host disease (GVHD) or they may be adversely affected by their ongoing medication. GVHD is a multisystem disease predominantly affecting the immune system, skin and liver, in the latter case causing cholestatic jaundice and coagulopathy.

In addition to routine screening, products should be CMV negative and irradiated or filtered to be lymphocyte depleted.

REFERENCES

1 Smith, C.E. and Hunter, J.M. Anesthesia for renal transplantation: relaxants and volatiles. In: Royston, D.R. and Feeley, T.W. (eds). *International Anesthesiology Clinics. Anesthesia for the Patient with a Transplanted Organ*. Boston, MA: Little Brown and Co., 1995: **33**(2): 69–92.

2 Lerman, J., Sikich, N., Kleinman, S. and Yentis, S. The pharmacology of sevoflurane in infants and children. *Anesthesiology* 1994; **80**: 814–24.

3 Duckett, J.W., Cangiano, T., Cubina, M., Howe, C. and Cohen, D. Intravesical morphine analgesia after bladder surgery. *Journal of Urology*. 1997; **157**: 1407–9.

4 Kohaut, E.C. and Tejani, A. The 1994 annual report of the North American Pediatric Renal Transplant Cooperative Study. *Pediatric Nephrology* 1996; **10**: 422–34.

5 Black, A.E. Anesthesia for pediatric patients who have had a transplant. In: Royston, D.R. and Feeley, T.W. (eds). *International Anesthesiology Clinics. Anesthesia for the Patient with a Transplanted Organ*. Boston, MA: Little Brown and Co., 1995: **33**(2): 107–23.

6 Henderson, A.M., Vallis, C.J. and Sumner, E. Anaesthesia in the prune-belly syndrome: a review of 36 cases. *Anaesthesia* 1987; **42**: 54–60.

7 Siegal, A.L., Snyder, H.M. and Duckett, J.W. Outpatient pediatric urological surgery: techniques for a successful and cost effective practice. *Journal of Urology* 1986; **136**: 879–881.

8 Kelleher, A.A., Black, A., Penman, S. and Howard, R. Comparison of caudal bupivacaine and diamorphine with caudal bupivacaine alone for repair of hypospadias. *British Journal of Anaesthesia* 1996; **77**: 586–90.

9 Cook, B. and Doyle, A.E. The use of additives to local anaesthetic solutions for caudal epidural blockade. *Paediatric Anaesthesia* 1996; **6**: 353–9.

10 Gadiyar, V., Gallagher, T.M., Crean, P.M. and Taylor, R.H. The effect of combiniation of rectal diclofenac and caudal bupivacaine on postoperative analgesia in children. *Anaesthesia* 1995; **50**: 820–2.

11 Howard, C.R., Howard, F.M., Garfunkel, L.C., de Blieck, E.A. and Weitzman, M. Neonatal circumcision and pain relief: current training practice. *Pediatrics* 1998; **101**: 423–8.

12 Taddio, A., Katz, J., Ilersich, A.L. and Koren, G. Effect of neonatal circumcision on pain response during routine vaccination. *Lancet* 1997; **349**: 599–603.

13 Zannette, C., Manani, G., Pittoni, G., Angelini, C., Trevisan, C.P. and Turra, S. Prevalence of unsuspected myopathy in infants presenting for clubfoot surgery. *Paediatric Anaesthesia* 1995; **5**: 165–70.

14 Cobb, J.R. Outline in the study of scoliosis. In: Edwards, J.W. (ed.). *Instructional Course Lectures. American Academy of Orthopedic Surgeons* 1948; **5**: 261–75.

15 Rawlins, B.A., Winter, R.B., Lonstein, J.E., *et al.* Reconstructive spine surgery in pediatric patients with major loss in vital capacity. *Journal of Pediatric Orthopedics* 1996; **16**: 284–92.

16 Milne, B. and Rosales, J.K. Anaesthetic considerations in patients with muscular dystrophy undergoing spinal fusion with Harrington rod insertion. *Canadian Anaesthetists Society Journal* 1982; **29**: 250–4.

17 Samra, S.K. Effects of isoflurane on human median nerve evoked potentials. In: Ducker, T.B. and Brown, R.H. (eds). *Neurophysiology and Standards of Spinal cord Monitoring*. Berlin: Springer, 1988: 147–56.

18 McPherson, R.W., Snell, B. and Traystman, RJ. Effects of intravenous anaesthetic induction agents on somatosensory evoked potentials: Thiopental, fentanyl and etomidate. In: Ducker, T.B. and Brown, R.H. (eds). *Neurophysiology and Standards of Spinal Cord Monitoring*. Berlin: Springer, 1988: 163–7.

19 Jones, S.J., Carter, L., Edgar, M.A., Morley, T., Ransford, A.O. and Webb, P.J. Experience of spinal cord monitoring in 410 cases. In: Schramm , J. and Jones, S.J. (eds). *Spinal Cord Monitoring*. Berlin: Springer, 1985: 215–20.

20 Manninen, P.H. Monitoring evoked potentials during spinal surgery in one institution. *Canadian Journal of Anaesthesia* 1998; **45**: 460–5.

21 Philips, W.A. and Hensinger, R.N. Control of blood loss during scoliosis surgery. *Clinical Orthopaedics and Related Research* 1988; **229**: 88–93.

22 de Ville, A. Blood saving in paediatric anaesthsia. *Paediatric Anaesthesia* 1997; **7**: 181–2.

23 Ferguson, R.L., Hansen, M.M., Nicholas, D.A. and Allen, B.L. Same day versus staged anterior–posterior spinal surgery in a neuromuscular scoliosis population: the evaluation of medical complications. *Journal of Pediatric Orthopedics* 1996; **16**: 293–303.

24 Shaw, B.A., Watson, T.C., Merzel, D.I., Gerardi, J.A. and Birek, A. The safety of continuous epidural infusion for postoperative analgesia in pediatric spine surgery. *Journal of Pediatric Orthopedics* 1996; **16**: 374–7.

25 Hamid, R.K.A. and Gordon, P.N. Anesthesia for pediatric spine procedures. In: Porter, S.S. (ed.). *Anesthesia for Surgery of the Spine*. New York: McGraw-Hill, 1995: 225–80.

Section 15.3. Anaesthesia for ophthalmic surgery

IAN JAMES

INTRODUCTION

Surgical procedures on the eye in adults can frequently be performed using local anaesthesia. This is not the case in small children, for whom general anaesthesia will always be required (Table 15.3.1). The most common ophthalmic surgical procedure in children is strabismus surgery; in addition, many children will require general anaesthesia to permit a full eye examination. Most of these children are ASA 1 or 2 and will be day cases, and anaesthesia is uncomplicated. However, many of the eye problems in children are associated with other anomalies which may have implications for the conduct of general anaesthesia, and it is necessary to be aware of these.

GENERAL PRINCIPLES

For the majority of ophthalmological procedures general anaesthesia is routine. Premedication and induction can follow usual practice. Spontaneous ventilation via a laryngeal mask airway (LMA) is satisfactory for most of the shorter procedures where a sterile operating field is not required, such as laser surgery, and in some cases in older children. However, because of the inaccessibility of the

Table 15.3.1 Procedures for which general anaesthesia may be required

Examination of the eye	General examination
	Measurement of intraocular pressure
	Retinoblastoma follow-up
Extraocular procedures	
On the lids	Excision of meibomian cysts/dermoids
	Steroid injection of haemangiomas
	Tarsorrhaphy
	Ptosis surgery
On the nasolacrimal apparatus	Syringing and probing of ducts
	Insertion of Crawford's tubes
	Dacryocystorhinostomy
On the eye	Laser surgery/cryotherapy
	Strabismus surgery
	Conjunctival surgery, e.g. dermoid excision
	Corneal surgery
	Enucleation
Intraocular procedures	To reduce intraocular pressure
	Goniotomy
	Trabeculectomy
	Cataract aspiration + artificial lens insertion
	Lensectomy

airway during surgery it is safer in the majority of other procedures to use a tracheal tube rather than a laryngeal mask airway. For procedures involving the globe the surgeon will require a still eye and this is most satisfactorily achieved using paralysis and controlled ventilation.

For many surgical procedures a dilated pupil is necessary and ophthalmologists frequently use mydriatic agents perioperatively. The most commonly used agents are cyclopentolate 0.5% or 1%, a parasympatholytic drug, or phenylephrine 2.5%, a sympathomimetic. These are normally administered topically in the preoperative period but when inadequate pupillary dilatation has been achieved further drops may be applied in the anaesthetic room. These are generally well tolerated, but serious systemic side-effects, including hypertension and pulmonary oedema consequent upon absorption of these agents, have been reported after subconjunctival injection.[1] On occasion, the surgeon may wish to inject mydricaine, a mixture of procaine, atropine and adrenaline, to obtain better pupillary dilatation. It is therefore prudent to avoid an anaesthetic technique utilizing a high concentration of volatile agent, particularly halothane, in these cases and to avoid hypercapnia, as dysrrhythmias may occur.

ASSOCIATED ANOMALIES

Many children who have eye problems have other problems as well, often as part of a chromosomal defect, or a metabolic or other congenital disorder. In many cases this may be limited to developmental delay, mental retardation and behavioural problems and the challenge lies in managing these patients in a sympathetic manner.

In other patients, the association may be of more direct anaesthetic relevance. For example, a number of syndromes in which there can be major difficulties with intubation may have cataracts, glaucoma or squints. These syndromes, described in detail in Chapters 1 and 20, include the mucopolysaccharidoses, craniofacial disorders such as Goldenhar syndrome, Pierre–Robin syndrome, Crouzon's disease and Smith–Lemli–Opitz syndrome, and Stickler's syndrome. Appropriate precautions and techniques for patients with potential intubation difficulties should be adopted. Glaucoma often occurs in Sturge–Weber syndrome, in which there may be seizures as well as mental retardation, and the airway can also be affected by haemangioma.

Dislocated lenses are common in homocystinuria, a metabolic disorder in which hypoglycaemia and thromboembolic episodes are common. It is important to ensure adequate hydration in these children perioperatively, and an intravenous glucose infusion should be started preoperatively. Patients with homocystinuria should be given aspirin in the perioperative period to minimize the risk of thromboembolic episodes. It is important to ensure that these patients are metabolically stable before proceeding with anaesthesia. Dislocated lenses are also common in patients with Marfan's syndrome, in whom there may be aortic root or valve problems.

Infants with congenital cataracts frequently present for surgery in the first few days of life. These cataracts may be part of a metabolic disorder, or may occur following intrauterine infection, with the attendant associated anomalies. In particular, they are common in the congenital rubella syndrome, now rare, in which there is frequently a cardiac anomaly.

BACTERIAL ENDOCARDITIS PROPHYLAXIS

Although many patients such as those with congenital rubella syndrome or Marfan's syndrome may have an associated cardiac anomaly, the vast majority of ophthalmic procedures do not produce a bacteraemia, and antibiotic prophylaxis is unnecessary. The exceptions are those children undergoing a procedure on the nasolacrimal ducts, in which there is a significant incidence of bacteraemia.[2] These patients should receive antibiotic prophylaxis if they have a structural cardiac lesion (see Appendix 4).

EXAMINATION OF THE EYES

Anaesthesia may be required in some children simply because they are too young or uncooperative to allow an adequate examination when awake. Normally, this can be carried out perfectly satisfactorily using an inhalational technique and a facemask. On occasion, it is easier for the surgeon if an LMA is inserted, particularly where it is necessary to use the operating microscope. Many of these children will require regular follow-up examinations and repeated anaesthetics, so it is essential that induction is made as gentle and atraumatic as possible.

Special consideration is required if the primary purpose of the examination under anaesthesia (EUA) is to measure intraocular pressure (IOP). Most anaesthetic agents reduce IOP and there is a risk that injudicious anaesthesia will lower the IOP to such an extent that a raised IOP will be masked, thereby delaying treatment. A gaseous induction using no more than 2% halothane or 5% sevoflurane will produce a lightly anaesthetized child with a minimal fall in IOP. If intravenous induction is planned, no more than the smallest dose needed to induce sleep should be given. Best results are achieved if the ophthalmologist is present or close by during induction and available to measure the IOP the instant the child stops moving, and while the eyes are still central. It is important to ensure that the facemask does not encroach on and compress the eye. IOP measurements should be taken before laryngoscopy or the use of suxamethonium (although this is now rarely used), as both of these will increase IOP.[3–5] Insertion of an LMA does not appear to raise IOP.[3]

An alternative technique is to use ketamine. A dose of 5–10 mg kg^{-1} intramuscularly will produce within a few minutes a child who is quiet and still enough to permit a thorough eye examination. It is essential to ensure that the airway is well maintained. There may be a slight increase in IOP using ketamine, although there are conflicting reports about this.[6,7] However, it is generally felt that it is safer to have a falsely high IOP than a falsely low one which might result in further IOP treatment being delayed.

Some centres prefer not to use ketamine because of a reluctance to administer intramuscular injections to small children, particularly as frequent follow-up measurements are often required. Unpleasant dreams following ketamine occur less frequently in small children than in adults. Nevertheless, both anaesthetic techniques are acceptable, but due account should be taken of the technique used when comparing IOP measurements over a period of time.

STRABISMUS SURGERY

This is the most common ophthalmic surgical procedure in children, with a squint occurring in up to 5% of non-premature infants. It is increasingly being performed on a day-stay basis, but the high incidence of postoperative nausea and vomiting (PONV) associated with this procedure results in a number of unplanned overnight admissions. The other significant anaesthetic complication that occurs during strabismus surgery is the oculocardiac reflex (OCR) and it has been postulated that these two events might be associated. Although very rare, there is an increased incidence of malignant hyperpyrexia in patients with a squint and suxamethonium should be avoided.

NAUSEA AND VOMITING FOLLOWING STRABISMUS SURGERY

Vomiting is a well recognized complication following strabismus surgery, particularly in children over the age of 2 years (see also p. 292). The precise mechanism of vomiting following squint surgery remains unknown but it is postulated to be part of an oculoemetic reflex, involving the ophthalmic division of the trigeminal nerve and the vomiting centre in the medulla.[8] There appear to be two distinct periods for vomiting, some children vomiting immediately or within the first few hours following surgery, and other groups in whom vomiting does not occur until several hours later, usually within 24 h but occasionally up to 40 h postoperatively.

Experience suggests that about two-thirds of children undergoing strabismus surgery vomit if no preventive measures are taken. This figure is supported by a systematic review of publications between 1981 and 1994 on vomiting in children following squint surgery, which established a mean incidence of vomiting within 6 h of 54% in children receiving no prophylactic antiemetic and of 59% within 48 h.[9]

Many different strategies have been attempted to reduce this incidence of vomiting. Most have involved the administration of prophylactic antiemetics such as metoclopromide, droperidol or ondansetron, or the use of anticholinergic agents or the putative antiemetic properties of propofol. It is possible to reduce the incidence of vomiting to around 30% using one or more of these techniques, but this remains unacceptably high, particularly as nausea, which is difficult to quantify and thus often unreported, can be equally distressing to the child.

It is not possible to compare these studies satisfactorily because they involve very different underlying anaesthetic techniques, in particular in the use or otherwise of anticholinergic agents and opioids. It has been shown,[10,11] however, that ondansetron 150 μg kg^{-1} is better than droperidol 75 μg kg^{-1} and metoclopramide 0.25 μg kg^{-1}. Concerns about the high cost of ondansetron have prompted others to try alternative techniques. Propofol may have antiemetic properties, and Splinter *et al.* have demonstrated that anaesthesia induced and maintained by propofol is as effective as ondansetron 150 μg kg^{-1} at reducing PONV following strabismus surgery.[12] Splinter and Rhine showed recently that using a lower dose of ondansetron (50 μg kg^{-1}) in conjunction with dexamethasone (150 μg kg^{-1}) was superior to ondansetron alone (150 μg kg^{-1}), with an incidence of vomiting of only 9%.[13] Dexamethasone may be more effective against the later vomiting.

Opioids should be avoided during squint surgery. They undoubtedly increase the incidence of vomiting and are unnecessary for adequate analgesia, which can be achieved satisfactorily using diclofenac, paracetamol or ketorolac 0.75–0.9 mg kg^{-1}.[14,15] Morton *et al.* showed that satisfactory postoperative analgesia can be obtained using either diclofenac 0.1%

or oxybuprocaine 0.4% eye drops alone.[16] If these are administered selectively to the operative site by the surgeon prior to suturing the conjunctiva, the problems of an anaesthetic cornea can be minimized. As an alternative, bupivicaine can be injected locally by the surgeon at the end of the procedure.

THE OCULOCARDIAC REFLEX

The OCR, which was described in 1908 independently by Aschner and Dagnini, is also common during squint surgery, occurring in approximately 60% of cases. It has been established that the OCR is a trigeminovagal reflex, the afferent pathway being the ophthalmic branch of the trigeminal nerve. It has been well described[17] and is evoked by traction on the extrinsic eye muscles or pressure on the globe, causing a sinus bradycardia.

The bradycardia reverts almost immediately once the stimulus is removed and it is very unusual to see a more serious rhythm disturbance. On occasion, however, it can produce major dysrhythmias or sinus arrest. Traction on any of the extraocular muscles can evoke the reflex but it is generally felt that it occurs most commonly when the medial rectus muscle is manipulated. This was not confirmed in one detailed study of the OCR.[17] The OCR can be successfully blocked by the prior administration of atropine or glycopyrrolate,[18] but the resultant tachycardia and the frequently benign nature of the reflex have led many anaesthetists to administer atropine only if the reflex occurs.

As the OCR and the vomiting associated with squint surgery may share the same trigeminal–vagal arc it has been suggested that preventing the OCR may reduce the incidence of vomiting. Chisakuta and Mirakhur studied this and concluded that while anticholinergic prophylaxis was effective at preventing the OCR, it did not prevent vomiting.[18] A more recent paper, however, found that children with a positive OCR were 2.6 times more likely to develop PONV than those with no measurable reflex.[19] It would seem sensible, therefore, to prevent the OCR if possible. Blocking the afferent limb of the reflex by subtenon infiltration of local anaesthetic is one way of achieving this, but this carries a risk of perforating the globe. The alternative is to administer atropine 20 μg kg^{-1}

at induction and to accept the resultant modest tachycardia. The administration of atropine is especially necessary if propofol, which has a bradycardic effect, is used.

It has been shown that hypercarbia doubles the incidence of significant bradycardia,[17] which suggests that controlled ventilation is more appropriate than allowing spontaneous ventilation during strabismus surgery.

A suitable anaesthetic technique for strabismus surgery is as follows. Premedication can be left to individual preference and is not necessary for co-operative patients. Either an intravenous induction with propofol 3–4 mg kg^{-1} or gaseous induction is appropriate. Where intravenous induction is planned a topical local anaesthetic cream should be applied. Following induction atropine 20 μg kg^{-1} and a relaxant of choice, depending on the speed of the surgeon, are given along with 50 μg kg^{-1} ondansetron and 150 μg kg^{-1} dexamethasone to minimize PONV. Analgesia is provided using diclofenac (not in early infancy) and paracetamol suppositories. Anaesthesia is maintained with oxygen in nitrous oxide and a volatile agent via a tracheal tube, with controlled ventilation to normocarbia. One or two drops of topical adrenaline 0.1% can help to reduce conjunctival bleeding. Topical anaesthetic drops should be administered by the surgeon at the end of the procedure.

Patients are often discharged home at around 3–4 h postoperatively. It is important to warn the parents or other carers that vomiting may start around this time. Restricting oral fluids prior to discharge has been shown to reduce vomiting[20] and limiting activity may also be helpful. If vomiting does occur it is usually self-limiting but additional antiemetics may be necessary. Very rarely, overnight admission and intravenous fluids may be required.

Anaesthetic management should be as for strabismus surgery, although the risks of PONV are much reduced.

SYRINGING AND PROBING OF NASOLACRIMAL DUCTS

Several children have blocked nasolacrimal ducts, which present usually within the first year of life. These can frequently be cleared by probing of the duct and irrigation with saline. This is a short procedure and traditionally has been managed with a tracheal tube and throat pack, although for a simple probing and irrigation a LMA would suffice.

On occasion, it is necessary for the surgeon to manipulate or 'fracture' the inferior turbinate to relieve any obstruction at the lower end of the duct. Where a simple probing has failed it may be necessary to pass a fine silicone catheter through the duct and leave it in place for a few weeks (Crawford's tubes). In both procedures there may be some minor bleeding in the nasopharynx and a tracheal tube and throat pack may be more satisfactory. Sometimes it is necessary to proceed to a dacryocystorhinostomy (DCR). This is a more extensive procedure which may produce bleeding, and a modest degree of hypotension will be of assistance to the surgeon. This can be obtained by posture, ventilation with isoflurane or the use of specific agents such as labetalol. Controlled ventilation with a tracheal tube and throat pack is necessary and opioid analgesia should be provided. These procedures can cause a bacteraemia, and antibiotic prophylaxis should be given to children with heart defects[2].

ENUCLEATION

Enucleation of the eye may be required because of retinoblastoma or for the removal of a blind eye for cosmetic reasons. As the surgical technique involves dissection of each of the extraocular muscles, the OCR may be evoked.

INTRAOCULAR SURGERY

The main requirement for all intraocular cases is a motionless eye, avoiding significant rises in IOP. With the possible exception of ketamine, all anaesthetic agents reduce IOP. Either intravenous or inhalational induction is appropriate. Anaesthesia should be maintained using muscle relaxation and controlled ventilation via a tracheal tube. Neuromuscular blockade should be monitored using a peripheral nerve stimulator.

It is important to try to reduce as far as possible the causes of a rise in IOP at the end of the procedure, such as coughing on the tube at extubation; the irritant properties of isoflurane on the airway make this a less satisfactory maintenance agent than halothane. Anaesthesia should be maintained until neuromuscular blockade has been reversed, the patient is breathing spontaneously and extubation has been performed. Some authorities recommend the intravenous administration of 1 mg kg^{-1} lignocaine prior to extubation. Another useful technique to obtain a smooth extubation is to give a small dose of propofol (0.5–1.0 mg kg^{-1}) immediately prior to extubation. In older children topical anaesthesia to the airway can be helpful. This should be avoided in infants, as the simplest way to avoid the elevated IOP associated with crying in the immediate post-operative period is to give them an early feed. It is important to avoid restlessness and crying at this stage, and adequate analgesia should be ensured. A combination of rectal paracetamol or diclofenac with 1–1.5 mg kg^{-1} codeine phosphate given intramuscularly during the procedure is usually satisfactory. Some authorities advocate the intraoperative administration of droperidol to prevent vomiting and to obtain some sedation postoperatively.

RETINOPATHY OF PREMATURITY

Despite meticulous neonatal care severe retinopathy of prematurity (ROP) still occurs and can lead to total blindness. Babies at risk for severe ROP are those of birth weight < 1500 g and/or < 31 weeks' gestational age. It has been shown that the outcome of disease beyond the threshold for treatment can be significantly improved by cryotherapy or laser. Early identification is essential and eye examinations in at-risk infants should take place between 6 and 7 weeks' postnatal age and continued two-weekly until the risk has passed.[21] Although the examinations, and in some centres the cryotherapy, will usually take place within the neonatal unit, these premature infants may be transferred to theatre for their cryotherapy. This is a painful procedure and warrants administration of opioid analgesia such as fentanyl. This has implications for the postoperative care of the patients who, because of their gestational age, will already be at risk of apnoeic episodes following anaesthesia. Provision should be made to provide postoperative ventilation with appropriate support. Many of these infants will have other systemic disorders consequent upon their extreme prematurity which may influence both the conduct of anaesthesia and the need for postoperative support, and they will need careful preoperative assessment.

EMERGENCY EYE SURGERY

Penetrating eye injury may require removal of any foreign bodies and early wound closure and often cannot be delayed to ensure an empty stomach. This has become one of the most contentious areas of anaesthesia because of two conflicting arguments. On the one hand, the possibility of a full stomach demands rapid intubation for airway protection which is conventionally achieved by the rapid induction–intubation sequence using suxamethonium. On the other hand, there is the need to protect the eye from a rise in IOP, since this may cause extrusion of ocular contents through even very small wounds, leading to total loss of vision in that eye. Suxamethonium, even in the absence of fasciculation, causes a transient but definite rise in IOP, which cannot be reliably prevented, and therefore theoretically it should not be used. Many authorities therefore recommend that intubation should be performed using a large dose of a non-depolarizing relaxant while cricoid pressure is maintained. The development of priming techniques to accelerate the onset of non-depolarizing blockade or its administration prior to the induction agent does not always provide good intubating conditions.

There are, of course, other factors which raise IOP and these must be taken into account. Crying, struggling or vomiting can raise IOP by as much as 40 mmHg, and there should be no attempt at passing a nasogastric tube before anaesthesia to empty the stomach. Prior to induction, attempts at securing venous access may not be well tolerated and gaseous induction may be appropriate. This is an acceptable alternative in experienced hands.

Laryngoscopy and intubation themselves produce a significant rise in IOP and this aspect requires further attention. Lignocaine 1.5 mg kg^{-1} i.v. attenuates the rise in IOP following intubation[22] and may be helpful. Alfentanil 20 μg kg^{-1} attenuates the hypertensive response and may limit the IOP rise,[23] and the other short-acting narcotics can be expected to have a similar effect. However, it is likely that changes in IOP are affected primarily by venous pressure and changes in arterial pressure probably have little effect.

In those difficult situations where the eye is at risk and regurgitation is a concern, the following technique has been shown to provide good early intubating conditions without raising IOP and should be considered. A secure intravenous line is established and fentanyl 2 μg kg^{-1} is given, followed by vecuronium 0.15 mg kg^{-1}. At the first sign of muscle weakness, thiopentone 5 mg kg^{-1} is given and cricoid pressure applied. Intubation can be performed 80–90 s after the vecuronium, which is approximately 60 s after loss of consciousness. Premature attempts at intubation provoke coughing, which significantly raises IOP and should be avoided. A nerve stimulator is essential in indicating when full relaxation has occurred.

The balance of opinion has fluctuated in recent years and the use of suxamethonium to provide optimal intubation conditions in a rapid induction sequence is now accepted again. One of the causes of this controversy stems from the desire to establish a rigid protocol for the management of patients with a penetrating eye injury, although this may not be in the best interests of the patients. Some patients may already have lost most of the vitreous, or have sealed the wound with lens or iris tissue and in these patients a rise in IOP is of much less importance. Unfortunately, this cannot always be assessed until the eye has been examined under anaesthesia. Equally, some patients may not be at risk of a full stomach or can be deferred for sufficient time to reduce the risks of aspiration, and intubation can be carried out with more confidence using a non-depolarizing relaxant. Gastric emptying may be considerably delayed following trauma and full consultation with the surgeons is required in making a decision about the timing of surgery.

Drugs used for the maintenance of anaesthesia are a matter for clinical judgement by the anaesthetist on a case-by-case basis since most general anaesthetic agents produce a modest decrease in IOP. The stomach should be emptied as much as possible before the end of anaesthesia. In order to prevent coughing on the tracheal tube it is helpful to maintain anaesthesia until relaxation has been reversed and the patient is breathing satisfactorily, and to extubate while the patient is still asleep. Because of the risk of regurgitation this should be performed with the patient on his or her side.

REFERENCES

1 Greher, M., Hartmann, T., Winkler, M., *et al.* Hypertension and pulmonary edema associated with subconjunctival phenylephrine in a 2 month old child during cataract extraction. *Anesthesiology* 1998; **88**: 1394–6.

2 Eppert, G.A., Burnstine, R.A. and Bates, J.H. Lacrimal-duct-probing-induced bacteremia: should children with congenital heart defects receive antibiotic prophylaxis? *Journal of Pediatric Ophthalmology and Strabismus* 1998; **35**: 38–40.

3 Watcha, M.F., White, P.F., Tychsen, L., *et al.* Comparative effects of laryngeal mask airway and endotracheal tube insertion on intraoular pressure in children. *Anesthesia and Analgesia* 1992; **75**: 355–60.

4 Joshi, C. and Bruce, D.L. Thiopental and succinylcholine: action on intraocular pressure. *Anesthesia and Analgesia* 1975; **54**: 471–5.

5 Dear, G.L., Hammerton, M., Hatch, D.J., *et al.* Anaesthesia and intraocular pressure in young children in young children. A study of three different techniques of anaesthesia. *Anaesthesia* 1987; **42**: 259–65.

6 Yoshikawa, K. and Murai, Y. The effect of ketamine on intraocular pressure in children. *Anesthesia and Analgesia* 1971; **50**: 199–202.

7 Ausinsch, B., Rayburn, R.L., Munson, E.S., *et al.* Ketamine and intraocular pressure in children. *Anesthesia and Analgesia* 1976; **55**: 773–5.

8 Van den Berg, A.A., Lambourne, A. and Clyburn, P.A. The oculo-emetic reflex: a rationalisation of postophthal-

mic anaesthesia vomiting. *Anaesthesia* 1989; **44**: 110–17.

9 Tramèr, M., Moore, A. and McQuay, H. Prevention of vomiting after paediatric strabismus surgery: a systematic review using the numbers-needed-to-treat method. *British Journal of Anaesthesia* 1995; **75**: 556–61.

10 Davis, A., Krige, S. and Moyes, D. A double-blind randomized prospective study comparing ondansetron with droperidol in the prevention of emesis following strabismus surgery. *Anaesthesia and Intensive Care* 1995; **23**: 438–43.

11 Rose, J.B., Martin, T.M., Corddry, D.H., *et al*. Ondansetron reduces the incidence and severity of poststrabismus repair vomiting in children. *Anesthesia and Analgesia* 1994; **79**: 486–9.

12 Splinter, W.M., Rhine, E.J. and Roberts, D.J. Vomiting after strabismus surgery in children: ondansetron vs propofol. *Canadian Journal of Anaesthesia* 1997; **44**: 825–9.

13 Splinter, W.M. and Rhine, E.J. Low-dose ondansetron with dexamethasone more effectively decreases vomiting after strabismus surgery in children than does high-dose ondansetron. *Anesthesiology* 1998; **88**: 72–5.

14 Munro, H.M., Riegger, L.Q., Reynolds, P.I., *et al*. Comparison of the analgesic and emetic properties of ketorolac and morphine for paediatric outpatient strabismus surgery. *British Journal of Anaesthesia* 1994; **72**: 624–8.

15 Mendel, H.G., Guarnieri, K.M., Sundt, L.M., *et al*. The effects of ketorolac and fentanyl on postoperative vomiting and analgesic requirements in children undergoing strabismus surgery. *Anesthesia and Analgesia* 1995; **80**: 1129–33.

16 Morton, N.S., Benham, S.W., Lawson, R.A., *et al*. Diclofenac vs oxybuprocaine eyedrops for analgesia in paediatric strabismus surgery. *Paediatric Anaesthesia* 1997; **7**: 221–6.

17 Blanc, V.F., Hardy, J.-F. and Milot, J., *et al*. The oculocardiac reflex: a graphic and statistical analysis in infants and children. *Canadian Anaesthetists Society Journal* 1983; **30**: 360–9.

18 Chisakuta, A.M. and Mirakhur, R.K. Anticholinergic prophylaxis does not prevent emesis following strabismus surgery in children. *Paediatric Anaesthesia* 1995; **5**: 97–100.

19 Allen, L.E., Sudesh, S., Sandramouli, S., *et al*. The association between the oculocardiac reflex and postoperative vomiting in children undergoing strabismus surgery. *Eye* 1998; **12**: 193–6.

20 Kearney, R., Mack, C. and Entwistle, L. Withholding oral fluids from children undergoing day surgery reduces vomiting. *Paediatric Anaesthesia* 1998; **8**: 331–6.

21 Royal College of Ophthalmologists; British Association of Perinatal Medicine. Report of a Joint Working Party. Retinopathy of Prematurity: Guidelines for Screening and Treatment. Royal College of Ophthalmologists, 1995.

22 Lerman, J. and Kiskis, A.A. Lidocaine attenuates the intraocuar pressure response to rapid intubation in children. *Canadian Anaesthetists Society Journal* 1985; **32**: 339–45.

23 Morton, N.S. and Hamilton, M.B. Alfentanil in an anaesthetic technique for penetrating eye injuries. *Anaesthesia* 1986; **41**: 1148–51.

Section 15.4. Dental anaesthesia

IAN JAMES

INTRODUCTION

Wherever possible, dental extractions or conservations in children should be performed using local anaesthesia. This is successful in the majority of children.[1] In some anxious or uncooperative patients it may be necessary to provide some sedation, the most commonly used agents being chloral hydrate or one of the benzodiazepines. Oral ketamine has also been shown to be effective[2] and there is still considerable use of nitrous oxide.[3] It is imperative that these sedative agents are given in doses sufficient only to achieve anxiolysis and co-operation rather than sleep, and facilities and equipment for resuscitation must be available.

A number of children is unable to co-operate with dental procedures being undertaken under local anaesthesia and will require general anaesthesia. Such patients may have a profound learning disability or behavioural disorder and need to be treated sympathetically. Others will require general anaesthesia because of the extent or nature of the dental work. It is totally unacceptable for these procedures to be performed by a sole operator/anaesthetist, and a trained anaesthetist must be present with all the appropriate monitoring, recovery and resuscitation facilities.

Many of these children will be outpatients without other significant health problems and anaesthesia is generally straightforward. The procedure may be undertaken in the dental chair or on a proper operating table. Unless there is clear clinical indication to do so there is little value in undertaking any preoperative haematological screening for patients requiring dental treatment.[4] Some patients may have an additional disease process with major anaesthetic implications such as a cardiac disorder or epidermolysis bullosa, in which dental caries is common, and appropriate anaesthetic techniques need to be adopted.

Patient preference and degree of co-operation will usually determine whether induction is intravenous or inhalational. Maintenance of anaesthesia is best achieved using sevoflurane, which has a significantly lower incidence of dysrrhythmias than halothane, although there may be a slightly slower recovery.[5,6] For procedures lasting for only a few minutes the Goldman nasal mask is commonly used, but a nasopharyngeal airway provides higher quality anaesthetic and operating conditions with better airway patency and fewer episodes of airway obstruction.[7]

For longer procedures the airway is best secured with a nasotracheal tube. If this is difficult to insert an orotracheal tube or a laryngeal mask airway will usually suffice, although this may make the procedure slightly more difficult for the surgeon. Some paediatric patients presenting for dental work under general anaesthesia can be difficult to intubate, including those with epidermolysis bullosa where there is a high incidence of restricted mouth opening.[8] In these situations full consultation with the dental surgeon is required to establish whether local anaesthesia may be more appropriate. If not, techniques for difficult intubation should be adopted. A throat pack will always be necessary, although it should be recognized that some aspiration can still occur.[9] Thorough examination and suction of the pharynx at the end of the procedure are essential.

Adequate analgesia can usually be provided for the extraction of carious deciduous teeth or the uncovering of teeth from the palate using paracetamol and diclofenac, although an opioid such as fentanyl may be needed in older children for extraction of molar teeth. Dexamethasone $0.1-0.2$ mg kg^{-1} can reduce the swelling and its associated pain following extraction of molar teeth.

Most procedures involved during conservative dentistry cause a significant bacteraemia, most commonly with species of *Streptococcus viridans*.[10] All patients at risk of bacterial endocarditis should therefore be given prophylactic antibiotics.

MAXILLOFACIAL PROCEDURES

Surgery to the maxilla or mandible may be required to correct congenital or developmental facial deformities. The surgical procedure involved will dictate whether an orotracheal or nasotracheal tube is required, although usually this is the latter. Great attention to detail is necessary in these cases, ensuring that the tracheal tube is well secured and the eyes are protected. The majority of these procedures is undertaken in older children and a cuffed endotracheal tube should be used. Apart from securing the airway, bleeding is the most significant anaesthetic problem. A nasogastric tube should be inserted to enable aspiration of swallowed blood in the postoperative period, which otherwise is a potent cause of nausea and vomiting. A throat pack is essential, but it is important to remind the surgeon to remove this before the end of the procedure if the jaws are being wired together. In some cases bone or cartilage grafts may be taken from the iliac crest or ribs, and opioid analgesia should be provided. An epidural catheter can be placed in the iliac crest wound to permit intermittent infiltration of bupivicaine for analgesia in the postoperative period. When a rib graft is used it is important to be aware of the possibility of a pneumothorax. Procedures and traction on the maxilla can evoke a bradycardia through the trigeminal–vagal reflex arc, similar to the oculocardiac reflex, and atropine may be required.

It is usually appropriate to extubate at the end of the procedure, even when the jaws are being wired together, unless surgery has been very prolonged and there has been extensive manipulation of the pharyngeal mucosa. In these cases there can be considerable soft tissue swelling with the potential for airway oedema, and it may be preferable to leave the patient intubated for $24-36$ h, and nursed in an intensive care area. Extubation should not be performed before the position of the wires has been noted. Wire cutters must be available. A nasopharyngeal airway is useful in maintaining an airway and providing reliable access to the pharynx for aspiration of blood and other secretions.

DIFFICULT INTUBATION

Many patients presenting for maxillofacial surgery may be very difficult to intubate, owing for example to limited mouth opening or mandibular hypoplasia. In some of these patients there may also be difficulties in maintaining a patent airway, and in patients with abnormal facial development it can be difficult to maintain a good seal with a facemask. In some patients with developmental defects, such as first arch syndromes, there can be increasing difficulty in intubation as the child gets older. It is important, therefore, not to be misled by a previous successful intubation.

Usually, potential difficulty is evident from merely looking at the child and it is exceedingly rare to be confronted with an unexpectedly difficult intubation. However, a thorough examination is essential to establish the limitation of mouth opening and to obtain a clearer picture of the likelihood of difficulty in maintaining the airway or in laryngoscopy. Micrognathia is the most common cause of difficult intubation and is associated with several developmental anomalies. It is important also to assess the patency and size of the nares. In older children the same screening tests used in adults should be applied,[11] such as the Mallampati, the ability to protrude the lower jaw beyond the upper, and the degree of head and neck movements. In cases of doubt it is wiser to plan for a difficult airway and intubation.

Opioid premedication should not be given to these patients, although it is important to give atropine or glycopyrrolate to obtain drying of the secretions. Monitoring and, where possible, a secure intravenous line should be obtained prior to inducing anaesthesia. A full range of laryngoscopes and airways should be available, together with expert assistance, preferably including a second anaesthetist.

Maintaining spontaneous ventilation is essential until the degree of difficulty has been established, so inhalational induction is generally most appropriate. If an intravenous induction is indicated propofol may be preferable as it can be titrated in slowly without causing apnoea, and it permits rapid recovery should the airway be difficult to maintain. If a patent airway can be maintained, anaesthesia can be deepened to permit laryngoscopy. It is generally preferable to intubate under deep anaesthesia maintaining spontaneous ventilation. If muscle relaxation is indicated this should not be administered until it has been demonstrated that it is possible to ventilate.

Owing to the greater mobility of tissues in the infant it is usually possible to intubate these patients using a malleable bougie and cricoid pressure. Infants desaturate more rapidly than adults and it is important to limit attempts at intubation to no more than 1 min before replacing the mask and restoring oxygenation. Several attempts at intubation may be necessary to achieve the right combination of laryngoscope blade, external laryngeal manipulation and angulation of bougie. It can sometimes be helpful if the laryngoscopist manipulates the larynx with their other hand while the assisting anaesthetist passes the tube.

In patients in whom conventional intubation proves impossible, the use of other instruments such as the McCoy laryngoscope, the Bullard laryngoscope[12] or a fibreoptic laryngoscope may be successful. Small-diameter fibreoptic laryngoscopes are now available which can be used even in small infants.[13,14] These are generally used to facilitate nasal intubation but in some patients this is not possible and the fibreoptic laryngoscope must be passed

orally.[15] Proper training should be obtained and experience gained in normal patients before utilizing these techniques in difficult patients.[16]

Intubation times are usually prolonged using fibreoptic laryngoscopes and there is an intubation failure rate even with their use.[14] This is said to occur because of impingement of the tube on the larynx. Rotation of the tube may overcome this, as may the use of a flexometallic tube. A useful technique has been described in which a fibreoptic scope is used to pass into the trachea a fine guide wire, over which a tube can subsequently be threaded.[17] An alternative technique is to use a lightwand (a lighted stylet). Success has been reported using this technique in infants as young as 3 weeks of age.[18] Factors contributing to successful intubation include the use of a shoulder roll and slight head extension, a conscientious alignment of the airway axes, and anterior jaw lift to elevate the epiglottis. These techniques are valuable for both conventional and fibreoptic intubation.

Where these all fail or are inappropriate, elective tracheostomy should be considered. This can be performed using inhalational anaesthesia and a facemask or laryngeal mask, and in older children can be carried out under local anaesthesia.

REFERENCES

1 Blain, K.M. and Hill, F.J. The use of inhalation sedation and local anaesthesia as an alternative to general anaesthesia for dental extractions in children. *British Dental Journal* 1998; **184**: 608–11.

2 Roelofse, J.A., Joubert, J.J., Swart, L.C., Stander, I. and Roelofse, P.G. An evaluation of the effect of oral ketamine and standard oral premedication in the sedation of paediatric dental patients. *Journal of the Dental Association of South Africa* 1996; **51**: 197–201.

3 Wilson, S. A survey of the American Academy of Pediatric Dentistry Membership: nitrous oxide and sedation. *Pediatric Dentistry* 1996; **18**: 287–93.

4 Mason, C., Porter, S.R., Mee, A., Carr, C. and McEwan, T. The prevalence of clinically significant anaemia and haemoglobinopathy in children requiring dental treatment under general anaesthesia: a retrospective study of 1000 patients. *International Journal of Paediatric Dentistry* 1995; **5**: 163–7.

5 Ariffin, S.A., Whyte, J.A., Malins, A.F. and Cooper, G.M. Comparison of induction and recovery between sevoflurane and halothane supplementation of anaesthesia in

children undergoing outpatient dental extractions. *British Journal of Anaesthesia* 1997; **78**: 157–9.

6 Paris, S.T., Cafferkey, M., Tarling, M., Hancock, P., Yate, P.M. and Flynn, P.J. Comparison of sevoflurane and halothane for outpatient dental anaesthesia in children. *British Journal of Anaesthesia* 1997; **79**: 280–4.

7 Bagshaw, O.N., Southee, R. and Ruiz, K. A comparison of the nasal mask and the nasopharyngeal airway in paediatric chair dental anaesthesia. *Anaesthesia* 1997; **52**: 786–9.

8 James, I. and Wark, H. Airway management during anesthesia in patients with epidermolysis bullosa dystrophica. *Anaesthesia* 1982; **56**: 323–6.

9 Davis, J., Alton, H. and Butler, J. Aspiration of foreign materials in children while under general anaesthesia for dental extractions. *Anaesthesia and Pain Control in Dentistry* 1993; **2**: 17–21.

10 Roberts, G.J., Holzel, H.S., Sury, M.R., Simmons, N.A., Gardner, P. and Longhurst, P. Dental bacteremia in children. *Pediatric Cardiology* 1997; **18**: 24–7.

11 Vaughan, R.F. Predicting a difficult intubation. In: Latto, I.P. and Vaughan, R.S. (eds). *Difficulties in Tracheal Intubation*. London: W.B. Saunders, 1997: 79–87.

12 Borland, L.M. and Casselbrant, M. The Bullard laryngoscope. A new indirect oral laryngoscope (paediatric version). *Anesthesia and Analgesia* 1990; **70**: 105–8.

13 Roth, A.G., Wheeler, M., Stevenson, G.W. and Hall, S.C. Comparison of a rigid laryngoscope with the ultrathin fibreoptic laryngoscope for tracheal intubation in infants. *Canadian Journal of Anaesthesia* 1994; **41**: 1069–73.

14 Wrigley, S.R., Black, A.E. and Sidhu, V.S. A fibreoptic laryngoscope for paediatric anaesthesia. A study to evaluate the use of the 2.2 mm Olympus (LF-P) intubating fibrescope. *Anaesthesia* 1995; **50**: 709–12.

15 Hakala, P., Randell, T., Meretoja, O.A. and Rintala, R. Orotracheal fibreoptic intubation in children under general anaesthesia. *Paediatric Anaesthesia* 1997; **7**: 371–4.

16 Erb, T., Marsch, S.C.U., Hampl, K.F. and Frei, F.J. Teaching the use of fiberoptic intubation for children older than two years of age. *Anesthesia and Analgesia* 1997; **85**: 1037–41.

17 Hasan, M.A. and Black, A.E. A new technique for fibreoptic intubation in children. *Anaesthesia* 1994; **49**: 1031–3.

18 Fisher, Q.A. and Tunkel, D.E. Lightwand intubation of infants and children. *Journal of Clinical Anesthesia* 1997; **9**: 275–9.

Section 15.5. The burned child

JOHN KENEALLY

INTRODUCTION

Burns are a major cause of injury in children and represent a significant management burden for hospitals caring for the victims. A typical figure from one hospital is that, while burns accounted for only 13% of trauma admissions, they resulted in 32% of bed days for these patients.[1] Two-thirds of these children were under 3 years of age, and scalding by hot fluids was the most common cause of thermal injury (Table 15.5.1). The in-hospital mortality was 0.8%.[2]

In principle, the management of burns in children is similar to that in adults, but variations in detail arise because of the differences in physiological parameters and the psychological and social effects of the injury. As a result of the greater surface area to body mass ratio, fluid and caloric demands are increased, as is the potential for heat loss. In small children, the risk of respiratory compromise is also magnified because of their smaller airways and increased oxygen requirements.

Table 15.5.1 Cause of thermal injury in 510 patients admitted to NSW Paediatric Burns Unit, 1995–1997

Mechanism of injury	%
Scald	63
Flame	20
Contact	11
Other	6

Consequently, critical burn size is less than in adults and burns of greater than 10% of body surface area (BSA), whether full or partial thickness, warrant admission to hospital. Burns are classified as being partial thickness when they involve the epidermis and part of the dermis, or full thickness when there is total skin destruction. Specialized paediatric burn care should be sought for children with more than 5% full thickness or 10% partial thickness injury. Differing bodily proportions, with a relatively larger head and smaller legs in younger children, affect the estimate of the percentage of BSA burned and resuscitation requirements (Table 15.5.2).

Special care is also needed for those patients with burns of the face, hands, feet or perineum, for electrical burns, which may result in extensive neurovascular damage, and for burns associated with respiratory injury.

Since most children who suffer thermal injury are less than 3 years of age, their inability to understand the painful and prolonged treatment will add to the already severe psychological problems. In some, these will be compounded because they have been the victims of abuse. Non-accidental injury should be suspected when presentation of the child to hospital is delayed, when the history is not consistent with the degree or nature of the burn or when there are other injuries. Whatever the circumstances, all parents feel a great deal of guilt over their child's suffering and both patients and their families will need support, often for a prolonged period. In addition, factors such as low educational levels and stress in the parents, disorganization and hazards in the home, and aggressive, uncontrolled behaviour in the child

Table 15.5.2 Body surface area estimations (%) and age

Region	Age (years)			
	0–1	1–3	3–8	> 8
Head and neck	20	18	12	10
Trunk	32	32	32	32
Both arms	20	20	20	20
Both lower limbs	28	30	36	38

are known to be aetiologically significant and may warrant assessment and treatment.

Anaesthetists are often involved in the care of burned children, in initial resuscitation, in definitive debridement and grafting procedures, and in later plastic surgery. They also have great expertise to offer in the management of both background and procedural pain.

PATHOPHYSIOLOGY OF BURNS

Major thermal injury not only results in local fluid loss through tissue injury and evaporation, but sets in train widespread physiological changes. Tissue damage initiates the local release of inflammatory mediators and subsequent cascades of reactions. There is also activation of leucocytes and endothelial cells, with alterations in circulating cytokines, leading to multiple systemic effects. These changes have recently been reviewed by Arturson.[3]

Of particular relevance to the acute stages of resuscitation, local vasodilatation, increased microvascular permeability and negative interstitial pressures result in fluid loss into the tissues, with the development of burns oedema in the hours following the initial injury. The initial fluid loss is proportional to the severity and extent of the injury and may result in hypovolaemic shock. This may be compounded by an, as yet, uncharacterized myocardial depressant factor, as well as by the effects of increased levels of catecholamines and other vasoactive substances which increase systemic vascular resistance, and cause tachycardia and

an increase in metabolic rate. Subsequently, hypoproteinaemia can result in continuing oedema in unburned areas of the body. By the third or fourth day after injury, cardiac output increases to match the increased metabolic rate; patients with only 15% burns increase their oxygen consumption by 50%.[4]

Loss of skin integrity results in large evaporative fluid losses and disruption of thermoregulation. In combination with the immunological changes, it also increases the risk of infection and sepsis.

The respiratory system may be compromised in a number of ways. Firstly, the upper airway may suffer direct injury with mucosal damage and this can result in the rapid onset of life-threatening airway obstruction due to oedema or sloughing. In practice, an artificial airway is necessary when stridor is associated with facial burns. Direct injury to the lower airway is occasionally caused by steam, but most lower airway problems arise from inhalation of toxic products of combustion, leading to chemical pneumonitis. Carbon monoxide and hydrogen cyanide are also produced in fires in closed spaces, and may lead to asphyxia. Even without inhalational injury of this nature, lung compliance falls in the first 12 h after a burn, probably because of mediator-induced bronchoconstriction[5] and the development of pulmonary oedema. Mechanical restriction of ventilation can be caused by circumferential chest burns, or even by deep burns involving the anterior aspect of the chest and abdomen.

Hypovolaemia, hypoxia, circulating vasoconstrictors, increased antidiuretic hormone levels and free plasma haemoglobin and myoglobin may affect renal function. Many of these factors will also affect the liver and gastrointestinal system. The introduction of early enteral feeding, if necessary by a transpyloric tube, has resulted in a great decline in the problems of gastric stress ulceration and ileus, and helps to maintain splanchnic blood flow and the normal mucosal barrier against gastrointestinal organisms.[6] It also assists in maintaining high caloric intake to meet the increased metabolic demands of the prolonged period following the acute injury and resuscitation.

RESUSCITATION

The burned child should be resuscitated in a heated area; infrared heaters may help to prevent hypothermia.

It is essential to carry out a rapid preliminary assessment of the airway, breathing and circulation. Respiration is likely to be compromised if the injury has resulted from a fire in an enclosed space, or if there are facial burns, hoarse cry, cough, stridor, soot in the mouth, dyspnoea or crepitus on examination of the chest. As rapidly developing oedema may make intubation difficult, early examination of the airway and nasotracheal intubation using a rapid sequence or inhalational induction of anaesthesia should be considered. Coma following asphyxiation or carbon monoxide poisoning is also an indication for airway intervention. Controlled ventilation should be commenced if there are signs of respiratory distress. While immediate monitoring includes pulse oximetry, carboxy-haemoglobin is registered as oxyhaemoglobin and a falsely optimistic reading may result. Oxygen must be given to all patients.

Tachycardia, reduced capillary return, and mottled or cool peripheries are important early signs of shock. Blood pressure should be recorded, and in a major injury an arterial cannula inserted, but hypotension is a relatively late sign of hypovolaemia in children. In fact, many children are hypertensive. One, or preferably two, large-bore intravenous cannulae should be inserted into an unburned area and resuscitation fluids commenced as quickly as possible. If venous cannulation cannot be achieved rapidly, an intraosseous needle should be used.

Resuscitation fluids are given in proportion to the area burned (see Table 15.5.2). The nature of these fluids has been the subject of some controversy over the years, with proponents arguing for the use of either crystalloid or colloid solutions. While the use of colloids increases blood volume more effectively and minimizes oedema in unburned areas,[7] it increases the extent of and prolongs oedema around the burn. Since capillary leak is maximal in the first 12 h and integrity improved by 24 h, many protocols now prescribe only crystalloids on day 1, but may introduce colloid on day 2. There have been no reports of the use of hypertonic saline in the resuscitation of children after burns; it has been suggested that children may be more liable to hypernatraemia and hyperosmolarity than adults with this therapy.[8] A typical protocol for fluid management is shown in Table 15.5.3.

Close monitoring of urine output is essential and insertion of a urinary catheter a priority. A

Table 15.5.3 Fluid management for burns

1. *First 24 h*
   3 ml kg^{-1} % BSA burn as Hartmann's solution:
   50% in first 8 h
   50% in next 16 h
   Plus maintenance fluids
   Achieve urine output $1 \text{ ml kg}^{-1} \text{ h}^{-1}$ (acceptable range $0.5–2 \text{ ml kg}^{-1} \text{ h}^{-1}$)
   Extra fluid to maintain urine output as Hartmann's solution (1-h requirement as bolus)
   If inadequate response to crystalloid, colloid may be given in second 12 h
2. *Second 24 h*
   $0.3–0.5 \text{ ml kg}^{-1}$% BSA burn as colloid
   Plus maintenance fluids
3. *Maintenance fluids*
   Nasogastric feeds
   Transpyloric tube if necessary
   Intravenous isotonic dextrose saline if necessary
4. *Increased fluid requirements*
   Delayed resuscitation
   Inhalational burns
   Young infants
   Hyperpyrexia
   Diarrhoea, vomiting

BSA, body surface area.
(Adapted from Protocol for General Management of Burns, New Children's Hospital, Sydney.)

nasogastric tube should also be inserted in the first stages of resuscitation, both to minimize the risk of acute gastric dilatation from air-swallowing and to facilitate early enteral alimentation.

Pain is treated by intravenous opioid administration. For example, an initial bolus dose of morphine 0.1–0.2 mg kg^{-1} (0.05 mg kg^{-1} for infants less than 6 months) can be followed by a morphine infusion at 30 μg kg^{-1} h^{-1} and further bolus doses of 20 μg kg^{-1} at intervals of 5 min (half these doses for infants) titrated against the patient's needs. The intramuscular administration of opioids is dangerous in these shocked patients because of unpredictable absorption and is contraindicated.

Once the initial assessment is completed and treatment commenced, further attention should be given to the history of the injury and patient, to assess significant factors such as the risk of carbon monoxide or cyanide poisoning and of child abuse. A complete physical examination should be undertaken to seek for signs of other injuries or illnesses. Investigations should include haematology, electrolytes and creatinine. A chest X-ray may indicate pulmonary oedema or adult respiratory distress syndrome resulting from smoke inhalation. Urine osmolality and electrolytes should also be measured, and haemoglobin and myoglobin levels determined if the urine is discoloured.

Limb ischaemia or restricted chest wall movement, caused by circumferential burns with oedema under eschar, may necessitate urgent escharotomy. Because of the depth of the burns which cause this complication, general anaesthesia is not usually necessary, although extension of the incision into unburned areas may require infiltration with local anaesthetic. However, further analgesia may be necessary to allow the initial cleaning and dressing of the burn wound with the application of an antibacterial cream, usually silver sulfadiazine.

ANAESTHESIA

EARLY SURGERY

Anaesthesia is only occasionally needed for procedures during the first day following burns. It may be required to allow assessment of airway injury, intubation or tracheostomy. The latter is uncommon, usually being avoided because of the risk of infection. However, it should be considered in children with severe anatomical damage to the supraglottic and glottic structures, or in those with gross facial burns and oedema which might make intubation very difficult if the nasotracheal tube were to be displaced. Surgery for other injuries, fasciotomy for electrical burns or the surgical insertion of central venous catheters to aid prolonged management are other indications for anaesthesia.

Patients with electrical burns are often the most severely burned. They will have gross fluid derangements and, potentially, gastric stasis and ileus, and airway management may be very difficult. Despite the risks of a full stomach, inhalational induction using halothane or sevoflurane may be preferred as this will allow spontaneous ventilation until the airway is secured.

Tangential excision of the burn on day 1, with coverage of the wound by skin graft or compatible membranes, is practised in some hospitals. While this may offer advantages in decreasing infection and reducing metabolic demands, it is accompanied by considerable blood loss at a time when intravascular volume is already unstable.

ELECTIVE DEBRIDEMENT AND GRAFTING

Excision and grafting of the burned area commonly commences between 3 and 7 days after the injury. It may be repeated at frequent intervals for some weeks, depending on the extent of the injury. While no longer hypovolaemic, the patients are commonly febrile and anaemic, have infected wounds, may be septic and can have residual pulmonary damage.

Other factors that affect the anaesthetic technique include:

- facial burns and access to the airway;
- positioning for surgery;
- extent of planned surgery;
- difficulty in venous access and monitoring;
- potential blood loss;
- temperature maintenance;
- altered pharmacology;
- analgesia, both before and after surgery;
- need to maintain high caloric intake and limit fasting.

Either a gaseous or an intravenous induction of anaesthesia may be appropriate, depending on the presence of facial burns and availability of veins. Commonly, anaesthesia is maintained with controlled ventilation and the use of non-depolarizing muscle relaxants, volatile agents and opioids. Secure fixation of the tracheal tube may be a problem, especially when there are facial burns and the patient is to be repositioned during surgery.

Given these problems, some units find ketamine of value.[9,10] An intramuscular dose of 4 mg kg^{-1} will usually allow the insertion of an intravenous cannula and may be followed by subsequent intravenous bolus doses. With this agent, laryngeal reflexes remain active and ventilation is not depressed. The necessity for equipment around the face is reduced, although supplemental oxygen should be given. Since ketamine is a vasoconstrictor, there may be less cardiovascular decompensation with acute blood loss or with changes in posture, and temperature maintenance is less of a problem than with vasodilating volatile agents. Postoperatively, the drug offers the advantages of causing less nausea and vomiting than other agents, a more rapid return to normal feeding and continuing analgesia. The dysphoric effects may be less common in children than in adults and can be reduced by premedication with a benzodiazepine. Despite these advantages, ketamine is not universally used; many anaesthetists are concerned that the airway is neither guaranteed nor protected and large doses, which result in prolonged sleep postoperatively, may be necessary to prevent movement during skin harvesting.

Venous access may create challenges in patients with extensive burns undergoing repeated procedures. While many children will have had central venous catheters inserted, their narrow lumens may be inadequate to allow rapid transfusion. A large-bore cannula should be inserted after induction, avoiding burned areas because of the risk of infection and difficulty with fixation.

Monitoring may also be a problem in these children. An oesophageal stethoscope and temperature probe may be inserted in intubated patients. There may be few locations to position a pulse oximeter probe. If the fingers are burned and legs are being used for donor sites, then a suitably protected probe can be attached to the tongue, cheek or nasal septum. An electrocardiograph is important both to detect arrhythmias and as an indicator of changes in serum calcium during rapid transfusion. Again, electrode placement may be difficult, but the use of crocodile-clip electrocardiogram (ECG) leads attached to skin staples provides an alternative.[10] Blood-pressure cuffs may need to be placed over a burned area not involved in the planned procedure. A light occlusive dressing between the cuff and the burn may reduce the accuracy of the measurement, but allows trends to be followed. For extensive procedures in ill patients, arterial cannulation should be considered.

Blood loss is a major concern. It may be reduced by the use of tourniquets on limbs, prior infiltration with a ornithine-8-vasopressin (POR-8) and the use of pads soaked in dilute adrenaline. POR-8 should be diluted to 0.05–0.2 U ml^{-1} and no more than 0.25 U kg^{-1} administered[11] at least 10 min before excision is carried out. This drug may cause generalized vasoconstriction with haemostasis continuing into the postoperative period. This can give the impression of central cyanosis; pulse oximetry is essential during this time. The immediate topical application of 1 : 10 000 adrenaline after harvesting decreases bleeding from donor sites. As the drug is minimally absorbed, no tachycardias or dysrhythmias result, at least during controlled ventilation.[12] Blood loss can also be limited by prompt diathermy or ligation of bleeding points and the application of firm dressings as soon as practicable on excised areas.

Accurate measurement of blood loss is impossible. There can be sudden episodes of heavy bleeding, much of which may be concealed in surgical drapes, so that weighing of packs and sponges often underestimates the total. Nevertheless, in association with other monitoring and clinical estimates, it is an essential guide to replacement. Rapid transfusion of citrated blood and fresh-frozen plasma can cause hypocalcaemia, resulting in hypotension. Calcium chloride may be necessary to correct this[13] and may be given prophylactically.

Exposure, evaporation from wounds, the use of wet sponges and administration of large volumes of fluid commonly result in hypothermia, even though patients are often febrile when they come to the operating theatre. Strategies to reduce this heat loss include increasing room temperature, using hot air mattresses and covers and overhead heaters, using heated humidifiers for inspired gases, heating intravenous fluids and blood, and retaining dressings or plastic wrapping on areas not involved in the surgery. Despite all these measures, some degree of hypothermia is common and active warming must often be continued into the postoperative period.

The pharmacology of many drugs is altered in burned patients, with increased glomerular filtration rate, decreased hepatic metabolism and alterations in plasma proteins (albumin decreased, α_1-acid glycoprotein increased) being the main factors.[14] The most important change for anaesthetists, however, is in the response to muscle-relaxant drugs. This appears to be related to an extension of acetylcholine receptor sites beyond the myoneural junction, similar to that which occurs in a number of other pathological conditions, including muscle trauma and immobilization.[15] Interestingly, it appears that the administration of d-tubocurarine may accentuate this process.[16]

As a result of this change, sensitivity to succinylcholine is increased and its administration can result in hyperkalaemia and cardiac arrest. The severity of the response varies with the extent of the injury and the time that has elapsed since it occurred, with the maximum increase in serum potassium at 4–12 days after the burn. However, this sensitivity may persist for some months and the drug should be avoided for this time.

In contrast, burned patients are resistant to the effects of most non-depolarizing relaxants, so that as much as two to three times the normal dose is required to achieve a given degree of relaxation.[17] Interestingly, sensitivity to mivacurium appears unaltered, although its duration of action is prolonged, perhaps because of reduced levels of plasma cholinesterase.[18] This resistance to non-depolarizers may be prolonged, even beyond apparent recovery from the injury.[19] To achieve rapid onset of relaxation while avoiding succinylcholine, large doses of non-depolarizing relaxants should be given.

Analgesia will be discussed later. In brief, any pain relief should be continued preoperatively and may need to be increased after surgery. Local anaesthetic techniques have a limited place in burns surgery in children, although femoral, lateral and posterior cutaneous nerve blocks of the thigh can provide excellent analgesia for donor sites for split skin harvesting. Central neuraxial blocks are usually avoided as they cause vasodilatation and may increase bleeding. Catheter techniques also carry the risk of sepsis.

Finally, anaesthetists must accept that an important element in recovery from burns is the provision of an adequate caloric intake. Many patients are on continuous gastric feeds and frequent, prolonged fasts before anaesthesia and surgery interfere with nutrition. Fasting times should be as short as possible, consistent with safe practice, and techniques which allow rapid wakening and resumption of feeds should be utilized.

ELECTIVE RECONSTRUCTIVE SURGERY

Reconstructive surgery can continue for months or even years after the original injury. There is some evidence that an abnormal response to both relaxants and induction agents may persist for some time.[20] Patients in this category should have their needs and preferences carefully listened to; they will often suggest particular premedications, induction methods, antiemetics and analgesics. Compliance with these reasonable requests is a part of the continuing psychological support that these experienced patients deserve. Severe facial scarring and neck contractures may make airway management difficult, although this has become less common with early surgery, vigorous physiotherapy and the introduction of pressure garments.

PAIN MANAGEMENT

Burns are accompanied by pain, almost from the time of injury until beyond the completion of treatment. There is usually some degree of background pain, which can worsen as tissues heal, and this can be associated with episodes of 'breakthrough', perhaps brought about by movement or posture changes. Procedural pain, caused by treatments such as dressing changes, bathing and physiotherapy, is usually much worse. Psychological factors, including anxiety and depression, also play a part in the patient's experience.[21]

Adequate analgesia must commence from the time of the initial resuscitation. As has already mentioned, intravenous opioids are required for major burns at this stage. These should be continued after the immediate resuscitation period and older children may benefit from patient-controlled analgesia (PCA). Once an effective opioid dose has been established, usually at about 48 h, it may be possible to change to a sustained-release oral morphine preparation. Since the bioavailability of oral morphine is about 50%, the dose should be commenced at twice the intravenous daily amount. Regular oral or rectal paracetamol (15 mg kg^{-1} every 4 h) should also be started as an adjunct, and breakthrough medication prescribed (morphine sulphate $0.2-0.3 \text{ mg kg}^{-1}$ or codeine sulphate 1 mg kg^{-1}, which may also be given at 4-h intervals). Very large doses of opioid are required for pain control in some patients and may cause excessive sedation and disturb gastrointestinal function. In these children the addition of other drugs, including intravenous lignocaine and clonidine, may be useful. A variety of non-pharmacological interventions, such as the teaching of relaxation techniques and hypnotherapy, can also help. Anxiolytics, commonly benzodiazepines or chlorpromazine, complement the action of analgesics, but are not a substitute for them.

Procedure-related pain is often undertreated, especially in children,[22] and is associated with a great deal of anxiety and even fear. This pain can usually be predicted and mitigated. The administration of additional opioid is the first step in this, but other techniques are also useful.

Nurse- or self-administered nitrous oxide relative analgesia, either from a constant flow, variable concentration device or as Entonox, has proved effective and safe.[23] Essentials of the technique include constant supervision and maintenance of age-appropriate verbal communication by a trained observer, other than the person carrying out the procedure. Nitrous oxide has the advantage of providing rapid onset and offset of action with good analgesia and some amnesia. The successful use of oral ketamine as an analgesic and sedative for burns dressing in children has been described recently.[24]

Intravenous opioids provide the basis for pain management in the postoperative period. Whether given as a continuous infusion or in the form of PCA, an adequate loading dose and continuing assessment of effectiveness, especially in the immediate postoperative period, are essential. As mentioned earlier, local anaesthetic techniques seem to have a relatively limited role.

Even with effective pain management, burned patients suffer a great deal of discomfort. Itching makes a major contribution to this, especially as the wounds heal. This may be a side-effect of opioid analgesics and respond to a change in the particular drug used or the infusion of a low dose of naloxone. Antihistamines, especially trimeprazine and cyproheptadine, may also be of benefit, but for many patients a complete solution remains elusive.

In conclusion, the anaesthetic management of burned children depends not only on an understanding of the alterations in physiology and pharmacology which accompany the injury, but also on an appreciation of the whole treatment process and the suffering and anxiety it entails. With this understanding, the anaesthetist can play an important role in the optimal care that these unfortunate children deserve.

REFERENCES

1 Cass, D.C., Armitage, K., Lamb, L., *et al. Trauma Admissions Report*. Sydney: New Children's Hospital, 1996.
2 *Burns Unit Data Base*. Sydney: New Children's Hospital, 1998.

3 Arturson G. Pathophysiology of the burn wound and pharmacological treatment. *Burns* 1996; **22**: 255–74.

4 Lalonde, C. and Demling, R.H. The effect of complete burn wound excision and closure on postburn oxygen consumption. *Surgery* 1987; **102**: 862–8.

5 Jin, L.J., Lalonde, C. and Demling, J.H. Lung dysfunction after thermal injury in relation to prostanoid and oxygen radical release. *Journal of Applied Physiology* 1986; **61**: 103–12.

6 McDonald, W.S., Sharp, C.W. and Deitch, E.A. Immediate enteral feeding in burn patients is safe and effective. *Annals of Surgery* 1991; **213**: 177–83.

7 Demling, R.H. Burns. *New England Journal of Medicine* 1985; **313**: 1389–98.

8 Palmisano, B.W. Anesthesia for plastic surgery. In: Gregory, G.A. (ed.). *Pediatric Anesthesia.* 3rd edn. New York: Churchill–Livingstone, 1994: 699–740.

9 Brown, T.C.K. and Fisk, G.C. (eds). Burns. In: *Anaesthesia for Children.* 2nd edn. Oxford: Blackwell, 1992: 281–90.

10 Irving, G.A.. and Butt, A.D. Anaesthesia for burns in children: a review of procedures practised at Red Cross War Memorial Children's Hospital, Cape Town. *Burns* 1994; **20**: 241–3.

11 Lamont, A.S.M. and York, P. Maximum safe dose of POR 8. *Anaesthesia and Intensive Care* 1987; **15**: 467.

12 Brezel, B.S., McKeever, K.E. and Stein, J.M. Epinephrine v thrombin for split thickness donor site haemostasis. *Journal of Burn Care and Rehabilitation* 1987; **8**: 132–4.

13 Cote, C.J., Drop, L.J., Hoaglin, D.C., *et al.* Ionized hypocalcemia after fresh frozen plasma administration to thermally injured children; effects of infusion rate, duration and treatment with calcium chloride. *Anesthesia and Analgesia* 1988; **67**: 152–60.

14 Martyn, J.A. Clinical pharmacology and drug therapy in the burned patient. *Anesthesiology* 1986; **63**: 67–75.

15 Martyn, J.A., White, D.A., Gronert, G.A., *et al.* Up-and-down regulation of skeletal muscle acetylcholine receptors. Effects on neuromuscular blockers. *Anesthesiology* 1992; **76**: 822–43.

16 Kim, C., Hirose, M. and Martyn, J.A. d-Tubocurarine accentuates the burn-induced upregulation of nicotinic acetylcholine receptors at the muscle membrane. *Anesthesiology* 1995; **83**: 237–40.

17 Mills, A.K. and Martyn, J.A. Neuromuscular block with vecuronium in paediatric patients with burn injury. *British Journal of Clinical Pharmacology* 1989; **28**: 155–9.

18 Werba, A.E., Neiger, F.X., Bayer, G.S., *et al.* Pharmacodynamics of mivacurium in severely burned patients. *Burns* 1996; **22**: 62–4.

19 Mills, A.K. and Martyn, J.A. Evaluation of atracurium neuromuscular blockade in paediatric patients with burn injury. *British Journal of Anaesthesia* 1988; **60**: 450–5.

20 Martyn, J.A.J., Matteo, R.S., Szyfelbein, S.K., *et al.* Unprecedented resistance to neuromuscular blocking effects of metocurine with persistence after complete recovery in a burned patient. *Anesthesia and Analgesia* 1986; **61**: 614–17.

21 Pal, S.K., Cortiella, J. and Herndon, D. Adjunctive methods of pain control in burns. *Burns* 1997; **23**: 404–12.

22 Ashburn, M.A. Burn pain: the management of procedure-related pain. *Journal of Burn Care and Rehabilitation* 1995; **16**: 365–71.

23 Keneally, J. Nitrous oxide analgesia. In: McKenzie, I., Gaukroger, P.B., Ragg, P. and Brown, T.C.K. (eds). *Manual of Acute Pain Management in Children.* London: Churchill Livingstone, 1997: 17–24.

24 Humphries, Y., Melson, M. and Gore, D. Superiority of oral ketamine as an analgesic and sedative for wound care procedures in the pediatric patient with burns. *Journal of Burn Care and Rehabilitation* 1997; **18**: 34–6.

Section 15.6. Anaesthesia for the neonate and infant

DAVID HATCH AND EDWARD SUMNER

BASIC TECHNIQUES

If neonatal anaesthesia is carried out in a specialized centre many of the basic principles upon which successful outcome depends, such as maintenance of adequate body temperature, will be followed automatically. It is nevertheless always important for the anaesthetist to check the operating environment and relevant equipment before embarking on any neonatal anaesthetic. A preoperative visit to the baby is essential so that the anaesthetist can be fully informed about the baby's condition, but also, where possible, to establish communication with the parents, explaining the procedures that are about to take place together with their risks and answering any previously unanswered questions. In some cases the mother will not have been able to accompany the child to the specialist centre and in these cases it is even more important to ensure that the father or other relative accompanying the baby should have enough information to pass on to the mother as soon as possible.

The sickest neonates, such as some with congenital diaphragmatic hernia, may already be receiving intensive care prior to surgery and will be transferred to the operating suite having already been intubated and ventilated and with full critical care monitoring. The majority of surgical neonates, however, will come from the neonatal surgical ward and are unlikely to have received significant preoperative therapy other than intravenous fluid and electrolyte manage-

ment. It is important to ensure that they do not lose heat during transfer to the operating theatre, but the time at which this is most likely to occur is during the period between induction of anaesthesia and commencement of surgery. During this period the anaesthetist must take meticulous care to ensure that the baby is covered with warm wrappings at all times and placed on a warm operating table with appropriate heating devices. Once general anaesthesia has been induced the neonate's metabolic response to cold will be suppressed. Skin preparation by the surgeon should preferably be carried out with warm fluids and drapes should be placed over the baby as soon as possible. Intravenous fluids should be warmed before administration.

INDUCTION OF ANAESTHESIA

If intravenous access has not been established prior to transfer of the baby it should be carried out before induction. After the patency of the intravenous line has been checked basic monitoring [electrocardiogram (ECG), pulse oximetry, temperature probe and precordial stethoscope] should be attached. A blood-pressure cuff can also be applied at this stage, although readings obtained before induction may not be particularly reliable and may disturb the child.

Induction of anaesthesia can be carried out either by an inhalational method using sevoflurane or halothane or by the intravenous administration of thiopentone or propofol. The median effective dose (ED_{50}) of intravenous induction agents is, however, significantly reduced in neonates.[1] Whichever method of induction is used it should be preceded by a short period of preoxygenation. Because of the relatively small functional residual capacity (FRC) alveolar oxygen tension rises rapidly during preoxygenation but since oxygen consumption is increased in the newborn, hypoxia will also develop rapidly when oxygen delivery is interrupted.

TRACHEAL INTUBATION

Since both tidal volume and FRC are significantly reduced by anaesthesia, neonates must be intubated and ventilated for all but the most trivial surgical procedures. The practice of awake intubation has now been almost completely replaced by intubation under general anaesthesia because of the rise in intracranial pressure (ICP) which occurs which may increase the risk of intraventicular haemorrhage, especially in preterm neonates and those with coagulation defects. Awake intubation may still be indicated in the presence of severe upper airway obstruction and some anaesthetists still favour its use for neonates with tracheo-oesophageal fistula.

Intubation is usually performed after administration of one of the newer short-acting non-depolarizing muscle relaxants such as atracurium or vecuronium. The advantages and disadvantages of the wide range of muscle relaxants now available are described in Chapter 5. The head should be placed in a neutral position for intubation with the shoulders lying flat on the operating table.[2] The best view of the infant larynx is usually obtained using a straight-bladed laryngoscope placed behind the epiglottis, although sometimes, particularly if the epiglottis is short, a better view may be obtained with the tip of the blade in the

vallecula in front of the epiglottis. Uncuffed tubes should always be used in the newborn and the correct size for anaesthesia is one which is easily inserted and preferably has a small but detectable leak of air around it when positive pressure is applied. This will ensure that it is not likely to cause pressure damage at the cricoid ring. Because of the shortness of the trachea in the newborn great care must be taken to ensure that the tracheal tube does not pass into one or other main bronchus. This should be confirmed by careful auscultation of the chest, followed by secure fixation of the tube. In the case of difficult intubation success may be achieved by the use of firm pressure applied to the front of the larynx either by the intubator or by an assistant. The use of an atraumatic but rigid bougie can also be extremely valuable in these cases.

MAINTENANCE OF ANAESTHESIA

Whilst halothane has traditionally been the most widely used inhalational anaesthetic agent for maintenance of anaesthesia in the newborn, isoflurane, sevoflurane or desflurane is a perfectly acceptable alternative. O'Brien *et al.* recently suggested that desflurane may give the most satisfactory recovery profile for neonates with a reduced incidence of postoperative respiratory problems, especially in the preterm.[3]

The lungs can be ventilated either by hand using a Jackson-Rees modification of Ayre's T-piece or by the use of a mechanical ventilator. Whilst some doubt has been cast on the value of the 'educated hand' in assessing changes in compliance or resistance of the respiratory system,[4,5] most paediatric anaesthetists revert to hand ventilation if there is any concern about the adequacy of chest-wall movement or of possible obstruction of the tracheal tube. The use of a mechanical ventilator allows better control of end-tidal CO_2 concentration and peak airway pressure, which should be kept as low as possible to minimize the risk of barotrauma. The use of up to 5 cm of positive end-expiratory pressure (PEEP) helps to maintain an adequate FRC. Inspired gas should reach the baby at a temperature not less than 33°C and should be fully humidified at that temperature to prevent damage to the mucosal lining of the respiratory tract.

The importance of providing adequate analgesia to the neonate during surgery and in the postoperative period is now universally accepted. This can often be achieved by simple skin infiltration with local anaesthetic or by the use of appropriate local, regional or central nerve blocks as described in Chapter 9. In other cases the use of opioids such as fentanyl in addition to the use of nitrous oxide and a low concentration of volatile anaesthetic agent may be the only way of providing satisfactory analgesia. In those babies who are expected to breathe spontaneously after surgery the dose of fentanyl should not exceed 3–5 μg kg^{-1}, and preterm infants usually need reduced doses. Babies who require postoperative ventilatory support can be given larger doses: a bolus of 10 μg kg^{-1} will last for at least 2 h.

FLUID AND ELECTROLYTE MANAGEMENT

In the absence of abnormal fluid losses, full-term neonates require reduced maintenance levels of fluids (40–60 ml kg^{-1}day on the first day of life) and the fluid used to dilute drugs administered during surgery may well be adequate to meet these requirements. Preterm neonates, however, have significantly increased insensible fluid losses and those of under 1000 g may require as much as 160 ml kg^{-1}day. Sodium and potassium balance seldom present problems in the full-term neonate at birth who has no abnormal losses but may become quite complex in low birth-weight or preterm infants or those with disturbances of fluid or electrolyte balance. Glucose and calcium levels should be carefully checked in all surgical neonates, particularly those at increased risk of hypocalcaemia or hypoglycaemia.

Blood loss can be extremely difficult to estimate in the newborn. There are few published papers on the relative merits of colloidal solutions available for volume replacement, although recent concern has been expressed about the cost–benefit ratio of the use of albumen.[6] Volume replacement should always be undertaken when losses are anticipated to exceed 5–10% of the blood volume. Because of the relatively high haematocrit at birth, red-cell replacement is seldom required and fortunately blood transfusion is seldom required for most routine neonatal surgical procedures when carried out by experienced surgeons. The concept of allowable blood loss (ABL) permits dilution to a haematocrit of between 35 and 40%:

$$ABL = weight(kg) \times EBV \times \frac{(Hm - He)}{Hm}$$

where EBV = estimated blood volume (50 + haematocrit ml kg^{-1}); Hm = measured haematocrit; He = lowest haematocrit.

TERMINATION OF ANAESTHESIA

In babies who are not critically ill or requiring postoperative ventilatory support, extubation is carried out when they are fully awake, opening their eyes and moving all limbs, with adequate respiratory depth and rate and no evidence of partial muscle paralysis or respiratory distress. With the newer muscle relaxants the possibility of reparalysis after reversal of neuromuscular block is slight. Most paediatric anaesthetists, however, still use anticholinesterase drugs to reverse the neuromuscular blockade and feel happier if there is evidence of partial recovery before reversal with at least one twitch being evident in response to train-of four nerve stimulation. Causes of poor respiratory function in the immediate postoperative period include pulmonary abnormalities such as the hypoplasia of the lungs which occurs with diaphragmatic hernia, tracheal aspiration in babies with tracheo-oesophageal fistula, hypothermia, acidosis, hypocalcaemia or prematurity. Babies should be assessed carefully in the recovery area before return to the neonatal ward or intensive care unit. They should be kept in the recovery area until they have been assessed to be fully recovered, warm, well perfused and pain free.

GENERAL SURGERY IN THE NEONATE AND INFANT

Most complex paediatric surgery in neonates and infants is carried out in specialized centres with fully trained and experienced medical, nursing and other personnel. Minor and intermediate procedures such as inguinal hernia repair, circumcision and orchidopexy often take place in District Hospitals, especially in children over 3 years of age.

Complex and specialized neonatal conditions such as congenital diaphragmatic hernia and tracheo-oesophageal fistula and their management are not discussed as they are outside the scope of this textbook.[7]

General surgery covers a wide range of abdominal and thoracic procedures, some of which are nowadays amenable to minimally invasive surgical techniques.[8] It is hoped that these techiques, such as for Nissen's fundoplication or a thorascopic approach to a mediastinal cyst, may result in a shorter hospital stay and the need for less postoperative analgesia, although this may not always be the case.[9]

The basic principles of anaesthesia and analgesia are discussed elsewhere, but include, whenever possible, regional anaesthesia with central or peripheral blocks or wound infiltrations, light general anaesthesia, an analgesia plan which starts intraoperatively but carries on for up to 48 h if necessary, full monitoring at all times in the perioperative period and intravenous fluids to cover deficits and perioperative losses.

INGUINAL HERNIA

In childhood, inguinal hernia is usually the result of a patent processus vaginalis (or canal of Nuck in a female) which is present in at least 90% of newborns. Fortunately, a clinical hernia presents in only 4–5% of newborns, but up to 20% of preterm babies. It is also common in patients with connective tissue disorders such as Ehler–Danlos syndrome and in patients with ventriculoperitoneal shunts.

The condition presents as a lump in the groin and while most are easily reducible, especially during the first 6 months of life, there is a risk of incarceration and inability to reduce the hernia. Surgery after urgent intravenous fluid is immediately indicated for strangulated hernias with intestinal obstruction. Occasionally, a testis or ovary becomes strangulated in the hernia. Many surgeons may postpone surgery in the preterm baby if the hernia is reducible to allow the child to become more mature, although this approach is controversial. Also controversial is whether the contralateral side is explored as well, because of the high incidence of bilateral hernias. If strangulation has occurred, the baby may rapidly become dehydrated from vomiting, with loss of water and electrolytes. Treatment is with intravenous fluids and nasogastric suction before surgery. If general anaesthesia is planned precautions against reflux of gastric contents and aspiration should be taken.

In premature and ex-premature babies the anxiety associated with anaesthesia and surgery is the occurrence postoperatively of apnoea. Liu *et al.* recommended that babies less than 46 weeks' postconception should be monitored for 24 h postoperatively for apnoea and other workers have suggested that the risk of apnoea persists for as long as 60 weeks.[10,11] Many babies have residual bronchopulmonary dysplasia with oxygen dependency, which is a predictor of likely postoperative problems and the need for intensive care and respiratory support, as well as the absolute weight and postconceptional age of the baby.[12]

The incidence of postoperative apnoea in ex-premature babies relates to gestational age and not postconceptional age and anaemia, and may be up to 5% in babies less than 50 weeks after conception, decreasing after that.[13,14] Allen *et al.* found that in ASA I–III babies all incidents of postoperative apnoea and bradycardia occurred within 4 h after surgery, even in those who had received intraoperative opioids.[15]

The incidence of postoperative apnoea may be less in babies given spinal anaesthesia without additional general anaesthesia or sedation and this technique is popular in many centres.[16,17] In countries such as the USA where tetracaine is available, 0–4 mg kg^{-1} with adrenaline will provide 60–80 min of anaesthesia.[18] Lignocaine and bupivacaine give shorter times and may not be satisfactory as the surgery can be difficult and prolonged, especially with bilateral hernias. A caudal epidural inserted with the baby awake is also recommended, although it requires a maximal dose of local anaesthetic agent (1 ml kg^{-1} bupivacaine 0.25%) and 15 min to become effective.[19]

For older babies less at risk from apnoea light general anaesthesia, together with a regional block such as a caudal or ilioinguinal–iliohypogastric block, will provide analgesia well into the postoperative period. Most babies below 5 kg will require tracheal intubation for general anaesthesia, although a laryngeal mask airway is suitable for babies over 5 kg. If a regional technique has been employed it is very unusual to require an opioid for postoperative pain relief, and simple analgesics such as paracetamol 20–30 mg kg^{-1} given as a suppository after the baby is anaesthetized are satisfactory. If stronger analgesia is required codeine phosphate 1 mg kg^{-1} can be given orally, rectally or intramuscularly. Most babies can feed soon after surgery. Intravenous caffeine 10 mg kg^{-1} or theophylline 8 mg kg^{-1} is recommended to decrease the incidence of apnoeas,[20] but does not change the need for close postoperative vigilance. The trend seems to be to allow ex-premature babies managed with spinal anaesthesia who have no apnoea or bradycardia within 4 h of surgery to be managed as day-stay cases. It is, however, wise to err on the side of caution.

PYLORIC STENOSIS

Pyloric stenosis is one of the most common gastrointestinal problems, occurring in between 1 : 300 and 1 : 400 live births and, even though the patients are infants, it is often treated in district hospitals, outside specialist neonatal surgical centres. In one series, 85% were males, 12% were premature and surgical correction took place at an average age of 5.6 weeks, with an average weight of 4 kg.[21] Recently, this classical group has been joined by a group of ex-premature babies who present with vomiting without a clear-cut clinical

diagnosis. Barium studies may be necessary in this group.

The pathological diagnosis is severe thickening of the pyloric smooth muscle which causes increasing obstruction to the passage of food from the stomach. A hard 'tumour' is formed which can be palpated in many cases, but is usually clearly seen on ultrasound imaging. There may be visible peristalsis, especially after a trial feed. Vomiting is the presenting symptom, but does not usually start before the 10th day, increasing in severity and becoming projectile. The baby loses weight and may become dehydrated. Loss of chloride in the vomitus produces hypochloraemic alkalosis and even tetany.

In the past, medical treatment with intravenous fluids was attempted before surgery was considered, but it is now standard practice to undertake surgical correction by pyloromyotomy in all cases.

Surgery is not an emergency, but complete correction of fluid and electrolyte abnormalities is urgent. With sodium, potassium and chloride being lost, the renal response is firstly to excrete bicarbonate (together with sodium) as an attempt to restore pH, and secondly to excrete potassium and retain sodium to minimize the reduction in extracellular fluid. The first phase produces an alkaline urine and the second an acid one.

The extent of the K^{+} loss is not usually well reflected in serum levels. A compensatory respiratory acidosis is also seen with hypoventilation, possibly to the point of apnoea, and in uncorrected patients, especially if they fall into an 'at-risk' group, apnoea is a significant risk postoperatively.[22]

Late diagnosis of cases is rare nowadays, so corrective fluid and electrolyte therapy is often not required for more than 6–12 h. In the past, extreme dehydration was not uncommon with prolonged vomiting, falling pH with ketoacidosis and the development of a vicious circle with falling cardiac output, increasing acidosis and hypoxia.

No surgery should be undertaken until the chloride is at least 90 mmol l^{-1}, the bicarbonate 24 mmol l^{-1} and the sodium 135 mmol l^{-1}; 0.9% sodium chloride may be given and up to 400 ml may be necessary. (Giving 2 ml kg^{-1} of 0.9% NaCl will raise the chloride by

1 mmol l^{-1}.) A urine flow of 1–2 ml kg^{-1} h^{-1} should be established as soon as possible. Maintenance fluids should be 2 ml kg^{-1} h^{-1} of 4% dextrose in 0.18% saline. Mild cases do not need potassium supplementation, but in others it should be given at a rate not exceeding 3 mmol kg^{-1} 24 h^{-1}. A large gastric residue is drained off and 4-hourly washouts of the stomach with physiological saline are carried out until the aspirate is clear and odourless (a secondary gastritis is often present). The nasogastric tube is aspirated before induction of anaesthesia and is left in place and opened because it does not reduce the effectiveness of cricoid pressure and will act as a valve if the intragastric pressure rises. There is a risk of reflux of stomach contents and subsequent aspiration during the induction of anaesthesia, although this is unlikely if the nasogastric tube is left open after aspiration. Induction of anaesthesia is by either inhalation or an intravenous method. Although there is no agreement on which method of induction of anaesthesia is the most appropriate, awake tracheal intubation is not and should not be used.[23] A survey of staff anaesthetists in the UK showed that two-thirds used an intravenous induction, but only half used cricoid pressure.[24] A short-acting relaxant such as atracurium is suitable. The surgery consists of delivering the pylorus through a very small periumbilical incision and splitting the muscle longitudinally down to, but not through the gastric mucosa. The surgeon often asks for air to be put into the stomach so a leak can be detected. Postoperative morbidity increases if the mucosal layer is incised by mistake. It is also possible to perform the surgery via a laparoscope.[8]

The baby is extubated awake in the lateral position. In one series recovery was faster and apnoea avoided when desflurane was used as the maintenance anaesthetic agent.[25] If the wound is infiltrated with bupivacaine 0.25% most babies are pain free on recovery and may not even require simple analgesics such as paracetamol for as long as 9 h postoperatively.[26] Oral feeding with clear fluids can usually be started 4–6 h after the operation, but an intravenous infusion of 4% dextrose in 0.18% saline (3 ml kg^{-1} h) should be maintained for the first 12–24 h until a normal oral intake has been re-established.

PULL-THROUGH SURGERY

Pull-through procedures are carried out for Hirschsprung's disease or anorectal anomaly.

Hirschsprung's disease causes a functional intestinal obstruction owing to the lack of ganglia in the distal colon and rectum and occurs at a frequency of between 1 : 5000 and 1 : 10 000 births. The condition may present soon after birth with failure to pass meconium, vomiting, reluctance to feed and abdominal distension. Barium enema and anorectal manometry studies help in the diagnosis, but this is confirmed by rectal suction biopsy. Rectal washouts temporarily relieve the situation, but a transverse colostomy is usually performed in the newborn with the definitive procedure being carried out at 6–9 months. The pull-through, which is a combined abdominal and perineal procedure, brings the ganglionated bowel through the preserved sphincter mechanisms to the perineum.

Surgery for high anorectal abnormalities is similar, but for low abnormalities a posterior sagittal anorectoplasty is carried out with the patient prone.

Epidural analgesia with the catheter introduced into the L4–5 space and directed caudad is very satisfactory. A bolus of up to 1 ml kg^{-1} bupivacaine 0.25% will block all the necessary segments and a continuous infusion of local anaesthetic agent and opioid can be continued postoperatively for 36–48 h. Particular attention must be paid to fluid replacement, as losses of blood and plasma can be high during the dissection in the pelvis. Peripheral temperature is a good guide to the adequacy of the circulating blood volume

NISSEN'S FUNDOPLICATION

Fundoplication is widely practised as an anti-reflux procedure with a high rate of success in children. The Nissen's fundoplication which is most often used involves a 360° wrap of the oesophagus by the fundus of the stomach and hopefully restores an intra-abdominal segment of oesophagus and augments the lower oesophageal sphincter.[27]

Reflux is very common in infancy, although in most cases the problem resolves within the first year of life as the lower oesophageal sphincter matures. Some babies require medical and surgical treatment. Reflux is associated with abnormalities such as oesophageal atresia and severe mental retardation, where the pain of acid reflux makes these children much harder to manage.[28] Other indications for surgery include oesophageal ulceration and stricture, apnoeic episodes and repeated chest infections from recurrent aspiration of gastric contents. Most patients have undergone a course of medical treatment with H_2 antagonists, cisapride, antacids and thickened feeds. Continuous monitoring of oesophageal pH is the most accurate means of documenting reflux and is used routinely. Nissen's fundoplication can also be performed using minimally invasive techniques.[29]

There is no agreement about which method of induction of anaesthesia is the most suitable for endoscopy and the definitive surgery for reflux. Many anaesthetists feel that in the presence of reflux there is a risk of pulmonary aspiration and a rapid sequence technique with cricoid pressure is mandatory.[30] However, reflux at this stage is extremely rare in children and other anaesthetists do not take these precautions, except in the case of the dilated oesophagus with acholasia.

A combination of epidural analgesia and light general anaesthesia has become the technique of choice for the procedure. The epidural catheter is best introduced at the L1–2 level after induction of anaesthesia. There is mounting anecdotal evidence that there are many fewer postoperative complications and a shorter hospital stay with this form of analgesia. Previously, the surgery, high under the diaphragm, often in children with chronic respiratory problems and poorly managed postoperative pain, would commonly result in basal collapse and pneumonia.

REFERENCES

1 Westrin, P., Jonmarker, C. and Werner, O. Thiopental requirements for induction of anesthesia in neonates and infants one to six months of age. *Anesthesiology* 1989; **71**: 344–6.

2 Creighton, R.E. The infant airway *Canadian Anaesthetists Society Journal* 1994; **41**: 174–6.

3 O'Brien, K., Robinson, D.N. and Morton, N.S. Induction and emergence in infants less than 60 weeks postconceptual age: comparison of thiopental, halothane, sevoflurane and desflurane. *British Journal of Anaesthesia* 1998; **80**: 456–9.

4 Spears, R.S., Yeh, A., Fisher, D.M., *et al.* The educated hand. Can anesthesiologists assess changes in neonatal pulmonary compliance manually? *Anesthesiology* 1991; **75**: 693–6.

5 Tan, S.S.W., Sury, M.R.J. and Hatch, D.J. The educated hand in paediatric anaesthesia – does it exist? *Paediatric Anaesthesia* 1993; **3**: 291–5.

6 Anon. Human albumin administration in critically ill patients: systematic review of randomised controlled trials. Cochrane Injuries Group Albumin Reviewers. *British Medical Journal* 1998; **317**: 235–40.

7 Hatch, D.J., Sumner, E. and Hellmann, J. *The Surgical Neonate: Anaesthesia and Intensive Care.* London: Arnold, 1995.

8 Alain, J.L., Grousseau, D., Longis, B., Ugazzi, M. and Terrier, G. Extramucosal pyloromyotomy by laparoscopy. *European Journal of Paediatric Surgery* 1996; **6**: 10–12.

9 Armstrong, T. and Martin, P.D. Anaesthetic management of a child undergoing thorascopic removal of a lung cyst. *Paediatric Anaesthesia* 1997; **7**: 159–61.

10 Liu, L.M.P., Cote, C.J., Goudsouzian, N.G., *et al.* Life-threatening apnea in infants recovering from anesthesia. *Anesthesiology* 1983; **59**: 506–10.

11 Kurth, C,D., Spitzer, A.R., Broennle, A.M. and Downes, J.J. Postoperative apnea in preterm infants. *Anesthesiology* 1987; **66**: 483–8.

12 Gollin, G., Bell, C., Dubose, R., *et al.* Predictors of postoperative respiratory complications in premature infants after inguinal herniorraphy. *Journal of Pediatric Surgery* 1993; **28**: 244–7.

13 Cote, C.J., Zaslavsky, A., Downes, J.J., *et al.* Postoperative apnea in former preterm infants after inguinal herniorraphy. A combined analysis. *Anesthesiology* 1995; **82**: 809–22.

14 Fisher, D.M. When is the ex-premature infant no longer at risk for apnea? *Anesthesiology* 1995; **82**: 807–8.

15 Allen, G.S., Cox, C.S., Jr, White, N., *et al.* Postoperative respiratory complications in ex-premature infants after inguinal herniorraphy. *Journal of Pediatric Surgery* 1998; **33**: 1095–8.

16 Abajian, J.C., Mellis, P.W., Browne, A.E., *et al.* Spinal anesthesia for surgery in the high risk infant. *Anesthesia and Analgesia* 1984; **63**: 359.

17 Welborn, L.G., Rice, L.J., Hannallah, R.S., *et al.* Postoperative apnea in former preterm infants: prospective comparison of spinal and general anesthesia. *Anesthesiology* 1990; **72**: 838–42.

18 Blaise, G.R. Spinal anesthesia in pediatric surgery. *Anesthesia and Analgesia* 1985; **64**: 196.

19 Gallagher, T.M. Regional anaesthesia for surgical treatment of inguinal hernia in preterm babies. *Archives of Disease in Childhood* 1993; **69**: 623–4.

20 Welborn, L.G., Hannallah, R.S., Fink, R., *et al.* High-dose caffeine suppresses postoperative apnea in former preterm infants. *Anesthesiology* 1989 71: 347–349.

21 Bissonnette, B. and Sullivan, P.J. Pyloric stenosis. *Canadian Journal of Anaesthesia* 1991; **38**: 668–76.

22 Andropoulos, D.B., Heard, M.B., Johnson, K.L., *et al.* Postanesthesia apnea in full-term infants after pyloromyotomy. *Anesthesiology* 1994; **80**: 216–19.

23 Cook-Sather, S.D., Tulloch, H.V., Cnaan, A., *et al.* A comparison of awake versus paralyzed tracheal intubation for infants with pyloric stenosis. *Anesthesia and Analgesia* 1998; **86**: 945–51.

24 Stoddart, P.A., Brennan, L., Hatch, D.J. and Bingham, R. Postal survey of paediatric practice and training among consultant anaesthetists in the UK. *British Journal of Anaesthesia* 1994; **73**: 559–63.

25 Wolf, A.R., Lawson, R.A., Dryden, C.M. and Davies, F.W. Recovery after desflurane anaesthesia in the infant: comparison with isoflurane. *British Journal of Anaesthesia* 1996; **76**: 362–4.

26 Habre, W., Schwab, C., Gollow, I. and Johnson, C. An audit of postoperative analgesia after pyloromyotomy. *Paediatric Anaesthesia* (in press).

27 Cilley, R.E. Management of gastro-esophageal reflux in children. *Current Opinion in Pediatrics* 1991; **3**: 483–8.

28 Spitz, L.R., Kiely, E.M., Brereton, R.J., *et al.* Operation for gastro-oesophageal reflux associated with severe mental retardation. *Archives of Disease in Childhood* 1993; **68**: 347–51.

29 Georgeson, K.E. Laparoscopic fundoplication. *Current Opinion in Pediatrics* 1998; **10**: 318–22.

30 Wetzel, R.C. Gastro-oesophageal reflux: theory over experience? *Paediatric Anaesthesia* 1998; **8**: 1–4.

Section 15.7. Anaesthesia for thoracic surgery

EDWARD SUMNER

THORACIC SURGERY

Surgical access to the chest may be required from very early in life for congenital lobar emphysema or repair of tracheo-oesophageal fistula, etc. Other pathology includes mediastinal masses, duplication cysts, pulmonary disease with bronchiectasis or cysts, which may be air or fluid filled.

The patients require very careful preoperative evaluation as many conditions have implications for the airway and cysts may burst to spill pus or other fluids into the normal lung areas of either side. Nitrous oxide should be avoided in patients with air-filled cysts as these will enlarge progressively, possibly increasing compression or displacement. Most patients will have computed tomographic or magnetic resonance imaging imaging to give clues to the degree and site of any respiratory obstruction, and whether masses are solid or fluid filled.

Minimally invasive surgical techniques are increasingly used for diagnosis and biopsy and for treatment of lung cysts, lobectomy, patent ductus ligation, treatment of empyema and anterior spinal fusions. The subject is comprehensively reviewed by Tobias.[1]

Nowadays, anaesthesia for most children undergoing some form of thoracic surgery would include the regional technique of thoracic epidural with the catheter placed at the required level or threaded up from the lumbar region (see Chapter 9) Other useful techniques include paravertebral or intercostal blocks or continuous interpleural analgesia. Invasive monitoring is usually undertaken with access to the internal jugular or subclavian vein on the side of the thoracotomy.

After induction of anaesthesia, patients with respiratory obstruction from a mediastinal mass are at risk from total obstruction, which can only be overcome by using a rigid bronchoscope to maintain the airway.

One-lung ventilation is not always necessary in children[2] but is mandatory if there is any risk of contralateral contamination with blood or pus. The smallest, conventional double-lumen tube is a 28FG (Mallinkrodt), which may be suitable for children above 35 kg. Marraro has described a small bilumen tube for selective bronchial intubation for use in surgery and intensive care, but this has not gained widespread acceptance.[3] The Univent tube (Juji) is a single lumen tracheal tube with a moveable bronchial blocker incorporated into the side of the tube, which is now widely used in adults[4] and has also been used in children.[5] This tube is easy to place and allows a change from one- to two-lung ventilation. The bronchus blocker contains a channel which enables suctioning or oxygen insufflation to take place. Although it is made in 3.5- and 4-mm sizes, the outside diameter of these is 7.5–8-mm, which makes them of use only in older children. For smaller children who require one-lung anaesthesia, selective bronchial intubation and bronchus blocking are the options. Left bronchial intubation for right-sided surgery is relatively easy to perform, either blind with the patient's head turned to the right and selecting a right bevelled tube or using a fibreoptic scope inserted through the tube as a guide.[6,7]

A Fogarty embolectomy catheter or, preferably, an atrioseptostomy catheter can be used for bronchus blocking. The latter has a central channel which allows suctioning of secretions and blood or oxygenation of the non-ventilated lung. Various methods of placing both the blocker and a tracheal tube have been described[8-12] but the preferred method is to use a fibreoptic scope, at least to check that correct placement has taken place. Blind, right-sided placement is easily achieved if the catheter is passed down a tracheal tube which has been advanced into the right main bronchus. The tracheal tube is then very carefully removed, leaving the blocker in place. The trachea is then reintubated so the bronchus blocker lies alongside the tracheal tube.

Postoperatively, patients require full analgesia, oxygen therapy and physiotherapy and are preferably nursed in a high-dependency or intensive care area. The site of the chest drain may be a source of pain or discomfort. There do not seem to be any differences in the analgesic requirements between those children having open thoracotomy and those having closed thoracoscopy.[12] The most satisfactory form of analgesia is the continuous epidural, although other techniques such as patient- or nurse-controlled analgesia with morphine or inter-pleural bupivacaine are acceptable alternatives.

REFERENCES

1 Tobias, J.D. Anaesthetic implications of thoracoscopic surgery in children. *Paediatric Anaesthesia* 1999; **1**: 103–10.

2 Gomola, G.O., Larroquet, M., Constant, I., *et al.* Video-assisted thorascopic surgery for right middle lobectomy in children. *Paediatric Anaesthesia* 1997; **7**: 215–20.

3 Marraro, G. Simultaneous independent lung ventilation in pediatric patients. *Critical Care Clinics* 1992; **8**: 131–45.

4 Gayes, J.M. Pro: one-lung ventilation is best accomplished with the Univent endotracheal tube. *Journal of Cardiothoracic and Vascular Anesthesia* 1993; **7**: 103–7.

5 Hammer, G.B., Brodsky, J.B., Redpath, J.H. and Cannon, W.B. The Univent tube for single-lung ventilation in paediatric patients. *Paediatric Anaesthesia* 1998; **8**: 55–7.

6 Baraka, A., Akel, S., Muallem, M., *et al.* Bronchial intubation in children: does the tube bevel determine the side of intubation? *Anesthesiology* 1987; **67**: 869–70.

7 Baraka, A. Right bevelled tube for selective left bronchial intubation in a child undergoing right thoracotomy. *Paediatric Anaesthesia* 1996; **6**: 487–9.

8 Dalens, B., Labbe, A. and Haberer, J.P. Selective endobronchial blocking versus selective intubation. *Anesthesiology* 1982; **55**: 555.

9 Vale, R. Selective bronchial blocking in a small child. *British Journal of Anaesthesia* 1986; **41**: 453–4.

10 Kaplan, R. and Guzzi, L. An aid in the placement of right sided bronchial blocker in small children. *Paediatric Anaesthesia* 1993; **3**: 263.

11 Cooper, M.G. Bronchial blocker placement in infants: a technique and some considerations. *Paediatric Anaesthesia* 1994; **4**: 73–4.

12 Turner, M.W.H., Buchanan, C.C.R and Brown, S.W. Paediatric one lung ventilation in the prone position. *Paediatric Anaesthesia* 1997; **7**: 427–9.

Neurosurgery

ANGELA MACKERSIE

INTRODUCTION

Neurosurgery in children requires that the anaesthetist has an intimate knowledge not only of the scientific basis of modern neuroanaesthesia, but also of the physiology and pathology of children and in particular of how they differ from adults. Current practice in neuroanaesthesia is based on the developing knowledge of cerebral physiology, hand in hand with a clear understanding of the specific pathology of each patient. In paediatric practice this is combined with an acute awareness of the potential problems that can arise at any time during major surgery in infants and small children, who have limited physiological reserves and small blood volumes. The techniques used may therefore sometimes be a compromise between the theoretical ideal for controlled neuroanaesthesia and a practical approach to the management of sick infants and children, from both a physiological and psychological point of view.

CENTRAL NERVOUS SYSTEM DEVELOPMENT

Knowledge of the embryology of the central nervous system (CNS) is essential for the understanding of the pathological processes involved in congenital neurological disease (see Chapter 1)

Cerebrospinal fluid (CSF) production commences between weeks 6 and 8, and between weeks 10 and 18 brain growth is mainly neuronal resulting from neuroblast multiplication. This explains the extreme sensitivity of the CNS to external noxious influences such as viral infections, drugs, toxins and X-rays during this stage in fetal development. At birth the number of neurons is almost complete, so that postpartum development is mainly glial, dendritic arborization with synaptic formation and myelination. At birth only about one-quarter of the number of all cells is present, reaching two-thirds by 6 months and with growth being completed during the second year of life.

Differential growth rates occur in different areas: the cerebellum is less developed at birth, but completes its development during the first year of life prior to the cortex and brainstem.

Nutrition both prenatally and postnatally is important for full cerebral development. Malnutrition results in a reduced number of cells and also dendritic connections with a reduction in cerebral lipid and protein content. The brain at birth weighs approximately 335 g, being approximately 10–15% of body weight. By 6 months it has doubled in weight and is about 900 g at 1 year and 1000 g at 2 years. The final adult weight of 1200–1400 g is reached at 12 years of age.

At birth the calvarium consists of ossified plates covering the dura which are separated by the fibrous sutures and fontanelles. The neonate has two recognizable fontanelles, the posterior which closes during the second or third month and the anterior fontanelle which usually closes between 10 and 16 months, with full ossification as growth finishes in the second decade.

Children with intracranial pathology differ from adults in certain ways which may be advantageous. The fontanelles and nonfused sutures, which can separate even in early adolescence, provide protection from gradual changes in intracranial volume, resulting in an increased head size prior to a rise in pressure. Acute changes are not absorbed in this way because of the rigidity of the fibrous tissue bridging the sutures and fontanelles. Children of all ages are fortunate in having healthy blood vessels devoid of atheroma and therefore are less likely to suffer focal ischaemia during treatment for intracranial pathology.

NEUROPHYSIOLOGY

Under normal physiological conditions the main source of energy for cerebral metabolism is glucose. The cerebral metabolic rate has been demonstrated to be higher in children. Glucose consumption in normal children (average age 6 years) is 6.8 mg min^{-1} 100 g^{-1}, compared with 5.5 mg in adults.[1] Kennedy and Sokoloff[2] showed that oxygen consumption is 5.8 ml min^{-1} 100 g^{-1}, compared with 3.5 ml in adults.

CEREBRAL BLOOD FLOW

Despite no definitive studies on cerebral blood flow (CBF) regulation in children, the same mechanisms as in adults are assumed. Between the ages of 3 and 12 years the CBF is maintained at approximately 100 ml min^{-1} 100 g^{-1}. Between the ages of 6 months and 3 years values of 90 ml min^{-1} 100 g^{-1} have been demonstrated.[3] However, values for newborns and premature infants are less, at 40–42 ml min^{-1} 100 g^{-1}. More recently, shifts in regional blood flow as development progresses have been demonstrated.[4] The lower limit of autoregulation is also unknown in small children but is assumed to be related to normal mean arterial blood pressure. Sick newborn infants with respiratory distress syndrome or birth asphyxia have impaired autoregulation with CBF following systemic pressure, which may explain the susceptibility of these infants to intraventricular haemorrhage.[5] The same effects of hypocarbia and hypercarbia on CBF have been assumed from clinical experience. Wyatt *et al.*[6] demonstrated the linear relationship between arterial carbon dioxide tension ($PaCO_2$) and changes in CBF using near infrared spectrophotometry in sick newborns. As in adults, hyperventilation has been demonstrated to restore autoregulation in the neonate.[7] Transcranial Doppler is increasing in popularity because of its noninvasive nature and ease of use. However, the results expressed as CBF velocity have not yet been clearly related to CBF or intracranial pressure (ICP).

INTRACRANIAL PRESSURE

Even in children the cranium can be regarded as a closed box occupied by the brain mass (70%), extracellular fluid (ECF; 10%), cerebral blood volume (CBV; 10%) and CSF (10%). In normal conditions 0.35 ml min^{-1} of CSF is produced in children[8] and ICP is more dependent on CBF and CBV than CSF production. The brain mass is relatively incompressible, with CSF volume changes acting as an initial buffer. The point at which the volume changes can no longer be absorbed results in a rise in ICP. As already stated, the paediatric patient is able to compensate for gradual increases in ICP by suture/

fontanelle expansion, but acute changes cannot be absorbed in this way.

ICP has been measured in neonates and infants and is usually in the range 2–4 mmHg,[9] whereas adult values are 8–18 mmHg.

Information about ICP in children of all ages has been obtained by the use of the Camino Bolt in patients with cranial abnormalities. In normal adults it has been shown that an increase in volume of approximately 25 ml is required to raise baseline ICP by 10 mmHg, while in infants this volume is only 10 ml,[10] which explains why children can demonstrate such rapid alterations in neurological function from the apparently normal to almost coning in 30 min.

Control of intracranial pressure

Good operative conditions for neurosurgery are produced by controlling the ICP. Raised pressure, caused by obstructive hydrocephalus and tumours associated with large cysts, is little affected by the anaesthetist's skills and therapeutic manoeuvres and conditions are only changed by removal of the encysted fluid. Reduction in the normal brain volume should be reserved for critical rises in ICP.

Steroids can provide a dramatic improvement in the clinical condition of patients with tumours by reducing the surrounding oedema. Dexamethasone 0.25 mg kg^{-1} as a loading dose with 0.1 mg kg^{-1} every 6 h is still used perioperatively for tumour surgery in most units, despite the lack of definite studies into its benefits. However, the hyperglycaemic response to steroids has stopped their routine use in head injury and after acute hypoxic insults.

Cerebral dehydration with reduction in both intracellular and extracellular fluid volume is achieved with diuretics. Apart from its use in the treatment of acute rises in ICP, 20% mannitol is usually reserved for operations where surgical access to small solid lesions is particularly difficult. Children have excellent renal function with small blood volumes so that a maximum dose of mannitol 1 g kg^{-1} is recommended with careful monitoring of urine output, using an indwelling urinary catheter. If urine output exceeds the infused volume plus 10% of the estimated blood volume, increased intravenous replacement will be urgently required. A vigorous and rapid response to the mannitol, leading to a marked reduction in intracerebral volume prior to opening the dura, may lead to tearing of the dural veins and haematoma formation. Cerebral dehydration can also be produced with frusemide 0.5 mg kg^{-1} which, despite its advantage of not providing an osmotic load to the circulation, has not replaced mannitol as the agent of choice in most units.

The development of stereotactic techniques, both frame and frameless varieties, has resulted in greatly improved access to deep-seated lesions and accurate surgery with minimal damage to surrounding tissues. This has reduced the requirement for cerebral dehydration for surgery, which is now more usually reserved for acute, life-threatening crises.

Hypertonic saline (3%) has been used to cause extracellular dehydration by increasing serum osmolality.[11] Considerable interest has also been shown in its use in resuscitation. In head trauma in children 3% saline has been shown to be effective in lowering raised ICP compared with normal saline, with a peak effect at 30 min, without significant changes in central venous pressure.[12] However, further investigation of the effect of the sodium load in young children is needed before its routine use is recommended.

CBV can be reduced by ensuring a low cerebral venous pressure. This results from good positioning of the patient, which is much harder to achieve in small children owing to their relatively short necks and large heads which may lead to kinking of the neck veins. A moderate head-up position should be used routinely but this is associated with an increased risk of venous air embolism (VAE), especially in the presence of hypovolaemia. The children also need to be supported in the chosen position using large sandbags and/or strapping to prevent movement during surgery. Otherwise, surgical manipulation, especially opening of the skull, can result in the child moving on the table, causing neck flexion and cerebral venous engorgement with potentially disastrous results.

VENTILATION

Moderate hyperventilation should be employed to control ICP. This may be difficult with ventilators of the T-piece occluder pattern, as increasing the rate results in rebreathing unless very high fresh gas flows are employed.[13] With larger tidal volumes the expiratory time needs to be increased to avoid rebreathing and the application of inadvertent positive end-expiratory pressure (PEEP). Children over 20 kg and those with abnormal lungs are better ventilated with a non-rebreathing system. More recently, the introduction of expensive volatile agents has increased the use of circle systems, which are ideal for neurosurgery.

PEEP, with its increase in mean intrathoracic pressure, is avoided during controlled ventilation of all neurosurgical patients except in those with inadequate respiratory function. Manual ventilation of neonates and small infants is still a recognized, although much less common, technique in general surgery. It should be avoided because of the difficulty in not applying PEEP and reserved only for high-risk infants with decreased compliance at times when further changes may be critical, for example in ex-premature patients with bronchopulmonary dysplasia, during tunnelling of the VP shunt system. Accumulation of water in circuits with humidifiers can result in PEEP being applied if, with positioning of the circuit, the water traps are not working effectively. This happens more commonly when the patient is supine. The routine use of a combined humidifier and microbial filters has removed this risk. Adequate oxygenation is essential at all times and there is some evidence from neurointensive care to suggest that hyperoxia [arterial oxygen tension (PaO_2) greater than 20 kPa] may have the beneficial effect of increasing tissue oxygenation in areas of poor flow from gross cerebral oedema.[14] During anaesthesia in patients with normal lungs and an inspiratory oxygen fraction (FiO_2) of 0.35 these levels are usually attained. However, care should be taken to avoid hyperoxia in newborns and ex-premature infants.

INDUCED HYPOTENSION

The use of induced hypotension is no longer popular. If it is used it must be associated with deep anaesthesia, adequate muscle relaxation, good oxygenation and normovolaemia. Hypotensive agents should not be administered to small children without direct arterial pressure monitoring, especially in a situation where sudden or heavy blood loss is expected. Good operative conditions are best achieved with a relatively slow heart rate for the particular size of patient. In a neonate 110 beats min^{-1} would be considered slow, but in an 8 year old tachycardic. If the heart rate is fast, priority should be given to deepening the anaesthesia, increasing the rate of intravenous fluid infusion and checking the blood gases. Control of heart rate with β-blockers either alone (propranolol incrementally up to 0.5 mg kg^{-1}) or in combination with an α-blocker (labetalol incrementally up to 1 mg kg^{-1}) is sufficient to provide moderate hypotension and improved surgical conditions. Where the patient already has a relatively slow heart rate or where more profound falls in pressure are required, vasodilator agents such as sodium nitroprusside 0.5 μg kg^{-1} min^{-1} can be used, with a maximum dose of 1 mg kg^{-1} 24 h^{-1}. Induced hypotension should only be used where surgical conditions are inadequate and where all other measures have failed to achieve the desired effect. In general, children are more resistant than adults to hypotensive agents.

In practice, the distinctive features of paediatric neuroanaesthesia stem directly from the small size of the patient, with an increased metabolic rate, greater oxygen demands and resultant rapid development of hypoxia during acute events. In addition, normal children have relatively large heads compared with adults (Table 16.1) and, as already described, children with intracranial pathology may have increased head sizes owing to separation of the sutures, so that in some neurosurgical patients the head may be almost half the total surface area, a factor which contributes to the increased blood losses and difficulty with temperature control.

Table 16.1 Surface area of the head of normal children

Age group (years)	Surface area of head (% of total)
0–1	19
1–4	17
5–9	13
10–14	11
Adult	7

PREOPERATIVE ASSESSMENT

All neurosurgical patients require an accurate assessment of their neurological status, including evidence of raised ICP, alteration in conscious level and any focal findings, in particular cranial nerve palsies. Bulbar palsies associated with brainstem lesions may result in reduced reflexes and impaired swallowing, causing aspiration with lung changes and hypoxaemia, especially in infants.

Raised ICP commonly presents with vomiting, which in a child is frequently diagnosed as originating from an infection. It may become sufficiently severe to cause dehydration, resulting in hypotension following induction of anaesthesia if not treated adequately.

Pathology in other systems is rare in children with CNS neoplasia. However, certain neurosurgical patients are likely to have multisystem disease, e.g. ex-premature patients with bronchopulmonary dysplasia and hydrocephalus, children with cerebral abscess and cyanotic heart disease or with renal disease and major spinal defects, and others with congenital syndromes undergoing craniofacial surgery.

Preoperative investigations should include a full blood count for all patients, and electrolyte estimation in those with a history of vomiting or with a ventricular drain. Children with chronic shunt infections frequently become severely anaemic as a result of poor oral intake and toxic bone marrow depression and may require preoperative transfusion. Lesser degrees of anaemia can be corrected perioperatively. In the presence of dehydration from vomiting the initial haemoglobin estimation may be falsely high, by 1–2 g dl^{-1}. All children having neurosurgical operations should have blood crossmatched because there is the possibility of sudden and catastrophic blood loss, particularly if sinuses or pathologically dilated veins from raised ICP are damaged. Therefore, despite altered attitudes to transfusion of blood and blood products since the early 1980s, blood should be immediately available for all small children.

During the preoperative visit, discussion should take place with children who are able to understand. The nature of their induction technique and postoperative course and monitoring equipment should be explained in simple terms, without frightening them about details of which they will be unaware. In younger children without verbal communication skills, alleviation of parental anxiety, as far as possible, will help in prevention of its transmission to the child.

PREMEDICATION

Sedative premedication should be avoided in all children undergoing intracranial surgery. Children with raised ICP, especially those with blocked ventricular shunts, may appear remarkably well apart from complaining of headache and occasional vomiting. However, many of these children have markedly raised ICP and minor triggers such as sedative premedication may cause a sudden spiralling effect, with increase in pressure and the possiblity of coning.

Children not undergoing intracranial surgery may receive standard sedative premedication such as midazolam 0.5 mg kg^{-1} (maximum dose 15 mg) or temazepam 0.5 mg kg^{-1} (maximum dose 20 mg).

With modern anaesthesia using sevoflurane for gaseous inductions and with the greater ease of intravenous inductions using topical analgesia, the use of antisialogogues in paediatric anaesthesia has decreased. However, high-risk infants, especially ex-premature infants, should probably receive atropine 20 μg kg^{-1} p.o. Children having anaesthesia in unusual positions such as prone or in the sitting position are also given atropine, both for drying and for cardiovascular stability. Dislodgement of the tracheal tube because of pooling of the secretions when the face is dependent is a disaster. Atropine is given orally for those going prone or for older children sitting (> 30 kg). However, younger children undergoing posterior fossa exploration in the sitting position have significantly fewer oropharyngeal secretions and better cardiovascular stability without tachycardia when atropine 20 μg kg^{-1} is administered intramuscularly, the advantages outweighing the disadvantages of this route of administration. Topical local anaesthetic cream, either Ametop or EMLA (eutectic mixture of local anaesthetics), is used routinely, applied over suitable veins.

The presence of a parent in the anaesthetic room, especially with an unsedated child, can provide great support and comfort to the young patient. However, with infants too small to be aware of their parent's presence or in situations where the parents are too distressed to support their child, it may be preferable to induce anaesthesia with the child alone. With the widespread practice of parents accompanying their children to theatre, the stress to the parents should not be underestimated.[15] Many of the children with brain tumours will have progressed from being a fit and an apparently well, normal child, to one with a diagnosis of a potentially lethal disease requiring major surgery within a few days or weeks.

ANAESTHESIA

Paediatric neuroanaesthesia requires a knowledge of the effects of the agents on the young child's CNS, in both healthy and pathological states. Such documentation as there is in this area suggests that these effects vary little between children and adults.

NITROUS OXIDE

There is still debate about the use of nitrous oxide as an adjunct to balanced neuroanaesthesia. Studies on CBF using transcranial Doppler in normal children have shown marked increases in blood flow using 60–70% nitrous oxide compared with an oxygen mixture in children lightly anaesthetized with fentanyl/diazepam and caudal analgesia.[16] Certainly in situations where ICP may be critically raised nitrous oxide should be avoided, but in other cases its analgesic properties and rapid elimination may outweigh the theoretical disadvantages. Pneumoencephalocoeles will enlarge if nitrous oxide is used, and this should be remembered in the acute postoperative period where there may be some intracranial air.

VOLATILE AGENTS

Isoflurane has been the gold-standard volatile agent for neuroanaesthesia for a number of reasons: its minimal effect on CBF, the fact that autoregulation is less affected than with halothane, and the minimal effect of isoflurane on cerebral reactivity to carbon dioxide. In animals sevoflurane has been shown to be similar to isoflurane in its effects on CBV, cerebral metabolic rate for oxygen and ICP,[17] and there is evidence that it may be more protective than fentanyl/nitrous oxide in incomplete ischaemia. At present, clinical studies in adults appear favourable and, in particular, the clinical characteristics with faster elimination may be particularly useful in adult neuroanaesthetic practice. Further research in both adults and children will need to be performed to find its ultimate role in clinical practice.[18]

INTRAVENOUS AGENTS

In adult neuroanaesthesia propofol is the principal agent for total intravenous anaesthesia (TIVA), supplemented by opioids. There is a variety of dosage regimes and it is also possible to interface with a portable computer.[19] A computerized monitoring system designed for paediatric neuroanaesthesia can be adapted for this use.[20] Because its use in children is discouraged following deaths or near deaths in children admitted with croup,[21] this technique has not developed widespread popularity in children. However, evidence is being gathered that in normal dosage use of propofol by infusion is safe.[22]

OPIOIDS

Fentanyl is probably the best narcotic in raised ICP[23] since, unlike alfentanil[24] and sufentanil,[25] it produces no increase in CBF or ICP. Remifentanil is increasingly popular in adult clinical neuroanaesthesia with its much shorter duration of action and the possibility of fine tuning to surgical stimuli.[26] However, its ultrashort action may be a disadvantage postoperatively, particularly in children, where further research needs to be published for its full clinical value to be evaluated.

TECHNIQUES

In clinical paediatric neuroanaesthesia, a compromise may need to be reached between theoretical advantages of certain agents in adult and animal studies and the disadvantages of their administration in small children. In a child with cerebral irritation an inhalational induction may have a less deleterious effect on the ICP than an intravenous injection, which is often associated with crying and breath-holding despite the use of local anaesthetic cream and sensitive handling of the young patient.

Sevoflurane has become the volatile agent of choice for induction of anaesthesia in children, replacing halothane, and in neuropractice the lack of CNS effects is a bonus. In the past, isoflurane had better theoretical properties as an inhalational agent in neuroanaesthesia than halothane, but the longer induction time and the potential for breath-holding and coughing, if not actual laryngeal spasm, precluded it from routine use as an induction agent.

Immediately following induction venous access can be secured and the concentration of volatile agent reduced. If necessary, a small dose of thiopentone or propofol 1–2 mg kg^{-1}/fentanyl 1–2 μg kg^{-1} can be administered to obtain deep anaesthesia prior to muscle relaxation and intubation.

In cases with critically raised ICP where there is likely to be a risk of vomiting because of a full stomach, suxamethonium may be used to achieve rapid intubation despite the theoretical risk of increasing ICP, which appears to be due to afferent stimulation of muscle spindles. Small children rarely demonstrate fasciculation with suxamethonium. The longer period of mask ventilation prior to the development of intubating conditions with non-depolarizing agents may lead to gastric distension, diaphragmatic splinting and reduced compliance in small children, and certainly moderate hyperventilation is harder to achieve.

The airway is secured with an uncuffed tracheal tube of a size which has only a small leak at cricoid level; too large a leak may cause hypoventilation. For neurosurgery a reinforced silastic tube may be used, which is slightly more difficult to insert but provides excellent security once in place. The tubes are sometimes thicker walled and therefore a smaller size may be required. After intubation it is essential to check for bilateral lung ventilation with the head both in a neutral position and in its position for surgery, as in a small child 1 cm may be the difference between a good position and bronchial intubation. Preformed, south-facing tubes such as Mallinkrodt RAE and Portex polar tubes are extremely popular in paediatric use, but their length is predetermined. They may be too long, with the risk of bronchial intubation, or they may be too short, which is especially dangerous for neurosurgery.[27] The Murphy eye may also complicate the issue, either by apparently giving bilateral ventilation when too long or by causing a leak when in the glottis.[28,29]

Maintenance of anaesthesia is with a balanced technique of muscle relaxation, analgesia and anaesthesia with mild to moderate hyperventilation ($PaCO_2$ approx. 3.8–4.2 kPa). The choice of muscle relaxant is one of personal preference based on experience. D-Tubocurarine 0.4–0.5 mg kg^{-1}, no longer available in the UK, has a place in paediatric anaesthesia for major surgery as significant falls in blood pressure are not seen in children, its use results in excellent cardiovascular stability and prolonged relaxation with no sudden end-point, and it is always easily reversible. For short procedures, especially in high-risk patients, e.g. ex-premature infants undergoing VP shunts insertion, atracurium 0.4–0.5 mg kg^{-1} is the agent of choice because of its very predictable metabolism. However, because of its abrupt spontaneous reversal neuromuscular function must always be monitored. Vecuronium 0.08–0.1 mg kg^{-1} provides excellent cardiovascular stability and has little histamine release, but in small children there may be an unpredictable dose response and therefore a peripheral nerve stimulator is recommended, especially if being administered by infusion.

Analgesia is provided with fentanyl in a total initial dose of 5 μg kg^{-1} with increments of 1 μg kg^{-1} h^{-1} after 2–3 h. Total doses should not exceed 7 μg kg^{-1} unless surgery is very prolonged (> 6 h) or postoperative ventilation is planned. Anaesthesia is provided with 0.5–1.0 MAC of isoflurane or sevoflurane in either air/oxygen or nitrous oxide/oxygen mixtures.

At the end of surgery residual muscle relaxation should be reversed with neostigmine

50 μg kg^{-1} and atropine 25 μg kg^{-1} or glyco-pyrrolate 10 μg kg^{-1}, unless postoperative ventilation is planned. Glycopyrrolate may have theoretical advantages with its lack of central effects and with less tachycardia, especially in older children and adolescents.

Extubation is performed when the child is breathing well and has a normal end-tidal carbon dioxide. The adult neurosurgical practice of leaving the tracheal tube *in situ* until the patient wakes is not applicable to paediatric neuroanaesthesia. With a balanced technique the child under 25 kg will reject both tube and airway soon after discontinuation of the anaesthesia and resumption of breathing. Older child/adolescents will take somewhat longer, but usually maintain their own airway patency with an oral airway *in situ* within 5 min of discontinuation of anaesthesia and reversal of residual muscle relaxation. There is no indication for tapering (gradual reduction) of anaesthesia until the head dressings are completed in children, as the movement of the head which occurs during this process will cause coughing and hypertension if anaesthesia is not adequate.

MONITORING

Routine monitoring as discussed in detail elsewhere in this book (Chapter 7) should always be used. It should include either precordial or oesophageal stethoscope, electrocardiogram, non-invasive blood pressure, pulse oximetry, capnography, both central and peripheral temperature probes, and peripheral nerve stimulator. The blood pressure cuff should be the largest that easily fits the upper arm of the child, making allowance for the relatively greater forearm and axillary subcutaneous fat, to provide an accurate reading. All major cases should have direct arterial pressure measurement.

Capnography has a dual role in neurosurgery, both to monitor for adequate moderate hyperventilation and for VAE. The latter can occur in all neurosurgical cases, especially if there is heavy blood loss and the patient becomes slightly hypovolaemic. Children with normal lungs and pulmonary blood flow have demonstrated a good correlation between arterial and end-tidal carbon dioxide.[30] Accuracy in many patients, compared with arterial levels, is within 0.5 kPa. However, while capnography is an excellent breath-to-breath monitor of adequate ventilation and a good trend monitor, if there is any doubt about absolute values arterial blood gas analysis must be performed.

Central venous pressure (CVP) lines are recommended for all major general surgery in children but the most reliable route for insertion in infants and children is via the internal jugular vein. This route might result in obstruction to the cerebral venous drainage in a small child when positioned with the neck flexed or extremely extended, or rotated as in neurosurgery. Percutaneous long lines inserted via the anticubital fossa are rarely successful in children under 5 years of age. The most appropriate route may be via the femoral vein. In experienced hands intraoperative fluid balance can be accurately assessed without CVP monitoring, by other cardiovascular parameters.[31] However, good venous access with at least two good peripheral cannulae is essential, for rapid transfusion if needed.

Urinary catheters are not used routinely as they cause great distress to young awake children postoperatively, but reserved for patients in whom a large urine output may produce fluid balance problems, either after diuretics in patients at risk for developing diabetes insipidus or in prolonged surgery.

TEMPERATURE CONTROL

The large surface area of most child neurosurgical patients contributes to heat losses. Heat losses by conduction, convection and radiation, and from the latent heat of vaporization must be minimized and active measures available for rewarming as required. Passive measures to prevent heat loss include wrapping the child in aluminium foil and covering in gamgee or a hot-air overblanket. If rapid transfusions are required, greater than 20% of blood volume per hour, an in-line blood warmer should be used. The introduction of the concentric water bath infusion line, 'Hot Line', has enabled body temperature to be maintained despite multiple exchange transfusions. Close monitoring of body temperature is essential, both central and peripheral. Hypothermia with peripheral circulatory shutdown and metabolic acidosis may be very difficult to reverse even with increased transfusion rates. Ideally, a temperature between 36 and 36.5°C should be maintained. However, when there are surgical difficulties a lower temperature may have a cerebral protective effect by lowering cerebral metabolism, enabling surgery to be completed while the cerebral perfusion is somewhat compromised. It has also been shown that moderate hypothermia postischaemia can have protective benefits.[32] Temperatures over 34.5°C may provide protection without placing the child in jeopardy from cardiac arrhythmias and metabolic changes.[33] This degree of hypothermia is usually achieved by cessation of warming and does not require active cooling in small children. The hot-air mattress gives the anaesthetist the ability to rewarm the patient if necessary.

A study in dogs showed significant changes in both postischaemic neurological function and cerebral histopathology with small (1–2°C) changes in temperature and suggested that all episodes of hyperthermia should be vigorously treated until the patient is no longer at risk for ischaemic injury.[34]

Postoperative hyperpyrexia is associated with certain neurosurgical procedures, e.g. craniopharyngioma resection and hypothalamic, pontine and midbrain manipulations and, if not treated vigorously, has a very poor prognosis, especially if the temperature exceeds 40.5°C. Initial active cooling methods include increased transfusion of room temperature fluids, fanning and administration of paracetamol 20 mg kg^{-1} rectally. If these measures are not successful peripheral vasodilatation can be achieved using small doses of chlorpromazine 0.1–0.2 mg kg^{-1} i.v. or other vasodilator drugs of choice, while closely monitoring and correcting any fall in blood pressure. If the temperature is still resistant to lowering and remains over 40°C other available steps include the use of icepacks placed over large vessels and the liver, and rectal, bladder or gastric washouts with ice-cold saline. Frequent blood gas analysis is required to ensure adequate ventilation during a period

of increased metabolism. Increased volumes of maintenance intravenous fluids are needed. Electrolyte imbalance is also likely, owing to both cellular dysfunction and rapid transfusion, and will require correction.

FLUID BALANCE

MAINTENANCE FLUIDS

Perioperative fluid balance is directed to the maintenance of circulating blood volume and cerebral perfusion. Fluid fluxes across the normal brain are primarily determined by osmotic forces,[35] whereas in the peripheral capillary bed fluxes are determined by colloid oncotic pressure. Therefore, minor falls in osmotic pressure by 5–10 mosmol kg^{-1} can have marked effects on water movement across the blood–brain barrier and result in cerebral oedema. Intraoperative maintenance fluid is with either lactated Ringer's or normal saline. If large volumes of fluid are to be administered, saline may be preferable as Ringer's is mildly hypo-osmolar and could cause oedema.

Hyperglycaemia in head injuries is known to be associated with an adverse outcome.[36] Adult neuroanaesthetists usually avoid glucose-containing infusions for the first 24 h. However, small children are more likely to develop perioperative hypoglycaemia, especially if there has been a prolonged period of vomiting and reduced food and fluid intake prior to surgery, which may have depleted reserves. Blood sugar should be monitored regularly during long operations and postoperatively, and glucose-containing infusions administered if required. A degree of fluid restriction is usual in neurosurgery to avoid cerebral oedema formation, but the first priority is to maintain an adequate circulating blood volume.

BLOOD LOSS

The major clinical problem in paediatric neurosurgery is posed by the larger blood losses from the relatively large size of the patient's head (Table 16.1), and this results in proportionately larger blood losses. In children under 20 kg undergoing craniotomy, blood transfusion is common even in the present climate of reduced blood transfusion, with optimal surgical conditions and the use of modern surgical techniques such as dissection using Colorado needles. However, when surgery is performed in the sitting position even in children under 10 kg, only 10% of patients require blood transfusion in the author's unit.

Blood loss in neurosurgery is difficult to measure, owing to contamination of the drapes and mixing of the blood with saline used during the bone work, as well as CSF. The use of the ultrasonic suction device with its continuous spray of saline adds to this difficulty. Accuracy of blood replacement is achieved by using all cardiovascular parameters, in particular heart rate and arterial pressure trace. Transfusions in excess of the blood volume are not unusual in small children and are well tolerated provided clotting factors, blood gases and potassium levels are checked regularly and normality maintained. Rapid transfusion of blood stored for more than 12 days combined with low cardiac output, a situation not that uncommon in small neurosurgical patients undergoing craniofacial or large tumour surgery, carries a high risk of hyperkalaemia and therefore the potassium level should be monitored.[37]

Fresh-frozen plasma at approximately 10% of the blood volume is administered for each exchange transfusion to ensure adequate clotting factors. Platelets are usually required after more than two exchange transfusions. Calcium supplements are usually only required with very rapid transfusions. Postoperatively, continuing blood losses should be expected and replaced. The definition of a massive transfusion is a blood volume transfused within 24 h. It is not uncommon for two or three exchange volumes to occur intraoperatively with a single exchange within 1 h and active intervention to maintain normal blood parameters is much more likely to be required in such situations.

POSTOPERATIVE CARE

Ventilation is reserved for patients who have particular indications. Airway problems from a craniofacial anomaly, or central causes such as bulbar lesions with obtunded reflexes are indications for intubation and possibly postoperative ventilation for the first 24 h. Otherwise, only if the operation has been particularly prolonged or if there has been cardiovascular instability or a particular neurosurgical indication are children ventilated in the author's unit.

All patients require close postoperative monitoring. Postcraniotomy patients have direct arterial pressure monitoring until the next day for easy blood sampling for testing clotting and electrolytes. Careful evaluation of the neurological status and cardiorespiratory function of the patient is carried out regularly, together with accurate assessment of fluid balance.

Analgesia has traditionally been administered as codeine phosphate 1 mg kg^{-1} i.m. every 4 h as in many adult neurosurgical units providing good pain relief without altering consciousness and pupil size. It should not be administered intravenously because of its potent cardiac depressant effect. Codeine can also be administered orally or rectally.[38] Recently, diclofenac 1.0–1.5 mg kg^{-1} rectally every 8–12 h starting at the end of surgery has provided excellent analgesia in craniotomy patients who subsequently only require simple analgesics, but it is not to be used where there is a high risk of bleeding or impaired renal function. Paracetamol 15–20 mg kg^{-1} with a maximum dose of 90 mg kg^{-1} day^{-1} administered orally or rectally is usually sufficient after the first 24 h.

Children ventilated postoperatively will require analgesia and sedation, usually provided by low-dose morphine infusion at a maximum rate of 10 μg kg^{-1} h^{-1}, which still allows neurological assessment. Additional sedation can be provided with either midazolam infusion 2–5 μg kg^{-1} min^{-1} or diazepam 0.1 mg kg^{-1} by bolus injection.. Children undergoing spinal surgery may receive morphine infusions as either patient-controlled or nurse-controlled analgesia, which has a higher background infusion level with a longer lock-out period. This latter is particularly effective in toddlers who are reluctant to lie flat after surgery unless well sedated.

Antiemetics are not routinely required in children under 5 years of age. Ondansetron 100–200 μg kg^{-1} i.v. or 50–100 μg kg^{-1} p.o. has become the antiemetic of choice.

ANAESTHESIA FOR SPECIFIC PROCEDURES

NEONATAL SURGERY

Neurosurgery in the neonatal period, which is now defined as less than 44 weeks' gestation, is usually performed for neural tube defects, especially spina bifida, encephalocoeles and hydrocephalus, or for elevation of depressed fractures caused during a traumatic delivery.

NEURAL TUBE DEFECTS

Neural tube defects occur around the 26th day of gestation at the time of anterior neural tube closure. Lesions involving meningeal structures only may occur at a later developmental stage. While much is known about the incidence of all these defects including anencephaly, many questions remain unanswered.[39] There is considerable geographical variation in incidence both within and between countries. Many areas have reported a spontaneous decrease in incidence which cannot be explained by early antenatal diagnosis and therapeutic abortion. Approximately 10% of neural tube defects may result from a genetic mutation or chromosomal abnormality, while the remainder has a multifactorial origin. This latter group gives rise to the geographic and racial variation, while genetic cases have a similar incidence worldwide. A 72% reduction has been achieved in the incidence of neural tube defects in subsequent pregnancies conceived after treatment with daily supplements of folic acid, but no such benefit from multivitamins has been shown.[40] The aetiology of these defects still requires considerable research. Antenatal diagnosis of neural tube defects is from maternal α-fetoprotein levels or by routine ultrasonography. The former is only reliable for open defects which are more common with anencephaly and meningomyelocoeles than encephalocoeles. Ultrasound provides not only the diagnosis but also some indication of the contents of the lesion and the presence of other abnormalities such as hydrocephalus. Early diagnosis by 12–14 weeks enables discussion of therapeutic abortion. Detection late in pregnancy allows

for discussion of the optimal mode of delivery and its timing. Non-vaginal delivery may be recommended to avoid rupture of flimsy meningeal sacs or the probability of pelvic disproportion with large, solid lesions. Early delivery is sometimes recommended where hydrocephalus is present to minimize the detrimental effect of the large ventricles on the cortical mantle and subsequent cerebral function. However, the risks of prematurity and the greater potential need for intensive care for complications may outweigh any advantage of an early planned delivery. Fetal surgery has potential for transamniotic aspiration of CSF, but the risk of infection has precluded its routine use. Emergency surgery for neural tube lesions is now thought to be unnecessary except for uncovered defects, allowing formal investigation of the lesion, at least with ultrasound, but preferably with computed tomography (CT) and/or magnetic resonance imaging (MRI) scans, and the ability to confirm the presence and magnitude of other CNS abnormalities. Early surgery is recommended for large lesions and those with very flimsy coverings where there is a risk of rupture and infection, but other lesions can have surgery deferred if necessary.

Preoperative assessment should include an assessment of the ease of intubation, especially for larger spinal lesions or occipital encephalocoeles. Traditionally, the left lateral position is used for intubation, but this author prefers the more common supine position with the lesion surrounded by a stack of 'doughnut' head rings; there is no pressure on the coverings and the remainder of the head and body is supported on foam pads or folded gamgee, so that the head, neck and thorax are in a neutral position and well supported. This position not only provides optimal conditions for intubation but also ensures an unobstructed airway during preoxygenation and induction of anaesthesia. Intravenous cannulation is performed preoperatively as many babies will require intravenous fluids prior to surgery to maintain blood glucose because of slow feeding secondary to their neurological state. A standard neonatal induction technique is used either with oxygen and sevoflurane or intravenously with thiopentone 2–3 mg kg^{-1}. A gaseous induction with muscle relaxant given with light anaesthesia may be better, as even with low-dose thiopentone there may be some residual depressant effect post-operatively. Anaesthesia should be maintained with nitrous oxide in oxygen with supplemental isoflurane as necessary, usually only during skin incision to avoid the stress response to surgery.[41] In this first of many papers Anand *et al.* have demonstrated an improved outcome when the stress response to surgery is blocked by either anaesthesia or analgesia. Opioids should be avoided in this very high-risk group of patients unless postoperative ventilation is planned.

Infants under 46 weeks' gestation are at risk of postoperative apnoea[42] and this will be much higher in a neurosurgical population who already have reduced cerebral activity. Since the operations are usually performed in the prone position, great care is needed to avoid IVC compression leading to engorgement of the paraspinal veins. Many neural tube defects have associated haemangiomas in the surrounding tissues and skin which may increase bleeding. Large lesions may need rotational flaps or, rarely, tissue expanders are used to produce adequate skin cover. The base of encephalo-coeles is frequently associated with a leash of vessels which may cause massive haemorrhage from dural veins; this can be very difficult to control because of the small size of the cranial defect.

HYDROCEPHALUS

Treatment of hydrocephalus is the most common procedure in paediatric neurosurgery. It is either primary or secondary to intraventricular haemorrhage (IVH), meningitis or the Arnold–Chiari malformation associated with spina bifida (see Chapter 1). There is evidence that primary or antenatal hydrocephalus is caused by intrauterine infection or haemorrhage. Progressive hydrocephalus is diagnosed by increasing head circumference. The clinical picture of the massively enlarged head, bulging fontanelles, engorged veins and 'sunsetting' eyes is rarely seen nowadays.

After a trial period of early shunt surgery for premature infants with hydrocephalus from IVH, these patients are now treated with repeated ventricular taps either direct or after insertion of a Rickham cap and ventricular catheter. The high surgical complication rate came from raised protein levels in the CSF and low shunt flow. Many infants will still be less than 44 weeks' gestation despite having survived for 3 months in the neonatal intensive care unit and may well have other complications of prematurity, such as bronchopulmonary dysplasia or incompletely resolved necrotizing enterocolitis. Ventriculoperitoneal shunts are the usual choice but coexisting inguinal hernias, very common in premature babies, have to be repaired to prevent CSF accumulating in the sacs. The peritoneal route is avoided if there is intra-abdominal pathology for which future surgical treatment is likely. Atrial shunts are no longer used routinely because of the rare but disastrous complication of bacterial endocarditis with pulmonary emboli and the resultant pulmonary hypertension. Alternatively, the pleural route can be used, but this is usually reserved for cyst or subdural fluid drainage. If large volumes drain into the pleural cavity, respiratory embarrassment can occur.

When inserting peritoneal shunts blood loss is usually less than 10 ml and transfusion is not required. With atrial shunts the blood loss may be greater but transfusion is still not routine. There is also a potential risk of air embolism as the catheter is inserted. Cross-matched blood should be available for all children having shunts in case the enlarged dural veins are damaged during burr hole drilling, when control can be difficult to achieve with limited access. CSF losses should also be kept to a minimum as a low ICP state can develop with circulatory and respiratory effects.

Central control of temperature may also be less efficient than with normal neonates and therefore every attempt to conserve heat is required. Surgical access is required to the head, thorax and abdomen, but the modern methods of heat conservation described in Chapter 6 can be applied to the rest of the body.

Preterm infants and those with neural tube defects will require very close postoperative monitoring, not only for apnoea but also for excessive drainage of CSF, which may affect cardiac stability and result in a low cardiac output. Any preoperative respiratory support either with oxygen therapy or with pressure support is likely to require upgrading, e.g. oxygen therapy to nasal continuous positive airway pressure (CPAP), nasal CPAP to intubation with pressure support or ventilation. The risks of hyperoxia should be remembered in preterm infants. Postoperative transcutaneous oxygen monitor or pulse oximetry should be used routinely, maintaining saturations between 90 and 92%. Infants under 5 kg should only be given intramuscular codeine phosphate with great caution. Paracetamol 10–15 mg kg^{-1} rectally can be used.

Overhead heating devices and open incubators enable the baby to be observed easily without heat loss and allow minimal handling, an advantage when the infants are irritable from blood in the ventricles.

TUMOURS

Malignancy is the second most common cause of death in children after accidents and CNS tumours are second only to the leukaemias in frequency in children. However, they are still rare, with fewer than 300 new cases diagnosed each year in the UK.[43] There have been no major changes in chemotherapy and radiotherapy. The latter is not recommended in younger patients because of the devastating effect on brain development.[44] Chemotherapy allows infants to reach an age when radiotherapy can be safely administered. Survival has improved largely as a result of better general care of the child and major advances in noninvasive imaging techniques leading to earlier diagnosis and treatment. More than 60% of children with medulloblastomas now survive more than 5 years, but younger children and those with spinal seedlings at presentation have a worse outcome.

Posterior fossa tumours

More than half of the brain tumours in children occur in the posterior fossa, with a higher incidence between 1 and 8 years. Histologically, 30% are astrocytomas, 30% medulloblastomas and 30% brainstem gliomas, with 7% ependymomas. They are also in the midline so that the sitting position is usually the surgical position of choice, producing excellent conditions. Less than half of 100 consecutive patients in the author's unit between 1980 and 1984 required blood transfusions, even in those weighing less than 15 kg, and only three patients required

more than 30% of their blood volume. Between 1984 and 1988, with greater caution about blood transfusion, only 20% of patients required intraoperative transfusions and only 3% postoperative top-ups. More recently, less than 10% of patients require transfusion.

Postural hypotension is rare in children unless they are dehydrated, in which case they respond rapidly to 5 ml kg^{-1} of crystalloid. Despite this, they should be moved gradually to the full sitting position over a period of 3–4 min while monitoring the blood pressure. Careful positioning is very important for maintaining the venous pressure, preventing air embolism and to ensure a free airway, as extremes of head flexion may result in bevelling of the end of the tracheal tube against the tracheal wall. The sitting position can be used in all ages but is harder to achieve in those infants who do not sit independently and have no secondary lumbar curve. The smaller children sit with flexed legs, the smallest cross-legged in a very natural and stable position on the seat of the chair; larger ones have flexed knees and feet supported at the same level as the buttocks. Only those approaching adult size are required to have their legs semidependent and the legs can then be strapped with elastic bandages. There are no antigravity devices available for small children.

VAE is the major disadvantage of the sitting position but it can also occur in other positions, although less commonly.[45,46] Most units in the UK monitor for VAE using end-tidal CO_2. Doppler is also used but tends to be oversensitive and noise interference during diathermy precludes its use during certain periods of the operation. There is some evidence that transoesophageal echocardiography may be helpful in the early detection of VAE and especially of paradoxical emboli.[47]

Significant VAE (i.e. those causing cardiovascular symptoms) are thought to be caused by emboli greater than 0.5 ml kg^{-1} min^{-1} and therefore more significant emboli could be expected in children. This was not confirmed either at the Mayo Clinic[48] or at Great Ormond Street Hospital. In an audit of 300 consecutive cases, the incidence of VAE was less than 9%, which compares well with other reported series. Significant emboli are those that cause falls in blood pressure > 15% or changes in heart rate and dysrhythmias. Only emboli associated with an end-tidal carbon dioxide of 2.5 kPa or less are likely to cause significant changes. This emphasizes the importance of minimizing the size of the embolus and the need for immediate action by both anaesthetist and surgeon to prevent more air entering the circulation and limiting the falls in end-tidal carbon dioxide less than 1 kPa. In the author's patients VAE had no adverse effect on outcome. The outcome of patients, both adults and children, who had posterior fossa craniectomies in the sitting or horizontal positions showed improved cranial nerve function in the sitting group, presumably owing to improved surgical conditions without increased morbidity or mortality.[49]

Craniopharyngioma

Craniopharyngioma is the most common intracranial tumour of non-glial origin in children but it is nevertheless very rare, with an incidence similar to that in adults. Despite its histologically benign nature, clinically the effects are progressive with neurological and endocrinological deterioration and death due to expansion into the hypothalamus, optic nerves and pituitary stalk. The optimal method of treatment remains controversial. After an era of more radical surgical removal followed by radiotherapy almost all children demonstrate major endocrinological defects and therefore some cases are now receiving less radical treatment until symptoms warrant intervention. Depending on the nature of the pressure effects the children tend to be either very small (growth failure) or very obese (hypothalamic dysfunction). The perioperative problems with radical surgery are related to fluid balance resulting from diabetes insipidus (DI). Both central venous pressure monitoring and a urinary catheter are essential as urine volumes up to 25% of the blood volume can be produced in 1 h. Synthetic vasopressin (DDAVP) is invariably required at some stage in the postoperative course in children.[50] The DI has been shown to be due to large amounts of inactive neurohypophyseal peptides excreted in the early postoperative phase.[51] More recently, evidence of a vasopressin antagonist has been shown by the same group.[52]

Hydrocortisone ($1–2$ mg kg^{-1} every 6 h) is given perioperatively until normal postoperative adrenal function has been confirmed.

There is also an increased incidence of hyperpyrexia and seizures after craniopharyngioma surgery.

Improved results from this complex lesion will require close involvement of paediatric endocrinologists and paediatric neurosurgeons with a particular interest in this type of surgery and anaesthetists aware of the major problems with fluid balance likely to occur in the perioperative period.

Other tumours

In infants primitive neuroectodermal tumours may be extremely vascular. Despite paying meticulous attention to the provision of optimal conditions there is still a small but significant operative mortality from these procedures, in even the best hands. Morbidity from massive transfusions in children is low provided good oxygenation is maintained both before and during periods of low cardiac output. Some lesions may be suitable for preoperative embolization of large feeding vessels, in order to reduce operative blood loss.

EPILEPSY SURGERY

The recent renewal of interest in epilepsy surgery has followed improved results[53] for patients with intractable epilepsy. Unlike adults, young children will not tolerate awake surgery. Developmental delay in most older children secondary to both epilepsy and drug treatment means that many are uncooperative and require general anaesthesia. If general anaesthesia is employed it is important that electrocorticography is not affected by the technique. Less than 1 MAC isoflurane minimizes effects on the electroencephalogram and enables the lesion to be mapped. Neuromuscular function must also be monitored as anticonvulsants usually increase tolerance to neuromuscular blockade.

For awake surgery a technique involving generous local infiltration with bupivacaine combined with propofol sedation/light anaesthesia is used until co-operation is required, when the propofol is discontinued. Low-dose fentanyl is also used to decrease the response to surgical stimulation.

NEW SURGICAL DEVELOPMENTS

STEREOTACTIC SURGERY

Stereotactic surgery gains access to small, deep-seated lesions with minimal neurological morbidity. In small children the application of the headframe requires general anaesthesia and therefore this type of surgery involves moving the patient anaesthetized between the CT scanner and the operating theatre, with all the associated risks. The airway is secured with a reinforced tracheal tube prior to application of the frame, as with most small children neither mask anaesthesia nor intubation can be performed after its application. Improved portable monitoring enables transport between sites to be safely achieved and either an intravenous infusion of propofol or a free-standing isoflurane vaporizer can be used to maintain anaesthesia during transfer.

Frameless stereotaxy enables intraoperative imaging of lesions to ensure total removal and also location of normal areas. It is essential that the head is immobilized with three-point pin fixation and that image correlation is carried out using the surface anatomy of the head prior to starting surgery. This can take some time, during which there is minimal stimulation, but hypotension is rarely a problem unless the child had reduced oral intake preoperatively.

ENDOSCOPY

Ventriculoscopy for either treatment of hydrocephalus or cyst puncture is a modern surgical development. The minimally invasive surgical technique requires little anaesthesia once the burr hole has been made. Periventricular tumours can also be biopsied by this route. While experience is being gained in this recently introduced technique, the possibility of complications, especially bleeding, should be remembered when preparing these cases.

CRANIOFACIAL SURGERY

Since the pioneering work of Tessier in Paris in the late 1960s,[55] there has been rapid development of the specialty of craniofacial surgery. This type of surgery is an example *par excellence* of the benefits of a team approach to both simple and very complex problems. Most large centres now have a comprehensive craniofacial team (Table 16.2). The centralization and regionalization of these units means that expertise can be accrued, developed and applied rapidly in the quest for optimal treatment in this young subspecialty. The development of specialist skills, especially among the nursing staff who care for the children postoperatively is an additional major advantage of centralization and enables highly complex procedures to be performed with minimal morbidity. The inclusion of geneticists in the team has enabled specific diagnoses and investigation of the abnormal gene site to be carried out.[55] Research into the molecular basis of the complex craniofacial syndromes has demonstrated dysostoses with abnormal bone growth.[56] Respiratory physiologists provide information[57] about the upper airway in craniofacial syndromes which enables surgical intervention to be both planned and timed to provide optimal benefit for the patient.

In 1979 a multicentre review[58] presented the pooled results of 793 patients, both adults and children, from six centres over a 10-year period. These figures from the start of the subspecialty showed that of the 13 deaths, nine were in intracranial or orbital operations and six were in children under 4 years of age. The complication rate was also much higher at 25% for the

Table 16.2 Craniofacial team

Surgeons	
Neuro	Respiratory physicians
Plastic	Neuroradiologists
Maxillofacial	Psychologists
ENT	Speech therapists
Ophthalmic	Geneticists
Orthodontic	Paediatric anaesthetists
	Specialist nurses

intracranial procedures and only 9% in extra-cranial cases. These figures demonstrate the potential for both morbidity and mortality in complex craniofacial surgery in children.

Craniofacial patients can be divided into two groups by diagnosis,[59] those with simple, usually single-suture synostosis occurring in otherwise normal children, and those with multiple-suture stenosis who represent the syndromic group with craniofacial lesions, often total cranial stenosis, maxillary hypoplasia and proptosis and some with limb abnormalities. These latter symptoms, along with the facial appearance, help to differentiate the different syndromes such as Apert's, Crouzon's and Pfeiffer's (Table 16.3). Jones[60] responded in an editorial to the recent apparent epidemic of occipital plagiocephaly which reached the lay press,[61] concluding that this apparent increase had resulted from confusion between positional distortion and craniosynostotic plagiocephaly, neither of which usually needs surgical correction. Only a very small number of these craniosynostotic deformities needs surgical correction, which is purely cosmetic and potentially dangerous, bearing in mind the proximity of dural venous sinuses.

Simple cases (Table 16.4) usually undergo surgery in the first 6 months of life, when the skull is more malleable and better cosmetic results are achieved. There is growing evidence of significant psychological disturbance in these patients if left untreated.[62] There is also a risk of raised ICP, but while this is more commonly associated with multiple suture involvement it is not infrequent in scaphiocephaly presenting later than 1 year.

Sagittal synostosis is usually treated by wide suture excision and, apart from blood loss, is not usually associated with major complications. Coronal fusion, either single or bilateral, and metopic synostosis are corrected with a 'floating forehead' procedure.[63] Again, blood losses may be large and oculocardiac reflexes may be triggered with orbital dissection.[64] Since abandoning routine tarsorrhaphies the incidence of bradycardia is much lower in the author's practice, presumably as the pressure from scalp traction is no longer transmitted to the orbital contents. Complex cases require considerable preoperative investigation and evaluation in order to provide optimal treatment for each individual patient. A preoperative assessment is carried out by the craniofacial team and the problems are identified. From the anaesthetist's point of view, airway assessment is paramount. In the early days this consisted of taking a good history, including difficulties with feeding, failure to thrive and sleep disturbance or deprivation, leading to daytime somnolence and developmental delay. With the formalized team approach, ear, nose and throat (ENT) and respiratory care is optimized and overnight sleep studies are performed to assess upper airway obstruction (UAO) with or without frank obstructive sleep apnoea (OSA), especially in patients with maxillary hypoplasia. This is combined with 24-h ICP measurement using a Camino bolt system.[65] Initial results[66] showed that patients with unicoronal synostosis may have raised ICP but do not suffer from UAO, while in syndromic patients, most of

Table 16.3 Craniofacial syndromes

Syndrome	Features
Crouzon	Bicoronal synostosis
	Maxillary hypoplasia
	Proptosis (including globe dislocation)
Apert	Bicoronal synostosis
	Maxillary hypoplasia
	Hypertelorism
	Complex syndactyly
Pfeiffer	Bicoronal synostosis
	Maxillary hypoplasia
	Curved great toe and thumb
Saethre Chotzen	Bicoronal synostosis
	Facial asymmetry
	Low hair line
	Ptosis
	Brachydactyly

Table 16.4 Simple craniosynostoses

Suture	Deformity
Sagittal	Scaphocephaly
Unilateral coronal	Plagiocephaly
Unilateral lamdoid	Plagiocephaly
Metopic	Trigonocephaly
Bilateral coronal	Brachycephaly

whom have an associated maxillary hypoplasia, the majority has UAO and more than 50% OSA, although 40% of patients have normal ICP. These results enable surgery to be directed at the specific problems, airway improvement or vault expansion or a combined procedure.

The airway can be improved by choanal dilatation with or without bony dissection, nasal stenting, nasopharyngeal airways and nocturnal nasal CPAP. The improvement in sleep quality can result in considerable improvement in the child's development and achievement of milestones. More recent studies by Gonsalez (personal communication) have shown low levels of cerebral perfusion pressure (approx. 20 mmHg) during peaks of raised ICP combined with UAO during rapid eye movement sleep. A monobloc craniofacial advance is now thought to be the optimal surgical intervention but midfacial retraction may become the optimal treatment in the future. Tracheostomy, while avoided if possible, may be necessary to ensure a patent airway in severe cases and can also provide time for growth before planned surgical interventions. The understanding of the abnormal bone growth and cellular function in the syndromic patients has explained the high relapse rate with surgical correction when surgery is performed early. As growth continues additional procedures will be required until it is completed in the mid-teens, at which time definitive corrections can be performed for improved cosmesis. For raised ICP, posterior vault expansion is the initial operation of choice. Modern developments with imaging of the cranial vault using three-dimensional reconstructions of CT scans and MRI have improved the understanding of the complex lesions,[67] and are essential to the planning of surgical correction. Following the operative death of a child with a clover leaf skull deformity in whom all the venous drainage was found to be via the cranium and scalp, and in whom the jugular foramina were occluded leading to uncontrolled haemorrhage and brain swelling, all complex patients should have a cerebral venogram as part of the preoperative work-up.[68] This policy has resulted in the identification of another patient with non-syndromic multiple cranial synostosis in whom all the intracranial blood drained via the dural sinuses and enlarged emissary veins to the external jugular and vertebral veins.[69] This situation is a contra-indication to vault expansion surgery.

ANAESTHESIA

The evolution of the craniofacial team has resulted from the pivotal roles of craniofacial (neuro and plastic) surgeons and anaesthetists. It is essential for the anaesthetist to understand the details of the surgical technique to be employed in the individual cases and to be prepared for the associated problems, in order to minimize complications and morbidity. Following standard preoperative assessment and investigations the infants are premedicated with atropine 20 μg kg^{-1} p.o.; older children have topical local analgesic cream applied if appropriate. Sedative premedication with benzodiazepines (midazolam 0.5 mg kg^{-1}, max. 15 mg, or temazepam 0.5 mg kg^{-1}, max. 20 mg) is reserved for older children without airway compromise or markedly raised ICP. In an audit of anaesthetic management of craniofacial patients,[70] only 12 children of 126 received intravenous inductions. This is because of the abnormal limbs which are part of many of the syndromes, and also because many patients will undergo multiple surgical procedures and intravenous induction is rarely easy. The agent of choice for gaseous induction is now sevoflurane, although previously halothane was used uneventfully. Children with maxillary hypoplasia often suffer airway obstruction with light anaesthesia and serially sized Guedel airways may be needed before full airway control is achieved. After intravenous cannulation it is advisable to check inflation with a facemask prior to using muscle relaxants. Although the syndromic patients usually have easy laryngoscopy (grade I–II), marked proptosis makes forming a seal with the facemask difficult to achieve, and either a much larger or smaller one can be used, either of which will avoid pressure on the eyes.

The type of tube used will depend on the planned surgery, with either a reinforced or preformed tube being commonly utilized. Secure fixation of the tube is essential and for maxillary osteotomies mandibular intradental wiring is the most secure. Accidental extubation is a disastrous complication in this form of surgery with mobile facial bones. A throat pack may also be needed.

A balanced neuroanaesthetic technique combining analgesia and anaesthesia is used, with controlled ventilation and mild hyperventilation. The surgical stimulus during this type of major reconstructive surgery varies considerably and there can be long periods of minimal stimulation while benchwork reconstruction is performed on the free bone flaps. This, combined with the potential for torrential haemorrhage from large abnormal veins, necessitates a balanced technique including a volatile agent which can be rapidly lightened and deepened to match the prevailing conditions and avoids surges and troughs in cardiovascular parameters. Hypotensive anaesthesia is not employed routinely, but a relatively slow heart rate for age is achieved by keeping the circulation well filled and avoiding hypovolaemia.

Venous access may be difficult, especially in Apert's syndrome with 'mitten-like' syndactyly. Owing to the high risk of massive transfusion at least two free-flowing cannulae must be used, although 22 G is usually sufficient in small babies. The long saphenous or femoral veins are the preferred access route. In the audit performed by Moylan[70] the average haemoglobin levels were the same preoperatively and postoperatively, except that the latter had a larger scatter. Haemoglobin was not affected whether or not CVP was used to aid volume replacement. Direct arterial monitoring is mandatory for these cases and again, depending on the limb abnormalities, radial artery puncture may be difficult. The radial pulses can appear to be located more medially and the ulnar artery may be easier to puncture. Alternatively, the femoral route can be employed.

Standard monitoring for major surgery is used and the comparison of central and peripheral temperature is an aid to adequate volume replacement.

As already implied, much of the perioperative morbidity and even mortality is related to intraoperative haemorrhage. Moylan showed that over half the patients received transfusions greater than 50% of estimated blood volume and over 20% had exchange transfusions. Positioning can be difficult if the head is very abnormally shaped, especially when combined with a short neck. Obsessional care must be taken to avoid cerebral venous congestion by neck rotation. A moderate head-up position is usually employed, and therefore VAE is a potential risk. In practice, this is kept very low by meticulous monitoring and maintenance of normovolaemia.

Improved surgical techniques using needlepoint diathermy for dissection and improved perioperative imaging have resulted in a reduction in blood loss. Other techniques, such as adrenaline infiltration, do not appear to reduce the loss.

Postoperatively, residual muscle relaxation is reversed and the patients are extubated when breathing well. Those who have undergone maxillary surgery will require airway maintenance for at least 48 h until facial swelling reduces. This can be achieved with bilateral nasopharyngeal airways. With improved investigation and care of the airway preoperatively most patients now return to their preoperative support. However, a small additional group may need a nasal airway for the acute phase of recovery. The development of a large specialized unit in the author's hospital has given both medical and nursing staff the confidence to allow the patients to self-ventilate. Earlier, a significant proportion of patients was electively ventilated for airway reasons and now the incidence is almost zero.

Analgesia is provided with simple analgesics, paracetamol, codeine and NSAIDS (provided clotting is normal and bleeding stopped) and pain scores are surprisingly low despite the presence of marked head and facial swelling and bilateral black eyes in most cases.

Blood loss may continue into the postoperative period and it is essential to confirm that clotting is normal and treat problems as they arise when continued transfusion is required.

The advent of specialized centres has meant not only that surgical treatments have been able to develop, but also that the morbidity and mortality for complex and major surgery in small children have been markedly reduced.

SPINAL AND CRANIOCERVICAL SURGERY

Congenital spinal abnormalities of the lumbar region are relatively common, frequently with cutaneous manifestations such as a hair tuft capillary or pigmented naevus or dermal pits as the only clinical feature. The lesions are delineated with MRI and myelography is very rarely used nowadays. Surgery is to untether the cord and debulk any subcutaneous lesions, with bony removal kept to a minimum in order to prevent further spinal distortion with growth. These lesions are usually avascular with minimal transfusion requirements. Spinal monitoring may be required but this is more usual with cervical and thoracic lesions. An anaesthetic technique which allows for accurate neurophysiological studies is essential with agents known to reduce evoked potential responses, such as isoflurane used in low doses only.

Spinal tumours in childhood can be either primary or secondary, are often extremely vascular and may require large transfusions, despite optimal positioning avoiding IVC compression and induced hypotension. All surgical manipulations of the spinal cord are very potent stimuli and may be associated with dysrrhythmias and hypotension if there is inadequate anaesthesia.

Another area of surgical development is craniocervical function surgery for congenital and acquired dislocations and instability. Many congenital cases of cervical instability present after minor trauma or even surgical positioning for neck surgery, especially lymph-node biopsy.[71] There is also the well-known association of atlanto occipital instability in children with Down's syndrome.[72]

The main problem for the anaesthetist initially is maintaining anaesthesia and intubation prior to fixation of the neck in a halo jacket or surgery. The neck is best stabilized by an assistant holding the head and preventing both flexion and extension during intubation. Once the child is in the halo jacket, what might have been a grade-I laryngoscopy may no longer be straightforward. The standard laryngeal handle normally hits either the lateral rods or the top of the jacket and therefore a polio handle is very useful. Fibreoptic intubation facilities should always be available when anaesthetizing these children in halo jackets. Simple procedures, such as adjustments to the halo and imaging, can be performed safely with a laryngeal mask. The laryngeal mask may also be needed as first-line airway management in the event of cardiorespiratory collapse prior to formal reintubation.

Depending on the lesion, the surgical approach will be either posterior lateral or transoral. Following the latter approach the child remains intubated until all oral swelling has settled, usually within 24–48 h.

NEUROIMAGING

This rapidly developing field with both non-invasive and invasive procedures can provide a considerable challenge in paediatric practice. In many paediatric specialist units, major investigative procedures are traditionally performed under sedation, which needs to be tailored to the specific procedure, for example to the type and likely duration. CT scans usually require lighter sedation than MRI scans. General principles should apply to all patients being sedated for investigations. They should be starved and must be observed by someone trained in paediatric resuscitation with the equipment readily available. Minimal monitoring should always be pulse oximetry, as the problems with oximetry in MRI scanners have now been overcome. Sedation is contraindicated for patients with raised ICP, airway obstruction (actual or potential), respiratory failure including potential failure due to muscle weakness or central causes, and severe hepatic or renal dysfunction, in whom recovery may be prolonged.

In units where fewer procedures are performed on children, the time involved in achieving a good working practice for sedation may be excessive to requirements and general anaesthesia is probably more appropriate. A simple technique of light anaesthesia using a laryngeal mask airway is usually suitable for most patients, using either propofol or a volatile agent. Tracheal intubation is only required if controlled ventilation is indicated. Angiography and myelography, if performed, usually require general anaesthesia, although those aged over 12 years and of normal intelligence may tolerate myelography under local analgesia and light sedation.

Invasive radiology and embolization techniques are areas of rapid development.[73] Intracranial vascular lesions are now routinely treated by embolization, in particular vein of Galen aneurysms. The latter are lesions associated with high mortality and morbidity rates whatever the treatment. They present at various stages depending on their size and blood flow. In the neonatal period they present as cardiac failure and initially high output, and on investigation have a normal heart but a loud cranial flow murmur or bruit. In infants there is increasing head size from associated hydrocephalus, or fitting due to ischaemia of the remainder of the brain. Older children usually present with neurological deficit, again from the effect of vascular steal.

In a 5-year period to 1989, 15 patients with vein of Galen aneurysm underwent 36 embolizations with variable results, but other vascular lesions had a better outcome. Since then considerably more experience has been gained with neonatal lesions as more patients are referred for this treatment. It is now obvious that some lesions are more amenable to treatment and cure than others. This observation is confirmed by the sporadic cases in the literature of good results from surgery. Greater experience of the techniques allows for better patient selection and reduced morbidity and mortality. The procedure itself can be hazardous, with risks of intracerebral bleeding or movement of the embolus material passing through the venous system into the lungs. Strict fluid balance is kept, with volume of contrast administered and blood loss estimated during sheath and catheter insertion during the investigation. Neonates may need blood transfusion and blood should always be cross-matched for all small patients.

The actual embolization may be associated with cardiovascular instability due to direct stimulation as the embolus is disconnected from the catheter or to dramatic alterations in blood flow to the malformation. The procedures are technically very demanding for the radiologist and can be very prolonged. These patients also make considerable demands on intensive care, both before and after treatment.

REFERENCES

1 Sokoloff, L. Circulation and energy metabolism of the brain. In: Siegel, G., *et al* (eds). *Basic Neurochemistry:*

Molecular, Cellular and Chemical Aspects. New York: Raven Press, 1989: 565–91.

2 Kennedy, C. and Sokoloff, L. An adaptation of nitrous oxide method to the study of the circulation in children: normal values for cerebral blood flow and cerebral metabolic rate in childhood. *Journal of Clinical Investigation* 1957; **36**: 1130–6.

3 Mehta, S., Kalsi, H.K., Nain, C.K., *et al.* Energy metabolism of brain in human protein calorie malnutrition. *Pediatric Research* 1977; **11**: 290–3.

4 Ogawa, A., Sakurai, Y. and Kayama, Y. Regional cerebral blood flow with age: changes in rCBF in childhood. *Neurology Research* 1989; **11**: 173.

5 Lou, H.C., Lassen, N.A. and Friis-Hansen, B. Impaired autoregulation of cerebral blood flow in the distressed newborn infant. *Journal of Pediatrics* 1979; **94**: 118.

6 Wyatt J.S., Cope, M., Delpy, D.T. *et al.* Quantification of cerebral oxygenation and haemodynamics in sick newborn infants by near infrared spectrophotometry. *Lancet* 1986; **ii**: 1063–6.

7 Gregory, G., Ong, B., Tweed, W., *et al.* Hyperventilation restores autoregulation in the cerebral circulation in the neonate. *Anesthesiology* 1983; **59**: 427.

8 Rubin, R.C., Henderson, E.S., Onimaya, A.K., *et al.* The production of cerebrospinal fluid in man and its modification by acetazolamide. *Journal of Neurosurgery* 1966; **25**: 430.

9 Welch, K. The intracranial pressure in infants. *Journal of Neurosurgery* 1980; **52**: 693.

10 Shapiro, K. and Marmarou, A. Mechanism of intracranial hypertension in children. In: McLauren, R., *et al.* (eds). *Pediatric Neurosurgery.* Philadelphia, PA: WB Saunders, 1989: 338–52.

11 Smerling, A. Hypertonic saline in head trauma. A new recipe for drying and salting. *Journal of Neurosurgical Anesthesiology* 1992; **4**: 1.

12 Fisher, B., Thomas, D., Peterson, B., *et al.* Hypertonic saline lowers raised ICP in children after head trauma. *Journal of Neurosurgical Anesthesiology* 1992; **4**: 4–10.

13 Nightingale, D.A., Richards, C.C. and Glass, A. An evaluation of rebreathing in a modified T-piece during controlled ventilation of anaesthetised children. *British Journal of Anaesthesia* 1965; **37**: 762–71.

14 Swedlow, D.B. Anesthesia for neurosurgical procedures. In: Gregory, G.A. (ed.). *Pediatric Anesthesia.* New York: Churchill Livingstone, 1983; **2**: 679–706.

15 Vessey, J.A., Bogetz, M.S., Caserza, L.C. *et al.* Parental upset associated with participation in induction of anaesthesia in children. *Canadian Journal of Anaesthesia* 1994; **41**: 276–80.

16 Leon, J.E. and Bissonnette, B. Transcranial Doppler sonography: nitrous oxide and cerebral blood flow velocity in children. *Canadian Journal of Anaesthesia* 1991; **38**: 974.

17 Scheller, M.S., Tateisha, A., Drummond, J.C., *et al.* The effect of sevoflurane on cerebral blood flow, cerebral metabolic rate for oxygen, intracranial pressure, and the electroencephalogram are similar to those of isoflurane in the rabbit. *Anesthesiology* 1988; **68**: 548.

18 White, M. and Kenny, G. Intravenous propofol anaesthesia using a computerised infusion system. *Anaesthesia* 1990; **45**: 204–9.

19 Sammartino, M., Pelosi, G., Pietrini, D., *et al*. Pediatric neuroanesthesia computerized monitoring system. *Acta Anaesthesiologica Belgica* 1989; **40**: 53–7.

20 Committee on Safety of Medicines. *Current Problems* 1992; 34.

21 Hatch, D.J. Propofol in paediatric intensive care. *British Journal of Anaesthesia* 1997; **79**: 274–5.

22 Moss, E., Powell, D., Gibson, R.M., *et al*. Effects of fentanyl on intracranial pressure and cerebral perfusion pressure during hypocapnia. *British Journal of Anaesthesia* 1978; **50**: 779–84.

23 Moss, E. Alfentanil increases intracranial pressure when intracranial compliance is low. *Anaesthesia* 1992; **47**: 134–6.

24 Marx, W., Shah, N., Long, C., *et al*. Sufentanil, alfentanil and fentanyl: impact on CSF in patients with brain tumors. *Anesthesiology* 1988; **69A**: 627.

25 Guy, J., Hindman, B.J., Baker, K.Z., *et al*. Comparison of remifentanil and fentanyl in patients undergoing craniotomy for supratentorial space occupying lesions. *Anesthesiology* 1997; **86**: 514–24.

26 Black, A. and Mackersie, A. Accidental bronchial intubation with RAE tubes. *Anaesthesia* 1991; **46**: 42–3.

27 Beasley, J. Difficulty with a preformed tube in a neonate. *Paediatric Anaesthesia* 1997; **7**: 431.

28 McDonald, D., McCormick, A., Mackerase, A., *et al*. Difficulty with a preformed tube in a neonate. *Paediatric Anaesthesia* 1997; **7**: 87.

29 Lindahl, S., Yates, A. and Hatch, D.J. Relationship between invasive and non-invasive measurements of gas exchange in anesthetized infants and children. *Anesthesiology* 1987; **66**: 168–75.

30 Uppington, J. and Goat, V. Anaesthesia for major craniofacial surgery: a report of 23 cases in children under 4 years of age. *Annals of the Royal College of Surgeons of England* 1987; **69**: 175–8.

31 Boris-Moller, F., Smith, M. and Siesjo, B.K. Effects of hypothermia on ischaemic brain damage: a comparison between pre ischaemic and post ischaemic cooling. *Neurosciences Research Committee* 1989; **5**: 87–93.

32 Berntman, L., Welsh, F.A., Harp, J.R. *et al*. Cerebral protective effect of low-grade hypothermia. *Anesthesiology* 1981; **55**: 495–8.

33 Wass, T., Lanier, W.L., Hofer, R.E., *et al*. Temperature changes of > 1°C alter functional neurologic outcome and opathology in a canine model of complete cerebral ischemia. *Anesthesiology* 1995; **83**: 325–35.

34 Zornow, M.H., Scheller, M.S., Todd, M.M., *et al*. Acute cerebral effects of isotonic crystalloid and colloid solutions following cryogenic brain injury in the rabbit. *Anesthesiology* 1988; **69**: 180–4.

35 Lam, A.M., Winn, R.H., Cullen, B.F., *et al*. Hyperglycaemia and neurological outcome in patients with head injury. *Journal of Neurosurgery* 1991; **75**: 545.

36 Brown, K.A., Bissonnette, B., McIntyre, B., *et al*. Hyperkalaemia during rapid blood transfusion and hypovolaemic cardiac arrest in children. *Canadian Journal of Anaesthesia* 1990; **37**: 747–54.

37 Sigston, P., Hack, H.A., Jenkins, A.M.C., *et al*. A comparison of rectal and intramuscular codeine phosphate in children following neurosurgery. *Paediatric Anaesthesia* 1999 (in press).

38 Sellars, M.J. Unanswered questions on neural tube defects. *British Medical Journal* 1987; **294**: 1–2.

39 MRC Vitamin Research Group. Prevention of neural tube defects: results of the Medical Research Council Vitamin Study. *Lancet* 1991; **338**: 131–5.

40 Anand, K., Sippell, W.G. and Aynsley-Green, A. Randomized trial of fentanyl anaesthesia in preterm babies undergoing surgery: effects on the stress response. *Lancet* 1987; **i**: 243–8.

41 Steward, D. Preterm infants are more prone to complications following minor surgery than are term infants. *Anesthesiology* 1982; **56**: 304–6.

42 Stiller, C.A. Population based survival rates for childhood cancer in Britain 1980–91. *British Medical Journal* 1994; **309**: 1612–16.

43 Duffner, P.K., Horowitz, M.E., Krischer, J.P., *et al*. Postoperative chemotherapy and delayed radiation in children less than 3 years of age with malignant brain tumors. *New England Journal of Medicine* 1993; **328**: 1725–31.

44 Harris, M., Strafford, M.A., Rowe, R.W, *et al*. Venous air embolism and cardiac arrest during craniectomy in a supine infant. *Anesthesiology* 1986; **65**: 547–50.

45 Kelleher, A. and Mackersie, A. Cardiac arrest and resuscitation of a six month old achondroplastic baby undergoing neurosurgery in the prone position. *Anaesthesia* 1995; **50**: 348–51.

46 Cucchiara, R., Nugent, M., Seward, J.B., *et al*. Air embolism in upright neurosurgical patients: detection and localization by two dimensional transesophageal echocardiography. *Anesthesiology* 1984; **60**: 353–5.

47 Cucchiara, R. and Bowers, B. Air embolism in children undergoing suboccipital craniectomy. *Anesthesiology* 1982; **57**: 338–9.

48 Harrison, E., *et al*. (in press).

49 Black, S., Ockert, D.B., Oliver, W.C., *et al*. Outcome following posterior fossa craniectomy in patients in the sitting or horizontal positions. *Anesthesiology* 1988; **69**: 49.

50 Yasargil, M., Curcic, M., Kis, M., *et al*. Total removal of craniopharyngiomas. *Journal of Neurosurgery* 1990; **73**: 3–11.

51 Seckl, J.R., Dunger, D.B., Lightman, S.L., *et al*. Neurophyphyseal function during early postoperative diabetes insipidus. *Brain* 1987; **110**: 737–46.

52 Seckl, J.R., Dunger, D.B., Bevan, J.S., *et al*. Vasopressin antagonist in early postoperative diabetes insipidus. *Lancet* 1990; **335**: 1353–6.

53 Sperling, M., O'Connor, M.J., Saykin, A.J., *et al*. Temporal lobectomy for refractory epilepsy. *Journal of the American Medical Association* 1996; **276**: 470–5.

54 Tessier, P., Guiot, G., Raigerie, J., *et al*. Osteotomies cranio-naso-orbito-facial. Hypertelorisme. *Annales de Chirogie Plastique* 1967; **12**: 103–18.

55 Reardon, W., Wilkes, D., Rutland, P., *et al*. Craniosynostosis associated with FGFR3 pro 250 arg mutation in a range of clinical presentations including unisutural sporadic craniosynostosis. *Journal of Medical Genetics* 1997; **8**: 632–6.

56 Reardon, W., Winter, R.M., Rutland, P., *et al*. Mutations in fibroblast growth factor receptor 2 gene caused Crouzon's syndrome. *Nature Genetics* 1994; **8**: 98–103.

57 Gonsalez, S., Lane, R.J., Stocks, J., *et al*. Upper airway obstruction and raised intracranial pressure in craniosynostosis. *European Respiratory Journal* 1997; **10**: 367–75.

58 Whitaker, L., Munro, I.R., Salyer, K.E., *et al*. Combined report of problems and complications in 793 craniofacial operations. *Plastic and Reconstructive Surgery* 1979; **64**: 198–203.

59 Thompson, D., Jones, B., Hayward, R., *et al*. Assessment and treatment of craniosynostosis. *British Journal of Hospital Medicine* 1994; **52**: 17–24.

60 Jones, B.M., Hayward, R., Erans, R., *et al*. Occipital plagiocephaly: an epidemic of craniosynostosis? *British Medical Journal* 1997; **315**: 693–4.

61 Ortega, R. Unkind cut. *Wall Street Journal* 1996; 29 Feb. **A:** 1–5.

62 Fehlow, P. Craniosynostosis as a risk factor. *Child's Nervous System* 1993; **9**: 325–7.

63 Marchac, D., Renier, D. and Jones, B.M. Experience with the 'floating forehead'. *British Journal of Plastic Surgery* 1988; **41**: 1–15.

64 Flandin-Blety, C. Anaesthesia and intensive care for craniofacial surgery in children. In: Marchac, D. and Renier, D. (eds). *Craniofacial Surgery for Craniosynostoses*. Boston, MA: Little Brown, 1982: 39–45.

65 Thompson, D.N.P., Harkness, W., Jones, B., *et al*. Subdural intracranial pressure monitoring in craniosynostosis. *Child's Nervous System* 1995; **11**: 269–75.

66 Mackersie, A., Gosalez, S., Lane, R.J., *et al*. The relationship between intracranial pressure and airway obstruction in craniofacial patients during sleep. *Proceedings of 9th European Congress of Anaesthesiologists*, 1994.

67 Hayward, R., Harkness, W., Kendall, B., *et al*. Magnetic resonance imaging in the assessment of craniosynostosis. *Scandanavian Journal Reconstructive Hand Surgery* 1992; **26**: 293–9.

68 Thompson, D. Lessons from a case of Kleeblattschadel. Case report. *Journal of Neurosurgery* 1995; **82**: 1071–4.

69 Anderson, P., Harkness, W., Taylor, W., *et al*. Anomalous venous drainage in a case of non-syndromic craniosynostosis. *Child's Nervous System* 1997; **13**: 97–100.

70 Moylan, S., Collee, G., Mackersie, A., *et al*. Anaesthetic management of paediatric craniofacial surgery. A review of 126 cases. *Paediatric Anaesthesia* 1993; **3**: 275–81.

71 Casey, A., O'Brien, M., Kumar, V., *et al*. Don't twist my child's head off: iatrogenic cervical dislocation. *British Medical Journal* 1995; **311**: 1212–13.

72 Mitchell, V., Howard, R. and Facer, E. Down's syndrome and anaesthesia. *Paediatric Anaesthesia* 1995; **5**: 379–84.

73 Taylor, W. and Rodesch, G. Interventional neuroradiology. *British Medical Journal* 1995; **311**: 789–92.

CHAPTER 17

Anaesthesia for ear, nose and throat surgery

ELIZABETH JACKSON AND ELSPETH FACER

INTRODUCTION

Minor ear, nose and throat (ENT) procedures in children are commonplace and frequently take place in centres where little other paediatric surgery is performed. Although many operations are short and simple, the potential for both anaesthetic and surgical complications is great, particularly in procedures where surgeon and anaesthetist share the airway. Diagnostic procedures in infants and small babies with upper airways obstruction require considerable anaesthetic expertise, and the importance of co-operation and understanding between surgeon and anaesthetist during these procedures cannot be overemphasized.

GENERAL CONSIDERATIONS

PREOPERATIVE CONSIDERATIONS

Many minor ENT operations are performed on a day-stay basis, often on dedicated day-surgery lists. Anaesthetic preadmission clinics are an alternative to performing full preoperative assessments on the day of surgery.

Particularly common in ENT practice is the child with the 'snuffly' nose.[1] This is often a feature of adenoidal hypertrophy and should not be a contraindication to surgery. It should be distinguished from an acute upper respiratory tract infection (URTI). General anaesthesia in the presence of an URTI, particularly if tracheal intubation is required, may result in an increased incidence of laryngeal spasm on induction and emergence, and an increased risk of postoperative lower respiratory tract infections.[2]

Upper airways obstruction of varying degrees at the nasal, pharyngeal or laryngeal level may be present in many patients, so it is particularly important for the anaesthetist to see all children to assess the degree of any respiratory obstruction. Anticipating a difficult airway problem and being suitably prepared in the anaesthetic room will go a long way to reducing anaesthetic complications.

The anaesthetist should also be alerted to any unusual conditions or syndromes known to be associated with airway and intubation difficulties. These include the Pierre Robin anomalad, hemifacial microsomia (Goldenhar syndrome), Treacher Collins syndrome and the mucopolysaccharidoses.

Bleeding from the tonsillar fossa or vascular tissues in the nose can result in serious morbidity. A history of a bleeding tendency in the child or the family is important, as a bleeding disorder may as yet be undiagnosed in a small child. If there is any doubt at all, coagulation studies should be carried out preoperatively.

Direct questioning about loose teeth is wise, as these can be dislodged during anaesthesia and accidentally inhaled or swallowed. It may be advisable to remove a very loose tooth following induction to prevent such accidents.

PREMEDICATION

Premedication should be tailored to suit the preoperative status of the patient and the intended anaesthetic technique. The special considerations in ENT surgery are the presence of upper airway obstruction and the need to control secretions if topical anaesthesia is to be used to facilitate endoscopy.

Most school-age children undergoing minor ENT surgery do not require sedation. Preschool children and older children who are particularly anxious or undergoing major surgery may benefit from an oral sedative such as midazolam. Sedatives should be avoided in patients with disturbed sleep patterns due to chronic upper airways obstruction and those with less severe obstruction due to pre-existing maxillofacial deformities. Sedation should also usually be avoided in patients for endoscopy, especially if they have signs of possible upper airways obstruction.

Many patients with airway pathology require repeat procedures at regular intervals over a prolonged period. Their preoperative preparation requires special attention. It is helpful if the same anaesthetist is involved each time so that he or she may get to know the patient and parents. Most families prefer a well-defined anaesthetic plan that does not vary from week to week. The precarious nature of the airway may be a contraindication to sedative premedication and this reinforces the need for meticulous psychological preparation.

Patients for endoscopy and those in whom airway difficulties are anticipated should receive an antisialogogue preoperatively. Atropine is the most frequently used drug and may be given orally or intramuscularly. As intramuscular administration results in a more predictable effect than oral administration[3] this route is often preferred, especially for small babies undergoing diagnostic endoscopy.

Topical anaesthetic cream should be considered for all children in whom an intravenous induction is planned.

MONITORING

Nowhere in paediatric anaesthetic practice is monitoring more important than in paediatric otolaryngology. Frequently, the theatre lighting is dimmed during use of the microscope or headlight. The patient may be almost totally covered in drapes, and when the airway is being shared there is always the potential for hypoxia, whether due to inadequate ventilation, kinking of a tracheal tube or accidental displacement of a tracheal tube or laryngeal mask airway.

Monitoring requires close clinical observation, including auscultation, combined with pulse oximetry, electrocardiography (ECG), blood pressure measurement and inspired and expired gas analysis. Airway pressure monitoring and a disconnect alarm are necessary if a mechanical ventilator is used. During endoscopic procedures capnography may be unreliable owing to difficulties in sampling expired gases.

POSTOPERATIVE CARE

As many ENT operations involve the airway, nursing care during the recovery period must be of the highest standard, so that danger signals are recognized early and appropriate action taken before serious complications occur. When there may be blood in the pharynx (e.g. after adenotonsillectomy and nasal operations) patients should be nursed not only on their side, but also with a pillow under the chest, so that any blood will run out of the mouth or nose. Blood running on to the larynx may result in laryngeal spasm or lead to obstruction by a blood clot. No patient should be returned to the ward until full recovery has taken place.

OPERATIONS ON THE EAR

MYRINGOTOMY AND INSERTION OF GROMMETS

The treatment of recurrent otitis media and persistent middle-ear effusions, with surgical myringotomies and insertion of ventilation tubes, is a very common surgical procedure and well suited to day-case surgery. Some patients, however, such as those with mucopolysaccharidoses or craniofacial anomalies, may require overnight stay.

Maintenance of anaesthesia with a laryngeal mask airway (LMA) provides good operating conditions.[4] Intubation is rarely required, even when the external auditory meatus is very narrow making surgical access difficult. Simple analgesics such as paracetamol or non-steroidal anti-inflammatory drugs (NSAIDs) are satisfactory for postoperative pain, which mainly results from trauma to the external auditory canal.

SURGERY FOR CONGENITAL DEFECTS OF THE EAR

Children with congenital defects of the external ears present for bone-anchored hearing aids and less commonly for surgery to form an external auditory meatus.[5] These congenital defects are associated with two important syndromes: Treacher Collins and Goldenhar syndrome (or hemifacial microsomia). Treacher Collins is an autosomal dominant mandibulofacial dysosto-

sis which includes severe mandibular hypoplasia and malformation of the pinna and external auditory meatus. In Goldenhar syndrome, in addition to unilateral hypoplasia of the malar, maxilla and mandible, there is deformity or absence of the pinna, external auditory meatus and middle ear. Congenital heart disease is common in Goldenhar syndrome.

These children are often difficult to intubate, although anaesthesia can usually be managed using laryngeal mask airway. The surgery is superficial and the procedures are uncomplicated.

MYRINGOPLASTY, EXPLORATION OF THE MIDDLE EAR AND MASTOIDECTOMY

Myringoplasty and exploration of the middle ear may be required when infection has badly damaged the tympanic membrane. Exploration of the mastoid air cells for removal of infected tissue or cholesteatoma is rare today. There are three special concerns with this type of surgery: bleeding, graft displacement and preservation of the facial nerve.

The operating microscope is used for these procedures, making even small amounts of blood troublesome. Venous bleeding due to raised venous pressure in the superior vena cava or internal jugular vein is usually the result of partial airways obstruction during spontaneous respiration, raised mean airway pressure during intermittent positive pressure ventilation (IPPV) or abdominal compression. Arterial bleeding in children is related more to heart rate and cardiac output than directly to peak systolic pressure. A stormy induction with crying, coughing and straining will increase catecholamine secretion, producing an increase in pulse rate and cardiac output which may last for up to 30 min. Meticulous attention to detail is therefore necessary if a bloodless field is to be obtained. Induction should be smooth, avoiding coughing, straining and hypertension at intubation. Agents that cause tachycardia should be avoided. The use of a muscle-relaxant, modest dose of opioid and IPPV with a volatile agent is recommended. The patient should be positioned in the 15–20° head-up position. With this approach a systolic pressure of 80–90 mmHg and good conditions are obtained in the majority of cases.

Hypotensive agents are seldom required. However, if necessary, labetolol in a dose of 0.2 mg kg^{-1} repeated to a maximum of 1 mg kg^{-1} may be given. Owing to its β-blocking effect it should be avoided in asthmatics.

Nitrous oxide is much more soluble than nitrogen; therefore, in closed body cavities it diffuses in and out much more rapidly than nitrogen. When nitrous oxide is discontinued, at the end of an anaesthetic, pressure in the middle ear will fall as nitrous oxide diffuses out more quickly than nitrogen diffuses in. As a result, a negative pressure will be applied to any tympanic membrane graft. If the surgeon wishes to avoid this, nitrous oxide should be avoided or discontinued 20 min before the middle-ear space is closed.

Where a postauricular incision is used for middle-ear surgery the surgeon has to take great care to avoid facial nerve damage and may wish to use a nerve stimulator. In this case neuromuscular function must be maintained while the facial nerve is identified.

Ear surgery is not usually very painful postoperatively and can usually be managed with codeine phosphate (1 mg kg^{-1}) and simple analgesics. Antiemetics should be prescribed.

COCHLEAR IMPLANTATION

Cochlear implants are used for the treatment of severe to profound sensorineural hearing loss in children who have not benefited from conventional hearing aids. A cochlear implant consists of an externally worn speech processor and headset and a surgically implanted receiver–stimulator that electrically stimulates the spiral ganglion cells of the cochlear nerve, resulting in auditory perception.[6]

The anaesthetic considerations are the same as for other middle-ear surgery, although the procedure is often quite prolonged. Monopolar diathermy must not be used in the vicinity of the implant as it destroys the device.

OPERATIONS ON THE NOSE, NASOPHARYNX AND PHARYNX

CHOANAL ATRESIA

Choanal atresia is a membranous or bony occlusions of the posterior nares and may be unilateral or bilateral. Some 60% of cases are associated with one or more congenital anomalies, including the CHARGE association.[7] As most neonates are obligate nose breathers bilateral atresia causes acute respiratory distress in the neonatal period. Unless an oral airway is inserted the baby may become hypoxic and may die. The airway is taped to the baby's cheeks and orogastric tube-feeding is provided until surgery is undertaken at 1–2 days (Figure 17.1).

After surgery, the stents provide a patent nasal airway and are removed after approximately 6–8 weeks. Patency must be maintained by careful suctioning. These children often require subsequent dilatations and may need

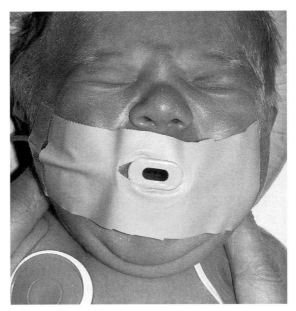

Figure 17.1 Neonate with bilateral choanal atresia showing oral airway and orogastric feeding tube taped in place.

further surgery in later infancy and childhood, although procedures present no special anaesthetic problems.

Acute respiratory distress is not a feature of unilateral choanal atresia, which usually presents later in childhood with persistent unilateral nasal discharge. Surgery can be performed electively and presents no special problems.

ADENOTONSILLECTOMY

Adenotonsillectomy is one of the most common operations carried out in children. The main indications for adenoidectomy and tonsillectomy are recurrent throat infections, adenotonsillar hypertrophy with upper airway obstruction and obstructive sleep apnoea (OSA). Occasionally, tonsillectomy is indicated during incision and drainage of a peritonsillar abscess (quinsy).

Adenotonsillar hypertrophy is the most common cause of upper airway obstruction in children. Children with congenital or acquired craniofacial abnormalities, including Down's syndrome, achondroplasia and the mucopolysaccharidoses, may have upper airway obstruction with lesser degrees of hypertrophy. Children with neuromuscular disease may have upper airway dysfunction that results from hypotonia or spasticity exacerbated by adenotonsillar hypertrophy.[8]

Severe adenotonsillar hypertrophy may cause OSA, which is characterized by restless sleep and snoring with apnoeic pauses. The sleep disturbance may result in behavioural problems. Occasionally, chronic upper airways obstruction leads to disordered central control of respiration[9–11] with hypoxia and hypercarbia that may, in turn, result in pulmonary vasoconstriction with right ventricular hypertrophy and, rarely, right heart failure.[12] Adenotonsillectomy is usually curative.[13] Children undergoing surgery for upper airway obstruction are generally younger than those undergoing surgery for recurrent infection.

Economic factors have seen day-case tonsillectomy established as standard practice in the USA and Canada. It has been shown to be a safe alternative to inpatient surgery provided there is careful patient selection, meticulous surgical technique and strict patient observation in the immediate postoperative period. In the early series observation periods of 6–12 h were usually recommended. More recent publications suggest that shorter periods of observation (5 h) are satisfactory.[14,15] Parents must be given clear instructions for homecare and support must be rapidly available if required. Although several centres in the UK have now established day-stay tonsillectomy services, it remains common practice for children to stay in hospital overnight after tonsillectomy. Many patients in the UK may prefer overnight stay or require overnight admission for social reasons.[16] Adenoidectomy is more commonly carried out on a day-care basis.

The preoperative assessment of children for adenotonsillectomy should include questioning about sleep pattern to identify children with OSA. Children with severe chronic symptoms require ECG and echocardiographic assessment for right heart changes. The diagnosis is usually clinical and sleep studies are seldom required. Children with sleep apnoea are at risk of apnoea and hypoxaemia in the postoperative period and require careful postoperative observation including pulse oximetry. The most severely affected children may require supplemental oxygen and a nasopharyngeal airway. Occasionally, nasal continuous positive airway pressure (CPAP) or even intubation is needed.[17] Overnight observation is recommended for patients under 2–3 years of age and for those with severe upper airway obstruction, cor pulmonale, craniofacial abnormalities affecting the airway, failure to thrive, hypotonia, morbid obesity or chronic medical problems.[8,17]

There is considerable variation in the anaesthetic technique chosen for adenotonsillectomy. Children with OSA should not receive sedation and they need to be wide awake at the end of the procedure. A technique using a muscle relaxant, tracheal intubation, intermittent positive pressure ventilation and minimal use of opioids is therefore appropriate. Children without OSA may be allowed to breathe spontaneously and extubated when deeply anaesthetized if preferred. A short-acting relaxant may be used to facilitate intubation. During induction, the airway of a child with nasal or pharyngeal obstruction due to large adenoids may be difficult to maintain, although it is helped by applying CPAP. Keeping the mouth slightly open under the mask will often help until the child is sufficiently anaesthetized to allow insertion of an oral airway.

Adenotonsillectomy requires a secure airway which must be protected from soiling by blood and debris. Prior to the introduction of the armoured LMA in 1990 tracheal intubation was standard for anaesthesia for adenotonsillectomy. Preformed plastic RAE tubes are satisfactory but may become compressed by the mouth gag if the gag is too short or opened excessively. The problem is greatest with the smallest tube sizes. Inability to remove the gag without extubating the patient due to wedging of the tube in the split in the blade has also been reported.[18]

The LMA can be placed without the aid of muscle relaxants, attains a gas-tight seal up to 2 kPa (20 cmH$_2$O) and has been shown to protect the larynx from dye placed in the pharynx. The LMA is usually well tolerated until the return of protective reflexes. A number of studies has claimed that the LMA has certain advantages over tracheal intubation for adenotonsillectomy.[19–21] These studies have been performed on ASA 1 and 2 patients. The major advantage of the LMA is that it can be left in place to secure and protect the airway during the recovery period until the return of the patient's reflexes. The choice between extubating at a deep plane of anaesthesia, leaving the airway unprotected, and extubating when the patient is awake, increasing the risk of coughing and postoperative laryngospasm, is thus avoided.[22]

If the LMA is to be used it is important to have the full co-operation of the surgeon. Although when correctly positioned the cuff is not visible with the gag *in situ* its presence means that positioning of the gag requires some additional skill. The success rate with the LMA for tonsillectomy increases with experience. Common problems include laryngospasm during placement of the mouth gag. This can be avoided by increasing the depth of anaesthesia prior to insertion of the gag and ensuring that manual inflation of the lungs is possible before allowing the operation to proceed. The mouth gag may cause obstruction. This is usually due to the LMA being too large or the surgeon using too long a blade. The blade either pushes the mask down into the pharynx or passes behind the mask and pushes it against the laryngeal inlet. Either repositioning of the gag or the use of a smaller gag is usually successful, otherwise tracheal intubation is required.

Airway problems can occur during recovery and removal of the mask. Problems are minimized if, at the end of surgery, a bite block is placed and the patient recovered in the lateral position. Excessive stimulation and suction should be avoided and the patient allowed to expel the LMA with the cuff still inflated so that any blood that has collected above the LMA is removed with it. Although the LMA may be satisfactory for many patients it may not be suitable for the smaller children with abnormal anatomy or other complicating factors.

Blood volume should be calculated (75 ml kg^{-1}) and a careful watch kept on blood loss. Blood loss depends on surgical technique. With modern cautery methods it is unusual for volume replacement to be necessary, even in small children. Intravenous access is always required and should be left *in situ* in case of bleeding in the immediate postoperative period.

It is sensible to give intravenous fluids in all children to counter the effects of preoperative fluid deprivation. Intravenous fluids are especially important when there is continuing bleeding, vomiting or excess insensible loss during hot weather. Very small children should receive fluids. Fluids are frequently given to children being managed as day cases.

Postoperative analgesia with a combination of paracetamol, NSAIDs (e.g. diclofenac or ibuprofen) and codeine phosphate started intraoperatively is satisfactory for most children. Codeine phosphate may be given intramuscularly or rectally intraoperatively. Intravenous opioids may be used intraoperatively but are associated with an increased incidence of postoperative nausea and vomiting. Opioid drugs should be avoided if possible in children with OSA. Increased blood loss after adenotonsillectomy has been demonstrated with NSAIDs in some studies but the clinical significance is not clear.[23] It is recommended that NSAIDs be avoided in patients where there is increased intraoperative blood loss or reduced platelet function and in children in whom postoperative bleeding poses special risks.[23] NSAIDs should be avoided in children with proven asthma receiving regular maintenance treatment or with a history of previous hospitalization, especially if associated with nasal polyps, severe eczema or atopy.[23] However, NSAIDs may reasonably be used in asthmatic children with a history of previous uncomplicated exposure to this class of drugs. Some centres advocate intraoperative infiltration of the tonsillar bed with 0.25% bupivacaine to reduce postoperative analgesic requirements.[24,25]

Postoperative nausea and vomiting can be a significant problem after adenotonsillectomy, especially for children receiving day care.[26–28] Prophylactic antiemetics should be considered, particularly if opioids are given. Ondansetron 100 μg kg^{-1} has been shown to be effective in reducing the incidence of nausea and vomiting after adenotonsillectomy.[26]

Patients undergoing adenotonsillectomy should be recovered in the classic 'tonsillar' position, head-down and on their side until awake. Postoperative care must be of a high standard, and the child should be returned to the ward fully awake, with no bleeding and with a good cough reflex.

POSTOPERATIVE BLEEDING

The incidence of primary haemorrhage requiring reoperation after adenotonsillectomy has been estimated at 0.5–1%.[29,30] The decision to return the child to theatre should be made promptly, as a delay of several hours to see whether the bleeding improves is a dangerous practice and will increase the chance of transfusion being required.

Early signs of blood loss include slow capillary refill, pallor and tachycardia. Restlesness, confusion and hypotension indicate severe losses. It is easy to underestimate losses as large amounts of blood may have been swallowed. Blood should be cross-matched early and volume replacement undertaken with crystalloid, colloid or blood, depending on the severity of the losses. A full blood count and coagulation screen should be performed in case there is an undiagnosed bleeding disorder.

Hypovolaemia should usually be fully corrected prior to induction of anaesthesia as induction of anaesthesia in the presence of hypovolaemia may precipitate cardiovascular collapse. Even if in the hypovolaemic child blood loss is so brisk that immediate surgery is necessary, resuscitation must precede induction of anaesthesia.

Once normovolaemia has been restored, the main anaesthetic problems to consider are that the child will have a full stomach as a result of swallowed blood and that the presence of blood may make laryngoscopy and intubation difficult. Preparation of the operating theatre should include checking that two suction devices with wide-bore tubing are available to remove blood clots. The first sucker may become blocked just when it is most needed. Spare laryngoscopes are necessary as the bulbs may become obscured with blood. Tracheal tubes of smaller sizes than the one used for the first operation should be prepared, as postoperative oedema may have reduced the size of the airway.

There is little agreement on the safest anaesthetic technique for a bleeding tonsil; whether an intravenous or inhalational technique should be used, whether the patient should be supine or lateral and whether relaxants should be used. Probably the most important factor is that the anaesthetist should be aware of the problems and use a technique with which he or she is familiar. Induction of anaesthesia is probably safest with the patient in the head-down, lateral position on the operating table, with the surgeon standing by. If the anaesthetist has never intubated a patient in the lateral position, the supine position may be justified.

Most anaesthetists recommend a rapid sequence induction using an intravenous induction agent and suxamethonium with preoxygenation and cricoid pressure. Others prefer inhalational induction with halothane or sevoflurane in oxygen. Once the child is anaesthetized a laryngoscope blade is gently introduced on to the tongue and the bleeding assessed. Provided it is not excessive and the patient is well oxygenated with no signs of obstruction, the mask is reapplied to ensure full oxygenation, then suxamethonium is given and cricoid pressure applied until the trachea is intubated. Ventilation via a facemask should be avoided as it may precipitate massive regurgitation of blood clot from the stomach. Intubation under deep volatile anaesthesia without relaxants may be used. However, cardiovascular collapse may occur if hypovolaemia has been inadequately corrected, and if intubation is attempted too soon laryngospasm may occur, resulting in dangerous hypoxia. During surgery the patient should be closely monitored and further fluids and blood transfused as necessary. Prior to extubation a wide-bore orogastric tube should be passed under direct vision to empty the stomach. Extubation should be in the lateral tonsillar position with the child fully awake.

Serious bleeding from the adenoid bed may require a postnasal pack to be left *in situ* for 24–48 h. In small children this necessitates that they remain sedated and intubated in an intensive care unit, as they are otherwise very restless and at risk of airway obstruction.

ENDOSCOPY

Most infants referred for diagnostic laryngoscopy and bronchoscopy, and treatment if indicated, have mild to moderate airway obstruction. Stridor is usually the presenting feature and the type of stridor, together with the history of onset and medical background give a clue as to the likely cause. A preoperative chest X-ray, lateral X-ray of the neck and barium swallow or echocardiogram may provide additional information (see Chapter 18)

Planning the anaesthetic requires a clear understanding of the patient's medical condition and the likely airway pathology. It is essential that there is close co-operation between the surgeon and the anaesthetist because, unless the surgical requirements are met, an accurate diagnosis, particularly of dynamic airway pathology is impossible.

Requirements for diagnostic laryngoscopy are a still, spontaneously breathing patient who can be maintained almost awake and without laryngospasm so that careful assessment of cord and cricoarytenoid movement can be made. To allow an unobstructed view of the larynx much of the examination must be made without the safety of a tracheal tube. Assisted or controlled ventilation may provide satisfactory conditions during bronchoscopy but spontaneous ventilation is necessary if bronchoma-

lacia or tracheomalacia are suspected. The most common technique uses spontaneous ventilation with a volatile anaesthetic agent in oxygen in combination with topical anaesthesia.

Before embarking on an endoscopy on a child with upper airways obstruction the anaesthetist, surgeon, operating theatre staff and equipment should be properly prepared. A wide range of tracheal tubes should be available, down to the smallest, together with introducers and bougies. The bronchoscopic equipment must be immediately available and the anaesthetist should understand how it functions and its hazards and limitations. Finally, instruments and personnel for emergency cricothyroid puncture and tracheostomy must be at hand in the event of total airway obstruction and inability to secure an artificial airway. A paediatric cricothyroidotomy needle with a 15-mm connector is commercially available (Figure 17.2). Emergency resuscitation drugs must be immediately available.

Patients should be premedicated with an anticholinergic agent to reduce secretions. Intramuscular atropine is the most effective. Control of secretions reduces the incidence of coughing, breath-holding and laryngospasm during induction and during endoscopy. It also avoids the need for repeated suctioning during the procedure and allows for more effective topical anaesthesia.[31] In general, sedative premedication should be avoided. Strict preoperative starvation is mandatory as the risk of aspiration of stomach contents is greater in the presence of airway obstruction where

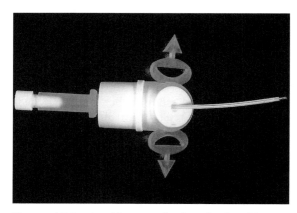

Figure 17.2 An 18-g paediatric cricothyroidotomy cannula and needle with 15-mm connector.

induction of anaesthesia may be prolonged and difficult, making gastric distension more likely.

The most important principle during induction of anaesthesia in children with airway obstruction is that spontaneous respiration should be maintained and relaxants avoided at least until it has been shown that IPPV is possible. It should be remembered that the site of obstruction may be below the glottis and it may not be possible to bypass it with a tracheal tube even if laryngoscopy is possible. Inhalational induction is safest using 100% oxygen and an increasing concentration of halothane or sevoflurane. Sevoflurane may provide a more pleasant and rapid induction. Although it causes more depression of minute ventilation than halothane, end-tidal carbon dioxide concentrations are similar, at least at 1 MAC.[32] One common practice is to use sevoflurane for induction and then to switch to halothane. Once consciousness is lost the application of continuous positive airway pressure by mask may help to improve gas exchange. The stridor of laryngomalacia will often improve or completely disappear, whereas the fixed biphasic stridor of subglottic stenosis will not improve.

In the presence of significant airway obstruction, induction of anaesthesia will be prolonged, taking several minutes to achieve sufficient depth of anaesthesia for intubation. Gently assisted ventilation or application of CPAP can speed up the process. During this time intravenous access is obtained, and a decision made whether to intubate the trachea using deep anaesthesia or a short-acting muscle relaxant. If mask ventilation is difficult relaxants should not be given. When the diagnosis is in doubt a preliminary look at the larynx to ensure that the laryngeal inlet is easily identifiable is wise. In some circumstances (e.g. supraglottic cysts), although ventilation is possible, intubation is easier if spontaneous ventilation is producing bubbles from the laryngeal inlet.

Although intubation is not essential, it gives a guide to subglottic size and provides a secure airway for transfer from the anaesthetic room and setting up of the suspension laryngoscope and microscope. A nasotracheal tube is usually more convenient as it can simply be withdrawn into the nasopharynx during endoscopy.

Topical anaesthesia, usually with lignocaine, is the key to avoiding coughing, breath-holding and laryngospasm during endoscopy, especially during emergence, when the assessment of cord and cricoarytenoid function is made. Laryngomalacia is usually only apparent at light planes of anaesthesia and paradoxical vocal cord movements only of pathological significance when the patient is nearly awake. The glottis, vallecula and trachea are sprayed depending on whether laryngoscopy, bronchoscopy or both are being performed. If a short-acting muscle relaxant is used the glottis is sprayed with lignocaine before intubation. In the presence of spontaneous respiration, however, the risk of laryngospasm is high, even in experienced hands, and it is safer to spray the glottis after intubation. This is particularly important if mask ventilation is difficult and relaxants are unsafe. Doses of lignocaine up to 4–5 mg kg^{-1} have been used in many large series without complications.[33] A metered-dose 10% lignocaine spray is suitable for most patients (the commonly used proprietary preparation contains 10 mg per aliquot). In very small patients more dilute preparations may be necessary, especially if it is necessary to spray the trachea as well as the glottis.

MICROLARYNGOSCOPY

Once the suspension laryngoscope and microscope are in position and the patient is breathing spontaneously with 100% oxygen and a volatile agent, usually halothane or sevoflurane, the tracheal tube can be withdrawn into the nasopharynx and anaesthesia maintained by insufflation. Techniques using propofol infusion have also been described, even in small babies. One-hundred per cent oxygen ensures that the oxygen reserve is as great as possible, and should be used even in premature babies where the dangers of hypoxia far outweigh the risks of retinopathy of prematurity. Bronchoscopy is performed if indicated (see below) and the patient is allowed to wake up with the tip of the laryngoscope in the vallecula to allow assessment of vocal cord and cricoarytenoid movement. It is often possible to obtain an adequate assessment of the subglottis and trachea using a telescopic rod alone while insufflation anaesthesia is continued. This minimizes the risk of postoperative subglottic oedema.

Close monitoring throughout the endoscopy is essential to detect hypoxia and hypoventilation so that prompt action may be taken to avoid serious consequences. A pulse oximeter whose pitch changes clearly as the oxygen saturation declines helps to alert the surgeon to the problem and the possible need to interrupt the procedure. The use of a camera and video display allows the anaesthetist to see what is happening to the airway during the procedure (Figure 17.3).

Postoperatively, the patient should be watched carefully until fully awake. Humidity and added oxygen may be required. If signs of increased airway obstruction develop nebulized adrenaline and steroids may be helpful. Up to 0.4 ml kg^{-1} of 1 : 1000 adrenaline to a maximum of 5 ml may be nebulized with air or oxygen. ECG monitoring is essential and administration should be discontinued if the heart rate increases markedly.[34] Dexamethasone may be used in a dose of 0.25 mg kg^{-1} i.v. followed by 0.1 mg kg^{-1} i.v. every 6 h for a further three doses. Occasionally, reintubation is required. Oral fluids should be withheld for 2 h after the larynx has been sprayed with lignocaine.

BRONCHOSCOPY

Bronchoscopy may be indicated for the diagnosis of upper and lower airway lesions or as a therapeutic manoeuvre, as for the removal of inhaled foreign bodies (see below) and treatment of refractory atelectasis. Almost all paediatric ENT surgeons use rigid Storz bronchoscopes (Figure 17.4). The scopes are used with Hopkins telescopic rods and have excellent optical characteristics. A side-arm allows attachment of an anaesthetic T-piece for ventilation. With the telescope in place a closed system exists, allowing controlled ventilation. However, the telescope narrows the lumen of the bronchoscope, increasing the resistance to airflow. The effect is greatest with the smallest bronchoscopes. Adequate gas exchange may require the frequent removal of the telescope to allow unimpeded ventilation. Adequate visualization of the proximal trachea may be possible with the telescopic rod alone.

Premedication and induction of anaesthesia are as described for diagnostic laryngoscopy, followed by full local anaesthesia of the respiratory tract. Some anaesthetists intubate all children having bronchoscopy, although it is not strictly necessary. It has the advantage of allowing the anaesthetist to advise the surgeon of a safe-size bronchoscope to use and preventing too large a scope being forced through the subglottis. Table 17.1 provides a guide to bronchoscope sizes.

When the surgeon is ready the tracheal tube is removed and the bronchoscope inserted. The anaesthetic T-piece is connected to the side-arm of the bronchoscope and anaesthesia continued with oxygen and a volatile agent. Assisted

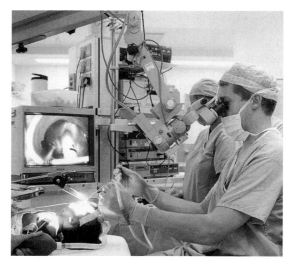

Figure 17.3 Operating theatre set-up for microlaryngoscopy with suspension laryngoscope, camera and television display.

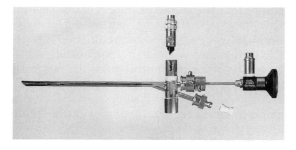

Figure 17.4 The Storz bronchoscope with Hopkins rod telescope. Light carrier above, 15-mm attachment for breathing system below and suction port.

ventilation is usually required to maintain adequate ventilation in infants, although paralysis is neither necessary nor advisable for diagnostic procedures where functional assessment is required. Constant communication with the operator is vital throughout the procedure and greatly improved by the use of a camera and video system. Alteration in the position of the bronchoscope and the prolonged use of suction may result in impaired ventilation. Hypoventilation, hypoxia and too light or too deep anaesthesia may all cause cardiac arrhythmias. Withdrawal of the bronchoscope into the trachea, temporary removal of the telescope and hyperinflation of the lungs with oxygen, adjusting the level of anaesthesia if necessary, will usually restore sinus rhythm. End-tidal carbon dioxide monitoring may be inaccurate owing to leaking of gases around the bronchoscope. Isoflurane or sevoflurane may be better tolerated than halothane in older children. Propofol as a bolus or infusion is an alternative technique.

Small fibreoptic endoscopes down to 2.2 mm external diameter are available and have been used for the evaluation of upper airway obstruction.[35] Fibreoptic bronchoscopes are more commonly used by respiratory physicians than by surgeons, either with sedation or with general anaesthesia. Anaesthesia may be better conducted with a laryngeal mask airway[36,37] or specially adapted facemasks than a tracheal tube as it allows passage of a larger fibreoptic scope which will have better optics. The smallest bronchoscopes have no suction channel.

Table 17.1 Guide to sizes of bronchoscopes

Size of bronchoscope [internal diameter (mm)]	External diameter (mm)	Age range
2.5	4.0	Premature to neonate
3.0	5.0	Neonate to 6 months
3.5	5.7	6–18 months
4.0	7.0	18 months–3 years
5.0	7.8	3–8 years
6.0	8.2	Over 8 years

REMOVAL OF INHALED FOREIGN BODY

Inhalation of foreign bodies is common in children. Foreign body impaction in the larynx or tracheobronchial tree most commonly occurs between the ages of 1 and 3 years and is the most common indication for airway endoscopy in this age group. Although many objects and foods have been inhaled, peanuts are encountered most often in the UK.[38] They are particularly dangerous as the oil in the nut produces mucosal irritation, oedema and often severe pneumonitis distal to the obstruction.

The majority of foreign body aspirations in children is witnessed and typically parents report an episode of choking followed by a variable period of coughing. Stridor, wheeze, dyspnoea and cyanosis may occur depending on the site of impaction. Hoarseness may occur if the foreign body is impacted in the larynx. If the object is small and passes beyond the main bronchi the child may quickly become asymptomatic and not present until changes due to local irritation and distal obstruction occur. Although the child may be taken to hospital straight away, in up to 30% of cases the patient does not present until more than a week after aspiration.[39,40] On examination there may be unilateral wheeze or decreased breath sounds. However, many children with bronchial foreign bodies have no obvious signs.[41]

The foreign body may be visible on chest X-ray but the majority is radiolucent. If the foreign body causes more obstruction to airflow during expiration than during inspiration there will be hyperinflation on the affected side. This will be more obvious on a film taken in expiration (Figure 17.5). The chest X-ray may show collapse and consolidation distal to an obstruction.

The principles of anaesthesia are the same as for diagnostic endoscopy, although removal of a foreign body often takes much longer. A Storz ventilating bronchoscope and forceps are usually used. It is common for the foreign body to be too large to pass through the bronchoscope and for the object, forceps and scope to be removed as a single unit. The biggest danger occurs when the foreign body is withdrawn into the trachea and falls out of the forceps, lodging just below the cords and totally obstructing the airway. If the foreign body cannot be quickly removed it should be pushed back down far enough to allow adequate ventilation and a second attempt made at its removal. Following removal of the foreign body endoscopy is performed to exclude a second foreign body.

In the absence of respiratory distress, endoscopy can wait until the child is starved. A technique including atropine premedication, topical anaesthesia of the airway and spontaneous respiration using a volatile agent in oxygen is usually satisfactory. It may be necessary to assist ventilation once the broncho-

scope is in place. Unless the foreign body is in the trachea, intubation prior to the passage of the bronchoscope may be helpful (see above). Techniques using muscle relaxants and manual IPPV via the ventilating bronchoscope are an alternative to deep inhalational anaesthesia but are better avoided if the foreign body is tracheal or causes ball-valve obstruction.

If the bronchoscope has been removed and reinserted several times dexamethasone should be considered to minimize the risk of airway oedema. Humidity, physiotherapy and antibiotics may all be required postoperatively, depending on the nature of the foreign body and whether pulmonary collapse and infection are present.

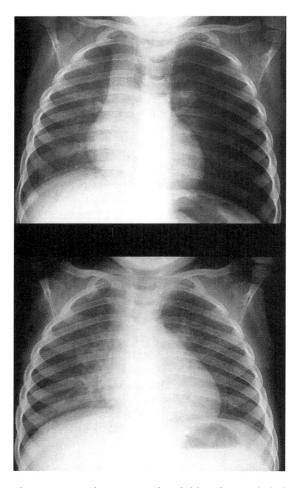

Figure 17.5 Chest X-ray of a child with an inhaled foreign body in the left main bronchus. Top: taken in expiration; bottom: taken in inspiration. Note that on the film taken in expiration the hyperinflation of the left lung is more marked and there is mediastinal shift. (Source: Hatch, 1985.[42])

OPERATIVE PROCEDURES ON THE LARYNX AND TRACHEA

With the introduction of the operating microscope and the advances in laser technology, operative airway procedures have become increasingly common. These procedures place special demands on the anaesthetist. The patients often present for repeated procedures and have significant airway obstruction. The airway must be shared with the surgeon and the use of lasers creates risks of injury to both the patient and operating theatre personnel.

For patients with airway obstruction the same principles for premedication and induction of anaesthesia apply as are outlined above for the management of diagnostic endoscopy. Intravenous induction is an alternative where there is no airway obstruction or obstruction is relieved by tracheostomy.

MICROLARYNGEAL SURGERY

Many minor surgical procedures can be performed using the suspension laryngoscope without the need for a tracheostomy. Various techniques for managing the airway in these cases have been used but none is ideal.

Endotracheal anaesthesia and insufflation

Spontaneous respiration with a volatile anaesthetic is combined with topical anaesthesia as for diagnostic endoscopy. As much surgery as possible is performed with a small tracheal tube in place, which is then withdrawn into the pharynx for the remainder of the operation. In practice, this technique is very satisfactory for short procedures and no special equipment is needed.

Apnoeic oxygenation

In this approach the surgeon and the anaesthetist take it in turns to use the airway. Muscle-relaxant drugs are used and anaesthesia is usually maintained with intravenous agents. The anaesthetist inserts a small tracheal tube and ventilates the patient with oxygen, then extubates the patient and delivers oxygen via a catheter in the nasopharynx. The surgeon has access to the airway until ventilation is needed. The tracheal tube is reinserted and the cycle repeats until surgery is completed. This technique has the major disadvantage that both surgery and ventilation are repeatedly interrupted and there is a risk of airway trauma from repeated intubations. Small children desaturate much more quickly than older children because their metabolic rate is high relative to their functional residual capacity.

Venturi jet ventilation

Venturi jet ventilation involves the delivery of boluses of gases through a narrow cannula. When each bolus of gas is released from the cannula it entrains surrounding air (Venturi effect), thereby increasing the volume and reducing the pressure of gas reaching the patient's lungs. The cannula used for delivery of the jet may be attached to the suspension laryngoscope[43] or placed in the trachea via the glottis.[44] Complete muscle paralysis is essential and anaesthesia must be maintained with intravenous agents. Jet ventilation in children requires the use of driving pressures well below standard pipeline pressures. Peak pressures of about 70–140 kPa (10–20 psi) supraglottically are reduced to 35 cmH$_2$O or less in the midtrachea.[45] When ventilation is adequate there should be visible movement of the chest and abdomen. An 18 or 16 gauge needle is suitable for jet ventilation of infants and children. It is important to monitor the position of the cannula at all times to ensure that it is aligned with the larynx. Serious gastric distension and injury may occur if proper alignment of the cannula is not maintained.[46] The glottis must be unobstructed at all times, otherwise serious barotrauma may occur. For this reason the technique is unsafe where there is pathology resulting in significant obstruction at the laryngeal level. Patients with lung pathology resulting in poor gas exchange and reduced pulmonary compliance are not candidates for jet ventilation.

High-frequency positive pressure ventilation

High-frequency positive pressure ventilation has been used for laryngoscopy and bronchoscopy either via a transglottic catheter[47,48] or via a percutaneous transtracheal catheter.[49,50] Again, muscle paralysis is essential to maintain an open glottis, but the risk of barotrauma is less than with Venturi jet ventilation as the peak inspiratory pressure is usually below that of conventional ventilation. This technique requires the use of a specially designed high-frequency jet ventilator. The adequacy of ventilation may be difficult to assess as conventional chest movements are not present. Close monitoring is therefore essential.

Laser endoscopy

The carbon dioxide laser was first introduced into clinical practice in the early 1970s and is now firmly established for the treatment of obstructive lesions of the paediatric airway-especially laryngeal papilloma, haemangiomas and cystic hygromas extending on to the base of the tongue. The CO$_2$ laser beam is transmitted through air with minimal absorption but is rapidly absorbed by fibreoptic systems and is therefore not amenable to fibreoptic transmission. It is used with an operating laryngoscope or rigid bronchoscope. More recently-potassium titanyl phosphate (KTP), neodymium : yttrium aluminium garnet (Nd :

YAG) and argon lasers which are transmitted through fibreoptic cables have been used to treat airway pathology in children.[51] The fibreoptic cables can be passed down the suction channel of a flexible or rigid bronchoscope.

The laser beam can be aimed very accurately and the depth of tissue destruction controlled precisely. The tissue destruction caused by the laser energy is a thermal process involving coagulation, carbonization and vaporization of the tissues. There is minimal bleeding and minimal damage to the surrounding tissues. Healing is good and almost pain free, with little postoperative oedema and scarring.[52] All of these advantages are especially valuable when dealing with the small dimensions of a child's airway.

All those involved in the use of lasers for airway surgery must be aware of the hazards. Anaesthesia for laser surgery has recently been reviewed by Rampil[53] and McCall.[54] The hazards can be subdivided into hazards to operating theatre personnel and hazards to the patient.

Personnel may be exposed to laser radiation by two mechanisms. Direct beam impact occurs as a result of misuse or gross misalignment of the laser. Indirect beam impact may result from reflection of laser energy from a shiny surface. The use of a matt finish on instruments in the operative field reduces this risk. The eyes are at particular risk and eye protection should be worn, which must be appropriate to the type of laser used. Personnel outside the theatre must be protected by keeping any windows covered and doors shut. The possibility that laser smoke contains viral particles has led some people to advocate the use of laser masks, at least when papilloma lesions are treated.[54]

The patient is also at risk from inadvertent laser burns to normal tissues. The eyes must be closed and covered with moist gauze swabs. Moist gauze swabs that will absorb the laser energy should be used to cover the patient's face, including the lips. The greatest risk to the patient is the risk of an airway fire. Airway fires arise from the ignition of non-metal materials, usually tracheal tubes, forgotten pledglets and excessively charred tissue that has not been removed from the airway. Both oxygen and nitrous oxide support combustion. However, gas mixtures do not absorb laser energy and

cannot be ignited. If the laser beam strikes metal it will be deflected and the energy scattered.

All tracheal tubes, tracheostomy tubes and cannulae for jet ventilation should be metallic. Small disposable metal tubes down to size 3.0 mm i.d. are now manufactured (Figure 17.6). As these tubes have a polyvinyl chloride (PVC) lining some form of ignition is still theoretically possible. The cuffed tubes also have PVC cuffs and these must be filled with saline. The use of an oxygen air mixture rather than 100% oxygen should be considered, especially when the airway is secured with a bronchoscope.

The choice of anaesthetic technique and method of airway management during laser treatment of the larynx depends on the child's age and size, the preferences of the surgeon and anaesthetist, and the pathology being treated. Some workers have claimed that paralysis is mandatory for laser surgery;[55] however, at Great Ormond Street Hospital for Children, London, this was not found to be necessary. Over 1000 anaesthetics have been administered using spontaneous respiration, without problems. Good topical anaesthesia is combined with oxygen-enriched air and a volatile agent, usually halothane, administered via a nasopharyngeal airway or laser-resistant tracheal tube. Spontaneous respiration is maintained throughout and the tube withdrawn into the pharynx to

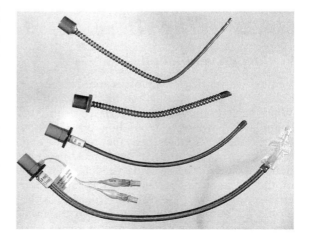

Figure 17.6 Paediatric laser tubes. From the top: neonatal and paediatric reusable linked metal tubes, disposable uncuffed 3.5-mm (i.d.) Laser-Flex (Mallinkrodt) tube and disposable cuffed 5.0-mm (i.d.) Laser-Flex (Mallinkrodt) tube.

allow areas previously obscured by it to be treated. There have been no serious complications attributable to this technique. McCall, based on his experience of over 500 procedures, also recommends spontaneous respiration (without tracheal intubation) using topical anaesthesia and insufflation of a volatile anaesthetic gas mixture.[54] Alternative techniques using paralysis and supraglottic or intratracheal jet ventilation have their advocates.[46,51,55–57]

Whenever laser surgery is performed on the paediatric airway, it is safest in the hands of an experienced team. Although risks should be minimized there should always be a plan to manage airway fires. In the event of an airway fire, a tracheal tube, if present, should be removed, the anaesthetic circuit disconnected and ventilation stopped. The fire should be extinguished with saline or water. Ventilation can then be resumed by mask and the damage assessed. Severe injuries may require prolonged intubation or tracheostomy.

ARYEPIGLOTTOPLASTY

Most infants with laryngomalacia will improve with age and do not require specific treatment. Where the symptoms are more severe aryepiglottoplasty may be performed. This is a form of supraglottoplasty in which the redundant mucosa over the arytenoids and aryepiglottic folds is excised using microlaryngeal instruments and the operating microscope.[58] The procedure can be performed with a nasotracheal tube *in situ*. Recovery is usually uncomplicated and postoperative steroids are seldom required.

SUPRAGLOTTIC CYSTS

These are rare and are normally single, but may be multiple. They give rise to intermittent episodes of upper airway obstruction, but for much of the time the patient may be asymptomatic. A good-quality lateral X-ray of the neck is usually diagnostic. Treatment is to deroof the cyst and marsupialize the base, using the suspension laryngoscope. The principles of anaesthesia are the same as for any child with upper airway obstruction. Muscle relaxants must be avoided prior to intubation as the cyst may act as a ball-valve over the glottic opening, making controlled ventilation imposs-

ible. If the larynx is unrecognizable it is useful to remember that its opening always lies behind the cyst, which is anteriorly placed arising from the vallecula. In the event of extreme difficulty the cyst may be aspirated with a needle attached to a suction unit. Following surgery the patient should be awake before extubation, but as there is little tissue damage or oedema, recovery is usually uncomplicated.

SURGERY FOR LARYNGOTRACHEAL STENOSIS

The surgical management of laryngotracheal stenosis has recently been reviewed by Lesperance and Zalzal.[59]

Anterior cricoid split

Anterior cricoid split is indicated in children with mild to moderate stenosis from a small, normally shaped cricoid ring. The procedure is unsuitable for infants with poor respiratory reserve.[59] With the head extended, a transverse cervical incision is made and the cricoid cartilage and the first and second tracheal rings are identified and split in the midline anteriorly. A tracheal tube is used as a stent for 5–14 days postoperatively. General anaesthesia with tracheal intubation, a muscle relaxant and manual IPPV is appropriate. Routine monitoring should be supplemented with a precordial stethoscope. It is usual to change the tracheal tube to a size larger prior to closing the neck. The tube tip should be positioned distal to the split. A securely fixed nasal tube is appropriate for postoperative intensive care. Meticulous attention to preventing plugging and maintaining the tracheal tube is essential, as reintubation in the early postoperative period may cause injury with the tube penetrating the anterior tissues of the neck. Extubation is performed with steroid cover.

Laryngotracheal reconstruction

This involves dividing the airway and distracting the edges with an interposed cartilage graft to widen the airway lumen. Anterior and posterior grafts may be required. Postoperatively the airway is stented. Single-stage laryngotracheal reconstruction refers to procedures performed for less severe cases which require only a short period of stenting, which is achieved with a tracheal tube and no covering tracheostomy. An existing tracheostomy may be closed at the same time. This technique is also used for suprastomal collapse.

The anaesthetic and intensive-care considerations for single-stage laryngotracheal reconstruction are similar to those for cricoid split. A postoperative chest X-ray is required to exclude pneumothorax after a rib graft is taken. Local anaesthetic infiltration of the graft site is useful in reducing postoperative pain. Stenting is for 1–2 weeks.

Children undergoing staged laryngotracheal reconstruction will already have a tracheostomy below the level of obstruction. Surgery is performed through a transverse cervical incision immediately above the tracheostome. Stenting is performed using a Teflon, silastic or PVC stent, which is sutured in place for at least 6 weeks. The patient returns to theatre for removal of the stent. Repeat endoscopy is undertaken about 2 weeks later to check the airway and remove any granulation tissue. When the airway is satisfactory decannulation can be attempted.

To allow good surgical access the head is extended and a south-facing tracheostomy is used. A cuffed armoured tube inserted into the tracheostome and strapped to the chest is the most satisfactory option. It is sometimes necessary for the surgeon to dilate the tracheostome before a tube of appropriate size for the child's age can be inserted. There are, however, problems associated with its use. It is important to ensure that the entire cuff is within the airway or it is likely to extrude or be damaged during the operation. The tip must be above the level of the carina. The tube position may be altered during the surgery as a result of surgical manipulations. A shortened, preformed plastic tube is an alternative but is far less satisfactory as it is uncuffed. The use of a cuffed tube prevents blood trickling into the trachea and prevents anaesthetic gases leaking into the operation site. Regardless of the tube chosen, close monitoring of airway patency during the procedure is essential. A precordial stethoscope is a useful supplement to routine minimal monitoring.

Anaesthesia is usually induced via the tracheostome and maintained using any technique that includes a muscle relaxant and IPPV. Tracheal suction should always be performed prior to changing the tracheostomy tube. Intravenous fluids are given as necessary and continued postoperatively until drinking is well established. Aspiration is common in the early postoperative period and occasionally necessitates revision of the stent. If the stent if too long it may give rise to glottic incompetence. If a rib graft is taken a postoperative chest X-ray is essential to exclude a pneumothorax and adequate postoperative pain relief must be provided.

Postoperatively, patients are nursed in humidified air, with added oxygen if necessary. Chest physiotherapy may be required as there is often a temporary increase in secretions.

Tracheal resection

Short segment stenoses of the upper trachea may be resected with primary anastomosis. Because of technical difficulties associated with the procedure reconstruction techniques with grafting are usually preferred in children. The surgeon may be able to work around a tracheal tube or jet ventilation cannula. Otherwise, cardiopulmonary bypass will be required. Tracheal transplantation has become a last-resort procedure in infants and children with previously untreatable tracheal pathology.

LARYNGEAL CLEFT

This is a condition that is often missed on direct laryngoscopy as the glottis appears superficially normal. A probe will reveal a deficiency posteriorly of interarytenoid tissue which prevents competent glottic closure during swallowing. The cleft may extend a variable distance into the trachea. These children may have other anomalies. The problem usually presents with episodes of aspiration and the longer the cleft the more severe the pulmonary problems. They usually require a low tracheostomy and a feeding gastrostomy, and repair of the cleft is achieved via either an anterior laryngofissure or a lateral pharyngotomy. Airway management is as for staged laryngotracheal reconstruction (see above). Minor forms can be closed by direct suture using the suspension laryngoscope. An oral tracheal tube is satisfactory.

TRACHEOSTOMY

The main indications for tracheostomy relate to the many causes of congenital and acquired upper airways obstruction. A smaller number of children requires tracheostomy to facilitate long-term respiratory support or for airway protection in the presence of a neurological abnormality.

Many patients present for tracheostomy already intubated, in which case anaesthesia may be induced via the tracheal tube. Unintubated children with upper airway obstruction are best premedicated with an antisialogogue and managed with an inhalational induction using halothane or sevoflurane in oxygen. Relaxants should be avoided in the presence of upper airways obstruction, at least until one has confirmed that IPPV with a mask is possible. If subglottic stenosis is suspected a wide range of cut and uncut tracheal tubes should be available, down to the smallest sizes. Occasionally, the stenosis is so severe that the smallest tube (2.5 mm i.d.) in common usage will not pass. In this situation, shouldered neonatal resuscitation tubes (Cole pattern) are useful. The 1.5-mm (i.d.) tube has an external diameter of just over 2.5 mm. This poses an unacceptably high resistance to spontaneous respiration. The rigid nature of the shouldered tubes makes them much more useful than the smallest Portex tube, which has an internal diameter of 2.0 mm. Where intubation is impossible the LMA may provide a good airway and spontaneous respiration with a facemask is occasionally an appropriate technique.

Local anaesthetic spray applied to the larynx and trachea prevents coughing or bucking when the trachea is being manipulated if a spontaneous respiration technique is used. An intravenous line and full monitoring are essential.

The patient is carefully positioned with a sandbag under the shoulders and the head fully extended to bring the trachea into prominence. Elastoplast strapping can be passed around the chin and secured to the table to help to maintain the position. The surgical technique is important if long-term complications are to be avoided.[60] Cartilage should never be excised, because of the risk of tracheal collapse and stenosis, and the incision in the trachea should always be below the level of the first tracheal ring to reduce the risk of stenosis. A vertical incision is made in the second and third tracheal rings. If the incision is too low there is a risk of dislodgement of the tube and bronchial intubation. Two 'stay' sutures are inserted, one on each side of the tracheal incision, and these are taped to the chest wall at the end of the operation.

Before the tracheal incision is made 100% oxygen is administered and the tracheostomy tube and connectors are checked. It is usual to select a tube one size larger than the anticipated tracheal tube size for the child's age. A wide range of tracheostomy tubes is available (Figure 17.7). Where the tube is required for controlled ventilation a tube with a standard 15-mm connector is generally convenient (e.g. Shiley and Portex). Where the tube is required for spontaneous breathing, alternatives include the Great Ormond Street plastic tracheostomy tube and Silver tracheostomy tubes. No British standard connectors exist for these tubes but an appropriate-size Portex tube connector can be placed in the tube. Bivona adjustable tubes can be useful in difficult circumstances. The length of the Bivona tube is adjustable and the extension will clear a very full chin.

When the tracheal wall is incised the tracheal tube is withdrawn into the upper trachea (it is safer not to remove it completely until the

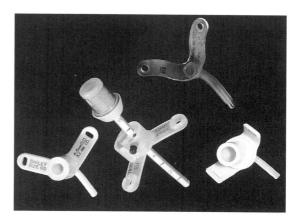

Figure 17.7 Paediatric tracheostomy tubes. From the top, clockwise: GOS pattern, Portex, Bivona adjustable and Shiley.

tracheostomy tube is taped in place). Once the tracheostomy tube is in position anaesthesia is continued via a sterile connector. Before the tube is tied in place the sandbag should be removed from behind the shoulders to allow the head to flex. Unless the head is flexed the ties will be too loose and the tube may fall out. It may be difficult to replace a dislodged tracheostomy tube in the first few days before a tract has formed and it is for this reason that tracheal stay sutures are inserted. Should the tube become accidentally dislodged the tracheal opening is more easily entered by pulling the sutures apart.

Postoperatively, a chest X-ray is taken to confirm correct positioning of the tube and to exclude a pneumothorax. The patient is nursed in humidified air, with added oxygen if necessary, using a tracheostomy mask. Regular suctioning using a sterile technique and the instillation of small aliquots of saline are necessary to prevent crusting of the tube with secretions. A spare tube, tapes and tracheal dilators should be at the bedside, in addition to oxygen and suction. During the early postoperative period the child requires very close observation. Babies are nursed more easily with a small roll behind the neck to prevent the chin obstructing the tracheostomy. Humidity can usually be discontinued after a week. Parents require appropriate training before discharge, including resuscitation training.

Complications of tracheostomy can be fatal. However, with careful management most should be avoidable. Bleeding, surgical emphysema, pneumothorax, pneumomediastinum, oesophageal injury and damage to the recurrent laryngeal nerve may all occur during surgery. Tube dislodgement, obstruction of the tube with crusted secretions, bleeding and local infection may occur in the first few days. Granuloma formation, vascular erosion, tracheo-oesophageal fistula, suprastomal collapse and tracheal stenosis are late complications.[61]

REFERENCES

1 Berry, F.A. The child with the runny nose. In: Berry, F.A. (ed.). *Anesthetic Management of Difficult and Routine Paediatric Patients*. New York: Churchill Livingstone, 1986: 349–67.

2 Cohen, M.M. and Cameron, C.B. Should you cancel the operation when a child has an upper respiratory tract infection? *Anesthesia and Analgesia* 1991; **72**: 282–8.

3 Gervais, H.W., El Gindi, M., Radermacher, P.R., *et al.* Plasma concentration following oral and intramuscular atropine in children and their clinical effects. *Paediatric Anaesthesia* 1997; **7**: 13–18.

4 Johnston, D.F., Wrigley, S.R., Robb, P.J. and Jones, H.E. The laryngeal mask airway in paediatric anaesthesia. *Anaesthesia* 1990; **45**: 924–7.

5 Granstrom, G. and Tjellstrom, A. The bone-anchored hearing aid (BAHA) in children with auricular malformations. *Ear, Nose & Throat Journal* 1997; **76**: 238–40.

6 Langman, A.W., Quigley, S.M. and Souliere, C.R., Jr. Cochlear implants in children. *Pediatric Clinics of North America* 1996; **43**: 1217–32.

7 Kaplan, L.C. Choanal atresia and its associated anomalies. Further support for the CHARGE association. *International Journal of Pediatric Otorhinolaryngology* 1985; **8**: 237–42.

8 Deutch, E.S. Tonsillectomy and adenoidectomy: changing indications. *Pediatric Clinics of North America* 1996; **43**: 1319–38.

9 Guilleminault, C., Tilkian, A. and Dement, W.C. The sleep apnea syndromes. *Annual Review of Medicine* 1976; **27**: 465–84.

10 Bradley, T.D. and Phillipson, E.A. Pathogenesis and pathophysiology of the obstructive sleep apnea syndrome. *Medical Clinics of North America* 1985; **69**: 1169–85.

11 Thach, B.T. Sleep apnea in infancy and childhood. *Medical Clinics of North America* 1985; **69**: 1289–315.

12 Macartney, F.J., Panday, J. and Scott, O. Cor pulmonale as a result of chronic nasopharyngeal obstruction due to hypertrophied tonsils and adenoids. *Archives of Disease in Childhood* 1969; **44**: 585–92.

13 Brouillette, R.T. and Fernbach, J. Obstructive sleep apnea in infants and children. *Journal of Pediatrics* 1982; **100**: 31–40.

14 Nicklaus, P.J., Herzon, F.S. and Steinle, M.S. IV. Short-stay outpatient tonsillectomy. *Archives of Otolaryngology, Head and Neck Surgery* 1995; **121**: 521–4.

15 Gabalski, E.C., Mattucci, K.F., Setzen, M. and Moleski, P. Ambulatory tonsillectomy and adenoidectomy. *Laryngoscope* 1996; **106**: 77–80.

16 Pringle, M.B., Cosford, E., Beasley, P. and Brightwell, A.P. Day-case tonsillectomy – is it appropriate? *Clinical Otolaryngology* 1996; **21**: 504–11.

17 Rosen, G.M., Muckle, R.P., Mahowald, M.W., Goding, G.S. and Ullevig, C. Postoperative respiratory compromise in children with obstructive sleep apnea syndrome: can it be anticipated? *Pediatrics* 1994; **93**: 784–8.

18 Wood, P. Difficulty in extubation. *Anaesthesia* 1987; **42**: 220.

19 Williams, P.J. and Bailey, P.M. Comparison of the reinforced laryngeal mask airway and tracheal intubation for adenotonsillectomy. *British Journal of Anaesthesia* 1993; **70**: 30–3.

20 Webster, A.C., Morley-Forster, P.K., Dain, S., *et al.* Anaesthesia for adenotonsillectomy: a comparison between tracheal intubation and the armoured laryngeal

mask airway. *Canadian Journal of Anaesthesia* 1993; **40**: 1171–7.

21 Nair, I. and Bailey, P.M. Review of uses of the laryngeal mask in ENT anaesthesia. *Anaesthesia* 1995; **50**: 898–900.

22 Parry, M., Glaisyer, H.R. and Bailey, P.M. Removal of LMA in children. *British Journal of Anaesthesia* 1997; **78**: 337–8.

23 Royal College of Anaesthetists. *Guidelines for the Use of Non-steroidal Anti-inflammatory Drugs in the Perioperative Period.* London: Royal College of Anaesthetists, 1998.

24 Molliex, S., Haond, P., Baylot, D., *et al.* Effect of pre- vs postoperative tonsillar infiltration with local anaesthetics on postoperative pain after tonsillectomy. *Acta Anaesthesiologica Scandinavica* 1996; **40**: 1210–15.

25 Wong, A.K., Bissonnette, B., Braude, B.M., Macdonald, R.M., St-Louis, P.J. and Fear, D.W. Post-tonsillectomy infiltration with bupivacaine reduces immediate postoperative pain in children. *Canadian Journal of Anaesthesia* 1995; **42**: 770–4.

26 Morton, N.S., Camu, F., Dorman, T., *et al.* Ondansetron reduces nausea and vomiting after paediatric adenotonsillectomy. *Paediatric Anaesthesia* 1997; **7**: 37–45.

27 Norinkavich, K.A., Howie, G. and Cariofiles, P. Quality improvement study of day surgery for tonsillectomy and adenoidectomy patients. *Pediatric Nursing* 1995; **21**: 341–4.

28 Sutters, K.A. and Miaskowski, C. Inadequate pain management and associated morbidity in children at home after tonsillectomy. *Journal of Pediatric Nursing* 1997; **12**: 178–85.

29 Myssiorek, D. and Alvi, A. Post-tonsillectomy hemorrhage: an assessment of risk factors. *International Journal of Pediatric Otorhinolaryngology* 1996; **37**: 35–43.

30 Schloss, M.D., Tan, A.K.W., Schloss, B. and Tewfik, T.L. Outpatient tonsillectomy and adenoidectomy: complications and recommendations. *International Journal of Pediatric Otorhinolaryngology* 1994; **30**: 115–22.

31 Whittet, H.B., Hayward, A.W. and Battersby, E. Plasma lignocaine levels during paediatric endoscopy of the upper respiratory tract. Relationship with mucosal moistness. *Anaesthesia* 1988; **43**: 439–42.

32 Yamakage, M., Tamiya, K., Horikawa, D., Sato, K. and Namiki, A. Effects of halothane and sevoflurane on the paediatric respiratory pattern. *Paediatric Anaesthesia* 1994; **4**: 53–6.

33 Byers, R.L., Kidd, J., Oppenheim, R. and Brown, T.C. Local anaesthetic plasma levels in children. *Anaesthesia and Intensive Care* 1978; **6**: 243–7.

34 Anon. Inhaled budenoside and adrenaline for croup. *Drugs and Therapeutics Bulletin* 1996; **34** (3): 23–34.

35 Wood, R.E. Spelunking in the pediatric airways: explorations with the flexible fiberoptic bronchoscope. *Pediatric Clinics of North America* 1984; **31**: 785–99.

36 Bandla, H.P.R., Smith, D.E. and Kieman, M.P. Laryngeal mask airway facilitated fibreoptic bronchoscopy in infants. *Canadian Journal of Anaesthesia* 1997; **44**: 1242–7.

37 Hinton, A.F., O'Connell, J.M., van Besouw, J.P. and Wyatt, M.E. Neonatal and paediatric fibre-optic laryngoscopy and bronchoscopy using the laryngeal mask airway. *Journal of Laryngology and Otology* 1997; **111**: 349–53.

38 Steen, K.H. and Zimmermann, T. Tracheobronchial aspiration of foreign bodies in children: a study of 94 cases. *Laryngoscope* 1990; **100**: 525–30.

39 Brown, T.C. Bronchoscopy for the removal of foreign bodies in children. *Anaesthesia and Intensive Care* 1973; **1**: 521–5.

40 Mu, L.H., He, P. and Sun, D. Inhalation of foreign bodies in Chinese children: a review of 400 cases. *Laryngoscope* 1991; **101**: 657–60.

41 Svedstrom, E., Puhakka, H. and Kero, P. How accurate is chest radiography in the diagnosis of tracheobronchial foreign bodies in children? *Pediatric Radiology* 1989; **19**: 520–2.

42 Hatch, D.J. Acute upper airway obstruction in children. In: Atkinson, R.S. and Adams, A.P. (eds). *Recent Advances in Anaesthesia and Analgesia*, Vol. 15. Edinburgh: Churchill Livingstone, 1985: 133–53.

43 Grasl, M.C., Donner, A., Schragl, E. and Aloy, A. Tubeless laryngotracheal surgery in infants and children. *Laryngoscope* 1997; **107**: 277–81.

44 Benjamin, B. and Gronow, D. A new tube for microlaryngeal surgery. *Anaesthesia and Intensive Care* 1979; **7**: 258–63.

45 Borland, L.M. and Reilly, J.S. Jet ventilation for laser laryngeal surgery in children. Modification of the Sanders jet ventilation technique. *International Journal of Pediatric Otorhinolaryngology* 1987; **14**: 65–71.

46 Borland, L.M. Airway management for CO_2 laser surgery on the larynx: Venturi jet ventilation and alternatives. *International Anesthesiology Clinics* 1997; **35**: 99–106.

47 Borg, U., Eriksson, I. and Sjostrand, U. High-frequency positive pressure ventilation (HFPPV): a review based on its use during bronchoscopy and for laryngoscopy and microlaryngeal surgery under general anesthesia. *Anesthesia and Analgesia* 1980; **59**: 594–603.

48 Hunsaker, D.H. Anesthesia for microlaryngeal surgery: the case for subglottic jet ventilation. *Laryngoscope* 1994; **104** (8 Part 2 Suppl. 65): 1–30.

49 Strashnov, V.I., Pluzhnikov, M.S. and Kolotilov, L.V. High frequency jet ventilation in endolaryngeal surgery. *Journal of Clinical Anesthesia* 1995; **7**: 19–25.

50 Depierraz, B., Ravussin, P., Brossard, E. and Monnier, P. Percutaneous transtracheal jet ventilation for paediatric endoscopic laser treatment of laryngeal and subglottic lesions. *Canadian Journal of Anaesthesia* 1994; **41**: 1200–7.

51 Rimell, F.L. Pediatric laser bronchoscopy. *International Anesthesiology Clinics* 1997; **35**: 107–13.

52 McGill, J., Friedman, E.M. and Healy, G.B. Laser surgery in the pediatric airway. *Otolaryngologic Clinics of North America* 1983; **16**: 865–70.

53 Rampil, I.J. Anesthetic considerations for laser surgery. *Anesthesia and Analgesia* 1992; **74**: 424–35.

54 McCall, J.E. Anesthetic techniques with laser endoscopy. In: Myer, C.M. III, Cotton, R.T. and Shon, S.R. (eds). *The Pediatric Airway: An Interdisciplinary Approach.* Philadelphia, PA: JB Lippincott, 1995: 307–26.

55 Simpson, G.T. II and Strong, M.S. Recurrent respiratory papillomatosis. The role of the carbon dioxide laser. *Otolaryngologic Clinics of North America* 1983; **16**: 887–94.

56 Norton, M.L. and DeVos, P. New endotracheal tube for laser surgery of the larynx. *Annals of Rhinology and Laryngology* 1978; **87**: 554–7.

57 Scamman, F.L. and McCabe, B.F. Evaluation of supra-glottic jet ventilation for laser surgery of the larynx. *Anesthesiology* 1984; **61:** A447.

58 Jani, P., Koltai, P., Ochi, J.W. and Bailey, C.M. Surgical treatment of laryngomalacia. *Journal of Laryngology and Otology* 1991; **105**: 1040–5.

59 Lesperance, M.M. and Zalzal, G.H. Assessment and management of laryngotracheal stenosis. *Pediatric Clinics of North America* 1996; **43**: 1414–27.

60 Shott, S.R. Pediatric tracheostomy. In: Myer, C.M. III, Cotton, R.T. and Shott, S.R. (eds). *The Pediatric Airway: An Interdisiplinary Approach.* Philadelphia, PA: JB Lippincott, 1995: 151–70.

61 Prescott, C.A.J. and Vanlierde, M.J.R.R. Tracheostomy in children – The Red Cross War Memorial Children's Hospital experience 1980–1985. *International Journal of Pediatric Otorhinolaryngology* 1989; **17**: 97–107.

CHAPTER 18

Airway obstruction: causes and management

JOSEF HOLZKI

INTRODUCTION

Respiratory obstruction can occur in the upper or the lower airways and is usually classified as congenital or acquired (Table 18.1). With any of these conditions there is the potential to develop hypoxaemia to a life-threatening degree and many children still die from these causes even although most are preventable. The anaesthetist should always be able to recognize and identify potential airway lesions which might present as an incidental finding during induction of anaesthesia for an unrelated condition. Recognition and treatment of airway obstruction requires knowledge of the normal anatomy and physiology of the airway during development and of the impact of various pathologies.

Children are predisposed to airway obstruction because of the enlarged base of the tongue relative to the mandible, the soft tissues of the pharynx and larynx and the more vulnerable mucous membranes of the upper airway being attached less firmly to the underlying structures than in adults. The critical diameter of the smallest part of their upper airway, the cricoid ring,[1] is easily occluded by infection as well as by oedema owing to injury according to Hagen–Poiseuille's law. The diameter of the airway is 3.5–4 mm at this level in the infant and 1 mm of oedema will cause a decrease in cross-sectional area of 75%.

The cartilaginous structures of the tracheobronchial tree and chest wall of the infant lack the rigidity of the older child or adult so that compression from outside will markedly decrease or distort the lumen. The flexible chest wall puts these children at a mechanical disadvantage from the respiratory point of view should obstruction occur.

In addition, many congenital conditions, such as Down's syndrome, cystic hygroma, Beckwith

Table 18.1. Common causes of upper airway obstruction in the paediatric patient

Congenital	Acquired
Choanal atresia	Infections
	Croup
	Epiglottis
	Abscess
	Adenotonsillar
	hypertrophy
	Diphtheria
	Ludwig's angina
Craniofacial malformations	Trauma
Pierre Robin syndrome	Foreign bodies
Treacher Collins syndrome	Thermal and
	chemical burns
	External trauma
	Postintubation
	Postoperative
Macroglossia	*Neurogenic*
Down's syndrome	Altered consciousness
Beckwith's syndrome	Muscular dystrophies
	Peripheral nerve
	lesions
Laryngeal	*Neoplastic*
Laryngomalacia	Tumours
Subglottic stenosis	Cysts
Webs	Nodes
Cleft (laryngeal-	
oesophageal)	
Cord palsies	
Tracheal	*Immunological*
Tracheomalacia	Angio-oedema
Congenital stenosis	Juvenile rheumatoid
Vascular rings	arthritis
Congenital tumours and	
cysts	
Haemangioma	
Lymphangioma	
Cystic hygroma	

tubes may occlude the airway more rapidly and unexpectedly than in the adult patient. Adenotonsillar hypertrophy, a common cause of obstructive sleep apnoea syndrome during childhood,[3] can lead to airway obstruction after induction of anaesthesia when artificial ventilation by face mask is begun. During intubation the cricothyroid membrane can be punctured as the tube passes the vocal cords. This is not possible in later life (see Figure 18.1).

(a) Adult

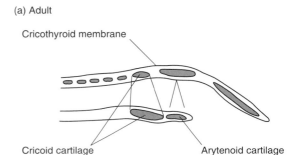

(b) Infant

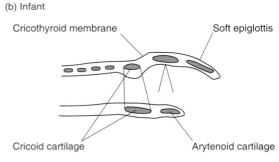

Figure 18.1. Difference in laryngeal structure between adults and infants, predisposing the infant to airway obstruction. (a) In the adult the narrowest part of the upper airway is located at the level of the vocal cords. For intubation a cuffed tracheal tube is needed. The cricothyroid membrane faces dorsally, permitting puncture for transcutaneous dilatation tracheostomy. (b) In the infant the cartilagenous structure of the larynx is softer than in the adult, frequently causing inspiratory stridor during crying or upper airway infection. The narrowest part of the upper airway is located at the subglottic level, formed by the cricoid cartilage. For intubation a non-cuffed tracheal tube is adequate. The cricothyroid membrane faces cephaled, predisposing it for perforation by the intubation manoeuvre. Transmembrane puncture of the trachea is difficult and dangerous.

syndrome, laryngotracheo-oesophageal cleft, the large group of craniofacial anomalies[2] and Pierre Robin anomalad, frequently incur airway obstruction. Many other diseases such as oesophageal atresia, congenital diaphragmatic hernia or the late stages of bronchopulmonary dysplasia involve dangers of airway obstruction which are not encountered in later life.

In paediatric ENT surgery, forgotten packs, kinking of tubes, clenching of teeth on the tube and oedema from inappropriately used cuffed

In the past, in particular before the clinical use of pulse oximetry, many of the above conditions were followed by mental retardation or growth impairment in later life, and this was often attributed to undefined neonatal cerebral disturbances. Retrospectively, it can be surmised that a considerable number of these handicaps is attributable to undetected airway obstruction with consequential brain hypoxia.

The predisposition of neonates and children to airway obstruction cannot be changed. However, it has been proved that the high incidence of intraoperative cardiac arrest in infancy can be reduced to almost zero by specially trained rather than with occasionally practising anaesthetists.[4] Bedside tests for predicting difficult intubation by measuring anatomical landmarks[5] have not been as practical in paediatric patients as in adults, but knowledge of typical syndromes and the particularities of the paediatric airway may reduce the incidence of airway obstruction by avoiding difficult intubation in unfavourable circumstances.

SIGNS OF RESPIRATORY OBSTRUCTION

Stridor and indrawing of the supraclavicular, intercostal and subdiaphragmatic areas are the true signs of upper airway obstruction. Inspiratory stridor indicates obstruction at or above the larynx. Hoarseness confirms vocal cord involvement. Biphasic (inspiratory and expiratory) stridor means that the obstruction is at or below the cords. Expiratory stridor alone indicates obstruction below the larynx, usually intrathoracic. The volume, pitch and tone of the stridor vary according to the type and extent of the obstructive lesion and the age of the child.

Retractions, especially in infancy, are the result of increased inspiratory effort to overcome the obstruction in the presence of a flexible chest wall. Stridor and indrawing occur when the diameter of the airway is reduced by 70% and are compounded by the development of an increased negative intrathoracic pressure below the level of the obstruction which, when combined with the baby's compliant respiratory structures, leads to a further decrease in the diameter of the trachea (Bernoulli effect)

As the infant matures the chest wall and supporting structures of the trachea become more rigid so that the indrawing and stridor, although always present in a major obstruction, may not be as severe.

If obstruction is severe, fatigue will occur, which is difficult to measure, although it can be assessed by the use of a scoring system such as that of Downes and Raphaely. This enables a baseline to be drawn and changes thereafter to be noted (Table 18.2).

Table 18.2 Clinical croup scores

	Score		
	1	2	3
Inspiratory breath sounds	Normal	Harsh with rhonchi	Delayed
Stridor	None	Inspiratory	Inspiratory and expiratory
Cough	None	Hoarse cry	Bark
Retractions and flaring	None	Flaring and supersternal retractions	As under 2, plus subcostal, intercostal retractions
Cyanosis	None	In air	In 40% O_2

From Downes and Raphaely.[6]

ACUTE AIRWAY OBSTRUCTION

ACUTE, LIFE-THREATENING COMPLETE AIRWAY OBSTRUCTION

In childhood, the causes of this unexpected event are quite different from those that apply in adulthood. They include birth asphyxia, sudden infant death syndrome (SIDS), foreign body aspiration or injury to the head, neck or chest.

When encountering such situations, clearing the airway without spending time looking for a diagnosis may solve the problem. Otherwise, it may be necessary to begin immediate artificial ventilation by the mouth-to-mouth technique or by using any resuscitation bag within reach until equipment for tracheal intubation is available.

In the delivery room adequate equipment is normally on hand for immediate use by obstetricians or nurses to clear and stabilize the airway until specialist help arrives. Instant ventilation with a mask and self-inflating bag, containing a pressure-relief valve which vents at 35 cmH$_2$O, should be instituted. If the neonate fails to breathe after birth, the relief valve must be occluded with a fingertip and a prolonged inspiration time of 0.5–0.8 s and a pressure of up to 40 cmH$_2$O applied to create a functional residual capacity (FRC) in the lung. Otherwise, the oxygenation remains grossly impaired. An exception should be made when thick meconium is seen in the pharynx. This has to be removed first, even in the presence of hypoxaemia, before passive breathing is instituted, since pushing thick meconium into the trachea and bronchi would harm the child.

For victims of SIDS, help often comes too late. These children, under 1 year of age, are usually found lifeless in their cubicle at home or in the hospital, but resuscitation must be attempted in order to rule out a 'near miss' SIDS or an apparent life-threatening event (ALTE) which may respond to resuscitation.[7] If foreign material is present in the pharynx, it has to be removed quickly and cardiopulmonary resuscitation begun. In the case of ALTE, results are encouraging, but investigation and, if appropriate, treatment for gastro-oesophageal reflux and congenital airway malformation must follow resuscitation immediately to prevent further attacks.[8]

In complete airway obstruction due to a foreign body, up to five abdominal thrusts are advocated when unconsciousness occurs, to dislodge the obstacle from the airway.[9] The danger of laceration of the liver in children under 1 year of age led the American Heart Association to advocate only five back blows and five chest thrusts in this age group to achieve the same result. This has been called into question by experimental data, showing that abdominal thrusts produce at least twice the pressure of back blows in infants.[10] Whatever procedure one chooses, rupture of the stomach, jejunum or oesophagus is an acceptable price for survival, as found with two preschool children who aspirated pieces from Chinese checkers. The first child died during an attempt to push the piece into the trachea by a tracheal tube; the second survived because the game piece could be pushed into the right main stem bronchus in the hypoxic child by the intubation manoeuvre, whence it could be surgically removed later. Immediate abdominal thrusts could have saved the first child and ameliorated the course of the second (see also Chapter 22).

Sometimes tracheal intubation cannot be performed owing to direct trauma to the larynx or pharynx, an impacted foreign body, or occlusion by a tumour or by the base of the tongue in micrognathia. A rigid bronchoscope with a telescopic lens, if available, is the most useful instrument to relieve this dangerous situation, provided the anaesthetist is experienced in its use.

In an ambulance, loss of the airway can only be overcome by puncturing the trachea with a large-bore intravenous needle in infants and small children or by a dilatation tracheostomy in school-aged children using a Seldinger technique. Although no systematic data from paediatric emergency treatment exist, data from adult emergency cricothyroidotomy show a high mortality and complication rate; however, some patients have been saved by this manoeuvre.[11]

Paediatric cardiopulmonary resuscitation following severe airway obstruction is described comprehensively elsewhere.[12]

UNEXPECTED AIRWAY OBSTRUCTION DURING ANAESTHESIA

The best way to prevent airway obstruction in patients where difficulties are anticipated is to ensure in advance the presence of experienced and appropriately equipped personnel (see Chapter 17). Algorithms for prediction and management of the difficult airway have been developed in adult anaesthesia,[13,14] which steer the practitioner through a series of choices not easily recalled in an emergency situation and are only partly applicable in neonates and infants.

Failure to maintain a patent airway may still occur during any stage of paediatric anaesthesia despite adequate experience and extreme prudence in difficult cases. If such an event cannot be managed within a few minutes, brain damage or death will inevitably occur. This is reflected in the many closed claims malpractice cases where unsuccessful management of airway obstruction is the cause of death.[15] In such emergency situations it is of the utmost importance to follow clinically valid rules in order to stabilize the airway by facemask ventilation, by the application of a laryngeal mask airway (LMA) or an oropharyngeal or nasopharyngeal airway until adequate aid arrives, to avoid oedema and injury to the larynx caused by unnecessary attempts at intubation.

Drawing on ample experience in airway endoscopy the author has developed a simple way of grading unexpected intubation difficulties. It can be remembered easily in emergency situations and avoids the continuation of unpromising attempts at intubation (Figure 18.2).

- Grade I: Visibility of tip of epiglottis and arytenoid cartilages only. Proceed with attempts at intubation, change of blades or tubes, consider use of LMA.
- Grade II: Visibility of backwardly tilted epiglottis only despite laryngeal thrust. Careful attempts at intubation using stylet or Magill forceps. Advancement of tube must be easy. Call for aid and endoscopy after four attempts. Secure airway by bagging, oropharyngeal airway or LMA.
- Grade III: No visibility of parts of larynx possible or extreme lateralization of larynx by pharyngeal masses. Call for aid and endoscopy after two attempts at intubation.

- Grade IV: Visibility of an apparently normal glottis. Advancement of tracheal tube not possible, despite stepping down with sizes. Call for assistance by endoscopy, the only way to diagnose subglottic airway obstruction.

All calls for aid presuppose simultaneous preparation of endoscopic equipment by an assistant. Even experienced anaesthetists should call for assistance in grade III and IV difficulties. Such guidelines prevent unnecessarily long attempts at intubation.

According to Katz's 25 years of experience of malpractice cases in paediatric anaesthesia, continuation of attempts at intubation under unfavourable circumstances were the leading cause of brain damage or death. Asking for aid after a defined period could have solved the airway problem in several cases, even without intubation.[16]

CONGENITAL RESPIRATORY OBSTRUCTION

Respiratory obstruction inevitably causes stridor, although children with congenital or acquired stridor are not encountered frequently. If children with stridor have to undergo anaesthesia without endoscopic diagnosis, they are at high risk of developing airway obstruction. After a case-by-case analysis of more than 150 infants the author believes that no child with stridor should be intubated before an X-ray of the chest and neck and a laryngotracheobronchoscopy are carried out.[17] Laryngeal malformation or residual scar tissue is found in a great number of patients, leading to the risk of airway occlusion during induction of anaesthesia (Figures 18.3–18.8).

STRIDOR

The primary causes of stridor are still thought to be a curled epiglottis and the caving-in of soft aryepiglottic folds or arytenoid cartilages during inspiration into the glottic opening (laryngomalacia),[18] but the use of functional endoscopy has revealed a surprisingly large variety of diag-

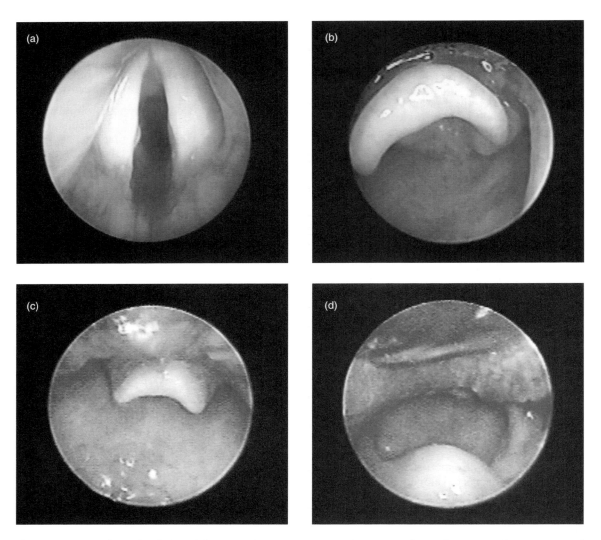

Figure 18.2 Grading of visibility of the larynx in emergency situations, according to laryngoscopic exposure and feasibility of tube advancement: (a) grade I; (b) grade II; (c) grade III; and (d) grade IV.

noses, with laryngomalacia being present only in about 5–7% of the cases.[17] Knowledge of this pathology is important for the paediatric anaesthetist to avoid airway obstruction or airway damage. Laryngomalacia, however, is not a well-defined anatomical entity. Aspiration of the curled epiglottis and the aryepiglottic folds is clinically different from an isolated aspiration of one or both arytenoid cartilages (Figures 18.3 and 18.4). Differentation between the affected parts of the larynx should be undertaken since treatment is different.

Intubation rarely poses a problem where structures of the larynx are soft. Sometimes a soft epiglottis and arytenoid cartilages are impacted into the glottis by ventilation with a bag, causing complete airway obstruction which requires a quick intubation procedure.[17] In these rare events reduction of the soft structure of the larynx by laser application might be justified.[19] Anaesthesia for laser surgery requires special tracheal tubes.

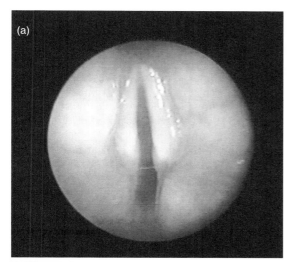

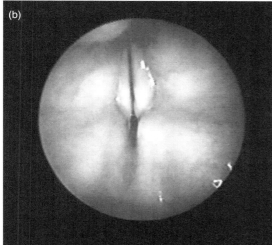

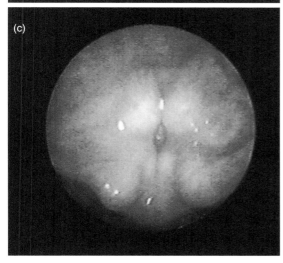

BILATERAL CHOANAL ATRESIA

Bilateral choanal atresia or severe nasal stenosis is a rare malformation in the neonate (1–4/ 10 000 live births) and is associated with APERT-, Treacher-Collins and CHARGE syndromes.[18] This malformation leads to serious respiratory problems after birth, including complete airway obstruction, and artificial ventilation is often only possible with an oral airway. The conscious infant may not tolerate such an irritating device for long. The unsuccessful passage of suction catheters through both nostrils, followed by X-ray with radiopaque dye, confirms the diagnosis. Immediate surgical repair is the most appropriate treatment, although unilateral atresia is not an indication for immediate surgery.

General anaesthesia with atropine premedication and tracheal intubation using a preformed tube, e.g. RAE, is required and is firmly secured to the chin in the midline. Ventilation is controlled using a muscle relaxant with all the precautions and monitoring appropriate to neonatal surgery. A throat pack is not usually used as the surgeon has a direct view to the larynx, even though there may be considerable bleeding. No split mouth gags are small enough for a newborn, so the tongue plate of the gag may compress or kink the tracheal tube.

During the operation the bony and occasionally membranous structures occluding the choa-

Figure 18.3. Glottic closure and laryngospasm. (a) Normal glottic opening. The vocal cords are moderately abducted; the false vocal cords are located laterally, hidden by the laryngeal mucosa. (b) Closure of the glottis (glottis spasm), not permitting adequate respiration. The vocal cords are pressed against each other, leaving a very small entrance open at the posterior commissure; the false vocal cords overlap the true vocal cords to some extent. Oxygen may be moved passively into the trachea by inflations of an anaesthesia bag and break the spasm. Intubation is possible by force, but not recommended (laryngeal trauma). (c) Laryngospasm. The false vocal cords have closed above the vocal cords; the paraglottis, the intralaryngeal part of the epiglottis, has moved dorsally; the base of the arytenoid cartilages anteriorly, being tilted backwards at the same time, thus occluding the larynx in an extremely effective way. Intubation is impossible during laryngospasm and should not be attempted.

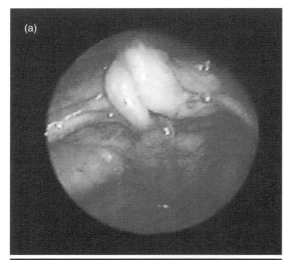

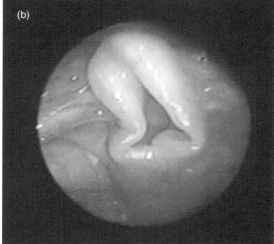

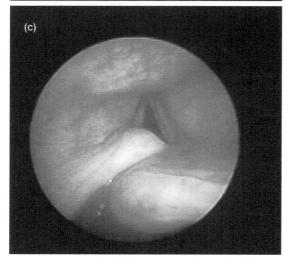

nae, including the posterior segment of the vomer, are removed by a burr. A twin drain is placed through the opened structures for about 8 weeks, stenting the operation site, permitting nasal breathing and restoring the choanal passages permanently.[20] Extubation should take place in the fully awake patient after thorough suctioning of the pharynx and when the stenting drains are clear. The surgery is painful and one dose of codeine phosphate 1 mg kg^{-1} i.m., together with rectal or oral paracetamol, is necessary.

Regular infusion of heparinized saline into the drains, humidified air and suctioning of coagulated blood prevent occlusion of the stents, but constant observation for several days is necessary to avoid obstructive apnoea, before the infants are sent home. Since only about 25% of mature neonates and 8% of premature infants are able to breathe by mouth in nasal airway occlusion,[21] apnoea remains a threat to patients during home treatment and they should be adequately monitored.

FACIAL DYSMORPHIC SYNDROMES

Facial dysmorphic syndromes such as Pierre Robin present easily recognizable dangers of airway obstruction before anaesthesia. Prudent

Figure 18.4. Structural abnormalities of the infantile larynx, causing airway obstruction. (a) Soft, folded epiglottis in an infant with severe stridor during inspiration. The epiglottis, together with the aryepiglottic folds, is aspirated with the inspiratory airstream and causes mild to severe stridor, but rarely severe airway obstruction, needing treatment. (b) The same larynx during expiration presenting clearly the abnormally winding aryepiglottic folds and the epiglottis in a more upright position. (c) Malacia of the posterior wall of the larynx. The arytenoid cartilages are positioned anteriorly in a sliding door manner during exhalation. During inspiration they are aspirated into the glottic opening and may occlude the larynx entirely, producing a severe snoring stridor, even apnoea. During ventilation by bag and mask, complete airway obstruction may occur, which can be overcome only by intubation. Surgical treatment is indicated. Although a curled, flaccid epiglottis, loose aryepiglottic folds and abnormally mobile arytenoid cartilages are summarized under the term 'laryngomalacia', a differentiation should be made between the parts of the larynx affected because treatment is different.

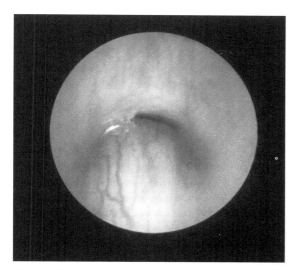

Figure 18.5. Subglottic haemangioma.

planning of the intubation procedure is the most important step to avoid obstruction of the airway in these patients (see Chapters 15 and 17).

EPIPHARYNGEAL FIBROMA

Epipharyngeal fibroma, hanging from a pedicle into the pharynx or oesophagus, can be impacted into the laryngeal opening like a foreign body and occlude it completely.[17] If no air at all can pass by mask ventilation, laryngoscopy should be carried out immediately (as is the case in any patient with suspected upper airway occlusion) and the obstacle removed by Magill forceps before intubation.

LARYNGEAL OR TRACHEAL STENOSIS

Laryngeal (subglottic) or tracheal stenosis can be detected clinically by stridor only if more than 70% of the lumen of the airway is obstructed.[22] Laryngeal obstruction occurs by compression of the entrance of the larynx by tumours, paravallecular cysts, scars, intrinsic connective tissue or viral papillomatosis. In the latter case, it is generally agreed that, where possible, a tube should not be introduced into the trachea because of the risk of seeding viruses below the vocal cords. Laser coagulation is the treatment of choice.

If a true stenosis of the subglottis or trachea is found unexpectedly, a decision must be made either to cancel or to continue the scheduled operation with a considerably smaller tube, an LMA or a tracheostomy. If a narrow subglottic space is detected during intubation, occluding less than 70% of the airway, and the patient has no clinical symptoms even during exercise, no operation is indicated to 'normalize' the airway, although it is recommended in the literature.[23] This operation has a high complication rate and the stenosis grows with the patient.[24]

Congenital subglottic stenosis in the neonate is mainly caused by a haemangioma (Figure 18.5) or cricoid chondroma, but sometimes endoscopy reveals cicatricial tissue after intubation injury.[17] It is surprising that many children are not compromised by significant subglottic stenosis. If stenosis is suspected from stridor, all preparations must be made to perform an emergency tracheostomy, in case obstruction of the airway occurs during endoscopy. If a stenosis is suspected before anaesthesia and a tracheal tube cannot pass the larynx, ventilation has to be maintained by mask/LMA until endoscopy makes the situation clear. In subglottic haemangioma a tracheal tube might be introduced into the airway; bleeding from a laceration of the haemangioma will be compressed by the tube as long as it is in place. In cricoid stenosis, tracheostomy is frequently needed because the rigid cartilage does not yield to the tracheal tube. Surgical resection of both malformations by laryngofissure usually causes little damage to the subglottic mucosa, thus reopening the subglottic space, sometimes even without the need to perform a tracheostomy.[25]

Ex-premature infants with ductal cysts,[26] scar bridging of the vocal cords or scar funicles crossing the upper airway frequently present with stridor (see Figures 18.6 and 18.9). Ventilation by a mask might be accompanied by air trapping and intubation can be impossible. The anaesthetist should be warned by the stridor and prepare a bronchoscope before induction of anaesthesia. If the tracheal tube cannot be advanced it should be immediately exchanged for one of a smaller size, carefully avoiding any force. Cautious rupture of the cyst or scar bridge by a stylet, armoured tube or the rigid endoscope should be attempted only after

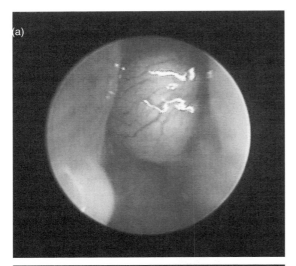

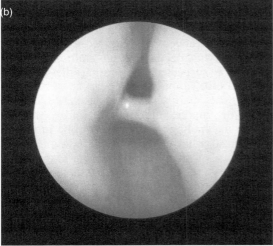

Figure 18.6. Typical upper airway obstruction in ex-premature infants after long-term artificial respiration. (a) Subglottic ductal cyst. The infant underwent several surgical interventions without any airway problems. After induction of anaesthesia at the age of 1 year, it was possible to pass a tracheal tube through the vocal cords only after endoscopy and perforation of the cyst. (b) Scar tissue bridging of vocal cords as a result of long-term tracheal intubation. After induction of anaesthesia, a tracheal tube could be passed through the vocal cords, only after endoscopy with separation of the scar tissue.

visualization of the anatomy (Figure 18.6). If this proves to be impossible, an emergency tracheostomy might be necessary.

In tracheal compression by bronchogenic cysts, tuberculous lymph nodes, mediastinal masses or in the cicatricially narrowed trachea, introduction of a rigid ventilating bronchoscope can overcome the obstruction in most cases, since there remains some elasticity of tissue. In congenital tracheal stenosis, however, formed by cartilaginous rings, the stenosis can be dilated neither by the advancing tube nor by a rigid bronchoscope. Injury to the mucosa by the intubation procedure might prove fatal. Therefore, the trachea should be inspected using a Hopkin's lens as soon as tracheal stenosis is suspected after induction of anaesthesia, and a decision made as to whether a tracheostomy should be performed or the recovery of the patient awaited. If no intubation trauma occurs in such a situation, major surgery with thoracotomy and cardiopulmonary bypass might be instituted later on.

COMPRESSION

Compression of the trachea by large vessels manifests itself mostly in infancy with episodes of stridor, wheezing and the inability to clear secretions from the trachea. It is sometimes accompanied by cyanosis as a late symptom before life-threatening apnoea occurs, necessitating urgent intervention. Narrowing of the trachea (and often the oesophagus as well) is frequently due to a double aortic arch, well described since 1949.[27,28] Sometimes an arteria lusoria or the ligamentum arteriosum is responsible for the obstruction of the trachea,[29] and is not visible in magnetic resonance imaging (MRI) or angiograms. Bronchoscopy is necessary for differentiating the symptoms; a double aortic arch shows an almost complete occlusion of the trachea with diffuse pulsation, whereas the more frequently encountered compression of the trachea by the innominate artery shows a flat lumen with heavy ventral pulsation (Figure 18.7). Anatomical obstruction is relieved by surgery but stridor may remain noticeable sometimes for months. Ventral pulsation of the tracheal wall is mostly related to the innominate artery in combination with oesophageal atresia[30] (see also Chapter 13).

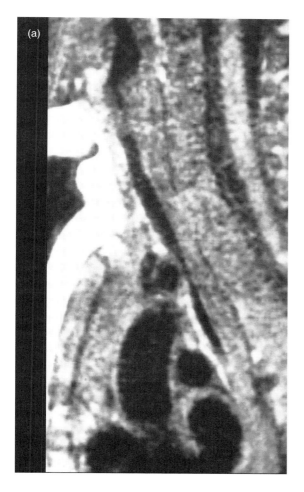

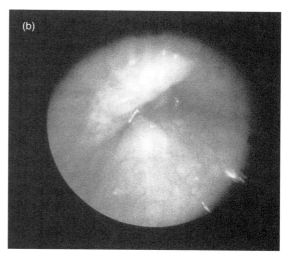

Figure 18.7. External compression of the trachea by an arterial vessel. (a) Magnetic resonance study of the mediastinum showing anterior compression of the trachea by innominate artery. The child had frequent attacks of apnoea after feeding, requiring resuscitation with tracheal intubation on several occasions. (b) Bronchoscopy showing complete collapse of the trachea with ventral pulsation at the site of compression by the innominate artery, opening up briefly during spontaneous inspiration. Granulation tissue developed at the narrowest part of the collapse because a tracheal tube was advance beyond this point. Aortopexy was indicated and carried out, relieving all respiratory symptoms.

CYSTIC HYGROMA

Cystic hygroma is a multilocular lymphangioma presenting at birth as a swelling in the neck and axilla. Involvement of the base of the tongue and oropharynx is common and may cause obstruction to breathing. Although the condition is benign and the swellings are soft, it invades tissues and can recur after surgery. Occasionally there is an intrathoracic extension.

An intraoral swelling may make inflation of the lungs and identification of the larnyx difficult. During induction of anaesthesia it is crucial to maintain spontaneous breathing since, in the worst cases, the only way to identify the larynx is to see the movement of bubbles as air passes in and out. Severe cases require tracheostomy. Surgical dissection of the tumour may be difficult as the cysts cross tissue planes.

OESOPHAGEAL ATRESIA

Patients with oesophageal atresia and tracheo-oesophageal fistulae show an associated abnormality of the respiratory tract in a very high proportion of cases and are candidates for airway obstruction during anaesthesia, not only in the neonatal period. Typical coarse stridor, caused by tracheomalacia in almost 70% of the patients, and an additional arterial compression of the ventral part of the trachea with pronounced pulsation in 16% of the cases are the most common findings.[31] Tracheoscopy should be carried out, preferably before primary anastomosis to inspect tracheal abnormalities which might be responsible for obstruction during anaesthesia and postoperatively. A proximal fistula can be excluded and the location of the distal fistula described in order to avoid advancement of the tube into the pouch-like remaining part of the fistula in subsequent intubations. If the tracheal tube is caught in tracheal pouches, ventilation is completely obstructed, and only pulling and twisting of the tube help to place it correctly.[31]

If only tracheomalacia exists, advancement of the tube to the carina might improve ventilation, but it might also induce injury to the mucosa of the distal trachea and make extubation impossible. Aortopexy is the treatment of choice[30] to alleviate symptoms and help towards normal respiration. Patients with an isolated tracheo-oesophageal fistula or oesophageal atresia type Vogt II show practically no anatomical airway abnormalities.[31]

LARYNGOTRACHEO-OESOPHAGEAL CLEFT

Patients with laryngotracheo-oesophageal cleft show signs of airway obstruction immediately after birth or when they choke during the first feed, but unfortunately diagnosis is frequently made only after months or years if the cleft involves the larynx and upper trachea only (Petterson types I and II) because the cleft is hidden in redundant, overlapping mucosa. Symptoms of obstruction are overcome by intubation. These patients cannot be extubated and may be treated for aspiration pneumonia, until bronchoscopy establishes the diagnosis and surgical treatment can be carried out.[32] If the cleft extends to the lower trachea (Petterson type III[33]), most patients die because ventilation is possible only via the oesophagus, causing inadequate oxygenation of the infant. Surgical closure by an anterior laryngofissure proves to be successful in most patients, although stage-I clefts may be closed via an endoscope.[32]

COLLAPSE

Collapse of the entire trachea and main stem bronchi, preventing spontaneous respiration in newborn infants, poses a very rare but desperate situation, because these infants have to remain intubated in the hospital until they die, since neither tracheostomy nor tracheal resection can provide unobstructed respiration. A new technique involving a bronchoscopically guided external tracheobronchial suspension by a tube-like prothesis has reportedly relieved collapse immediately in 11 patients and permitted spontaneous respiration.[34]

MYELOMENINGOCELE

The incidence of myelomeningocele (MMC) is relatively high and often complicated by the Arnold–Chiari malformation. Passive movements of the vocal cords because of the impact of the medulla into the spinal canal and subsequent cranial nerve invovlement may produce severe stridor with problems in spontaneous respiration or during ventilation by a facemask. More importantly, the impact of the medulla into the foramen magnum may lead eventually to irreversible cardiac arrest.[35] This is sometimes attributed to airway obstruction. A possible lethal outcome has to be explained to the parents in patients with attacks of stridor and MMC before surgical interventions.

ACQUIRED RESPIRATORY OBSTRUCTION

OCCLUSION OF THE PHARYNX

Occlusion of the pharynx by relaxation of the muscles of the tongue, which is large in relation to the oral cavity, is the most frequent airway obstruction in childhood. This occurs during sleep in predisposed children with craniofacial anomalies or adenotonsillar hypertrophy, when it is known as obstructive sleep apnoea,[2,3] and in all comatose states, but most frequently during induction and maintenance of anaesthesia and during emergence from anaesthesia in the recovery room. Placing the head in a sniffing position, pushing the mandible firmly forward with two fingers behind the angles of the jaw and simultaneously opening the mouth by depressing the tip of the mandible (triple airway manoeuvre) detaches the tongue from the posterior wall of the pharynx and reopens the airway immediately, as shown in studies using lateral radiographs.[36] However, in neonates and infants, the tongue is often tightly attached to the palate and can only be removed by the blade of the laryngoscope or by the insertion of an oropharyngeal tube. Owing to the large occiput in infants, the sniffing position is achieved by laying the head flat on the operating table into an inflatable ring or placing a small pad under the shoulders. Overextension of the head to move the tongue forward is ineffective; this movement itself may cause airway obstruction. Chin lift in children with enlarged tonsils may worsen airway patency.[37] Gentle, but frequent strokes with an anaesthesia bag move sufficient air through the larynx, re-establishing spontaneous or assisted breathing.

Intravenous induction with thiopentone often causes apnoea, sometimes with involuntary muscular movements similar to clonic seizures which impede assisted ventilation briefly, but should not be confused with mechanical airway obstruction.

LARYNGOSPASM

Laryngospasm is the most frequently encountered airway obstruction during anaesthesia, especially in early infancy, because of immature co-ordination of laryngopharyngeal movements.[38] The incidence of laryngospasm was investigated in a large cohort study in 1984;[39] 17 events in 1000 anaesthetics were found in children aged up to 9 years. This number increased to 64/1000 in children with obstructive lung disease and to 96/1000 in those with acute upper respiratory tract infection. Similar results are described in another study,[40] showing children with an active upper respiratory infection, young age or supervision by less experienced anaesthetists to be at higher risk of laryngospasm.

Laryngospasm is defined as complete closure of the larynx caused by external stimulation. The ventricular cords (false vocal cords) are tightly occluded, the paraglottis (intralaryngeal part of the epiglottis) moves posteriorly and the arytenoid cartilages both perform a ventral movement, thus effectively sealing the larynx (Figure 18.3). This also applies to patients with bilateral vocal cord paralysis, which is often

forgotten. Attempts at intubation during laryngospasm can only damage the larynx and maintain the stimulus of spasm, prolonging the dangerous situation.

Closure of the glottis (glottic spasm) is anatomically quite different from laryngospasm: both vocal cords are firmly pressed against each other, leaving a small lumen open at the posterior commissure which allows minimal ventilation by the anaesthetist (see Figure 18.3b). Intubation is technically possible but not recommended because it inevitably leads to intubation trauma. Although it is difficult to differentiate clinically between glottic spasm and laryngospasm, the dynamics of laryngospasm can easily be studied in patients with a tracheostomy or during investigation of stridor, using halothane anaesthesia. The slow emergence from halothane anaesthesia helps greatly in functional descriptions of laryngeal movements and the different clinical approach to glottic spasm compared to laryngospasm can clearly be demonstrated for educational purposes.

Prevention of laryngospasm depends almost entirely on the attentiveness and experience of the anaesthetist, particularly in neonatal anaesthesia. Strategies to avoid laryngospasm have been discussed frequently in the literature[41–43] and during training of residents. The incidence of laryngospasm may be higher without the use of premedication. Laryngospasm has been seen in recent clinical studies with the new inhalational anaesthetic agent, desflurane, where it occurred in more than 50% of cases. One group using this drug discontinued their study because of a high incidence of laryngospasm[44] and this agent is not recommended for inhalation induction in children.

Is laryngospasm 'a neglectible minor incident in paediatric anaesthesia, since it always resolves in the healthy, awake child after a short period of hypoxia?' Obviously not, since laryngospasm can lead to deep cyanosis, a drop in arterial blood pressure and cardiac arrest, not only in sick patients. For these reasons high priority should be given to strategies of prevention.

Laryngospasm occurs most frequently at the beginning and the end of anaesthesia. During induction, preventive measures include: (1) a reduction in mucus production through adequate premedication; (2) the slow injection of intravenous induction agents; (3) no handling of the patient during induction; (4) no forced bagging after apnoea by thiopentone, opioids, propofol; (5) the cancellation of operations on patients with proven upper airway infection; (6) and no inhalational induction with isoflurane or desflurane.

Laryngospasm during induction of anaesthesia without noticeable external irritation of the larynx can be the first clinical sign of reflux of gastric contents and imminent vomiting. The attentive anaesthetist, with the precordial stethoscope in place and hearing sounds of heavy retroperistalsis, may turn the child to one side and thus prevent aspiration.

If ketamine is used for induction by intramuscular injection in doses greater than 6 mg kg^{-1}, there is a four-fold increase in laryngospasm compared with doses less than 3.5 mg kg^{-1} which are also adequate for induction.[45]

Local anaesthesia of the larynx prevents laryngospasm, but may promote aspiration, when the larynx is exposed to reflux or vomiting after early extubation, so it is not generally used in paediatric anaesthesia except in diagnostic laryngoscopy.

Laryngospasm during emergence from anaesthesia occurs more frequently than during induction; for that reason prevention during this particular stage of anaesthesia is clinically most important, and is best achieved by: (1) the presence of heated and humidified gases during anaesthesia; (2) the suctioning of pharyngeal or tracheal secretions before extubation; (3) extubation in the awake patient after full reversal of muscle relaxation; (4) extubation after deep inspiration; and (5) the administration of atropine to prevent recurrence of laryngospasm

However, tracheal suction before extubation may itself provoke bronchospasm. It is preferable to clear secretions from the tracheobronchial tree at a deeper level of anaesthesia. Atropine helps to prevent laryngospasm and bronchospasm only if administered at least 10 min before the intended procedure. In contrast to the quick action of atropine on heart rate, its effect on laryngeal reflexes and reduction of mucus secretion is most effective after about 30 min.

Treatment of laryngospasm involves applying oxygen via a mask well sealed to the face with continuously applied, not too vigorous positive pressure with the anaesthesia bag up to a pressure of 20–40 cmH$_2$O. After this it is a matter of waiting. If there is some air movement through the vocal cords discernible by the precordial stethoscope within 20–30 s, laryngospasm is broken. If spasm continues, a vigorous forward pull of the mandible is helpful to cause a painful stimulus and stretch the geniohyoid muscle to ventralize the paraglottis. Both manoeuvres, accompanied by rapid bagging, solve laryngospasm instantly in many patients. If these measures do not help or if severe laryngospasm recurs, immediate injection of 0.1 mg kg^{-1} atropine and 2.0 mg kg^{-1} succinylcholine resolves the spasm and makes ventilation possible. If secretions are present in the larynx or trachea, suctioning during the time of muscular paralysis is necessary to prevent a second attack. In patients with heart disease and laryngospasm, waiting should be limited to 15 s and then atropine and succinylcholine given because these patients are liable to have a cardiac arrest after short periods of hypoxia. Sustained forceful ventilation from an anaesthesia bag to overcome laryngospasm is very ill advised, because high intrapharyngeal pressure overextends the piriform fossae, pressing both aryepiglottic folds against each other and sealing the entrance to the larynx above the false vocal cords, compounding the problem of laryngospasm and causing gastric distension.

If a patient becomes rapidly hypoxic and severely bradycardic during laryngospasm, it is too late for the administration of succinylcholine since this may cause cardiac arrest and prolong the period of hypoxia. In this exceptional situation it may be advantageous to wait until laryngospasm is eventually resolved by hypoxia and to ventilate the hypoxic patient before cardiac arrest occurs. The role of propofol in such a situation has not been defined; it seems to be slower than succinyl choline in relieving laryngospasm, but it leaves the heart rhythm unaffected (see also Chapter 5).

Differential diagnosis of laryngospasm

Inhibitory reflexes such as the Hering–Breuer and the intercostal phrenic reflex frequently mimic laryngospasm. They are classic protective reflexes to protect the lung from overdistension. The Hering–Breuer reflex is frequently produced in childhood by forceful bagging of the lung and results in apnoea or a profound exhalation which is repeated if attempts at forceful ventilation are continued. FRC is lost rapidly and hypoxia ensues. Succinylcholine helps immediately but is not indicated since careful observation of chest movements alone may lead to the correct diagnosis. The intercostal phrenic inhibitory reflex occurs only in newborn infants[46] and terminates inspiration as a response to chest wall distortion or forceful ventilation. It resolves more easily than the Hering–Breuer reflex by gentle bagging, but is sometimes treated by giving succinylcholine as well. Since succinylcholine resolves both reflexes immediately, many anaesthetists are not aware of having encountered this type of inhibitory reflex.

Complications after laryngospasm

Hypoxic brain damage can be avoided in almost all patients by following the above guidelines, but in patients with impaired cardiac function, cardiac arrest may be induced by laryngospasm and damage the heart or brain, in particular during hyperglycaemia.[47]

When intubation is attempted during laryngospasm, trauma to the supraglottic structures can be expected. Fortunately, these structures tend to recover spontaneously, but in severe injuries special treatment has to be instituted.[17]

On rare but regular occasions, negative pressure pulmonary oedema occurs owing to intense respiratory movements against the closed glottis. A high negative pressure builds up in the intrapleural space, venous return increases enormously, the left heart lacks volume, the alveoli fill rapidly with fluid, moist rales are heard and pink froth pours out of the tracheal tube. This condition, first described in 1927,[48] has been rediscovered[49] and is often mistaken for aspiration, with disadvantageous consequences for the patient as suctioning of the supposedly aspirated matter from the airway prolongs oedema and hypoxaemia. Ventilation with increased inspiratory times and positive end-expiratory pressure (PEEP) brings an end to this dangerous event. Although athletic

adolescents are supposed to be most at risk for this condition, it occurs in all age groups, including healthy neonates.

DISLODGEMENT

Dislodgement of an accurately placed tracheal tube should not occur during intraoperative postural changes, fixation of the tube, manipulations in the oropharynx or in facial burns. Accidental extubation is usually quickly recognized by auscultation with the precordial stethoscope and the loss of the end-tidal CO_2 signal, but incomplete retraction of the tube, with the tip remaining in the entrance of the larynx, permitting some air to be exhaled and to produce a CO_2 signal, and some air to inflate the stomach, may cause a hazardous situation. If there is any doubt about the position of a tracheal tube, only visualization of the glottis by laryngoscopy, showing the tube between the vocal cords, and the presence of a regular CO_2 signal give evidence of an intratracheal placement of the tube. Nevertheless, the tracheal tube may be pushed too far down into one of the main stem bronchi and cause cyanosis and bradycardia. The breath sounds in small children are often misleading, making the diagnosis of a dislodged tube by auscultation difficult. The marking of the ventral side of tracheal tubes in centimetres, as in those from Portex and Rusch, helps in gauging the depth of the tracheal tube below the vocal cords during laryngoscopy. Marking the tracheal tube at the lips or nostril after intubation helps to prevent subsequent incidents. In situations where there is no access to the pharynx, the tube position can only be determined by a chest X-ray.

OCCLUSION

If occlusion of the tube by secretions or blood clots occurs, saline lavage and vigorous suctioning are the only way to clear the airway. Otherwise the tube must be changed during the operation, which is a difficult procedure, in particular during thoracotomies. Fibreoptic endoscopy is limited for technical reasons to children with internal tube diameters > 3.5 mm. With smaller instruments, although they are useful for determining the location of the tip of the tube, it is rarely possible to remove tenacious secretions because they have an extremely narrow or even non-existent suction channel.

CHEST RIGIDITY BY OPIOIDS

Opioids such as fentanyl and alfentanil, in doses above 20 μg kg^{-1}, and sufentanil have been thought to reduce significantly chest-wall compliance in children by muscle rigidity.[50] At induction of anaesthesia, ventilation may be impossible, as in complete airway obstruction, and may cause hypercarbia.[51] This well-known complication is circumvented by precurarization with 1/10th of the paralysing dose of a competitive muscle relaxant or by induction of anaesthesia by propofol. However, recently, fibreoptic observation of the larynx during induction of anaesthesia with sufentanil revealed vocal cord closure as the major cause of difficult ventilation,[52] which might be true for all opioids and explain convincingly the quick reaction to muscle relaxants.

MEDIASTINAL MASSES

Patients with mediastinal masses who are scheduled for biopsies deserve special attention because their life virtually depends on the careful planning and co-operation of all the physicians involved in their surgical treatment. These patients may seem to have little airway compromise before the operation, but patency of the airway might be due to compensatory efforts which are obtunded by induction of anaesthesia or even by awake sedation for needle biopsy. This has been well recognized since 1976,[53] with lethal outcomes documented since 1981.[54] If the patient shows dyspnoea lying down local anaesthesia without sedation should be considered instead of general anaesthesia,[55] but airway obstruction may still occur and all prerequisites for securing the airway must be in place (see below). Patients are only safe if computed tomographic (CT) scans in anterior masses (lymphoma, teratoma) or MRI studies in posterior masses (neurogenic tumours) are carried out before anaesthesia, and the anaesthetist, endoscopist and thoracic surgeon have discussed the anatomy relating to the airway and are present at induction. A rigid ventilation bronchoscope and a number of tracheal tubes of different sizes and types (e.g.

incompressible ones) should be prepared for securing the airway. If airway obstruction occurs and the surgeon cannot remove the tumour from the mediastinum, the tracheal tube ought to stay in place until radiation or chemotherapy shrinks the tumour and release the pressure from the trachea. In rare cases venous return via the superior vena cava is markedly impaired during surgery by traction of the tumour at the mediastinal vessels, in particular after intubation with a bronchoscope. Volume administration and quick replacement of the rigid scope by an incompressible tube are mandatory. Sometimes the surgeon is forced to remove as much of the tumour as possible to restore venous return.

If there is any doubt about the patency of the airway before extubation, a tracheoscopy under spontaneous respiration should be carried out. This strict approach has kept many patients safe in the author's institution over the past 20 years and was reinforced by a near miss fatal obstruction when a small mediastinal mass was thought to be irrelevant to airway obstruction and inadequate precautions were taken. Conversely, one teenaged patient with Hodgkin's disease was extubated after radiotherapy in an institution without an anaesthetist standing by; severe airway obstruction after awake extubation could not be treated in time, which resulted in brain damage.

INTUBATION TRAUMA

Intubation trauma is encountered in more than 50% of infants with acquired stridor.[17] Laryngeal injury is probably the price to pay for the survival of increasing numbers of extremely low birth-weight neonates and stems chiefly from the long exposure of immature laryngotracheal structures to tracheal tubes over weeks or even months. Scar-tissue formation and obstruction of the larynx and upper trachea are aggravated by gastro-oesophageal reflux disease,[17,56] a frequent problem in ex-premature infants.

Airway obstruction due to intubation trauma consists mainly of masses of granulation tissue occluding the glottis and subglottis, and the bridging of the vocal cords and the lumen of the subglottis and upper trachea by funicles of scar tissue (Figures 18.6, 18.8, 18.9). Centric cicatricial stenosis of the subglottis, trachea or one

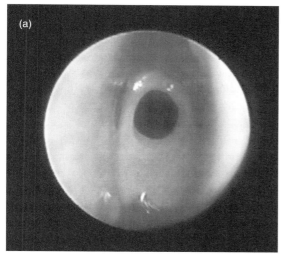

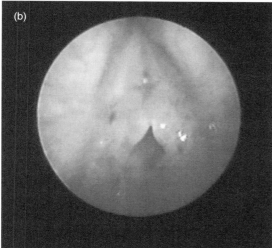

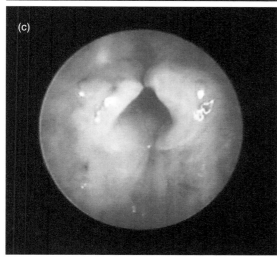

of the main stem bronchi is the most complicated injury of the airway and is very difficult to treat.[57,58] Glottic and subglottic lesions are caused by injury during the intubation procedure in less than 10% of cases; in the majority, the choice of a tube with too large a bore is responsible.[59] Tracheal and bronchial stenoses are frequently caused by traumatic suctioning in patients with a highly inflamed mucosa or by too far advanced tracheal tubes.

The location of an intrathoracic or extrathoracic airway stenosis can be differentiated clinically. The intrathoracic stenosis opens during inspiration by the negative intrathoracic pressure and closes during expiration, when positive pressure is exerted on the airway, producing expiratory stridor and some degree of air trapping. The extrathoracic stenosis generates stridor during inspiration because movable structures are aspirated by the negative intrathoracic pressure into the upper airway (Figure 18.8b) and open up during expiration (Figure 18.8c).

Combined inspiratory and expiratory stridor indicates a combination of deformities of the airway, a severe or fixed obstruction or an unusual form of stenosis (Figure 18.9).

Airway obstruction must be anticipated by the paediatric anaesthetist in all patients after closure of a tracheostomy, regardless of whether it was undertaken because of laryngotracheal reconstruction, cricoid split, trauma or infection. Supraglottic stenosis/collapse has been found in a remarkably high number of such patients.[60]

In some patients with a history of previous long-term intubation or laryngeal surgery a surprisingly narrow subglottic space has been found many years later, requiring intubation with tubes 30–50% less diameter than calculated, although these patients may present only mild symptoms of stridor perioperatively. In

Figure 18.8. Laryngeal airway obstruction caused by intubation trauma with too large-bore tracheal tubes. (a) Acute necrosis of the subglottic mucosa by application of a too large-bore tube during an emergency intubation. (b) Copious granulation tissue in the vocal cords of a preschool child after long-term intubation. Stridor and airway obstruction during inspiration. (c) Same larynx during expiration, showing no clinical signs of airway obstruction.

some centres microlaryngoscopy is undertaken routinely in patients with this history before anaesthesia for other surgery.

Once considerable airway obstruction is diagnosed by endoscopy and the patient shows little airway compromise clinically, the least invasive technique for securing the airway for anaesthesia should be used, such as an oropharyngeal airway with assisted mask ventilation or the application of an LMA. If tracheal intubation is really unavoidable, it should be carried out after careful selection of the smallest tube possible.

The LMA is a useful tool to circumvent tracheal intubation in selected cases. Although complications are rare, vocal cord palsy by compression of the recurrent laryngeal nerve and the external branch of the superior laryngeal nerve has been described, even after short day-case surgery.[61,62]

Prevention of intubation trauma by avoiding inadequate intubation techniques, too large-bore tubes and cuffed tubes in small children should be an important goal in paediatric anaesthesia. Controversies arise about cuffed intubation even in neonates, because studies to prove the innocuousness of cuffed intubation in

early childhood would have to comprise thousands of patients. The devastating effect of cuffed intubation on the larynx and trachea, regularly seen in paediatric endoscopy, cannot be justified by minor advantages of cuffed intubation in a few hundred patients under ideal conditions.[17,59,63]

CROUP, EPIGLOTTITIS AND BACTERIAL TRACHEITIS

POSTINTUBATION LARYNGEAL OEDEMA

Postintubation laryngeal oedema (postintubation croup) is mostly benign oedema of the glottis or subglottic region, primarily caused by the use of too large-bore tubes, or by appropriately sized tubes in patients with upper airway infection, or after intubation of patients with poor peripheral perfusion or following a chemical reaction of the laryngeal mucosa to aspirated gastric acid in patients with gastro-oesophageal reflux.[56] It is only rarely caused by the intubation procedure itself.[59] This condition seldom needs special treatment and disappears within hours. In severe cases, nebulization of racemic adrenaline and systemic steroids is indicated. If stridor does not subside within a day, pronounced intubation trauma must be suspected and laryngotracheoscopy should be performed (see Chapter 17).

LARYNGOTRACHEOBRONCHITIS (VIRAL CROUP)

Croup (from Scottish *kropan*, to cry, to make a croaking noise),[64] is characterized primarily by the symptom of a croaking or barking cough. This specific noise is produced by a subglottic narrowing of the larynx by trauma (e.g. post-intubation croup) or more commonly by specific infections (diphtheria, parainfluenza viruses) which cover the larynx and upper trachea with layers of thickened secretions composed of fibrin and necrotic cells, sometimes referred to as pseudomembranes. Since the disappearance

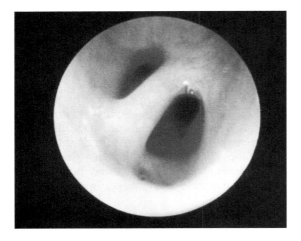

Figure 18.9. Intubation trauma caused by a cuffed tracheal tube. The healthy infant had been intubated with a cuffed tracheal tube for a short, elective procedure presenting with a hoarse voice and breathing difficulties postoperatively. A tracheostomy was performed without bronchoscopy several days after surgery; bronchoscopy showed a scar funicle in the upper trachea 1 year later.

of diphtheria thanks to vaccination, the term 'croup' is generally used as a synonym for viral laryngotracheobronchitis. Unless compliance with vaccination programmes is maintained, however, diphtheria may re-emerge as a cause of airway obstruction.

This most common cause of obstructive airway disease between the ages of 6 months and 5 years begins with upper respiratory tract infection, followed by a barking cough and, in more severe cases, by inspiratory stridor. Diagnosis can be confirmed by X-ray, showing typical subglottic narrowing (steeple sign). Sedation, humidified respiratory gases and nebulized racemic adrenaline relieve symptoms in the majority of cases. Although the effectiveness of dexamethasone, 0.6 mg kg^{-1}, has been well documented since 1980,[65] the attitude of most physicians towards the use of steroids has changed only in the late 1990s, in large measure as a result of the excellent effect of the nebulized steroid budesonide.[66] This dramatic change in therapeutic approach has decreased considerably the number of patients seen by the paediatric anaesthetist.

In contrast to the patient with supraglottitis, the patient with croup tires slowly and intubation, necessary only in 0.1–1.0% of children hospitalized for croup,[67] can be carried out under optimal conditions, which include a laryngotracheoscopy after induction of anaesthesia. Patients scheduled for intubation show severe dyspnoea, inspiratory and often expiratory stridor despite sedation. Anaesthesia can easily be induced by thiopentone or a similar drug preceded by atropine if tachycardia is not too pronounced. Assisted ventilation with 100% oxygen and halothane, avoiding nitrous oxide, deepens the level of anaesthesia until the larynx can be inspected. Some slowing of expiration is noticeable during mask ventilation, but since total exhaustion of muscular strength is the main cause of respiratory insufficiency, the majority of patients shows far better ventilation after induction of anaesthesia than before, encouraging the view that muscle paralysis can safely be used. After exposure of the larynx, a thin Hopkins rod lens is introduced into the larynx, not touching the inflamed mucosa.

All differential diagnoses of upper airway obstruction are ruled out by this inspection (atypical epiglottitis, subglottic stenosis or haemangioma, foreign body of larynx, pharynx or oesophagus). In some cases adhesive coatings of fibrin can be removed by a forceps and intubation avoided. The latter findings relate to later stages of the disease and explain why neither nebulized adrenaline nor steroids produce the desired effect in all cases.

Intubation has to be performed with extremely narrow tubes, not just 'a size smaller than usual', and often neonatal sizes have to be used. In older children neonatal tubes are not long enough for nasotracheal intubation; therefore, 'croup-tubes' are available with outer diameters of 4.2 and 4.8 mm, equivalent to 3.0 and 3.5 mm internal diameter, respectively (Blue Line Tracheal Tube, extra length 250 mm, size 3.0 and 3.5 mm; Portex Co., UK). Only by avoiding significant pressure on the laryngeal structures during intubation can the danger of intubation injury and subsequent tracheostomy be prevented. Intubation is needed for 2 or 3 days, the best test for extubation being the development of a small air leak around the tube.

In rare cases the disease progresses to a purulent stage with difficulty in clearing adhesive, membranous formations, probably caused by bacterial overgrowth, from the trachea.

The peak of the disease is commonly reached after 2–4 days, with symptoms disappearing after 7–10 days, although this varies considerably.

Children are sometimes admitted for bronchoscopy after weeks of continuous symptoms of croup to rule out different obstructions, still showing inflammation of the subglottic region with layers of fibrin.

EPIGLOTTITIS

Epiglottitis is the traditional term for a severe, bacterial inflammation of the supraglottic structures (supraglottitis), the extremely swollen, cherry-red epiglottis being the main cause of a life-threatening airway obstruction.[68] This disease has almost disappeared from clinical practice since vaccination against *Haemophilus influenzae*, the most frequent bacterial agent, was introduced in 1990. In the author's children's tertiary care centre the incidence of three to six annual cases decreased to one case in 2 years.

However, epiglottitis can occur in vaccinated children (personal observation), demonstrating that various micro-organisms are able to cause this life-threatening condition, and there is an increase of epiglottitis in adolescents and adults.[69]

Because of the inevitable loss of expertise in treating this disease, it is of particular importance to describe the clinical appearance and treatment of this disease of brief duration in otherwise healthy children. Even in intensive care units patients die from supraglottitis.[70]

Epiglottitis first causes a high fever with moderate signs of a common cold, leading after a few hours to symptoms of dysphagia which end in difficulty in swallowing and talking. Children present with tachycardia, tachypnoea, moderate dyspnoea, drooling and speaking, if at all, in a low clear voice, and are usually sitting, leaning forward and exhibiting acute anxiety. Inspiratory stridor appears to be a late symptom, warning of incipient total airway obstruction.

If symptoms are not convincing or if there is a suspicion that a foreign body is occluding the pharynx, a lateral X-ray of the neck is an extremely helpful diagnostic tool with almost no false-positive results.[71] Otherwise, X-rays should not be taken for risk of respiratory obstruction and instead, reliance placed on a clinical diagnosis.

Urgent intubation after diagnosis is the treatment of choice since the airway may become totally and unexpectedly obstructed. Diagnosis is established by laryngoscopy, performed under controlled conditions, after which the trachea is intubated. An ENT surgeon stands by, should the need for immediate bronchoscopy and/or tracheostomy become necessary. The process of laying the child down or the painful stimulus from the intravenous access can cause immediate occlusion of the glottis so that emergency intubation has to be performed, which would be challenging even for experts. Induction takes place with the child sitting and the intravenous infusion only started after the inhalational induction is underway. The technique of choice is induction with halothane in oxygen in the operating theatre, but occasionally the urgency of symptoms may force the anaesthetist to intubate in an emergency room. The tracheal tube has to be considerably smaller than usual because of the extreme vulnerability of the inflamed supraglottic region. If possible, the trachea is intubated with

the patient deeply anaesthetized as the respiratory movements of secretions provide a clue as to the location of the larynx among swollen and abnormal tissues. If it is possible to ventilate the lungs via the facemask it is usually safe to administer a dose of muscle relaxant to achieve the intubation. After intubation the patients require sedation and analgesia. Older children who have experienced supraglottitis mainly recall the intense pain when swallowing saliva.

In several patients who had respiratory arrest before controlled conditions for intubation could be procured, ventilation by bag and mask was successfully carried out, although with many difficulties such as inflation of the stomach, until tracheal intubation could be performed (personal observation). The entrance to the laryngeal opening could sometimes be visualized only by air bubbles coming out of amorphous tissue at the base of the tongue when the thorax was compressed by a nurse. In such a critical situation, intravenous diazepam and thiopentone or intramuscular ketamine, together with atropine, can be used. Orotracheal instead of nasotracheal intubation in unfavourable situations is an adequate approach; the tube can be changed later under safer, controlled conditions. The advantage of intubation over tracheostomy in acute epiglottitis has been convincingly demonstrated.[72,73]

At present, with a low incidence of epiglottitis it seems mandatory to rely on the extensive past experience, using the safest way of securing the airway, i.e. immediate intubation as soon as the diagnosis is established.

Treatment of epiglottitis after intubation consists of antibiotics, analgesia and sedation, humidification of inspired gases and the avoidance of accidental extubation. If this occurs during the first day of treatment, immediate reintubation is of utmost importance, because obstruction recurs within minutes. Planned extubation can be carried out after 2 days in the majority of cases after inspection of the epiglottis and presence of a leak around the tube, although some units think it unwise to bronchoscope the patient at this stage. Previously, the antibiotic given initially was chloramphenicol, but nowadays a third-generation cephalosporin would be used.

BACTERIAL TRACHEITIS

This unusual, severe, sometimes toxic disease with a high mortality[74] has undergone several shifts of nomenclature during the few last decades, from membranous laryngotracheo-bronchitis via non-diphtheritic laryngitis to bacterial tracheitis, the most frequently used term in textbooks of paediatric anaesthesia and in the paediatric literature today, although there would be good reasons to include the larynx in the terminology[75] since laryngotracheoscopic findings always show involvement of the larynx. The high incidence of preventable airway obstruction makes it an important disease for the paediatric anaesthetist.

Primarily, it is an independent acute airway infection, mainly caused by *Staphylococcus aureus*, *H. influenzae* and anaerobic bacteria,[76] and it may follow an episode of viral croup. Leading symptoms are copious mucopurulent secretions, persisting high fever and a tendency to shock and toxicity. Fluid resuscitation and, frequently, inotropic support are needed as emergency measures. Application of anti-biotics is the only treatment to prevent toxin formation.[77]

Nebulization of racemic adrenaline is widely used in paediatric intensive care units if stridor is present, but if the racemic solution is not available, ordinary adrenaline can be used. Thickening of secretions and membranous casts of the trachea, which progress to pro-nounced airway obstruction, may necessitate the intervention of a paediatric anaesthetist to perform an intubation or to clear the secretions from the trachea. In this case the chosen tube has to be considerably smaller than the pre-dicted one, but still the tracheal tube may push a cast of fibrin towards the bifurcation and occlude the trachea completely. In the author's experience only a rigid bronchoscope can clear the trachea by curettage mechanisms to re-establish the airway quickly enough.

AIRWAY OBSTRUCTION DURING BRONCHOSCOPY

In the paediatric patient, bronchoscopy, whether rigid or flexible, is mostly performed under general anaesthesia. Rigid bronchoscopy with telescope lenses obstructs the airway considerably in small infants. This requires excellent co-operation between the anaesthetist and endoscopist; sometimes ventilation has to be stopped for critical manipulations. Flexible bronchoscopy faces the same problem when the instrument has to pass through narrow tracheal tubes. In case the field of vision becomes extremely limited during flexible investigation, it may be prudent to change to rigid broncho-scopy with short periods of apnoea for instru-mentation. Flexible bronchoscopy under sedation only, stimulates the child to buck against the instrument and fight for breath, causing numerous artefacts, in particular erro-neous diagnosis of tracheal and bronchial collapse; such an important diagnosis should be double checked by application of a rigid instrument during apnoea.

Bronchoscopy is frequently carried out for removal of foreign bodies.[78] A considerable amount of airway obstruction is present in these patients before anaesthesia begins. Premedica-tion should include anticholinergic agents. Many paediatric anaesthetists would still use halothane in preference to other agents for the same reasons as described in the treatment of bronchospasm (see p. 502).

During bronchoscopy the use of short-acting opioids has a favourable effect in the control of reflexes and postoperative coughing. Extraction of foreign bodies might be followed by erup-tions of pus from behind the obstacle or profuse bleeding from granulation tissue and injured mucosa. A strong suction device has to be on hand to remove thick material rapidly. The best way to stop bleeding from granulation tissue around a foreign body which has been in place for days or weeks can be accomplished by advancing the rigid bronchoscope into the bleeding bronchus and waiting. Topical adrena-line is useful for local vasoconstriction, short-ening the time for coagulation and drying of the wound bed.

A foreign body can be lost during extraction and occlude the trachea or both main stem bronchi. Such situations can be the most critical ones for anaesthetists and endoscopists and lead to a situation where neither intubation nor ventilation seems possible. Only quick reactions, pushing the foreign body into one of the main stem bronchi, can save the patient. If large pieces of nut are found in the tracheobronchial tree, it is often possible to break them down to several pieces, as extraction in one piece might prove impossible or create a subglottic obstruction.

Bronchography in patients with impaired lung function and the use of large amounts of radiopaque dye may cause obstruction of large parts of the lung, with oxygen desaturation, cyanosis and bradycardia. Therefore, intermittent suction of the material must be carried out during the study, from areas where the contrast medium is not needed.

Children admitted to hospital after a choking crisis should not be sent home without at least a chest X-ray being carried out, even when there are no clinical signs of airway obstruction. A choking event with heavy coughing, although it may have subsided after several minutes, still points to the strong possibility of a foreign body in the airway. Late extractions have a high morbidity, leading to bronchial stenosis in about 7% of the cases.[79]

AIRWAY OBSTRUCTION FROM BURNS, SMOKE INHALATION OR CHEMICAL BURNS

Mortality in children with burns depends to some degree on the presence of smoke inhalation.[80,81] Patients with smoke inhalation without cutaneous burns have a mortality higher than 3%, in particular when soot deposits are found in the pharynx.[82] For the paediatric anaesthetist involved in an endoscopy service, it is very surprising how seldom airway endoscopy is used to evaluate the depth and extension of laryngeal, tracheal and bronchial involvement[83] (see also Chapter 17).

All children with facial burns, superheated air and smoke inhalation, and those who swallowed hot fluids or food or caustic material should be evaluated for airway damage by bronchoscopy. Endoscopic evaluation serves to remove soot and tissue debris in the first place and, secondly, defines the injury accurately, to assist in decision making for intubation, tracheostomy or long-term artificial ventilation. Radioaerosol lung scintigraphy may evaluate the severity of lung involvement in acute inhalation injury in fire victims and monitor the course of the disease.[84]

Combustion of plastic material in closed rooms or cars causes extremely severe airway obstruction by forming sulphur and nitrogen dioxides, which combine with water of the mucosa to form highly corrosive acids, affecting the entire tracheobronchial tree and damaging bronchioles and alveoli.[85] When children are dragged out of a space where combustion of plastic or toxic material occurred, immediate intubation of the frequently severely hypoxic patients should be undertaken in order to oxygenate the victim rapidly and to secure the airway, which can easily be lost through rapid swelling of the bronchial mucosa, preventing the later passage of a tracheal tube. Vigorous advancing of the tracheal tube may cause sloughing of the mucosa, with further obstruction.

The same type of damage, although less pronounced, may happen in accidents where jets of flames hit the face or in the presence of open fires producing great amounts of soot, which will penetrate the upper airways.

Circumferential burns to the chest and abdomen may produce a shell of rigid tissue, preventing excursions of the thorax and diaphragm; ventilation can only be accomplished after escharotomy. However, these patients frequently die early after the accident.

Although there is little question about the indication of early intubation in smoke inhalation, the author prefers to perform a bronchoscopy before intubation in all patients with suspected airway injury or if the indication of intubation remains questionable, except in patients with profound shock. Soot or debris can be suctioned from the tracheobronchial tree, the extension and depth of the injury evaluated and an adequately sized tracheal tube chosen for intubation. In patients with burns to large body surfaces with symptoms of shock, bronchoscopy is postponed, but great care should be taken to choose a tube with a noticeable leak during moderate inflation pressures. If this leak disappears during the following days, changing the tube to one of a smaller size is advisable to prevent subglottic ulceration. In extreme swelling of the face, a tube exchanger may be used or the procedure be postponed for a short period.

Securing the tube in a severely burned face can prove a problem. Strings of cloth and tape attached to the facial drapes may fix the tube securely, but during wound dressing accidental extubation must be prevented by extreme care on the part of the anaesthetist.

Swallowing of hot food may cause blisters at the posterior part of the larynx; the involvement of the arytenoid cartilages is followed by severe stridor, sometimes leading to supraglottic obstruction, necessitating intubation. This type of lesion heals normally within several days. Hot, even boiling fluids are swallowed by toddlers, but fortunately only the ventral facing part of the epiglottis and adjacent part of the tongue are usually injured, and they heal within a few days.

Similarly, if caustic material is swallowed, it rarely enters the larynx and trachea, but the severely affected anterior part of the epiglottis frequently becomes attached to the base of the tongue, forming scar tissue which fixes the epiglottis inseparably to the tongue. Aspiration of fluids occurs for several weeks, but finally these children become adapted to this anatomical change and swallow without problems. If caustic material enters the larynx, tracheostomy is inevitable.

MANAGEMENT OF INHALATION INJURY

The first and most important step in treatment is to secure the airway before swelling of the mucosa makes intubation difficult or impossible. If small airways are affected with severely impaired lung compliance, artificial ventilation with high inspiratory pressures becomes necessary. Pronounced air trapping may lead to respiratory insufficiency as in severe bronchos-

pasm. The application of PEEP up to 8 cmH_2O with vigorous physiotherapy may improve oxygenation and facilitate exhalation. The application of nitric oxide (NO), which has marked effects in pulmonary hypertension, has shown only moderate effects, not reaching statistical significance.[86]

Since children with severe inhalation injury are rarely encountered in paediatric burn centres, no systematic investigations of advanced treatment have been published. Paediatric anaesthetists, being familiar with the treatment of bacterial tracheitis and croup, frequently use nebulization of adrenaline in patients with smoke inhalation, which seems to be helpful as long as perfusion of the mucosa is maintained. In involvement of small airways, when exhalation of trapped air is scarcely possible and terminal respiratory insufficiency is to be expected, nebulization of budesonide, of proven effect in the treatment of croup[66] and in asthmatic patients,[87] seems promising in the author's experience, but no references to this have been found in the literature.

In two desperate situations with severe toxic airway injury from combustion of plastic material, leading to respiratory insufficiency with air trapping, not reacting to β_2 stimulants, budesonide was used in the paediatric burn centre of the Cologne Children's Hospital. Halothane was not used because of symptoms of shock. After inhalation of budesonide every hour for 12 h, a dramatic improvement in lung function was seen in both patients. One patient died from cerebral hypoxia after improvement of lung function, while the second survived and regained normal lung function.

LOWER RESPIRATORY OBSTRUCTION

BRONCHOSPASM AND STATUS ASTHMATICUS

Asthmatic children make up about 10% of the patients dealt with by paediatric anaesthetists, but there is great regional variety and the percentage is rising.[88,89] A history of frequent wheezing bronchitis or asthmatic attacks should be well documented on the anaesthetic chart. Some of these patients show smooth muscle hypertrophy, interstitial oedema and some inflammation of the bronchial wall, depending on the time of the year. The differential diagnosis of wheezing, especially in an infant, must include an inhaled foreign body and rarely an extrinsic compression on the lower trachea such as a double aortic arch.

Most asthmatics do not show any clinical signs of obstruction during anaesthesia. However, overwhelming bronchoconstriction during anaesthesia is one of the most frightening situations the anaesthetist has to deal with, especially in patients with cardiovascular compromise. This event will remain thankfully rare, with careful preoperative assessment, adequate premedication and smooth induction of anaesthesia.

Preoperative assessment has to concentrate on present medication and possible infection. The surgical intervention in an asthmatic child should definitely be an elective one. Current medical treatment should be continued, in particular cromolyn sodium and β-adrenergic agents as well as anticholinergic agents (ipratropium bromide). Theophylline, a frequently used bronchodilator, should be well below the toxic level of 20 μg ml^{-1}, because in combination with high doses of halothane it has proved arrhythmogenic in experimental animals[90] and is today considered to be of tertiary value.[91]

Premedication should include a sedative, atropine and possibly opioids, because stimulation of the irritable mucous membranes of the predisposed patient during light anaesthesia is considered to be the main cause of bronchospasm.[92] Potent premedication can easily be accomplished by intramuscular injection in the many children who are well able to tolerate the procedure. In patients who are afraid of the needle, very slow intravenous injection of the premedicating agents (after venepuncture through anaesthetized skin) and a wait of at least 10 min provide adequate conditions for induction.

Bronchoconstriction is triggered by one of three possible mechanisms or by a combination of all three: (1) direct stimulation by an irritant; (2) stimulation by an antigen mediator; or (3) stimulation by reflex activity.

Lignocaine prevents irritant-induced airway constriction (1 mg kg^{-1}, therapeutic level 1–4 μg ml^{-1}), but has no effect on mediator-induced bronchospasm in clinically achievable concentrations.[92] It may be given in severe cases immediately before induction of anaesthesia. Atropine reduces antigen-induced bronchoconstriction.[93] Potent inhalation anaesthetics such as halothane, isoflurane and enflurane act directly and indirectly in a complex way on airway smooth muscles, thus preventing and treating bronchoconstriction.[93] In the predisposed patient, induction of anaesthesia is best accomplished by a mask with halothane in a well premedicated child, because halothane prevents and treats irritant-induced, mediator-activated and reflex airway constriction, the latter by direct action on the airway smooth muscles.

Sevoflurane does not irritate the smooth muscles of the airway, but compared with halothane it is in some ways a more potent ventilatory depressant, reducing diaphragmatic contractility to a greater extent and attenuating anaphylaxis-induced increase in pulmonary resistance less,[94] and it prevents increases in lung resistance and decreases in dynamic compliance during histamine challenge less than halothane.[95] In the author's experience of this extremely safe agent, gained over four decades, the greatest advantages of halothane for asthmatic patients lie in its predictable sedative effect during emergence from anaesthesia and the smooth postanaesthetic period. The most disturbing effect of sevoflurane is the high incidence of postoperative delirium,[96] which may cause personality changes for hours and can be effectively treated only by opioids, often less desirable in the postoperative period because of respiratory depression (Trieschmann, U., Holzki, J., Laschat, M. and Stratmann, C., unpublished data). Possibly irritant substances are also formed by sevoflurane with dry soda-lime in highly exothermic reactions up to 130C,[97] producing considerable amounts of methanol and larger quantities of compounds A–D.[98] Reactions between halothane and dry soda-lime also occur, but reactions are less exothermic and have proved innocuous in children.

One patient with latex allergy undergoing sevoflurane anaesthesia developed severe bronchospasm despite latex-free equipment, and needed full treatment of status asthmaticus including halothane, which solved the spasm. The same patient exhibited no bronchospasm during repeat anaesthesia with halothane, and only a moderate decrease in compliance and increase in oxygen consumption was noted. A similar event was observed in a patient with Prader–Willi syndrome.[99]

Comparisons between halothane and sevoflurane in paediatric anaesthesia are discussed in Chapter 3, although arguments for and against may not be based on scientific data.[100] Only independent investigations, similar in quality to those of Hirshman and co-workers,[92,93,101] may solve the question of whether sevoflurane or halothane will be more appropriate for anaesthesia in children with asthma. There seems to be no hurry in discarding halothane from clinical use in exchange for a less thoroughly investigated agent.

If an intravenous induction in the asthmatic child is preferred, ketamine is still the drug of choice and it can also be used in treating postoperative bronchoconstriction.[101,102] Propofol reduces histamine-induced contraction in human isolated airway smooth muscles that were passively sensitized with asthmatic serum, but no clinical studies have been carried out comparing it with ketamine.[103]

Treatment of bronchospasm should begin with an increase in the proportion of inspired oxygen and a deepening of the anaesthetic level with halothane as a true bronchodilator of the constricted airway.[92] Ketamine, easily available in the operating theatre, is very helpful in the cardiac-compromised patient where high doses of inhalational agents are disadvantageous. It may be used routinely in asthmatic attacks, but the well-known dysphoria during and after emergence might be frightening to the patient and the parents, so it is only used in severe cases with the addition of diazepam.

The second step involves using some of the wide variety of bronchodilating drugs which, until recently, were quite confusing as to choice and dosage. An international consensus group has reached agreement since 1992 on a rather rigid, but scientifically well-supported schedule of treatment of status asthmaticus,[91] which has proved to be helpful for the paediatric anaesthetist in intraoperative bronchospasm as well:

- nebulization of salbutamol into the anaesthesia circuit;
- infusion of salbutamol 1 mg kg^{-1} h^{-1}, increasing every 15 min until effective;
- steroids in increasing doses, starting with prednisolone 1 mg kg^{-1};
- aminophylline 1 mg kg^{-1} h^{-1} (loading 5 mg kg^{-1}/30 min), only if all previous medication has failed and control of serum levels is necessary.

Intravenous lignocaine has no effect, once bronchospasm has occurred, nor do lignocaine aerosols, which fail to prevent bronchospasm even if applied before the release of mediators.[104]

In the author's experience, all patients with bronchospasm during anaesthesia, treated according to the above schedule, have responded to therapy. Non-steroidal analgesics should be avoided in children symptomatic with asthma.

MECONIUM ASPIRATION

Meconium aspiration occurs in approximately 5% of all deliveries,[105] predominantly in postmature neonates and almost never before the 34th week of gestation. Since meconium seldom penetrates into the smaller airways before birth, meconium aspiration syndrome (MAS) can usually be prevented by suctioning of the upper airways after delivery of the head, before the delivery of the shoulders. Most infants stay well after the presence of thick meconium in the amniotic fluid. If MAS develops, all surgical interventions should be postponed until persistent fetal circulation has resolved, as in patients with congenital diaphragmatic hernia (CDH).

However, if a patient with meconium aspiration has to undergo urgent surgery, (gastroschisis, omphalocele, oesophageal atresia), the paediatric anaesthetist is faced with a patient with an overinflated thorax as a clinical sign of diminished aeration with air trapping and a high probability of a pneumothorax during artificial ventilation, which should include only moderate PEEP. Antibiotic treatment is advisable, although hydrocortisone showed no benefit in one study.[106] Repeated application of surfactant causes a dramatic improvement in lung function.[107] If surgery is urgent, administration of surfactant before or even during anaesthesia is helpful. Tracheal lavage with saline and suctioning with minimal interruption of oxygenation frequently produces considerable amounts of meconium, hopefully shortening the course of the pulmonary disease. Patients should not be extubated after surgery because lung function is unpredictable.

PULMONARY AIR LEAK

Pulmonary air leak is far more likely in the neonatal period than in any other period of life. The incidence of pneumothorax is approximately 1% of all live births.[108] This low incidence makes it necessary for the paediatric anaesthetist always to bear it in mind as a possibility when oxygen desaturation occurs during anaesthesia of critically ill neonates. If a neonate suddenly deteriorates during anaesthesia, extra-alveolar air should be suspected. A tension pneumothorax might occasionally be recognized by auscultation but generally a chest X-ray is necessary to detect pneumothorax or pneumomediastinum. The latter may be accompanied by a pneumopericardium; a rapidly dropping blood pressure may indicate such a complication. Interruption of the operation for a chest X-ray is the only way to make the diagnosis and perform emergency treatment (thoracocentesis or pericardiocentesis).

Air leaks occur occasionally in accidental tube displacement into one of the main stem bronchi, the premature neonate again being the most frequent victim of interstitial gas accumulation because of the fragility of the elastic tissue of the lung and the shortness of the trachea (3.5–4.0 cm), predisposing to deep bronchial intubation. Unilateral overinflation of a lung in infancy may remain visible on X-ray for months.

On rare occasions unilateral barotrauma may lead to cystic transformation of the lung tissue with progressive air trapping, shift of the mediastinum to the contralateral side and great difficulty in ventilating the patient. Chest X-ray and CT scan may not differentiate between lobar emphysema, cystic adenomatous malformation, isolated parenchymal lung cysts and bronchogenic cysts, and may not show interstitial emphysema. After bronchoscopy, which should rule out a flap valve mechanism, the lung may be erroneously resected.[109] With the diagnosis so much in doubt and before embarking on lung resection, selective contralateral intubation should be performed during bronchoscopy, occluding the hyperinflated lung from ventilation. Improvement of lung function within hours proves the diagnosis of interstitial emphysema and avoids the loss of the organ.

PULMONARY HAEMORRHAGE

The incidence of pulmonary haemorrhage which obstructs the airway has decreased in clinical practice since the treatment of hyaline membrane disease by surfactant. Obstructing pulmonary haemorrhage can be seen after suctioning of patients with severe sepsis, cardiac failure or coagulation disorders. All patients respond to lavage with adrenaline, diluted 1 : 10 000 with normal saline. In the neonate, pulmonary haemorrhage frequently occurs after severe hypoxia.

REFERENCES

1 Eckenhoff, J.E. Some anatomic considerations of the infant larynx influencing endotracheal anesthesia. *Anesthesiology* 1951; **12**: 401–10.
2 Perkins, J.A., Sie, K.C., Milczuk, H. and Richardson, M.A. Airway management in children with craniofacial anomalies. *Cleft Palate Craniofacial Journal* 1997; **34**: 135–40.
3 Marcus, C.L. and Loughlin, G.M. Obstructive sleep apnea in children. *Seminars in Pediatric Neurology* 1996; **3**: 23–8.
4 Keenan, R.L., Shapiro, J.H., Kane, F.R. and Simpson, P.M. Frequency of cardiac arrests in infants: effect of pediatric anesthesiologists. *Journal of Clinical Anesthesia* 1991; **3**: 433–7.
5 Cobby, T.F., Wrench, I.J. and Girling, K.J. Assessment of a combination of different bed side techniques in predicting difficult intubation. *British Journal of Anaesthesia* 1997; **78** Suppl. 1; A34.
6 Downes, J.J. and Raphaely, R.C. Pediatric intensive care. *Anesthesiology* 1975: **43**: 238–50.
7 Brooks, J. Apparent life threatening event. *Clinical Perinatology* 1992; **19**: 809–39.
8 Kahn, A., Souttiaux, M. and Appelboom-Fondu, I. Long-term development of children monitored as infants for an apparent life threatening event during sleep: a 10 year follow-up study. *Pediatrics* 1989; **83**: 668–73.

9 Heimlich, H.J. and Patrick, E.A. The Heimlich manoeuver: best technique for saving any choking victim's life. *Postgraduate Medicine* 1990; **87**: 38–53.

10 Day, R.L., Crelin, E.S. and DuBois, A.B. Choking; the Heimlich abdominal thrust vs back blows: an approach to measurement of inertial and aerodynamic forces. *Pediatrics* 1982; **70**: 113–19.

11 Isaacs, J.H. and Pedersen, A.D. Emergency cricothyroidotomy. *American Surgeon* 1997; **63**: 346–9.

12 Richmond, C.E. and Bingham, R.M. Paediatric cardiopulmonary resuscitation. *Paediatric Anaesthesia* 1995; **5**: 11–27.

13 Cormack, R.S. and Lehane, J. Difficult tracheal intubation in obstetrics. *Anaesthesia* 1984; **39**: 1105–11.

14 Benumof, J.L. Management of the difficult adult airway: with special emphasis on the awake tracheal intubation. *Anesthesiology* 1991; **75**: 1087–110.

15 Caplan, R.A., Posner, K.L., Ward, R.J. and Cheney, F.W. Adverse respiratory events in anesthesia: a closed claims analysis. *Anesthesiology* 1990; **72**: 828–33.

16 Katz, R.L. Medicolegal issues. *29th Clinical Conference in Pediatric Anesthesiology 1991*. Children's Hospital of Los Angeles.

17 Holzki, J., Laschat, M. and Stratmann, C. Stridor in the neonate and infant. *Paediatric Anaesthesia* 1998; **8**: 221–7.

18 Miller, M.J., Fanaroff, A.A. and Martin, R.J. Airway obstruction. In: Fanaroff, A.A. and Martin, R.J. (eds). *Neonatal–Perinatal Medicine*, 5th edn. St Louis, MO: Mosby Year Book, 1992: 855–7.

19 Roger, G., Denoyelle, F., Triglia, J.M. and Garabedian, E.N. Severe laryngomalacia: surgical indications and results in 115 patients. *Laryngoscope* 1995; **105**: 1111–17.

20 Knegt-Junk, K.J., Bos, C.E., Berkovits, R.N.P. Congenital nasal stenosis in neonates. *Journal of Laryngology and Otology* 1988; **102**: 500–2.

21 Miller, M.J., Carlo, W.A., Kingman, P., et al. Effect of maturation on oral breathing in sleeping premature infants. *Journal of Pediatrics* 1986; **109**: 515–19.

22 Cotton, R.T. Pediatric laryngotracheal stenosis. *Journal of Pediatric Surgery* 1984; **19**: 699–704.

23 Chhibber, A.K., Hengerer, A.S. and Fickling, K.B. Unsuspected subglottic stenosis in a two-year-old. *Paediatric Anaesthesia* 1997; **7**: 65–7.

24 Hoeve, L.J., Eskici, O. and Verwoerd, C.D.A. Therapeutic reintubation for post-intubation laryngo-tracheal injury in preterm infants. *International Journal of Pediatric Otorhinolaryngology* 1995; **31**: 7–13.

25 Berkovits, R.N.P., Bos, C.E., Pauw, K.H. and Gee, A.W.J. Congenital cricoid stenosis. Pathogenesis, diagnosis and method of treatment. *Journal of Laryngology and Otology* 1978; **92**: 1083–100.

26 Bauman, N.M. and Benjamin, B. Subglottic ductal cysts in the preterm infant: association with larygeal intubation trauma. *Annals of Otology, Rhinology and Laryngology* 1995; **104**: 963–8.

27 Grob, M. Über Anomalien des Aortenbogens und ihre entwicklungsgeschichtliche Genese. *Helvetica Paediatrica Acta* 1949; **3/4**: 274–93.

28 Gross, R.E. Arterial malformations which cause compression of the trachea or esophagus. *Circulation* 1955; **11**: 124–34.

29 Gharieb, M. and Ebel, K.D. Kongenitaler Stridor durch Gefä?anomalien. *Zeitschrift für Kinderchirurgie* 1970; **9**: 161–74.

30 Slany, E., Holzki, J., Holschneider, A.M., et al. Trachealinstabilität bei tracheoösophagealen Fehlbildungen. *Zeitschrift für Kinderchirurgie* 1990; **45**: 78–85.

31 Holzki, J. Bronchoscopic findings and treatment in patients with tracheo-oesophageal fistula. *Paediatric Anaesthesia* 1992; **2**: 297–303.

32 Berkovits, R.N.P., Bax, N.M.A. and van der Schans, E.J. Surgical treatment of congenital laryngo-tracheo-oesophageal cleft. *Progress in Pediatric Surgery, Berlin*. Heidelberg: Springer, 1987; **21**: 36–46.

33 Petterson, G. Laryngo-tracheo-oesophageal cleft. *Z Kinderchir* 1969; **7**: 43–9.

34 Hagl, S., Jakob, H., Sebening, C., et al. External stabilization of long segment tracheobronchomalacia guided by intraoperative bronchoscopy. *Annals of Thoracic Surgery* 1997; **64**: 1412–21.

35 Worley, G., Schuster, J.M. and Oakes, W.J. Survival at 5 years of a cohort of newborn infants with myelomeningocele. *Developmental Medicine and Child Neurology* 1996; **38**: 816–22.

36 Safar, P., Aguro-Escarraga, L. and Chang, F. A study of upper airway obstruction in the unconscious patient. *Journal of Applied Physiology* 1959; **14**: 760–5.

37 Reber, A., Paganoni, R. and Frei, F.J. Chin lift may worsen airway patency in children. *Anesthesiology* 1997; **V87**: A1042.

38 Suzuki, M. and Sasaki, C.T. Laryngeal spasm: a neurophysiologic redefinition. *Annals of Otology, Rhinology and Laryngology* 1977; **86**: 150–5.

39 Olson, G.L. and Hallen, B. Larygospasm during anaesthesia. A computer aided incidence study in 136 929 patients. *Acta Anaesthesiologica Scandinavica* 1984; **28**: 567–75.

40 Schrelner, M.S., O'Hara, I., Markakis, D.A. and Politis, G.D. Do children who experience laryngospasm have an increased risk of upper respiratory tract infection? *Anesthesiology* 1996; **85**: 475–80.

41 Keating, V. Laryngeal and bronchial spasm during anaesthesia. In: *Anaesthetic Accidents*. London: Lloyd-Luke, 1961: 103–8.

42 Salem, M.R. *Pediatric Anesthesia: Current Practise*. New York: Academic Press, 1981: 109–10.

43 Fink, B.R. The etiology and treatment of larygospasm. *Anesthesiology* 1956; **17**: 569–73.

44 Bunting, H.E., Kelly, M.C. and Milligan, K.R. Effect of nebulized lignocaine on airway irritation and haemodynamic changes during induction of anaesthesia with desflurane. *British Journal of Anaesthesia* 1995; **75**: 631–3.

45 Zsigmond, E.K., Kocacs, V. and Fekete, G. A new route, jet-injection for anesthetic induction in children – II. ketamine dose-range finding studies. *International Journal of Clinical Pharmacology and Therapeutics* 1996; **34**: 84–8.

46 Knill, R. and Bryan, A.C. An intercostal–phrenic inhibitory reflex in human newborn infants. *Journal of Applied Physiology* 1976; **40**: 352–6.

47 Longstreth, W.T., Jr and Inui, T.S. High glucose level on hospital admission and poor neurological recovery after cardiac arrest. *Annals of Neurology* 1984; **15**: 59–63.

48 Moore, R.L. and Binger, C.A. The response to respiratory resistance: a comparison of the effects produced by partial obstruction in the inspiratory and expiratory phases of respiration. *Journal of Experimental Medicine* 1927; 1065–80.

49 Lang, S.A., Duncan, P.G., Shephard, D.A.E., *et al.* Pulmonary oedema associated with airway obstruction. *Canadian Journal of Anaesthesia* 1990; **37**: 210–18.

50 Koehntop, D.E., Rodman, J.H., Brundage, D.M., *et al.* Pharmacokinetics of fentanyl in neonates. *Anesthesia and Analgesia* 1986; **64**: 227–32.

51 Comestock, M., Scamman, F., Moyers, J. and Stevens, W. Rigidity and hypercarbia associated with high dose fentanyl induction of anesthesia. *Anesthesia and Analgesia* 1981; **60**: 362–3.

52 Bennett, J.A., Abrams, J.T., Van Riper, D.F. and Horrow, J.C. Difficult or impossible ventilation after sufentanil-induced anesthesia is caused primarily by vocal cord closure. *Anesthesiology* 1997; **87**: 1070–4.

53 Todres, I.D., Reppert, S.M., Walker, P.F. and Grillo, H.C. Management of critical airway obstruction in a child with a mediastinal tumour. *Anesthesiology* 1976; **45**: 100–2.

54 Keon, T.P. Death on induction of anesthesia for cervical node biopsy. *Anesthesiology* 1981; **55**: 471–2.

55 Neuman, G.G., Weingarten, A.E., Abramowitz, R.M., *et al.* The anesthetic management of the patient with an anterior mediastinal mass. *Anesthesiology* 1984; **60**: 144–7.

56 Contencin, Ph. and Narcin, Ph. Gastropharyngeal reflux in infants and children. A pharyngeal pH monitoring study. *Archives of Otolaryngology, Head and Neck Surgery* 1992; **118**: 1028–130.

57 Bos, C.E., Berkovits, R.N.P. and Struben, W.H. Wider application of prolonged nasotracheal intubation. *Journal of Laryngology and Otology* 1973; **87**: 263–79.

58 Monnier, Ph., Lang, F. and Savary, M. Krikoidteilresektion mit primärer laryngotrachealer Anastomose bei subglottischen Stenosen im Kindesalter. *Oto-Rhino-Laryngologica Nova* 1993; **3**: 26–34.

59 Holzki, J. Die Gefährdung des Kehlkopfs durch Intubation im frühen Kindesalter. *Deutsches Ärzteblatt* 1993; **90B**: 1131–4.

60 Walner, D.L. and Holinger, L.D. Supraglottic stenosis in infants and children. *Archives of Otolaryngology, Head and Neck Surgery* 1997; **123**: 337–41.

61 Daya, H., Fawcett, W.J. and Weir, N. Vocal cord palsy after use of laryngeal mask airway. *Journal of Laryngology and Otology* 1996; **110**: 383–4.

62 Lloyd Jones, F.R. and Hegab, A. Case report. Recurrent laryngeal nerve palsy after laryngeal mask airway insertion. *Anaesthesia* 1996; **51**: 171–2.

63 Khine, H.H., Corddry, D.H., Kettrick, R.G., *et al.* Comparison of cuffed and uncuffed endotracheal tubes in young children during general anesthesia. *Anesthesiology* 1997; **86**: 27–31.

64 *Roche Lexikon Medizin.* München: Urban & Schwarzenberg, 1993.

65 Tunessen, W.W. and Feinstein, A.R. The steroid-croup controversy: an analytical review of methodologic problems. *Journal of Pediatrics* 1980; **96**: 751–6.

66 Geelhoed, G.C. Croup. *Pediatric Pulmonology* 1997; **23**: 370–4.

67 Berry, F.A. Laryngotracheobronchitis. In: Berry, F.A. (ed.). *Anesthetic Management of Difficult and Routine*

Pediatric Patients. New York: Churchill Livingstone, 1986: 265–9.

68 Miller, A.H. Acute epiglottitis. *American Academy of Ophthalmology and Otolaryngology* 1948; **53**: 519–23.

69 Park, K.W., Darvish, A. and Lowenstein, E. Airway management for adult patients with acute epiglottitis. A 12-year experience at an academic medical center (1984–1995). *Anesthesiology* 1998; **88**: 254–61.

70 Mayo-Smith, M. Fatal respiratory arrest in adult epiglottitis in the intensive care unit: implications for airway management. *Chest* 1993; **104**: 964–5.

71 Nemzek, W.R., Katzberg, R.W., Van Slyke, M.A. and Bickley, L.S. A reapraisal of the radiologic findings of acute inflammation of the epiglottis and supraglottic structures in adults. *American Journal of Neuroradiology* 1995; **16**: 495–502.

72 Oh, T.H. and Motoyama, E.K. Comparison of nasotracheal intubation and tracheostomy in management of acute epiglottitis. *Anesthesiology* 1977; **46**: 214–16.

73 Schloss, M.D., Gold, J.A., Rosales, J.K. and Baxter, J.D. Acute epiglottitis: Current management. *Laryngoscope* 1983; **93**: 489–5.

74 McKenzie, M., Norman, M.G., Anderson, J.D., *et al.* Upper respiratory tract infection in a 3-year-old girl. *Journal of Pediatrics* 1984; **105**: 129–33.

75 Nelson, W.E. Bacterial croup: a historical perspective. *Journal of Pediatrics* 1984; **105**: 52–5.

76 Brook, I. Aerobic and anaerobic microbiology of bacterial tracheitis in children. *Pediatric Emergency Care* 1997; **13**: 16–18.

77 Britto, J., Habibi, P., Walters, S., *et al.* Systemic complications associated with bacterial tracheitis. *Archives of Disease in Childhood* 1996; **74**: 249–50.

78 Barrios Fontaba, J.E., Gutierrez, C., Lluna, J., *et al.* Bronchial foreign body: should bronchoscopy be performed in all patients with a choking crisis? *Pediatric Surgery International* 1997; **12**: 118–20.

79 Wildermann, G.U.M. Die Fremdkörperaspiration im Kindesalter. Inaugural-Dissertation, Universität Köln, 1998.

80 Wolf, S.E., Rose, J.K., Desai, M.H., *et al.* Mortality determinants in massive pediatric burns. An analysis of 103 children with more than 80% TBSA burns (or more than 70% full thickness). *Annals of Surgery* 1997; **225**: 554–65.

81 Demirdjian, G. Adjusting a prognostic score for burned children with logistic regression. *Journal of Burn Care and Rehabilitation* 1997; **18**: 313–16.

82 Hantson, P., Butera, R., Clemessy, J.L., *et al.* Early complications and value of initial clinical and paraclinical observations in victims of smoke inhalation without burns. *Chest* 1997; **111**: 671–5.

83 Strekalovskii, V.P., Alekseev, A.A. and Kurbanov, S.A. Bronchoscopy in inhalation burns (English abstract). *Khirurgiia* 1997; **1**: 9–12.

84 Lin, W.Y., Kao, C.H. and Wang, S.J. Detection of acute inhalation injury in fire victims by means of technetium-99m DTPA radioaerosol inhalation lung scintigraphy. *European Journal of Nuclear Medicine* 1997; **24**: 125–9.

85 Sherwin, R.P. and Richters, C. Lung capillary permeability: nitrogen dioxide exposure and leakage of nitritiated serum. *Archives of Internal Medicine* 1971; **128**: 61–5.

86 Sheridan, R.L., Hurford, W.E., Kacmarek, R.M., *et al.* Inhaled nitric oxide in burn patients with respiratory failure. *Journal of Trauma* 1997; **42**: 629–34.

87 Booms, P., Cheung, D., Timmers, M.C., *et al.* Protective effect of inhaled budesonide against unlimited airway narrowing to methacholine in atopic patients with asthma. *Journal of Allergy and Clinical Immunology* 1997; **99**: 330–7.

88 Williams, H. and McNichol, K.N. Prevalence, natural history, and relationship of wheezing bronchitis and asthma in children. An epidemiological study. *British Medical Journal* 1969; **4**: 321–7.

89 Burr, M.L., Butland, B.K., King, S. and Vaughan-Williams, E. Changes in asthma prevalence: two surveys 15 years apart. *Archives of Disease in Childhood* 1989; **64**: 1452–6.

90 Stirt, J.A., Berger, J.M., Roe, S.D., *et al.* Halothane-induced cardiac arrhythmias following administration of aminophylline in experimental animals. *Anesthesia and Analgesia* 1981; **60**: 515–19.

91 Warner, J.O. Asthma: a follow up statement from an international paediatric asthma consensus group. *Archives of Disease in Childhood* 1992; **67**: 240–8.

92 Hirshman, C.A. Airway reactivity in humans. *Anesthesiology* 1983; **58**: 170–7.

93 Hirshman, C.A., Edelstein, G., Peetz, S., *et al.* Mechanisms of action of inhalational anesthesia on airways. *Anesthesiology* 1982; **56**: 107–11.

94 Green, W.B. The ventilatory effects of sevoflurane. *Anesthesia and Analgesia* 1995; **81**: 23–6.

95 Katoh, T. and Ikeda, K. A comparison of sevoflurane with halothane, enflurane and isoflurane on bronchoconstriction caused by histamine. *Canadian Journal of Anaesthesia* 1994; **41**: 1214–19.

96 Kataria, B., Epstein, R., Bailey, A., *et al.* A comparison of sevoflurane to halothane in paediatric surgical patients: result of a multicentre international study. *Paediatric Anaesthesia* 1996; **6**: 283–92.

97 Wissing, H., Kuhn, I. and Dudziak, R. Heat production from reaction of volatile anaesthetics with dried soda lime (English abstract). *Anaesthesist* 1997; **46**: 1064–70.

98 Förster, H. and Dudziak, R. Causes for the reaction between dry soda lime and the degradation products of inhalation anaesthetics (English abstract). *Anaesthesist* 1997; **46**: 1054–63.

99 Kawahito, S., Kitahata, H., Kimura, H. and Kohyama, A. Bronchospasm in a patient with Prader–Willi syndrome. *Masusi* 1995; **44**: 1675–9.

100 Haynes, S.R., Bolton, D.T. and Smith, J.H. Is there still a place for halothane in paediatric anaesthesia? (Correspondence). *Paediatric Anaesthesia* 1998; **8**: 181.

101 Hirshman, C.A., Downes, H., Farbood, A., *et al.* Ketamine block of bronchospasm in experimental canine asthma. *British Journal of Anaesthesia* 1979; **51**: 713–17.

102 McGrath, J.C., MacKenzie, J.E. and Millar, R.A. Effects of ketamine on central sympathetic discharge and the baroreceptor reflex during mechanical ventilation. *British Journal of Anaesthesia* 1975; **47**: 1141–7.

103 Quedraogo, N., Roux, E., Forestier, F., *et al.* Effects of intravenous anesthetics on normal and passively sensitized human isolated airway smooth muscle. *Anesthesiology* 1998; **88**: 317–26.

104 Downes, H. and Hirshman, C.A. Lignocaine aerosols do not prevent allergic bronchoconstriction. *Anesthesia and Analgesia* 1981; **60**: 28–32.

105 Gregory, G.A., Gooding, C.A., Phibbs, R.H. and Tooley, W.H. Meconium aspiration in infants; a prospective study. *Journal of Pediatrics* 1974; **85**: 848–52.

106 Miller, M.J., Fanaroff, A.A. and Martin, R.J. Meconium aspiration syndrome. In: Fanaroff, A.A. and Martin, R.J. (eds). *Neonatal–Perinatal Medicine*, 5th edn. St Louis, MO: Mosby Year Book, 1992: 834–7.

107 Findlay, R.D., Taeusch, H.W. and Walther, F.J. Surfactant replacement therapy for meconium aspiration syndrome. *Pediatrics* 1996; **97**: 48–52.

108 Miller, M.J., Fanaroff, A.A. and Martin, R.J. Pneumothorax and other air leak syndromes. In: Fanaroff, A.A. and Martin, R.J. (eds). *Neonatal–Perinatal Medicine*, 5th edn. St Louis, MO: Mosby Year Book, 1992: 840–5.

109 Wilson, J.M. and Mark, E.J. A preterm newborn triplet with diffuse cystic changes in the lung. *New England Journal of Medicine* 1997; **337**: 916–26.

Day-stay surgery

LIAM BRENNAN

INTRODUCTION

The past 20 years have seen an enormous increase in the amount of children's surgery performed in day-case facilities. Over 60% of paediatric surgery in the USA is performed on an ambulatory basis.[1] In the UK, the Royal College of Surgeons of England has estimated that 50% of all elective surgery, especially that in children, can be performed as day surgery.[2]

Although the main impetus for this expansion has been economic, health-care professionals and parents have generally embraced this innovation, as ambulatory care has been shown to have many advantages for children. The key benefits are the minimization of parental separation, avoidance of the stress of inpatient admission and decreased disruption for the family.

Good-quality day surgical care in children is judged by minimal postoperative morbidity, high child and parental satisfaction and low inpatient admission rates. Achievement of these goals requires a multidisciplinary team approach with the services of experienced and enthusiastic clinicians. Furthermore, concise selection criteria, appropriate anaesthesia, scrupulous postoperative symptom control and clear communication with parents will ensure a consistently successful outcome.

HISTORICAL PERSPECTIVES

It is a popular misconception that day-case surgery only evolved in the second half of the twentieth century. This is not the case since day-stay management is as old as general anaesthesia itself. Many of the early general anaesthetics administered in the 1840s were for dental and other minor surgical procedures. The patients, many of whom were children, recovered rapidly from light ether or nitrous oxide anaesthesia and left their doctor's premises soon afterwards.

However, the first major landmark in the history of paediatric day-case surgery was the work of J.H. Nicoll. Nicoll, a Glasgow surgeon, reported a series of 8988 children managed as day cases over a 10-year period from 1899 to 1908.[3] His series included 406 cleft lip and palate corrections, 220 inguinal and umbilical hernia repairs and 18 congenital pyloromyotomies. Nicoll made some observations about day surgery that are still pertinent today. He commented that much of the surgery performed in hospital was a waste of resources and that the same caseload could be managed on an outpatient basis for one-tenth of the inpatient costs. He also suggested that children were better managed in their own homes after minor surgery, trusting to the common-sense of their parents supported by visiting nurses from the hospital. Finally, he voiced what were radical opinions for his day: that separation of the child from its mother was harmful and that prolonged inpatient bed rest after surgery in children was unnecessary.

In 1916, Ralph Waters opened his Downtown Anaesthesia Clinic in Sioux City, Iowa. This facility provided care for dental and minor surgical cases, including many children. It is generally regarded as the prototype for the modern free-standing day-case unit.[4]

Outside the USA, the early enthusiasm of Nicoll was not sustained. The increasing availability of hospital services in the UK and heightened expectations of the community saw the pendulum swing firmly in the direction of inpatient care. Consequently, few reports appear in literature describing experiences with day surgery for the next 50 years.

Modern day-case surgery dates from the 1960s. The escalating costs of health care in the USA prompted the development of formal outpatient surgical programmes in several cities (e.g. Los Angeles in 1962 and Rhode Island in 1968). In the UK, the first purpose-built day-care unit opened at the Hammersmith Hospital in 1967.[5] The first free-standing day unit opened in Phoenix, Arizona, in 1970 – the Downtown Surgicentre.[6]

Subsequent developments in paediatric day surgery have been prompted as much by benefits for the child and their family as by economic advantages. In the UK, these clinical benefits were emphasized by the organization 'Caring for Children in the Health Service'. This group, consisting of clinicians, nurses and parents, produced a seminal report on paediatric day-case management which is the current blueprint for good practice in the UK.[7] It contains a wealth of practical advice and sets out 12 quality standards for the care of paediatric day cases (Table 19.1).

FACILITIES FOR DAY SURGERY

A key aspect of providing high-quality paediatric day-case management is the location of the service. Several types of facility can deliver optimal care but much depends on the numbers

Table 19.1 Quality standards for paediatric day care

1	An integrated admission plan should be formulated to include preadmission, day of admission and postadmisssion care, with planned transfer of care to community services
2	The child and parent should be offered preparation before and during the day of admission
3	Parents should be provided with specific written information
4	The child should be admitted to a designated day-case area and not mixed with acutely ill inpatients
5	Children should not be admitted or treated alongside adults
6	Specifically designated day-case staff should care for the child
7	Only staff with paediatric and day-care experience should manage the child
8	Care should be organized so that every child is likely to be discharged within the day
9	The building, equipment and furnishings should comply with children's safety standards
10	The environment should be child friendly
11	Essential documentation should be completed before the child's discharge to ensure efficient aftercare and follow-up
12	Paediatric nursing support should be available to children at home

(From Thornes, 1991.[7])

of children to be treated, staffing levels and economic considerations. Whichever type of facility is used, however, it is essential that the 12 quality standards noted previously (Table 19.1) are adhered to when designing the environment for paediatric use.

PURPOSE-BUILT CHILDREN'S DAY UNIT

This is undoubtedly the best pattern if the numbers of children are sufficient. The design of the unit should ensure that children circulate so that preoperative and postoperative patients are separated (Figure 19.1). The environment should be cheerful, safe and child friendly in all areas of the unit where conscious children are managed. Adequately sized play areas must be provided for children preoperatively. Other potential uses of the paediatric day unit should also be considered. For example, a treatment room for medical day cases can be incorporated at the design stage.

CHILDREN IN ADULT DAY UNITS

Many purpose-built day-surgery units admit both children and adults. However, the nursing of children alongside adults has been considered unacceptable in all health-care systems for many years. This is not only because of the difficulties in maintaining child-centred care in such an environment, but also because adult patients, particularly women, find the proximity of distressed children in the recovery phase very upsetting. These problems can be overcome by having dedicated children's days or sessions in the adult unit according to demand. The unit can be made child friendly for these sessions and appropriately trained children's nurses and play

specialists can be brought in to ensure the best-quality care.

CHILDREN'S DAY CASES THROUGH INPATIENT FACILITIES

Despite the expansion in day-case management it has been estimated that 60% of hospitals still admit paediatric day patients to inpatient wards.[7] Although this model ensures that appropriate nursing and support personnel are available and the environment is optimal for children, it has many disadvantages. Children who are basically healthy are mixed with acutely ill inpatients. This is potentially psychologically harmful.[8] In addition, ward staff are often more focused on the management of the sicker inpatients. The result is that day cases can become second-class patients with a failure to provide the appropriate supportive care for children and their parents.[7] The operating facility is also often distant from the children's wards, which may result in a slow turnover of cases.

If this model is to be used successfully a separate part of the inpatient ward should be dedicated for day-case use, with nursing staff assigned to this area with no other responsibilities. The admission procedures, nursing protocols and information for parents in this area should be distinct from those used for inpatients and be appropriate for day-case management.

PERSONNEL

A multidisciplinary team is required to provide high-quality day care. All staff involved should be experienced in the management of children as well as having expertise in day surgery.

SURGEONS AND ANAESTHETISTS

These clinicians should be of consultant status and have specific training and regular ongoing paediatric experience.[9,10] Trainees in anaesthesia or surgery should only work in paediatric

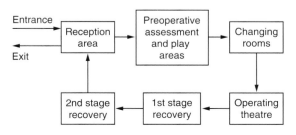

Figure 19.1 Essential components of a paediatric day-case unit.

day care under senior supervision. A clinician of consultant status usually takes the role of director in large units. The director develops an effective operational policy and trouble-shoots administrative problems in conjunction with the unit's operational manager.

NURSING STAFF

All nursing staff working in the day unit should be experienced in day-case management. In addition, a proportion of the nursing establishment should be trained paediatric nurses. The number of children's trained nurses allocated to the day-care service will depend on the paediatric workload as well as on the availability of suitably trained personnel. There is currently a shortage of working children's nurses in the UK, with the result that only 49% of UK day units have any paediatric trained staff.[11] Strategies for overcoming this problem include offering flexible employment to nurses to entice them back from a career break and rotating inpatient children's nurses to the day unit as part of their working week.

PLAY SPECIALISTS

Play staff, ideally with specialist training, should be available to provide a play service for children of all ages.[7] Through the medium of structured play, play specialists can provide a relaxed atmosphere which helps to allay the anxieties of children (and their parents), most of whom are unpremedicated. Play staff can start to gain a rapport with the child and their family at preadmission visits and help to provide appropriate explanations of anaesthetic and surgical procedures. They can also alert the anaesthetist to the overly anxious child who might benefit from sedative premedication. Despite the clear benefits it is disappointing to note that only 21% of UK day units have play specialist services.[11]

ADMINISTRATIVE STAFF

Good clerical assistance is essential if the day unit is to function efficiently. An operational manager should be appointed (usually an enthusiastic senior nurse) to take charge of the day-to-day administration of the unit.

COMMUNITY NURSING SERVICES

Many units arrange follow-up visits by community paediatric nurses. Home visits serve a useful audit function, alerting the unit staff to any significant complications[12] as well as providing specific nursing care.

ADVANTAGES OF DAY CARE

It is becoming increasingly apparent that managing children on a day-stay basis confers major benefits for the child and their family as well as for the providers of health care.

The main advantages for the child and family are the minimization of parental separation, decreased disruption to family routine and avoidance of the psychological stress of inpatient admission. Short-term behavioural problems, sleeping problems, nocturnal enuresis and regression of developmental milestones are common after inpatient hospital stay.[8] These problems, more common in anxious children less that 6 years old who come from discordant homes, are decreased by day-stay management. From a purely medical viewpoint, exposure to hospital-acquired infection is minimized by day stay. Thus, cross-infection rates may be significantly decreased[13] and the risks to immuno-compromised children are lessened (making day care particularly attractive for oncological patients).

Paediatric day-care surgery confers many operational benefits. In the UK public health-care system waiting lists have been reduced by an expansion of day care allowing contractual obligations and central government targets for surgical care to be more easily met. Transferring cases to the day unit also releases inpatient resources for those requiring more complex surgical procedures. Alternatively, major cost savings may accrue in larger institutions if increased day surgery is combined with closure of inpatient beds.[14] Even without bed closures major savings can be made when common children's procedures are switched from inpatient to day care.[15] For example, in the Cambridge unit, the costs for day-case circumcision are only 46% of the inpatient equivalent.

SELECTION CRITERIA

Successful day-care surgery requires unambiguous selection criteria protocols to be developed by the day unit's director in conjunction with admitting clinicians (Table 19.2). These proto-

Table 19.2 Exclusion criteria for paediatric day care

Patient-related factors
    Preterm or ex-preterm baby < 60 weeks' postconceptional age
    Poorly controlled systemic disease (e.g. asthma, cardiac disease, epilepsy)
    Inborn errors of metabolism and diabetes mellitus
    Uninvestigated cardiac murmur
    Sickle cell disease (not trait)
    Active infection (especially of respiratory tract)

Anaesthetic and surgical factors
    Inexperienced anaesthetist or surgeon
    Prolonged procedure (> 1 h)
    Opening of a body cavity
    High risk of perioperative haemorrhage
    Postoperative pain unlikely to be relieved by oral analgesics
    Difficult airway (including sleep apnoea)
    Malignant hyperpyrexia susceptibility?
    Siblings of victims of sudden infant death syndrome?

Social factors
    Parent unable or unwilling to care for child postoperatively
    Single parent with several other children and no home support
    Poor housing conditions
    No telephone
    Excessive journey time (> 1 h)
    Inadequate postoperative transport arrangements

cols, which should be periodically updated in the light of local audit and peer-reviewed developments in day surgery, should focus on four key areas: the patient, the type of operative procedure, specific anaesthetic considerations and the social circumstances of the child and family.

THE PATIENT

The vast majority of children are healthy and free of chronic disease, making them particularly suitable for day care. However, children with well-controlled systemic disease, e.g. asthma, epilepsy or malignant disease may still be suitable candidates.[16] Even some children in ASA class 3 may be eligible.

Chronic medical conditions

Children with inborn errors of metabolism make poor candidates for day surgery because of the dangers of symptomatic hypoglycaemia associated with perioperative fasting.[17] Similarly, glycaemic control may be difficult to manage on a day-stay basis for children with insulin-dependent diabetes.

Complex congenital heart disease is always a contraindication to day surgery. However, asymptomatic children with uncomplicated lesions, e.g. small VSD, can be safely managed on an ambulatory basis provided suitable antibiotic prophylaxis against bacterial endocarditis is used. Children with surgically corrected cardiac lesions, who are well, are also suitable with antibiotic prophylaxis as appropriate. Close liaison with cardiological colleagues will ensure appropriate case selection in this context.

A previously undiagnosed heart murmur is a common dilemma in paediatric day surgery. Fortunately, a comprehensive review of this subject gives useful guidance in this area.[18] It is clear from this review that it is difficult on clinical grounds to differentiate an innocent murmur from one caused by a significant cardiac abnormality, particularly in children under 1 year of age in whom a potentially serious lesion may not yet have declared itself.

Careful assessment by experienced staff is therefore essential in this situation, with deferment of the operative procedure sometimes being necessary to allow full cardiological appraisal.

Respiratory tract infections

Deciding on the appropriate management of the child with a respiratory infection is one of the most controversial areas of day-surgical practice. It has been estimated that 20–30% of children have a runny nose for a significant part of the year.[19] Many of these children have a benign, non-infectious seasonal rhinitis or their symptoms are due to infected adenoids which are perennial. Cancelling these patients confers no clinical benefit.

However, coryza may be a prelude to more severe upper or lower respiratory tract infections or life-threatening problems such as meningitis. Anaesthesia in the presence of significant respiratory infection may produce an increased incidence of perioperative respiratory complications including airway obstruction, laryngeal spasm, vagally mediated bronchoconstriction and atelectasis.[20] These complications are increased 11-fold if the trachea is intubated[21] and are worse and more common in the infant age group.[22] The other concern, which has not been quantified, is the incidence of myocarditis associated with the viraemic phase of some coryzal illnesses.[23]

It is clear that there is no one correct approach to this problem and each child must be assessed on an individual basis by an experienced anaesthetist. If the respiratory infection is mild with non-purulent secretions and non-productive cough, and the child is constitutionally well then it may be reasonable to proceed. However, even with mild respiratory symptoms the indications for considering postponement are: age under 1 year, associated bronchospasm and the possible need for tracheal intubation. All children with moderate or severe respiratory infections should be postponed. Clinical indicators of severity include productive cough, purulent nasal secretions and systemic features of viraemia/bacteraemia including fever, malaise and irritable behaviour.

If the procedure is postponed, several authors recommend deferment for 2 weeks if the upper respiratory tract alone is affected but 4 weeks if there is evidence of lower respiratory tract involvement.[17,19] However, others recommend greater caution with a 6-week postponement.[20] Special considerations should be given to children following measles, pertussis or respiratory syncytial virus infection. A delay of 6 weeks is advisable as respiratory tract irritability can be troublesome.[24]

Age

In theory there is no minimal age at which a term infant may not be managed on a day-care basis. Procedures such as examination of the eyes for retinoblastoma may be appropriate for ambulatory care, provided suitably qualified anaesthetic and surgical personnel are involved[17] and there is access to inpatient neonatal care if required.[25]

Preterm or ex-preterm infants are not suitable candidates for day surgery because of the potential for complications, such as apnoeas and problems with body-temperature homeostasis. The age at which an ex-preterm infant may be safely anaesthetized on a day-stay basis is unknown and each child should be assessed individually. Factors such as the history of apnoeic episodes, the presence of anaemia and bronchopulmonary dysplasia are important in the decision-making process. However, most authorities in this area will not anaesthetize children younger than 50 weeks' postconceptional age, or even older if the ex-premature infant still exhibits evidence of chronic lung disease.[26]

Outside specialist paediatric centres the lower age limit for day surgery is usually much higher: common thresholds in UK practice are less than 6 months or even 1 year old, regardless of physical status. This often reflects the experience of the staff in paediatric management, the availability of appropriate facilities and equipment for infants as well as the paediatric workload.

THE PROCEDURE

Surgical procedures over a wide range are suitable for day-care management (Table 19.3). In addition, many medical interventions and radiological procedures can be managed through the day unit. When deciding whether a procedure is suitable for day care, the clinician may consider using the following criteria.

Table 19.3 Examples of procedures suitable for paediatric day care

General surgery
     Herniotomy (inguinal, umbilical, epigastric)
     Upper and lower gastrointestinal tract
     endoscopy ± biopsy
     Lymph node excision/biopsy
Urology
     Cystoscopy
     Orchidopexy
     Preputial adhesions and circumcision
     Minor hypospadias
ENT
     Myringotomy ± grommets
     Nasal fracture reduction
     Adenotonsillectomy?
Dental
     Extractions
     Conservations
Ophthalmology
     Examination under anaesthesia
     Lacrimal duct probing
     Strabismus correction
Plastic surgery
     Otoplasty
     Excision skin lesions
     Scar revisions
Orthopaedics
     Change of plastercast
     Removal of metalwork
     Arthroscopy
Medical
     Imaging techniques, e.g. CT, MRI scanning
     Interventional radiology/cardiology
     Bone marrow sampling
     Lumbar puncture ± intrathecal medication

1 The procedure should take no more than 1 h to complete.
2 The procedure should not involve major encroachment on a body cavity.
3 The procedure should not be associated with a significant risk of a large perioperative haemorrhage.
4 The procedure should not result in postoperative pain that cannot be adequately relieved by oral analgesics.

Besides these criteria there are other contentious areas that should be resolved at local level. For example, some clinicians are unhappy to perform bilateral procedures (e.g. orchidopexy) because of potentially excessive postoperative pain.

Adenoidectomy and tonsillectomy

Tonsil and adenoid surgery is a highly controversial area of day-case practice. Although these procedures have been performed on a day-stay basis in North America for many years, the UK, Australia and some other European countries have been more reticent. In 1985 the Royal College of Surgeons of England published guidelines for day surgery in which they concluded that adenotonsillar surgery was an unsuitable day-care procedure owing to the risk of haemorrhage.[27] However, attitudes have changed in recent years, with increasing reports in the UK literature testifying to the safety of day-case adenoidectomy[28] and tonsillectomy.[29]

Haemorrhage is the most feared complication and several studies have established that this is most likely to occur within 4–8 h postoperatively.[30] These same authors recommend a 6-h observation period in the day unit prior to discharge. Pain and postoperative nausea and vomiting are also major concerns after adenotonsillectomy. Successful management of these problems by liberal use of non-steroidal anti-inflammatory drugs (NSAIDs), judicious use of opioids and prophylactic antiemetics has recently been reported.[31]

Scrupulous patient selection is essential to the success of a day-case adenotonsillectomy programme. Patel and Hannallah[32] have suggested the following exclusion criteria: (1) patients less than 3 years old; (2) history of obstructive sleep apnoea; (3) coexisting medical condition; (4) social limitation (home more than 1-h drive from hospital; lack of private car or telephone).

Although adenoidectomy alone is being increasingly performed on a day-case basis in the UK and Europe,[25] there is still concern expressed about same-day tonsillectomy or adenotonsillectomy. It may be that the move towards 23-h overnight stay will be the model of care that has the most widespread acceptance.

ANAESTHETIC CONSIDERATIONS

Prolonged general anaesthesia, even with modern agents, is associated with protracted recovery and complications such as nausea and vomiting which may result in increased rates of inpatient admission. For this reason, many units avoid procedures that consistently take more than 1 h to complete.

Children with potentially difficult airways, e.g. Pierre Robin, Treacher Collins and Goldenhar's syndromes, should not be managed as day cases. However, the anaesthetist must be adequately trained and equipped to deal with the unanticipated problem airway.

Concern has been expressed about the problems associated with tracheal intubation of day-surgery patients. Postextubation stridor in children under 6 years old may occur up to 6 h postoperatively, by which time the child would normally have been discharged home.[33] However, this is much less of a problem in contemporary practice with modern tracheal tubes which are less likely to induce mucosal oedema. In addition, the increasing use of the laryngeal mask airway (LMA) has superseded many of the previous indications for intubation (see below).

Several conditions which are of particular concern to the anaesthetist should be considered at this point. Some authorities consider children who are susceptible to malignant hyperthermia (MH) to be unsuitable for day care.[34] However, this view has been challenged by a retrospective review of MH-susceptible children which concluded that ambulatory care in this condition can be safe.[35] Finally, although there is no evidence implicating anaesthesia with sudden infant death syndrome (SIDS), siblings of SIDS victims are best managed as inpatients to minimize the understandably heightened parental anxieties.[17]

THE FAMILY

Although the advantages of day care for the child and their family have been emphasized, there are some families for which this model of care is unsuitable. The parent must be able to cope with the postoperative instructions and with the care of the child after treatment. Single parents with several other children may find day care difficult to contend with, as may very nervous parents. Both of these groups may be supported by community nurses postoperatively, thus avoiding the need for inpatient admission.[17]

Other social considerations are also important to ensure successful day care. Thus, poor housing conditions (e.g. lack of an easily accessible lavatory) and no private telephone are considered by many to contraindicate day surgery. Transport home postoperatively must be by either private vehicle or taxi. Ideally, a second adult should care for the child other than the driver.[7] Excessive journey times after surgery should be avoided to minimize wound pain and emetic symptoms. In this respect many units arbitrarily preclude patients with more than a 1-h journey time home postoperatively. The use of public transport is controversial.[36]

PREOPERATIVE ASSESSMENT

Assessing children well in advance of day surgery is advantageous for the patient, the family and the efficient running of the day-care service. Preventable cancellation of children on the day of surgery is minimized. This limits wastage of operating time and resources and more importantly avoids distress for children and parents. Preadmission assessment also provides the opportunity to optimize a child's condition, which may then make the case suitable for day care. An effective assessment system also improves efficiency and decreases stress for the child on the day of surgery by speeding the admission process.

The following methods of assessing patients have been used successfully.

PATIENT QUESTIONNAIRES AND NURSE-LED ASSESSMENT

Having been seen by the surgeon in the outpatient department the child and parent are sent to the day unit. The parent completes a questionnaire detailing the child's medical history (Figure 19.2) This is reviewed with the parent by an experienced day-surgery nurse who then triages the children into those who are fit, those needing further assessment and those who can immediately be recognized as being unsuitable for day care. Nurse-led assessment works very well in day-care practice; it has been

ADDENBROOKES HOSPITAL DAY SURGICAL UNIT
CHILDREN'S PRE-OPERATIVE QUESTIONNAIRE:

DAY_____ AM PM_____ DATE_____

SURGICAL
    CONSULTANT_____

OPERATION_____

Name

No

D.O.B.:

PLEASE TICK CORRECT ANSWERS

	No	Yes
Has your child had anything to eat or drink in the last 6 hours?		
Will this be your child's first operation?		
Has your child had any serious illness?		
Has your child had any problems with anaesthetics?		
Has any of your family had any problems with anaesthetics?		
Has your child got a cough, cold or nose trouble?		
Has your child had heart disease or rheumatic fever?		
Has your child had bronchitis, asthma or other chest problem?		
Has your child had convulsions or fits?		
Does your child faint easily?		
Does your child have anaemia or other blood problems?		
Does your child bruise or bleed excessively?		
Does your child have allergies or reactions to medicines, etc?		
Is your child on any medicines now? (tablets, capsules, injections, inhalers etc)		
Has your child ever been jaundiced?		
Has your child ever had urinary or kidney trouble?		
Has your child ever had diabetes or sugar in the urine?		
Has your child any loose teeth at present?		

Nursing Observations:

Pulse   bpm

B.P.   mm hg

Wt.   Kg.

Temp.   deg.C

LIST ALLERGIES HERE:

LIST DRUGS HERE:

R   L

PARENTS PLEASE NOTE THAT AFTER YOUR CHILD'S ANAESTHETIC HE/SHE SHOULD NOT RIDE A BICYCLE NOR UNDERTAKE ANY OTHER DANGEROUS ACTIVITIES ON THE SAME DAY

Consent forms signed?   Yes No

Identification bracelets   Yes No

PARENTS SIGNATURE: _____

REF DES CS

SP7301

Figure 19.2   Example of a paediatric preoperative questionnaire.

validated in adult practice[37] and is used for children and adults in the Cambridge unit.[38]

Suitable children can be given a date for surgery and parents can be given preoperative instructions and an information leaflet which emphasizes important issues such as preoperative fasting (Figure 19.3). Unsuitable patients are referred back to the surgeon. Borderline cases will require further assessment by a clinician (see below).

TELEPHONE SCREENING

If the surgeon sees the child at a site remote from the day unit, telephone screening by unit staff utilizing the questionnaire method described above is appropriate. Contact with parents is improved by calling in the evening.[39] Borderline cases can attend the day unit for further assessment.

A second telephone call made within 24 h of surgery has also been shown to be advantageous.[19] The child's current state of health can be assessed (particularly the presence of respiratory infections), starvation instructions reinforced and practical issues such as car parking discussed.

CLINICIAN ASSESSMENT

Arbitration over borderline cases requires assessment by an experienced clinician. Most equivocal cases involve decisions regarding anaesthetic suitability; a consultant anaesthetist who works in the unit should perform this task.

Finally, all children must be seen by the operating surgeon and anaesthetist on the day of surgery. Both should perform a relevant clinical examination, with the anaesthetist focusing on any recent illnesses such as respiratory tract infection which may contraindicate proceeding that day.

PREPARING FOR YOUR CHILD'S APPOINTMENT

■ **DO NOT** let your child eat anything (including sweets and chewing gum) for **SIX HOURS** before your appointment.

■ **THREE HOURS** before their appointment your child **SHOULD** have a clear drink which does not contain milk (ie water, squash, black tea or coffee)

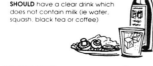

NO FOOD FROM .... a.m. / p.m.

NO DRINK FROM .... a.m. / p.m.

■ Make up and Nail Varnish needs to be removed before your child's appointment.

■ Your child may bring a dressing gown and slippers, but this is optional as we can provide it if necessary. Your child may also bring a favourite doll, teddy bear, or book.

■ **DO NOT** bring large sums of money or jewellery with you as we are unable to accept any responsibility for loss or damage to your property.

■ **YOU MUST** arrange for a parent or responsible adult to take your child home and to stay with them for 24 hours following their operation.

Public transport should not be used to take your child home

■ Please bring details of current or recent medications. Please give your child all regular medications as usual on the day of surgery with a sip of water unless otherwise instructed

WHAT WILL HAPPEN ON THE DAY?

■ Parents are encouraged to stay with their child in the Unit.

■ When you arrive, you will meet your nurses who will prepare your child for surgery and anaesthesia.

■ If you have not already done so, you will be asked to complete a pre-operative questionnaire and sign a consent form.

■ Your child's anaesthetic will be selected to ensure rapid recovery and as few after effects as possible. It may be given by mask or injection.

■ At the discretion of the anaesthetist you may be able to stay with your child while they are being given their anaesthetic.

■ After about one hour, most children are ready to enjoy a drink.

■ If necessary your child will be prescribed pain killers to take.

■ Arrangements will be made for any follow up treatment your child may require.

■ Post-operative information will be given to you before leaving the unit.

DISCHARGE

■ Morning Patients should be ready to return home at about 1 p.m.

■ Afternoon Patients should be ready to return home at about 5 p.m.

■ Discharge times may vary according to the nature of your child's operation.

FOR 24 HOURS AFTER YOUR CHILD'S OPERATION

■ Remember any operation no matter how minor requires **AFTERCARE**.

■ Rest is advised especially if nausea or dizziness occurs.

■ No school or playgroup on the day following your child's operation. It may be necessary to keep your child at home longer depending on the type of operation.

■ **DO NOT** allow your child to cycle or go on busy roads or playgrounds.

■ Observe any special precautions which the surgeon or anaesthetist have advised.

■ If you are worried about your child's condition, contact your general practitioner first.

SPECIAL INFORMATION

Addenbrooke's NHS Trust is a teaching hospital. This means we are responsible for teaching medical and nursing students who are always under the direct supervision of senior experienced staff. To facilitate their education our operating theatres have a camera link to a seminar room within the Day Surgery Unit.

If you have any objection to your child being involved in these education issues please let the staff know on your arrival. This will not prejudice their treatment in any way

Privacy, dignity and confidentiality of your child is carefully protected at all times

Figure 19.3 Example of an information leaflet for children's day surgery.

PREOPERATIVE PREPARATION

In order that the entire clinical episode can be successfully completed within a day, careful consideration needs to be focused on the preoperative preparation of the child and the parents.

PSYCHOLOGICAL

Although day surgery avoids the emotional trauma of inpatient admission, children and parents require careful psychological preparation for what is still a stressful life event.

Preparation should begin at the initial outpatient surgical consultation. Careful explanation of the intended procedure and its aftermath should be provided and the parents (and child as appropriate) given the opportunity to ask questions. If the child is then seen for assessment in the day unit (see above) this opportunity can also be used to answer further questions and allay anxieties. Options for immediate pain relief, including the use of rectal suppositories and the management of late pain occurring after discharge home, should be discussed at this stage.

Preadmission programmes which utilize play simulation, photograph albums, video presentation or visits to the day unit out of hours (e.g. Saturday clubs) have been found to be very useful in preparing the child for day surgery. Long-term behavioural benefits have been demonstrated in children who have received an interactive teaching book prior to day surgery.[40] However, the view has been expressed that the parents who usually take advantage of these preoperative programmes are often those whose level of education, motivation and understanding renders such formal processes unnecessary.[41]

On the day of surgery, stress levels can be decreased by ensuring a child-friendly environment in the day unit with plenty of toys and activities co-ordinated by a play specialist. Younger children should be encouraged to bring a favourite soft toy. The needs of older children and teenagers should not be neglected. An appropriate adult-style approach is required, with access to activities such as personal CD players or computer games.

Separation of child from parent should be minimized; parents should be encouraged to accompany their child during anaesthetic induction. However, anxious parents should not be pressurized into coming to theatre as they may transfer their anxiety to the child.[42]

PREOPERATIVE FASTING

Prolonged preoperative starvation at best produces an irritable, uncooperative child and at worst may result in significant hypoglycaemia in young infants. Parents also commonly suffer from the effects of prolonged fasting, with one study showing that 85% of parents fast alongside their children.[43]

It is now well established that liberalization of fasting regimens for clear fluids (but not milk or solids) improves perioperative behaviour and maintains normoglycaemia without increasing the risk of pulmonary aspiration.[44,45]

A well-established starvation regimen used in the Cambridge unit and elsewhere is as follows:

- 6 h for solids, milk (including formula feeds for infants);
- 4 h for breast-fed infants;
- 3 h for clear fluids (includes water, squashes, carbonated drinks, black tea or coffee).

Clear written and verbal instruction need to be given to parents emphasizing that prolonged preoperative starvation can be harmful and that clear fluids should, rather than can, be given until 3 h preoperatively.

PREOPERATIVE INVESTIGATIONS

Indiscriminate preoperative investigations of children prior to day surgery are unjustified on clinical, economic and humanitarian grounds.[46] However, in the USA 27% of patients scheduled for day care were having routine haemoglobin measurement as late as 1993.[47] Although the incidence of mild anaemia is higher in the infant age group there is a paucity of evidence that this affects perioperative morbidity or management, particularly for day-case procedures.[48,49]

The need for routine sickle-cell testing in racially susceptible groups has been challenged in adult practice.[50] However, sickle-cell testing remains one of the few commonly performed investigations in UK paediatric day-case practice.[17] This is because there is concern that in younger children the manifestations of sickle-cell disease may not have become apparent.

SEDATIVE PREMEDICATION

Routine preoperative sedation of day-care children is unnecessary. Good psychological preparation, as outlined above, combined with parental presence at anaesthetic induction, minimizes the need for this approach. (< 5% of children are given sedation in the Cambridge unit). However, selected groups of children benefit from preoperative sedation. These include the unduly anxious child, the child who has had a previously traumatic perioperative experience, some children attending for repeated procedures and those children with mental handicap with whom it is difficult to gain a rapport.

Traditional sedative premedicants are unsuitable for day surgery as they produce excessive postoperative sedation and delay discharge.[51] Opioids as premedicants are suboptimal as they increase postoperative emesis, an important cause of morbidity after day surgery. This problem also extends to the oral transmucosal fentanyl preparation (presented as a lollipop), which has been used in North America in recent years.[52]

Considerable interest has focused on midazolam for premedication of day-care children. The oral route is particularly promising, with several studies showing that a dose of 0.5–0.75 mg kg^{-1} acts within 10–30 min to produce a calm, co-operative child without delaying recovery.[53,54] However, other workers have more recently suggested that higher doses (0.75 mg kg^{-1}) may delay recovery and produce postoperative agitation.[55]

In the Cambridge unit and at other UK centres 0.5 mg kg^{-1} is the established regimen. The standard formulation of midazolam is very bitter and to make it more acceptable to children it should be added to a suitable vehicle such as paracetamol elixir or a small volume of a sweet drink (e.g. lemonade). Other routes of administration for midazolam have been described, including rectal[56] and intranasal.[57] Although these routes have their advocates they often involve a degree of restraint of the child to administer them and may be associated with unacceptable side-effects (e.g. nasal stinging and coughing[58]).

ANTICHOLINERGIC PREMEDICATION

The use of anticholinergic premedication for day cases is also an area of controversy. Whilst many anaesthetists are happy to administer anticholinergic medication as required intraoperatively, some still insist on its routine preoperative use, particularly prior to inhalational induction in smaller children. Oral atropine (up to 40 μg kg^{-1}) may be useful in the infant or young child undergoing mask anaesthesia, although its routine use in older children may not improve induction conditions.[53]

CUTANEOUS ANAESTHESIA FOR VENEPUNCTURE

The introduction of local anaesthetic skin preparations has made it possible to perform painless venepuncture in children and has increased the use of intravenous induction for paediatric day cases. The two available products in the UK are amethocaine gel (Ametop®) and a eutectic mixture of lignocaine and prilocaine (EMLA®). The use of EMLA requires careful planning since at least 60 min of contact time under an occlusive dressing is needed to ensure adequate cutaneous analgesia.[59] Amethocaine gel has some advantages over EMLA, with a quicker onset time (45 min) and less tendency to produce venoconstriction.[59]

PREINDUCTION TECHNIQUES

Occasionally, very unco-operative children may require last-minute premedication in order to facilitate anaesthetic induction. In this situation, and with parental consent, it may be appropriate to impose an intramuscular sedative on the child. Low-dose ketamine (2 mg kg^{-1}) can be used in young children, with an onset time of around 3 min. Recovery is not prolonged and postoperative delirium does not seem to be a problem.[60]

However, careful consideration needs to be given before using such techniques in older, rational children. Clearly, there is a risk that significant physical restraint may be required in this situation despite the support of the parents. In the UK, the law has recognized the concept of emerging competence by which children may achieve sufficient understanding and maturity to enable them to give consent to treatment.[61] A recent review of this topic advises that if an older child absolutely refuses to co-operate with treatment the procedure should be cancelled and counselling of the child and parents should ensue.[62] Imposing treatment on such a child may lead to a charge of assault.

ANAESTHETIC MANAGEMENT

INDUCTION

Providing smooth, atraumatic induction of anaesthesia in the unpremedicated child is one of the biggest challenges for the day-case anaesthetist. The choice of technique should be tailored to the needs of the individual child. Consequently, the anaesthetist must be versatile and able to use both intravenous and inhalational techniques as the situation dictates. Whichever technique is used, encouraging parents to be present during induction can be very helpful for the child and the anaesthetist.[63,64] However, as already indicated careful parent selection and education are essential for the success of this approach,[65] as anxious parents may make their children even more upset during the induction period.[42]

Inhalational techniques

The inhalational route is particularly suitable in the needle-phobic child or the child with poor venous access. Co-operation from the child can be enhanced by allowing him or her to sit on the parent's lap during induction and by the use of transparent anaesthetic face masks. Some workers have described success using masks painted with food flavourings of the child's choice. Halothane has been the most commonly used inhalational induction agent for many years. However, sevoflurane has now become the first choice volatile agent in the USA and Europe owing to its pleasant smell, non-irritating properties and rapid onset of action.[66]

Intravenous techniques

Intravenous induction has become increasingly popular since the introduction of local anaesthetic skin preparations (see above). In the Cambridge unit, 87% of children are induced intravenously.

The choice of intravenous induction agent for day care rests between thiopentone and propofol. When thiopentone is used a relatively large dose (5–6 mg kg^{-1}) is required in unpremedicated children to ensure a satisfactory induction. Barbiturate induction is associated with slightly delayed initial recovery from anaesthesia compared with propofol usage, but discharge times in children aged under 5 years are similar.[67]

Propofol induction has several advantages for children's day-case anaesthesia. Induction is usually smooth provided a sufficiently large dose (up to 4 mg kg^{-1}) is used in unpremedicated children.[68] The ability of propofol profoundly to obtund upper airway reflexes facilitates early insertion of a LMA.[68] Propofol induction is also associated with quicker, clearheaded recovery, particularly in older children, in whom it may allow more rapid discharge home than if thiopentone is used.[67] One drawback of propofol is that it can be painful on injection, although this problem can be minimized by adding lignocaine 0.2 mg kg^{-1} to the propofol immediately before induction.[69]

MAINTENANCE

For the majority of children's day-case procedures maintenance of anaesthesia with nitrous oxide, oxygen and a volatile agent is entirely satisfactory. Of the well-established volatile agents none has any clear advantages. Although isoflurane has a slightly lower blood–gas solubility coefficient than halothane, this does not result in any clinically significant difference in speed of recovery for shorter procedures. Of the newer volatile agents, early recovery after sevoflurane anaesthesia is reported to be 33% quicker than with halothane, but the time to discharge home is similar for both anaesthetics. This is apparently due to a three-fold greater incidence of emergence agitation necessitating more frequent use of sedation during recovery.[70] Similar findings of problems with emergence agitation have been described for desflurane maintenance,[71] although it has been suggested that these problems can be minimized by ensuring good local analgesia before emergence from anaesthesia.[72]

For patients at high risk of vomiting, a total intravenous technique using a propofol infusion has been shown to be highly beneficial in decreasing emetic symptoms, e.g. for strabismus correction.[73] Others have demonstrated that infants experience faster emergence and fewer airway and respiratory side-effects with propofol induction and maintenance, compared with a thiopentone–halothane combination.[74] Differences in the pharmacokinetics of propofol in children compared with adults (increased-clearance and higher volume of distribution) mean that higher infusion rates (125–300 μg kg^{-1} min^{-1}) are required in younger children during the early part of maintenance.[75]

AIRWAY MANAGEMENT

The LMA has many advantages for children's day-case anaesthesia (Table 19.4). Many of the problems associated with tracheal intubation (e.g. use of muscle relaxants and extubation stridor) are avoided by the use of the LMA. In experienced hands even many of the previous mandatory indications for tracheal intubation (adenotonsillectomy,[76] strabismus correction,[77] dental surgery and prominent ear correction) can be successfully fulfilled by the reinforced version of the LMA. Several studies have demonstrated that the reinforced LMA protects the airway from contamination during adenotonsillectomy, oral surgery and a variety of other procedures.[78,79]

Although the LMA can be inserted successfully following any form of anaesthetic induction, problems can occur if thiopentone has been used, as barbiturates heighten the sensitivity of laryngeal reflexes. Deepening the anaesthesia with volatile agents or combining the thiopentone with fentanyl and midazolam

Table 19.4 Advantages of the laryngeal mask airway

Quick and easy to insert
Insertion does not require muscle relaxants
Faster turnaround time
Allows for hands-free anaesthesia
Less sore throat
Avoids tracheal intubation

can overcome this problem.[80] However, the majority of studies have concluded that LMA insertion conditions are best following propofol induction, making it the agent of choice for this form of airway management.[81]

Deciding the optimal time to remove the LMA in children is contentious. Some workers have shown that fewer complications (such as laryngeal spasm) occur if the LMA is removed with the child deeply anaesthetized.[82] However, others have found that following procedures in which blood and secretions are likely to be present in the mouth, e.g. adenotonsillectomy, leaving the LMA *in situ* with the cuff still fully inflated is the safest option.[76]

MONITORING AND EMERGENCY EQUIPMENT

Perioperative monitoring equipment should be appropriate for children and adhere to the same standards as for inpatient anaesthesia, as defined by national regulatory bodies. In addition, the full range of resuscitation equipment, adjuncts for dealing with an unexpected difficult intubation and essential drugs, such as dantrolene, must be immediately available.

FLUID THERAPY

The goal of perioperative fluid management is to correct preoperative deficits and to replace intraoperative losses. On this basis the majority of children do not require parenteral fluids as most day-case procedures are not associated with significant fluid losses and modern, liberalized starvation regimens avoid preoperative dehydration.

However, perioperative intravenous fluids are indicated in specific circumstances in day-case practice:

1 procedures known to be associated with a high vomiting risk (e.g. strabismus surgery);
2 procedures associated with intraoperative haemorrhage or an increased risk of post-operative bleeding (e.g. adenotonsillectomy);
3 young children who have been fasted excessively.

For the majority of cases where intravenous fluids are indicated, a balanced salt solution is appropriate. As the incidence of hypoglycaemia associated with day care is low (less than 1%),[83] the routine use of glucose-containing solutions is unnecessary.

ANALGESIA

Scrupulous attention to pain control is essential to the success of children's day surgery. Effective analgesia requires a balanced approach utilizing NSAIDs, local anaesthesia and, when appropriate, judicious use of opioids.

NON-STEROIDAL ANTI-INFLAMMATORY DRUGS AND PARACETAMOL

NSAIDs are effective analgesics which are particularly suitable for day-case surgery. Their main advantages are lack of emetic side-effects, opioid-sparing properties and minimal sedation. The most commonly used agents in UK practice are diclofenac (1 mg kg^{-1} p.o. or rectally), ibuprofen (10 mg kg^{-1} orally) and ketorolac (0.5 mg kg^{-1} i.v.). Oral NSAIDs can usefully be given as premedication and topical diclofenac eye drops, commenced intraoperatively, provide good analgesia after strabismus surgery.[84] When rectal dosing is being considered, it should preferably occur after induction of general anaesthesia. If the rectal route is used in the conscious child, the consent of the parents and child, if appropriate, should be obtained.[85] Aspirin (but no other NSAID) is associated with Reye's syndrome and should not be administered to children less than 12 years old. The lower age limit for NSAID use is generally accepted as 1 year, although some centres routinely administer these drugs to

children of 6 months. The potential adverse effects of NSAIDs are well known; of these, gastrointestinal and renal side-effects are rarely a problem in well-hydrated, healthy children presenting for day surgery. Controversy surrounds the potential for NSAIDs to increase postoperative haemorrhage via their platelet-inhibitory effects. Although some studies have shown an increased incidence of wound haematoma in children given diclofenac,[86] this has not been a consistent finding[87] and has not deterred day-care anaesthetists from using NSAIDs for body-surface surgery. However, concern has been expressed regarding increased post-tonsillectomy bleeding associated with NSAIDs, particularly ketorolac.[88] A recent comprehensive review of NSAID usage recommends that NSAIDs should be avoided for adenotonsillectomy in patients with increased perioperative blood loss or reduced platelet function.[85]

Many anaesthetists are hesitant to administer NSAIDs to asthmatic children. However, if NSAIDs were withheld from all children who have experienced asthmatic symptoms it would exclude very effective analgesia from a large section for the paediatric day-case population. The majority of asthmatic children are not NSAID sensitive as NSAID sensitivity is much more common in adult-onset non-allergic type asthma (5–10% of adult asthmatics).[89] However, NSAIDs should certainly be avoided in children who exhibit the triad of NSAID sensitivity, asthma and nasal polyps and in those children with proven severe asthma requiring regular hospitalization, especially admission to an intensive care unit.[85] In children with lesser symptomatology, careful judgement of the relative risks and benefits of the use of NSAIDs is required by experienced personnel.

Paracetamol is also universally used and can be given as an oral loading dose preoperatively (20 mg kg^{-1}). If rectal dosing is used intraoperatively higher doses are recommended (as much as 50 mg kg^{-1} in some computer-simulation studies[90]) in order to achieve analgesic plasma concentrations. This is due to the poor and erratic absorption of rectally administered paracetamol.

OPIOIDS

The indiscriminate and repeated use of long-acting opioids in children's day-case surgery is to be deprecated as it is associated with excessive morbidity. Although remifentanil may have a place intraoperatively as an analgesic, as a general principle, if a procedure is found to necessitate repeated opioid analgesia it should not be performed on a day-stay basis. Increased vomiting and prolonged postoperative sedation are the major problems associated with opioid use which may result in the need for inpatient admission. For example, the incidence of vomiting in paediatric day cases without opioids is 1–15% and this rises to 19–56% when children receive morphine.[91]

However, accepting these potential side-effects, single doses of opioids in the perioperative period are useful in some children undergoing day surgery. Fentanyl (up to 2 μg kg^{-1}) intravenously is particularly useful to obtain rapid pain control in the immediate postoperative period if NSAIDs and local anaesthetic techniques are inadequate. Codeine (1mg kg^{-1}) orally, rectally or very rarely intramuscularly may also be useful in the immediate postoperative period.

LOCAL ANAESTHETIC TECHNIQUES

Local anaesthetic techniques are extensively used in children's day surgery. Intraoperative local anaesthesia as part of a balanced technique decreases general anaesthetic requirements, provides excellent postoperative analgesia and allows opioids to be avoided (with a concomitant decrease in postoperative morbidity).

The route of administration will depend on the skill and experience of the anaesthetist as well as the requirements of the operative procedure. However, guiding principles are that the local anaesthetic technique should be quick and simple to perform, have minimal potential for side-effects and should not interfere with motor function and early ambulation.[19] Full details of local anaesthetic techniques, particularly peripheral nerve blocks are found elsewhere in this book (see Chapter 9) and in a recent monograph.[92]

Topical

EMLA has been used prior to injection of local anaesthetic in older children undergoing minor cutaneous procedures without general anaesthesia as well as to facilitate painless venepuncture. In addition, EMLA has been used as the sole anaesthetic technique prior to myringotomies[93] and division of preputial adhesion.[94]

Topical local can also very effectively provide postoperative analgesia. Amethocaine 1% eye drops instilled at the conclusion of strabismus surgery provide very effective analgesia for up to 3 h postoperatively[95] and lignocaine gel is a useful analgesic applied to the penis after circumcision.[96] Both of these techniques can be continued by the parents after the child is discharged home.

Infiltration

Infiltration of local anaesthetic is simple to perform and very effective and the opportunity to use this technique should never be overlooked in children's day-case surgery. Bupivacaine with or without adrenaline is the agent most frequently utilized.

It can be used to supplement general anaesthesia, and selected older children can have superficial procedures performed with local anaesthesia alone, e.g. naevi and wart removal. Even more extensive procedures, such as otoplasty, can be successfully performed under infiltrative anaesthesia.

Increased acceptance of infiltrative anaesthesia in conscious children can be achieved by using EMLA cream well in advance of infiltration, using very fine needles (27 or 25G), warming the local anaesthetic solution to body temperature prior to use and injecting the local anaesthetic slowly so as to avoid discomfort from tissue distension.

Peripheral nerve blockade

Although a wide variety of peripheral nerve blocks is feasible in paediatric day care, only a few are commonly utilized in practice. Since the topic is discussed in detail elsewhere in this book (see Chapter 9), only those blocks which the author finds particularly useful will be mentioned here.

Ilioinguinal/iliohypogastric nerve block

Blockade of the ilioinguinal and iliohypogastric nerves very effectively provides analgesia after inguinal herniotomy and for the groin incision performed for orchidopexy. The block is easily performed by infiltrating local anaesthetic (usually bupivacaine 0.25%, 1 mg kg^{-1}) medial to the anterior superior iliac spine immediately beneath the external oblique aponeurosis. If only one injection is made then there is an increased incidence of inadequate pain relief after groin surgery. This is because in 50% of patients the subcostal nerve accompanies the iliohypogastric nerve and contributes to the innervation of the inguinal region. Consistently effective blockade of the whole area is achieved by a second injection directed laterally to contact the inside wall of the ileum and infiltrating local anaesthetic as the needle is slowly withdrawn.

Timing of blockade to ensure successful postoperative analgesia is controversial. In one study no difference in postoperative analgesia was demonstrated whether the block was administered by the anaesthetist percutaneously before surgery or by the surgeon under direct vision intraoperatively.[97] However, with a swift surgeon, blockade performed intraoperatively may not be fully functional as the child emerges from anaesthesia and the author's preference is therefore to perform the block before surgery starts.

Two further practical points are worthy of consideration here. Firstly, for orchidopexy, ilioinguinal/iliohypogastric blockade must be combined with local infiltration of the scrotum to provide adequate postoperative analgesia. This is because the inferior part of the scrotum is innervated by the pudendal nerve and therefore the scrotal incision (performed to facilitate testicular fixation) is not covered by the inguinal block. Secondly, inadvertent femoral nerve block can occur if the local anaesthetic injection is made too near to the inguinal ligament. This may result in leg weakness with delayed mobility in older children.[98]

Penile block

This block is becoming the favoured local analgesic technique after circumcision, minor hypospadias surgery and other penile pro-cedures. Various techniques for blocking the dorsal penile nerves are described, including midline and paramedian approaches.[92] Both methods involve depositing bupivacaine 0.5% without adrenaline deep to Buck's fascia at the base of the penis.

The single-injection midline technique is associated with an increased incidence of failed block because of the inability of local anaesthetic to diffuse across the space in the subfascial compartment. Damage to dorsal penile vessels and intravascular/intracorporeal injection of local anaesthetic (with risk of toxicity) may also occur. These problems are much less frequent with the paramedian approach, whereby injections are made either side of the midline. A simpler approach to penile block is subcutaneous infiltration of plain bupivacaine around the base of the penis. Excellent results have been reported with this technique, with no reports of significant complications.[99]

Greater auricular nerve block

Blockade of this nerve which innervates most of the pinna provides excellent analgesia (and decreased vomiting) after otoplasty. The block is easily performed by subcutaneous infiltration of local anaesthetic between the mastoid process and the descending ramus of the mandible.

Caudal extradural block

Caudal blockade is probably the most common block performed in paediatric day surgery. Its popularity stems from its reliability and technical ease of performance in young children. It is also the most versatile block available as it can be used to provide analgesia for most day-case procedures below the level of the umbilicus.

However, despite these advantages caudal block is associated with potential complications which have made the technique less attractive to some working in the day-unit environment.[92] Many feel that if a peripheral block can provide equal or superior analgesia over caudal blockade then it is more appropriate for day-case use.

Although urinary retention is perceived as a problem, several large series have failed to demonstrate that this is a significant problem after caudal blockade.[99,100] Lower limb weakness can be a problem, particularly in older children who may find the inability to bear weight distressing. This problem may be minimized by using weaker local anaesthetic solutions for caudal block (e.g. bupivacaine 0.125%).[101] Interestingly, some studies have suggested that vomiting may be more common after caudal block.[102] This may be due to an increase in cerebrospinal fluid pressure.

One of the main disadvantages of single-shot caudal block with local anaesthetic alone is that reliable analgesia is only provided for a few hours. Recently, prolongation of caudal analgesia has been achieved by addition of opioids, N-methyl-d-aspartate antagonists and α_2-agonists to bupivacaine. Opioid supplementation is probably inappropriate for day-case use because of the risk of delayed respiratory depression,[103] although ketamine and clonidine look useful.[104] Clonidine $(1-2 \mu g \ kg^{-1})$ will double the duration of bupivacaine-initiated analgesia without significant cardiorespiratory effects or sedation. Similarly, ketamine $(0.5 \ mg \ kg^{-1})$ may quadruple the duration of analgesia without cardiorespiratory or psychological effects. Preservative-free preparations of these drugs must be used.

POSTOPERATIVE MANAGEMENT

RECOVERY PARAMETERS

Initial recovery from general anaesthesia should be in a fully equipped recovery area with one-to-one nursing by staff experienced in the management of unconscious paediatric patients. Discharge from this first stage area is usually swift and without complications but occasionally serious cardiorespiratory compromise occurs which means that an anaesthetist must be available immediately to deal with this eventuality.

Timing of transfer from the first-stage recovery facility is often decided intuitively by experienced recovery staff, but some day units utilize the Steward score, which assesses the safe return of protective reflexes.[105] Wakefulness,

airway control and movement are assessed and assigned a score of 0, 1 or 2.

DISCHARGE CRITERIA

Once transferred from the first-stage recovery area, children should be reunited with their parents. The timing of discharge home from the day unit will depend on anaesthetic, surgical and social factors and the adequacy of postoperative symptom control (Table 19.5).

Assessment of vital signs and conscious level should take into account the age of the child and pre-existing conditions, such as mental handicap. If children have been intubated this does not preclude discharge even in the infant age group, but day-unit staff must watch carefully for any signs of respiratory distress or stridor. Some units require all children who have been intubated to stay a minimum of 2 h before discharge.[106] Careful assessment should be made of the child's ability to move and ambulate before discharge. Although lower limb weakness after caudal block (or occasionally inguinal block) may not contraindicate discharge in the infant or toddler age group, it may pose a problem for older children.

No mention in these criteria has been made of the need to drink or pass urine prior to discharge. Although it is desirable that children should drink before leaving the day unit, it is not essential. A child who is well hydrated may be safely discharged without drinking, provided other discharge criteria are met. This view is supported by a large, well-conducted study

Table 19.5 Discharge criteria

Vital signs and conscious level normal for age and preoperative condition of the child
Protective airway reflexes fully regained
No respiratory distress or stridor
No unexpected intraoperative anaesthetic events
No bleeding or surgical complications
PONV absent or mild
Pain absent or mild
Appropriate ambulation for age of the child
Written/verbal instructions issued and lines of contact emphasized
Escort home by responsible adult in private car or taxi

which demonstrated that when children received perioperative intravenous fluids they could be discharged home without being required to drink and this policy did not result in any readmissions for vomiting or dehydration.[107] Ability to void urine is also not an absolute requirement prior to discharge in many institutions. Urinary voiding intervals were identical in a study comparing caudal and inguinal blocks in day surgery with no cases of urinary retention.[100] However, some units still insist on a child passing urine before discharge on surgical grounds, particularly after penile surgery.

It is essential that parents are given clear verbal and written instructions regarding aspects of postoperative care prior to discharge. This should include details of wound care, analgesia, diet, mobilization and resumption of normal activities such as return to school (Figure 19.4). These instructions will vary according to the procedure but should always

include a telephone number to report complications and seek advice as appropriate.

Finally, although medical staff may delegate the final discharge of patients to experienced nursing staff utilizing locally agreed criteria, both the surgeon and anaesthetist must see the child and their parents postoperatively.[7] They must subsequently continue to be available to deal with any complications until the child has left the day-surgery facility.

POSTOPERATIVE PAIN CONTROL

Provided local anaesthetics and NSAIDs are used appropriately the majority of children should have minimal or no pain in the immediate postoperative period. In Cambridge, 10% of children experience mild or moderate pain and only 1% severe pain whilst in the day unit.[108] However, other authors report a higher incidence of severe pain after day surgery.[109] This probably reflects differences in case mix and the inherent difficulties of assessing pain levels in young children. Despite these difficulties, pain assessment is essential to ensure quality control in this area. A variety of pain-scoring systems is available, each with its own advantages and disadvantages.[110] The overriding principles, whichever scoring system is used, are that assessment should be repeated regularly, appropriate analgesic interventions prescribed and their effectiveness in reducing the pain score monitored.

Severe pain in the immediate postoperative period usually requires rescue opioid analgesia

---

SQUINT SURGERY
POST-OPERATIVE INSTRUCTIONS

SPECIAL ADVICE

1. ANALGESIA
    CALPOL (PARACETAMOL) WILL BE PRESCRIBED FOR YOU TO TAKE HOME THE NURSE WILL ADVISE YOU ON HOW AND WHEN TO GIVE THIS .

2. EYE DROPS
    THESE WILL BE PRESCRIBED TO BE INSTILLED INTO YOUR CHILDS EYE OVER THE NEXT FEW DAYS. PLEASE CHECK WITH THE NURSE ON HOW AND WHEN TO ADMINISTER THE DROPS

3. NO SWIMMING FOR 6 WEEKS

4. PLEASE KEEP EYES DRY WHEN HAIR WASHING

5. NO PLAYSCHOOL, NURSERY OR SCHOOL UNTIL YOU HAVE BEEN BACK TO YOUR CHILDS OUTPATIENT APPOINTMENT.

6. YOUR CHILD SHOULD HAVE A RESTFUL FEW DAYS. THEY MAY FEEL RATHER UNDER PAR AT TIMES AND MAY SUFFER DOUBLE VISION AT TIMES. THIS MAY LAST FOR A FEW DAYS FOLLOWING SURGERY.

7. IF YOU FIND IT DIFFICULT TO INSTIL THE EYEDROPS - TRY TO LAY YOUR CHILD FLAT AND PUT A DROP IN THE INSIDE CORNER OF THE EYE AND IT SHOULD RUN IN.

8. IF YOUR CHILD DOES NOT OPEN THEIR EYE FOR THE FIRST TWELVE HOURS AFTER SURGERY DO NOT WORRY. AFTER TWELVE HOURS THEY SHOULD GRADUALLY BEGIN TO OPEN THEIR EYES. IF THIS DOES NOT HAPPEN DO NOT HESITATE IN CONTACTING THE REGISTRAR ON CALL BY RINGING 01223 245151 AND ASKING FOR THE OPHTHALMIC REGISTRAR ON CALL

9. IF YOUR CHILD APPEARS TO HAVE A STICKY EYE OVER THE NEXT FEW DAYS THEN YOU MAY CLEAN THE EYE WITH COOLED BOILED WATER.

10. IF YOUR CHILD WEARS SPECTACLES THEY SHOULD CONTINUE TO DO SO ONCE THEIR EYES ARE OPEN.

IF YOU HAVE ANY CONCERNS DO NOT HESITATE IN CONTACTING DAY SURGERY UNIT ON 01223 216545 BETWEEN 8AM AND 6PM
OR
THE REGISTRAR ON CALL BY CONTACTING 01223 245151 AND ASKING FOR THE OPHTHALMIC REGISTRAR ON CALL

Figure 19.4 Example of a postoperative information sheet for parents.

Table 19.6 Oral analgesics for use at home

Age group	Analgesics
< 1 year old	Paracetamol 15 mg kg^{-1} p.o. every 6 h
> 1 year old	Paracetamol 15 mg kg^{-1} p.o. every 6 h $\pm$ ibuprofen 10 mg kg^{-1} p.o. every 6 h Codeine elixir 0.5 mg kg^{-1} p.o. every 6 h
Older children (> 10 years)	Compound paracetamol/codeine preparations, e.g. co-codamol $\pm$ ibuprofen 200–400 mg p.o. every 6 h

NB. Analgesia given regularly, **not** as required.

with fentanyl or codeine, as discussed previously. Failure to decrease pain scores to the mild range is a common indication for inpatient admission. Once the child has returned home, the mainstay of pain relief is oral analgesia (Table 19.6). In addition to oral medication, topically applied analgesics can be very effective, such as lignocaine gel after circumcision and diclofenac eye drops after strabismus surgery. Whichever analgesic regimen is used it is very important that parents are taught to give pain relief regularly for 24–48 h postoperatively, starting before any local anaesthetic block has worn off. This will ensure optimal pain relief at home and decreases the number of referrals to general practitioners because of analgesic problems.[108]

POSTOPERATIVE NAUSEA AND VOMITING

Postoperative nausea and vomiting (PONV), covered in detail elsewhere in this book (see Chapter 10), is potentially a major problem after children's day surgery. In a series of over 15 000 children's day cases from the USA, PONV was the most common reason for unexpected inpatient admission.[111] Many of the common day-case procedures are associated with a high incidence of PONV. In this respect, adenotonsillectomy has an incidence of around 70%,[112] prominent ear corrections 60%[113] and strabismus surgery as high as 80%.[114]

The key to decreasing the impact of PONV is recognizing the at-risk child (Table 19.7). Subsequently, a range of strategies should be used to minimize the problem. General measures include avoiding too long a preoperative fast, maintaining good hydration, avoiding

Table 19.7 Preoperative risk factors for PONV

History of previous PONV
History of motion sickness
Gender (females > males after menarche)
Age (> 1 year old)
Surgical procedure
e.g. Adenotonsillectomy
    Strabismus correction
    Otoplasty
    Orchidopexy

rapid postoperative mobilization and discouraging early postoperative oral intake.[115]

Pharmacological strategies should include avoidance of emetic agents perioperatively (especially opioids) and considering the use of total intravenous anaesthesia with propofol for the very high-risk patient, e.g. strabismus surgery.[116] The role for nitrous oxide is controversial, with some studies reporting an increased incidence of PONV[117] and others reporting no increase in emetic symptoms.[118]

Effective prophylactic antiemetic drugs should be used for the high-risk case.[119] Many of the traditional antiemetics have been disappointing in conventional dosage, with low efficacy and unacceptable high incidences of side-effects, such as sedation and extrapyramidal reactions.[115] Droperidol in low dosage (20 μg kg^{-1}) has been shown to decrease PONV prior to discharge of day cases without adverse effects.[120] 5-Hydroxytryptamine-3 antagonists are being increasingly used for PONV management in children. Ondansetron (0.1 mg kg^{-1}) is effective in prophylaxis[121] and treatment of established PONV in children.[122] The main advantages of ondansetron are the lack of sedation associated with its use and freedom from dystonic reactions.

In conclusion, although more effective antiemetics are becoming available they are unlikely to be the sole answer to the problem of PONV in day-case surgery. PONV in children is a complex issue and minimizing its impact in day-case practice requires a multifaceted approach from all personnel involved in day care based on a thorough knowledge of the problem.

REASONS FOR HOSPITAL ADMISSION

Even in centres with well-established day-case units, a small proportion of children will require inpatient admission because of unexpected complications. A widely quoted figure for inpatient admission is 1–2% of the unit's caseload, although a leading North American unit reports an overnight admission rate of only 0.3%.[111]

The reasons for unexpected admission are varied (Table 19.8) but the most common problems are PONV, complicated surgery and severe pain. Postextubation stridor is a not infrequent indication in North American prac-

Table 19.8 Reasons for unexpected admission

Problem	Examples
Persistent PONV	
Severe pain	
Surgical problems	Complicated surgery
	Protacted surgery
	Bleeding
Anaesthetic problems	Abnormal vital signs
	Postextubation stridor
	Excessive sedation
	Persistent motor blockade
	in older children
	Miscellaneous, e.g. allergic
	reactions, aspiration,
	suxamethonium apnoea

tice,[111] but this is an uncommon problem in the UK with the increased use of the laryngeal mask for airway management.

It is important that the possibility of inpatient admission is discussed with parents preoperatively so that disruption of family routine is minimized. Free-standing day units should ensure that they have the capability to transfer children to inpatient facilities if the need arises.

FOLLOW-UP AND COMMUNITY LIAISON

The responsibilities of the paediatric day-care service do not end with the discharge of the child. In order to ensure that continuity of patient care is achieved, day-unit staff must liaise closely with community-based medical and nursing colleagues. In addition, follow-up of children after discharge home fulfils a vital audit function and also enhances professional satisfaction for day-unit staff.

These important aims can be achieved by the following means.

DISCHARGE LETTER

Prior to discharge, medical staff should complete a brief letter stating the operation per-

formed, anaesthesia type, discharge drugs, complications and arrangement for subsequent follow-up. This letter should be either posted or faxed to the general practitioner or passed to the parents for immediate delivery.

POSTOPERATIVE HOME VISIT

The advantages of a visit from community nursing services was recognized by Nicoll at the beginning of the twentieth century[3] and reiterated more recently as an integral part of a modern children's day-care programme.[12] It is impractical and unnecessary for every child to receive a home visit. However, this service should be targeted at those whose needs have been identified prior to discharge. The community paediatric nurse may provide advice and reassurance for children and parents, assess and provide pain relief and assist in wound care and suture removal. Provision of community nursing services may also reduce general practitioner callouts.[12]

POSTDISCHARGE TELEPHONE CALLS

Many units contact families by telephone on the day after surgery and subsequently if necessary. This not only enables parents to ask questions and receive advice from experienced nursing staff, but is also a means of obtaining feedback from the parents of the care provided. This important audit function of the telephone call is enhanced if a standard questionnaire is completed concerning problems, such as postoperative pain, PONV, bleeding, and whether these problems necessitated contacting the general practitioner.

Some units have experimented with a 24-h helpline utilizing mobile telephones held by nursing staff.[123] The majority of calls in this study were for basic advice and reassurance, concerns about pain relief and wound problems.

REFERENCES

1 Hannallah, R.S. and Epstein, B.S. The pediatric patient. In: Wetchler, B.V. (ed.). *Anesthesia for Ambulatory*

Surgery, 2nd edn. Philadelphia, PA: JB Lippincott, 1991: 131–95.

2 *Guidelines for Daycase Surgery*. London: Royal College of Surgeons of England, 1992.

3 Nicoll, J.H. The surgery of infancy. *British Medical Journal* 1909; **ii**: 753–6.

4 Waters, R.M. The downtown anesthesia clinic. *American Journal of Surgery* 1919; **33**: 71–3.

5 Calnan, J. and Martin, P. Development and practice of an autonomous minor surgery unit in a general hospital. *British Medical Journal* 1971; **iv**: 92–6.

6 Reed, W.A. and Ford, J.L. Development of an independent outpatient surgical centre. *International Anesthesiology Clinics* 1976; 14–30.

7 Thornes, R. *Just for the Day*. London: NAWCH, 1991.

8 Scaife, J.M. and Johnstone, J.M. Psychological aspects of day care surgery for children. In: Healy, T.E. (ed.). *Anaesthesia for Day Case Surgery*. London: Bailliere Tindall, 1990: 759–79.

9 *National Confidential Enquiry into Perioperative Deaths*. Report 1989. London: NCEPOD, 1990.

10 Morris, S.P. Paediatric day case anaesthesia. *British Journal of Anaesthesia* 1992; **68**: 3–4.

11 Ghosh, S. Is the development of UK day surgery good enough? *Journal of One-Day Surgery* 1996; **5**(4): 14–16.

12 Atwell, J.D. and Gow, M.A. Paediatric trained district nurse in the community; expensive luxury or economic necessity? *British Medical Journal* 1985; **291**: 227–9.

13 Otherson, A.B. and Clatworthy, H.W. Outpatient herniorraphy for children. *American Journal of Disease in Children* 1968; **116**: 78–80.

14 Ogg, T.W. Day case surgery. *Drugs and Therapeutics Bulletin* 1990; **28**: 22–85.

15 Sadler, G.P., Richards, H., Watkins, G., *et al.* Daycase paediatric surgery: the only choice. *Annals of the Royal College of Surgeons of England* 1992; **74**: 130–3.

16 Berry, F.A. Outpatient anesthesia should not be limited to ASA 1 patients. *Anesthesiology* 1984; **60**: 620.

17 Arthur, D.S., Morton, N.S. and Fyfe, A.H. Patient selection, assessment and preoperative preparation. In: Morton, N.S. and Raine, P.A. (eds). *Paediatric Day Case Surgery*. Oxford: Oxford University Press, 1994: 10–20.

18 McEwan, A.I., Bingham, R. and Birch, M. The preoperative management of the child with a heart murmur. *Paediatric Anaesthesia* 1995; **5**: 151–6.

19 Hannallah, R.S. Anesthetic considerations for pediatric ambulatory surgery. *Ambulatory Surgery* 1997; **5**: 53–9.

20 Van der Walt, J. Anaesthesia in children with viral respiratory tract infections. *Paediatric Anaesthesia* 1995; **5**: 257–62.

21 Cohen, M.M. and Cameron, C.B. Should you cancel the operation when a child has an upper respiratory tract infection? *Anesthesia and Analgesia* 1991; **72**: 282–8.

22 Liu, L.M., Ryan, J.F., Cote, C.J., *et al.* Influence of upper respiratory infection on critical incidents in children under anaesthesia. *9th World Congress of Anaesthesiologists Abstracts* 1988; **2**: A0786.

23 Block, E.C. Anaesthetic death of a child with a cold. *Anaesthesia* 1993; **48**: 171.

24 Keneally, J.P. Day stay surgery in pediatrics. *Clinics in Anesthesiology* 1985; **3**: 679–96.

25 Morton, N.S. Practical paediatric day case anaesthesia and analgesia. In: Millar, J.M., Rudkin, G.E. and Hitch-cock, M. (eds). *Practical Anaesthesia and Analgesia for Day Surgery*. Oxford: Bios, 1997: 141–52.

26 Cote, C.J., Zaslovsky, A., Downes, J.J., *et al.* Postoperative apnoea in former preterm infants after inguinal herniorraphy. *Anesthesiology* 1995; **82**: 809–22.

27 *Guidelines for Daycase Surgery*. London: Royal College of Surgeons of England 1985.

28 Mahmoud, N.A. Day case adenoidectomy – safety and cost effectiveness. *Ambulatory Surgery* 1995; **3**: 31–5.

29 Teway, A.K. The science in daycase tonsillectomy. *Ambulatory Surgery* 1993; **1**: 165–7.

30 McGoldrick, K.E. Outpatient tonsilloadenoidectomy: avoiding complications. *Ambulatory Surgery* 1994; **2**: 23–6.

31 Church, J.J. Daycase tonsillectomy for children. *Journal of One-Day Surgery* 1996; **5**(4): 8–9.

32 Patel, R. and Hannallah, R.S. Ambulatory tonsillectomy. *Ambulatory Surgery* 1993; **1**: 89–92.

33 Koka, B.V., Jeon, I.S. and Andre, J.M. Post-intubation croup in children. *Anesthesia and Analgesia* 1977; **56**: 501–5.

34 Morton, N.S. and Herd, D. General principles of paediatric day-case anaesthesia. In: Whitwam, J.G. (ed.). *Day-Case Anaesthesia and Sedation*. Oxford: Blackwell Scientific Publications, 1994: 303–12.

35 Yentis, S.M., Levine, M.F. and Hartley, E.J. Should all children with suspected or confirmed MH susceptibility be admitted after surgery? A 10 year review. *Anesthesia and Analgesia* 1992; **75**: 345–50.

36 *Arrangements for Care of Persons Attending for Surgical Procedures as Day Patients*. London: DHSS, 1973: HM(73)32.

37 Koay, C.B. and Marks, M.J. A nurse-led preadmission clinic for elective ENT surgery. *Annals of the Royal College of Surgeons of England* 1996; **78**: 15–19.

38 Penn, S. Nursing and unit organisation. In: Whitwam, J.G. (ed.). *Day-Case Anaesthesia and Sedation*. Oxford: Blackwell Scientific Publications, 1994: 369–80.

39 Patel, R.I. and Hannallah, R.S. Preoperative screening for pediatric ambulatory surgery: evaluation of a telephone questionnaire method. *Anesthesia and Analgesia* 1992; **75**: 258–61.

40 Margolis, J.O., Ginsberg, B., Dear, G.D., *et al.* Paediatric preoperative teaching: effects at induction and postoperatively. *Paediatric Anaesthesia* 1998; **8**: 17–23.

41 Rosen, D.A., Rosen, K.R. and Hannallah, R.S. Preoperative characteristics which influence the child's response to induction of anesthesia. *Anesthesiology* 1985; **63**: A462.

42 Bevan, J.C., Johnston, C. and Haig, M.J. Preoperative parental anxiety predicts behavioural and emotional responses to induction of anaesthesia in children. *Canadian Journal of Anaesthesia* 1990; **37**: 177–82.

43 Vessey, J.A., Caserza, C.L. and Bogetz, M.S. In my opinion another Pandora's box? Parental participation in anesthetic induction. *Children's Health Care* 1990; **19**: 116–18.

44 Splinter, W.M., Stewart, J.A. and Muir, J.G. The effect of preoperative apple juice on gastric contents, thirst and hunger in children. *Canadian Journal of Anaesthesia* 1989; **36**: 55–8.

45 Phillips, S., Daborn, A.K. and Hatch, D.J. Preoperative fasting for paediatric anaesthesia. *British Journal of Anaesthesia* 1994; **73**: 529–36.

46 Hannallah, R.S. Preoperative investigations. *Paediatric Anaesthesia* 1995; **5**: 325–9.

47 Patel, R.I. and Hannallah, R.S. Patients'selection criteria for ambulatory surgery. *Ambulatory Surgery* 1993; **1**: 183–8.

48 Baron, M.J., Guter, J. and White, P. Is the pediatric preoperative hematocrit determination necessary. *Southern Medical Journal* 1992; **85**: 1187–9.

49 Meneghini, L., Zandra, N., Zannette, G., *et al.* The usefulness of routine preoperative laboratory tests for one day surgery in healthy children. *Paediatric Anaesthesia* 1998; **8**: 11–15.

50 Eichorn, J.H. Preoperative screening for sickle cell trait. *Journal of the American Medical Association* 1988; **259**: 907.

51 Steward, D.J. Anaesthesia for paediatric outpatients. *Canadian Anaesthetists Society Journal* 1980; **27**: 412–16.

52 Friesen, R.H. and Lockhart, C.H. Oral transmucosal fentanyl citrate for preanesthetic medication of pediatric day surgery patients with and without droperidol as a prophylactic antiemetic. *Anesthesiology* 1992; **76**: 46–51.

53 Weldon, B.C., Watcha, M.F. and White, P.F. Oral midazolam in children–effect of time and adjunctive therapy. *Anesthesia and Analgesia* 1992; **75**: 51–5.

54 Parnis, S.J., Foale, J.A., Van der Walt, J.H., *et al.* Oral midazolam is an effective premedication for children having day stay anaesthesia. *Anaesthesia and Intensive Care* 1997; **20**: 9–14.

55 Cray, S.H., Dixon, J.L., Heard, C.M., *et al.* Oral midazolam premedication for paediatric day case patients. *Paediatric Anaesthesia* 1996; **6**: 265–70.

56 De Jong, P.C. and Verburg, M.P. Comparison to rectal to intramuscular administration of midazolam and atropine for premedication in children. *Acta Anaesthesiologica Scandinavica* 1988; **32**: 485–9.

57 Davis, P.J., McGowan, F.X. and Tome, J.A. Preanesthetic medication with intranasal midazolam for brief pediatric surgical procedures: effect on recovery and hospital discharge times. *Anesthesiology* 1995; **82**: 2–5.

58 Landsman, I.S. and Davis, P.J. Pharmacologic and physiologic pediatric considerations. In: White, P.F. (ed.). *Ambulatory Anesthesia and Surgery*. Philadelphia, PA: WB Saunders, 1997: 541–58.

59 Freeman, J.A., Doyle, E., Ng, T.I., *et al.* Topical anaesthesia of the skin: a review. *Paediatric Anaesthesia* 1993; **3**: 129–38.

60 Hannallah, R.S. Low dose intramuscular ketamine for anesthesia preinduction in young children undergoing brief outpatient procedures. *Anesthesiology* 1989; **70**: 598–600.

61 *The Children's Act.* London: HMSO, 1989.

62 Stokes, M.A. and Drake-Lee, A.B. Children who withdraw consent for elective surgery. *Paediatric Anaesthesia* 1998; **8**: 113–15.

63 Hannallah, R.S. Who benefits when parents are present during anaesthetic induction in their children? *Canadian Journal of Anaesthesia* 1994; **41**: 271–5.

64 Ryder IG. and Spargo PM. Parents in the anaesthetic room. A questionnaire survey of parents'reactions. *Anaesthesia* 1991; **46**: 977–9.

65 Vessey, J.A., Bogetz, M.S., Caserza, C.H., *et al.* Parental upset associated with participation in induction of anaesthesia in children. *Canadian Journal of Anaesthesia* 1994; **41**: 276–80.

66 Conran, A.M. and Hannallah, R.S. Paediatric outpatient anaesthesia and perioperative care. *Current Opinion in Anaesthesiology* 1997; **10**: 205–8.

67 Runcie, C.J., MacKenzie, S., Arthur, D.S., *et al.* Comparison of recovery from anaesthesia induced in children with propofol or thiopentone. *British Journal of Anaesthesia* 1993; **70**: 192–5.

68 Morton, N.S., Johnstone, G., White, M., *et al.* Propofol in paediatric anaesthesia. *Paediatric Anaesthesia* 1992; **2**: 89–97.

69 Cameron, E., Johnston, G., Crofts, S., *et al.* Minimum effective dose of lignocaine to prevent injection pain due to propofol in children. *Anaesthesia* 1992; **47**: 604–6.

70 Herman, J., Davis, P.J., Welborn, L.G., *et al.* Induction, recovery and safety characteristics of sevoflurane in children undergoing ambulatory surgery. *Anesthesiology* 1996; **84**: 1332–40.

71 Welborn, L.G., Hannallah, R.S. and Norden, J.M. Comparison of emergence and recovery characteristics of sevoflurane and halothane in ambulatory pediatric patients. *Anesthesia and Analgesia* 1996; **83**: 917–20.

72 Murat, I. New inhalational agents in paediatric anaesthesia: desflurane and sevoflurane. *Current Opinion in Anaesthesiology* 1996; **9**: 225–8.

73 Watcha, M.F., Simeon, R.M., White, P.F., *et al.* Effect of propofol on the incidence of post operative vomiting after strabismus surgery in pediatric outpatients. *Anesthesiology* 1991; **75**: 204–9.

74 Schrum, S.F., Hannallah, R.S., Verghese, P.M., *et al.* Comparison of propofol and thiopentone for rapid anesthetic induction in infants. *Anesthesia and Analgesia* 1994; **78**: 482–5.

75 Hannallah, R.S. Pediatric general anaesthetic considerations. In: White, P.F. (ed.). *Ambulatory Anesthesia and Surgery*. Philadelphia, PA: WB Saunders, 1997: 573–82.

76 Williams, P.J. and Bailey, P.M. Comparison of the reinforced laryngeal mask airway and tracheal intubation for adenotonsillectomy. *British Journal of Anaesthesia* 1993; **70**: 30–3.

77 Haynes, S.R. and Morton, N.S. The LMA: a review of its use in paediatric anaesthesia. *Paediatric Anaesthesia* 1993; **3**: 65–73.

78 Goodwin, A.P., Ogg, T.W. and Lamb, W.T. The reinforced LMA in dental day surgery. *Ambulatory Surgery* 1993; **1**: 31–5.

79 Brimacombe, J. and Berry, A. The LMA for ENT, head and neck surgery. *Journal of Otolaryngology* 1995; **24**: 125–33.

80 Bapat, P., Joshi, R.N., Yound, E., *et al.* Comparison of propofol versus thiopentone with midazolam or lignocaine to facilitate LMA insertion. *Canadian Journal of Anaesthesia* 1996; **43**: 564–8.

81 Scanlon, P., Carey, M., Power, M., *et al.* Patient response to LMA insertion after induction of anaesthesia with propofol or thiopentone. *Canadian Journal of Anaesthesia* 1993; **40**: 816–18.

82 Verghese, A., McCullock, D., Lewis, M., *et al.* Removal of the LMA in children awake or asleep? *Anesthesiology* 1994; **81**: A1321.

83 Stuart, J.C. and Morton, N.S. A clinical audit of day case surgery for children. *Journal of One-Day Surgery* 1991; **1**: 8–15.

84 Morton, N.S., Benham, S.W., Lawson, R.A., *et al.* Diclofenac versus oxybuprocaine eyedrops for analgesia in paediatric strabismus surgery. *Paediatric Anaesthesia* 1997; **7**: 221–6.

85 *Guidelines for the Use of NSAIDs in the Perioperative Period*. London: Royal College of Anaesthetists, 1998.

86 Ryhanen, R., Adamski, J. and Puhakka, K. Postoperative pain relief in children: a comparison between caudal bupivacaine and intramuscular diclofenac. *Anaesthesia* 1994; **49**: 57–61.

87 Kenny, G.N. Potential renal haematological and allergic effects associated with NSAIDs. *Drugs* 1992; **44** Suppl. 5: 31–7.

88 Hall, S.C. Tonsillectomies, ketorolac and the march of progress. *Canadian Journal of Anaesthesia* 1996; **43**: 544–8.

89 Frew, A. NSAIDs and asthma. *Prescriber's Journal* 1994; **34**(2): 74–7.

90 Anderson, B.J. and Holford, N.H. Rectal paracetamol dosing regimens: determination by computer simulation. *Paediatric Anaesthesia* 1997; **7**: 451–5.

91 Roberts, N. and Goresky, G. Management of postoperative pain. In: White, P.F. (ed.). *Ambulatory Anesthesia and Surgery*. Philadelphia, PA: WB Saunders, 1997: 607–16.

92 McNicol, L.R. Peripheral nerve blocks. In: Morton, N.S. and Raine, P.A. (eds). *Paediatric Day Case Surgery*. Oxford: Oxford University Press, 1994: 38–53.

93 Bingham, R., Hawke, M. and Halik, J. The safety and efficacy of EMLA cream for myringotomy and ventilation tube insertion. *Journal of Otolaryngology* 1991; **20**: 193–5.

94 Mackinlay, G.A. Save the prepuce. Painless separation of preputial adhesions in the outpatient clinic. *British Medical Journal* 1988; **297**: 590–1.

95 Watson, D.M. Topical amethocaine in strabismus surgery. *Anaesthesia* 1991; **46**: 368–70.

96 Tree-Trakern, T. and Piryavarapern, S. Postoperative pain relief for circumcision in children: a comparison among morphine, nerve block and topical anesthesia. *Anesthesiology* 1985; **62**: 519–22.

97 Trotter, C., Martin, P. and Youngson, G. A comparison between ilioinguinal iliohypogastric nerve block performed by anaesthetist or surgeon for postoperative analgesia after groin surgery in children. *Paediatric Anaesthesia* 1995; **5**: 363–7.

98 Hannallah, R.S., Broadman, L.M. and Belman, A.B. Comparison of caudal and ilioinguinal/iliohypogastric nerve blocks for control of post orchidopexy pain in pediatric ambulatory surgery. *Anesthesiology* 1987; **66**: 832–4.

99 Broadman, L.M., Hannallah, R.S., Belman, B., *et al.* Postcircumcision analgesia – a prospective evaluation of subcutaneous ring block of the penis. *Anesthesiology* 1987; **67**: 99–102.

100 Fisher, Q.A., Mccomiskey, C.M., Hill, J.L., *et al.* Postoperative voiding intervals and duration of analgesia following peripheral or caudal nerve blocks in children. *Anesthesia and Analgesia* 1993; **76**: 173–7.

101 Wolf, A.R., Valley, R.D., Fear, D.W., *et al.* Bupivacaine for caudal analgesia in infants and children: the optimal effective concentration. *Anesthesiology* 1988; **69**: 102–6.

102 Martin, L.V. Postoperative analgesia after circumcision in children. *British Journal of Anaesthesia* 1982; **54**: 1263–6.

103 Krane, E.J. Delayed respiratory depression in a child after caudal epidural analgesia. *Anesthesia and Analgesia* 1988; **67**: 79–82.

104 Cooke, B. and Doyle, E. The use of additives to local anaesthetic solution for caudal epidural blockade. *Paediatric Anaesthesia* 1996; **6**: 353–9.

105 Steward, D.J. A simplified scoring system for the postoperative recovery room. *Canadian Anaesthetists Society Journal* 1975; **22**: 111–13.

106 Patel, R.I. Postoperative morbidity and discharge criteria. In: White, P.F. (ed.). *Ambulatory Anesthesia and Surgery*. Philadelphia, PA: WB Saunders, 1997: 617–31.

107 Schreiner, M.J., Nicolson, S.C., Martin, T., *et al.* Should children drink before discharge from day surgery? *Anesthesiology* 1992; **76**: 528–33.

108 Radhakrishnan, D., Brennan, L.J., Watson. B., *et al.* Audit of current practice in paediatric day surgery at Addenbrooke's Hospital, Cambridge. In: *Proceedings of the 7th British Association of Day Surgery Annual Scientific Meeting*. British Association of Day Surgery, 1996.

109 Tan, S.G., May, H.A. and Cunliffe, M. An audit of pain and vomiting in paediatric day case surgery. *Paediatric Anaesthesia* 1994; **4**: 105–9.

110 Morton, N.S. Pain assessment in children. *Paediatric Anaesthesia* 1997; **7**: 267–72.

111 Patel, R.I. and Hannallah, R.S. Complications following pediatric ambulatory surgery. *Ambulatory Surgery* 1995; **3**: 83–6.

112 Grunwald, Z. Droperidol decreases the incidence and severity of vomiting after adenotonsillectomy in children. *Paediatric Anaesthesia* 1994; **4**: 163–7.

113 Ridings, P. and Gault, D. Reduction in postoperative vomiting after surgical correction of prominent ears. *British Journal of Anaesthesia* 1994; **72**: 592–3.

114 Abramowitz, M.D. The antiemetic effect of droperidol following strabismus surgery in children. *Anesthesiology* 1983; **59**: 579–83.

115 Baines, D. Postoperative nausea and vomiting in children. *Paediatric Anaesthesia* 1996; **6**: 7–14.

116 Watcha, M.F., Simeon, R.M., White, P.F., *et al.* Effect of propofol on the incidence of postoperative vomiting after strabismus surgery in pediatric outpatients. *Anesthesiology* 1991; **75**: 204–9.

117 Wilson, I.G. and Fell, D. Nitrous oxide and postoperative vomiting in children undergoing myringoplasty as a day case. *Paediatric Anaesthesia* 1993; **3**: 283–5.

118 Pandit, U., Pryn, S., Randel, G., *et al.* Nitrous oxide does not increase postoperative vomiting in pediatric outpatients undergoing adenotonsillectomy. *Anesthesiology* 1990; **73**: A1245.

119 Brennan, L.J. Nausea and vomiting after surgery. *Family Medicine* 1997; **1**(10): 14–15.

120 Lunn, D.V., Lander, G.R. and Williams, A.R. Low dose droperidol reduces postoperative vomiting in paediatric day case surgery. *British Journal of Anaesthesia* 1995; **74**: 509–11.

121 Paxton, L.D., Taylor, R.H., Gallagher, T.M., *et al.* Postoperative emesis following otoplasty in children. *Anaesthesia* 1995; **50**: 1083–4.

122 Khalil, S., Roderte, A., Weldon, B.C., *et al.* Intravenous ondansetron in established postoperative emesis in children. *Anesthesiology* 1996; **85**: 270–6.

123 Mukumba, S., Wright, M. and Punchihova, V.G. Notes on an unlimited telephone helpline. *Journal of One-Day Surgery* 1997; **6**(3): 14.

CHAPTER 20

Unusual conditions in paediatric anaesthesia

ANNE LYNN AND STEVEN SASAKI

INTRODUCTION

Since it is impossible to discuss comprehensively every congenital syndrome that might affect anaesthetic management, this chapter will present an approach to the evaluation of children with congenital syndromes. It will include those anomalies with obvious implications for anaesthesia management or monitoring, and some syndromes with subtle or hidden potential problems. After a general presentation of preoperative evaluation, some specific congenital syndromes, their anaesthetic-related problems and alternatives for management will be discussed. A more complete list of syndromes grouped by area of potential anaesthetic impact appears in Table 20.1, which expands and reorganizes the indices of Jones and Pelton[1] and Steward.[2] Many are summarized in Rai-

zen's text.[3] A discussion of malignant hyperthermia (MH), its presentation, diagnosis and treatment will follow, and the chapter will end with a section on latex allergy.

PREOPERATIVE EVALUATION

Thorough preoperative evaluation is essential to ensure optimum perioperative monitoring and care, and to identify the patient needing subspecialty consultation prior to surgery.

Past anaesthetic records can provide a wealth of information concerning airway, respiratory, cardiovascular and metabolic function. Unsuspected problems may have been identified and treated, and a previous anaesthetic plan may

Table 20.1 Congenital syndromes affecting anaesthesia[a]

(a) Airway (difficult intubation or mask fit: J, micrognathia; C, cervical spine instability or limited motion; M, soft tissue mass or macroglossia; L, small larynx; S, increased secretions; F, facial configuration hinders mask fit)

Aaskog–Scott C	Kabuki cleft, J
*Achondroplasia C, F	Klippel–Feil C
Aglossia–adactylia J	Kniest's C
Anderson's midface hypoplasia, F	Larsen's C
Angioneurotic oedema L (swelling)	*Meckel's J
*Apert's J, F	Median cleft face J, cleft
*Arthrogryposis multiplex C, J	Miller's J, F
*Beckwith–Wiedemann M	Moebius J
*Behçet's ulcers of pharynx	*Morquio C
Carpenter's J	*Multiple mucosal neuroma M
*CHARGE association J; choanal atresia	*Myositis ossificans C
*Cherubism M, F	Najjars J, F
*Christ–Siemens–Touraine J, F	Noack's J
Chotzen J, F	*Noonan's C
*Cretinism M	*Opitz–Frias J, L, cleft
*Cri du chat M, J, F	*Orofacial–digital cleft
Crouzon J, occasionally	Pallister Hall J
Cystic hygroma M	*Patau (trisomy 13) J, cleft
Diastrophic dwarfism C, J	Pendred M
*Down's (trisomy 21) C, M	Pierre Robin J, cleft, F
Dyggue–Melchior–Clausen's C	*Pompe's disease M
*Edward's (trisomy 18) J	*Prader Willi F, J
*Epidermolysis bullosa see text, L	Rieger abnormal teeth
*Farber's disease L	Russell–Silver dwarf J
Freeman–Sheldon small mouth	*Scleroderma-small mouth
*Goldenhar (hemifacial microsomia) J, F	*Smith–Lemli–Opitz J
Goltz–Gorlin abnormal teeth, C	Spondylometaphyseal dysplasia C
Hallermann–Strief J, small mouth	Spondyloepiphyseal dysplasia C
Hallervorden–Spatz torticollis, trismus	Sprengel's C
*Hand–Schuller–Christian L	Treacher Collins J, small mouth, F
*Hunter's S, M	*Turner's-C, J
*Hurler's S, M	Urbach–Wiethe disease L
*I-cell disease C, J	*Velocardiofacials syndrome F, cleft, J
Juvenile rheumatoid arthritis C	von Recklinghausen's disease M
	Weaver J

(b) Ventilation problems (L, intrinsic lung disease; W, muscle weakness; C, chest wall deformity)

*Achondroplasia C	*Maroteaux–Lamy C
Amyotonia congenita W, see text	*McArdle's disease W
Central core myopathy W	Morquio's C
Chronic granulomatous disease L	Myasthenia congenita W
*Cretinism W	Myasthenia gravis W
*Cutis laxa L	*Myositis ossificans C (stiff)
*Cystic fibrosis L	*Myotonic dystrophy see text
*Duchenne muscular dystrophy W	*Niemann-Pick disease L

Table 20.1 Continued

*Ehlers–Danlos L (pneumothorax)
*Familial periodic paralysis W
Gaucher's disease L (aspiration)
*Guillain–Barré W
*Hand–Schüller–Christian L
*I-cell disease L, C (stiff)
Jeune's C
Kartagener's L
*Kearnes–Sayre syndrome W
Kugelberg–Welander muscular atrophy W
*Leigh syndrome W
*Letterer–Siwe disease L
*Marfan's L, C

*Opitz–Frias syndrome L
*Osler Weber Rendu pulmonary AVMs
*Osteogenesis imperfecta C
*Polcystic kidneys L (cysts in 33%)
*Pompe's diseaseW
*Prader–Willi W (in infancy)
*Prune belly W
*Riley–Day L
*Rubinstein L
*Scleroderma L
*Smith–Lemli–Opitz L
*VATER L
Werdnig–Hoffman disease W
Wilson–Mikity L

(c) Cardiovascular (C, congenital heart disease; M, cardiomyopathy; A, autonomic or arrhythmias; I, ischaemic; T, thrombotic risk)

Albright's osteodystrophy A
*Apert's C
Asplenia (Ivemark) C
CHARGE association C
*Cherubism C
Conradi's C
Cretinism M
*Cri du Chat C
*DiGeorge's C
Down's (trisomy 21) C
Duchenne muscular dystrophy M
Edward's (trisomy 18) C
Ehlers–Danlos T
Ellis–Van Creveld C
Fabry's disease I
*Farber's disease M
Freidreich's ataxia M
*Gullain–Barré A
*Goldenhar C
Groenblad–Strandberg T
Holt–Oram C
*Homocystinuria T
*Hunter's M
*Hurler's M
*I-cell disease C (valvular)
Ivemark C
Jervell–Nielson A
*Kearns–Sayre syndrome A

*Laurence–Moon–Biedl C
*Leigh syndrome M
Leopard C
*Marfan's C
*Maroteaux–Lamy M
*Meckel's C
*Myotonic dystrophy M
*McArdle disease M
*Noonan C
*Opitz–Frias syndrome C
*Patau (trisomy 13) C
Polysplenia C
*Pompe's disease M
Progeria I
*Riley–Day A
*Rubinstein C
Sebaceous naevi C
Shy–Drager A
Sipple A
*Stevens–Johnson M
Tangier's disease I
*TAR C
*Turner syndrome C
*VATER C
*Velocardiofacial (Shprintzen syndrome) C
*Werner I
*William's C
Wolff–Parkinson–White A

Table 20.1 Continued

(d) Endocrine (S, steroid coverage perioperatively; P, phaeochromocytorna; T, thyroid)

*Adrenogenital S
*Behcet's S (often)
*Blackfan–Diamond S
*Chediak–Higashi S

Collagen vascular diseases S (often)
  Dermatomyositis
  Juvenile rheumatoid arthritis
  *Scleroderma
  Lupus
  Periarteritis nodosa
*Cretinism T
*Down's syndrome T

Epidermolysis bullosa S (often)
*Hand–Schuller–Christian S
*Kasabach–Merrit syndrome S
Multiple mucosal neuroma (multiple endocrine adenomatosis type 11b) P
Myositis ossificans S (often)

Pendred T
Sipple T, P

*von Hippel–Lindau P
Von Recklinghausen disease P

(e) Metabolic (G, glucose; E, electrolyte; C, calcium problems)

*Adrenogenital E
*Albers–Schönberg C
Albright's osteodystrophy C
Albright–Butler E
Alström G
Andersen's disease G
Bartter's E
*Beckwith–Wiedemann G
*Cretinism G, E
*Cystic fibrosis E (in hot climates)
*DiGeorge's C
*Down's syndrome G
*Familial periodic paralysis E
*Fanconi E

*Hand–Schüller–Christian E

Homocystinuria G
*Laurence–Moon–Biedl E (diabetes insipidus)
Leprechaunism G
Lesch–Nyhan uric acid
*Lipodystrophy G
Lowe C
Maple syrup urine disease E, G
*McArdle's disease G
*Paramyotonia congenita E
Phenylketonuria G
Prematurity G, E, C
*Prader–Willi G
Von Gierke's disease G
*Wermer syndrome (multiple endocrine adenomatosis I) G, C
*Werner G, C
*William's syndrome C

(f) Skin problems (careful positioning, intravenous access may be difficult and/or temperature regulation may be problematic)

*Behçet's ulcers in mouth
*Christ–Siemens–Touraine
*Cutis laxa
*Down's syndrome
*Ehler–Danlos
*Epidermolysis bullosa mucosal and skin ulcers

Groenblad–Strandberg
*Osler–Weber–Rendu
Ritter's disease
*Scleroderma
*Stevens–Johnson

(g) Orthopaedic (limited joint mobility or fragile bones)

*Albers–Schönberg disease
Ollier's
*Osteogenesis imperfecta

Marfan's
Scheie disease

Table 20.1 Continued

(h) Haematological (anaemia, platelet decrease or dysfunction, or clotting disturbance)

*Albers–Schönberg	*Letterer–Siwe disease
*Blackfan–Diamond	*Lipodystrophy
*Chediak–Higashi	*Maroteaux–Lamy
Christmas disease	Moschkowitz disease
Collagen vascular diseases	*Niemann–Pick disease
Favism	Sickle cell disease avoid pneumatic tourniquets
Gaucher's disease	Tangier disease
*Hand–Schüller–Christian	*TAR
Hermansky	von Willebrand's disease
*Homocystinuria	Wiskott–Aldrich
*Kasabach–Merrit	Wolman's disease
Klippel–Trenaunay	

(i) Renal (renal dysfunction affects use of drugs such as muscle relaxants, morphine, pethidine)

Alport	Lesch–Nyhan
Alström	Lowe
Bowen's (cerebrohepatorenal)	Meckel's
Chotzen's	Orofacial–digital
Conradi's	Polycystic kidneys
Denys Drash	*Prune belly syndrome
*Edward's (trisomy 18)	Tuberous sclerosis
Fabry's disease	*VATER
*Fanconi	*von Hippel–Lindau
*Farber's disease	*Wermer
*Laurence–Moon–Biedl	*Wilson's disease

(j) Pharmacology (S, avoid succinylcholine; M, careful use of muscle relaxants or barbiturates; H, avoid halothane; B, avoid barbiturates)

Amyotonia congenita M	Lesch–Nyhan S
*Arthrogryposis multiplex M	*Lipodystrophy H
Bowen's M	*McArdle's disease S
*Central core myopathy M, S, H	*Mytonia congenita M, S
*Duchenne's muscular dystrophy M, S, H	*Myotonic dystrophy S, H, M
*Familial periodic paralysis M	*Paramyotonia congenita S, H, M
*Guillain–Barré S	Phenylketonuria M
Hallervorden–Spatz disease S	Porphyria B
King syndrome S, H	*Wilson's disease M

[a]Listed by system: *many syndromes are listed in several sections.

have resolved potential problems during past anaesthetics.

The general health of the child may be assessed by reviewing height and weight, including percentiles from growth grids. Many syndromes cause alterations in overall growth as in the syndromes associated with dwarfing;[4] most will be associated with growth failure, but several are distinctive for excessive size or weight such as the multiple X or multiple Y syndromes, Beckwith–Wiedeman, Prader–Willi or Soto syndromes.

Evaluation of the upper airway seeks to identify conditions that will modify anaesthesia planning. If abnormalities are found, parents may be informed of potential problems and therapeutic plans. A history of snoring which wakens the child or causes daytime somnolence reveals significant airway obstruction. The child with micrognathia who may present difficulties during induction and intubation can be identified if the child's face, especially in profile, is examined (Figure 20.1). Stehling reported in adults that if the distance from the lower border of the mandible to the thyroid notch, measured with the neck extended, is less than 6 cm, visualization of the larynx by direct laryngoscopy will be impossible.[5] A distance of 6.5 cm, if associated with prominent upper teeth or limited cervical or temporomandibular motion, will also lead to difficult direct laryngoscopy. The equivalent distance in paediatric patients has not been reported. The child should also be assessed for asymmetry of facial contours which may make mask fit problematic.

A complete history and physical examination of the respiratory system will identify patients with poor pulmonary reserve. A history of either infant respiratory distress syndrome requiring mechanical ventilation, cystic fibrosis, recurrent pneumonia, asthma or muscular dystrophy will identify patients at risk for intraoperative or postoperative respiratory problems. Pulmonary function testing in older children with advanced pulmonary disease, as in those with cystic fibrosis or with weakness, as in Duchenne's muscular dystrophy, may guide perioperative care and family counselling.

The cardiovascular assessment is guided by enquiries about congenital heart disease, the use of cardiac medications (digoxin, diuretics, propranolol or antiarrhythmics), the exercise tolerance of the child or a history consistent with

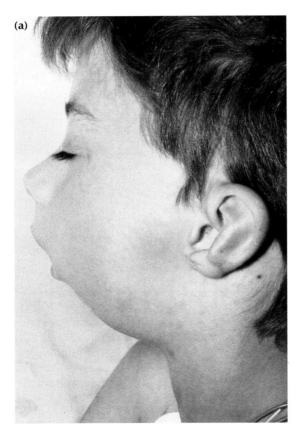

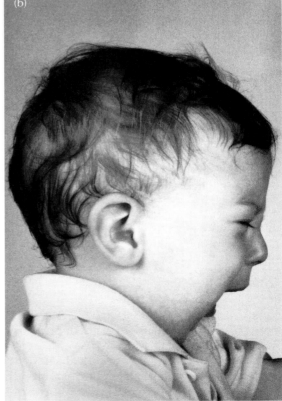

Figure 20.1 Profiles of children demonstrating (a) micrognathia and (b) retrognathia.

arrhythmias (syncopal episodes or paroxysmal tachycardia). The signs and symptoms of congestive heart failure in infants are non-specific and can be subtle. Tachypnoea, nasal flaring or grunting respirations are often present.The infant may feed slowly, tire during feeding or sweat profusely and weight gain is often poor. The older child may tire more quickly than playmates. Physical examination may reveal a cardiac murmur, tachycardia at rest or irregular rhythms, hepatomegaly, cyanosis or clubbing of the fingers. Recent cardiological evaluations should be reviewed or obtained to aid perioperative care. Cardiac evaluation should be considered when major anomalies are present in other systems, such as gastrointestinal (e.g. omphalocoele, duodenal atresia), or with extremity malformations

Table 20.2 Congenital syndromes frequently found to have associated congenital heart defects

Syndrome	Findings	Congenital cardiac lesion	Incidence (%)
Alagille	Intrahepatic cirrhosis, vertebral anomalies	Peripheral pulmonary stenosis	
Apert	Craniosynostosis, midfacial hypoplasia, syndactyly of extremities	VSD, TOF	
Blackfan–Diamond	Anaemia in infancy	VSD	
Carpenter	Synostosis of coronal, sagittal or lambdoid sutures Brachydactyly and partial syndactyly of hands and feet, polydactyly of feet	PDA, VSD	
CHARGE association	Coloboma, choanal atresia, retarded growth, retarded mental development, microphallus, cryptorchidism, micrognathia/cleft palate, ear anomalies/deafness	Vascular ring or interrupted aortic arch, AV canal, TOF, truncus arteriosus, DORV with AV canal, VSD, PDA	60–70
Cri du chat	Slow growth, mental deficiency, microcephaly, hypertelorism, strabismus, simian crease	VSD, ASD	25
Crouzon	Craniostenosis, shallow orbits	Coarctation of aorta	
DiGeorge	Hypoparathyroidism, hypocalcaemia, deficient T-cell-mediated immunity thymic hypoplasia, micrognathia, cleft palate, hypertelorism	Truncus arteriosus, double aortic arch (vascular ring), right aortic arch, TOF, interr. aortic arch, VSD	13–30 TA, 8–25 VSD, 14–26 R Ao arch, 20–30 TOF, 30–56 IAA
Down's syndrome	(see Trisomy 21)		
Duchenne's muscular dystrophy	Myopathy with progressive weakness, scoliosis, at risk for aspiration, malignant hyperthermia risk, progressive respiratory insufficiency	Cardiomyopathy Mitral valve prolapse	eventual 100 25
Ehlers–Danlos	Hyperextensible joints, blue sclerae, easy bruising, parchment scars, scoliosis, hernias, pes planus	Mitral insufficiency	50

Table 20.2 continued

Syndrome	Findings	Congenital cardiac lesion	Incidence (%)
Ellis–van Creveld	Short distal extremities, polydactyly, hypoplastic nails, dysplastic teeth, small thorax	ASD	50
Fetal alcohol	Microphthalmos, microcephaly, mental retardation, growth failure	VSD, PDA	
Goldenhar	See text	TOF, VSD	33
Holt–Oram	Radial club hand or hypoplasia, proximal thumb placement	ASD, VSD	
Homocystinuria	Lens dislocation (downward), slender, pectus, osteoporosis, malar flush	Thrombotic events	
Hurler	See text	Aortic insufficiency, mitral insufficiency	
Ivemark (asplenia)	Absent spleen, infection risk increased, situs inversus of abdominal viscera	Dextrocardia, complex cyanotic heart disease (e.g. TGA; single ventricle) AV canal defects	100
Kartageners	Ciliary dyskinesis with sinusitis, male Infertility	Dextrocardia and situs inversus	
Marfan	Long thin limbs and fingers, joint laxity with scoliosis, pectus excavatum, tall stature, upward lens dislocation	Aortic aneurysm, aortic regurgitation, mitral valve prolapse	60
Multiple lentigines (Leopard)	Hypertelorism, dark lentigenes especially on face or trunk, prominent ears, sensorineural deafness, retardation	PS	95
Noonan	See text Cardiomyopathy	PS, ASD, Hypertrophic cardiomyopathy	62 (PS) 20
Rubella	Cataract, deafness, retardation, Cryptorchidism	PDA, PS (peripheral), VSD	
Scimitar	Hypoplasia right lung and right pulmonary artery	Right pulmonary veins into IVC	
Smith–Lemli–Opitz	Retardation, microcephaly Ptosis, strabismus, micrognathia hypospadias, cryptorchidism	ASD, VSD, TOF	
TAR (thrombocytopenia, absent radius)	Decreased platelets and megakaryocytes, bilateral radial hypoplasia/aplasia	TOF	
Trisomy 13	Small-for-age, severe retardation, deafness, microcephaly, retinal dysplasia, cleft lip/palate (80%), polydactyly, parieto-occipital scalp, skin defects	VSD, dextroversion	90

Table 20.2 continued

Syndrome	Findings	Congenital cardiac lesion	Incidence (%)
Trisomy 18	Growth deficiency, retardation, low-set ears, micrognathia, short sternum, clenched hand	VSD, PDA, PS	99
Trisomy 21	See text	AV canal, ASD, VSD	50
		TOF	8
Tuberous sclerosis	Adenoma sebaceum, ash-leaf spots, Cafe-au-lait spots, hamartoma of brain, seizures, mental deficiency	Rhabdomyomas	
Turner	Pterygium colli, infantile lymphoedema, short stature, webbed neck, low hairline	Coarctation, AS	35
VATER	Vertebral anomalies, anal atresia, T-O fistula, radial dysplasia	VSD	20–30
Velocardiofacial syndrome (overlap with DiGeorge syndrome)	Hypotonia, slender fingers high arch or cleft palate retardation (variable) long face with deficient malar area, micrognathia	VSD	75
		TOF	20
		Rt aortic arch	50
Williams	Prominent lips, hoarse voice, mental deficiency, talkative, hypercalcaemia in infancy (20%), blue eyes with stellate pattern	AS, PS	

VSD, ventricular septal defect; TOF, tetralogy of Fallot; PDA, patent ductus arteriosus; AV, arterio venous; ASD, atrial septal defect; TGA, transposition of great arteries; PS, pulmonic stenosis; AS, aortic stenosis; DORV c̄ AV canal, double outlet right ventricle with atrio-ventricular canal; T-O, tracheo-oesophageal; IAA, interrupted aortic arch.

(Holt–Oram syndrome, VATER syndrome; see Table 20.2), since cardiac development occurs concurrently with gastrointestinal and extremity formation, and anomalies may be present in both.

In congenital syndromes known to include metabolic abnormalities (Table 20.1), laboratory studies are needed and should include evaluation of glucose levels, acid–base status, electrolytes or calcium concentrations. General neurological development needs to be assessed in more detail in children with congenital anomalies than in the normal population, since it affects anaesthetic plans. Focal findings such as spastic diplegia or hemiparesis may affect the placement of intravenous or arterial catheters or choice of anaesthesia (general compared with regional techniques). Positioning of these children to avoid pressure areas can be more challenging. The infant with hydrocephalus requires a smooth induction and intubation to avoid potential problems from increases in intracranial pressure.

Musculoskeletal abnormalities may also affect anaesthesia choices. In the myotonia syndromes, succinylcholine is avoided; Duchenne's muscular dystrophy may be associated with MH and requires the use of a non-triggering anaesthetic technique which avoids succinylcholine or potent inhalational agents. Children with unusual facies or defects in multiple systems can be identified and seen by genetic or dysmorphology consultants to aid preoperative diagnosis before elective surgical procedures.

SYNDROMES AFFECTING AIRWAY MANAGEMENT

The infant or child with a congenital syndrome, which includes compromise of the airway, can be identified at the preoperative examination by the presence of an obstructing mass (e.g. cystic hygroma or a large tongue), micrognathia, limited mouth opening or neck mobility, or by symptoms such as stridor. In these children, preoperative sedation should be avoided or only given in small incremental doses in the presence of the anaesthesiologist, since its effect on airway patency is unpredictable. Drying of oral secretions and blockade of vagal stimulation during laryngoscopy can be achieved using an anticholinergic agent such as atropine (0.01–0.02 mg kg^{-1}). The intravenous route ensures absorption and eliminates an unnecessary intramuscular injection for the child. A variety of facemasks, laryngeal mask airways (LMAs), laryngoscope blades, tracheal tubes and stylets should be assembled, along with functioning suction equipment. Fibreoptic bronchoscopes are available in sizes of 2.2, 3.5 and 4.5 mm, the smallest of which will pass through a 2.5-mm tracheal tube if the tube connector is removed. In many centres, including the present authors' in Seattle, all of this airway equipment is stored in a difficult airway equipment cart. The components of this cart are shown in Table 20.3. The anaesthesia mask should have a soft air-filled cushion to facilitate mask fit when distortions of facial anatomy are present. Use of an oxyscope in infants allows delivery of oxygen into the pharynx during laryngoscopy through a channel welded to the laryngoscope blade, giving an additional 30–60 s for visualization during direct laryngoscopy. A modified oxyscope may be made for older children by taping a feeding tube or suction catheter to the back of the laryngoscope blade. A 3.0-mm tracheal tube adapter is inserted into the end of the catheter and connected to the anaesthesia circuit, allowing oxygen to be delivered to the pharynx in the same manner.

In cases where airway involvement is expected to be severe, the equipment needed to perform an emergency cricothyrotomy or tracheostomy and an otolaryngologist or surgeon experienced in performing tracheostomy should be present before anaesthesia induction is undertaken. Awake laryngoscopy is the usual procedure in infants under 6 weeks of age and may be used in the co-operative older child or adolescent, although this is not universal practice. Application of cotton swabs soaked in 1% lignocaine to the anterior tongue can make laryngoscopy less troubling for the infant, but care must be exercised so that lignocaine is applied only to the tongue, not the posterior pharynx. Lack of understanding and co-operation, which increases struggling and the risk of damage to oral or pharyngeal tissues, usually mandate another approach in the young or retarded child.

An inhalation induction with spontaneous ventilation may be used in the unco-operative child presenting for elective surgery. It is often modified in children with associated congenital heart disease who may develop hypotension or an increase in right-to-left shunting under deep inhalation anaesthesia with the associated systemic vasodilatation. When inhalation induction is elected, halothane or sevoflurane are the agents used, and the induction is begun with the child positioned comfortably (often sitting or lying laterally). Sevoflurane has a shorter induction time than halothane and a pleasant non-irritating odour, providing a smooth inhalation induction even when its concentration is increased rapidly.[6] Sevoflurane better preserves cardiac output[7] but causes more profound respiratory depression than halothane, as measured by decreased tidal volume and respiratory rate.[8] Relaxation of upper airway muscles resulting in upper airway obstruction may be more pronounced with sevoflurance than with halothane.[9] An airtight mask fit allows the application of a constant distending pressure or assisted ventilation during induction if increasing airway obstruction occurs when the child is positioned supine. Demonstration of the ability to ventilate with a mask must precede the use of any muscle relaxants. Airway obstruction during early induction may be decreased by

Table 20.3 Difficult intubation cart supply list

Drawer 1a	Drawer 2b	Drawer 5 (O_2 delivery supplies)

Drawer 1a

Fibreoptic laryngoscope
Blades:
   Miller 0, 1, 2, 3
   Mac 2, 3, 4
   Miller 0-oxyscope
   Wis Hippel 1–1/2
   Phillips 1, 2
Handles:
   Large × 2
   Small × 2
   Adjustable × 1

Drawer 1b

Batteries:
   Size C × 6
   Size AA × 8
Magill forceps:
   Small × 1
   Large × 1

Drawer 2a

2% lignocaine 5 ml × 2
4% lignocaine 10 ml × 2
2% viscous lignocaine × 2
2% lignocaine jelly × 2
0.05% oxymetalozone × 2
0.25% neosynephrine × 1
Defogger × 1
Silicone fluid × 2

Drawer 2b

Syringes: Needles:
TBs × 5   20 g × 10
3 cc × 5   19 g × 19
5 cc × 5
Angiocaths:
20 g × 5
22 g × 5
3 × 3 non-sterile gauze

Drawer 3

Cass needles × 2
Tongue depressors × 5
Cotton-tipped applicators × 10
Atomizers: Devilbliss × 1
Duo-trach kit × 1
Nebulizer set × 1

Drawer 4

Angiocath: 14 g × 2
Stylets:
   Small – uncoated (blue) × 1
   Large – uncoated (green) × 1
Retrograde supplies:
   14 g Touhy × 1
   18 g Touhy × 1
   18 g Crawford × 1
Wires:
   035 inch diameter 150 cm
   fixed straight (spring guide wire)
   018 inch diameter 125 cm
   spring guide wire
Lightwands:
   Metal × 1
   Plastic × 1
Emergency cricothyroidotomy kit:
   Catheter set kit × 1
   Cricothyroid kit × 1

Drawer 5 (O_2 delivery supplies)

In-line medication adapters × 2
Airway connector for broncho-scopy × 2
Manometer
ETT adapter for NIF and DIP tubing w/o connector
Connecting tubing × 1

Drawer 6

Nasal airways:
One of each size:
   12, 14 ... 32 Fr.
Oral airways:
   3 of each: 00, 5.5, 6, #2/7
   2 of each: #3/8, #4/10
Ovassapian airway × 2
Masks for fibreoptic intubation
   Infant × 1   Child × 1
   Toddler × 1   Adult × 1
LMAs:
   1 of each: #1, $1\frac{1}{2}$, 2, 2–1/2, 3, 4

Drawer 7

ET CO_2 detector × 1
Emergency bag system with: bag with pop-off elbow, O_2 bowing
Biopsy valves

On cart

O_2 tank – full
Jet delivery system
Eschmann Stylets
   5 Ch. 50 cm × 2
   10 Ch. 70 cm × 2
   15 Ch. 60 angled tip × 2
   15 Ch. 70 cm × 2

the use of a nasopharyngeal airway, which is tolerated at lower anaesthetic concentrations than oral airways. Induction with titrated doses of propofol can also be used to allow spontaneous ventilation.

If laryngoscopy under deep inhalational anaesthesia allows visualization of the vocal cords, intubation under direct vision may be accomplished. If the vocal cords are not visible but the epiglottis is, the use of a stylet to direct the tracheal tube just below the epiglottis may allow intubation if the tube can be gently advanced into the trachea. The importance of an assistant holding the child's head in the midline, 'sniffing' position cannot be overemphasized. Placement of a folded towel under the occiput may align the pharnygeal and tracheal planes allowing visualization of an anteriorly placed larynx. If the larynx cannot be visualized directly, alternative methods of intubation are employed. There are several reviews on optimizing the conditions for fibreoptic bronchoscope intubations.[10] Ventilation and intubation are often possible through an LMA where laryngoscopy is unsuccessful.

Blind nasotracheal intubation may be attempted by those experienced in its use following topical vasoconstriction to the nares with oxymetolazone. Because of its lack of systemic effects, oxymetalozone is preferred to neosynephrine which can cause hypertension. The pharynx and larynx are sprayed with 4% lignocaine to a maximum dose of 3 mg kg^{-1}. Intravenous sedation is obtained with propofol (1–2 mg kg^{-1}), thiopentone (1–2 mg kg^{-1}), diazepam (0.1–0.2 mg kg^{-1}), midazolam (0.05–0.1 mg kg^{-1}) and/or fentanyl (1–2 μg kg^{-1}) in doses carefully titrated to maintain spontaneous ventilation while allowing maximal patient comfort.[11] With the child sitting tilted head-up at 60° and with the chin lifted in the 'sniffing' position, the nasal tube is advanced while listening at the tracheal tube adapter for maximal breath sounds. Entry into the oesophagus causes loss of breath sounds. The availability of fibreoptic bronchoscopes has greatly decreased the use of 'blind' techniques. A tracheal tube greater than a 2.5–3.0-mm internal diameter and an operator experienced in the use of fibreoptic laryngoscopes are prerequisites.[5] Alfery *et al.* reported the use of the fibreoptic laryngoscope via one nostril for visualization, while a tracheal tube was manipulated into the trachea via the other nostril in an infant.[12] When fibreoptic laryngoscopy is considered, it is best used early before attempts at intubation obscure the pharynx with secretions or blood.

If inhalational induction with a mask is possible, it may be followed by laryngeal nerve block with 2 mg kg^{-1} of lignocaine to each side of the neck, with passage of a guide wire retrogradely through the cricothyroid membrane into the oropharynx or nasopharynx. A tracheal tube may then be advanced into the trachea while the guide wire is held taut. Once the tracheal tube enters the proximal trachea, the guide wire is pulled through the tracheal tube while the tube is advanced into a more secure position in the trachea.[13] This procedure has been fairly, but not uniformly, successful in children over 6 years in Seattle. It is not a procedure recommended for use in infants since the cricothyroid membrane is closer to the thyroid isthmus and anatomic landmarks may be more difficult to palpate in infants. If mask ventilation can be established, tracheostomy can be carried out in this manner.

Finally, tracheostomy with local anaesthesia is possible with a co-operative patient. A more complete approach to the difficult airways may be found in Chapters 17 and 18.

PIERRE ROBIN SYNDROME

Pierre Robin syndrome or the Robin anomalad includes micrognathia, glossoptosis and a U-shaped cleft palate (Figure 20.2). *In utero*, mandibular hypoplasia displaces the tongue posteriorly, interfering with closure of the soft palate. These children may present in infancy for glossopexy or tracheostomy if the tongue and small mandible cause severe airway obstruction with cyanosis and apnoea. This condition is seen in otherwise normal children, and growth of the mandible in the first year of life is possible, resulting in a normal jaw in later childhood. However, the Robin anomalad may be seen as part of other syndromes, including Stickler, DeLange, Hallerman–Streiff or femoral hypoplasia syndromes. Most of these infants used to be cared for with prone

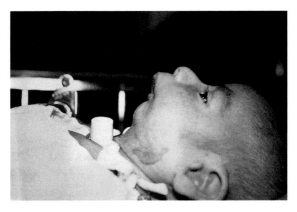

Figure 20.2 Pierre–Robin anomalad; severe airway obstruction necessitated tracheostomy.

positioning for their first weeks or months of life, but many feel that the use of nasopharyngeal airways is safer. Severe airway compromise may necessitate surgery to improve airway patency (Figure 20.2).

GOLDENHAR SYNDROME

Goldenhar syndrome (hemifacial microsomia) occurs as a defect in development of the first and second branchial arches (Figure 20.3). These children show asymmetric hypoplasia of malar, maxillary and mandibular development, which may include soft tissues and the tongue. Goldenhar's is the diagnosis if epibulbar dermoids, congenital heart disease or cervical vertebral defects accompany the facial defects. If involvement is primarily facial, then hemi-

facial microsomia is the diagnosis given, but these probably represent gradations of the same defect in morphogenesis.[14] The mouth often has a cleft-like extension on the affected side, making mask fit during anaesthesia a problem. A deformed to absent external pinna or a preauricular skin tag is often associated with unilateral deafness. Cardiac defects, especially ventricular septal defect (VSD) or tetralogy of Fallot (TOF), are associated conditions in the Goldenhar syndrome. These children present for reconstructive surgery of their mandibles or external ear. Induction of general anaesthesia may present difficulties in maintaining a patent airway and in laryngoscopy and intubation, particularly if the right side is affected. The facial asymmetry may worsen as the child ages, increasing airway problems during anaesthetic induction.

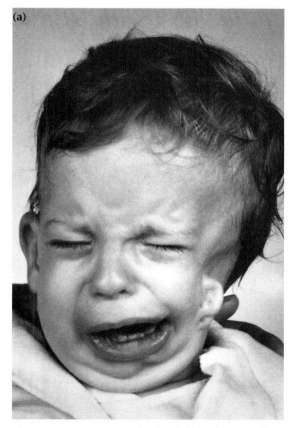
(a)

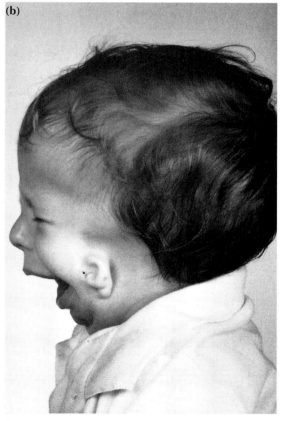
(b)

Figure 20.3 A 16-month-old child with severe hemifacial microsomia. His profile from the unaffected side is shown in Figure 20.1b.

TREACHER COLLINS' SYNDROME

This is an autosomal dominant, mandibulofacial dysostosis with down-slanting palpebral fissures, eyelid colobomata, bilateral malar and mandibular hypoplasia and malformation of the external pinna and ear canal (Figure 20.4). Conductive deafness is seen in 40% of these children. Mandibular and pharyngeal hypoplasia in these children are significant contributors to apnoea during awake and sleep states, as well as to difficult intubations during anaesthesia.[15] The risk of apnoea does not improve and may even worsen with age, unlike most other craniofacial syndromes which often improve with age. Mandibular and maxillary advancement osteotomies, which reorientate growth in a more normal direction, provide functional as well as aesthetic benefits.[16] Mental development is normal. Miller and Nager syndromes share the facial features of Treacher Collins' syndrome, in association with limb defects.

KABUKI SYNDROME

This syndrome was first described in Japan in 1981 and consists of five characteristics, including a peculiar face resembling the make-up used in Kabuki theatre, skeletal anomaly, dermatoglyphic abnormality, moderate mental retardation and short stature. Other manifestations of anaesthetic importance include retrognathia (36%), cardiac defects such as ventricular and

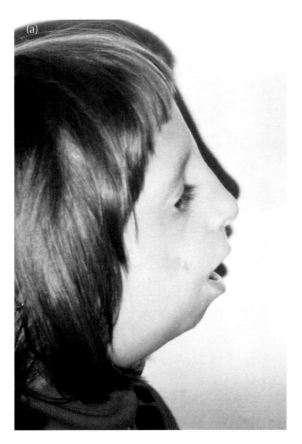

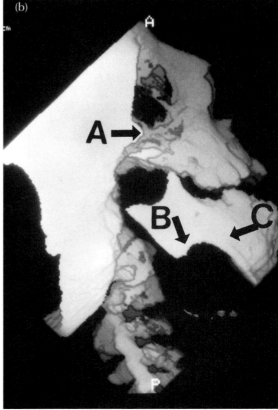

Figure 20.4 (a) An 8-year-old female with Treacher–Collins' syndrome, with (b) corresponding three-dimensional computed tomographic scan showing complete absence of zygoma (A), characteristic mandibular deformity with prominent antigonial notch (B), and severe mandibular retrusion (C). (Photographs courtesy of Dr Joseph Gruss.)

atrial septal defect (VSD and ASD; 32%)[17] and, in non-Japanese patients, neonatal hypotonia (33%) and seizures (29%).[18]

MOEBIUS SYNDROME

This rare defect results from agenesis or hypoplasia of cranial nerve nuclei, in particular cranial nerves VI and VII. The facial nerve palsies can be associated with poor mandibular growth and secondary micrognathia; XII nerve involvement may limit tongue movement. A small number (approximately 10%) of affected children has other brain anomalies. Difficulties in intubation in these children relate mainly to the degree of micrognathia or limited mouth opening.

KLIPPEL–FEIL ANOMALAD

The Klippel–Feil anomalad shows fusion of cervical vertebrae causing a short neck with limited mobility. This may interfere with positioning for intubation, making visualization of the larynx difficult. Frequently associated findings in these children include neurological defects, deafness, congenital heart disease (VSD) and scoliosis. The limited neck motion can be easily missed, resulting in unanticipated intubation difficulties.

ARTHOGRYPOSIS MULTIPLEX CONGENITA

This results from a number of neuropathic or myopathic problems in utero, which lead to limited fetal joint mobility and cause congenital joint contractures. The immobile joints are most obvious in the extremities, but these children cause most concern to anaesthetists when limited temporomandibular and cervical spine movement make intubation difficult. These patients are discussed in detail by Hall;[19] two-thirds of them have a good prognosis for mental development, but one-third will have severe central nervous abnormalities and most of the latter group die in infancy. Whether these patients are at risk for MH remains an area of dispute.[20–23] Similar limitations in joint mobility in the jaw and neck may be seen in children with juvenile rheumatoid arthritis.

MUCOPOLYSACCHARIDOSES

The mucopolysaccharidoses are lysosomal storage disorders characterized by the progressive diffuse accumulation of mucopolysaccharides in lysosomes in bone, muscle, visceral organs and in the soft tissues of the mouth and pharynx. Classification of these disorders is based on clinical, biochemical and/or genetic differences.

Hurler's syndrome, mucopolysaccharidosis type I, shows the most severe involvement with coarse facies, macroglossia, infiltration of pharyngeal and laryngeal soft tissues, short neck, kyphosis, corneal opacities, claw hand and limited cardiac function as distinctive features (Figure 20.5). Profuse secretions from upper and lower airways are usual, and severe mental retardation is obvious by 3 years of age. Hunter's syndrome, mucopolysaccharidosis type II, differs only in the more gradual onset of symptoms, lack of corneal opacities and presentation only in males. The combination of mental deficiency with a limited ability to co-operate, profuse airway secretions and increasing soft-tissue infiltration with the mucopolysaccharide tissue makes airway management and intubation a major anaesthetic problem, particularly in the child past infancy.

Baines and Keneally reported their experience with these children: some 50% of their patients had difficulties with airway management during anaesthesia.[24] Profuse secretions occluding a tracheostomy, coughing spasms, difficulty maintaining a patent airway during mask anaesthesia and failed intubation were problems they described. Inhalation inductions were used in the majority, with small amounts of intravenous agents to aid induction in unco-operative children. Maintaining spontaneous ventilation until airway control is secured and preoperative atropine were recommended. Moores *et al.* summarize recent experience with these patients, including cardiac and ventilatory difficulties.[25]

Morquio syndrome, mucopolysaccharidosis type IV, presents fewer problems with soft-tissue infiltration of the upper airway and mental development is usually normal (Figure 20.6). Chest-wall deformities result in limited ventilatory reserve. These children also have odontoid hypoplasia, putting them at risk of anterior dislocation of the C1 vertebra with

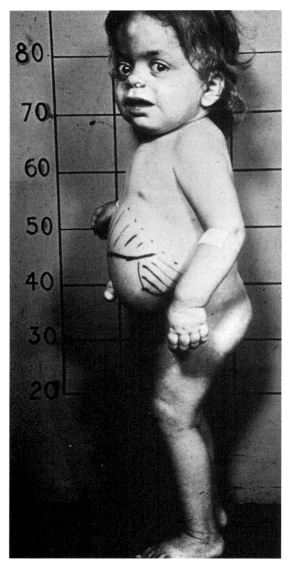

Figure 20.5 Hurler's syndrome (mucopolysaccharidosis type 1). Note thickened facial features, short neck and nasal secretions. (Courtesy of Dr V.A. McKusick.)

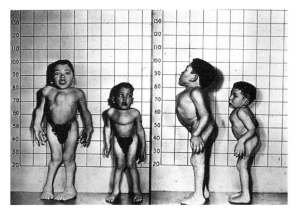

Figure 20.6 Morquio syndrome in two brothers. (Courtesy of Dr V.A. McKusick.)

CLEFT LIP AND/OR PALATE

Cleft lip and/or palate may be seen as part of many syndromes, including the CHARGE association, fetal hydantoin, fetal trimethadione, Robert's, 4P⁻, Mohr, orofacial–digital and velocardiofacial syndromes and trisomy 18, but it is an isolated defect in 90–95% of affected children. Isolated cleft palate is more commonly associated with other congenital anomalies than cleft lip/palate. Airway management and intubation are usually straightforward, but may be difficult if the cleft displaces intraoral tissues so that palatal tissues mechanically interfere with placing the tracheal tube at the glottis. Visualization of the larynx is usually not a problem. Following palate closure, the tongue may cause airway obstruction, so these children should be extubated when they are fully awake after removal of pharnygeal packs and inspection for tongue swelling from the mouth gag. Practical management of these patients is covered more fully on p. 383.

HAEMANGIOMAS AND LYMPHANGIOMAS

Haemangiomas and lymphangiomas (cystic hygromas) are congenital benign tumours but can cause significant airway problems, particularly if intraoral extension limits airway access or their large size causes extrinsic tracheal compression (Figure 20.7). Haemangiomas, if present elsewhere, can provide a clue to their

resultant spinal cord compression. This can occur during head positioning for tracheal intubation, so extreme flexion should be avoided by having an assistant to hold the head in the neutral position during laryngoscopy. Several other congenital syndromes associated with odontoid hypoplasia have been included in Table 20.1a.

presence in the trachea and, like laryngeal webs or cysts, may present with stridor or other symptoms of airway obstruction.

BECKWITH–WIEDEMANN SYNDROME

This syndrome includes omphalocoele, macroglossia, large size and neonatal hypoglycaemia (Figure 20.8). Because omphalocoeles are also seen in 10–50% of infants with trisomy 13 or 18, chromosomal studies are indicated in all infants with omphalocoeles.[14] Congenital heart disease is seen in 20% of infants with omphalocoeles and genitourinary defects, including exstrophy of the bladder, have been reported frequently.[26] Because of the Beckwith–Wiedemann association of omphalocoele and neonatal hypoglycaemia, anaesthesia in these infants should include frequent blood sugar determinations. Extubation is attempted only when the infant has demonstrated adequate spontaneous ventilation following repair, since limitation of diaphragmatic excursion often necessitates a period of postoperative mechanical ventilation.

SYNDROMES AT RISK FOR RAPID INTRAOPERATIVE BLOOD LOSS

Craniostenosis, premature fusion of one or more of the skull sutures, is a major component of several congenital syndromes, including Crouzon (Figure 20.9), Saethre–Chotzen, Pfeiffer, Carpenter and Apert syndromes (Figure 20.10a, b). All but Crouzon syndrome have associated syndactyly; most patients with these disorders are of normal intellect or mildly delayed. These children present at several months of age for craniectomy or for more extensive revision of the skull and orbital area. The anaesthetic management of these syndromes is discussed on p. 452.

Many other congenital anomalies carry a high risk of blood loss, including separation of conjoined twins,[27,28] correction of kyphoscoliosis in a child with Morquio's syndrome or resection of a sacrococcygeal teratoma. Ade-

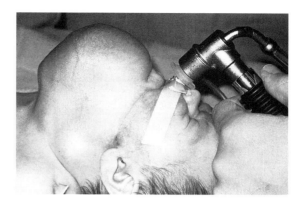

Figure 20.7 Infant with large cystic hygroma.

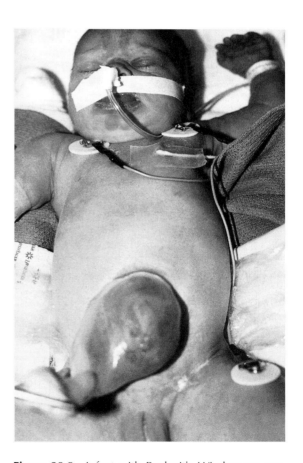

Figure 20.8 Infant with Beckwith–Wiedemann syndrome showing omphalocoele, macroglossia and large size (birth weight 4.1 kg). Hypoglycaemia responded to intravenous 10% dextrose solution.

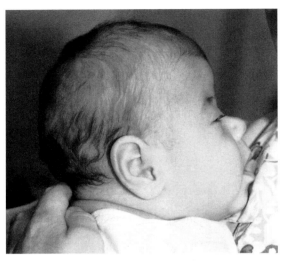

Figure 20.9 Profile of infant with Crouzon syndrome, showing small cranial vault in relation to normal size of facial features. Craniectomy is performed to prevent intracranial pressure problems during the infant's period of rapid brain growth.

quate intravenous access is necessary, cross-matched blood must be present in the operating room or immediate environment and checked so that transfusion can be immediately given, and intra-arterial catheters for continuous blood pressure monitoring must be available. Urinary catheters are a helpful adjunct to assess the adequacy of fluid resuscitation.

SYNDROMES ASSOCIATED WITH VENTILATORY PROBLEMS

Ventilation difficulties may be present before surgery, or may develop intraoperatively or in the postoperative period. They may be caused by intrinsic lung disease, chest-wall deformities or muscular weakness (Table 20.1).

MYOTONIC DYSTROPHY

This autosomal dominant disorder is characterized by myotonia (the inability to relax muscles), cataracts, frontal baldness, testicular atrophy in males and the expressionless 'myopathic' facies. Presentation in late adolescence is most common, with progressive muscle weakness and swallowing difficulties, but subtle symptoms have been reported in childhood. Cardiac conduction abnormalities are present in over 50% of patients.

Myotonia congenita, another autosomal dominant disorder, shows hypertrophied muscle and more severe myotonia but no weakness or cardiac involvement. Paramyotonia presents as myotonia and weakness induced by exposure to cold; potassium levels should be evaluated in these patients since myotonia may be seen in patients with familial periodic paralysis where episodes of weakness may be seen in association with abnormal serum potassium. Hypokalaemia-related episodes tend to be longer (up to 36 h), while in the hyperkalaemia type duration is several hours.

Anaesthetic management in the myotonia syndromes is influenced by several special considerations. Since cold or shivering increases myotonia, a warm environment is essential and some authors avoid halothane to minimize postoperative shivering.[29] The depolarizing muscle relaxants are absolutely contraindicated, since generalized myotonia has been seen following succinylcholine, making ventilation difficult or even impossible for several minutes.[30] Non-depolarizing muscle relaxants may be used safely with a transcutaneous nerve stimulator to titrate dosage, but are ineffective if local manipulation causes myotonia. Muscle relaxants should be avoided if possible, especially in familial periodic paralysis. Minimal fasting and avoiding hypoglycaemia are important in the hyperkalaemic type, while glucose loading can precipitate weakness in the hypokalaemic type. Direct injection of local anaesthetic into the affected muscle has been suggested to treat local myotonia.[31] Demonstration of adequate spontaneous ventilation prior to extubation should include an inspiratory effort greater than -30 cmH$_2$O and a tidal volume greater than 5 ml kg^{-1}. Postoperative monitoring should last for several hours or overnight to observe for delayed episodes of weakness.

Inadequate ventilation may be seen in congenital neuromuscular syndromes associated

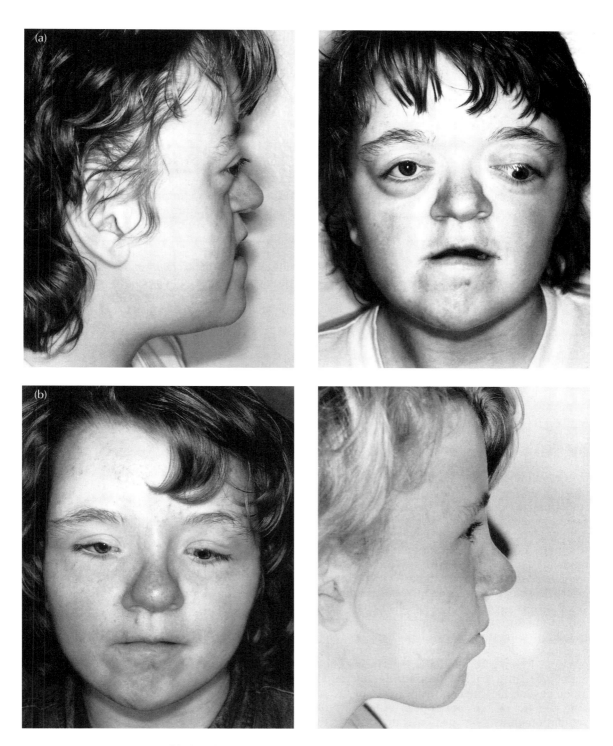

Figure 20.10 A 14-year-old female with Apert's syndrome (craniosynostosis, midface hypoplasia): (a) preoperative and (b) post-Lefort III mid-face advancement, performed by Dr Joseph Gruss. (Photographs courtesy of Dr Joseph Gruss.)

with weakness or inadequate cough, such as Werdnig–Hoffmann, myasthenia gravis, nemaline myopathy, central core disease or the muscular dystrophies, Duchenne's being the most common and most severe. Careful titration of muscle relaxants, if any are used, and assisted or controlled ventilation intraoperatively guide care. Assessment of chest-wall and diaphragmatic function should include inspiratory effort (normal > -30 cmH_2O) and vital capacity ($= 15$ ml kg^{-1}) prior to extubation. Children with central core disease, nemaline myopathy and Duchenne's muscular dystrophy are at risk for MH (see Malignant hyperthermia section for anaesthetic management).

CYSTIC FIBROSIS

This autosomal recessive disorder, whose gene locus on chromosome 7 has been isolated, involves abnormal sweat and mucus production and pancreatic insufficiency with diffuse effects, but it is the pulmonary involvement which impinges most directly on anaesthetic management. The ventilatory problems include inspissated secretions, ventilation–perfusion mismatching with resultant hypoxaemia, and infection of large and small airways with multiple organisms, often including *Pseudomonas* species. Advanced pulmonary disease results in cor pulmonale. The use of chest percussion, postural drainage and antibiotics preoperatively to optimize pulmonary function has been generally recommended.[31] Atropine will cause drying of secretions and is usually omitted. Ketamine is best avoided because of its stimulation of airway reflexes with exacerbation of coughing. General anaesthesia with tracheal intubation allows intraoperative suctioning of secretions as needed, and controlled or assisted ventilation is used to minimize atelectasis. Inhalation anaesthesia with halothane or sevoflurane is well tolerated, but induction may be prolonged owing to ventilation–perfusion mismatching. Intra-arterial monitoring for serial blood gases is indicated in the presence of severe lung disease or cor pulmonale. Adequacy of ventilation must be demonstrated prior to extubation, as detailed above, with inspiratory effort and tidal volume and, in the severely affected child, by blood gas measurement during spontaneous ventilation. Postoperative chest physiotherapy and close observation remain necessary, since deterioration in lung function has been reported following general anaesthesia.[32] Information on postoperative analgesia is limited; regional techniques have been used with good results.[33]

PRUNE BELLY SYNDROME

This syndrome results from a congenital deficiency of the abdominal musculature, associated with genitourinary anomalies (Figure 20.11).[34] The long-term prognosis in these children is determined by the degree of compromise of their renal function. The abdominal musculature deficiency raises the potential problem of inadequate cough and breathing before, during or after anaesthesia (see p. 403 for anaesthetic management).

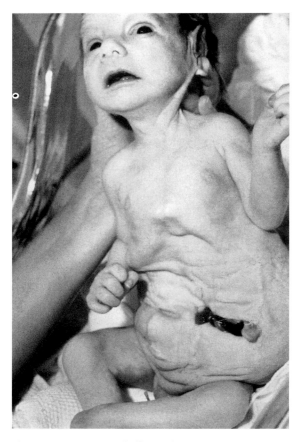

Figure 20.11   Prune belly syndrome with air hunger.

SYNDROMES ASSOCIATED WITH CARDIOVASCULAR PROBLEMS

An extensive discussion of congenital heart disease and its implications for anaesthesia is beyond the scope of this chapter. Recent literature presents discussion in depth.[31,35–37] Table 20.3 lists syndromes frequently associated with congenital heart disease. The anaesthetic management of cardiovascular problems is discussed in Chapter 13.

TRISOMY 21 (DOWN'S SYNDROME)

Down's syndrome is a chromosomal disorder involving all body systems. The characteristic flat facies, protruding tongue, inner canthal folds, up-slanting palpebral fissures, hypotonia and hyperflexible joints, mental retardation and short broad hand with simian creases are easily recognized. Some 50% of these children have congenital heart disease, most commonly endocardial cushion defects or VSD. The hyperflexible joints necessitate careful intubation, since cervical dislocation with spinal cord damage has been reported.[38,39]

TURNER'S SYNDROME

This should be suspected in any female with short stature. Ovarian dysgenesis with failure of sexual maturation at puberty and infertility, as well as short neck, low hairline with posterior webbing or pterygium and widely spaced nipples, are additional findings (Figure 20.12). Thirty per cent of these children have cardiac defects, usually coarctation of the aorta. Chromosome studies demonstrate the XO karyotype.

Noonan's syndrome represents the phenotype of Turner's syndrome with normal chromosomal studies. Short stature, webbed neck and cryptorchidism in males are findings similar to Turner's; mental retardation and pectus excavatum are more common in Noonan's and the congenital heart disease seen is commonly pulmonary stenosis rather than coarctation.[40]

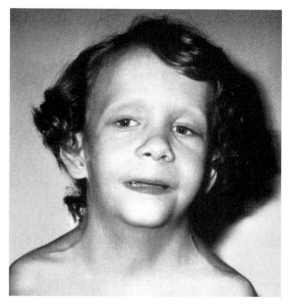

Figure 20.12 Female child with Turner syndrome. Past surgical scars from resection of nuchal lymphoedema can be seen.

WILLIAM'S SYNDROME

This sporadic disorder includes prominent lips, wide mouth, elfin facies, mild growth retardation and mental deficiency, hypercalcaemia in infancy (20%), and valvular or supravalvular aortic stenosis. These children have a distinctive hoarse voice and most have a talkative manner but 10% have severe behaviour problems.

ARRHYTHMIAS

Arrhythmias are the major feature in Romano–Ward syndrome (prolonged QT), Jervell–Lange–Nielsen (prolonged QT and deafness) and Wolff–Parkinson–White syndrome (aberrant arteriovenous conduction, with a short PR interval and delta waves on the electrocardiogram). Placement of a transvenous pacemaker for perioperative care is the safest course for the prolonged QT syndromes, but left stellate ganglion block has also been used with success.[41,42] In patients with Wolff–Parkinson–White syndrome, avoidance of tachycardia and excitation is recommended. If supraventricular tachycardia appears, the use of esmolol 0.01 mg kg^{-1} increments i.v. or adenosine

0.05 mg kg^{-1} i.v., with doubling of the dose if no effect is seen, has been successful in converting the rhythm to normal sinus rhythm. Verapamil (0.1 mg kg^{-1}) use is suggested by some, but discouraged by others. In recalcitrant cases, synchronized d.c. cardioversion should be available for intraoperative use.

TUBEROUS SCLEROSIS

Tuberous sclerosis is characterized by hamartomatous lesions that may involve multiple systems and is dominantly inherited, with many cases representing fresh mutations. The skin changes appear in early to mid-childhood, have been called adenoma sebaceum (a misnomer) and prominently affect nasolabial folds. Affected children have ash-leaf spots (hypopigmented areas) and café-au-lait spots are visible from infancy. Seizures and mental deficiency are seen in most affected children. Intracranial hamartomas can present in some children. Cardiac involvement with rhabdomyomas may present with arrhythmias or signs of obstruction to blood flow. Anaesthetic management should avoid possible arrhythmogenic agents, e.g. halothane, and should maintain normal intravascular volume to minimize ventricular outflow obstruction.

Children with congenital heart disease should be examined for other anomalies. If abnormalities of the vertebrae, anus (imperforate) or arms (radial dysplasia) are found, careful evaluation for the presence of tracheo-oesophageal fistula is mandatory; this symptom complex represents the VATER association: **v**ertebral anomalies, imperforate **a**nus, **t**racheo-oesophageal fistula, **r**adial or renal anomalies.[43] Congenital heart disease is seen in 20–30% of these children.

FAMILIAL DYSAUTONOMIA (RILEY–DAY SYNDROME)

Disturbances of autonomic function with this condition have profound anaesthetic implications.[44] There may be a defect in the formation of noradrenaline from levodopa which is manifest clinically by cardiovascular and temperature instability, hypotonia, no tear production and insensitivity to pain. Recurrent pulmonary aspiration after gastro-oesophageal reflux is common, so that lung function deteriorates as the child ages and is usually the eventual cause of death. Nissen fundoplication and feeding jejunostomy are frequently required.[45]

The absence of compensatory cardiovascular reflexes may make anaesthesia hazardous. Respiratory-depressant analgesics should be used with great care and in reduced doses. Premedication with a benzodiazepine is satisfactory, but atropine should be avoided where possible. There is no contraindication to the use of muscle relaxants, but inhalational agents must also be used with care. Hypovolaemia is poorly tolerated. Hypotension may be controlled by fluid administration and hypertension by increasing the dose of inhalational agent. Where appropriate, epidural anaesthesia is recommended.[46] Postoperative respiratory support may be necessary.

SYNDROMES THAT REQUIRE SPECIAL CARE IN PATIENT MOVEMENT OR POSITIONING

Difficulties with positioning occur in the infant with meningomyelocoele or in thoracopagus conjoined twins. Intubation is usually possible with these infants in a lateral position.

EPIDERMOLYSIS BULLOSA

Epidermolysis bullosa is a genetically inherited group of skin disorders which result in vesicles and bullae, occurring either spontaneously or with minimal trauma or friction. Both dominant and recessively inherited forms of the disorder have been described. The most severely involved are the recessive forms, where bullae heal with scarring that can result in significant contractures and syndactyly. Involvement of oral mucosa in these patients can result in microstomia and involvement of mucosa in the larynx and pharynx has been reported.[47] James and

Wark reported no tracheal or laryngeal problems after anaesthesia with tracheal intubation in 131 patients with epidermolysis bullosa dystrophica.[48] Stomal ulcers, strictures, reduced mouth opening and limited neck movement can contribute to difficult laryngoscopy as well as acquired microstomia and poor dentition.[49] Special care is essential to prevent trauma to skin or mucosa. Tape is avoided; soft cotton padding under the blood pressure cuff, needle electrodes for electrocardiogram monitoring and securing the tracheal tube with umbilical tape help to protect skin. Lubricating the facemask, laryngoscope and face with hydrocortisone ointment and using a tracheal tube of 0.5–1 mm internal diameter smaller than predicted have been recommended.[31] Ketamine and halothane have both been used successfully. When tracheal tubes have been used the pharynx and vocal cords should be visualized prior to extubation to look for bullae formation. A carefully inserted, well-lubricated LMA has proved satisfactory in many cases.

No problems have been reported with the use of suxamethonium but unpredictable sensitivity to non-depolarizing neuromuscular relaxants demands strict monitoring if these drugs are used.

Regional anaesthesia is gaining in popularity despite theoretical risks of sepsis and infective complications. Skin condition needs careful assessment prior to percutaneous needle placement as typical landmarks and 'tissue feel' are often altered.

Children with ectodermal dysplasia (Christ–Siemens–Touraine syndrome) have no sebaceous or sweat glands, absent hair and absent teeth (partial or complete). Full expression of this sex-linked recessive disorder is seen in males, and the facial features include depressed nasal bridge, deformed external ears, thick lips and underdeveloped maxilla and mandible. Airway management may be a problem in these children. Thermoregulation is defective because of the lack of sweat glands; therefore, cooling measures should be available (cooling mattress, cool intravenous solutions) and temperature should be closely monitored. Anticholinergic medication is avoided because of its effect on temperature.

OSTEOGENESIS IMPERFECTA

Patients with osteogenesis imperfecta or with osteopetrosis are at risk of fractures and joint dislocations with minimal trauma. Care in moving and positioning these patients extends to intubation, since their teeth are more fragile than normal.

MALIGNANT HYPERTHERMIA

MH is a rare, potentially lethal hypermetabolic disorder most commonly triggered by anaesthetic agents. Some children with congenital syndromes mentioned above are at risk of this reaction during anaesthesia (Table 20.4).

MH is an inherited disorder of skeletal muscle characterized by intermittent hypermetabolic crises. It may be triggered by the potent inhalational anaesthetics (halothane, enflurane, isoflurane, sevoflurane) and succinylcholine. Although stress alone is a trigger in the swine model, this rarely applies in humans. Its incidence is reported as 1 : 15 000 in children and 1 : 50 000 in adults.

A clinical diagnosis of MH is made when the signs and symptoms listed in Table 20.5 appear during anaesthesia. The earliest signs are given in italic and are always present; the others appear in fulminant cases or when diagnosis is delayed. All reflect the hypermetabolism seen; hence, tachycardia and tachypnoea with immediate rise in end-tidal CO_2 are the earliest and most sensitive signs. Temperature increases may

Table 20.4 Congenital syndromes associated with malignant hyperthermia (MH) or signs and symptoms of MH

Central core disease
Duchenne's muscular dystrophy
King–Denborough syndrome
Nemaline myopathy
Osteogenesis imperfecta*
Myotonia congenita
Schwartz–Jampel syndrome
Arthrogryposis*

*Controversial if true association with MH.

be rapid or more insidious. If succinylcholine has been used, masseter spasm may be the first sign of a MH reaction. Children with any of the myotonic syndromes (myotonia congenita, myotonic dystrophy, paramyotonia) may develop masseter spasm following succinylcholine, but whether this represents a MH reaction or myotonia is unclear. Current controversy exists about how to classify and treat patients who develop masseter muscle spasm following succinylcholine, which may occur in up to 1% of paediatric patients.[50] Schwartz reported positive muscle biopsy results in 100% of such patients;[51] others report 50–65% incidence.[52–54] When metabolic demands exceed supply, venous desaturation, lactic acidosis and hyperkalaemia develop. A high index of suspicion will stimulate blood gas and potassium determinations in the event of unexpected tachycardia, tachypnoea, temperature rise ($> 0.5°C$) or masseter spasm.

No single laboratory screen is available; serial (at least three) serum creatine phosphokinase (CPK) determinations will show elevated baseline levels in 70% of susceptible patients. Following a MH reaction CPK levels rise, with peak values reached 8–12 h after the reaction begins. Muscle biopsy testing is the best diagnostic test currently available, as susceptible muscle shows contracture to halothane and to low concentrations of caffeine. Unfortunately, the contracture testing is technically difficult, performed only in selected centres, is invasive (requiring fresh muscle) and is not usually undertaken in prepubertal subjects. In both Europe and the USA, uniform criteria for performing and interpreting the results are being established.[55]

MH is an inherited disorder and genetic evaluation is usually consistent with an autosomal dominant pattern of inheritance. Molecular medicine has made great strides since 1990 when McCarthy *et al.* first identified the human ryanodine receptor gene on chromosome 19 which codes for the RYR1 peptide, a protein integral to the regulation of calcium in skeletal muscle.[56] Nine different RYR1 MHS mutations have been published, and seven more have been identified but await characterization.[57] About half of susceptible families do not show linkage of MH to chromosome 19 but, rather, link to other chromosomes such as 1, 3 and 17. Therefore, since MH is genetically heterogeneous, a future simple genetic screening test is not likely.

The pathophysiology of the disorder is incompletely understood. Research has been facilitated by the presence of an animal model (several breeds of pig), which undergoes a similar hypermetabolic crisis in response to stress. Current understanding is that the hypermetabolism is related to a defect in calcium metabolism in susceptible skeletal muscle. This leads to high levels of intracellular calcium and stimulates actin–myosin coupling, causing sustained contraction. The contraction generates heat and metabolic byproducts, eventually leading to muscle degeneration with release of myoglobin, potassium and CPK.

Larach *et al.* have created a clinical grading scale (a six-point likelihood scale from 1 = almost never to 6 = almost certain) to standardize and define qualitatively the decision process in diagnosing MH retrospectively.[58] It is noted by the authors that, at present, because this scale tends to underestimate the MH likelihood it is not intended for clinical decision making. Priority should be given to starting appropriate treatment rather than calculating the clinical indicator score. The real utility of this clinical grading scale is that by providing a clinical gold standard, caffeine–halothane contraction tests, which were standardized in 1989, could be adjusted for optimal sensitivity (88%) and specificity (81%). Since the consequences of a false-negative test could be disastrous, the

Table 20.5 Signs and symptoms of malignant hyperthermia

Symptoms	Signs
Tachycardia	Venous oxygen saturation
Tachypnoea	Venous hypercarbia
Arrhythmias	Metabolic acidosis
Cyanosis	Respiratory acidosis
Mottling of skin	Hyperkalaemia
Fever	Myoglobinaemia/myoglobinuria
Rigidity	Elevated creatine phosphokinase
Sweating	Disseminated intravascular coagulation
Labile blood pressure	Masseter spasm (after succinylcholine)

MHAUS group set the criteria for positive and equivocal categories to accept false-positives to avoid any false-negative diagnoses.[55]

Patients at risk for MH include: (1) those with a past history of a MH event or with a positive muscle biopsy; (2) first-degree relatives of patients with MH, if CPK is elevated; and (3) patients with muscular dystrophy, central core myopathy or perhaps osteogenesis imperfecta (see Table 20.4). These patients are given anaesthesia with non-triggering agents. Nitrous oxide, thiopentone, propofol, droperidol, morphine, fentanyl, pethidine (demerol), fentanyl derivatives such as sufentanil, alfentanil or remifentanil, and non-depolarizing muscle relaxants such as pancuronium, vecuronium or atracurium may be used safely in such patients. Careful monitoring of the electrocardiogram for heart rate and rhythm, blood pressure, end-tidal CO_2 and temperature are mandatory with blood sampling for blood gas and electrolytes if any signs of MH occur.

Pretreatment with dantrolene is no longer recommended.[59] The side-effects are serious and include muscle weakness (24%), phlebitis (9%), respiratory failure (6%) and gastrointestinal upset (6%).[60]

Treatment of a MH event must include:

1 elimination of the triggering agents, i.e. stop halothane, isoflurane or sevoflurane, change anaesthesia circuit (tubing, CO_2 absorber) and machine, if possible, converting to nitrous oxide–narcotic–relaxant technique and stop surgery as soon as possible;
2 drawing blood gas, potassium and initial CPK level to corroborate diagnosis;
3 hyperventilation with 100% O_2 and the use of $NaHCO_3$ intravenously to treat respiratory and metabolic acidosis;
4 cooling measures for fever (cooling mattress, cold saline for bladder, gastric or, in rare cases, even peritoneal lavage, cool intravenous solutions);
5 aborting the muscle hypermetabolism with dantrolene, which is continued until the patient has been asymptomatic and afebrile for 24 h;
6 maintaining good urine output with fluid therapy, and mannitol or frusemide if necessary;
7 repeating CPK level at 8 and 24 h after the event (levels over 20 000 units are diagnostic; over 10 000 are highly suggestive).

Close cardiovascular and temperature monitoring (usually in an intensive care unit) are necessary for 24–48 h following an event.

MH was first recognized in 1960, and the mortality was greater than 50%. With the development of intravenous dantrolene in 1979 and the rising alertness of the anaesthesia community, especially through the service of the Malignant Hyperthermia Association of the United States (MHAUS), established in 1982, this mortality rate had decreased to less than 4% in 1996. Of the 985 consultations for acute management of MH, 24% were outpatient ENT cases. The patients were 0–10 years old in 81%, 57% were male, halothane was used in 69% and succinylcholine in 75%. The most common signs and symptoms were jaw rigidity in 57%, followed by fever in 33%. The diagnosis made most commonly by the consultants were masseter muscle rigidity (MMR) in 40%, not MH in 23%, suspect or mild MH in 15%, MMR/acute MH in 15% and acute MH in 5%. In treating a crisis, dantrolene increments of 1 mg kg^{-1} (up to 10 mg kg^{-1}) may be necessary to reverse the hypermetabolism. Lerman *et al.* reported dantrolene kinetics in children and found more rapid clearance than in adults.[61] Blood levels in children remain protective (> 3.0 μg.ml^{-1}) for 5 h following an intravenous bolus of 2.4 mg kg^{-1}. Indeed, nearly 25% of patients relapsed at some point and, thus, supplemental doses may be needed more frequently in children than in adults.[60]

LATEX ALLERGY

With the development of universal precautions in the early 1980s, the increased incidence of latex allergy was inevitable. Latex is a milky sap harvested from the commercial rubber tree *Hevea brasiliensis* in South America and Malaysia, and contains 65% water, 31% rubber, 2% resin and 2% protein. Certain individuals develop immunoglobulin E (IgE)-mediated responses to these proteins, which remain after the sap has been chemically processed into 40 000 medical and household products. There are four types of hypersensitivity reaction, of which this section will focus on the type-I IgE-mediated anaphylactic reactions involving degranulation of mast cells and basophils. An early case report of this type-I reaction appeared in the anaesthesia literature in 1989.[62] More than 1100 severe allergic reactions, including 15 deaths from anaphylaxis, were reported to the Food and Drug Administration of the United States (FDA) between 1988 and 1992. All of these deaths were associated with the use of latex-containing barium enema catheters, which were recalled in 1990.

Risk factors for latex allergy in children include multiple surgeries, history of myelodysplasia with a neurogenic bladder or bowel, genitourinary anomalies, atopy including asthma, eczema or allergic rhinitis, or allergies to balloons, bananas, avocados and chestnuts. Porri *et al.* found that three or more surgeries rather than spina bifida per se increased the sensitization to latex as determined by skin-prick tests.[63] The incidence of actual anaphylaxis is increased after more than six to nine surgeries.[64–65] Latex is thought to be responsible for 70% of anaphylactic reactions occurring in anaesthetized children. A recent study using the AlaSTAT latex allergy test preoperatively found IgE antibodies in 6.7% of 996 day-surgery patients. In these same patients, no systemic allergic reactions occurred by retrospective chart review. This study illustrates that sensitization is common in the general population, although only a small portion actually manifests anaphylaxis.[66] Interestingly, most patients with spina bifida and latex allergy have IgE specific for 14-, 20- and 27-kDa peptides, while the IgE of health-care workers with latex allergy usually recognizes only the 20-kDa peptide.

Minimizing latex exposure is the only reliable method of preventing latex anaphylaxis. Holzman has outlined a preoperative, intraoperative and postoperative checklist (Table 20.6).[67] One must begin with having a high suspicion in individuals at risk. Asking for specific symptoms of clinical latex allergy such as lip swelling with latex balloons or sneezing/rhinitis with dental procedures may reveal those with the potential for intraoperative anaphylaxis. At the authors' institution patients with a meningomyelocoele or cloacal exstrophy are identified as requiring latex precautions from their first surgery. This creates a latex-free environment to avoid sensitizing the patient. Allergy testing

is not necessarily required but may be useful if the anaphylactic trigger is unclear. *In vitro* tests such as the AlaSTAT latex allergy test mentioned earlier are recommended by the FDA because they are safe, reproducible, practical, and highly sensitive (> 90%) and specific (> 90%).[66,68] Luckily, the link between sensitization to latex and the development of anaphylaxis with exposure is rare.

Chemoprophylaxis against latex allergy with H_1- (diphenhydramine 1 mg kg^{-1} to 50 mg i.v. maximum) and H_2-blockers (ranitidine 1 mg kg^{-1} or 50 mg i.v. maximum) and steroids (hydrocortisone 1 mg kg^{-1}) has been advocated by some.[69] However, there are case reports of failure to prevent anaphylaxis with such prophylaxis. Latex exposure may be minimal with exuberant reactions, as reported in a patient with known latex allergies who received prophylaxis for two doses but developed a severe reaction immediately upon entering the operating room.[70] Swanson *et al.* found that the operating room area where powdered latex gloves are used had a 10–100-fold higher concentration of latex aeroallergen.[71] This led to the recommendation for scheduling a severely allergic patient as the first case in the morning. Since latex-safe equipment is now more readily available, Holzman does not advocate chemoprophylaxis.[67] He recently reviewed 267 anaesthetics given without chemoprophylaxis to 162 children with latex allergy, established by clinical history, allergy testing, or both, revealing a single case of an allergic reaction after an epidural injection with bupivacaine from a syringe prepared 1.5 weeks earlier. He feels that regular syringes may be used if medications are not drawn up more than 6 h before use (latex-free plastic syringes and tourniquets are available), and that the most important factor is avoidance of human error breaching this latex-free environment. Violation of the latex-safe environment accounted for three out of five anaphylactic reactions in another published series.[72] Thoroughly rinsing a latex device such as a balloon cardiac catheter with sterile saline prior to use may be sufficient if latex-free products are not available.

The presenting time and signs and symptoms of the allergic reaction vary. Time of onset can be from minutes to hours into a surgical case and severity of symptoms may vary from grade

Table 20.6 Checklist for latex-allergic patients

Preoperative

Solicit specific history of latex allergy or risk for latex allergy

History of chronic care with latex products

History of spina bifida, urological reconstructive surgery

History of repeated surgical procedures (e.g. > 3)

History of intolerance to latex-based products: balloons, rubber gloves, condoms, dental dams, rubber urethral catheters

History of allergy to tropical fruits

History of intraoperative anaphylaxis of uncertain aetiology

Health-care workers, especially with a history of atopy or hand eczema

Consider allergy consultation

In vitro testing

In vivo testing

Minimize latex exposure for at-risk patients

Latex alert: patients with significant risk factor for latex allergy but no overt signs or symptoms

Latex allergy: patients with or without significant risk factors for latex allergy and positive history, signs, symptoms or allergy evaluation

Carefully co-ordinate care between anaesthesia and nursing teams

Have lists available of non-latex product alternatives

First case of the day is preferable to decrease aeroallergen concentration

Display 'latex allergy' or 'latex alert' signs inside and outside the operating room

Postoperative

Medical alert tag

Warning sign posted on chart

Warning sign posted on bed

Intraoperative

Anaesthesia equipment

Latex-free gloves, airways, tracheal tubes

Masks: polyvinyl chloride if available, or old, well-washed, black rubber masks

Rebreathing bags: neoprene if available, or old, well-washed, black rubber bags

Ventilator bellows: neoprene or silicone if available, or old, well-washed, black rubber bellows

Breathing circuit: disposable, poly-vinyl chloride, packaged separately from a latex rebreathing bag

Remove rubber stoppers from multidose vials

Beware of latex intravenous injection ports, penrose-type tourniquets and rubber bands; use non-latex glove as tourniquet; tape latex injection ports or use silicone injection ports or stopcock

Blood-pressure cuffs: if new latex, cover with soft cotton

Ambu-type bag: ensure that bag and valve do not have latex components (alternative is silicone self-inflating bag)

Check syringe plungers; reconstitute medications every 6 h

Dilute concentration of adrenaline (0.01 mg ml^{-1} or $1{:}100\ 000$) available

Surgical equipment

Avoid latex surgical gloves

Avoid latex drains (e.g. penrose)

Avoid latex urinary catheters

Avoid latex instrument mats

Avoid rubber-shod clamps

Avoid latex vascular tags

Avoid latex bulb syringes for irrigation

Avoid rubber bands

(Used with permission from Holzman, 1997.[67])

I (non-systemic with urticaria or rash) to grade IV [severe systemic reactions with cardiovascular compromise often exhibited by tachycardia (30% increase), hypotension (25–45% decreases in systolic or diastolic pressure), increased airway resistance and decreased oxygen saturations].[65]

Treatment for anaphylaxis requires small bolus doses of adrenaline 0.1–1 mg kg^{-1} (vs 10 mg kg^{-1} for cardiac arrest) and crystalloid infusions for hypotension. An adrenaline infusion at 0.1–0.3 μg kg^{-1} min^{-1} may be required, depending on the severity of the reaction and amount of latex exposure. Surgeons should immediately change to non-latex gloves if the route of exposure is thought to be surgical. Inhaled albuterol, subcutaneous or intravenous terbutaline and intravenous isoproterenol are useful adjuncts for treating bronchospasm. High inspired oxygen concentrations are usually necessary, at least until the reaction abates. Steroids, H$_1$- and H$_2$-histamine blockers are also indicated. All medical records should indicate latex allergy and Medic Alert bracelets and self-injectable adrenaline should be provided, along with patient and family education.

REFERENCES

1 Jones, A.E.P. and Pelton, D.A. An index of syndromes and their anaesthetic implications. *Canadian Anaesthetists Society Journal* 1976; **23**: 207–26.
2 Steward, D.J. *Manual of pediatric anesthesia*, 4th edn. New York: Churchill Livingstone, 1995.
3 Roizen, M.F. and Fleisher, L.A. (eds) *Essence of Anesthesia Practice*, 1st edn. Philadelphia, PA: W.B. Saunders, 1997.
4 Berkowitz, I., Raja, S., Bender, K., et al. Dwarfs: pathophysiology and anesthetic implications. *Anesthesiology* 1990; **73**: 739–59.
5 Stehling, L.C. The difficult intubation and fiberoptic techniques. In: *ASA Annual Refresher Course Lectures*. American Society of Anesthesiologists, 1984: 230.
6 Baum, V., Yemen, T. and Baum, L. Immediate 8% sevoflurane induction in children: a comparison with incremental sevoflurane and incremental halothane. *Anesthesia and Analgesia* 1997; **85**: 313–16.
7 Wodey, E., Pladys, P., Copin, C., et al. Comparative hemodynamic depression of sevoflurane versus halothane in infants – an echocardiographic study. *Anesthesiology* 1997; **87**: 795–800.

8 Yamakage, M., Yamita, K., Horikawa, D., et al. Effects of halothane and sevoflurane on the paediatric respiratory pattern. *Paediatric Anaesthesia* 1994; **4**: 53–6.
9 Motoyama, E. Sevoflurane in pediatric ear, nose and throat procedures. In: Borland, L. (ed.) *International Anesthesiology Clinics. Airway Management in Pediatric Anesthesia*. Philadelphia, PA: Lippincott-Raven, 1997: **35**: 93–7.
10 Roberts, J.T. Optimizing FOB. Fiberoptics in anesthesia. *Anesthesiology Clinics of North America* 1991; **9**: 1–192.
11 Lynn, A.M., Morray, J.P. and Furman, E.B. Short-acting barbiturate sedation: effect on arterial pH and PaCO$_2$ in children. *Canadian Anaesthetists Society Journal* 1988; **35**: 76–9.
12 Alfery, D.D., Ward, C.F., Harwood, I.R., et al. Airway management for a neonate with congenital fusion of the jaws. *Anesthesiology* 1979; **51**: 340.
13 Lopez, N.R. Mechanical problems with the airway. *Clinical Anesthesia* 1968; **3**: 16.
14 Jones, K.L. *Smith's Recognizable Patterns of Human Malformation*, 4th edn. Philadelphia, PA: W.B. Saunders, 1988.
15 Roa, N. and Moss, K. Treacher–Collins syndrome with sleep apnea: anesthetic considerations. *Anesthesiology* 1984; **60**: 71–3.
16 Arvystas, M. and Shprintzen, R. Craniofacial morphology in Treacher Collins syndrome. *Cleft Palate–Craniofacial Journal* 1991; **28**: 226–31.
17 Niikawa, N., Kuroki, Y., Kajii, T., et al. Kabuki make-up (Niikawa–Kuroki) syndrome: a study of 62 patients. *American Journal of Medical Genetics* 1988; **31**: 565–89.
18 Schrander-Stumpel, C., Meinecke P., Wilson, G., et al. The Kabuki (Niikawa–Kuroki) syndrome: further delineation of the phenotype in 29 non-Japanese patients. *European Journal of Pediatrics* 1994; **153**: 438–45.
19 Hall, J. Arthrogryposes. In Emery, A.E.H., Rimoin, D.L. (eds). *Principles and Practice of Medical Genetics*. Philadelphia, PA: Churchill Livingstone, 1983: 781–811.
20 Kanaya, N., Nakayama, M., Nakae, Y., et al. Hyperthermia during sevoflurane anaesthesia in arthrogryposis multiplex. congenita with central nervous system dysfunction (Letter). *Paediatric Anaesthesia* 1996; **6**: 428–9.
21 Hopkins, P.M., Ellis, F.R. and Halsall, P.J. Hypermetabolism in arthrogryposis multiplex congenita. *Anaesthesia* 1991; **46**: 374–5.
22 Froster-Iskenius, U.G., Waterson, J.R. and Hall, J.G. A recessive form of congenital contractures and torticollis associated with malignant hyperthermia. *Journal of Medical Genetics* 1988; **25**: 104–12.
23 Baines, D.B., Douglas, I.D. and Overton, J.H. Anaesthesia for patients with arthrogryposis multiplex congenita: what is the risk of malignant hyperthermia? *Anaesthesia and Intensive Care* 1986; **14**: 370–2.
24 Baines, D. and Keneally, J. Anaesthetic implications of the mucopolysaccharidoses: a 15-year experience in a children's hospital. *Anaesthesia and Intensive Care* 1983; **11**: 198–202.
25 Moores, C., Rogers, J.G., McKenzie, I.M., et al. Anaesthesia for children with mucopolysaccharidoses. *Anaesthesia and Intensive Care* 1996; **24**: 459–63.

26 Stehling, L.C. and Zauder, H.L. *Anesthetic Implications of Congenital Anomalies in Children.* New York: Appleton-Century-Crofts, 1980.

27 Furman, E.B., Roman, D.G., Hairabet, J., *et al.* Management of anesthesia for surgical separation of newborn conjoined twins. *Anesthesiology* 1971; **34**: 95–101.

28 Towey, R.M., Kisia, A.K.L., Jacobacci, S., *et al.* Anaesthesia for the separation of conjoined twins. *Anaesthesia* 1979; **34**: 187–92.

29 Kaufman, J., Friedman, J.M. and Sadowsky, B. Myotonic dystrophy: surgical and anesthetic considerations during orthognathic surgery. *Journal of Oral and Maxillofacial Surgery* 1983; **41**: 667–71.

30 Ellis, F.R. Neuromuscular disease and anaesthesia. *British Journal of Anaesthesia* 1974; **46**: 603–12.

31 Gregory, G.A. *Pediatric Anesthesia*, 3rd edn. New York: Churchill-Livingstone, 1994.

32 Richardson, V.F., Robertson, C.R., Mowat, A.P., *et al.* Deterioration in lung function after general anaesthesia in patients with cystic fibrosis. *Acta Paediatrica Scandinavica* 1984; **73**: 75–9.

33 Cain, J.C., Lish, M.C. and Passannante, A.N. Epidural fentanyl in a cystic fibrosis patient with pleuritic chest pain. *Anesthesia and Analgesia* 1994; **78**: 793–4.

34 Henderson, A.M., Vallis, C. and Sumner, E. Anaesthesia in the prune belly syndrome. *Anaesthesia* 1987; **42**: 54–60.

35 Hickey, P.R. and Hansen, D.D. Fentanyl and sufentanil–oxygen–pancuronium anesthesia for cardiac surgery in infants. *Anesthesia and Analgesia* 1984; **63**: 117–24.

36 Lake, C.L. (ed.) *Pediatric Cardiac Anesthesia*, 2nd edn. Norwalk, CT: Appleton Lange, 1993.

37 Nichols, D.G., Cameron, D.E., Greeley, W.J., *et al.* (eds) *Critical Heart Disease in Infants and Children.* St Louis, MO: Mosby-Year Book, 1995.

38 Kobel, M., Creighton, R.E. and Steward, D.J. Anaesthesia considerations in Down's syndrome; experience with 100 patients and a review of the literature. *Canadian Anaesthetists' Society Journal* 1982; **29**: 593–9.

39 Mitchell, V., Howard, R. and Facer, E.K. Down's syndrome and anaesthesia. *Paediatric Anaesthesia* 1995; **3**: 379–84.

40 Noonan, J. Noonan syndrome. An update and review for the primary pediatrician. *Clnical Pediatrics* 1994; **33**: 548–55.

41 Callaghan, M.L., Nichols, A.B. and Sweet, R.B. Anaesthetic management of prolonged Q-T syndrome. *Anesthesiology* 1977; **47**: 67–9.

42 Joseph-Reynolds, A.M., Anden, S.M. and Sobczyzk, W.L. Perioperative considerations in a newly described subtype of congenital long QT syndrome. *Paediatric Anaesthesia* 1997; **7**: 237–41.

43 Quan, L. and Smith, D.W. The VATER association. Vertebral defects, anal atresia, T-E fistula with esophageal atresia, radial and renal dysplasia: a spectrum of associated defects. *Journal of Pediatrics* 1973; **82**: 104–7.

44 Stenqvist, O. and Sigurdsson, J. The anaesthetic management of a patient with familial dysautononoma. *Anaesthesia* 1982; **37**: 929–32.

45 Cox, R.G. and Sumner, E. Familial dysautonomia. *Anaesthesia* 1983; **38**: 293.

46 Challands, J.F. and Facer, E.K. Epidural anaesthesia and familial dysautonomia (the Riley Day syndrome). Three case reports. *Paediatric Anaesthesia* 1998; **8**: 83–8.

47 Stehling, L.C. *Common Problems in Pediatric Anesthesia*, 2nd edn. New York: C.V. Mosby, 1992.

48 James, I. and Wark, H. Airway management during anesthesia in patients with epidermolysis bullosa dystrophica. *Anesthesiology* 1982; **56**: 323–6.

49 Griffin, R.P. and Mayou, B.J. The anaesthetic management of patients with dystrophic epidermolysis bullosa. A review of 44 patients over a 10 year period. *Anaesthesia* 1993; **48**: 810–15.

50 Orr, R. and Ramamoorthy, C. Controversies in pediatric ambulatory anesthesia. In: Orr, R. and Pavlin, J. (eds). *Anesthesiology Clinics of North America.* Philadelphia, PA: W.B. Saunders, 1996; **4**: 767–80.

51 Schwartz, L., Rockoff, M.A. and Koka, B.V. Masseter spasm with anesthesia: incidence and implications. *Anesthesiology* 1984; **61**: 772–5.

52 Flewellen, E.H. and Nelson, T.E. Masseter spasm induced by succinylcholine in children; contracture testing for malignant hyperthermia. *Canadian Anaesthetists Society Journal* 1982; **129**: 432–49.

53 Ellis, F.R. and Halsall, P.J. Suxamethonium spasm – a differential diagnostic conundrum. *British Journal of Anaesthesia* 1984; **56**: 381–4.

54 Rosenberg, H. and Fletcher, J.E. Masseter muscle rigidity and malignant hyperthermia susceptibility. *Anesthesia and Analgesia.* 1986; **65**: 161–4.

55 Allen, G., Larach, M. and Kunselman, A. The North American Malignant Hyperthermia Registry of MHAUS The sensitivity and specificity of the caffeine–halothane contracture test. *Anesthesiology* 1998; **88**: 579–88.

56 McCarthy, T.V., Healy, J.M.S., Heffron, J., *et al.* Localization of the malignant hyperthermia susceptibility locus to human chromosome 19q12–13.2. *Nature* 1990; **343**: 562–4.

57 Hogan, K. Molecular medicine and malignant hyperthermia. *Anesthesiology* 1997; **86**: 511–13.

58 Larach, M., Localio, A., Allen, G., *et al.* A clinical grading scale to predict malignant hyperthermia susceptibility. *Anesthesiology* 1994; **80**: 771–9.

59 Wedel, E., Pladys, P., Copin, C., *et al.* Comparative hemodynamic depression of sevoflurane versus halothane in infants – an echocardiographic study. *Anesthesiology* 1997; **87**: 795–800.

60 Larach, M., Simon, L., Allen, G., *et al.* Safety and efficacy of dantrolene sodium for the treatment of malignant hyperthermia events. *Anesthesiology* 1993; **79**: A1079.

61 Lerman, J., Derdemezi, J., Strong, H.A., *et al.* Pharmacokinetics of intravenous dantrolene in malignant hyperthermia susceptible pediatric patients. *Anesthesia and Analgesia* 1988; **67**: S133.

62 Gerber, A. Severe intraoperative anaphylaxis to surgical gloves: latex allergy, an unfamiliar condition. *Anesthesiology* 1989; **71**: 800–2.

63 Porri, F., Pradal, M., Lemiere, C., *et al.* Association between latex sensitization and repeated latex exposure in children. *Anesthesiology* 1997; **86**: 599–602.

64 Kwittken, P.L., Sweiberg, S.K., Campbell, D.E., *et al.* Latex hypersensitivity in children: clinical presentaiton and detection of latex-specific immunoglobulin E. *Pediatrics* 1995; **95**: 693–9.

65 Kelly, K., Pearson, M., Kurup, V., *et al*. A cluster of anaphylactic reactions in children with spina bifida during general anesthesia: epidemiologic features, risk factors, and latex hypersensitivity. *Journal of Allergy and Clinical Immunology* 1994; **94**: 53–61.

66 Lebenbom-Mansour, M.H., Oesterle, J.R., Ownby, D.R., *et al*. The incidence of latex sensitivity in ambulatory surgical patients: a correlation of historical factors with positive serum immunoglobin E levels. *Anesthesia and Analgesia* 1997; **85**: 44–9.

67 Holzman, R.S. Clinical management of latex-allergic children. *Anesthesia and Analgesia* 1997; **85**: 529–33.

68 Ownby, D. and McCullough, J. Testing for latex allergy. *Journal of Clinical Immunoassay* 1993; **16**: 109–17.

69 Slater, J.E. Allergic reactions to natural rubber. *Annals of Allergy* 1992; **68**: 203–9.

70 Setlock, M. Latex allergy; failure of prophylaxis to prevent severe reaction. *Anesthesia and Analgesia* 1993; **76**: 650–2.

71 Swanson, M.C., Bubak, M.E., Hunt, L.W., *et al*. Quantification of occupational latex aeroallergens in a medical center. *Journal of Allergy and Clinical Immunology* 1994; **94**: 445–51.

72 Birmingham, P., Dsida, R. and Grayhack, J. Do latex precautions in children with myelodysplasia reduce intraoperative allergic reactions? *Journal of Pediatric Orthopedics* 1996; **16**: 799–802.

CHAPTER 21

Anaesthesia and sedation outside the operating room

MICHAEL SURY

INTRODUCTION

The recent increase in the numbers of investigations and interventions by paediatricians and radiologists has created an enormous demand for anaesthesia and sedation services. This chapter covers sedation and anaesthesia for a wide range of procedures outside operating rooms.

The most difficult issue associated with sedation is safety. In adult patients safety is virtually guaranteed if verbal contact is preserved, whereas usually in children procedures can only be carried out if they are asleep. Anaesthesia resources are limited so it is inevitable that non-anaesthetists must give sedation. Sedation is less reliable than anaesthesia and is often falsely considered to be cheaper and safer. Drugs and techniques are important, and those in common use are detailed, but the safety of sedation is dependent on the sedationist and this problem is discussed in depth. The general and specific requirements for both sedation and anaesthesia, including facilities, equipment and personnel, are examined and, finally, the economic, safety and quality factors are considered for planning services outside the operating room.

WHICH PROCEDURES CAN TAKE PLACE OUTSIDE THE OPERATING ROOM?

Awake adult patients should be co-operative enough to tolerate most minor procedures but for many children success can only be achieved with either sedation or anaesthesia. Recently, because medical investigations and interventions have increased, the problems of providing high-quality, safe sedation or anaesthesia services have become prominent.[1–7] In the past, procedures were often carried out under sedation using a technique relying on intramuscular drugs, local anaesthesia and physical restraint, whereas now these sometimes painful and unpleasant procedures are often repeated, and children and parents demand a higher quality service. The sheer numbers of children involved are so large that, inevitably, there is debate about whether certain procedures justify sedation and anaesthesia.[8,9]

Operating rooms are a scarce resource and are used most efficiently for procedures that need the operating personnel and equipment. Any procedure, therefore, that could be performed safely outside the operating room is considered in this chapter. Table 21.1 lists the main procedures that either cannot or may not be done in operating rooms, and together they represent a considerable workload in paediatric hospitals.

DEFINING SEDATION AND ANAESTHESIA

As an individual becomes progressively more deeply unconscious a point is reached at which respiratory reflexes fail to maintain a patent airway and adequate breathing, and as a consequence hypoxia occurs. The glottic reflexes which prevent pulmonary aspiration of gastric contents also fail eventually, as do the control of heart rate and vascular tone. The level of consciousness is difficult to measure and define

Table 21.1 Common paediatric procedures performed outside the operating room requiring sedation or anaesthesia

Imaging	Magnetic resonance imaging (MRI), cardiac angiography, interventional radiology, neuro- and general angiography, computed tomography (CT), ultrasound, echocardiography
Medical procedures	Minor oncology procedures, lumbar puncture (LP), intrathecal injections and bone marrow aspiration (BMA), oesophagogastroscopy, colonoscopy, renal and hepatic biopsy, electroencephalography (EEG), brainstem evoked potentials (BSER), muscle and joint injections, eye examinations, wound care, insertion of intravenous lines, intensive care procedures
Dental treatment	Extractions, conservation, periodontal surgery, oral biopsy

and consequently the precise point at which these important protective reflexes are affected is unknown. It is clear, however, that there is considerable variation in the effects of sedation, not only between drugs and between patients but also with respect to the arousal stimulus of the procedure.

It is generally understood that sedation is a state of depression of the central nervous system from which the subject can be roused, whereas anaesthesia is an unrousable sleep state in which protective reflexes are lost. If non-anaesthetists (i.e. those without anaesthetic skills) use sedation which causes unintentional anaesthesia and they are unable to give prompt attention to the airway and breathing, death or cerebral damage can follow. Sadly, this avoidable situation has been known to occur and is probably under-reported.[1,10] In order to prevent sedation disasters safety guidelines and recommendations have been published by paediatricians,[11] radiologists,[12] anaesthetists,[12,13] surgeons,[14] dentists,[15–17] gastroenterologists[18] and accident and emergency physicians.[19] On the whole, these publications are helpful for children but there is a problem concerning the definition of safe sedation in children as opposed to adults.

CONSCIOUS SEDATION IS IMPRACTICAL IN CHILDREN

The Royal Colleges of Anaesthetists and Radiologists[12] have defined a state of conscious sedation which is 'depression of the nervous system – during which verbal contact is maintained'. Sedation deeper than this is an unconscious state which, in the UK at least, is considered to be equivalent to anaesthesia and should be administered only by anaesthetists. This concept of conscious sedation is usually practical for adults but not often for children.

Maintaining 'verbal contact' is very safe because it ensures that protective reflexes are maintained, but it is only useful in co-operative patients, and children – particularly ill children – are rarely in this category. Children do not lie still during uncomfortable or frightening procedures unless they are asleep. While it is true that it should be possible to rouse the sleeping child if necessary, trying to prove rousability during the procedure itself is impractical, especially if the procedure requires immobility. Conscious sedation for magnetic resonance imaging (MRI), for example, is not possible for the vast majority of small children.[20,21]

If it is accepted that sedation deeper than conscious sedation requires an anaesthetist, then a great many anaesthetists and support staff will be required. World-wide, in large paediatric hospitals where the demand for services has been greatest, this has been difficult to achieve and because of this problem, sedation services have been developed involving non-anaesthetists having to use sedation deeper than conscious sedation.

DEEP SEDATION

The American Academy of Pediatrics has suggested a defined state of 'deep sedation', which is deeper than conscious sedation but not anaesthesia, as:[11]

A medically controlled state of depressed consciousness or unconsciousness from which the patient is not easily roused. It may be accompanied by a partial or complete loss of protective reflexes and includes the inability to maintain a patent airway independently and respond purposefully to physical stimuli.

The problem with this definition is that it can be difficult to demonstrate the difference between deep sedation and anaesthesia and, for a patient in either state, respiratory depression and hypoxia can occur.

Obviously, what matters is that the sleeping patient can control the airway and breathing to maintain oxygen saturations and carbon dioxide levels, but it may not be possible to predict from one moment to the next whether this will continue. For imaging, children must be asleep to be still enough and yet defining their level of sedation is impractical. Whatever the depth, sleep must be safe. One suggested working definition of deep sedation for children is:

A technique in which the use of a drug or drugs produces a state of depression of the nervous system such that the patient is not easily roused but which has a safety margin wide enough to render the loss of airway and breathing reflexes unlikely.

PROBLEMS WITH SEDATION DRUGS

Sedatives such as benzodiazepines, major tranquillizers and opioids, given in standard doses, do not usually cause unconsciousness because they are not sufficiently potent. They will, however, cause an unrousable state if the dose is increased but the difference between the sedative and the anaesthetic dose is large enough to allow safe use by non-anaesthetists. Anaesthetic drugs are potent and although they can be given in subanaesthetic doses the difference between sedation and anaesthetic doses is small. If, therefore, a non-anaesthetist used subanaesthetic doses of potent drugs, anaesthetic skills would be required too often. In the UK recommendations emphasize that for sedation 'drugs and techniques should carry a margin of safety wide enough to render unintended loss of consciousness unlikely'.[12] Consequently, safe sedation drugs for use by non-anaesthetists are those which are not potent and consequently will not always succeed. Any truly sedative drug regimen therefore will have a failure rate and although increasing the doses can reduce the failure rate, more children will sleep too deeply. Moreover, sedation drugs have a long action and children will sleep for too long. Finally, the effect of a sedative is unpredictable and so even for standard doses there is a small risk of deep and prolonged sedation.

WHICH SEDATION DRUGS ARE SAFE?

Determining a new drug regimen for 'safe sleep' sedation by non-anaesthetists can be hazardous and hospitals have therefore developed their own unique drug regimen based on years of experience and usually by adapting anaesthesia sedative premedication. Because major complications of sedatives are uncommon the safety of a regimen can only be defined adequately by hundreds or thousands of cases and not by short clinical trials. Which regimen is best? Retrospective analyses aside, prospective and randomized comparisons of 'successful' regimens have not been undertaken because large numbers of cases would be needed to establish robust conclusions. Individual drugs are examined later, as are the drug regimen and techniques used for specific procedures. Nevertheless, the safety and success of sedation depends almost entirely on the use of protocols and on the medical and nursing staff who administer them.

ANAESTHETISTS OR NON-ANAESTHETISTS?

An anaesthetist has the benefit of both standard medical training and specialist anaesthetic training and can therefore combine particular knowledge and skills with judgement based on considerable experience. Non-anaesthetists can be taught about drugs and techniques and be trained to have relevant skills, but it takes years to achieve experience and good judgement. Anaesthetists also have a formal system of training, assessment by examination, specialist registration and collegiate recommendation and regulation. In contrast, non-anaesthetists must rely on standard medical training and informal sedation training and experience, which is extremely variable; there are no national courses or qualifications in paediatric sedation. There are few well-organized sedation units staffed by senior and experienced doctors and it is not unusual for sedation to be administered by unsupervised trainees. Nurses have an extremely valuable role in sedation since they can achieve a good level of judgement and experience over time.

Considering all the problems of non-anaesthetists and the restricted number of drugs that they are permitted to use, anaesthesia by anaesthetists seems a better option. The insurmountable problem with this approach is that the anaesthetist human resource is limited and, whenever it is overwhelmed, a sedation service by non-anaesthetists must be considered. Protocols or guidelines should be developed which suit the specific requirements of the procedure; for example, procedures such as colonoscopy require analgesia, whereas imaging is painless and requires immobility.

DEVELOPING SAFE AND SUCCESSFUL SEDATION BY NON-ANAESTHETISTS

Protocols must be both safe and successful. The following principles have been helpful in developing sedation protocols at Great Ormond Street Children's Hospital in London (GOSH) and have been based on local experience as well as on reports and recommendations from the elsewhere in the UK and from the USA.[11,12,15,19,22] Other paediatric hospitals have produced their own protocols and guidelines and, although there are differences in detail, the general theme of safety is common to all.[7,23-25] In defining these principles it must be understood that, in general, safety reduces success and vice versa. A success rate of near 100% probably means that some children are anaesthetized, whereas principles of safety are designed to prevent sedation becoming too deep and they therefore reduce the success rate. Sedation protocols must also balance safety with success.

PRINCIPLES OF SAFETY

CONTRAINDICATIONS

Children with the conditions listed in Table 21.2 are more at risk of hypoxia than others and they must therefore be managed by anaesthetists. The list covers common contraindications and cannot be fully comprehensive: inevitably there will be children who have unusual problems which make sedation unwise. Whenever there is doubt an anaesthetist should be consulted.

PATIENT ASSESSMENT

The responsibility for patient assessment is shared between the referring doctor and the sedationist. Assessment should take place before admission by the referring clinician, who should relay all relevant clinical details to the sedationist. The patient must be reassessed on admission (Table 21.3).

DRUG POINTS

The drugs must be unlikely to cause unrousable sleep, apnoea or airway obstruction.

The chosen drug regimen should have a proven safety record in paediatric sedation.

Drug regimen doses must not be exceeded and a failure rate must therefore be accepted. Increasing the doses may not necessarily achieve successful images and can make a child sleepy for hours. Occasionally, sedation must be abandoned because of a distress reaction with crying and aggressive behaviour caused perhaps by dizziness, anxiety or hallucinations.

Table 21.2 Common contraindications for sedation in children

Patients should not be sedated by non-anaesthetists if they have any of the following:

1. Airway problems
   Any actual or potential airway obstruction, e.g. snoring or stridor, blocked nose, small mandible, large tongue
2. Apnoeic spells
   Related to brain damage or previous drug treatment
3. Respiratory disease
   SpO_2 less than 94% in air, respiratory failure (high respiratory rate, oxygen treatment), inability to cough or cry
4. High intracranial pressure
   Drowsiness, headache, vomiting
5. Epilepsy
   Generalized convulsions requiring rectal diazepam within the last 24 h or rectal diazepam used more frequently than once in 2 weeks
   Previous adverse reaction to sedation, i.e. exacerbation of seizures
   Children requiring resuscitation during a convulsion within the last month
   Children who not only have convulsions but also have other major neurological or neuromuscular disease, e.g. apnoeic spells or hypotonia as part of global neurological disease; intracranial hypertension due to cerebral tumour or encephalitis.
   Generalized convulsions with cyanosis more frequent than once per day
   Children who have had a convulsion less than 4 h before sedation
   Failure to regain full consciousness and mobility after a recent convulsion
6. Risk of pulmonary aspiration of gastric contents
   Abdominal distension, appreciable volumes draining from NG tube, vomiting
7. Severe metabolic, liver or renal disease
   Requiring i.v. fluids or dextrose, jaundice or abdominal distension, requiring peritoneal or haemodialysis

Table 21.3   Presentation checklist for nurses

History
Age and weight
Scan required
Indication for scan
Diseases/syndromes: check for contraindications to sedation
Drugs
Allergies
Previous sedation
Previous problems with anaesthesia
Intercurrent disease, e.g. upper respiratory tract infections or gastroenteritis
Children must return another day if:
tempadot > 38°C (that day), nasal secretions (capable of blocking nose), generally unwell, productive cough, rash or earache

Physical examination	
General	Weight, heart rate, respiratory rate, temperature: check within normal limits
Airway	Clear nasal breathing, easy mouth opening, normal mandible and tongue
Breathing	No cough, wheeze, or oxygen requirement
	$SpO_2 > 93\%$ in air
Circulation	Not dehydrated
	If appropriate, check BP within normal limits
Abdomen	No abdominal distension

Special investigations
Check notes for recent blood tests: inform doctor of abnormal results
Hb > 9 g dl^{-1}, no sickle cell disease

Anaesthesia should not be administered soon after sedation has failed because combined effects could cause prolonged recovery. Unless the imaging is urgent, patients should return for anaesthesia another day.

PERSONNEL

Each sedated child must be attended by a nurse or doctor until awake enough to respond easily to verbal command. The doctor or nurse must have suitable paediatric experience and be trained in paediatric resuscitation.

An assistant, either a nurse or a doctor, trained in paediatric resuscitation must be available immediately.

The procedure for which the sedation is given should be carried out by someone who is not the sedationist, i.e. a doctor or nurse should concentrate solely on the sedation and wellbeing of the patient. (in adult practice the operator–sedationist principle has been accepted for conscious sedation, at least in dentistry).

Either a doctor or a nurse should take a lead role in the organization and administration of the sedation.

An experienced doctor must be available to assist with sedation problems and resuscitation promptly.

Sedation should not take place 'out of hours' when skilled staff are not available.

FACILITIES

There must be sufficient space for a trolley, a chair, sedation monitoring and resuscitation equipment. There must be space for four adults (a parent, a sedationist, an operator and an assistant)

For MRI there must be an area close to the scanner which is free from all magnetic restrictions. This area can be used for induction, recovery and resuscitation.

There must be a facility for overnight admission if recovery is prolonged.

EQUIPMENT

The following equipment must be available for each patient under sedation: a pulse oximeter, and equipment for monitoring electrocardiogram (ECG), non-invasive blood pressure, oxygen, airways and suction, and a tipping patient trolley; capnography should also be available for remote monitoring of breathing.

The following equipment must be available in the sedation unit or ward: a resuscitation trolley with airways, tracheal tubes and laryngoscopes of all sizes, T-piece breathing system, self-inflating bags (large and small), tracheal suction tubes and resuscitation drugs. A drug cupboard and refrigerator containing relevant sedation, reversal and muscle-relaxant drugs (sedation regimen drugs, naloxone, flumazenil, atropine and suxamethonium) and a defribrillator.

FASTING BEFORE SEDATION

Pulmonary aspiration of gastric contents can occur if the protective reflexes of the glottis are obtunded during deep sedation. For most situations when deep sedation is planned fasting guidelines should be the same as for general anaesthesia: food or milk should not be taken later than 6 h before sedation and clear fluid 2 h beforehand.

RECOVERY AND DISCHARGE CRITERIA

Children should be easily roused and be able to drink unaided before discharge. A few children will recover slowly and need overnight admission.

PRINCIPLES OF SUCCESS

SELECTION OF PROCEDURE

Sedation is least likely to be successful for procedures which are painful and prolonged. Many procedures are therefore best managed by anaesthetists (see section under Specific procedures).

SEDATION AREA

Sedation provides a window of time when the child is asleep and therefore children should be sedated as near to the procedure as possible to reduce wasting time in transport. For imaging, the area must be as quiet as possible to encourage sleep.

FAST SCANNING, FAST PROCEDURES

Modern, fast, quiet scanners will reduce the sedation failure rate. Scanning protocols should minimize the time of routine scans; non-routine scans should be planned by a radiologist. Any procedure should be performed as quickly and

skilfully as possible by experienced doctors or nurses.

SELECTION OF CHILDREN

Sedation is unlikely to be successful in children with severe behavioural disorders, severe epileptics and children older than 8 years or larger than 30 kg with developmental delay. These children, as well as those who have failed sedation previously, should have a general anaesthetic.

DRUGS

The following drugs are valuable for sedation of children. Drug doses and technique descriptions are summarized only and the reader is encouraged to consult the relevant references for more detail. Later, drugs and techniques relevant to specific procedures are discussed.

CHORAL HYDRATE AND TRICLOFOS

Both of these drugs are effective sedatives and can be administered by mouth, are well absorbed and are metabolized to the active metabolite trichloroethanol. Chloral hydrate has an unpleasant taste and causes gastric irritation but can be given rectally. There has been concern over chloral hydrate being a liver carcinogen in mice, although there is no evidence of this problem in humans.[26]

The literature contains a wealth of chloral hydrate studies in which large numbers of infants and children have been successfully sedated for non-painful imaging.[23,25,27–31] In one study, approximately 2000 children under 18 months received up to 100 mg kg^{-1} chloral hydrate without respiratory complications and 99% were successfully sedated.[23] In another, 854 children were sedated (dose up to 132 mg kg^{-1}), four children had airway obstruction, 11 vomited and the failure rate was 3% (six children had paradoxical reactions with excitement and agitation).[27] The younger the children the greater the success, although desaturations (5.4% of cases) were more common in infants.[27]

Triclofos is more palatable than chloral but is less potent (1 g triclofos = 600 mg chloral hydrate). In a respiratory laboratory setting infants over 6 months old sedated with 100 mg kg^{-1} triclofos and infants less than 6 months receiving 75 mg kg^{-1} fall asleep within 10–80 min without significant respiratory depression.[32] Triclofos in 'subsedation' doses, and probably also choral hydrate, has the advantage of reducing distressed behaviour[33] without altering conscious level.

BENZODIAZEPINES

Midazolam

Midazolam is water soluble, can be administered by many routes and causes anxiolysis, sedation and amnesia. Compared with diazepam in adults it is four to five times more potent, and in children has both a shorter elimination half-life and a much shorter action.[34,35] Intravenously, its sedative effect can be increased by careful titration but its effect on conscious level is variable, unpredictable and depends largely on the discomfort of the procedure. Sedation for oesophagoscopy can be satisfactory in children over 8 years after 0.05–0.1 mg kg^{-1} titrated over 5 min.[36] For minor oncology procedures an intravenous bolus of 0.05 mg kg^{-1} repeated to a maximum dose of 0.2 mg kg^{-1} has been used for conscious sedation safely and recovery is usual by 1 h.[37] At these doses mild desaturation related to the degree of sedation occurs but is easily corrected by stimulation or by oxygen treatment. The intravenous dose sufficient for deep sedation or anaesthesia is unpredictable but is usually greater than 0.5 mg kg^{-1}.[38] Although apnoea or airway obstruction is unlikely, it must always be expected as a possibility, especially when it is used in combination with other sedatives whose effects are also unpredictable.[37,39–41] Unconsciousness has occurred after 0.5 mg kg^{-1} (orally) in association with intravenous erythromycin, which has an hepatic enzyme-inhibiting effect.[42] Amnesia, an important property for children who must undergo repeated procedures, can occur in up to 90% of children.[37] As with diazepam, occasionally midazolam can cause paradoxical distressed behaviour[43] and sedation may have to be abandoned.

Midazolam is absorbed well enterally and via the mucosa of the mouth and nose. By mouth, 0.5 mg kg^{-1} prevents crying before anaesthesia in most children if administered 30 min beforehand,[44,45] but there are children who still cry[46] and higher doses are associated with loss of balance and dysphoria.[47] Its taste is extremely bitter and the intravenous preparation must therefore be mixed with a sweetening agent such as cola, fruit juice (1 ml kg^{-1}) or paracetamol syrup to make it palatable.

Intranasal midazolam drops, 0.2 mg kg^{-1}, repeated once 5–15 min later if necessary, effectively calm small children and infants for cardiac echocardiography and other imaging,[48,49] but this route is unpleasant and causes crying, coughing and sneezing.[49] The absorption via the nose is rapid and the pharmacokinetic profiles of intranasal and intravenous midazolam are similar:[35] apnoea and desaturation occur occasionally.[49] Sublingual administration is more pleasant, as well as rapid and equally effective, although it requires co-operation.[50]

Rectal midazolam is useful: 0.3–1 mg kg^{-1} causes conscious sedation[51,52] and doses up to 5 mg kg^{-1} have been used but without significant benefit.[52] Unconsciousness has occurred in a child after 4.5 mg kg^{-1}.[52]

Diazepam

In its lipid formulation (diazemuls), diazepam is useful intravenously for its longer action than midazolam. Doses of 0.1–1 mg kg^{-1} have been used but, as with midazolam, titration to effect must be by small doses (0.1 mg kg^{-1}) with 30–60 s between each dose. Despite its prolonged elimination half-life, recovery is usually sufficient after 2 h or so, even in combination with other drugs.[53] Nevertheless, residual and prolonged sedation occasionally occurs.

Flumazenil

Residual benzodiazepine sedation can usually be reversed by flumazenil, either 20–30 μg kg^{-1} i.v.[54] or 20–40 μg kg^{-1} per rectum.[55] It should be remembered that the half-life of flumazenil is shorter than that of some benzodiazepines, so that resedation can, at least in theory, occur.

BARBITURATES

Thiopentone and methohexitone

Barbiturates are extremely effective sedatives. Thiopentone and methohexitone are short-acting intravenous agents which have been used successfully in single-drug techniques. They are so potent that respiratory effects are to be expected; they must therefore be used only by anaesthetists. Thiopentone 6 mg kg^{-1} i.v. reliably induces unconsciousness and immobility[3,56] which lasts for approximately 20–30 min provided there are no painful stimuli: airway support is required in 1% of cases.[56] Methohexitone intravenously has a shorter action and, unlike thiopentone, it can, if necessary, be used intramuscularly (10 mg kg^{-1} of 3.5 or 5% solution[57] or 8 mg kg^{-1} of 5% solution[58]).

Both drugs are effective after rectal administration but there is a risk of respiratory depression. Thiopentone 25–50 mg kg^{-1} causes sleep within 30 min and lasts for approximately 45 min.[24,59] Methohexitone 30 mg kg^{-1} achieved sleep in 85% of a series of 648 patients, but two children required airway interventions by an anaesthetist.[60] Sleep begins approximately 10–15 min after 30 mg kg^{-1} methohexitone and lasts for a variable time between 30 and 90 min.[61–63] Defaecation after rectal administration can be prevented by holding the buttocks together or by introducing the drug via a balloon-tipped catheter, which is held in place for 10–15 min. Further doses can then be added if necessary.

Pentobarbitone and secobarbitone

Pentobarbitone can be administered enterally as well as intravenously and intramuscularly. By mouth or rectum its effect is less predictable, causing sedation in 15–60 min and lasting for 1–4 h. It is usually given intravenously, its effect starting in 1 min and lasting for 15 min. As with other potent barbiturates, airway events and apnoeas may occur and are more likely at higher doses and with fast administration. In a technique using 2–6 mg kg^{-1} i.v. (slow boluses of 2.5, 2.5 and 1 mg kg^{-1}, separated by at least 30 s) in 225 children, sedation for imaging was successful in all but two children.[64] Oxygen saturation decreased to 80% in 17 cases, of which three had airway obstruction and one had 2 min of apnoea: all were treated by moving the head position and with stimulation. Pentobarbitone is not available in the UK but in the USA and Canada it is used by non-anaesthetists, particularly in radiology settings.[24,65]

Secobarbitone, in a report of 300 cases, has been used successfully per rectum; a dose of 5–7 mg kg^{-1} causes sleep in 10–15 min and recovery is usual 45 min after painless imaging.[66]

PROPOFOL

The short action and lack of side-effects make propofol the best of all the intravenous agents. Propofol has been used as a single drug to cause deep sedation or anaesthesia for painless procedures and imaging.[65,67–73] Initial and transient mild desaturation is common (5%) and oxygen treatment is usually effective. Occasionally, airway obstruction occurs which may need more than extension of the head and for this reason propofol is not recommended for use by non-anaesthetists. After sleep has been induced by 2–4 mg kg^{-1} of propofol it is usually maintained by an infusion of 6–8 mg kg^{-1}h;[3,65,71,73] recovery is pleasant and can occur within a few minutes.

It is not recommended for children younger than 3 years. In a few children propofol does not reliably cause immobility and in this respect it is not as reliable as inhalational anaesthesia.[74] Tolerance and behavioural disturbances are also described with propofol and methohexitone has been used successfully in these children instead.[75]

OPIOIDS

Used alone, opioids are not effective for causing immobility or sleep. In small doses, however, and used in combination with sedatives, they provide necessary analgesia for uncomfortable or painful procedures. This requires more care than single-drug techniques since the combined respiratory depressant effects of sedatives and opioids are well known to be supra-additive and unpredictable.[39] Opioids have a long history of safe use for sedative premedication before anaesthesia and are known to calm children without necessarily affecting conscious level.[76] Of all the sedatives, only opioids, midazolam and triclofos (and probably chloral hydrate) have this useful property.[33,76]

Morphine

Intramuscular papaveretum (the active component being morphine) has a safe record in children over 15 kg for imaging when combined with hyoscine, trimeprazine and diazepam.[77] For short, painful procedures 60 μg kg^{-1} of morphine has been used combined with 0.05 mg kg^{-1} midazolam i.v. (additional midazolam used if necessary up to 0.15 mg kg^{-1}) without major respiratory effects in a series of 35 children, except for one child who desaturated to 67%.[37]

Fentanyl

Intravenously, this potent drug has a much shorter action than morphine but is more likely to cause apnoea. In combination with i.v. midazolam, 1–6 μg kg^{-1} fentanyl has been used for upper gastrointestinal endoscopy in a series of 61 children, of whom three had prolonged desaturation requiring naloxone.[41] A smaller dose may be safe, as 0.6 μg kg^{-1} of fentanyl has been added to 0.05 mg kg^{-1} midazolam i.v. (additional midazolam used if necessary up to 0.15 mg kg^{-1}) to provide successful conscious sedation for lumbar puncture and bone marrow aspiration.[37] Combined with ketamine, 1 μg kg^{-1} of fentanyl has been used for cardiac angiography in 202 children, of whom five needed controlled ventilation either because of apnoea or because of laryngospasm.[78]

Fentanyl is absorbed from the mucosa of the mouth and oral transmucosal fentanyl citrate has been prepared both as a lozenge (15–20 μg kg^{-1}) and in the form of a palatable lollipop (20–25 μg kg^{-1}). These doses cause effective analgesia and sedation for painful procedures, but side-effects include vomiting (30%) and desaturation (10%).[79,80]

Pethidine

Combined with 0.05–0.1 mg kg^{-1} of i.v. midazolam (max. dose 0.4 mg kg^{-1} or 10 mg), 0.5–1 mg kg^{-1} of i.v. pethidine (max. dose 50 mg kg^{-1}) is effective sedation for upper gastrointestinal endoscopy, and of 553 children in one study, 16 had prolonged oxygen desaturation.[41] Of 30 children given 2 mg kg^{-1} of pethidine and 0.1 mg kg^{-1} of diazepam i.v. for endoscopy, none had respiratory depression but four had prolonged sedation for up to 6 h afterwards.[53]

Naloxone

Whenever opioids are used for sedation, naloxone must be available. An i.v. dose of 40 μg kg^{-1} should reverse respiratory depression but may need to be repeated.

MAJOR TRANQUILLIZERS

Trimeprazine

This oral sedative, in doses of 3–4 mg kg^{-1}, causes sleep in approximately 50% of children before anaesthesia but at these doses there have been reports of hypotension and unconsciousness, and as a consequence the maximum recommended dose is 2 mg kg^{-1}. At this dose it has a long and safe history of being combined with intramuscular morphine for sedation of children over 15 kg for MRI.[77]

Chlorpromazine and promethazine

These two drugs have been combined together with pethidine to form a 'lytic cocktail' also known as DPT (demerol, phenergan, thorazine), MPC (meperidine, promethazine, chlorpromazine) and pethidine compound. One millilitre of the mixture contains 25 mg pethidine, 6.25 mg chlorpromazine and 6.25 mg promethazine. It combines analgesia, anxiolysis and sedation and effective doses are between 0.06 and 0.1 ml kg^{-1} i.m. With the addition of oral triclofos and intravenous diazmuls, pethidine compound is a useful technique for sedation of children under 15 kg for MRI.[77] Pethidine compound can be effective enough for diagnostic cardiac angiography in small children but it occasionally causes respiratory depression[81].

Droperidol

Used alone, droperidol has the reputation for causing adults to appear calm while being extremely anxious. Dystonic reactions may also occur but are rarely seen at an oral dose of 0.25 mg kg^{-1} (max. dose 5 mg). Combined with temazepam 1 mg kg^{-1} orally, 0.25 mg kg^{-1} of droperidol (i.v. diazemuls up to 1 mg kg^{-1} may be given) sedates over 95% of children successfully for MRI (see Table 21.4).

NITROUS OXIDE

Nitrous oxide provides valuable pain relief and sedation for dental treatment. The method of application (relative analgesia) has been described by Roberts:[82] he recommends gradual increases in inspired concentration from 30% up to 70% in oxygen via a nasal mask because high concentrations too quickly result in loss of verbal contact. Combining nitrous oxide with 0.5 mg kg^{-1} midazolam orally reduces the inspired concentration requirement to 15%.[83] Desaturation due to the Fink effect does not occur.[84] Entonox, delivered via a demand valve, may be useful for short, painful procedures and can be used provided the child is big enough and co-operative enough to hold a facemask or a mouth piece.[85] The higher concentration of 70% is more effective than 50% but is more likely to cause excitement, dysphoria, nausea and restlessness.[86]

Table 21.4 Intramuscular sedation drug regimen for MR scans (given on ward, remote from scanner)

< 45 weeks' gestation	Nil, feed only
> 45 weeks but < 5 kg	Triclofos 50 mg kg^{-1} p.o.
5–15 kg	Triclofos 50 mg kg^{-1} p.o. and Inj. pethidine compound[a] 0.06 ml kg^{-1} i.m. (to be given 45 min before scan; check with MR staff for timing)
> 15 kg	Trimeprazine 2 mg kg^{-1} (max. dose 80 mg) p.o. and morphine 0.2 mg kg^{-1} (max. dose 10 mg) i.m. (to be given 1 h before scan; check with MR staff for timing)

Additional sedation, i.v. diazemuls (0.2–0.3 mg kg^{-1} i.v.) may be given in the MR unit

[a]1 ml of Inj. pethidine compound contains 25 mg pethidine, 6.25 mg chlorpromazine and 6.25 mg promethazine.

KETAMINE

This unique anaesthetic drug has the ability to cause sedation or anaesthesia (depending on the dose) and potent analgesia. In addition to these properties, its lack of effects on airway patency and breathing, and its ability to cause mild tachycardia and hypertension, make ketamine an extremely useful drug when other methods of anaesthesia are either not available or not practical.[87] It has, however, several drawbacks. It causes pharyngeal secretions which can provoke laryngospasm, although in a series of 11 589 administrations tracheal intubation was required only twice.[88] Apnoea can also occur and although this is probably less likely at low doses it has been described following 4 mg kg^{-1} i.m.[89,90] If ketamine is combined with opioids, apnoea is more likely.[91] Ketamine has a reputation for safety, to the extent that it has been suggested that it is safe enough for use by non-anaesthetists.[90,92–95] The author believes that non-anaesthetists would require special training and protocols to ensure safe practice and, in any case, ketamine anaesthesia is neither as pleasant nor as safe as other available techniques.[96]

Two lesser but still important side-effects are nausea and vomiting, which may be as frequent as 15–33%,[96,97] and distressing hallucinations,[98,99] which still occur in 3% of cases even when ketamine is combined with midazolam.[92] Distressing hallucinations may be less common in small children.

Orally, ketamine is absorbed well; 6 mg kg^{-1} causes sedation between 10 and 20 min[100] and recovery after 10 mg kg^{-1} is usual by 2 h.[101] Ketamine is also effective after rectal[102] and intranasal[103,104] administration.

SPECIFIC PROCEDURES AND THEIR REQUIREMENTS FOR SEDATION AND ANAESTHESIA

The greatest demand for sedation and anaesthesia outside operating rooms is for MRI, minor oncology procedures, cardiac angiography, interventional radiology, gastrointestinal endoscopy and dental treatment.

MAGNETIC RESONANCE IMAGING

Procedure details

Routine brain imaging requires perfect immobility for at least 20 min, although scanners are becoming faster. Other scanning sequences can take up to 90 min. Although the procedure is not painful, it is often difficult to persuade children to lie still in the noisy, frightening and enclosed environment. Infants less than 3 months should sleep naturally after a feed and children older than 8 years may be co-operative enough but, otherwise, the vast majority of other children need drug-induced sleep. An intravenous injection of the 'magnetic contrast' gadalinium is sometimes required.

Sedation strategy

Table 21.5 presents a general protocol in which most children undergo sedation and anaesthesia is reserved for children in whom sedation is contraindicated or in whom sedation has already failed. At GOSH, from 1989 to 1996, sedation for MRI was based on intramuscular sedation administered on the ward (Table 21.5) and had a success rate of 80–85%. Since 1996 an oral sedation regimen has been used (Table 21.6), modified from a regimen developed in

Birmingham. It is administered next to the scanner, an important factor in achieving its success rate of over 95%. Other hospitals have their own sedation regimens and also achieve high success; chloral hydrate, in particular, is used widely.[23–25,28,29] Two potent intravenous drugs, ketamine and pentobarbitone, have been suggested for use by non-anaesthetists. Ketamine, although preserving airway and breathing, does not prevent patient movement unless given in high doses, when it can cause airway events such as salivation and apnoea. Intravenous pentobarbitone can cause about 1 h of sleep in almost all children and is therefore successful.[23,24,64] It is used by non-anaesthetists in Canada and the USA but is not available in the UK because of concerns about barbiturate misuse.

Points of safety and success

To avoid sedation failure children must be sedated in a quiet area next to the scanner and it is crucial for safety reasons that this area is free of all magnetic restrictions (see Anaesthesia section). At GOSH a nurse-led service provides a safe and high-quality sedation service. Experienced radiology nurses follow a protocol, in which they assess and check children (Table 21.3) and both chart and administer the

Table 21.6 Birmingham oral sedation drug regimen for MRI (modified by GOSH and given in sedation area next to scanner)[129]

< 45 weeks' gestation	Nil, feed only
> 45 weeks but < 5 kg	Chloral hydrate 50 mg kg^{-1} p.o.
< 10 kg	Chloral hydrate 100 mg kg^{-1}
10–20 kg	Temazepam 1 mg kg^{-1} with droperidol 0.25 mg kg^{-1}
> 20 kg	As directed by radiologist (droperidol max. dose 5 mg)

Intravenous sedation top-up to be considered if oral sedation is not effective after 20–30 min [diazemuls up to 1 mg kg^{-1} (max. dose 20 mg); slowly i.v. 30% to 60% to 100%]. Sedation reversal if necessary: flumazenil 10–20 μg kg^{-1}

Table 21.5 General protocol: how to keep children still for imaging

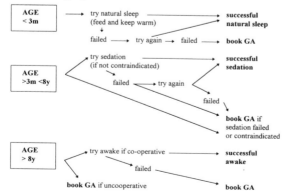

sedation drugs, including intravenous diazemuls (Table 21.6). Training within the hospital maintains their resuscitation and airway skills (Table 21.7) and a radiologist is always nearby. Often a radiologist must decide whether the images are satisfactory and whether it is necessary and safe to continue with sedation. Hungry and thirsty children are irritable and resist sedation, and so with the nurse-led service the fasting policy has been modified so that children are allowed a light meal or milk up to 3 h before sedation. Clear fluid in small volumes is unrestricted and 5 ml kg^{-1} is administered with the oral sedation. If sedation fails in an infant or small child, food, given an hour or so later, may make them sleepy enough for imaging to be successful (good judgement by experienced medical and nursing staff is essential).

Children should be comforted by their parents and as soon as the child falls asleep, pulse oximetry monitoring should start and continue until recovery. A nurse stays with each child throughout the sedation and imaging and watches the breathing. A fibreoptic pulse oximeter is used during imaging (see section on Equipment for anaesthesia in MRI) and its display can be seen from the scanning room through a screen. Other monitors may rouse the child but capnography may be helpful if catheters are placed carefully next to the nose or mouth.

Anaesthesia

Technical problems with monitoring and equipment in MRI[105–108] are presented in Table 21.8. It is extremely important to have an area next to the scanner where patients can be sedated, recovered and, if necessary, resuscitated without any magnetic restriction. Any metal on or within a patient may prevent safe and accurate imaging and radiology departments have a responsibility to check patients for incompatible implants and attachments: cerebral arterial clips and cardiac pacemakers are unsafe for MRI, although they are unusual in children. Technical problems are greater the stronger the magnetic field; for example, weak ferric magnets with a field of 0.3 Tesla may be compatible with conventional pulse oximetry but superconducting magnets can generate 1.5–3 Tesla and require fibreoptic pulse oximetry. Before purchase of the scanner the manufacturers should

Table 21.7 Sedation training for nurses

Nurses are considered suitable to sedate children if they are experienced with children, can demonstrate the necessary skills and show good clinical judgement during a period of supervised work. The Radiology Director, with agreement from the nursing and anaesthesia departments, decides whether a nurse can be a designated sedationist.

Skills training

The nurse sedationist must be able to demonstrate:
Skill 1   Maintenance of a clear airway, including insertion of an oropharyngeal airway
Skill 2   Chest inflation using self-inflating bag
Skill 3   Recovery from anaesthesia using the T-piece
These skills are taught as follows:
A Resuscitation Training Officer teaches:
(a) Basic life-support training, which is a 3-h multidisciplinary session covering theoretical aspects of paediatric resuscitation (no equipment training) and
(b) Paediatric resuscitation workshop, which is a full-day session especially for nurses, concentrating on practical skills and equipment (skills 1 and 2)
In theatre:
One day in the operating theatre for training and assessment of skills 1 and 2 by a Consultant Anaesthetist
Two days in the Theatre Recovery Ward, where skill 3 will be taught and assessed by the Recovery Nurses

Training record and assessment

There must be a good record of training. Airway skills must be maintained and assessed every 3 months; this can be done during GA lists by a Consultant Anaesthetist. Also, whenever possible, there should be instruction in intravenous cannulation.

give advice on compatible monitoring. Broadly, however, there are two solutions to the problem of equipment and monitoring during MRI.

The first option is that fully compatible and comprehensive monitoring is available and can be used next to the patient in the magnetic field to allow the anaesthetist to stay in the room. This monitoring is expensive but is essential if

Table 21.8 Technical problems with monitoring and equipment for MRI

Technical problem	Details
Ferromagnetic equipment may be attracted to the strong magnetic field	Special equipment or strict policy with ferromagnetic equipment required Steel gas cylinders are dangerous: use piped gas only Non-ferromagnetic patient trolleys
Conventional electrical monitoring produces electromagnetic noise which disrupts image acquisition	Powerful MR scanners are screened by a copper shield within the walls, ceiling and floor of the scanning room Conducting cables passing through the screen to the scanning room will transfer electromagnetic interference and disrupt imaging
During scanning, the changing magnetic gradients induce electric current	Conventional electrical monitoring inside the scanning room may not function Coiled wires can burn skin Metallic implants must be checked for compatibility

anaesthesia and recovery areas which are free of magnetic restrictions are not available.

Alternatively, the anaesthetist stays out of the scanning room and observes the patient via a screen. Blood-pressure, airway gas analysis, pulse-oximetry and ECG monitors stay with the anaesthetist in the observation room and are connected to the patient by extended tubes and cables (up to a distance of 10 m) through a hole in the copper shield. Blood-pressure and gas-analysis machines can be conventional and connecting tubes pose no problem because they are non-conducting. In small infants, however, non-invasive blood-pressure measurement at range is not easy because the frequency and small amplitude of the pressure changes may be damped by the length of tubing. Conventional pulse oximetry needs to be replaced with monitors with fibreoptic cables which, although less robust, give a good signal at range and neither affect nor are affected by magnetic fields. ECG electrodes and cables are alloy and carbon fibre and the electrical signals need to pass through filters to remove frequencies which distort the image; the ECG and filters should be provided by the manufacturer.

Anaesthesia machines do not pose major problems provided gas pipelines are installed. Steel gas cylinders are extremely dangerous and aluminium substitutes hold a much lower pressure. MR-compatible machines are not expensive and conventional machines can be secured to the wall at a safe distance. Vaporizers are made of high-grade steel which is not magnetic and the bimetallic strip is not affected significantly by the magnetic field. Extending the length of breathing systems need not adversely affect their resistance or performance. In critically ill children, extensions of intravenous tubing allow the infusion of cardiac drugs at range but care must be taken not to allow infusion pumps too close to the magnetic field since they can malfunction.[74]

Anaesthesia techniques vary according to patient requirements. Many children have neurological or other abnormalities which require a technique to control the airway and breathing. Others (those in whom sedation is not contraindicated) can be managed using a propofol infusion or thiopentone with or without airway support,[65,67,68,70–72,109] although in a small number of children the intravenous techniques fail to prevent movement during scanning.[74] Rectal thiopentone is another alternative.[59] Critically ill children can be managed in MRI with careful planning,[108] but the value of imaging must be balanced against the risks of remote anaesthesia and transportation of unstable patients.

MINOR PAINFUL ONCOLOGY PROCEDURES (LUMBAR PUNCTURE, INTRATHECAL INJECTIONS AND BONE MARROW ASPIRATION)

Procedure details

These short, painful procedures often have to be repeated, frequently in children who may be very distressed by their illness and who do not tolerate discomfort.[8]

Sedation strategy

Conscious sedation in older children using midazolam or fentanyl or nitrous oxide can be successful and local anaesthesia skin cream also helps.[8,37,79] Some older children can be taught coping strategies for these procedures which are probably an integral part of the psychological management of the illness.[110] Nevertheless, uncooperative, anxious and younger children need deep sedation or anaesthesia to undergo these procedures without causing excessive distress.[8] Anaesthesia is also feared by many but, on balance, it is best for most of these patients because it removes all memory of the procedure itself.

Points of safety and success

In the USA ketamine is used successfully by non-anaesthetists as it provides short periods of dissociative sedation or anaesthesia with analgesia.[92,93] It is remarkably safe in small doses (1–2 mg kg^{-1}), although laryngospasm and apnoea are recognized complications.[88] Oral ketamine is an alternative but 10 mg kg^{-1} makes 50% of children unconscious and recovery can take up to 2 h.[101]

Anaesthesia

Many children have indwelling central venous lines which make the administration of intravenous anaesthesia such as propofol very easy. Sevoflurane has also reduced the distress of inhalational induction and, being short acting, allows rapid recovery.

CARDIAC ANGIOGRAPHY

Procedure details

Femoral arterial and venous catheters can be inserted almost without pain if local anaesthesia is used skilfully but this is often technically challenging. Angiography requires immobility for both imaging and measurement of intravascular pressures which are dependent on a steady-state cardiorespiratory function. Many procedures are prolonged and some involve interventional work such as balloon dilatations and insertion of coils and stents, which can be hazardous. Cyanosis and cardiac failure are obvious hazards to consider. The number of purely diagnostic scans has reduced in recent years because of advances in echocardiography.

Sedation strategy

Almost all cardiac angiography should be conducted under general anaesthesia because it provides optimum steady-state conditions with maximum safety. Sedation can be successful in a few children providing the investigation is short and diagnostic, although every sedative technique risks hypoxia.[78,81,91,111] Nasal midazolam can be helpful in infants and small children.

Points of safety and success

Sedation by non-anaesthetists is difficult, unpredictable and, if used at all, must be used by an experienced sedationist in selected cases.

Anaesthesia

Contrast media cause diuresis and care should be taken to ensure hydration, especially in children with polcythaemia who may be at risk of thrombosis. After angiography some children will need either intensive care or surgery.

INTERVENTIONAL RADIOLOGY

Procedure details

Biplanar X-ray angiography, fast computed tomographic (CT) scanning, ultrasound and colour Doppler mapping of blood flow all provide a radiologist with the means to intervene in the management of diseases managed previously by surgeons in operating room. Percutaneous biopsy of solid organs and tumours, drainage of abscesses and cysts, dilatation of stenoses and strictures, insertion of gastrostomy and nephrostomy tubes, and central venous catheters are now within the service capability of radiology departments. It is expected that in the near future, procedures will be required during MRI. All of these procedures are likely to be painful, unpredictable and of variable length.

Sedation strategy

Anaesthesia is preferable for all of these procedures. If the patient is very co-operative and the pain can be prevented by local anaesthetic, conscious sedation is possible, although there are very few children in this category. Ketamine has been considered for use by non-anaesthetists in the USA but, as already stated, it must be administered by a sedationist who is not the operator and who has had specific training in airway management.[90,94,112,113] Ketamine delivered by a non-anaesthetist is a poor substitute for shorter acting and more pleasant anaesthesia by an anaesthetist.

Points of safety and success

Any sedation is likely to cause sleep and should therefore be supervised by a sedationist who is not the operator.

Anaesthesia

The anaesthetic technique must be chosen to suit the patient and procedure, although most patients will require intubation and controlled ventilation because the procedure can be prolonged.

OESOPHAGOGASTROSCOPY AND COLONOSCOPY

Procedure details

Endoscopy is uncomfortable and can be extremely painful. Oesophagogastroscopy usually lasts for about 10–20 min and colonoscopy takes about 40 min, although either procedure can take a variable length of time. Oesophago-gastroscopy is only successful under sedation if the gag reflex is sufficiently suppressed. At this level of sedation airway and breathing reflexes are affected and the endoscope can mechanically obstruct the upper airway:[114,115] if too large, the endoscope can compress the trachea.

Sedation strategy

Oesophagogastroscopy is best managed under anaesthesia,[116] although skilled and experienced physicians can provide a sedation service. Episodes of desaturation are less likely during anaesthesia via a tracheal tube than during sedation with an unprotected airway.[117] Colonoscopy under sedation is more feasible than oesophagoscopy.

Points of safety and success

The advantages of anaesthesia for upper endoscopy are not challenged but, where anaesthesia services are unavailable, non-anaesthetists use a sedation combination of an opioid and benzodiazepine.[21,41,53] At GOSH pethidine and midazolam is the current sedation regimen. The failure rate is approximately 10% but depends on careful patient selection by experienced practitioners. Occasionally, apnoea occurs and naloxone is used regularly. Colonoscopy can traumatize the large bowel and cause perforation occasionally; for this reason, sedation may be safer than anaesthesia because the patient can give warning by complaining of pain.

DENTAL PROCEDURES

Procedure details

Even with the use of local anaesthesia dental procedures can be painful and cause much anxiety in many children. Conservative dentistry can take approximately 1 h, whereas extractions of primary teeth can take just a few minutes. The airway must be protected from blood, teeth and other debris with adequate suction: dental gauze can cause gagging.

Sedation strategy

Behavioural management and local anaesthesia should be attempted in most children and if this fails conscious sedation can be tried[16]. Patient co-operation is essential and treatment can be spread over several visits, allowing the child to adjust and become less anxious. If patients are not co-operative, either because they are too young, too ill or have behavioural problems, deep sedation is required. This must be administered and monitored by an experienced sedationist and, in this situation, a short anaesthetic by an anaesthetist is safer and more predictable.[118,119] Ill children should not be deeply sedated or anaesthetized in isolated sites and are best managed in operating rooms.

Points of safety and success

Guidelines on the administration of dental sedation and anaesthesia have been specified in the UK[15,16] and the USA.[17] Conscious sedation can be given by the dentist providing there is a trained assistant, but deep sedation and anaesthesia is not suitable for use by the operator alone; a separate qualified person must be responsible.[16] When using conscious sedation with nitrous oxide, a specific safety point to note is that a mouth gag must not be used, because to open the mouth wide is a voluntary action, and as soon as the mouth begins to close the sedation may be becoming too deep.[82] The nasal mask requires co-operation but, with skill and patience, 90% of children can benefit.[120] Exposure of female staff to nitrous oxide exceeding 5 h per week may decrease fertility and increase miscarriage rates; in these circumstances scavenging and room ventilation reduces pollution.[121,122]

MULTIPLE PROCEDURES

Procedure details

Often, clinicians request that more than one procedure be undertaken under the same sedation or anaesthetic. A frequent request is for a lumbar puncture to be combined with an MRI.

Sedation strategy

All procedures have to be planned sensibly with the most important procedures going first. Local anaesthesia creams are helpful but, if appreciable pain is anticipated, anaesthesia will be more successful. If imaging is likely to lead to surgery then the effects of sedation combined with anaesthesia may cause prolonged recovery and therefore scanning under anaesthesia is preferable.

Points of safety

Multiple scanning could mean that a child is sedated for long periods and could be transferred between several sites, with obvious safety concerns. The transfer of anaesthetized children between scanning sites is not recommended unless all investigations are crucial. Two short anaesthetics may be safer than a long one involving transport.

COMPUTED TOMOGRAPHY

CT has become much faster in recent years, allowing many scans to be completed in 5 min. The environment can be made child friendly and most well children do not need sedation. If a child cannot be persuaded to lie still, either oral chloral hydrate, trichlofos or midazolam is usually effective. If this fails anaesthesia is indicated.

NEURO- AND GENERAL ANGIOGRAPHY

Most angiograms are prolonged and in sick children the vast majority should be conducted under general anaesthesia. The clinical condition of the patient predicts the specific risks of the procedure. Embolization of vascular malformations can be hazardous because of pulmonary artery emboli. Haemostasis must be checked beforehand to ensure that embolization will be successful. Cerebral or spinal vascular embolization risks ischaemia to vital areas. If the malformation is large, these children can be in high-output cardiac failure.

RENAL AND HEPATIC BIOPSY

These are painful procedures, even with local anaesthesia, and require the child to remain immobile. They occasionally need to be carried out under radiological guidance. Most renal biopsies can be performed under sedation with a combination of opioid and benzodiazepine, but one should beware of the small risk of apnoea. Liver biopsies require both immobility and control of breathing, and without excellent patient co-operation they are best carried out under anaesthesia. Haemorrhage is a specific risk with hepatic biopsy.

ECHOCARDIOGRAPHY AND ULTRASOUND

Many infants are too irritable even for these short, painless procedures.

Parental comforting and short-acting light sedation are usually sufficient to stop excessive movement. Two drugs are currently used successfully; either oral triclofos or chloral hydrate,[31] which takes at least 20–30 min to work, or nasal midazolam, which usually causes crying but is effective within 5 min.[48] Oral midazolam could be used but is bitter and infants may spit it out. For transoesophageal echocardiography, anaesthesia is almost always required because the probes are too large to tolerate under sedation.

ELECTROENCEPHALOGRAPHY AND BRAINSTEM EVOKED RESPONSES

Both of these procedures require immobility for approximately 20 min but usually this can only be achieved with sleep. Electroencephalography is an investigation for convulsions, and brainstem evoked responses, a test of deafness, measures the electrical changes at the level of the brainstem resulting from noise. Children taking high doses of anticonvulsants and those with behavioural disturbances are resistant to sedatives and need anaesthesia. Deaf children usually need sedation and an MRI sedation regimen is suitable. More sensitive electrical tests may require a special room insulated from sound and electrical interference.

WOUND CARE

Wound procedures are a common problem in busy accident and emergency departments[19] and on the postoperative wards. Fortunately, many small wounds need only tissue adhesive and tape rather than sutures. Deep sedation is not recommended; therefore, if conscious sedation is insufficient, anaesthetists should manage the patient. Midazolam is probably the most common drug used, although its effect will be variable.[123] Most small children can be restrained while local anaesthesia is skilfully inserted. In postoperative wards, the removal of drains and catheters requires analgesia and either opioids or nitrous oxide can be helpful.

RADIOTHERAPY

Radiotherapy, most commonly for solid tumours such as retinoblastoma, requires perfect immobility for approximately 10–20 min and is repeated each day for 2 or more weeks. Either deep sedation or anaesthesia is required for all but the most co-operative of children and, because the treatment is repeated, short-acting anaesthesia is preferred. Staff cannot be exposed to radiation and therefore remote monitoring is mandatory. Anaesthesia using propofol alone, with or without an airway, provides a smooth technique but tolerance and behavioural changes have occurred and methohexitone provides an alternative.[75] Propofol is not recommended for children younger than 3 years and although ketamine or methohexitone has been used in the past[58,124] an inhalational technique with sevoflurane and laryngeal mask may be shorter acting and more pleasant.

EYE EXAMINATIONS

Eye examinations which do not involve any surgery can be performed under sedation and local anaesthesia. Chloral hydrate is usually successful for small children.[125]

MUSCLE AND JOINT INJECTIONS

Spasticity in children with cerebral palsy can be treated with botulinum toxin muscle injection and children with arthritis may benefit from steroid injections to the joints. One or two injections can be achieved with conscious sedation using midazolam and local anaesthesia, but anaesthesia is usually required for multiple injections.

INSERTION OF INTRAVENOUS CATHETERS

Almost all children object to intravenous catheters but, since the numbers are so large, few can be sedated. Local anaesthetic cream is helpful and in older children nitrous oxide may have a role, especially for children who need repeated procedures.[86,126]

GENERAL REQUIREMENTS FOR ANAESTHESIA OUTSIDE OPERATING ROOMS

STAFF

The anaesthetist should be senior, experienced and able to choose a technique to suit the patient and the procedure rather than be dependent on protocols. The anaesthetist must have a trained anaesthetic assistant and, in order to minimize anaesthesia time between procedures, consideration should be given to having a recovery nurse and a second anaesthetist, who could be a trainee.

EQUIPMENT

Full anaesthetic equipment and monitoring must be available, including gas analysis and temperature measurement. As well as oxygen and nitrous oxide, piped air should be installed as it may be indicated in the management of the critically ill. A separate oxygen outlet should be available so that non-anaesthetists have a source of oxygen which is not via the anaesthetic machine. Scavenging of anaesthetic gases must be available. A defibrillator must be nearby. Consideration must be given to the management of difficult intubation. Access to hospital computer systems should be considered since computerized records will soon become readily available and standard. All electrical equipment should comply with appropriate safety standards to prevent microelectrical shock (Hospital Technical Memorandum no. 8 in the UK).[127]

SPACE

In the UK the recommendation for floor space required for an anaesthetic room is at least 16.7 m^2 and the space per recovery bed is 9.3 m^2.[128]

LIGHTING AND ACCESS TO THE PATIENT

For some procedures, such as MRI or radiotherapy, the patient may be neither visible nor accessible for long periods, and therefore it is reasonable for the anaesthetist to stay in an observation room provided the patient is adequately monitored. MRI sequences last for 5–10 min and can be interrupted at any stage. Adequate lighting must be available to ensure visibility of the equipment and monitoring.

TEMPERATURE

Consideration must be given to the control of ambient temperature and air movement, especially for small infants.

STERILITY

Procedures with open wounds need a sterile environment and are best carried out in theatres.

NOISE

There should be a peaceful setting for the induction of and recovery from anaesthesia.

PLANNING CONSIDERATIONS FOR SEDATION AND ANAESTHESIA OUTSIDE OPERATING ROOM

Although each procedure should be examined for its specific requirements, there are general issues of economy, safety and quality in planning sedation and anaesthesia services outside operating rooms. All three depend heavily on the training, capabilities and experience of doctors and nurses.

ECONOMICS

Anaesthesia, if available, is expensive because of the cost of anaesthetists and their assistants. Equipment costs are small by comparison and similar to those required for sedation. Throughput of cases may be quicker with anaesthesia, but only if two anaesthetists are working together, allowing one patient to be anaesthetized while the other is being scanned. Sedation services need nurses and doctors with paediatric skills and this too is very expensive. Sedation is probably cheaper, but will depend on the ability to prepare enough patients for a fast throughput. Finally, failed sedation is expensive since patients usually have to return for anaesthesia on another day, depending on the availability of an anaesthetist and the urgency of the investigation.

SAFETY

Which is safer, sedation or anaesthesia? An unproven view is that both methods are equally safe provided they are done to a high standard. High standards in anaesthesia are ensured through regulation and recommendation but sedation is not as well regulated and establishing safe standards for non-anaesthetists is crucial. Non-anaesthetists can be taught resuscitation skills, but can they achieve sufficiently good judgement? Some paediatric hospitals may have enough experienced doctors and nurses

and could develop a safe sedation service, but small hospitals may not. In a small hospital which has a manageable demand for paediatric medical procedures, an anaesthesia service is likely to be safer, but in larger institutions, where the demand may be too great for anaesthesia services, replacing sedation with anaesthesia is impossible without considerable expense and reorganization. If appropriate procedures are followed, as outlined in this chapter, sedation can be made as safe as anaesthesia.

QUALITY

Sedation by non-anaesthetists is less reliable than anaesthesia by anaesthetists, and anaesthesia drugs are shorter acting and have fewer after effects than sedatives. Nevertheless, sedation, particularly oral sedation, is preferred by many children and parents since it engenders less anxiety and seems less complicated. Having an experienced anaesthetist provides the flexibility to choose the sedation or anaesthetic technique to suit the patient and the procedure.

SEDATION TEAMS AND SEDATION UNITS

In bringing together the skills and experience of physicians, sedation nurses and anaesthetists to form sedation teams, a flexible and efficient service can be provided.[129] One solution is a mobile service, although it can only cope with a low demand[130]. With planning, sedation and anaesthesia services can be centralized to form a medical procedures unit (MPU) and this solution suits hospitals with a high demand for procedures both in and out of operating rooms. Many minor surgical procedures can be moved to an MPU to make the use of operating rooms more efficient.

REFERENCES

1 Cohen, M.D. Pediatric sedation. *Radiology* 1990; **175**: 611–12.
2 Nelson, M.D. Guidelines for the monitoring and care of children during and after sedation for imaging studies. *American Journal of Roentgenology* 1993; **160**: 581–2.
3 Spear, R.M. Deep sedation for radiological procedures in children: enough is enough. *Paediatric Anaesthesia* 1993; **3**: 325–7.
4 Sury, M.R.J. The pros and cons of anaesthesia for children who need radiological procedures. *Paediatric Anaesthesia* 1993; **3**: 329–31.
5 Hall, S. Paediatric anaesthesia outside the operating room. *Canadian Journal of Anaesthesia* 1995; **42**: R68–72.
6 Wouters, P.F. and Van Aken, H. Magnetic resonance imaging in children. *European Journal of Anaesthesiology* 1997; **14**: 236–8.
7 Morton, N.S. and Oomen, G.J. Development of a selection and monitoring protocol for safe sedation of children. *Paediatric Anaesthesia* 1998; **8**: 65–8.
8 Berde, C. Pediatric oncology procedures: to sleep or perchance to dream? *Pain* 1995; **62**: 1–2.
9 Proctor, L.T. The peripatetic anesthesiologist. *Current Opinion in Anaesthesiology* 1998; **11**: 283–4.
10 Cote, C.J. Sedation disasters: adverse drug reports in pediatrics FDA, USP and others. *Anesthesiology* 1995; **83**: A1182.
11 Committee on Drugs. Guidelines for monitoring and management of pediatric patients during and after sedation for diagnostic and therapeutic procedures. *Pediatrics* 1992; **89**: 1110–15.
12 Royal College of Anaesthetists and Royal College of Radiologists. Sedation and anaesthesia in radiology. Report of a joint working party. London, 1992.
13 American Society of Anesthesiologists Task Force on Sedation and Analgesia by Non-Anesthesiologists. Practice guidelines for sedation and analgesia by non-anesthesiologists. *Anesthesiology* 1996; **84**: 459–71.
14 Royal College of Surgeons Working Party. Guidelines for sedation by non-anaesthetists. London, 1993.
15 Report of an Expert Working Party. General anaesthesia, sedation and resuscitation in dentistry. Standing Dental Advisory Committee: Department of Health, UK, 1990.
16 British Society of Paediatric Dentistry. A policy document on sedation for paediatric dentistry. *International Journal of Paediatric Dentistry* 1996; **6**: 63–6.
17 American Academy of Pediatric Dentistry. Guidelines for the elective use of pharmacologic conscious sedation and deep sedation in pediatric dental patients. *Pediatric Dentistry* 1993; **15**: 297–301.
18 Bell, G.D., McCloy, R.F., Charlton, J.E., *et al.* Recommendations for standards of sedation and patient monitoring during gastrointestinal endoscopy. *Gut* 1981; **151**: 385–8.
19 Sacchetti, A., Scafermeyer, R. and Geradi, M. Pediatric analgesia and sedation. *Annals of Emergency Medicine* 1994; **23**: 237–50.

20 Maxwell, L.G. and Yaster, M. The myth of conscious sedation. *Archives of Pediatrics and Adolescent Medicine* 1996; **150**: 665–7.
21 Murphy, M.S. Sedation for invasive procedures in paediatrics. *Archives of Disease in Childhood* 1997; **77**: 281–6.
22 Cote, C.J. Sedation protocols – why so many variations? *Pediatrics* 1994; **94**: 281–3.
23 Egelhoff, J.C., Ball, W.S., Jr, Koch, B.L. and Parks, T.D. Safety and efficacy of sedation in children using a structured sedation program. *American Journal of Roentgenology* 1997; **168**: 1259–62.
24 Boyer, R.S. Sedation in pediatric neuroimaging: the science and the art. *American Journal of Neuroradiology* 1992; **13**: 777–83.
25 Vade, A., Sukhani, R., Dolenga, M. and Habisohn-Schuck, C. Chloral hydrate sedation of children undergoing CT and MR imaging: safety as judged by American Academy of Pediatrics guidelines. *American Journal of Roentgenology* 1994; **165**: 905–9.
26 American Academy of Pediatrics Committee on Drugs and environmental health. Use of chloral hydrate for sedation of children. *Pediatrics* 1993; **92**: 471–3.
27 Malviya, S., Voepel-Lewis, T. and Tait, A.R. Adverse events and risk factors associated with the sedation of children by nonanesthesiologists. *Anesthesia and Analgesia* 1997; **85**: 1207–13.
28 Neuman, G.G., Kushins, L.G. and Ferrante, S. Sedation for children undergoing magnetic resonance imaging and computed tomography. *Anesthesia and Analgesia* 1992; **74**: 931–2.
29 Greenberg, S.B., Faerber, E.N., Aspinall, C.L. and Adams, R.C. High-dose chloral hydrate sedation for children undergoing MR imaging: safety and efficacy in relation to age. *American Journal of Roentgenology* 1993; **161**: 639–41.
30 Hubbard, A.M., Markowitz, R.I., Kimmel, B., Kroger, M. and Bartko, M.B. Sedation for pediatric patients undergoing CT and MRI. *Journal of Computer Assisted Tomography* 1992; **16**: 3–6.
31 Napoli, K.L., Ingall, C.G. and Martin, G.R. Safety and efficacy of chloral hydrate sedation in children undergoing echocardiography. *Journal of Pediatrics* 1996; **129**: 287–91.
32 Jackson, E.A., Rabbette, P.S., Dezateux, C., Hatch, D.J. and Stocks, J. The effect of triclofos sodium sedation on respiratory rate, oxygen saturation and heart rate in infants and young children. *Pediatric Pulmonology* 1991; **10**: 40–5.
33 Page, B. and Morgan-Hughes, J.O. Behaviour of small children before induction. The effect of parental presence and EMLA and premedication with tricoflos or a placebo. *Anaesthesia* 1990; **45**: 821–5.
34 Kupietzky, A. and Houpt, M.I. Midazolam: a review of its use for conscious sedation of children. *Pediatric Dentistry* 1993; **15**: 237–41.
35 Rey, E., Delaney, L., Pons, G., *et al.* Pharmacokinetics of midazolam in children: comparative study of intranasal and intravenous administration. *European Journal of Clinical Pharmacology* 1991; **41**: 355–7.
36 Tolia, V., Brennan, S., Aravind, A.K. and Kauffman, R.E. Pharmacokinetic and pharmacodynamic study of midazolam in children during esophagogastroduodenoscopy. *Journal of Pediatrics* 1991; **119**: 467–71.

37 Sievers, T.D., Yee, J.D., Foley, M.E., Blanding, P.J. and Berde, C.B. Midazolam for conscious sedation during pediatric oncology procedures: safety and recovery parameters. *Pediatrics* 1991; **88**: 1172–9.

38 Salonen, M., Kanto, J. and Iisalo, E. Midazolam as an induction agent in children: a pharmacokinetic and clinical study. *Anesthesia and Analgesia* 1987; **66**: 625–8.

39 Yaster, M., Nichols, D.G., Deshpande, J.K. and Wetzel, R.C. Midazolam–fentanyl intravenous sedation in children: case report of respiratory arrest. *Pediatrics* 1990; **86**: 463–7.

40 Diament, M.J. and Stanley, P. The use of midazolam for sedation of infants and children. *American Journal of Roentgenology* 1988; **150**: 377–8.

41 Chuang, E., Wenner, W.J., Jr, Piccoli, D.A., Altschuler, S.M. and Liacouras, C.A. Intravenous sedation in pediatric upper gastrointestinal endoscopy. *Gastrointestinal Endoscopy* 1995; **42**: 156–60.

42 Hiller, A., Olkkola, K.T., Isohanni, P. and Saarnivaara, L. Unconsiousness associated with midazolam and erythromycin. *British Journal of Anaesthesia* 1990; **65**: 826–8.

43 Doyle, W.L. and Perrin, L. Emergence delirium in a child given oral midazolam for conscious sedation. *Annals of Emergency Medicine* 1994; **24**: 1173–5.

44 McCluskey, A. and Meakin, G.H. Oral administration of midazolam as a premedicant for paediatric day-case anaesthesia. *Anaesthesia* 1994; **49**: 782–5.

45 Karl, H.W. Midazolam sedation for pediatric patients. *Current Opinion in Anaesthesiology* 1993; **6**: 509–14.

46 Feld, L.H., Negus, J.B. and White, P.F. Oral midazolam: optimal dose for pediatric premedication. *Anesthesiology* 1989; **71**: A1054.

47 McMillan, C.O., Spahir-Schopfer, I.A., Sikich, N., Hartley, E. and Lerman, J. Premedication of children with oral midazolam. *Canadian Journal of Anaesthesia* 1992; **39**: 545–50.

48 Latson, L.A., Cheatham, J.P., Gumbiner, C.H., *et al.* Midazolam nose drops for outpatient echocardiography sedation in infants. *American Heart Journal* 1991; **121**: 209–10.

49 Harcke, H.T., Grissom, L.E. and Meister, M.A. Sedation in pediatric imaging using intranasal midazolam. *Pediatric Radiology* 1995; **25**: 341–3.

50 Karl, H.W., Rosenberger, J.L., Larach, M.G. and Ruffle, J.M. Transmucosal administration of midazolam for premedication of pediatric patients: comparison of the nasal and sublingual routes. *Anesthesiology* 1993; **78**: 885–91.

51 Saint-Maurice, C., Meistelman, C. and Rey, C. The pharmacokinetics of rectal midazolam for premedication in children. *Anesthesiology* 1986; **65**: 536–8.

52 Spear, R.M., Yaster, M., Berkowitz, I.D., *et al.* Preinduction of anesthesia in children with rectally administered midazolam. *Anesthesiology* 1991; **74**: 670–4.

53 Nahata, M.C., Murray, R.D., Zingarelli, J., Li, B.U., McClung, H.J. and Lininger, B. Efficacy and safety of a diazepam and meperidine combination for pediatric gastrointestinal procedures. *Journal of Pediatric Gastroenterology and Nutrition* 1990; **10**: 335–8.

54 Jones, R.D.M., Lawson, A.D., Andrew, L.J., Gunawardene, W.M.S. and Bacon-Shone, J. Antagonism of the hypnotic effect of midazolam in children: a randomised, bouble blind study of placebo and flumazenil administered after midazolam-induced anaesthesia. *British Journal of Anaesthesia* 1991; **66**: 660–6.

55 Carbajal, R., Simon, N., Blanc, P., Paupe, A., Lenclen, R. and Oliver-Martin, M. Rectal flumazenil to reverse midazolam sedation in children. *Anesthesia and Analgesia* 1996; **82**: 895.

56 Spear, R.M., Waldman, J.Y., Canada, E.D., Worthen, H.M., Fraierman, A.H. and Rodart, A. Intravenous thiopentone for CT and MRI in children. *Paediatric Anaesthesia* 1993; **3**: 29–32.

57 Varner, P.D., Ebert, J.P., McKay, R.D., Nail, C.S. and Whitlock, T.M. Methohexital sedation of children undergoing CT scan. *Anesthesia and Analgesia* 1985; **64**: 643–5.

58 Jefferies, G. Radiotherapy and childrens anaesthesia. *Anaesthesia* 1988; **43**: 416–26.

59 Beekman, R.P., Hoorntje, T.M., Beek, F.J. and Kuijten, R.H. Sedation for children undergoing magnetic resonance imaging: efficacy and safety of rectal thiopental. *European Journal of Pediatrics* 1996; **155**: 820–2.

60 Audenaert, S.M., Montgomery, C.L., Thompson, D.E. and Sutherland, J. A prospective study of rectal methohexital: efficacy and side effects in 648 cases. *Anesthesia and Analgesia* 1995; **81**: 957–61.

61 Liu, L.M.P., Goudsouzian, N.G. and Liu, P.C. Rectal methohexital premedication in children, a dose comparison study. *Anesthesiology* 1980; **53**: 343–5.

62 Griswold, J.D. and Liu, L.M.P. Rectal methohexital in children undergoing computerized cranial tomography and magnetic resonance imaging scans. *Anesthesiology* 1987; **67**: A494.

63 Manuli, M.A. and Davis, L. Rectal methohexital for sedation of children during imaging procedures. *American Journal of Roentgenology* 1993; **160**: 577–80.

64 Strain, J.D., Campbell, J.B., Harvey, L.A. and Foley, L.C. IV. Nembutal: safe sedation for children undergoing CT. *American Journal of Roentgenology* 1988; **15**: 975–9.

65 Bloomfield, E.L., Masaryk, T.J., Caplin, A., *et al.* Intravenous sedation for MR imaging of the brain and spine in children: pentobarbital versus propofol. *Radiology* 1993; **186**: 93–7.

66 Montecinos, S. Sedation for children undergoing diagnostic procedures. *Anesthesia and Analgesia* 1993; **77**: 198.

67 Valtonen, M. Anaesthesia for computerised tomography of the brain in children: a comparison of propofol and thiopentone. *Acta Anaesthesiologica Scandinavica* 1989; **33**: 170–3.

68 Lefever, E.B., Potter, P.S. and Seeley, N.R. Propofol sedation for pediatric MRI. *Anesthesia and Analgesia* 1993; **76**: 919–20.

69 Martin, L.D., Pasternak, L.R. and Pudimat, M.A. Total intravenous anesthesia with propofol in pediatric patients outside the operating room. *Anesthesia and Analgesia* 1992; **74**: 609–12.

70 Burke, A. and Pollock, J. Propofol and paeadiatric MRI. *Anaesthesia* 1994; **49**: 647.

71 Frankville, D.D., Spear, R.M. and Dyck, J.B. The dose of propofol required to prevent children from moving during magnetic resonance imaging. *Anesthesiology* 1993; **79**: 953–8.

72 Vangerven, M., Van Hemelrijck, J., Wouters, P., Vandermeersch, E. and Van Aken, H. Light anaesthesia

with propofol for paediatric MRI. *Anaesthesia* 1992; **47**: 706–7.

73 Scheiber, G., Ribeiro, F.C., Karpienski, H. and Strehl, K. Deep sedation with propofol in preschool children undergoing radiation therapy. *Paediatric Anaesthesia* 1996; **6**: 209–13.

74 MacIntyre, P.A. and Sury, M.R.J. Is propofol infusion better than inhalational anaesthesia for paediatric MRI? *Anaesthesia* 1996; **51**: 517.

75 Metriyakool, K. Methohexital as alternative to propofol for intravenous anesthesia in children undergoing daily radiation treatment: a case report. *Anesthesiology* 1998; **88**: 821–2.

76 Morgan-Hughes, J.O. and Bangham, J.A. Pre-induction behaviour of children. A review of placebo-controlled trials of sedatives. *Anaesthesia* 1990; **45**: 427–35.

77 Shepherd, J.K., Hall-Craggs, M.A., Finn, J.P. and Bingham, R.M. Sedation in children scanned with high-field magnetic resonance; the experience at the Hospital for Sick Children, Great Ormond Street. *British Journal of Radiology* 1990; **63**: 794–7.

78 Rautiainen, P. and Meretoja, O.A. Ketamine boluses with continuous low-dose fentanyl for paediatric sedation during diagnostic cardiac catheterization. *Paediatric Anaesthesia* 1993; **3**: 345–51.

79 Schechter, N.L., Weisman, S.J., Rosenblum, M., Bernstein, B. and Conard, P.L. The use of oral transmucosal fentanyl citrate for painful procedures in children. *Pediatrics* 1995; **95**: 335–9.

80 Goldstein-Dresner, M.C., Davis, P.J., Kretchman, E., Siewers, R.D., Certo, N. and Cook, D.R. Double-blind comparison of oral transmucosal fentanyl citrate with oral meperidine, diazepam, and atropine as preanesthetic medication in children with congenital heart disease. *Anesthesiology* 1991; **74**: 28–33.

81 Nahata, M.C., Clotz, M.A. and Krogg, E.A. Adverse effects of meperidine, promethazine, and chlorpromazine for sedation in pediatric patients. *Clinical Pediatrics* 1985; **24**: 558–60.

82 Roberts, G.J. Relative analgesia: an introduction. *Dental Update* 1979; **6**: 271–84.

83 Litman, R.S., Berkowitz, R.J. and Ward, D.S. Levels of consciousness and ventilatory parameters in young children during sedation with oral midazolam and increasing concentrations of nitrous oxide. *Anesthesiology* 1995; **83**: A1182.

84 Dunn-Russell, T., Adair, S.M., Sams, D.R., Russell, C.M. and Barenie, J.T. Oxygen saturation and diffusion hypoxia in children following nitrous oxide sedation. *Pediatric Dentistry* 1993; **15**: 88–92.

85 Evans, J.K., Buckley, S.L., Alexander, A.H. and Gilpin, A.T. Analgesia for the reduction of fractures in children: a comparison of nitrous oxide with intramuscular sedation. *Journal of Pediatric Orthopedics* 1995; **15**: 73–7.

86 Henderson, J.M., Spence, D.G., Komocar, L.M., Bonn, G.E. and Stenstrom, R.J. Administration of nitrous oxide to pediatric pateints provides analgesia for venous cannulation. *Anesthesiology* 1990; **72**: 269–71.

87 Friesen, R.H. and Morrison, J.E. The role of ketamine in the current practice of paediatric anaesthesia. *Paediatric Anaesthesia* 1994; **4**: 79–82.

88 Green, S.M. and Johnson, N.E. Ketamine sedation for pediatric procedures: Part 2. Review and implication. *Annals of Emergency Medicine* 1990; **19**: 1033–46.

89 Smith, S.M. and Santer, L.J. Respiratory arrest following intramuscular ketamine injection in a 4-year old child. *Annals of Emergency Medicine* 1993; **22**: 613–15.

90 Green, S.M., Rothrock, S.G., Lynch, E.L., *et al.* Intramuscular ketamine for pediatric sedation in the emergency department: safety profile in 1022 cases. *Annals of Emergency Medicine* 1998; **31**: 688–97.

91 Greene, C.A., Gillette, P.C. and Fyfe, D.A. Frequency of respiratory compromise after ketamine sedation for cardiac catheterization in patients less than 21 years of age. *American Journal of Cardiology* 1991; **68**: 1116–17.

92 Parker, R.I., Mahan, R.A., Giugliano, D. and Parker, M.M. Efficacy and safety of intravenous midazolam and ketamine as sedation for therapeutic and diagnostic procedures in children. *Pediatrics* 1997; **99**: 427–31.

93 Dachs, R.J. and Innes, G.M. Intravenous ketamine sedation of pediatric patients in the emergency department. *Annals of Emergency Medicine* 1997; **29**: 146–50.

94 Cotsen, M.R., Donaldson, J.S., Uejima, T. and Morello, F.P. Efficacy of ketamine hydrochloride sedation in children for interventional radiologic procedures. *American Journal of Roentgenology* 1994; **169**: 1019–22.

95 Harari, M.D. and Netzer, D. Genital examination under ketamine sedation in cases of suspected sexual abuse. *Archives of Disease in Childhood* 1994; **70**: 197–9.

96 Barst, S., McDowall, R. and Pratila, M. Anesthesia for pediatric cancer patients: ketamine, etomidate or propofol? *Anesthesiology* 1990; **73**: A1114.

97 Hollister, G.R. and Burn, J.M.B. Side effects of ketamine in pediatric anesthesia. *Anesthesia and Analgesia* 1974; **53**: 264–7.

98 Donahue, P.J. and Dineen, P.S. Emergence delirium following oral ketamine. *Anesthesiology* 1992; **77**: 604–5.

99 Gingrich, B.K. Difficulties encountered in a comparative study of orally administered midazolam and ketamine. *Anesthesiology* 1994; **80**: 1414–15.

100 Gutstein, H.B., Johnson, K.L. and Heard, M.B. Oral ketamine preanesthetic medication in children. *Anesthesiology* 1992; **76**: 28–33.

101 Tobias, J.D., Phipps, S., Smith, B. and Mulhern, R.K. Oral ketamine premedication to alleviate the distress of invasive procedures in pediatric oncology patients. *Pediatrics* 1992; **90**: 537–41.

102 Saint-Maurice, C., Laguenie, G., Couturier, C. and Goutail-Flaud, F. Rectal ketamine in paediatric anaesthesia. *British Journal of Anaesthesia* 1979; **51**: 573–4.

103 Foesel, T., Hack, C., Knoll, R., Kraus, G.B. and Larsen, R. Intranasally administered midazolam in children: plasma concentrations and the effect on respiration. *Anesthesiology* 1992; **77**: A1171.

104 Fuks, A.B., Kaufman, E., Ram, D., Hovav, S. and Shapira, J. Assessment of two doses of intranasal midazolam for sedation of young pediatric dental patients. *Pediatric Dentistry* 1994; **16**: 301–5.

105 Menon, D.K., Peden, C.J., Hall, A.S., Sargentoni, J. and Whitwam, J.G. Magnetic resonance for the anaesthetist. Part 1: Physical principles, applications, safety aspects. *Anaesthesia* 1992; **47**: 240–55.

106 Peden, C.J., Menon, D.K., Hall, A.S., Sargentoni, J. and Whitwam, J.G. Magnetic resonance for the anaesthetist. Part II: Anaesthesia and monitoring in MR units. *Anaesthesia* 1992; **47**: 508–17.

107 Sury, M.R.J., Johnstone, G. and Bingham, R. Anaesthesia for magnetic resonance imaging of children. *Paediatric Anaesthesia* 1992; **2**: 61–8.

108 Tobin, J.R., Spurrier, E.A. and Wetzel, R.C. Anaesthesia for critically ill children during magnetic resonance imaging. *British Journal of Anaesthesia* 1992; **69**: 482–6.

109 Barst, S.M., Merola, C.M., Markowitz, A.E., Albarracin, C., Lebowitz, P.W. and Bienkowski, R.S. A comparison of propofol and chloral hydrate for sedation of young children during magnetic resonance imaging scans. *Paediatric Anaesthesia* 1994; **4**: 243–7.

110 Jay, S., Elliott, C.H., Fitzgibbons, I., Woody, P. and Siegel, S. A comparative study of cognitive behavior therapy versus general anesthesia for painful medical procedures in children. *Pain* 1995; **62**: 3–9.

111 Lebovic, S., Reich, D.L., Steinberg, G., Vela, F.P. and Silvay, G. Comparison of propofol versus ketamine for anesthesia in pediatric patients undergoing cardiac catheterization. *Anesthesia and Analgesia* 1992; **74**: 490–4.

112 Vade, A. and Sukhani, R. Ketamine hydrochloride for interventional radiology in children: is it sedation or anesthesia by the radiologist. *American Journal of Roentgenology* 1998; **171**: 265–6.

113 Green, S.M., Nakamura, R. and Johnson, N.E. Ketamine sedation for pediatric procedures: Part 1, A prospective series. *Annals of Emergency Medicine* 1990; **19**: 1024–32.

114 Casfeel, H.B., Fiedorek, S.C. and Kiel, E.A. Arterial blood oxygen desaturation in infants and children during upper gastrointestinal endoscopy. *Gastrointestinal Endoscopy* 1992; **36**: 489–93.

115 Bendig, D.W. Pulse oximetry and upper intestinal endoscopy in infants and children. *Journal of Pediatric Gastroenterology and Nutrition* 1991; **12**: 39–43.

116 Stringer, M.D. and McHugh, P.J.M. Paediatric endoscopy should be carried out under general anaesthesia. *British Medical Journal* 1995; **311**: 452–3.

117 Dubreuil, M., Da Conceicao, M., Lamireau, T., Meymat, Y. and Bidalier, I. Oxygen desaturation in children during gastrointestinal endoscopy: general anaesthesia versus sedation. *Anesthesiology* 1995; **83**: A1184.

118 Schwartz, S., Bevan, J.C., Roberts, G. and Dean, D.M. Midazolam sedation and local anaesthesia compared with general anaesthesia for paediatric outpatient dental surgery. *Paediatric Anaesthesia* 1992; **2**: 309–15.

119 Barr, E.B. and Wynn, R.L. IV sedation in pediatric dentistry: an alternative to general anesthesia. *Pediatric Dentistry* 1992; **14**: 251–5.

120 Shaw, A.J., Meechan, J.G., Kilpatrick, N.M. and Welbury, R.R. The use of inhalation sedation and local anaesthesia instead of general anaesthesia for extractions and minor oral surgery in children: a prospective study. *International Journal of Paediatric Dentistry* 1996; **6**: 7–11.

121 Cohen, E.N., Brown, B.W. and Wu, M.L. Occupational disease in dentistry and chronic exposure to trace anesthetic gases. *Journal of the American Dental Association* 1998; **101**: 21–31.

122 Rowland, R.S., Baird, D.D., Weinberg, C.R., Shore, D.L., Shy, C.M. and Wilcox, A.J. Reduced fertility among women employed as dental assistants exposed to high levels of nitrous oxide. *New England Journal of Medicine* 1992; **327**: 993–7.

123 Theroux, M., West, D., Corddry, D., Kettrick, R. and Bachrach, S. Efficacy of midazolam administered nasally for suturing lacerations in emergency rooms. *Anesthesiology* 1992; **77**: A1172.

124 Cronin, M.M., Bousefield, J.D., Hewitt, E.B., McLellan, I. and Boulton, T.B. Ketamine anaesthesia for radiotherapy in small children. *Anaesthesia* 1972; **27**: 135–42.

125 Judisch, G.F., Anderson, S. and Bell, W.E. Chloral hydrate sedation as a substitute for examination under anesthesia in pediatric ophthalmology. *American Journal of Ophthalmology* 1980; **89**: 560–3.

126 Mjahed, K., Sadraoui, A., Benslama, A., Idali, B. and Benaguida, M. Association creme EMLA et protoxide d'azote pour l'abord veineax chez l'enfant. *Annals Francais Anesthesie et Reanimation* 1997; **16**: 488–91.

127 Hull, C.J. Electrocution hazards in the operating theatre. *British Journal of Anaesthesia* 1978; **50**: 647–57.

128 Department of Health and Social Security. Operating theatres, hospital building note 26. London: HMSO, 1967.

129 Sury, M.R.J., Hatch, D.J., Deeley, T., Dicks-Mireaux, C. and Chong, W.K. Development of a nurse-led sedation service for paediatric magnetic resonance imaging. *The Lancet* 1999; **353**: 1667–71.

130 Gozal, C.V., Kadri, A. and Gozal, Y. A paediatric sedation unit in a university hospital: a one year survey. *British Journal of Anaesthesia* 1998; **80**: A500.

CHAPTER 22

Resuscitation

DAVID ZIDEMAN

INTRODUCTION

Paediatric resuscitation is a crucial element in the practice of paediatric anaesthesia. It is fundamental that all who treat infants and children are well versed in simple basic life support and that those who are required to perform the more complex skills are taught and regularly practise advanced life-support procedures.

The epidemiology of paediatric resuscitation is different from that in adults. Ventricular fibrillation and ventricular tachycardia, the most common causes of cardiac arrest in adults, are reported in less than 10% in the paediatric age groups.[1–3] In infants and children there is usually an initial airway or respiratory event resulting in profound hypoxia, the final event being cardiac arrest if the initial episode has not been recognized and treated promptly.[1–5] The 'prearrest' phase is therefore vitally important. It must be recognized promptly and treatment commenced immediately to prevent the event progressing to circulatory collapse and cardiac arrest. Many of the long-term permanent effects of paediatric resuscitation can be attributed to a prolonged prearrest hypoxic phase. Trauma is the most common cause of death in the first four decades of life, yet trauma and its consequences should be regarded as preventable. Certainly, cardiac arrest secondary to trauma should be preventable by the careful and correct management of the airway, breathing and circulation in the prehospital and early hospital phases.

The outcome of paediatric life support is poor. Survival rates are quoted at between 3 and 17%[1,2,5–14] and can be considered even more dismal when the majority is reported as showing significant neurological impairment after arrest. Outcome is related to the aetiology of the initial event. Better outcomes have been reported when the primary event was respiratory[7,14,15] rather than cardiac in nature.[7,8,16]

The reporting and analysis of paediatric resuscitation events is complex. Resuscitation of infants and children is relatively uncommon and most studies have had to collect data over several years to reach an acceptable sample size. In the BRESUS study, analysing over 3000 cardiac arrests in 12 hospitals in the UK in one year, only 2% of the subjects were less than 14 years of age.[17] During these long data-collection periods staff change, techniques advance and resuscitation protocols are often modified. Sometimes the only way to achieve meaningful conclusions is to group studies into prehospital and in-hospital incidents and to separate the latter into ward, specialized area and intensive-care resuscitation occurrences. Definitions used in evaluating such events vary and are often inconsistent, thus invalidating comparisons between reported studies. Success rates varying between 51 and 96% have been reported for paediatric ward resuscitation events (survival rates 9–65%) and between 12 and 80% for paediatric intensive area resuscitation (survival rates 9–33%).[18]

In an effort to standardize definitions and improve the reporting of paediatric resuscitation a reporting template, the Paediatric Utstein template, was devised.[19] It is hoped that by using this reporting format and the intrinsic specific definitions it uses studies will become comparable and future guidelines may be derived from acceptable evidence based practice.

In a study from Copenhagen, 79 consecutive paediatric prehospital cardiac arrests were analysed using the Utstein template.[20] The study took 8 years to complete. Sudden infant death syndrome was the leading cause of cardiac arrest, followed by trauma, airway-related events and near drowning. Asystole was the most common initial rhythm (78.9%) in the 52 children considered for resuscitation. Ventricular fibrillation was only seen in 3.8%. The overall survival rate was 9.6%. Only 34 of the 79 patients were considered for resuscitation and in this group survival rates rose to 14.7%. They rose further to 25% when resuscitation was attempted after a witnessed event. There were no survivors, even for attempted resuscitation, when the initial arrest was of primary cardiac origin.

infants and children in 1998.[21,22] The foundation of the European recommendations was the International Liaison Committee in Resuscitation (ILCOR) advisory statement on Paediatric Life Support.[23] The ILCOR recommendations were based on the specific evidence where available, or supported on the basis of common sense or ease of teaching and skill retention.

The resuscitation process is classically divided into basic life support, simple initial resuscitation procedures, and advanced life support, complex technical procedures requiring the use of drugs and equipment. This division between basic and advanced procedures is artificial as both should run concurrently, with the advanced procedures providing definitive treatment to support basic life support.

AGE DEFINITION

Before resuscitation can begin, it is essential that an assessment be made of the victim's age. Age will determine the finer details of the procedures to be performed especially in basic life support.

- An infant is a child under the age of 1 year.
- A child is aged between 1 and 8 years.
- Children over the age of 8 years should still be treated as younger children but may require different techniques to attain adequate chest compressions.

Adult resuscitation protocols have also been modified by the European Resuscitation Council to dovetail with the above definitions.[24,25] They require the rescuer to determine the cause of the arrest and where this is not primarily of cardiac origin, for example trauma or drowning, to use a protocol that more closely aligns to the paediatric recommendations.

PAEDIATRIC LIFE SUPPORT

The European Resuscitation Council published its revised recommendations for resuscitation of

BASIC LIFE SUPPORT

Before beginning basic life support, it is essential to ensure the safety of the casualty and rescuer. Although this is often performed in a clinical environment, a rapid assessment of the cause of the cardiorespiratory arrest (for example electrocution, drowning, etc.) must be made and the necessary safety precautions taken to prevent a recurrence of the event.[21]

The next stage is to check the responsiveness of the child. Gentle stimulation together with shouting 'Wake up!' or 'Are you alright?' will establish a conscious level and the response to stimulation. This forms a timed baseline for the assessment of the conscious level of the casualty. If there is no response (unconsciousness) then proceed without further delay to the ABC (airway, breathing and circulation) sequence of resuscitation.

AIRWAY

The airway is opened by gently tilting the head back and lifting the jaw up and forward. This simple measure will extend the neck and displaces the tongue from the back of the pharynx. A recent study has shown that there is no compromise of the airway by hyperextension of the neck.[26] In cases where trauma has been the cause, great care must be taken in moving the head and neck because of a possible cervical spine injury. Therefore, in trauma cases, the neck must be carefully stabilized by in-line immobilization, the head-tilt manoeuvre should not be used and the airway should be opened by the jaw thrust manoeuvre only.

A brief visual inspection of the airway must be made and any visible obstruction removed. Clearing an airway obstruction of a foreign body beyond the line of sight should not be attempted blindly as this may cause trauma, impaction and further airway obstruction.

BREATHING

Initially, by checking for breathing, the rescuer assesses the patency of the child's airway and looks at the chest to see whether it is moving with a normal pattern. The rescuer should look, listen and feel for breath sounds at the mouth and nose. Not only will this assess airway patency, but it will give an indication of the cause of any residual airway obstruction (croup, epiglottitis). Any intercostal recession, sternal recession or see-saw movement of the chest and abdomen may indicate residual airway obstruction that can be improved by repositioning the airway. The nares should be inspected to see whether flaring is occurring, also indicating residual airway obstruction.

If the child is not breathing and the airway is clear, then expired air resuscitation should be initiated. Holding the airway open, the rescuer covers the mouth and nose of the infant or the mouth of the child with his own mouth. By breathing out gently into the child and watching the chest move upwards, the rescuer can judge the correct amount of ventilation. When the chest has expanded as if the child has taken a deep breath the rescuer should stop breathing into the child's airway. Although expired air resuscitation is described as a hyperventilation technique, this can only be achieved in children by varying the ventilatory rate and not the tidal volume. Raising the latter could result in a pneumothorax. Excessive ventilation, either in volume or airway pressure, will result in air entering the stomach rather than the lungs.[27,28] This can cause gastric distension and regurgitation of the stomach contents and soiling of the airway.[29]

Because of the probable hypoxic aetiology of the event, five expired air ventilations are considered the optimal number of breaths to oxygenate an infant or a child.

If the chest does not rise when attempting ventilation or excessive pressure is needed to achieve ventilation then the airway should be realigned or an attempt be made to clear it using the procedures described in the Foreign body airway obstruction section below.

CIRCULATION

Conventionally, the circulation is assessed by checking the pulse. Assessment of the brachial pulse is recommended for infants[30] and the carotid pulse for children. Alternatively, the femoral pulse can be palpated. The pulse check should take no longer than 10 s and if a pulse is not felt, or the pulse rate is below 60 beats min^{-1} in an infant, then resuscitation should continue immediately with chest compressions.

Despite the apparent simplicity of a pulse check, studies have shown that both the lay rescuer and the experienced health-care professional have difficulty in making an accurate pulse check.[31–34] The inaccuracy of the procedure has led to the validity of a pulse check in paediatric life support being challenged.[35] The concept of not performing a pulse check at all before commencing chest compressions is considered difficult to accept by some, as it may appear to be illogical not to establish cardiac arrest formally before commencing chest compressions. Therefore, the guidelines now include the statement that starting chest compressions should be considered without delaying for a pulse check in an unresponsive child who does not show obvious signs of recovery after expired air ventilation.

Chest compressions are performed on the lower half of the sternum. In the infant, compression is performed using two fingers placed one finger's breadth below an imaginary line joining the nipples. In the child, the heel of one hand is used and positioned one finger's breadth up from the xiphisternum. In the older child (over the age of 8 years) and in the larger young child, this one-handed compression technique may be found to be inadequate. In these situations, a two-handed overlapping compression technique (as used in adult resuscitation) may be required to produce an effective depth of chest compression.

The depth of compression should be judged in relative rather than absolute terms. For infants and small children, the chest is compressed to one-third of its resting diameter. The efficacy of chest compression can be judged by palpation of the femoral vessels but this may reflect venous and not arterial blood pulsation.[36] Analysis of the arterial waveform or evaluation of the expired carbon dioxide tracing is a more effective assessment.

The compression rate for infants and children is 100 compressions min^{-1}. After every five compressions a single expired air ventilation is given. This ratio of 5 : 1 provides adequate circulation, ventilation and oxygenation for the infant or child. In the older child, where two hands are required for effective chest compression, the adult ratio of 15 compressions to two ventilations can be used, compressing the chest at a rate of 100 compressions min^{-1}.

ACTIVATION OF EMERGENCY MEDICAL SYSTEM

A call for help is usually made during the initial assessment of the conscious level of the child. This may activate the local emergency systems but it is essential, in view of the aetiology of paediatric cardiac arrest, to establish an airway rapidly, to commence effective ventilation and to circulate oxygenated blood. Therefore, if the initial call has not elicited a local response, then a definitive direct call to the emergency medical system must be made after approximately 1 min of resuscitation. The infant or small child can be carried to the telephone, thereby continuing life-support procedures, but the older child may have to be left whilst help is summoned.

Basic life support must continue without further interruption until experienced help arrives or until signs of life return.

FOREIGN BODY AIRWAY OBSTRUCTION

Aspiration of food or vomit, or the inhalation of a foreign body will compromise the paediatric airway. Spontaneous coughing to clear the material should be encouraged but if this fails back blows and chest thrusts in infants and back blows together with alternate cycles of chest thrusts and abdominal thrusts in children may provide vibration to loosen the material and enough expiratory force to expel the obstruction. Abdominal thrusts are not recommended in infants under the age of 1 year as damage to the abdominal contents may occur. The importance of checking the mouth, formally opening the airway and attempting expired air ventilation after each cycle has been highlighted by the need to ensure that the airway is actually obstructed. These checks are also required to assess whether the clearing manoeuvres have dislodged the material enough to allow some air to pass the obstruction.

PAEDIATRIC ADVANCED LIFE SUPPORT

The basic life support sequence provides the fundamental treatment of an infant or child that collapses in cardiopulmonary arrest. Advanced life support is the definitive management of the condition using complex techniques, drugs and equipment.[22] As in basic life support, advanced life support protocols emphasize the importance of establishing an airway, oxygenation and ventilation from the outset. Although it includes a pathway for the management of ventricular fibrillation and ventricular tachycardia, the emphasis is on non-ventricular fibrillation and non-ventricular tachycardia (asystole and pulseless electrical activity) as these are the rhythms found in the majority of paediatric events. Ventricular fibrillation has been documented in less than 10% of paediatric events.[6,7,20,37–39]

AIRWAY

The simple manoeuvre of opening the airway by head tilt and chin lift/jaw thrust may be sufficient to maintain an adequate airway. In some cases, where maintaining an effective position may be difficult, the airway can be improved by inserting an oropharyngeal (Guedel) airway. An oropharyngeal airway can be correctly sized by measuring its length against the distance from the centre of the mouth to the angle of jaw. The airway is initially inserted concave size upwards and rotated through 180° (concave size down) as it is advanced along the hard palate into the oropharynx. Attempts at inserting too large a size airway will cause trauma to the oropharynx. Nasopharyngeal airways are also useful; the correct size is that which fits comfortably through the anterior nares. A tracheal tube of suitable size, cut short, can often be substituted as an effective nasopharyngeal airway (a safety pin through the distal end will ensure that the tube does not disappear into the nose).

The laryngeal mask airway has been assessed as an effective airway adjunct in adult resuscitation. It is a technique that can be taught easily to doctors, nurses and paramedic staff.[40–45]

Small-sized laryngeal masks are available for infants and children but their effectiveness in paediatric resuscitation has yet to be established. They will probably have their most significant effect where intubation is difficult or where the health-care provider is not proficient in paediatric tracheal intubation.

Tracheal intubation is the most effective method of securing the paediatric airway. Using a straight-bladed laryngoscope and a plain plastic tracheal tube of the appropriate size [internal diameter (mm) = (age in years/4) + 4] is a technique that requires skills only developed by formal training and regular practice. Intubation must be achieved rapidly and accurately without a prolonged delay to basic life support. Any attempt lasting for longer than 30 s should be abandoned and the child reoxygenated before a further attempt at intubation is made. Having achieved tracheal intubation, the position of the tube needs to be checked by auscultating both sides of the child's chest for equal breath sounds. The tracheal tube needs to be fixed carefully in place to prevent its accidental removal or displacement.

OXYGENATION

Ventilation using a self-inflating bag-valve-mask with supplemental oxygen will provide higher levels of inspired oxygen than the expired air ventilation of basic life support. Concentrations up to 90% can be achieved if the self-inflating resuscitation bag is fitted with an oxygen reservoir system. Facemasks, for use with a self-inflating bag, should be made of clear plastic so that the proximal airway can be observed through the mask. The circular facemask with a soft seal rim has been found to be the most efficient design, especially in the hands of a less experienced operator. Although many anaesthetists are skilled in the use of the Ayre's T-piece with the Jackson–Rees modification for paediatric ventilation, this circuit is not recommended for the less experienced and should not be part of the routine resuscitation equipment. Furthermore, this system does require a constant reliable source of gas supply to function and this may not always be immediately available. The self-inflating resuscitation bag can function independently and has the advantage of being capable of being operated safely and effectively by a much wider range of operators.

CIRCULATION

Circulatory access is of prime importance to effective advanced life support[46,47] and yet this technical procedure is more fraught with difficulty than any other in resuscitation. Direct intravenous access is preferable, but in cases where this may not be possible intraosseous access is the next best choice. The decision as to which venous access site is to be attempted must be balanced against the resuscitation skills of the team, its relative technical difficulty and the risks of the technique. Experimental data have shown that drugs given via the inferior vena cava take longer to reach the heart than those given into the superior vena cava. Therefore, vascular access points draining into the superior vena cava from peripheral or central routes are preferable.[48–50] Furthermore, centrally administered drugs act more rapidly than those given by a peripheral route.[49,51–53] Drugs administered peripherally must be followed by a fluid bolus flush to move them into the central circulation.[54] The final choice of venous access site must also reflect the practical facts that central access above the diaphragm is a difficult, skilled technique and most operatives find peripheral venous access simpler.

Intraosseous access to the circulatory system is a relatively simple technique that provides rapid access when the direct venous approach has failed[55–57] (see Chapter 6). Any drug or fluid can be given via the intraosseous route. Drugs and fluids administered through the intraosseous route reach the heart in a time comparable with direct peripheral venous access.[57–60] Intraosseous puncture is usually performed on the anterior surface of the tibia, one finger's breadth below the tibial tuberosity, although access can also be gained directly into the distal femur. Successful entry into the marrow cavity must be confirmed by loss of resistance as the marrow cavity is entered, the needle should remain upright without support, bone marrow can be aspirated and there is free flow of drugs and fluid without subcutaneous infiltration around the entry point.[61–63] Marrow aspiration samples can be used for estimation of haematological and electrolyte results. Complications

of intraosseous access include osteomyelitis, long bone fractures,[64] subcutaneous drug extravasation[65,66] and compartment syndrome, but are rare.[67–69]

Tracheal drug administration should only be used when there is likely to be a significant delay in the administration of the core resuscitation drugs. The route is considered unreliable[70] and postresuscitation hypertension and tachycardia have been reported as a result of the depot storage effect of adrenaline in the lungs.[71–73] Severe hypertension resulting from the depot effect of drugs stored in the lungs may be an underlying cause of poor cerebral outcome.[74] None the less, it can be argued that because of the simplicity of the technique and the speed of access of the route, essential resuscitation drugs should be administered via the tracheal tube whilst direct venous access is being established.[75,76]

DRUGS

Although many drugs have been tried in paediatric life support, few have retained their place in the resuscitation treatment protocols.

Adrenaline (epinephrine)

Adrenaline is the mainstay of paediatric life support. It is used mainly for its α-adrenergic activity, causing peripheral vasoconstriction, raising the peripheral vascular resistance, increasing the end-diastolic filling pressure and thereby improving coronary blood flow.[11,77] Adrenaline's β-adrenergic activity is also useful as it has a direct inotropic and chronotropic effect on the myocardium.

The recommended initial dose of adrenaline is $10 \ \mu g \ kg^{-1}$ when administered via the intravenous or intraosseous route ($10 \ \mu g \ kg^{-1}$ is $0.01 \ mg \ kg^{-1}$ or $0.1 \ ml \ kg^{-1}$ of a $1:10\ 000$ solution). Recent studies in infants and children have suggested the benefit of a higher dose of adrenaline for the unresponsive asystolic child.[78] Therefore, should the child not respond to the initial dose of adrenaline then a second dose of $100 \ \mu g \ kg^{-1}$ ($0.1ml \ kg^{-1}$ of a $1:1000$ solution) is recommended. If the child does not respond to this and further $100 \ \mu g \ kg^{-1}$ doses of adrenaline then the eventual outcome is likely to be poor; the results of several studies show that no children have survived to discharge who have received more than two doses of adrenaline.[5,6,13]

Atropine

Atropine is a parasympathetic blocking drug that will block the cardiac activity of the vagus nerve. It is used to treat bradycardia in a dose of 20 μg kg^{-1}. Atropine should be considered in the periarrest scenario, especially as it will prevent bradycardias of vagal origin before they progress to cardiopulmonary collapse. Atropine is not recommended during resuscitation as the adrenergic effects of adrenaline are considered to override the parasympathetic bradycardic effects on the heart.

Bicarbonate

Sodium bicarbonate is an alkalysing agent used to correct the acidosis often associated with resuscitation. However, sodium bicarbonate is a solution with a high osmolarity containing a high level of sodium. The recommended dose is 1 mmol kg^{-1} (1 ml kg^{-1} of an 8.4% solution). Sodium bicarbonate should only be given if the child is being effectively ventilated, as any carbon dioxide that is released by the process of acid neutralization must be removed from the body via the lungs or paradoxical intracellular acidosis will result.

TREATMENT ALGORITHMS

It is important when performing paediatric life support to use a recognized and an efficient treatment pathway. Algorithms have been developed for basic and advanced life support.

BASIC LIFE SUPPORT (FIGURE 22.1)

This simple but effective algorithm guides the health-care professional through the important steps of establishing an airway, initiating breathing and commencing chest compressions. The algorithm provides for cases where attempts at ventilation have failed by suggesting repositioning of the airway before the rescuer

proceeds to an obstructed airway procedure. The basic life-support algorithm provides the core of paediatric life support. It should be taught and made available to all those involved with the care of infants and children.

ADVANCED LIFE SUPPORT (FIGURE 22.2)

The advanced algorithm starts with the reminder that basic life support must be ongoing. Establishing venous access and ventilating with oxygen are the next steps. The algorithm then divides into two pathways according to the underlying rhythm: non-ventricular fibrillation (or tachycardia) or ventricular fibrillation (or tachycardia).

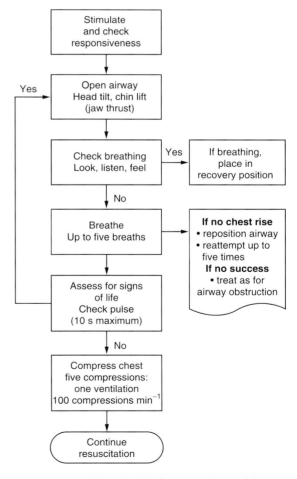

Figure 22.1 Algorithm for basic paediatric life support.[21]

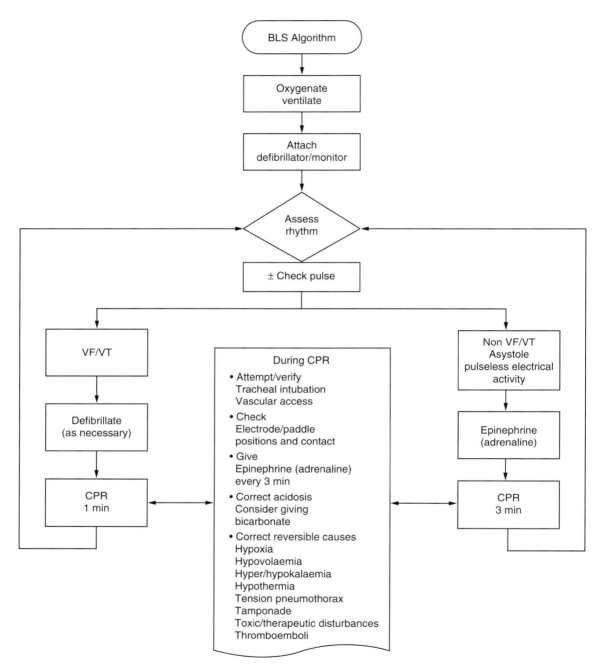

Figure 22.2 Algorithm for paediatric advanced life support.

Non-ventricular fibrillation or tachycardia

A profound bradycardia or asystole is the most common rhythm associated with cardiac arrest in infants and children. A profound bradycardia (described as being a pulse rate of less than 1 beat s^{-1}) may precede asystole but in itself the bradycardia does not produce an adequate cardiac output. A profound bradycardia should therefore be treated in the same way as an asystole. The treatment of asystole is an initial dose of adrenaline at 10 μg kg^{-1} given by the intravenous or intraosseous route (or 10 times this dose via the tracheal tube if venous access has not been established). Second and subsequent doses of adrenaline should be at 100 μg kg^{-1}. Where there is a cardiac rhythm but no cardiac output (pulseless electrical activity) it is also necessary to treat any of the underlying reversible causes of cardiac arrest. These are the four Hs and four Ts of cardiac arrest: hypoxia, hypovolaemia, hyper/hypokalaemia and hypothermia; and tension pneumothorax, tamponade, toxic/therapeutic disturbances and thromboemboli.

Again, adrenaline should be administered every 3 min according to the schedule described previously and resuscitation should not be abandoned until a reasonable attempt has been made to correct these potentially reversible causes of cardiac arrest.

Ventricular fibrillation and ventricular tachycardia

These rhythms, although common in adults, are relatively rare in infants and children. Although one study[8] reported an incidence of 23% ventricular fibrillation in children most other studies report an incidence of between 0 and 10%.[7,9,14,79,80] None the less, the physician must always be aware of the occasional need to treat ventricular fibrillation in children by defibrillation.

The recommended sequence is to give two rapid defibrillatory shocks of 2 J kg^{-1}, followed immediately by a third single shock at 4 J kg^{-1}. All further defibrillation attempts should then be made at 4 J kg^{-1} in a rapid repeated series of three shocks. Following the first cycle of three defibrillation attempts adrenaline 10 μg kg^{-1} should be given and, in accordance with previous explanations, further doses of 100 μg kg^{-1} should be given following the second cycle of three shocks and between all subsequent cycles. When ventricular fibrillation occurs in children the possibility of a correctable underlying cause such as hypothermia, drug overdose (tricyclic antidepressant overdose) and electrolyte imbalance (hyperkalaemia) should be considered.

RESUSCITATION OF THE NEWBORN

Newborn resuscitation specifically refers to the resuscitation procedures at or immediately after the delivery of a newly born infant.[81] There is a specific sequence of events centred on the respiratory and circulatory changes that occur in relation to the 'first breath'. Therefore, the recommended resuscitation procedures (Figure 22.3) emphasize the airway and breathing manoeuvres, whilst the management of the circulation is left to the trained health-care provider. Resuscitation of the newborn is unique in that it is, in most cases, predictable. It is only rarely an unexpected emergency procedure. Careful assessment of maternal and fetal factors, the mode of delivery and the obstetric care will predict the majority of newborns that will require resuscitation procedures.

It has been estimated that the use of simple airway measures could prevent newborn asphyxia occurring in 900 000 infants per year world-wide. Of the 5 million newborn deaths per year world-wide, 56% of which occur in 'out of hospital births', 19% have 'birth asphyxia' as a cause.[82] In the UK newborn mortality is much lower but with the increase in home deliveries it has become increasingly important for the birth attendants and other health-care professionals to be not only conversant with obstetric problems but also proficient in newborn resuscitation techniques.

The majority of newborn infants cry within a few minutes of birth and require little more than careful drying and then wrapping in a warm towel to prevent heat loss. If the baby does not cry, it should be gently stimulated by more vigorous drying with a towel or flicking the soles of the feet. More vigorous stimulation is contraindicated and can be potentially dangerous. Of those that do not cry, most will only need the airway clearing and ventilation; very few will need full resuscitation including intubation, circulatory access and drug administration.

The newborn baby's initial cry and subsequent efforts at breathing must be assessed carefully to ensure that they result in adequate and sustained oxygenation of the lungs. Gasp-

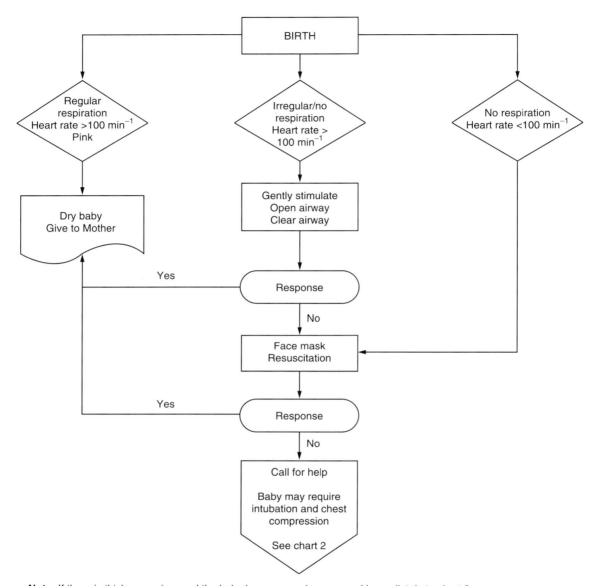

Note: If there is thick meconium and the baby is unresponsive, proceed immediately to chart 2

Figure 22.3 Algorithm of resuscitation of babies at birth (chart 1).[81]

ing without additional efforts at breathing is usually considered inadequate. Abnormal or absent ventilatory patterns will require immediate active intervention.

The initial assessment of the neonate is based on respiratory activity, colour and heart rate. These three parameters have been shown to be more accurate in the assessment of the newborn than the total Apgar scoring system.[83,84]

The newborn can be classified into three groups.

1 *Fit and healthy baby:*
- vigorous effective respiratory efforts;
- centrally pink;

- heart rate > 100 min^{-1}.

This baby requires no intervention other than drying, wrapping in a warm towel and, where appropriate, handing to the mother. The baby will usually remain warm by skin to skin contact with mother and may be put to the breast at this stage.

2 *Breathing inadequately or apnoeic:*
- central cyanosis;
- heart rate > 100 min^{-1}.

This group of babies may respond to tactile stimulation and/or facial oxygen but often need basic life support.

3 *Breathing inadequately or apnoeic:*
- pale or white owing to poor cardiac output and peripheral vasoconstriction;
- heart rate < 100 min^{-1} or no detectable heart rate (although this was documented up to 15–20 min before delivery.)

These babies sometimes improve with initial basic life support but normally require immediate intubation and positive pressure ventilation progressing to chest compressions, and full advanced life support including resuscitation drugs if they fail to respond.

NEWBORN BASIC LIFE SUPPORT (FIGURES 22.3 AND 22.4)

AIRWAY

The airway is opened by tilting the head into the neutral position and lifting the jaw upwards by gentle pressure on the mandible (Figure 22.3). The airway can be cleared of residual debris and fluid by gentle suction of the mouth and nares. Aggressive pharyngeal suction can delay the onset of spontaneous breathing and cause laryngeal spasm and vagal bradycardia.[85] It is not indicated unless the amniotic fluid is stained with thick meconium or blood. If suction is required, a 10FG (or if preterm, 8FG) suction catheter should be connected to a suction source not exceeding -100 mmHg. This should not continue for longer than 5 s in the absence of meconium. The catheter should normally not be inserted further than about 5 cm from the lips.

BREATHING

Check for breathing by looking, listening and feeling for respiratory effects. The inspired air can be supplemented with oxygen from a loose-fitting facemask or funnel. Effective ventilation can only be carried out by using a well-fitting facemask that covers the mouth and nose but does not cover the eyes or overlap the chin.[86]

Self-inflating resuscitation bags refill independently of adjuvant gas flow. They should incorporate a pressure limited pop-off valve preset at 20–30 cmH$_2$O. In a minority, this pressure may be inadequate to achieve lung expansion at birth and the facility to override this is useful for a few babies. The volume of the bag should be at least 500 ml, so that the inflation pressure can be maintained for at least 0.5 s. Facemask T-piece resuscitation uses compressed air/oxygen fed to one arm of a T-piece attached to the facemask.[87] The baby's lungs are inflated by occluding the open arm of the T-piece. It is essential to have a safety pressure-release system (set at 20–30 cmH$_2$O) incorporated in the gas supply tubing. A method for monitoring the peak pressures will also be required. This system has the advantage that it requires only one hand for normal operation and the inflation pressures can be maintained for longer than with the self-inflating bags. It has been traditional to use 100% oxygen as the ventilating gas for resuscitation but there are data indicating that, in term babies, 100% inspired oxygen has little advantage and may increase oxygen free-radial damage. Furthermore, there is evidence that newborn resuscitation is as effective with air as with 100% inspired oxygen.[88–91] If gas-mixing facilities are available then a 40% inspired oxygen is recommended as the ventilating gas to expand the newborn lungs, but if cyanosis persists or the heart rate falls the inspired oxygen level should be raised.

The first five or six breaths require an inspiration held for 1–2 s. This prolonged inspiration will double the inspiratory volume and is more likely to establish the functional residual capacity needed by the baby to

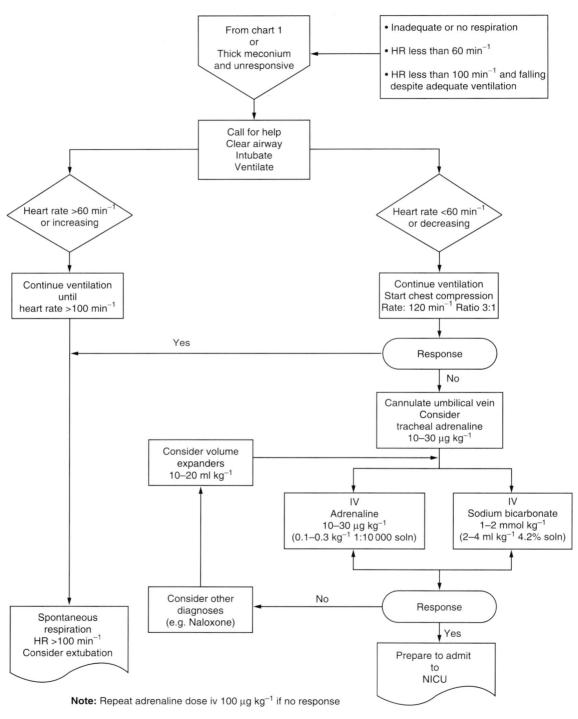

Figure 22.4 Algorithm of resuscitation of babies at birth (chart 2).[81]

continue to breath spontaneously.[92] After these initial breaths a normal ventilatory pattern can be used, ventilating at a rate of approximately 30–40 breaths min^{-1} until spontaneous respiration is established.

If the baby does not respond to these initial facemask resuscitation manoeuvres or the heart rate falls below 100 beats min^{-1}, the health-care professional must proceed to tracheal intubation and advanced life-support procedures immediately.

NEWBORN ADVANCED LIFE SUPPORT (FIGURES 22.3 AND 22.4)

Tracheal intubation is a skilled technique that requires training and practice. It is achieved using a straight-blade laryngoscope and an appropriate size of tracheal tube (Table 22.1). These are only guidelines and tubes 0.5 mm larger and smaller should always be available.

Once the tracheal tube is passed through the vocal cords its position must be checked carefully to ensure that there is equal ventilation of both lungs. The tube should then be fixed securely in position. Ventilation is continued using the self-inflating bag or T-piece system.

When there is any doubt about the position or patency of the tube remove the tracheal tube immediately and reintubate after a brief period of oxygenation using face mask ventilation.

CIRCULATION

The initial attempts at establishing a viable circulation are made using chest compressions.

Table 22.1 Guidelines for tracheal tube size

Tracheal tube size (mm i.d.)	Weight (g)	Gestation (weeks)
2.5	< 1000	< 28
3	1000–2500	28–36
3.5	> 2500	> 36

Chest compressions should be performed if: the heart rate is less than 60 beats min^{-1}, or the heart rate is less than 100 beats min^{-1} and falls despite adequate ventilation.

The optimal technique is to place the two thumbs side by side over the lower one-third of the sternum with the fingers encircling the torso and supporting the back.[93–95] The lower third of the sternum[96] is compressed 2–3 cm in a term baby at a rate of approximately 120 compressions min^{-1}. The compressions should be smooth and not jerky and each compression should last 50% of the compression/relaxation cycle. An alternative technique is to use the index and middle finger of one hand to compress the lower half of the infant's sternum. This allows the operator's free hand to perform simple resuscitation procedures whilst maintaining external chest compressions. A single ventilation should be performed after every three chest compressions. The pulse should be checked periodically and chest compressions only discontinued when the spontaneous heart rate of greater than 100 beats min^{-1} is established.

If the infant fails to respond to active ventilation following intubation and chest compressions then venous access must be established. Failure of the infant to respond is usually a result of inadequate ventilation and it is therefore essential to check the seal of the facemask or the position of the tracheal tube. If, in spite of optimal airway control there continues to be no improvement, the umbilical vein should be catheterized using a 4.5–5FG umbilical catheter. This is achieved by transecting the cord 1–2 cm away from the abdominal skin and inserting the umbilical catheter until there is a free flow of blood up the catheter.

An initial dose of intravenous adrenaline, 10–30 μg kg^{-1} (0.1–0.3 ml kg^{-1} of 1 : 10 000 solution), should be given via the umbilical venous catheter, flushing the adrenaline through the catheter with 2 ml of saline. If venous access fails, an intraosseous needle can be inserted into the proximal tibia and this route temporarily used instead of the venous umbilical catheter. If there is a delay in establishing umbilical vein catheterization or intraosseous access then the same dose of adrenaline, 10–30 μg kg^{-1}, can be given through the tracheal tube. Despite the tracheal administration of adrenaline being widely practised there is little evidence that it is effective.[76,97,98] It may be least effective if given before the lungs are fully inflated.

If there is still no response the baby should be given $1–2$ mmol kg^{-1} body weight of sodium bicarbonate slowly over $2–3$ min. Either a 4.2% bicarbonate solution is used, or a volume of 8.4% sodium bicarbonate solution is mixed with an equal volume of 5 or 10% dextrose or sterile water. This results in a concentration of 0.5 mmol ml^{-1} solution. Basic life support must be continued. Sodium bicarbonate is a hyperosmolar solution and should be administered by slow infusion in preterm babies below 32 weeks because of the risk of inducing intracerebral bleeding. Further doses of bicarbonate are best given in response to the results of arterial blood-gas analysis data.

Repeat doses of adrenaline should be given if the newborn continues to fail to respond. Subsequent larger doses, up to 100 μg kg^{-1}, may be considered, but there is evidence that the need for adrenaline during resuscitation is associated with a poor prognosis.[99]

Hypovolaemia in the newborn requires active volume replacement. Indications for intravenous fluid therapy are: evidence of acute fetal blood loss, pallor which persists after oxygenation, and faint pulses with a good heart rate and poor response to resuscitation including adequate ventilation. Fluid replacement, at $10–20$ ml kg^{-1}, can be given as 4.5% albumin, whole blood or plasma.

Finally, intramuscular naloxone (100 μg kg^{-1}) should be considered in the apnoeic newborn who rapidly becomes pink and who obviously has a satisfactory circulation on resuscitation. Naloxone is a narcotic antagonist and is specifically indicated where there is a history of recent therapeutic administration of opioids to the mother.

In conclusion, paediatric life support is an essential part of the care of newborns, infants and children. The protocols described in this chapter all follow the simple airway, breathing and circulation outline. To be effective, healthcare professionals practising these resuscitation techniques must be properly trained, formally accredited and frequently practised in the skills of the procedure. Delay or hesitation in recognizing the need for life support will have disastrous consequences.

REFERENCES

1 Hickey, R.W., Cohen, D.M., Strausbaugh, S. and Dietrich, A.M. Pediatric patients requiring CPR in the prehospital setting. *Annals of Emergency Medicine* 1995; **25**: 495–501.

2 Innes, P.A., Summers, C.A., Boyd, I.M. and Molyneaux, E.M. Audit of paediatric cardiopulmonary resuscitation. *Archives of Disease in Childhood* 1993; **68**: 487–91.

3 Teach, S.J., Moore, P.E. and Fleisher, G.R. Death and resuscitation in the pediatric emergency department. *Annals of Emergency Medicine* 1995; **25**: 799–803.

4 Thompson, J.E., Bonner, B. and Lower, G.M. Pediatric cardiopulmonary arrests in rural populations. *Pediatrics* 1990; **86**: 302–6.

5 Zaritsky, A., Nadkarni, V., Getson, P. and Kuehl, K. CPR in children. *Annals of Emergency Medicine* 1987; **16**: 1107–11.

6 Dieckmann, R.A. and Vardis, R. High-dose epinephrine in pediatric out-of-hospital cardiopulmonary arrest. *Pediatrics* 1995; **95**: 901–13.

7 Isenberg, M., Bergner, L. and Hallstrom, A. Epidemiology of cardiac arrest and resuscitation in children. *Annals of Emergency Medicine* 1983; **12**: 672–4.

8 Friesen, R.M., Duncan, P., Tweed, W.A. and Bristow, G. Appraisal of paediatric cardiopulmonary resuscitation. *Canadian Medical Association Journal* 1982; **126**: 1055–8.

9 Losek, J., Hennes, H., Glaeser, P.W., Smith, D.S. and Hendley, G. Prehospital countershock treatment of pediatric asystole. *American Journal of Emergency Medicine* 1989; **7**: 571–5.

10 Mogayzel, C., Quan, L., Graves, J.R., Tiedeman, D., Fahrenbruch, C. and Herndon, P. Out-of-hospital ventricular fibrillation in children and adolescents: causes and outcomes. *Annals of Emergency Medicine* 1995; **25**: 484–91.

11 O'Rourke, P.P. Outcome of children who are apneic and pulseless in the emergency room. *Critical Care Medicine* 1986; **14**: 466–8.

12 Ronco, R., King, W., Donley, D.K. and Tilden, S.J. Outcome and cost at a children's hospital following resuscitation for out-of-hospital cardiopulmonary arrest. *Archives of Pediatric and Adolescent Medicine* 1995; **149**: 210–14.

13 Schindler, M.B., Bohn, D., Cox, P., *et al.* Outcome of out-of-hospital cardiac or respiratory arrest in children. *New England Journal Medicine* 1996; **335**: 1473–9.

14 Torphy, D.E., Minter, M.G. and Thompson, B.M. Cardiorespiratory arrest and resuscitation of children. *American Journal of Diseases of Children* 1984; **138**: 1099–102.

15 Lewis, J.K., Minter, M.G., Eshelman, S.J. and Witte, M.K. Outcome of pediatric resuscitation. *Annals of Emergency Medicine* 1983; **12**: 297–9.

16 Otto, C.W., Yakaitis, R.W. and Blitt, C.D. Mechanism of action of epinephrine in resuscitation from cardiac arrest. *Critical Care Medicine* 1981; **9**: 321–4.

17 Tunstall-Pedoe, H., Bailey, L., Chamberlain, D.A., Marsden, A.K., Ward, M.E. and Zideman, D.A. Survey of 3765 cardiopulmonary resuscitations in British hospi-

tals (the BRESUS Study): methods and overall results. *British Medical Journal* 1992; **304**: 1347–51.

18 Berg, R. and Goetting, M. Pediatric sudden death. In: Paradis, N., Halperin, H. and Nowak, R. (eds). *Cardiac Arrest*. Baltimore, MD: Williams & Wilkins, 1996: 671–94.

19 Zaritsky, A., Nadkarni, V., Hazinski, M.F., *et al.* Recommended guidelines for uniform reporting of pediatric advanced life support: the Pediatric Utstein Style. *Resuscitation* 1995; **30**: 95–116.

20 Kuisma, M., Suominen, P. and Korpela, R. Pediatric out-of-hospital cardiac arrests – epidemiology and outcome. *Resuscitation* 1995; **30**: 141–50.

21 European Resuscitation Council. Pediatric Basic Life Support. *Resuscitation* 1998; **37**: 97–100.

22 European Resuscitation Council. Pediatric Advanced Life Support. *Resuscitation* 1998; **37**: 101–2.

23 Nadkarni, V., Hazinski, M.F., Zideman, D.A., *et al.* Pediatric life support: an advisory statement by the Paediatric Life Support Working Group of the International Liaison Committee on Resuscitation. *Resuscitation* 1997; **34**: 115–27.

24 European Resuscitation Council. Working group on Basic Life Support. *Resuscitation* 1998; **37**: 67–80.

25 European Resuscitation Council. Working Group on Advanced Life Support. *Resuscitation* 1998; **37**: 81–90.

26 Wheeler, M., Roth, A., Dunham, M., Rae, B. and Cote, C. A bronchoscopic, computer-assisted examination of the changes in dimension of the infant tracheal lumen with changes in head position. *Anesthesiology* 1998; **88**: 1183–7.

27 Melker, R.J. Asynchronous and other alternative methods of ventilation during CPR. *Annals of Emergency Medicine* 1984; **13**: 758–61.

28 Melker, R.J. and Banner, M.J. Ventilation during CPR: two-rescuer standards reappraised. *Annals of Emergency Medicine* 1985; **14**: 397–402.

29 Bowman, F., Menegazzi, J., Check, B. and Duckett, T. Lower esophageal sphincter pressure during prolonged cardiac arrest and resuscitation. *Annals of Emergency Medicine* 1995; **26**: 216–19.

30 Cavallaro, D.L. and Melker, R.J. Comparison of two techniques for detecting cardiac activity in infants. *Critical Care Medicine* 1983; **11**: 198–200.

31 Brearley, S., Simms, M.H. and Shearman, C.P. Peripheral pulse palpation: An unreliable sign. *Annals of the Royal College of Surgeons of England* 1992; **74**: 169–72.

32 Mather, C. and O'Kelly, S. The palpation of pulses. *Anaesthesia* 1996; **51**: 189–91.

33 Monsieurs, K.G., De Cauwer, H.G. and Bossaert, L.L. Feeling for the carotid pulse: is five seconds enough? *Resuscitation* 1996; **31**: S3.

34 Monsieurs, K.G., De Cauwer, H.G. and Bossaert, L.L. Obesity of the victim negatively influences carotid pulse checking performance. *Resuscitation* 1996; **31**: S6.

35 Connick, M. and Berg, R.A. Femoral venous pulsations during open-heart cardiac massage. *Annals of Emergency Medicine* 1994; **24**: 1176–9.

36 Berg, R.A., Kern, K.B., Sanders, A.B., Otto, C.W., Hilwig, R.W. and Ewy, G.A. Bystander cardiopulmonary resuscitation. Is ventilation necessary? *Circulation* 1993; **88**: 1907–15.

37 Appleton, G.O., Cummins, R.O., Larson, M.P. and Graves, J.R. CPR and the single rescuer: at what age

should you 'call first' rather than 'call fast'? *Annals of Emergency Medicine* 1995; **25**: 492–4.

38 Gillis, J., Dickson, D., Rieder, M., Steward, D. and Edmonds, J. Results of inpatient pediatric resuscitation. *Critical Care Medicine* 1986; **14**: 469–71.

39 Walsh, C.K. and Krongrad, E. Terminal cardiac electrical activity in pediatric patients. *American Journal of Cardiology* 1983; **51**: 557–61.

40 Alexander, R., Hodgson, P., Lomax, D. and Bullen, C. A comparison of the laryngeal mask airway and guedel airway, bag and facemask for manual ventilation. *Anaesthesia* 1993; **48**: 231–4.

41 Davies, P.R.F., Tighe, S.Q.M., Greenslade, G.L. and Evans, G.H. Laryngeal mask airway and tracheal tube insertion by unskilled personnel. *Lancet* 1990; **336**: 977–9.

42 De Mello, W.F. and Ward, P. The use of the laryngeal mask airway in primary anaesthesia. *Anaesthesia* 1990; **45**: 793–4.

43 Martin, P.D., Cyna, A.M., Hunter, W.A., Henry, J. and Ramayya, G.P. Training nursing staff in airway management for resuscitation. *Anaesthesia* 1993; **48**: 133–7.

44 Pennant, J.H. and Walker, M. Comparison of the endotracheal tube and the laryngeal mask in airway management by paramedical personnel. *Anesthesia and Analgesia* 1992; **74**: 531–4.

45 Samarkandi, A.H., Seraj, M.A., El Dawlathy, A., Mastan, M. and Bahamces, H.B. The role of the laryngeal mask airway in cardiopulmonary resuscitation. *Resuscitation* 1994; **28**: 103–6.

46 Brunette, D.D. and Fischer, R. Intravascular access in pediatric cardiac arrest. *American Journal of Emergency Medicine* 1988; **6**: 577–9.

47 Kanter, R.K., Zimmerman, J.J. and Strauss, R.H. Pediatric emergency intravenous access: evaluation of a protocol. *American Journal of Disease in Children* 1986; **140**: 132–4.

48 Dalsey, W.C., Barsan, W.G. and Joyce, S.M. Comparison of superior vena caval access using a radioisotope technique during normal perfusion and cardiopulmonary resuscitation. *American Journal of Emergency Medicine* 1984; **13**: 881–4.

49 Emerman, C.L., Pinchak, A.C., Hancock, D. and Hagen, J.F. Effect of injection site on circulation times during cardiac arrest. *Critical Care Medicine* 1988; **16**: 1138–41.

50 Rosa, D.M., Griffen, C.C., Flanagan, J.J. and Machiedo, G.W. A comparison of intravenous access sites for bolus injections during shock and resuscitation after emergency room thoracotomy with and without aortic crossclamping. *Annals of Surgery* 1990; **56**: 566–70.

51 Barsan, W.G., Levy, R.C. and Weir, H. Lidocaine levels during CPR: differences after peripheral venous, central venous, and intracardiac injections. *Annals of Emergency Medicine* 1981; **10**: 73–8.

52 Hedges, J.R., Barsan, W.B. and Doan, L.A. Central versus peripheral intravenous routes in cardiopulmonary resuscitation. *American Journal of Emergency Medicine* 1981; **10**: 417–19.

53 Kuhn, G.J., White, B.C. and Swetman, R.E. Peripheral versus central circulation time during CPR: a pilot study. *Annals of Emergency Medicine* 1981; **10**: 417–19.

54 Emerman, C.L., Pinchak, A.C., Hancock, D. and Hagen, J.F. The effect of bolus injection on circulation times

during cardiac arrest. *American Journal of Emergency Medicine* 1990; **8**: 190–3.

55 Heinild, S., Sondergard, T. and Tudvad, F. Bone marrow infusion in childhood: experiences from a thousand infusions. *Journal of Pediatrics* 1947; **30**: 400–11.

56 Pillar, S. Re-emphasis on bone marrow as a medium for administration of fluid. *New England Journal of Medicine* 1954; **251**: 846–51.

57 Rosetti, V.A., Thompson, B.M., Miller, J., Mateer, J.R. and Aprahamian, C. Intraosseous infusion: an alternative route of paediatric intravascular access. *Annals of Emergency Medicine* 1995; **14**: 885–8.

58 Andropoulos, D., Soifer, S. and Schreiber, M. Plasma epinephrine concentrations after intraosseous and central venous injection during cardiopulmonary resuscitation in the lamb. *Journal of Pediatrics* 1990; **116**: 312–15.

59 Orlowski, J.P., Porembka, D.T., Gallagher, J.M., Lockren, J.D. and Van Lente, F. Comparison study of intraosseous, central intravenous and peripheral intravenous infusions of emergency drugs. *American Journal of Diseases in Children* 1990; **144**: 112–17.

60 Valdes, M.M. Intraosseous fluid administration in emergencies. *Lancet* 1977; **i**: 1235–6.

61 Berg, R.A. Emergency infusion of catecholamines into bone marrow. *American Journal of Diseases in Children* 1984; **138**: 810–11.

62 Fiser, D. Intraosseous infusion. *New England Journal of Medicine* 1990; **322**: 1579–81.

63 Spivey, W.H. Intraosseous infusions. *Journal of Pediatrics* 1987; **111**: 639–43.

64 LaFleche, F.R., Slepin, M.J., Vargas, J. and Milzman, D.P. Iatrogenic bilateral tibial fractures after intraosseous infusion attempts in a 3-month-old infant. *Annals of Emergency Medicine* 1989; **18**: 1099–101.

65 Christensen, D.W., Vernon, D.D., Banner, W.J. and Dean, J.M. Skin necrosis complicating intraosseous infusion. *Pediatric Emergency Care* 1991; **7**: 289–90.

66 Simmons, C.M., Johnson, N.E., Perkin, R.M. and Van Stralen, D. Intraosseous extravasation complication reports. *Annals of Emergency Medicine* 1994; **23**: 363–6.

67 Galpin, R.D., Kronick, J.B., Willis, R.B. and Frewen, T.C. Bilateral lower extremity compartment syndromes secondary to intraosseous fluid resuscitation. *Journal of Pediatric Orthopedics* 1991; **11**: 773–6.

68 Moscati, M. and Moore, G.P. Compartment syndrome with resultant amputation following intraosseous infusion. *American Journal of Emergency Medicine* 1990; **8**: 470–1.

69 Rimar, S., Westry, J. and Rodriguez, R. Compartment syndrome in an infant following emergency intraosseous infusion. *Clinical Pediatrics* 1988; **27**: 259–60.

70 Orlowski, J.P., Gallagher, J.M. and Porembka, D.T. Endotracheal epinephrine is unreliable. *Resuscitation* 1990; **19**: 103–13.

71 Hahnel, J.H., Lindner, K.H. and Ahnefeld, K.F.W. Endobronchial administration of emergency drugs. *Resuscitation* 1989; **7**: 261–72.

72 Hornchen, U., Schuttler, J., Stoeckel, H., Eichelkraut, W. and Hahn, N. Endobronchial instillation of epinephrine during cardiopulmonary resuscitation. *Critical Care Medicine* 1987; **15**: 1037–9.

73 Hornchen, U., Schuttler, J. and Stoekel, H. Influence of the pulmonary circulation on adrenaline pharmacokinetics during cardiopulmonary resuscitation. *European Journal of Anaesthesiology* 1992; **9**: 85–91.

74 Bleyaert, A.L., Sands, P.A., Safar, P., *et al.* Augmentation of postischemic brain damage by severe intermittent hypertension. *Critical Care Medicine* 1980; **8**: 41–5.

75 Greenberg, M.I., Roberts, J.R. and Baskin, S.I. Use of endotracheally administered epinephrine in a pediatric patient. *American Journal of Diseases in Children* 1981; **135**: 767–8.

76 Lindemann, R. Resuscitation of the new-born: endotracheal administration of epinephrine. *Acta Paediatrica Scandinavica* 1984; **73**: 210–12.

77 Kosnik, J.W., Jackson, R.E., Keats, S., Tworek, R.M. and Freeman, S.B. Dose-related response of centrally administered epinephrine on the change in aortic diastolic pressure during closed chest massage in dogs. *Annals of Emergency Medicine* 1985; **14**: 204–8.

78 Patterson, M., Boenning, D. and Klein, B. High dose epinephrine in pediatric cardiopulmonary arrest. *Pediatric Emergency Care* 1994; **10**: 310.

79 Fiser, D.H. and Wrape, V. Outcome of cardiopulmonary resuscitation in children. *Pediatric Emergency Care* 1987; **3**: 235–7.

80 Nichols, D.G., Kettrick, R.G., Swedlow, D.B., Lee, S., Passman, R. and Ludwig, S. Factors influencing outcome of cardiopulmonary resuscitation in children. *Pediatric Emergency Care* 1986; **2**: 1–5.

81 European Resuscitation Council. Recommendations on resuscitation of babies at birth. *Resuscitation* 1998; **37**: 103–10.

82 World Health Organization. World Health Report. Geneva: *World Health Organization*, 1995: 21.

83 Chamberlain, G., Banks, J. Assessment of the Apgar score. *Lancet* 1974; **ii**: 1225–8.

84 Apgar, V. and James, L.S. Further observations of the newborn scoring system. *American Journal of Diseases in Children* 1962; **104**: 419–28.

85 Codero, L. and How, E.H. Neonatal bradycardia following nasopharyngeal suction. *Journal of Pediatrics* 1971; **78**: 441.

86 Palme, C., Nystrom, B. and Tunell, R. An evaluation of the efficiency of face masks in the resuscitation of the newborn infants. *Lancet* 1985; **i**: 207–10.

87 Hoskyns, E.W., Milner, A.D. and Hopkin, I.E. A simple method of face mask resuscitation at birth. *Archives of Disease in Childhood* 1987; **62**: 376–9.

88 Lundstrom, K.E., Pryds, O. and Greisen, G. Oxygen at birth and prolonged cerebral vasoconstriction in preterm infants. *Archives of Disease in Childhood* 1995; **73**: F81–6.

89 Svenningsen, N.W., Stjernquist, K., Stavenow, S. and Hellstrom-Vestas, L. Neonatal outcome of extremely low birth weight liveborn infants below 901g in a Swedish population. *Acta Paediatrica Scandinavica* 1989; **78**: 180–8.

90 Ballot, D.E., Rothberg, A.D., Davies, V.A., Smith, J. and Kirste,n G. Does hypoxemia prevent brain damage in birth asphyxia? *Medical Hypotheses* 1993; **41** Suppl. 4: 344–7.

91 Ramji, S., Ahuja, S., Thirupuram, S., Rootwelt, T., Rooth, G. and Saugstad, O.D. Resuscitation of asphyxic new-

born infants with room air or 100% oxygen. *Pediatric Research* 1993; **34** Suppl. 6: 809–12.

92 Vyas, H., Milner, A.D., Hopkin, I.E. and Boon, A.W. Physiologic responses to prolonged slow rise inflation in the resuscitation of the asphyxiated newborn infant. *Journal of Pediatrics* 1981; **99**: 635–9.

93 Thaler, M.M. and Stobie, G.H.C. An improved technique of external cardiac compression in infants and young children. *New England Journal of Medicine* 1963; **269**: 606–10.

94 Todres, I.D. and Rogers, M.C. Methods of external cardiac massage in the newborn infant. *Journal of Pediatrics* 1975; **86**: 781–2.

95 David, R. Closed chest cardiac massage in the newborn infant. *Pediatrics* 1988; **81**: 552–4.

96 Phillips, G. and Zideman, D.A. Relation of infant heart to sternum: its significance in cardiopulmonary resuscitation. *Lancet* 1986; **i**: 1024–5.

97 Lucas, V.W., Preziosi, M.P. and Burchfield, D.J. Epinephrine absorption following endotracheal administration: effects of hypoxia-induced low pulmonary blood flow. *Resuscitation* 1997; **27**: 31–4.

98 Mullett, C.J., Kong, J.Q., Romano, J.T. and Polak, M.J. Age related changes in pulmonary venous epinephrine concentration and pulmonary vascular response after intratracheal epinephrine. *Pediatric Research* 1992; **31**: 458–61.

99 Sims, D.G., Heal, C.A. and Bartle, S.M. The use of adrenaline and atropine in neonatal resuscitation. *Archives of Disease in Childhood* 1994; **70**: F3–10.

CHAPTER 23

Organization of paediatric anaesthesia

DAVID HATCH AND ANNA-MARIA ROLLIN

INTRODUCTION

Parents understandably expect the best possible care for their children, and are often prepared to travel considerable distances to obtain it. Paediatric anaesthetic services must therefore be organized to ensure that this reasonable parental expectation can be met. Whilst this chapter reviews the way in which attempts are being made to address this challenge in the UK, the issues are of global importance. The UK experience may provide a template which can be adapted according to local circumstances for use elsewhere.

THE NEED FOR CHANGE

We live in a rapidly changing world where patients are becoming much better informed and have higher expectations of doctors. With increased access to the Internet they are in a better position to evaluate the competence of professional health workers and to ask searching questions about their training and experience as well as about the risks and outcomes of treatment. Parents increasingly expect to be involved in the decisions affecting their children's treatment, including the best place to have that treatment carried out. In the past doctors have not been accustomed to their advice or decisions being questioned in this way and for some this provides a major challenge. It is therefore increasingly important for anaesthetists, surgeons and other health-care workers to work together in clinical teams with well-defined values and standards. Once these have been developed and agreed the limitations of the team should become quite clear so that the indications for referral to other centres of children whose needs cannot be met satisfactorily should also become apparent. Standards should be regularly reviewed in the light of continuing developments in medicine, the availability of national clinical guidelines, systematic audit and risk management. Anaesthetic departments with clearly defined operational policies and practices for maintaining professional standards may wish to invite occasional external clinical review. Communications between clinical staff and patients' families should be full and open and questions about the performance of the team should be answered honestly. This will not only lead to the maintenance of good practice but also reduce the incidence of complaints and the likelihood of medicolegal claims being made.

CODIFYING CHANGES AT NATIONAL LEVEL

Whilst every anaesthetist has a personal responsibility as an individual to maintain his or her professional standards, and whilst clinical teams have a corporate responsibility for the performance of the team as outlined above, the framework in which we all work is defined at a national level. In the UK training is supervised by the Royal Colleges, who are increasingly expected to play a leading role in continuing medical education and continuing professional development. National guidelines are produced not only by the Colleges but also by the specialist associations and other professional bodies, and the overall ethical framework for the profession is set by the General Medical Council in its document *Good Medical Practice*.

THE MOVE TOWARDS INCREASING SPECIALIZATION

Dr G. Jackson Rees was one of the first British anaesthetists to plead the case for specialist anaesthetists for children. Editorials in British scientific journals in the late 1970s supported this plea and pointed out the lack of specialist paediatric anaesthetic training or experience of anaesthetists giving most of the children's anaesthetics at that time.[1,2] On the basis of figures derived in 1984 from 1975 data, it was estimated that 70% of anaesthetics for children less than 3 years old were at that time given in District Hospitals as opposed to specialist children's centres.[2] More recent data suggest that this figure was approximately 60% in 1989.[3,4] Although the question of who should anaesthetize children remains a subject for debate,[5,6] there is no reason why the majority should not be treated outside the specialist centres, as long as agreed standards are maintained.

The issue received wider attention with the publication of the 1989 Report of the National Confidential Enquiry into Peri-Operative Deaths (NCEPOD), which reviewed the surgical and anaesthetic care of children in hospital.[3] This Report reviewed all deaths of children under 10 years old occurring in the UK within 30 days of a surgical operation.

The most widely publicised of this Report's recommendations was that:

> Surgeons and anaesthetists should not undertake 'occasional paediatric practice'.
> The outcome of surgery and anaesthesia in children is related to the experience of the clinicians involved.

Safe and satisfactory care of children requiring surgery depends not only on the quality of surgeons and anaesthetists. Other appropriately trained and experienced support staff are required, including paediatricians, radiologists, pathologists, nurses and other non-medical staff, working together to form an effective clinical team. Appropriate facilities and resources are also essential, as defined in the

Department of Health document, *The Welfare of Children and Young People in Hospital.*[7]

While few would disagree with the NCEPOD recommendation, which has been endorsed by the Audit Commission[8] and incorporated in the Royal College of Anaesthetists' guidelines for purchasers,[9] its implementation is not entirely straightforward. Problems of definition of 'childhood' and 'occasional practice' arise immediately.

WHAT IS A CHILD?

While the NCEPOD Report studied children aged under 10 years, the most challenging anaesthetic problems usually arise in younger children. Based on a review of the literature, Atwell and Spargo recommended that general surgery in children under 3 years should be carried out in specialist centres, especially if the admission is for an emergency rather than for an elective procedure.[10] The British Association of Paediatric Surgeons suggested that the eventual aim should be to transfer all children under 5 years of age, but that given current resources, transferring those under 3 years was a more practical possibility. There appears to be a consensus of opinion in the UK that trained anaesthetists should be capable of dealing with the common surgical problems that arise in children over 5 years.

In a Report published in 1993, a joint working party of the then British Paediatric Association (BPA), involving paediatricians, surgeons and anaesthetists, focused on children under 3 years old requiring emergency surgery, since these children are at the highest risk. The report recommended their transfer unless consultant surgical and anaesthetic staff with relevant training and experience are available in the district hospital.[11] The relatively small numbers of children involved appear to make this a practical possibility.

Age is clearly not the only consideration. The multidisciplinary liaison group of the Royal College of Paediatrics and Child Health has published recommendations from all the specialist associations about which procedures should fall into the category of 'specialist practice' and which are likely to require intensive care.[12] Most anaesthetists and ear, nose and throat (ENT) surgeons would feel competent to deal with insertion of grommets in infants and young children but might not, for example, be familiar with elective surgery for upper airway obstruction in an 8-year-old child.

WHAT IS ADEQUATE TRAINING?

All anaesthetists must be capable of providing first-line, life-saving care to critically ill children who may present at the local hospital and stabilizing their condition until more expert help is available. The Royal College of Anaesthetists therefore expects all trainees to receive a minimum of 3 months' training in paediatric anaesthesia. At the other end of the spectrum, comprehensive training in paediatric anaesthesia is essential for all intending to specialize in this field on either a part-time or a full-time basis. Those aiming at general career posts with an interest in paediatric anaesthesia should receive at least 6 months' further training and those planning to make a major commitment to the specialty require at least 12 months.[13] National moves towards improvements in continuing medical education and continuing professional development are to be welcomed and may increase the opportunities for anaesthetists working in general hospitals to visit specialist centres for short periods of further training.

WHAT IS OCCASIONAL PRACTICE?

However well trained, without ongoing clinical experience most people's skills deteriorate with time. Lunn suggested that a regular annual caseload of 12 infants under 6 months, 50 infants and children under 3 years, and 300 children under 10 years old might reasonably be accepted as regular and frequent practice.[4] However, results of a postal survey of UK consultants suggested that less than 20% of those anaesthetizing children met these criteria, so a radical change in practice would be required, with far fewer anaesthetists dealing with children, if those who did were to achieve this level of continuing experience.[14] Forty-one per cent of respondents had a regular paediatric practice equivalent to at least one operating session each week, as recommended by the BPA joint working party, and this seems a more realistic figure at which to aim.

OBSTACLES TO IMPLEMENTATION OF NATIONAL GUIDELINES

Although the publication of the above national guidelines has influenced the organization of paediatric anaesthetic services in many hospitals, in some it appears to have had little or no impact. This may be partly due to a natural reluctance among the medical staff involved to refer out of their care some of their most interesting clinical cases. There are, however, other more justifiable obstacles to implementing change. In some parts of the country, particularly remote areas or those in which transportation is poor, geographical considerations become significant. The need to maintain a basic level of skill in the local hospital and to have access to clinical material for teaching purposes are also factors put forward by those opposed to transferring children out of the local hospital environment. Although there is undoubtedly validity in these arguments, they should not take precedence over the safety and welfare of individual children.

Probably the most important obstacle to the increased referral of children to more specialized centres is the suggestion that there is no evidence that outcome is improved by such a policy. NCEPOD data are at best anecdotal and suffer from the lack of a known denominator, as do reports from medicolegal closed claims studies. Other evidence, although sparse, exists in relation to both surgical and anaesthetic outcome. Atwell and Spargo reported a sevenfold increase in mortality and 20-fold increase in morbidity when surgery for congenital pyloric stenosis was undertaken occasionally, and a fall in mortality for neonatal surgery from 75% to 25% within 5 years when it was concentrated into a single unit.[10] These authors also found that of 33 deaths due to intussusception in England and Wales during the period 1984–1989, only one patient was being cared for in a specialized unit and this patient had been transferred there from a district hospital for the management of multisystem failure. They point out that morbidity following inguinal hernia repair in the best centres can be as low as 0.4%, whilst in the NCEPOD report five infants died from complications related to surgery for this condition. In one centre the incidence of testicular atrophy after orchidopexy fell from 35% to 9.4% following the appointment of a surgeon with interest, training and experience in paediatric surgery.[10] Keenan *et al.*, reviewing over 4000 anaesthetics in children less than 1 year old, found no anaesthesia-related cardiac arrests in the group of 2310 patients supervised by paediatric anaesthetists compared with four anaesthetic cardiac arrests in the 2033 patients whose anaesthetist had not received paediatric fellowship training or the equivalent.[15] The frequency of hypoxaemia during induction of anaesthesia in neonates has been shown to be reduced when an anaesthetist with regular paediatric experience is present.[16] In the related area of interhospital transport of critically ill children, Edge *et al.* found that specialized paediatric teams could significantly reduce transport morbidity.[17]

IMPLEMENTING CHANGE LOCALLY

Historically, and certainly prior to the publication of the 1989 NCEPOD report,[3] the organization of children's surgery within general hospitals in the UK tended to be an *ad hoc* affair. Children were often booked on to operating lists to suit the convenience of the staff or in a random fashion. It was assumed that surgery and anaesthesia could be carried out by anybody assigned to the list. Minor operations on children were often used as 'fillers' on general lists.

The publication of the NCEPOD Report has changed all that. The central recommendation of the Report, that surgeons and anaesthetists should not undertake occasional paediatric practice, has been so widely accepted that it now seems axiomatic. Nevertheless, the implementation of the organizational changes needed to fulfil this recommendation is complex and requires the agreement and co-operation of many different departments throughout a hospital.

Often, change is driven by outside forces, such as standards set by Colleges and other professional bodies, or purchasers or the increasing consumer-power of parents. Whatever the incentive, those involved must understand the need for change and be willing to accept corporate responsibility for making it work.

ASSESSMENT OF CURRENT PRACTICE

The first step to effecting change is to assess current workload, practice and resources.

WORKLOAD

Figures for overall numbers of cases, age distribution of patients, case mix by specialty and within each specialty, and the elective/emergency split are required for rational planning. There is probably a critical mass below which it is not safe or economically viable to provide certain services.

RESOURCES

The most important resource is, of course, human. Lunn has defined the caseload required for an anaesthetist to remain 'up to date and competent'.[4] Although it is possible to argue with specifics (that one infant per month is not sufficient to maintain competence, whilst one 10-year-old per day is more than is necessary), his general recommendation that workload should be equivalent to at least one full operating list per week has been widely accepted, not only by anaesthetists but also by surgeons.[12]

It is necessary to assess the available numbers of 'competent' surgeons and anaesthetists, and of other medical staff, including paediatricians, radiologists and pathologists. In addition, nurses, physiotherapists, technical staff including operating department assistants and practitioners (ODAs and ODPs), teachers, play

leaders and others must be built into the equation.

Non-human resources essential to the provision of adequate services include suitable theatre facilities, ward space, intensive and/or high-dependency care as appropriate, X-ray and pathology facilities.

REALISTIC AIMS

Once current practice and workload have been assessed, it is possible to set realistic aims for what can be achieved with current resources. It can also be encouraging and motivating to set targets for what could be achieved with increased resources.

'COMPETENT' SURGICAL SERVICES: NATIONAL GUIDELINES

The NCEPOD report was followed by reports and documents from a large number of learned bodies, defining 'best practice' and setting standards for what might be regarded as 'competent' surgical services for children.[3,7,9,11–13,18,19] They provide guidance on staffing, and the training, experience, minimum numbers and skill mix required, as well as defining lines of responsibility. They also delineate the infrastructure that should be in place to permit surgery at various levels of complexity.

There is consensus on the following requirements.

NAMED CONSULTANTS

In any hospital which admits children, named consultants, both in anaesthesia and in surgery, should be responsible for leading children's services.[3,11] It is now a requirement of the Royal College of Anaesthetists that each anaesthetic department has such a named consultant.

His or her role will include representing anaesthetic interests and concerns on any hospital planning group responsible for children's surgery. The lead consultant should ensure that services are staffed appropriately and that suitable anaesthetic equipment and facilities are available.

Training programmes for both junior and senior anaesthetists should be co-ordinated by the lead consultant in conjunction with the College Tutor. They should take into account College requirements as well as targeting individual and departmental needs.

Information for parents and children, especially with regard to preoperative procedures, consent, preparation for and induction of anaesthesia, and postoperative analgesia, should be based on national guidelines modified to take account of local practice (see Chapter 2).

Clearly, it is neither possible nor appropriate for the named consultant to administer all children's anaesthetics. It is important that as many anaesthetists as practicable retain paediatric skills. Nevertheless, children under 5 years of age should normally be anaesthetized by, or under the supervision of, consultants who have appropriate training and continuing experience[4,12] and a sufficient workload to maintain those skills.

PAEDIATRIC SERVICES

All children admitted to hospital as inpatients should be under the supervision of a children's physician or surgeon.[7] This requirement presupposes a paediatric department which is fully staffed 24 h a day, in accordance with guidelines issued by the former British Paediatric Association.[18] These require an on-call team made up, at minimum, of a consultant and a resident doctor with at least 12 months' experience.

OTHER MEDICAL SUPPORT SERVICES

Radiology and pathology services will be required for children in any hospital dealing with anything other than the most minor cases. The specialists providing these services should have relevant training and experience, and the facilities, often rather frightening, should be rendered as child friendly as possible. The same applies to Accident and Emergency Departments that accept children.[12]

SPECIALIST NURSES

Children should, ideally, be nursed by children's nurses. In any unit which undertakes inpatient surgery, there should be at least two Registered State Children's Nurses (RSCNs) on duty throughout the whole (24-h) day.[7]

Suitably trained and experienced nurses or ODAs/ODPs will also be required in the anaesthetic room, the operating theatre and the recovery room. Postoperative care, high-dependency and intensive care, and postoperative analgesia all demand skilled staff.

Preoperative and postoperative care should be carried out by nursing staff to the standards set out in *Welfare of Children and Young People in Hospital*.[7]

DEDICATED CHILDREN'S OPERATING LISTS

Dedicated children's operating lists should be established in each specialty. In most district general hospitals, unless the workload is exceptional, this will mean that one surgeon in each specialty will be the designated children's surgeon. Although there is consensus that dedicated lists are essential for a high-quality service, surgeons are understandably reluctant to lose what they see as an enjoyable and valued part of their work, and this change is often the most difficult to achieve in practice.

Fortunately, anaesthetists, ODPs and nurses may form a paediatric team which works across specialties, enabling the workload and therefore the experience to be shared by a greater number of people. This, in turn, increases the number of adequately trained staff available for emergencies.

It may well be necessary to recruit staff, especially for the children's service in operating theatres. Apart from providing a high level of service themselves, they can be expected to assist in training existing staff to appropriate standards, thereby increasing the pool of competence.

EQUIPMENT

A full range of equipment (Chapter 6) especially designed for children is required. This includes breathing systems, masks and airways, tracheal tubes of various designs, laryngeal mask airways, connectors, laryngoscopes and suitable ventilators.

Monitoring during anaesthesia and recovery, which should conform with the standards recommended by the Association of Anaesthetists of Great Britain and Ireland,[19] will require a range of blood-pressure cuffs, precordial and oesophageal stethoscopes, temperature probes, electrocardiograms, pulse oximeters and capnographs. If the planned surgery requires it, appropriate invasive monitoring must be available.

DEDICATED WARDS AND FACILITIES

Children should be treated in facilities appropriate to their age and should not be admitted to adult wards.[7]

Ideally, a dedicated children's day care or surgical ward should be provided, to concentrate available expertise and provide optimal conditions for care before and after surgery.

Where it is not possible to establish a separate unit, a day-care ward normally used for adults may be dedicated to children on set days of the week. Although theoretically possible, this is a difficult and potentially unsatisfactory option.

PAEDIATRIC SURGERY COMMITTEE

The establishment of competent children's surgical services in an institution which has previously provided them on an *ad hoc* basis requires a change in culture and the involvement of staff from most departments within the hospital. A multidisciplinary working party, with representation from all groups who will be required to agree and implement change, should oversee children's surgical services. In order to be effective this committee must link into other parts of the hospital's management structure and must have executive as well as advisory powers.

The Paediatric Surgical Committee should cover the following functions.

STANDARD SETTING

There is no shortage of published national guidelines.[3,7,9,11–13,18,19] The committee should review these and adopt those which are relevant, with such modification as local circumstances require.

It is for this group to consider and define the limits of the hospital's competence to provide children's surgical services, assessing the expertise and resources available and comparing them with standards of best practice. In the current climate, in a developed country like the UK, the same single standard of care should apply wherever surgery is carried out. That does not mean that all district general hospitals should be capable of carrying out complex major surgery in children. It does mean, however, that a tonsillectomy or appendicectomy should be performed to the same high standard in any hospital which accepts the responsibility of care.

The committee should set out guidelines for what should and should not be undertaken and by whom. The limits of competence of the hospital will vary from time to time, depending on current staffing and facilities, and they should be subject to periodic review.

The group will need the facilities to monitor standards and the power to enforce them.

AUDIT

'The outcome of surgery and anaesthesia in children is related to the experience of the clinicians involved.'[3]

In the light of this statement from the NCEPOD report, the committee should audit both the quality (outcome) and quantity (available experience) of children's surgery within the unit, and act on the results.

Suitable subjects for audit would include quality of preoperative information, preoperative fasting times, postoperative analgesia and patient/parent satisfaction surveys.

A system for regular critical incident reporting and review should be in place, as part of a comprehensive risk-management strategy.

CONTINUING MEDICAL EDUCATION (CME)/CONTINUING PROFESSIONAL DEVELOPMENT (CPD)

Specialty-specific training will be provided within individual departments, but the multidisciplinary committee is well placed to take an overview of the needs of the service as a whole, and to organize or co-ordinate training accordingly.

Paediatric advanced life support courses should be made available, either locally or at a regional centre, to all staff working with children.

EMERGENCIES

Surgical emergencies in very young children are relatively rare. However, when they do arise, children under the age of 3 years are most in need of an expert team with a full supporting infrastructure.[11] Consultants in general hospitals should be capable of dealing with common surgical problems arising in children over the age of 5 years. Uncommon or complicated problems are properly the province of specialist centres.

In most district general hospitals, there are usually insufficient numbers of appropriately trained consultants to allow a separate on-call rota for children, although many departments operate satisfactory informal schemes. If a consultant with relevant training and continuing experience is not available, the child should be transferred to a specialist unit.

Local guidelines for emergency surgery should be drawn up by the Paediatric Surgery Committee. Audit of the emergency workload may show that the number of babies and very young children needing emergency surgery is so small that the paediatric team cannot maintain its skills. It may then be wise for the hospital to set a lower age limit below which all infants should be transferred for emergency surgery.

The criteria for transfer to a specialist unit should be agreed in advance, as should the routes and mechanisms of such transfers.

The 'competence' of the emergency service may vary from day to day, depending on the skills of the staff on call, and local guidelines should be flexible enough to reflect this. However, children under the age of 5 years should not be operated on by doctors in training without close supervision.[11]

In a life-threatening emergency where transfer is not feasible, anaesthesia should be undertaken by the most senior appropriately experienced anaesthetist available.

TRANSFER AND REFERRAL ARRANGEMENTS

Clearly, neonates and very young infants who require surgery should be referred to a specialist centre. Similarly, older children with rare or complicated conditions requiring major surgical intervention should be treated in large hospitals with a concentrated workload, appropriately expert staff and sophisticated facilities.

The Paediatric Surgery Committee, in close consultation with the clinicians involved, should establish guidelines for referral of cases to a specialist centre using criteria such as the facilities and expertise available in relation to those required, the age of the child, the rarity of the condition and the complexity of the treatment.

A hub-and-spoke arrangement between the specialist centre and its surrounding district general hospitals can provide a satisfactory organizational model. Consultants from the centre visit the peripheral hospital to conduct outreach clinics. Children can be seen and assessed close to home and can then have their operation performed locally if appropriate, or be transferred to the specialist hospital if necessary.

Specialist and general surgeons and anaesthetists thus have the opportunity to work together, and to establish co-operation and two-way traffic between their institutions. There are obvious benefits for postgraduate training and continuing professional development.

Patients benefit because they have access to both the convenience of the local hospital (often especially important for children and families) and the expertise of the specialist centre when their condition requires it.

Good working relationships between specialist centres and general hospitals are potentially beneficial to all those involved. The Paediatric Surgery Committee should encourage close communication and foster both clinical and academic links.

REFERENCES

1 Paediatric anaesthesia (Leading article). *British Medical Journal* 1978; **ii**: 717.
2 Hatch, D.J. Anaesthesia for children. *Anaesthesia* 1984; **39**: 405–6.
3 Campling, E.A., Devlin, H.B. and Lunn, J.N. *The Report of the National Confidential Enquiry into Perioperative Deaths 1989.* London: NCEPOD, Royal College of Surgeons of England, 1990.
4 Lunn, J.N. Implications of the National Confidential Enquiry into Perioperative Deaths for paediatric anaesthesia. *Paediatric Anaesthesia* 1992; **2**: 69–72.
5 Rollin, A.-M. Paediatric anaesthesia – who should do it? The view from the district general hospital. *Anaesthesia* 1997; **52**: 515–16.
6 McNicol, R. Paediatric anaesthesia – who should do it? The view from the specialist hospital. *Anaesthesia* 1997; **52**: 513–15.
7 Department of Health. *Welfare of Children and Young People in Hospital.* London: HMSO, 1991.
8 Audit Commission. *Children First – A Study of Hospital Services.* London: HMSO, 1993.
9 *Guidelines for Purchasers of Paediatric Anaesthetic Services.* London: Royal College of Anaesthetists, 1994.
10 Atwell, J.D. and Spargo, P.M. The provision of safe surgery for children. *Archives of Disease in Childhood* 1992; **67**: 345–9.
11 *The Transfer of Infants and Children for Surgery – the Report of the Joint Working Group.* London: British Paediatric Association, 1993.
12 Children's Surgical Services. *Report of an Ad-hoc Multi-disciplinary Children's Surgical Liaison Group.* Royal College of Paediatrics and Child Health, 1996.
13 *The Pattern of Medical Services for Children: Medical Staffing and Training.* London: Joint Consultants' Committee, BMA, 1997.
14 Stoddart, P.A., Brennan, L., Hatch, D.J. and Bingham, R. Postal survey of paediatric practice and training amongst consultant anaesthetists in the UK. *British Journal of Anaesthesia* 1994; **73**: 559–63.
15 Keenan, R.L., Shapiro, J.H. and Dawson, K. Frequency of anesthetic cardiac arrests in infants: effective pediatric anesthesiologists. *Journal of Clinical Anesthesia* 1991; **3**: 433–7.
16 Kong, A.S., Brennan, L., Bingham, R. and Morgan-Hughes, J. An audit of induction of anaesthesia in neonates and small infants using pulse oximetry. *Anaesthesia* 1992; **47**: 896–9.
17 Edge, W.E., Kanter, R.K., Reigle, C.G.M. and Walsh, R.F. Reduction of morbidity in inter-hospital transport by specialized pediatric staff. *Critical Care Medicine* 1994; **22**: 1186–91.
18 *Future Configuration of Paediatric Services.* London: British Paediatric Association, 1996.
19 *Recommendations for Standards of Monitoring during Anaesthesia and Recovery.* Rev edn. London: Association of Anaesthetics of Great Britain and Ireland, 1994.

Normal physiological values in the neonate and adult

	Neonate	Adult
Hb	18–25 g dl^{-1}	15 g dl^{-1}
Haematocrit (PCV)	50–60%	45%
Blood volume	70–125 ml kg^{-1}	70 ml kg^{-1}
WBC	9.4–15 × 10^9 l^{-1}	4.5–44 × 10^9 l^{-1}
ESR	0–10 mm h^{-1}	0–20 mm h^{-1}
Extracellular fluid (% of body weight)	35%	20%
Water turnover per 24 h (% of body weight)	15%	9%
Serum K$^+$	5–8 mmol l^{-1}	3–5 mmol l^{-1}
Serum Na$^+$	136–143 mmol l^{-1}	135–148 mmol l^{-1}
Serum Cl$^-$	96–107 mmol l^{-1}	98–106 mmol l^{-1}
Serum HCO$^-$	20 mmol l^{-1}	24 mmol l^{-1}
Blood urea nitrogen	1.3–3.3 mmol l^{-1}	6.6–8.6 mmol l^{-1}
Creatinine	27–88 μmol l^{-1}	53–106 μmol l^{-1}
pH	7.35	7.40
$PaCO_2$	4.7 kPa (35 mmHg)	4.7–6.0 kPa (35–45 mmHg)
PaO_2	8.7–10.7 kPa (65–80 mmHg)	10.7–12.7 kPa (80–95 mmHg)
Base excess	−5	0
Total bilirubin	100 μmol l^{-1}	2–14 μmol l^{-1}
Total Ca^{2+}	1.0–1.7 mmol l^{-1}1	2.13–2.6 mmol l^{-1}
Calcium (ionized)	1.0–1.7 mmol l^{-1}	1.12–1.23 mmol l^{-1}
Mg^{2+}	0.7–1.1 mmol l^{-1}	0.6–1.0 mmol l^{-1}
Phosphate	1.15–2.8 mmol l^{-1}	1.0–1.4 mmol l^{-1}
Glucose	2.7–3.3 mmol l^{-1}	2.4–5.3 mmol l^{-1}
Total proteins	46–74 g l^{-1}	60–80 g l^{-1}
Albumin	36–54 g l^{-1}	35–47 g l^{-1}
Cortisol	28–662 nmol l^{-1}	27–276 nmol l^{-1}
Creatine kinase	68–580 μmol l^{-1}	10–80 μ l^{-1}
Serum osmolality	270–285 mmol l^{-1}	270–295 mmol l^{-1}
Urine osmolality	50–600 mmol l^{-1}	20–1400 mmol l^{-1}
Urine Na$^+$	50 mmol l^{-1}	30 mmol l^{-1}
Specific gravity	1005–1020	1005–1035

Resuscitation charts and guidelines

Tracheal Tube	
Length (cm)	Int. Dia (mm)
18–21	7.5–8.0
18	7.0
17	6.5
16	6.0
15	5.5
14	5.0
13	4.5
12	4.0
	3.5
10	3.0–3.5

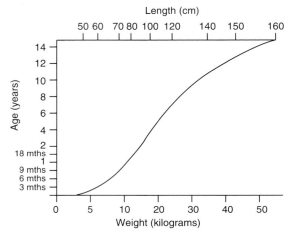

Adrenaline ml of 1:10 000	iv/et	0.5	1	2	3	4	5
Atropine mg	iv/et	0.1	0.2	0.4	0.6	0.6	0.6
Bicarbonate ml of 8.4%	iv	5	10	20	30	40	50
Calcium chloride* mmol	iv	1	2	4	6	8	10
Diazepam mg	iv / pr	1.25 / 2.5	2.5 / 5	5 / 10	7.5 / –	10 / –	10 / –
Glucose ml of 50%	iv	10	20	40	60	80	100
Lignocaine mg	iv/et	5	10	20	30	40	50
Salbutamol micrograms	iv/et	25	50	100	150	200	250
Initial D.C.defibrillation joules		10	20	40	60	80	100
Initial fluid infusion in hypovolaemic shock ml		50	100	200	300	400	500

*1ml of calcium chloride 1 mmol·ml^{-1} = 1.5 ml of calcium chloride 10%
= 4.5 ml of calcium gluconate 10%

From Oakley, P. Inaccuracy and delay in decision making in paediatric resuscitation, and a proposed chart to reduce error. *British Medical Journal* 1988; **297**: 817–9.

Latex allergy protocol

Three groups of patients exist:

1 with a history of anaphylaxis to latex;
2 with a history of allergy to latex or rubber;
3 high-risk group: no previous reaction, but:
  - spina bifida
  - genitourinary anomalies
  - multiple surgical procedures
  - known reactions to intravenous drugs

PREMEDICATION

Groups 1 and 2 should be treated identically.

INTRAVENOUS MEDICATION

(i) Methylprednisolone: 1 mg kg^{-1} 6 hourly i.v., Max. dose: 50 mg dose^{-1}
(ii) Ranitidine: 1 mg kg 6 hourly i.v. over 20 min
(iii) Chlorpheniramine: 1 month–1 year, 250 μg kg^{-1}; 1–5 years, 2.5–5 mg; 6–12 years, 5–10 mg.

All doses i.v. 6 hourly given slowly. Note that at least two doses must be given preoperatively and continued 24 h postoperatively, and diluents must not be added to vials through rubber bungs. The bung must be removed or dispensing pin with filter (Braun) should be used.

PATIENTS WITH ASTHMA

Salbutamol inhaler, 6 hourly, 2 doses preoperatively.

GROUP 3 (HIGH-RISK PATIENTS)

No special precautions. Maintain high index of suspicion during and after case.

AIM OF MANAGEMENT IS TO PREVENT ANY CONTACT OF THE PATIENT WITH ANY LATEX-CONTAINING PRODUCT

Many manufacturers state whether their products contain latex.
  The following equipment is safe:

GLOVES: LATEX FREE

- Ansell: dermaprene

RESPIRATORY EQUIPMENT

- Clear silicone masks (e.g. King Systems Laerdal)
- Tracheal tubes (Portex)
- Airways (Guedel)
- Filter should be placed at patient end of the breathing circuits
- Polythene bags should be placed over reservoir bag of Bain circuit if used (in group-1 patients only)
- Laryngeal masks

INTRAVENOUS EQUIPMENT

- i.v. cannulae (Jelco, Venflon, Neoflon)

- Latex-free syringes (BD Discardit)
- Latex-free giving sets (DOSFIX; Braun)
- i.v. giving sets with latex port can be used but injections should not be made through these parts and they should be covered with tape-Temperature probes (disposable probes can be used)
- Dispensing pin with filter (Braun) used to draw or mix drugs held in ampoule with rubber bung
- Do not mix drugs by injecting through rubber bungs
- Do not draw up drugs through rubber bungs
- CVP (Cook, Vygon, Arrow). Avoid injecting through rubber bungs
- Syringe pump infusions, e.g. PCA/NCA/epidurals. Use ordinary syringes with an epidural filter between syringe and giving set

MONITORING EQUIPMENT

- ECG electrodes (Nelcor, Medicotest)
- BP cuff hoses to be covered with tape or use Disposa Cuff (J&J)
- Operating table and trolley (avoid contact with mattress by covering with sheet)
- Tape/dressings: avoid elastoplast (Transpore, 3M; Micropore, 3M; Hyperfix, Smith & Nephew; Tegaderm, 3M; Steri-Strips, J&J)
- NG Tubes (Vygon-Portex)
- Suction catheter (Penine)
- Suction tubing (Penine)
- Yankauer sucker (Argyle)
- Epidural catheter (Portex)
- Diathermy (3M place and lead safe)

OTHER POINTS

- Avoid touching latex products and then touching patient

TREATMENT OF ANAPHYLAXIS TO LATEX

The onset may be insidious and the diagnosis difficult. A smaller dose of adrenaline should be used if the reaction is not severe.

1 Maintain 100% oxygen
2 Adrenaline 5–10 μg kg^{-1} (0.05–0.1 ml kg^{-1} of 1 : 10 000)
3 Intravascular volume expansion: repeat 10–20 ml kg^{-1} as necessary (Hartmann's or saline).

In addition, give:

(i) Methylprednisolone: 1 mg kg^{-1} i.v.
(ii) Chlorpheniramine: 1 month–1 year, 250 μg kg^{-1} i.v.; 1–5 years, 2.5–5 mg i.v.; 6–12 years, 5–10 mg i.v.
(iii) Ranitidine: 1 mg kg^{-1} slowly i.v.

This is the current protocol in use at the Great Ormond Street Hospital for Children, London.

Guidelines for drug dosages in children

All drugs given on a body-weight basis (kg).

SEDATIVES

(e.g. night-time preoperatively): all given *orally*

1 Chloral hydrate
 Dose: up to 30 mg kg^{-1}; not more than 1 g in a single dose (chloral mixture BPC 100 mg ml^{-1})
2 Diazepam (e.g. as pre-premedication 4 h preoperatively)
 Dose: 0.4 mg kg^{-1}: use rectally if nil by mouth
3 Promethazine
 Dose: 0.5–1.0 mg kg^{-1} to a max. of 50 mg (elixir BPC 5 mg 5 ml^{-1})
4 Temazepam
 Dose: 0.5 mg kg^{-1} (max dose: 10 mg)
5 Triclofos syrup
 Dose: about 30 mg kg^{-1}. *Preparation*: 100 mg ml^{-1}
6 Trimeprazine tartrate (Vallergan)
 Dose: 2 mg kg^{-1} (Vallergan Forte 6 mg ml^{-1})

PREMEDICATION

Routine (not cardiac, ENT or neurosurgery)

1 Requirements depend on patient and surgery
2 Avoid i.m. injections if possible
3 Infants below 5 kg: avoid sedatives
4 EMLA/Ametop routinely. (NB. Be careful with EMLA in small infants: prilocaine may cause methaemoglobin)

ATROPINE

0.02 mg kg^{-1} i.m.	
min. dose 0.1 mg	45 min preop.
max. dose 0.5 mg	(ENT only)
0.04 mg kg^{-1} p.o.	60 min preop.
min. dose 0.1 mg	
max. dose 0.5 mg	

ORAL

Triclofos	50–75 mg kg^{-1}	30–45 min
(5–10 kg)	(max. dose 1 g)	preop.
Midazolam	0.5 mg kg^{-1}	20–40 min
(over 10 kg)	(max. dose	preop.
	15–20 mg)	
Temazepam	0.5 mg kg^{-1}	
(older children)	(max. dose 20 mg)	
Trimeprazine	2–3 mg kg^{-1}	90–120 min
(Vallergan)		preop.

I.M.

Pethidine compound injection (Inj. Peth. Co.). *Dose*: 0.06–0.08 ml kg^{-1} i.m. 1 h preoperatively (this has a pethidine content of 1.5–2 mg kg^{-1}). *Preparation*: Pethidine, 25 mg in 1 ml; Promethazine, 6.25 mg in 1 ml; Chlorpromazine, 6.25 mg in 1 ml. Max. dose: 1.5 ml.

Morphine: 0.2 mg kg^{-1} (max. 10 mg) (tetralogy of Fallot). Hyoscine: 0.01 mg kg^{-1} (max. 0.4 mg).

For cardiac catheters under sedation give 30 min preop.

SPECIAL CIRCUMSTANCES

CARDIAC INVESTIGATIONS

May be performed under basal sedation with local anaesthesia supplemented if required by i.v. injection of diazepam or midazolam 0.1–0.2 mg kg^{-1}.

Sedation the night before catheter: Triclofos 30 mg kg^{-1} p.o. nocte

Age	Weight	Drug	Dose	Route	Comments
Tetralogy of Fallot		Morphine	250 μg kg^{-1}	i.m.	30 min precatheter
For all other patients:					
Newborns up to 1 month + infants	< 5 kg	Inj. Peth. Co.	0.05 ml kg^{-1}	i.m.	30 min precatheter
Older children	All weights	Trimeprazine	2 mg kg^{-1} Max. dose: 100 mg	p.o.	3 h precatheter
Followed by:	5 kg to 15 kg	Inj. Peth. Co.	0.1 ml kg^{-1} Max. dose: 1.5 ml	i.m.	30 min precatheter. Smaller babies in poor condition should have a reduced dose
Or:	> 15 kg	Morphine	200 μg kg^{-1} Max. dose: 10 mg	i.m.	30 min precatheter
		Hyoscine	100 μg kg^{-1} Max. dose: 500 μg	i.m.	Sick children (e.g. transplant assessments) may need reduced doses

Children > 2.5 years who are just under 15 kg body weight are usually best sedated with morphine and hyoscine rather than Inj. Peth. Co.
Most children require the full dose of sedation.
Timing is very important because of patient preparation time and the duration of the investigation.
Supplementary sedation to be given only by doctor skilled in paediatric resuscitation: diazemuls 200–300 μg kg^{-1} i.v. in increments of 100 μg.
NB: EMLA/Ametop should be applied to all children

CARDIAC SURGERY

Age	Weight	Drug	Dose	Comments
< 4 weeks		Atropine		
Between 4 weeks and	6 kg	Triclofos	50–75 mg kg^{-1}	
	6–15 kg	Triclofos	50–75 mg kg^{-1}	
	> 15 kg	Midazolam syrup	500 μg–1 mg kg^{-1}	Max. dose: 15 mg
		Temazepam	500 μg–1 mg kg^{-1}	Max. dose: 20 mg Use tablets not elixir

Larger doses may be required in some patients.

CLEFT PALATE

Atropine only

Never prescribe sedation preoperatively for any child with micrognathia or other anatomical deformity of the respiratory tract.

ENT

Endoscopy, laser surgery

Atropine only (usually i.m.)

- no sedation
- pre-existing tracheostomy
  - atropine
  - older children may have midazolam

ADENOTONSILLECTOMY

	Drug	Dose	Route	Comments
Premedication				
Children with upper airway obstruction	Atropine ONLY	40 μg kg^{-1} Max. dose: 500 μg	p.o.	These children must not have a sedative premed
Children without airway problems	Midazolam	500 μg kg^{-1} Max. dose: 15 mg	p.o.	Larger doses may be required in some patients
Analgesia				
All children	Codeine phosphate and	Loading dose: 1 mg kg^{-1}	i.m.	Before leaving theatre
	diclofenac and	Loading dose: 1 mg kg^{-1}	p.r.	
	paracetamol	Loading dose: 30 mg kg^{-1}	p.r.	

NB. Paracetamol can be given orally 1 h preoperatively.

NEUROINVESTIGATIONS

Angiography– embolization and myelography: atropine only. CT and MRI: either GA or sedation. Body scans: normal premedication

CT AND MRI

Sedation protocols

MRI: sedation on the ward 40–60 min prescan

Age	Weight	Drug	Dose	Route	Comments
< 45 weeks postconceptional age	< 5 kg	Nil			Feed and keep warm
> 45 weeks postconceptional age	< 5 kg	Triclofos	50 mg kg^{-1}	p.o.	
	5–15 kg	Triclofos + Inj. Peth. Co.	50 mg kg^{-1} 0.06 ml kg^{-1}	p.o. i.m.	
	> 15 kg	Trimeprazine + morphine	2 mg kg^{-1} 200 μg kg^{-1}	p.o. i.m.	Max. dose: 100 mg Max. dose: 10 mg

NB. EMLA/Ametop should be applied to all children. Supplementary sedation to be given by doctor skilled in paediatric resuscitation: Diazemuls 200 μg kg^{-1} i.v. in increments of 100 μg.

MRI (sedation administered in sedation unit by trained nurses)*

Weight	Drug	Dose	Route	Comments
< 5 kg	Nil			Feed and keep warm
5–10 kg	Chloral hydrate	100 mg kg^{-1}	p.o.	
>10–20 kg	Temazepam	1 mg kg^{-1}	p.o.	
	Droperidol	250 μg kg^{-1}	p.o.	
> 20 kg	As directed by radiologist			

NB. Intravenous diazemuls may be used as supplementary sedation up to 1 mg kg^{-1}. The drugs are prescribed and administered by the sedation nurses; a radiologist must be close by.

CT scan (sedation administered on ward) 40–60 min prescan

Age	Weight	Drug	Dose	Route	Comments
< 45 weeks postconceptional age	< 5 kg	Nil			Feed and keep warm
>45 weeks postconceptional age	< 5 kg	Triclofos	50 mg kg^{-1}	p.o.	
	5–15 kg	Inj. Peth. Co.	0.08–0.1 ml kg^{-1}	i.m.	
	> 15 kg	Trimeprazine + Morphine	2 mg kg^{-1} 200 μg kg^{-1}	p.o. i.m.	Max. dose: 100 mg Max. dose: 10 mg

Patients with raised ICP or potentially raised ICP should be sedated with great care or not at all.
Patients with airways obstruction (actual or potential) should not be sedated, e.g. some craniofacial abnormalities.
Ex-premature babies should not receive opioids until over 2 months' corrected gestational age and should receive other sedation with great caution because of the risk of apnoea.
Severe epilepsy is usually a contraindication to sedation in MRI and CT.
No sedation for patients with severe metabolic, liver or renal disease.

*Sury, M.R.J., Hatch, D.J., Deeley, T., Dicks-Mireaux, C. and Chong, W.K. Development of nurse-led sedation service for paediatric magnetic resonance imaging. *Lancet* 1999; **353**: 1667–71.

NEUROSURGERY

Sedatives are contraindicated in the presence of raised ICP

Operation	Drug	Dose	Route	Comments
Intracranial operations Sitting cases:	Atropine ± EMLA/Ametop	20 μg kg$^-$1	p.o./i.m.	As indicated
Posterior fossa < 30 kg	Atropine	20 μg kg^{-1}	i.m.	Almost all posterior fossa explorations and those going prone require an antisialogogue
Posterior fossa 30 kg + prone cases	Atropine	20 μg kg^{-1} Max. dose: 500 μg	p.o.	
Craniofacial (without airway obstruction)	EMLA/Ametop			May receive oral sedation as appropriate
Thoracolumbar spinal procedures	EMLA/Ametop			May receive oral sedation as appropriate

NB. Care should be taken sedating children with generalized muscle weakness

STEROID COVER FOR SURGERY

The Anaesthetic Department should be responsible for prescribing steroid cover for the operation and subsequent 24 h, but further management of the dosage should be the responsibility of the clinician in charge of the patient.

1   On steroids at present

Hydrocortisone 1 mg kg^{-1} i.v. at induction
– 6-hourly postop.
– reduce to maintenance level after 1–4 days depending on type of surgery.

2   Off steroids within preceding 2 months

Hydrocortisone 1 mg kg^{-1} i.v. at induction
– 6-hourly postop. 1–2 days

3   Off steroids longer than 2 months

No cover, but hydrocortisone should be available.

ANAESTHETIC AGENTS

All are given intravenously.

Induction	Dose	Preparation
1. Etomidate	0.3 mg kg^{-1}	
2. Ketamine	induction: i.v. 2 mg kg^{-1}; i.m. 5–10 mg kg^{-1} (increments i.v. 1 mg kg^{-1}) (may also be given rectally or orally 10 mg kg^{-1})	
3. Methohexitone	1.5–2 mg kg^{-1}	10 mg ml^{-1}
4. Propofol	2–3 mg kg^{-1}	10 mg ml^{-1}

(Unpremedicated children may require up to 5 mg kg^{-1}. Add lignocaine 1 mg for each 10 mg propofol to prevent pain on injection)

5. Thiopentone	4–6 mg kg^{-1}	25 mg ml^{-1}
—neonates	2 mg kg^{-1}	

Relaxants	Dose	Preparation
1. Atracurium	0.5 mg kg^{-1} (increments 0.25 mg kg^{-1}) infusion: 8 μg kg.$^{-1}$ min^{-1}	10 mg ml^{-1}
2. Cis-atracurum	0.1–0.4 mg kg^{-1} increments 0.05 mg kg^{-1}	2 mg ml^{-1}
3. Mivacurium	0.1–0.2 mg kg^{-1} increments 0.1 mg kg^{-1} infusion 10–15 μg kg^{-1} min^{-1}	2 mg ml^{-1}
4. Pancuronium		
(a) Infants and children	0.1 mg kg^{-1}	2 mg ml^{-1}
(b) Neonates	0.06 mg kg^{-1}	
5. Rocuronium	0.6 mg kg^{-1} increments 0.1–0.2 mg kg^{-1}	10 mg ml^{-1}
6. Suxamethonium intubation	1–2 mg kg^{-1}	50 mg ml^{-1}
7. Vecuronium	0.1 mg kg^{-1} infusion 1.5–2 μg kg^{-1} min^{-1}	2 mg ml^{-1}

ANALGESICS (INTRAOPERATIVE)

	Preparation	Dilution	Dose
Alfentanil	500 μg ml^{-1}		30–50 μg kg^{-1}
Codeine	30 mg ml^{-1}		i.m.: 1–1.5 mg kg^{-1}.dose^{-1}
			6-hourly prn
			Never give intravenously
Fentanyl	50 μg ml^{-1}	10 μg ml^{-1}	2–5 μg kg^{-1}
			Cardiac surgery:
			Up to 25 μg kg^{-1}
Morphine sulphate	10 mg ml^{-1}	1 mg ml^{-1}	50–200 μg kg^{-1}
	30 mg ml^{-1}		Cardiac surgery:
			Up to 1 mg kg^{-1} total dose
Remifentanil	1, 2, 5 mg	300 μg kg^{-1} in 50 ml	Loading dose:
		5% glucose	1–2 μg kg^{-1}
			Infusion:
			0.1–2 μg kg^{-1} min^{-1} as clinically
			indicated

REVERSAL

1. Atropine   0.02 mg kg^{-1}
2. Glycopyrrolate   0.04–0.08 mg kg^{-1}
                        (max. dose 0.2 mg)
3. Neostigmine   0.05 mg kg^{-1}

NEBULIZED AGENTS

Epinephine (adrenaline)   5 ml 1 : 1000 (1 mg ml^{-1}); monitor ECG and heart rate
Ipratropium   0.5 ml in 2 ml saline
Lignocaine spray   (10% solution) metered dose 10 mg
                        Max. dose to trachea 5 mg kg^{-1}

OTHER DRUGS

Adenosine	30–40 μg kg^{-1} i.v.
Aminophylline	5 mg kg^{-1} bolus i.v.
	0.8 mg kg^{-1} h^{-1} infusion
Amiodarone	5 mg kg^{-1} i.v. slowly
Aprotinin	1 ml kg^{-1} bolus (after 1-ml test dose)
	1 ml kg^{-1} h^{-1} infusion
	1 ml kg^{-1} to pump prime
Caffeine (for apnoea of prematurity)	12.5 mg kg^{-1} of caffeine base i.v. slowly
	Then 5 mg kg^{-1} daily
	Check blood levels weekly (therapeutic range 5–40 mg l^{-1})
Captopril	0.1 mg kg^{-1} orally: gradually increase dose
	0.3–3 mg kg^{-1} day^{-1}
Cardioplegia	20–30 ml kg^{-1}; half-doses after 30 min
Chlorpromazine	1-mg increments up to 0.5 mg kg^{-1}
Dantrolene	
pretreatment	2.5 mg kg^{-1} i.v.
malignant hyperthermia	1–10 mg kg^{-1} i.v.
Dexamethasone	0.25 mg kg^{-1} i.v., then 0.1 mg kg^{-1} 6-hourly i.v., i.m. for three doses
for cerebral oedema	up to 0.5 mg kg^{-1}
Dextrose/insulin	dextrose 1 g kg^{-1} + insulin 0.25 u kg^{-1}
Digoxin	Total digitalizing dose: 0.05 mg kg^{-1}
	one-third stat
	one-third 4–6 h
	one-third 8–12 h
	Maintenance: one-tenth digitalizing dose b.d.
	For premature babies, total dose: 0.03 mg kg^{-1}
Droperidol	0.3 mg kg^{-1}
Flumazenil	1–2 μg kg^{-1} bolus
	1–5 μg kg^{-1} h^{-1} infusion
Furosemide (frusemide)	Up to 1 mg kg^{-1} repeatable
	Infusion 50 mg in 50 ml 0.9% saline 1 mg kg^{-1} h^{-1}
Heparin	bypass: 3 mg kg^{-1}
(1 mg 100 U)	shunts: 1 mg kg^{-1}
	infusion: 1.5–4 mg kg^{-1}.h^{-1}
Hydralazine	0.2 mg kg, then 1.5–3 mg kg^{-1} day^{-1}
Hydrocortisone	1 mg kg^{-1}
Indomethacin	0.2 mg kg^{-1} $\times$ 3
Labetalol	Increments of 0.02 mg kg^{-1} up to 1 mg kg^{-1}
	Infusion 1–3 mg kg^{-1} h^{-1}
Lignocaine	1 mg kg^{-1}
Mannitol	Up to 1 g kg^{-1}
Methoxamine	dilution to 0.5 mg ml^{-1}
	increments of 0.25 mg to achieve desired result
Methylprednisolone	30 mg kg^{-1}
Naloxone	4 μg kg^{-1} (repeat after 20 min if necessary)
	0.5 μg kg^{-1} for itching, urinary retention
Nifedipine	0.5 mg kg^{-1} day^{-1} in divided doses

Propranolol	dilution to 0.1 mg ml^{-1}; max. dose of 0.05 mg kg^{-1}
Prostacyclin	4–20 ng kg^{-1} min^{-1}
Prostaglandin E$_2$	90 μg in 50 ml 5% dextrose – 1 ml kg^{-1} h^{-1}
Protamine	6 mg kg^{-1} *slowly*
Ranitidine	0.5–1 mg kg^{-1} *slowly* (diluted to 5 ml) 6-hourly
Salbutamol	0.2–4 μg kg.$^{-1}$ min^{-1} i.v.
	increase from low dose *slowly*
Verapamil	0.1 mg kg^{-1} *slowly*

POSTOPERATIVE AGENTS

Analgesia is given with caution in the neonate after individual assessment.

ANALGESICS

Codeine phosphate	1 mg kg^{-1} 4–6-hourly. Do NOT give i.v. because it causes a severe fall in cardiac output.
	i.m., oral or rectal
Fentanyl	infusion: 100 μg kg^{-1} in 50 ml 5% dextrose
	2 ml h^{-1} = 4 μg kg^{-1} min^{-1}
Morphine	0.2 mg kg^{-1} i.m. or i.v.
	Infusion 1.0 mg kg^{-1} in 50 ml
	5% dextrose run at 1 ml h^{-1}
	(Fentanyl and morphine to be used with great caution in spontaneously breathing babies)
Paracetamol	Oral: 20 mg kg^{-1} (15 mg kg^{-1} in neonates)
	Then 15 mg kg^{-1} doses 4–6 hourly
	Rectal: 30 mg kg^{-1} (20 mg kg^{-1} in neonates)
	Then 20 mg kg^{-1} doses 6 hourly
	(15 mg kg^{-1} in neonates)
	Maximum dose: 90 mg kg^{-1} (60 mg kg^{-1} in neonates)
Diclofenac	1–3 mg kg^{-1} day^{-1} in divided doses 8-hourly
	not below 6 months
Ibuprofen	< 25 kg: 5 mg kg^{-1} 6-hourly
	> 25 kg: 200 mg kg^{-1} 8-hourly

NCA AND PCA

i.v. up to 50 kg
Morphine 1 mg kg^{-1} in 50 ml SD = 20 μg kg ml^{-1}
Max. dose: 400 μg kg in 4 h

	Loading dose	Background	Bolus	Lockout
NCA	50–100 μg kg^{-1}	0.5 ml h^{-1}	0.5 ml	20
PCA	50–100 μg kg^{-1}	0–0.4 ml h^{-1}	up to 1 ml	5–10

EXTRADURAL

Bupivacaine	0.125%, 100 ml
Morphine (preservative free)	1 mg in 100 ml
	0.1– 0.4 ml kg^{-1} h^{-1}

SEDATIVES

Baclofen	5–15 mg 6-hourly	orally
Chloral	30 mg kg^{-1}	orally
Diazepam	0.2 mg kg^{-1}	orally
Midazolam	Bolus 20 μg kg^{-1} i.v.	10 mg in 2 ml
	infusion 2–5 μg kg^{-1} min^{-1}	dilute in dextrose
Phenobarbitone	1–2 mg kg^{-1} to control seizures (4-hourly if necessary)	
Promethazine	0.5–1 mg kg^{-1}	orally
Triclofos elixir	30 mg kg^{-1}	orally

ANTIEMETICS

Not used routinely except in high-risk cases (strabismus, adenotonsillectomy, middle-ear surgery) and patients with previous history.

Ondansetron	0.1–0.2 mg kg^{-1} i.v. 6–8-hourly
	or oral 0.05–0.1 mg kg^{-1} preoperatively
	in younger children use metoclopramide first

Others

Dexamethasone	0.15 mg kg^{-1} i.v. 6-hourly
Droperidol	0.025 mg kg^{-1} i.v.
Metoclopramide	0.015 mg kg^{-1} i.v., i.m. or orally 8-hourly
	(max. total daily dose 0.5 mg kg^{-1})
Prochlorperazine (over 10 kg only)	0.18–0.25 mg kg^{-1} i.m., orally or rectally 8-hourly (max 12.5 mg)

Tablets 2.5 mg, 5 mg
Syrup 5 mg in 5 ml
Suppository 5 mg

CAUDAL ANALGESIA

1. Sacral roots
   e.g. circumcision, hypospadias: up to 0.5 ml kg^{-1} 0.25% bupivacaine (plain)
2. Lumbar roots
   e.g. inguinal hernia: up to 1.0 ml kg^{-1} 0.25% bupivacaine (plain)
3. Up to T10
   e.g. orchidopexy: up to 1.25 ml kg^{-1} of 0.25% bupivacaine diluted with saline to give 0.175%
   Higher doses not recommended
   Maximum dose in any 4-h period should not exceed 2 mg kg^{-1}

LUMBAR/THORACIC EPIDURAL

Bupivacaine 0.25% plain 0.5–0.75 ml kg^{-1}

SPINAL ANALGESIA

Heavy bupivacaine 0.13 ml kg^{-1} (to allow for dead space of the needle)

WOUND INFILTRATION

Bupivacaine 0.25% plain 0.5 ml kg^{-1}

INOTROPIC AGENTS

DILUTIONS ONLY ARE GIVEN. The effect of administration must be monitored. The strength may be increased if fluid restriction is necessary.

Adrenaline, isoprenaline, noradrenaline	60 μg kg^{-1} in 100 ml 5% dextrose 1 ml h^{-1} = 0.01 μg kg^{-1} min (dose 0.01–0.5 μg kg^{-1} min)
Dobutamine	6 mg kg^{-1} in 100 ml 5% dextrose 1 ml.h^{-1} = 1 μg kg^{-1} min^{-1}
Dopamine	6 mg kg^{-1} in 100 ml 5% dextrose 1 ml h^{-1} = 1 μg kg^{-1} min^{-1} At a dose not exceeding 10 μg kg^{-1} min^{-1} there is little α-adrenergic activity
Enoximone	100 mg in 40 ml water bolus 0.5–1 mg kg^{-1} slowly i.v. infusion 10–15 μg kg^{-1} min^{-1}

VASODILATORS

Nitroglycerine	3 mg kg^{-1} in 50 ml 5% dextrose; 1 ml h^{-1} = 1 μg kg^{-1} min^{-1} Dose: 1–6 μg kg^{-1} min^{-1}
Nitroprusside	3 mg kg^{-1} in 100 ml 5% dextrose 1 ml h^{-1} = 0.5 μg kg^{-1} min^{-1} Do not exceed 1–1.5 mg kg^{-1} total dose per 24 h Dose: 0.5–8 μg kg^{-1} min^{-1}

ANTIBIOTICS

Amikacin	10 mg kg^{-1}	12-hourly
Amoxycillin	25 mg kg^{-1}	6-hourly
Ampicillin	up to 50 mg kg^{-1}	6-hourly for severe infections
Cefuroxime	25 mg kg^{-1}	6-hourly
Flucloxacillin	25 mg kg^{-1}	6-hourly
Erythromycin	12.5 mg kg^{-1}	by i.v. infusion over 30 min.
Gentamicin	2 mg kg^{-1}	8-hourly
Metronidazole	7.5 mg kg^{-1}	6-hourly
Penicillin	25 mg kg^{-1}	6-hourly
Piptazobactam	90 mg kg^{-1}	12-hourly
Teicoplanin	10 mg kg^{-1}	12-hourly
Vancomycin	20 mg kg^{-1}	by i.v. infusion over 1 h (12-hourly)

PROPHYLAXIS FOR CARDIAC SURGERY: GIVE ON INDUCTION

First-time surgery, no penicillin allergy

0–4 weeks	Amikacin	10 mg kg^{-1}	i.v. stat
> 4 weeks	Amikacin	10 mg kg^{-1}	i.v. 12-hourly
0–4 weeks	Flucloxacillin	25 mg kg^{-1}	i.v. 8-hourly
> 4 weeks	Flucloxacillin	25 mg kg^{-1}	i.v. 6-hourly

Reoperations (same admission) and penicillin allergy

0–4 weeks	Amikacin	10 mg kg^{-1}	stat
> 4 weeks	Amikacin	10 mg kg^{-1}	12-hourly
0–8 weeks	Teicoplanin	16 mg kg^{-1}	i.v. stat
> 8 weeks	Teicoplanin	10 mg kg^{-1}	12-hourly

Bypass cases

Give extra dose of flucloxacillin after bypass (cautiously; can cause hypotension)

PREVENTION OF BACTERIAL ENDOCARDITIS: RECOMMENDATION BY THE AMERICAN HEART ASSOCIATION

The 1997 approach for endocarditis prophylaxis considers:

1 the apparent risk of bacteraemia with the procedure;
2 the potential adverse reactions of the prophylactic antimicrobial agent to be used;
3 the cost–benefit aspect of the prophylactic regime.

CARDIAC CONDITIONS

High risk, prophylaxis recommended

- Prosthetic cardiac valves
- Previous history of endocarditis
- Complex cyanotic congenital heart disease
- Surgically constructed systemic pulmonary shunts or conduits

Moderate risk, prophylaxis recommended

- Most other uncorrected cardiac conditions, patent ductus arteriosus, ventricular septal defect, primary atrial septal defect, coarctation of the aorta, bicuspid aortic valve
- Acquired valvular dysfunction, rheumatic heart disease
- Collagen vascular disease
- Hypertrophic cardiomyopathy
- Mitral valve prolapse (not needed if there is no regurgitation on echocardiographic findings)

Negligible risk, prophylaxis not needed

- Risk of endocarditis development is not higher than in the general population
- Functional heart murmur
- Satisfactory surgically repaired atrial septal defect, ventricular septal defect or patent ductus ateriosus

- Previous coronary artery bypass graft surgery
- Previous rheumatic heart disease without valvular dysfunction
- Patients with cardiac pacemaker

DENTAL AND ORAL PROCEDURES

High risk patients, prophylaxis recommended

- Procedures associated with significant bleeding, e.g. dental extraction, periodontal surgery, professional teeth cleaning where bleeding is anticipated

Negligible risk, prophylaxis not recommended (bleeding not expected)

- Restorative dentistry (filling cavities)
- Local anaesthetic injection
- Postoperative suture removal
- Shedding of primary teeth

RESPIRATORY TRACT PROCEDURES

High risk, prophylaxis recommended

- Surgical procedure involving the respiratory tract
- Tonsillectomy and/or adenoidectomy
- Rigid bronchoscopy (possible mucosal damage)

Negligible risk, prophylaxis not recommended

- Tracheal intubation
- Flexible bronchoscopy
- Tympanostomy tube insertion

Table 1 Prophylactic regimens for dental, oral, respiratory tract and oesophageal procedures

Situation	Agent	Dose		Mode of administration
		Adults	Children[a]	
Standard general prophylaxis	Amoxycillin	2.0 g	50 mg kg^{-1}	p.o.[b]
Unable to take oral medications	Ampicillin	2.0 g	50 mg kg^{-1}	i.m./i.v.[c]
	Clindamycin or	600 mg	20 mg kg^{-1}	p.o.[b]
	cephalexin or cefadroxil[d]	2.0 g	50 mg kg	p.o.[b]
Allergic to penicillin	Azithromycin or clanthromycin	500 mg	15 mg kg^{-1}	p.o.[b]
Allergic to penicillin and unable	Clindamycin	600 mg	20 mg kg^{-1}	i.v.[c]
to take oral medications	Cefazolin[d]	1.0 g	25 mg kg^{-1}	i.m./i.v.[c]

[a]Total children's dose should not exceed adult dose; [b]p.o. medication are given 1 h before the procedure; [c]i.m. or i.v. within 30 min before the procedure; [d]Cephalosporins should not be used in individuals with immediate-type hypersensitivity reaction (urticaria, angio-oedema, or anaphylaxis) to penicillins.

Table 2 Prophylactic regimens for genitourinary and gastrointestinal (excluding oesophageal) procedures

Situation	Agent	Dose		Mode of administration
		Adults	Children[a]	
		2 g	50 mg kg^{-1}	i.m./i.v.[b]
High-risk patients	Ampicillin plus gentamicin	1.5 mg kg^{-1}	1.5 mg kg^{-1}	i.m./i.v.
High-risk patients allergic to	Vancomycin[d]	1.0 g	20 mg kg^{-1}	i.v./i.m.[c]
ampicillin/amoxycillin	plus gentamicin	1.5 mg kg^{-1}	1.5 mg kg^{-1}	i.v./i.m.
		2.0 g	50 mg kg^{-1}	p.o.
Moderate-risk patients	Amoxycillin or ampicillin	2.0 g	50 mg kg^{-1}	i.m./i.v.
Moderate-risk patients allergic to ampicillin/amoxycillin	Vancomycin[d]	1.0 g	20 mg kg^{-1}	i.v.

[a]Total children's dose should not exceed adult dose, i.v. drugs are given within 30 min before the procedures; [b]repeat half the dose of ampicillin 6 h later i.m./i.v. or amoxycillin p.o.; [c]no second dose of vancomycin or gentamicin is recommended; [d]Vancomycin i.v. given slowly over 1–2 h.
(From Dajani, A.S., Tambert, K.A., Wilson, A.F. *et al.* Prevention of bacterial endocarditis. Recommendations of the American Heart Association. *Journal of the American Heart Association* 1997; **227**: 1794–801.

GASTROINTESTINAL PROCEDURES

Prophylaxis recommended

- Surgery of intestine and biliary tract
- Endoscopic cholangiography with biliary obstruction
- Sclerotherapy for oesophageal varices and oesophageal dilatation

Prophylaxis not recommended

- Endoscopy with or without biopsy

GENITOURINARY TRACT

Prophylaxis recommended

- Cystoscopy, prostate surgery
- Urethral dilations, especially in the presence of urinary tract infection

Prophylaxis not recommended

- Vaginal hysterectomy or vaginal delivery (prophylaxis optional in high risk patients)
- Caesarian section
- Catheterization in the absence of urinary tract infection
- Therapeutic abortion, dilatation and curettage
- Sterilization procedures, circumcision

PROPHYLACTIC REGIMENS

General principles

- Effective prophylactic therapy should be given perioperatively to assure adequate antibiotic concentration. It should be initiated shortly before the procedure and preferably not be continued for more than the 6–8 h to avoid the likelihood of microbial resistance.
- For dental, oral respiratory tract or oesophageal procedures prophylaxis is directed toward *Streptococcus viridans* (α-*haemolytic streptococci*). For such conditions a single dose of ampicillin, penicillin V or amoxycillin is adequate. Amoxycillin is preferred because of its better gastrointestinal absorption and more sustained serum concentrations.
- For genitourinary and non-oesophageal gastrointestinal procedures the prophylaxis is aimed to prevent endocarditis from enterococci (*Enterococcus faecalis*).

Index